The ESC Textbook of
Sports Cardiology

European Society of Cardiology publications

The ESC Textbook of Cardiovascular Medicine (Third Edition)
Edited by A. John Camm, Thomas F. Lüscher, Gerald Maurer and Patrick W. Serruys

The ESC Textbook of Intensive and Acute Cardiovascular Care (Second Edition)
Edited by Marco Tubaro, Pascal Vranckx, Susanna Price, and Christiaan Vrints

The ESC Textbook of Cardiovascular Imaging (Second Edition)
Edited by Jose Luis Zamorano, Jeroen Bax, Juhani Knuuti, Udo Sechtem, Patrizio Lancellotti, and Luigi Badano

The ESC Textbook of Preventive Cardiology
Edited by Stephan Gielen, Guy De Backer, Massimo Piepoli, and David Wood

The EHRA Book of Pacemaker, ICD, and CRT Troubleshooting: *Case-based learning with multiple choice questions*
Edited by Haran Burri, Carsten Israel, and Jean-Claude Deharo

The EACVI Echo Handbook
Edited by Patrizio Lancellotti and Bernard Cosyns

The ESC Handbook of Preventive Cardiology: *Putting prevention into practice*
Edited by Catriona Jennings, Ian Graham, and Stephan Gielen

The EACVI Textbook of Echocardiography (Second Edition)
Edited by Patrizio Lancellotti, José Luis Zamorano, Gilbert Habib, and Luigi Badano

The EHRA Book of Interventional Electrophysiology: *Case-based learning with multiple choice questions*
Edited by Hein Heidbuchel, Mattias Duytschaever, and Haran Burri

The ESC Textbook of Vascular Biology
Edited by Robert Krams and Magnus Bäck

The ESC Textbook of Cardiovascular Development
Edited by José M. Pérez-Pomares and Robert Kelly

The EACVI Textbook of Cardiovascular Magnetic Resonance
Edited by Massimo Lombardi, Sven Plein, Steffen Petersen, Chiara Bucciarelli-Ducci, Emanuela Valsangiacomo Buechel, Cristina Basso, and Victor Ferrari

The ESC Textbook of Sports Cardiology
Edited by Antonio Pelliccia, Hein Heidbuchel, Domenico Corrado, Mats Börjesson, and Sanjay Sharma

Forthcoming

The ESC Handbook on Cardiovascular Pharmacotherapy
Edited by Juan Carlos Kaski and Keld Kjeldsen

For a full listing of all ESC Educational Publications please visit:
https://www.escardio.org/Education/Textbooks

The ESC Textbook of Sports Cardiology

Edited by

Antonio Pelliccia

Hein Heidbuchel

Domenico Corrado

Mats Börjesson

Sanjay Sharma

OXFORD
UNIVERSITY PRESS

EAPC
European Association
of Preventive Cardiology
European Society of Cardiology

OXFORD
UNIVERSITY PRESS

Great Clarendon Street, Oxford, OX2 6DP,
United Kingdom

Oxford University Press is a department of the University of Oxford.
It furthers the University's objective of excellence in research, scholarship,
and education by publishing worldwide. Oxford is a registered trade mark of
Oxford University Press in the UK and in certain other countries

Published in the United States of America by Oxford University Press
198 Madison Avenue, New York, NY 10016, United States of America

British Library Cataloguing in Publication Data
Data available

Library of Congress Control Number: 2018951253

ISBN 978–0–19–877974–2

Printed and bound by CPI Group (UK) Ltd, Croydon, CR0 4YY

Contents

Abbreviations *viii*

Contributors *xi*

SECTION 1
Physiology of cardiovascular response to exercise and cardiac remodelling

1.1 Cardiovascular response induced by exercise *3*

1.1.1 Physiology of exercise *3*
Andrew D'Silva and Sanjay Sharma

1.2 Long-term adaptation to exercise: athlete's heart and vascular adaptations *9*

1.2.1 Structural and functional adaptations in the athlete's heart *9*
Antonio Pelliccia and Stefano Caselli

1.2.2 Impact of sporting discipline, gender, ethnicity, and genetics on the athlete's heart *20*
Nabeel Sheikh

1.2.3 The athlete's heart in children and adolescents *32*
Graham Stuart and Guido E. Pieles

1.2.4 Vascular remodelling *41*
Stephan Gielen, M. Harold Laughlin, and Dirk J. Duncker

SECTION 2
Clinical evaluation of the athlete's heart

2.1 History and physical examination *51*

2.1.1 History and physical examination *51*
Maurizio Schiavon, Alessandro Zorzi, and Domenico Corrado

2.2 The electrocardiogram in the athlete *57*

2.2.1 The electrocardiogram in the athlete *57*
Alessandro Zorzi and Domenico Corrado

2.2.2 Common ECG patterns in the athlete's heart *68*
Ricardo Stein and Victor Froelicher

2.2.3 Overlap ECG patterns in the athlete's heart and cardiomyopathies *77*
Harshil Dhutia and Michael Papadakis

SECTION 3
Additional testing in the evaluation of the athlete's heart

3.1 Exercise testing *87*

3.1.1 Protocols of exercise testing in athletes and cardiopulmonary testing: assessment of fitness *87*
Marco Guazzi and Paolo Emilio Adami

3.1.2 Evaluation of ischaemia, blood pressure, QT interval, and arrhythmias *98*
Frédéric Schnell and François Carré

3.2 Arrhythmia registration *107*

3.2.1 Ambulatory (24-hour Holter monitoring, event recorders) and signal-averaged ECG for arrhythmia registration in the athlete's heart *107*
Mahdi Sareban and Josef Niebauer

3.2.2 Class 1 anti-arrhythmic drug provocation test *114*
Matthias Antz

3.2.3 Electrophysiological study *116*
Matthias Antz

3.3 Imaging the athlete's heart: anatomical and functional *120*

3.3.1 Echocardiogram: morphological and functional evaluation including new echocardiographic techniques *120*
Stefano Caselli and Flavio D'Ascenzi

3.3.2 Cardiac magnetic resonance imaging *140*
Guido Claessen and André La Gerche

3.3.3 Coronary computed tomography *153*
Stefan Möhlenkamp

3.3.4 Nuclear imaging *159*
Stefan Möhlenkamp

3.3.5 Coronary angiography *162*
Stefan Möhlenkamp

3.4 Genotyping *166*

3.4.1 Indications for genetic testing in athletes and its application in daily practice *166*
Andrea Mazzanti, Katherine Underwood, and Silvia G. Priori

SECTION 4
Cardiac diseases of interest in sports cardiology

4.1 Myocardial and coronary diseases *179*

4.1.1 Hypertrophic cardiomyopathy in athletes *179*
Aneil Malhotra and Sanjay Sharma

4.1.2 Arrhythmogenic cardiomyopathy and sudden death in young athletes: causes, pathophysiology, and clinical features *184*
Gaetano Thiene, Kalliopi Pilichou, Stefania Rizzo, and Cristina Basso

4.1.3 Myocarditis in athletes *201*
Martin Halle

4.1.4 Differentiating athlete's heart from left ventricular non-compaction cardiomyopathy *209*
Andrew D'Silva and Sanjay Sharma

4.1.5 Congenital coronary artery anomalies *217*
Cristina Basso, Carla Frescura, Stefania Rizzo, and Gaetano Thiene

4.2 Valvular and aortic disease *226*

4.2.1 Mitral valve prolapse in relation to sport *226*
Christian Schmied and Sanjay Sharma

4.2.2 Bicuspid aortic valve disease and competitive sports: key considerations and challenges *233*
Benjamin S. Wessler and Natesa G. Pandian

4.2.3 The athlete with congenital heart disease *238*
Guido E. Pieles and Graham Stuart

SECTION 5
Rhythm disorders of interest in sports cardiology

5.1 Channelopathy in athletes *253*
Nicole M. Panhuyzen-Goedkoop and Arthur A.M. Wilde

5.2 Ventricular tachyarrhythmias *265*
Eduard Guasch and Lluís Mont

5.3 Supraventricular tachyarrhythmias *277*
Matthias Wilhelm

5.4 Pre-excitation and conduction abnormalities *288*
Pietro Delise

SECTION 6
Sudden cardiac death in athletes

6.1 Incidence of sudden cardiac death in athletes *299*
Jonathan A. Drezner and Kimberly G. Harmon

6.2 Cardiovascular causes of sudden death in athletes *309*
Cristina Basso, Stefania Rizzo, and Gaetano Thiene

6.3 The risk, aetiology, clinical features, management, and prevention of exercise-related sudden cardiac death and acute cardiac events in adult athletes *321*
Paul D. Thompson

6.4 Less frequent causes of sudden cardiac death *328*

6.4.1 Less frequent causes of SCD (commotio cordis): non-cardiac causes (drug abuse, hyperpyrexia, rhabdomyolysis, sickle cell anaemia)—Part 1 *328*
Erik Ekker Solberg and Paolo Emilio Adami

6.4.2 Less frequent causes of SCD (aortic rupture): non-cardiac causes (asthma, extreme environmental conditions (heat, cold, altitude))—Part 2 *332*
Erik Ekker Solberg and Paolo Emilio Adami

6.5 Pre-participation screening of young competitive athletes *339*
Domenico Corrado and Alessandro Zorzi

6.6 Cardiovascular screening of adult/senior competitive athletes *352*
Luc Vanhees and Mats Börjesson

6.7 Cardiovascular screening of children and adolescent athletes (<14 years) *359*
Massimo Chessa, Werner Budts, and Javier Fernandez Sarabia

SECTION 7
Sports eligibility in athletes with cardiac abnormalities

7.1 **Criteria and considerations relative to safe participation in sport for athletes with cardiac abnormalities** *369*
Antonio Pelliccia, Hein Heidbuchel, Domenico Corrado, Sanjay Sharma, and Mats Börjesson

SECTION 8
Exercise prescription for cardiovascular health

8.1 **Physical activity and leisure-time exercise prescription for sedentary/untrained individuals** *381*
Massimo F. Piepoli, Mikael Dellborg, and Mats Börjesson

8.2 **Monitoring exercise programmes and improving cardiovascular performance** *389*
Stephan Mueller, Flavia Baldassarri, Julia Schoenfeld, and Martin Halle

SECTION 9
Cardiac safety at sports facilities

9.1 **Resuscitation on the field: basic and advanced life support and automatic external defibrillators** *403*
Mark S. Link and Mark Estes III

9.2 **Cardiac safety at sports events: the medical action plan** *411*
Luis Serratosa, Efraim Kramer, and Mats Börjesson

9.3 **Cardiac safety at fitness centres** *419*
Erik Ekker Solberg, Jakob Johansson, and Alessandro Biffi

SECTION 10
Cardiovascular effects of substances of abuse/doping

10.1 **World Anti-Doping Agency (WADA) and International Olympic Committee (IOC) list of prohibited substances and methods and their cardiovascular effects** *427*
Josef Niebauer and Carl Johan Sundberg

10.2 **Nutrition and ergogenic aids prescription for competitive athletes** *433*
Ronald J. Maughan and S.M. Shirreffs

SECTION 11
Hypertension in athletes

11.1 **Diagnosis and management of hypertension in athletes** *447*
Stefano Caselli and Josef Niebauer

Index *453*

Abbreviations

AAS	androgenic anabolic steroids
AC	arrhythmogenic cardiomyopathy
ACC	American College of Cardiology
ACE	angiotensin-converting enzyme
ACEi	angiotensin convertase inhibitor
ACS	acute coronary syndrome
ACSM	American College of Sports Medicine
AECVP	Association for European Cardiovascular Pathology
AED	automated external defibrillator
AF	atrial fibrillation
AFL	atrial flutter
AHA	American Heart Association
ALCAPA	anomalous left coronary artery from the pulmonary artery
ALS	advanced life support
AMI	acute myocardial infarction
AMS	acute mountain sickness
ANS	autonomic nervous system
Ao	aorta
AoV	aortic valve
APB	atrial premature beat
APMHR	age-predicted maximal heart rate
ARB	angiotensin receptor blocker
ARVC	arrhythmogenic right ventricular cardiomyopathy
ARVD/C	arrhythmogenic right ventricular dysplasia/cardiomyopathy
AS	aortic stenosis
ASCAD	arteriosclerotic coronary artery disease
ASD	atrial septal defect
ASR	anaerobic speed reserve
AT	anaerobic threshold, atrial tachycardia
ATP	adenosine triphosphate
AV	atrioventricular
AVN	atrioventricular node
AVNRT	atrioventricular nodal re-entrant tachycardia
AVR	aortic valve replacement
AVRT	atrioventricular re-entrant tachycardia
BAV	bicuspid aortic valve
BLS	basic life support
BMI	body mass index
BP	blood pressure
bpm	beats per minute
BrS	Brugada syndrome
BSA	body surface area
bSSFP	balanced steady state free precession
BTPS	body temperature and pressure, saturated
BW	body weight
CA	competitions area
CAA	coronary artery anomaly
CAC	coronary artery calcium, coronary artery calcification
CAD	coronary artery disease
CBF	coronary blood flow
CC	commotio cordis
CCT	coronary computed tomography
CCTA	CCT angiography
ccTGA	congenitally corrected transposition of the great arteries
CHD	congenital heart disease
CI	confidence interval
CK	creatine kinase
CMJ	counter-movement jump
CMR	cardiac magnetic resonance
CO	cardiac output
COPD	chronic obstructive pulmonary disease
CP	chest pain
CPET	cardiopulmonary exercise testing
CPR	cardiopulmonary resuscitation
CPVT	catecholaminergic polymorphic ventricular tachycardia

CRY	Cardiac Risk in the Young
CT	computed tomography
CVD	cardiovascular disease
CW	continuous wave
DBP	diastolic blood pressure
DCM	dilated cardiomyopathy
DGE	delayed gadolinium enhancement
DJ	drop jump
EACPR	European Association for Cardiovascular Prevention and Rehabilitation
EAPC	European Association of Preventive Cardiology
ECC	external chest compression
ECG	electrocardiography, electrocardiogram
ECV	extracellular volume
EDV	end-diastolic volume
E-EPS	endocavitary electrophysiological study
EF	ejection function
EHRA	European Heart Rhythm Association
ELR	external loop recorder
EMB	endomyocardial biopsy
EMS	emergency medical service
eNOS	endothelial NO synthase
EP	electrophysiology, electrophysiological
EPO	erythropoietin
EPS	electrophysiological study
ER	early repolarization
ESC	European Society of Cardiology
ET	exercise testing, exercise test
FA	fascicular tachycardia
FFR	fractional flow reserve
FIFA	Fédération Internationale de Football Association
FMD	flow-mediated dilation
GLS	global longitudinal strain
GP/PN	genotype positive/phenotype negative
HACE	high altitude cerebral (o)edema
HAPE	high altitude pulmonary (o)edema
HCM	hypertrophic cardiomyopathy
HDL	high density lipid
HGH	human growth hormone
HIIT	high intensity interval training
HIT	high intensity training
HR	heart rate
HRR	heart rate reserve
HU	Hounsfield unit(s)
ICD	implantable cardioverter defibrillator
ICDUS	intra-coronary Doppler ultrasound
ICU	intensive care unit
IGF-1	insulin-like growth factor 1
IOC	International Olympic Committee
IRAD	International Registry of Aortic Dissection
IRBB	IR incomplete right bundle branch block
IVRT	isovolumic relaxation time
IVUS	intra-vascular ultrasound
LA	left atrium, left atrial
LAD	left anterior descending artery, left axis deviation,
LAE	left atrial enlargement
LAFB	left anterior fascicular block
LAH	left anterior hemiblock
LBBB	left bundle branch block
LCC	left coronary cusp
LCX	left circumflex artery
LDL	low density lipid
LPFB	left posterior fascicular block
LQTS	long QT syndrome
LT	lactate threshold
LTPA	leisure-time physical activity
LV	left ventricle, left ventricular,
LVH	left ventricular hypertrophy
LVNC	left ventricular non-compaction cardiomyopathy
LVOTO	left ventricular outflow tract obstruction
LVRI	left ventricular remodelling index
MAP	medical action plan
MCT	mobile cardiac telemetry
MDI	mass dispersion index
MET	metabolic equivalent
MFS	Marfan syndrome
MMT	mobile medical team
MR	mitral regurgitation
MS	maximum strength
MTU	muscle–tendon unit
MV	maximal ventilatory volume
MVC	maximal voluntary contraction
MVP	mitral vave prolapse
MVV	maximal voluntary ventilation
NAEMSP	National Association of Emergency Medical Services Physicians
NCA	non- competitions area
NCC	non-coronary cusp
NOAC	novel oral anticoagulant
NSAID	non-steroidal anti-inflammatory drug
NSVT	non-sustained ventricular tachycardia
NYHA	New York Heart Association
O-AVRT	orthodromic atrioventricular re-entrant tachycardia
OHCA	out-of-hospital cardiac arrest
OT-VT	outflow tract-ventricular tachycardia

PA	physical activity
PAH	pulmonary artery hypertension
PCr	phosphocreatine
PDA	patent ductus arteriosus, patent arterial duct
PEA	pulseless electrical activity
PES	programmed electrical stimulation
PKC	protein kinase C
PPAR	peroxisome proliferator-activated receptor
PPS	pre-participation screening
PVC	premature ventricular contraction
PW	pulse wave
PWV	pulse wave velocity
RA	right atrium, right atrial
RAD	right axis deviation
RAE	right atrial enlargement
RAS	renin–angiotensin system
RBBB	right bundle branch block
RC	respiratory compensation
RCC	right coronary cusp
RCT	randomized controlled trial
RE	running economy
RER	respiratory exchange ratio
RF	radiofrequency
ROSC	return of spontaneous circulation
RPE	rating of perceived exertion
RPP	rate pressure product
RSS	repeated sprint sequences
RV	right ventricle, right ventricular
RVOT	right ventricular outflow tract
SAM	systolic anterior motion
SARM	selective androgen receptor modulator
SBP	systolic blood pressure
SCA	sudden cardiac arrest
SCA/D	sudden cardiac arrest and death
SCD	sudden cardiac death
SCT	sickle cell trait
SD	standard deviation
SJ	squat jump
sPAP	systolic pulmonary artery pressure
SPECT	single photon emission computed tomography
SQTS	short QT syndrome
SSA	spectator seating area
SSC	stretch–shortening cycle
STE	speckle-tracking echocardiography
STPD	standard temperature and pressure, dry
SVT	supraventricular tachyarrhythmia
TAPSE	tricuspid annular plane systolic excursion
TCFA	thin-cap fibroatheroma
TDI	tissue Doppler imaging
TdP	torsades de pointes
T-EPS	trans-oesophageal electrophysiological study
TGA	transposition of the great arteries
TLOC	transient loss of consciousness
TOE	trans-oesophageal echocardiography
TUE	therapeutic use exemption
TV	tricuspid valve
TWI	T-wave inversion
VA	ventricular arrhythmia
VCO_2	carbon dioxide production
Vd	ventilatory dead space
VE	minute ventilation
VO_2	oxygen consumption
VOC	venue operations centre
VPB	ventricular premature beat
VR	virtual reality
VSD	ventricular septal defect
Vt	tidal volume
VT	ventilatory threshold, ventricular tachycardia
VUS	variant of uncertain significance
WADA	World Anti-Doping Agency
WPW	Wolff–Parkinson–White

Contributors

Paolo Emilio Adami
Sports Medicine and Science Institute of the Italian Olympic Committee, Rome, Italy

Matthias Antz
Department of Electrophysiology, Hospital Braunschweig, Braunschweig, Germany

Flavia Baldassarri
Department of Prevention, Rehabilitation and Sports Medicine, Technical University of Munich (TUM), Munich, Germany

Cristina Basso
Cardiovascular Pathology Unit, Department of Cardiac, Thoracic, and Vascular Sciences, University of Padua Medical School, Padua, Italy

Alessandro Biffi
Institute of Sport Medicine and Science, Rome, Italy

Mats Börjesson
Institute of Neuroscience and Physiology and Institute of Food and Nutrition, and Sports Science, University of Gothenburg, and Sahlgrenska University Hospital/Östra, Gothenburg, Sweden

Werner Budts
Cardiovascular Diseases, University Hospitals Leuven, Leuven, Belgium

François Carré
Department of Sports Medicine, Pontchaillou Hospital, Rennes, and Department of Physiology, Rennes 1 University, Rennes, France

Stefano Caselli
Institute of Sports Medicine and Science, Rome, Italy

Massimo Chessa
Paediatric and Adult Congenital Heart Centre, IRCCS-Policlinico San Donato University Hospital, Milan, Italy

Guido Claessen
Department of Cardiovascular Medicine, University Hospital Leuven, Leuven, Belgium

Domenico Corrado
Department of Cardiac, Thoracic, and Vascular Sciences, University of Padua Medical School, Padua, Italy

Flavio D'Ascenzi
Department of Medical Biotechnologies, Division of Cardiology, University of Siena, Siena, Italy

Pietro Delise
Department of Cardiovascular, Neurological, and Kidney Diseases, Division of Cardiology, Hospital of Conegliano, Veneto, Italy

Mikael Dellborg
Department of Medicine, Sahlgrenska Academy, University of Gothenburg, and Adult Congenital Heart Unit, Sahlgrenska University Hospital/Östra, Gothenburg, Sweden

Harshil Dhutia
Cardiovascular and Cell Sciences Research Centre, St George's University of London, London, UK

Jonathan Drezner
Center for Sports Cardiology, Department of Family Medicine, University of Washington, Seattle, WA, USA

Andrew D'Silva
St George's University of London and St George's University Hospital NHS Foundation Trust, London, UK

Dirk J. Duncker
Department of Cardiology, Thoraxcenter, Erasmus University Medical Centre, Rotterdam, The Netherlands

Mark Estes III
University of Pittsburgh Medical Center, Pittsburgh, PA, USA

Javier Fernandez Sarabia
Paediatric and Adult Congenital Heart Centre, IRCCS-Policlinico san Donato University Hospital, Milan, Italy

Carla Frescura
Cardiovascular Pathology Unit, Department of Cardiac, Thoracic, and Vascular Sciences, University of Padua Medical School, Padua, Italy

Victor Froelicher
Sports Cardiology Clinic and Center for Inherited Cardiovascular Disease, Stanford School of Medicine, Stanford, CA, USA

Stephan Gielen
Department of Cardiology, Angiology, and Intensive Care Medicine, Klinikum Lippe, Detmold, Germany, and Martin-Luther-University Halle/Wittenberg, Medical Faculty, Halle/Saale, Germany

Eduard Guasch
Hospital Clínic de Barcelona—IDIBAPS, University of Barcelona, Barcelona, Spain

Marco Guazzi
University of Milan, Italy

Martin Halle
Department of Prevention, Rehabilitation, and Sports Medicine, Technical University of Munich (TUM), Munich, Germany; and DZHK (German Centre for Cardiovascular Research), partner site Munich Heart Alliance, Munich, Germany

Kimberly Harmon
Center for Sports Cardiology, Department of Family Medicine, University of Washington, Seattle, WA, USA

Hein Heidbuchel
Antwerp University and Department of Cardiology, Antwerp University Hospital, Antwerp, Belgium, and Hasselt University, Hasselt, Belgium

Jakob Johansson
Institute of Medicine and Sports Science, Rome, Italy

Efraim Kramer
University of the Witwatersrand, Johannesburg, South Africa

André La Gerche
Department of Cardiovascular Medicine, University Hospital Leuven, Leuven, Belgium; Department of Sports Cardiology, Baker IDI Heart and Diabetes Institute, Melbourne, Australia, and Department of Cardiology, Alfred Hospital, Melbourne, Australia

M. Harold Laughlin
Departments of Biomedical Sciences and Medical Pharmacology and Physiology, University of Missouri, Columbia, MO, USA

Mark Link
UT Southwestern Medical Center, Dallas, TX, USA

Aneil Malhotra
St. George's University of London, Cardiology Clinical Academic Group, London, UK

Ronald J. Maughan
School of Medicine, University of St Andrews, St Andrews, UK

Andrea Mazzanti
Molecular Cardiology, IRCCS Salvatore Maugeri Foundation, Pavia, Italy

Stefan Möhlenkamp
Clinic of Cardiology and Intensive Care Medicine, Bethanien Hospital Moers, Moers, Germany

Lluís Mont
Hospital Clínic de Barcelona—IDIBAPS, University of Barcelona, Barcelona, Spain

Stephan Mueller
Department of Prevention, Rehabilitation, and Sports Medicine, Technical University of Munich (TUM), Munich, Germany

Josef Niebauer
Institute of Sports Medicine, Prevention and Rehabilitation and Research Institute of Molecular Sports Medicine and Rehabilitation, Paracelsus Medical University Salzburg; Institute of Sports Medicine of the State of Salzburg; and Sports Medicine of the Olympic Centre Salzburg-Rif, Salzburg, Austria

Natesa G. Pandian
Tufts Medical Center, Tufts University School of Medicine, Boston, MA, USA, and Hoag Hospital, Newport Beach, CA, USA

Nicole M. Panhuyzen-Goedkoop
Heart Centre, Department of Clinical and Experimental Cardiology, Amsterdam University Medical Centre, Amsterdam, The Netherlands

Michael Papadakis
Cardiovascular and Cell Sciences Research Centre, St George's University of London, London, UK

Antonio Pelliccia
Institute of Sport Medicine and Science, Rome, Italy

Guido E. Pieles
Congenital Heart Unit, Bristol Royal Hospital for Children/Bristol Heart Institute, University Hospital Bristol NHS Trust, Bristol, UK

Massimo F. Piepoli
Heart Failure Unit, Cardiology Department, G. Da Saliceto Hospital, ASL Piacenza, Italy

Kalliopi Pilichou
Department of Cardiac, Thoracic, and Vascular Sciences, Cardiovascular Pathology Unit, University of Padua Medical School, Padua, Italy

Silvia G. Priori
Molecular Cardiology, IRCCS Salvatore Maugeri Foundation, Pavia, Italy; Department of Molecular Medicine, University of Pavia, Pavia, Italy; and Fundación Centro Nacional de Investigaciones Cardiovasculares, Madrid, Spain

Stefania Rizzo
Cardiovascular Pathology, Department of Cardiac, Thoracic and Vascular Sciences, University of Padua, Padua, Italy

Mahdi Sareban
Paracelsus Medical University, Salzburg, Austria

Maurizio Schiavon
Sports Medicine and Physical Activities Unit, National Health Service—ULSS 6 Euganea of Padua, Italy

Christian Schmied
Department of Cardiology, University Hospital Zurich, Switzerland

Frédéric Schnell
Department of Sports Medicine, Pontchaillou Hospital, Rennes, and Department of Physiology, Rennes 1 University, Rennes, France

Julia Schoenfeld
Department of Prevention, Rehabilitation, and Sports Medicine, Technical University of Munich (TUM), Munich, Germany

Luis Serratosa
Hospital Universitario Quironsalud Madrid, Spain; and Ripoll & De Prado Sport Clinic, FIFA Medical Centre of Excellence, Spain

Sanjay Sharma
St George's University of London, Cardiology Clinical Academic Group, London, UK

Nabeel Sheikh
Department of Cardiology and Division of Cardiovascular Sciences, Guy's and St Thomas' Hospitals and King's College London, UK

S.M. Shirreffs
School of Medicine, University of St Andrews, St Andrews, UK

Erik Ekker Solberg
Diakonhjemmet Hospital, Oslo, Norway

Ricardo Stein
Internal Medicine Division, Hospital de Clínicas de Porto Alegre - Universidade Federal do Rio Grande do Sul, Porto Alegre, Brazil

Graham Stuart
Congenital Heart Unit, Bristol Royal Hospital for Children/Bristol Heart Institute, University Hospital Bristol NHS Trust, Bristol, UK

Carl-Johan Sundberg
Department of Physiology and Pharmacology, Karolinska Institutet, Stockholm, Sweden

Gaetano Thiene
Cardiovascular Pathology Unit, Department of Cardiac, Thoracic, and Vascular Sciences, University of Padua Medical School, Padua, Italy

Paul D. Thompson
Hartford Healthcare Cardiovascular Institute, Hartford, CT, USA

Katherine Underwood
Molecular Cardiology, IRCCS Salvatore Maugeri Foundation, Pavia, Italy

Luc Vanhees
Department of Rehabilitation Sciences, Biomedical Sciences, University of Leuven, Leuven, Belgium

Benjamin S. Wessler
Tufts Medical Center, Tufts University School of Medicine, Boston, MA, USA

Arthur A.M. Wilde
Heart Centre, Department of Clinical and Experimental Cardiology, Amsterdam University Medical Centre, Amsterdam, The Netherlands

Matthias Wilhelm
Department of Cardiology, Interdisciplinary Center for Sports & Exercise Medicine, University Hospital Bern, Bern, Switzerland

Alessandro Zorzi
Department of Cardiac, Thoracic, and Vascular Sciences, University of Padua Medical School, Padua, Italy

SECTION 1

Physiology of cardiovascular response to exercise and cardiac remodelling

1.1 Cardiovascular response induced by exercise *3*

1.1.1 Physiology of exercise *3*
Andrew D'Silva and Sanjay Sharma

1.2 Long-term adaptation to exercise: athlete's heart and vascular adaptations *9*

1.2.1 Structural and functional adaptations in the athlete's heart *9*
Antonio Pelliccia and Stefano Caselli

1.2.2 Impact of sporting discipline, gender, ethnicity, and genetics on the athlete's heart *20*
Nabeel Sheikh

1.2.3 The athlete's heart in children and adolescents *32*
Graham Stuart and Guido E. Pieles

1.2.4 Vascular remodelling *41*
Stephan Gielen, M. Harold Laughlin, and Dirk J. Duncker

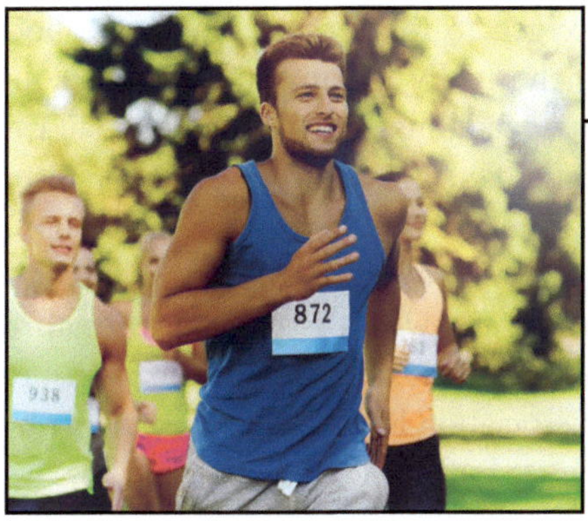

1.1

Cardiovascular response induced by exercise

Contents

1.1.1 **Physiology of exercise** Andrew D'Silva and Sanjay Sharma 3

1.1.1 Physiology of exercise

Andrew D'Silva and Sanjay Sharma

Introduction

Exercise physiology incorporates the study of both the acute responses and chronic adaptation of the human body to physical activity. The normal resting cardiac output is approximately 5L/min. The liver, kidneys, muscle, and brain account for the largest consumption of blood volume at approximate proportions of 27%, 22%, 20%, and 14%, respectively. The situation changes dramatically during strenuous exercise when the cardiac output is capable of increasing up to 25–35L/min. Skeletal muscle demands approximately 84% of this blood volume when exerting strenuously, and this is critical to satisfy the oxygen demand for ATP generation and carbon dioxide removal necessary for acid–base homeostasis [1]. Athletes capable of sustaining the highest cardiac outputs during prolonged exercise achieve this through chronic adaptation, particularly of the heart and cardiovascular system. Through training, the heart is capable of adapting in structure and function to meet the demands of an increasing workload. Despite this, maximal cardiac output remains a major limitation on oxygen delivery and therefore limits exercise capacity. For the purposes of this chapter, the heart should be considered as both a pump for delivering oxygen to the tissues and carbon dioxide to the lungs, and a highly specialized striated muscle with substantial energy demands.

We begin by outlining the respiration requirements of every muscle cell, including cardiac and skeletal muscle and how the demands of exercise are met.

Exercise and the muscle cell

Fundamentally, exercise is an energetic process that reflects an upregulation of the essential oxidation of metabolic substrate to support physical activity. Oxygen facilitates oxidative chemical reactions to create high energy bonds in compounds, chiefly in the terminal phosphate bond of ATP, which is the cellular currency for energy transformation. Exercise demands that chemical energy is converted into kinetic energy at a high rate and mass scale. When energy is borrowed from alternative anaerobic sources it must also be repaid.

At the level of striated muscle, ATP is split to release energy to generate mechanical force through the interaction between the myosin head and actin. Occurrence of this process on a large scale, throughout the entire muscle, results in fibre shortening and muscle contraction downstream. Exercise demands high levels of ATP and therefore high oxygen consumption, which is necessary to power this contractile machinery.

Even when physical activity is initiated abruptly there is no delay in achieving sufficient ATP levels, as one would anticipate if ATP were sourced from the oxidation of metabolic substrates. From an evolutionary perspective it is prudent to be able to summon energy immediately to escape an unanticipated threat. This is achieved by having stores of high energy phosphate bonds in the form of phosphocreatine, which are rapidly hydrolysed in early exercise by creatine kinase to release inorganic phosphate and generate ATP. However, as this becomes rapidly depleted, sustained exercise depends on the aerobic oxidation of metabolic substrates, predominantly glycogen and fatty acids for the continued regeneration of ATP.

Human skeletal muscle contains approximately 15–18g of glucose per kilogram stored as glycogen, which can be broken down into glucose for utilization through glycogenolysis. The liver also has a fluctuating glycogen reserve that can be converted into glucose and released into the bloodstream when required. In addition, during severe and prolonged exercise the liver ensures that plasma glucose levels do not fall and maintains a constant glucose supply from the conversion of non-carbohydrate precursors through gluconeogenesis. Both glycogenolysis and gluconeogenesis are stimulated by a rise in circulating adrenaline. When glucose is metabolized as the metabolic fuel for energy, through glycolysis, the net yield is 36 molecules of ATP per molecule of glucose. Six oxygen molecules are consumed and six carbon dioxide molecules are produced for every single glucose molecule, and the result is a respiratory quotient of 1.0 for the oxidation of glucose:

$$C_6H_{12}O_6 + 6O_2 \rightarrow 6CO_2 + 6H_2O + 36ATP \quad (1.1.1.1)$$

Fatty acids are also catabolized as an energy substrate. Fat metabolism provides more energy and greater storage economy than carbohydrate; however, it is more expensive in terms of oxygen consumption. Therefore, during conditions of strenuous exercise where oxygen transport is a limiting factor, muscle metabolism preferentially utilizes carbohydrate as a fuel, which yields ATP at a rate four times faster than the oxidation of fatty acids [2].

When exercise is sufficiently intense and prolonged, oxygen delivery to the muscle mitochondria becomes a limiting factor and is unable to match the rate of ATP consumption. At this point, the body is able to continue to generate energy for muscle contraction in the absence of oxygen through anaerobic glycolysis, albeit at a lower yield of ATP and at greater metabolic cost due to the development of lactic acidosis. Muscle groups experiencing inadequate oxygen flow to meet demand will initiate anaerobic cellular metabolism to augment ATP production once aerobic metabolism reaches maximal capacity. The net gain of ATP is only three molecules from each molecule of glucose metabolized into two lactate molecules. This pales in comparison with the 36 ATP molecules generated from the complete oxidation of glucose to carbon dioxide and water via the aerobic pathway.

Acid–base homeostasis is of vital importance in the cell as acidosis can denature proteins, altering their molecular structure and affecting enzymatic activity. Severe acidosis reduces myocardial contractility directly and by causing resistance to beta-adrenergic stimulation. Although the effects of acidosis are predominantly negative, mild acidosis promotes aerobic cellular respiration by allowing oxygen to dissociate from haemoglobin more readily and increasing the availability of oxygen to the muscle. Hence the body regulates pH extremely tightly through the use of multiple buffering systems, including bicarbonate ions, and by elimination of carbon dioxide from the lungs. When bicarbonate ions accept protons from acid they form carbonic acid, which is catalysed to carbon dioxide and water by the enzyme carbonic anhydrase, which is present in erythrocytes. Elimination of carbon dioxide from the lungs ensures that carbonic acid dissociation leaves water as the only by-product. The bicarbonate buffer system is described by

$$H^+ + HCO_3^- \leftrightarrow H_2CO_3 \leftrightarrow CO_2 + H_2O \quad (1.1.1.2)$$

In the early stages of exercise, energy is generated by the most efficient method, aerobic glycolysis, where oxygen consumption is coupled to ATP production. As exercise progresses, a point is reached where oxygen transport to muscle cells is insufficient to meet the demands required to maintain energy production and anaerobic metabolism begins to contribute. Beyond this anaerobic threshold, an oxygen debt accumulates and lactic acid is generated. In this phase, oxygen uptake continues to rise throughout exercise, persisting into the recovery phase where the oxygen debt must be repaid. The ceiling value of oxygen uptake achieved at exhaustive exercise is termed the peak oxygen consumption, or peak VO_2. Peak oxygen consumption is a key determinant of exercise performance and reflects the integrative function of muscle metabolism, oxygen transport through the cardiovascular system, and pulmonary ventilation. An impediment in any of these systems will limit peak oxygen consumption, which can be expressed as the product of cardiac output (CO) and systemic arteriovenous oxygen difference ($C(a\text{-}v)O_2$), described in the Fick equation:

$$VO_2 = CO \times C(a\text{-}v)O_2 \quad (1.1.1.3)$$

The Fick equation defines the entire oxygen transport and utilization capacity of the system. The principles discussed here, at the cellular level, are fundamental to understanding and interpreting cardiopulmonary exercise tests. In a cardiopulmonary exercise test, the respiratory exchange ratio is a useful parameter for assessing whether maximal effort was achieved. At rest, the body metabolizes both carbohydrate and fat to generate ATP. As fat metabolism yields a respiratory quotient of 0.71, this means that, at rest, oxygen consumption (VO_2) is slightly greater than carbon dioxide production (VCO_2), resulting in a respiratory exchange ratio of 0.8–0.9. On commencing exercise, active muscle exclusively metabolizes carbohydrate for the generation of ATP. As the respiratory quotient of carbohydrate is balanced at 1.0, carbon dioxide production is equal to oxygen consumption in early exercise, when glycolysis is entirely aerobic. This results in a rise of the respiratory exchange ratio to 1.0. With more prolonged and strenuous exercise anaerobic glycolysis of carbohydrate ensues, generating lactic acid which must be buffered to maintain cellular pH. Ultimately, bicarbonate ions accept protons to form carbonic acid, which upon dissociation results in a substantial rise in carbon dioxide relative to oxygen consumption, and this requires ventilatory elimination. In this phase of exercise, the respiratory exchange ratio rises above 1.0 and a ratio of greater than 1.15 indicates excellent effort with confidence that the anaerobic threshold was exceeded.

Understanding these principles permits calculation of the ventilatory anaerobic threshold (AT); the point during exercise where anaerobic metabolism contributes to energy production and lactic acid is produced. The AT can be determined by plotting oxygen consumption (VO_2) against carbon dioxide production (VCO_2) and determining the point of intersection of two lines of best fit. This is known as the V-slope method and is commonly used in cardiopulmonary exercise testing to determine the AT (➲ Fig. 1.1.1.1). The AT usually occurs at 50–60% of the peak oxygen consumption in normal individuals, although it can be increased to 80% of peak oxygen consumption in endurance-trained athletes.

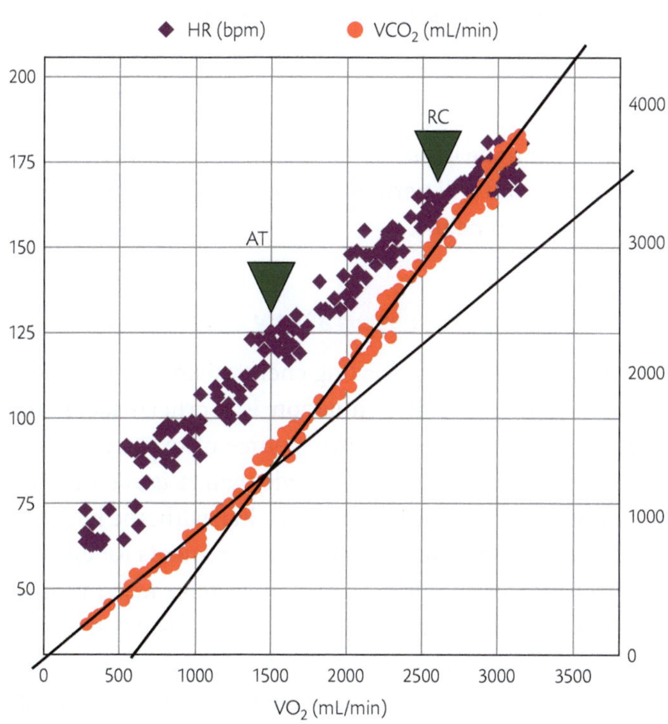

Fig. 1.1.1.1 Carbon dioxide output (VCO_2) and heart rate (HR) vs oxygen uptake (VO_2). Carbon dioxide output increases linearly with oxygen uptake with a slope of 1 up to the anaerobic threshold. After the anaerobic threshold carbon dioxide output increases more rapidly, with steepening of the slope depending on the rate of lactic acid buffering. Heart rate increases linearly with oxygen uptake. The V-slope method of determining ventilator anaerobic threshold (AT) is demonstrated by intersecting lines. The respiratory compensation threshold is indicated by RC.

Exercise and the cardiovascular system

At rest, a proportion of muscle capillaries have little or no blood flow. The role of these dormant capillaries and arterioles is to vasodilate during strenuous exercise, allowing greater diffusion of oxygen and nutrients into contracting muscles. Vasodilatation is triggered by local tissue depletion of oxygen, which is rapidly consumed by active muscle. Oxygen deficiency stimulates the release of vasodilator substances including adenosine, which promotes vasodilatation in early exercise, and potassium ions, ATP, lactic acid, and carbon dioxide maintain this process throughout the rest of exercise.

Local vasodilatation is accompanied by activation of the sympathetic nervous system, which results in a sustained increase in cardiac output and arterial pressure. At the onset of exercise, the brain initiates movement from the motor cortex and simultaneously recruits the vasomotor centre which activates the sympathetic nervous system. Sympathetic activity on the heart results in greater contractile force (inotropy) and an increase in heart rate (chronotropy). As cardiac output is the product of stroke volume and heart rate, adequate function of the sympathetic nervous system is essential to achieving high performance exercise. Sympathetic vasoconstrictor nerves exert their action through the release of noradrenaline at their nerve endings and innervate most arterioles of the peripheral circulation. In concert with this, the adrenal medulla secretes large amounts of noradrenaline and adrenaline into the circulation during exercise, and the consequence is widespread vasoconstriction of peripheral blood vessels except for arterioles in active muscles, which are overwhelmed by the local vasodilator effects described above. This diversion of blood is responsible for increasing muscle blood flow by approximately 2L/min. The coronary and cerebral circulations are central circulatory systems, vital for sustaining prolonged exercise, and are spared this vasoconstrictor effect as they possess little vasoconstrictor innervation. Approximately two-thirds of the total blood volume resides within the veins and their distensible capacitance vessels. This vascular bed is the seat of the most profound vasoconstrictor effects. Vasoconstriction of the muscular venous walls produces a significant rise in the systemic venous filling pressure, which increases venous return of blood to the heart that is critical for increasing cardiac output and eliminating carbon dioxide. These combined effects of the sympathetic nervous system raise the systemic arterial pressure, which drives muscle perfusion. Considering the circulation as a closed hydraulic circuit, in order to enhance oxygen transport blood flow rates to exercising muscles must be increased. A high flow rate within the arteries and arterioles supplying muscle is maintained by an elevated systemic arterial pressure, which also stretches the vessel walls, increasing vessel cross-sectional area to further augment blood flow. Elevation of systemic blood pressure during exercise and arterial distensibility are crucial for those endurance athletes who demand up to 35L/min of cardiac output over a sustained period to maintain physical activity at a high level.

With respect to the heart, cardiac output is increased by increasing stroke volume and raising the heart rate. Stroke volume is regulated during exercise by intrinsic forces and extrinsic factors. The intrinsic force is governed by the Frank–Starling relationship. During exercise venous return rises, resulting in an increase in ventricular volume loading and an increased diastolic filling pressure. The magnitude of myocardial fibre stretch in diastole governs the contractile force and stroke volume. Therefore intrinsic regulation of the myocardial contractile force allows automatic adjustment of stroke volume to match venous return. In addition, extrinsic factors also increase the myocardial contractile force, generating positive inotropy independent of myocardial fibre tension, which is achieved by the sympathetic nervous system. The myocardium has a high proportion of β_1-adrenoreceptors, which become activated by circulating adrenaline and noradrenaline. On cardiopulmonary exercise testing, the oxygen pulse is a surrogate of stroke volume. Oxygen pulse is calculated by dividing oxygen uptake by heart rate and therefore represents the stroke volume multiplied by the arteriovenous blood oxygen content difference:

$$\frac{VO_2}{HR} = SV \times C(a\text{-}v)O_2 \qquad (1.1.1.4)$$

When initial rises in stroke volume alone are insufficient to meet the demands of intense exercise, sympathetic nerves arising from the thoracic sympathetic chain stimulate an increase in heart rate. Whilst the heart rate is capable of rising substantially during exercise, efficiency at higher rates is compromised due to shortening of ventricular filling time in diastole, which results in an impairment of stroke volume. In health, heart rate rises in direct proportion to oxygen uptake to the point of exhaustion, where the physiological limit to heart rate is reached. Achievement of an estimated maximum predicted heart rate based on age can provide some supportive evidence of exhaustive effort during exercise (➲ Fig. 1.1.1.2).

Positive chronotropy is achieved by noradrenergic stimulation of the sinoatrial node, which increases the permeability of the pacemaker cells to sodium and calcium ions. This results in an increase in the slope of the action potential, allowing the sinoatrial node pacemaker cells to reach the activation threshold more quickly and the interval between successive action potentials to be reduced. The atrioventricular node is also under the influence of sympathetic innervation and will permit faster conduction when stimulated by noradrenaline.

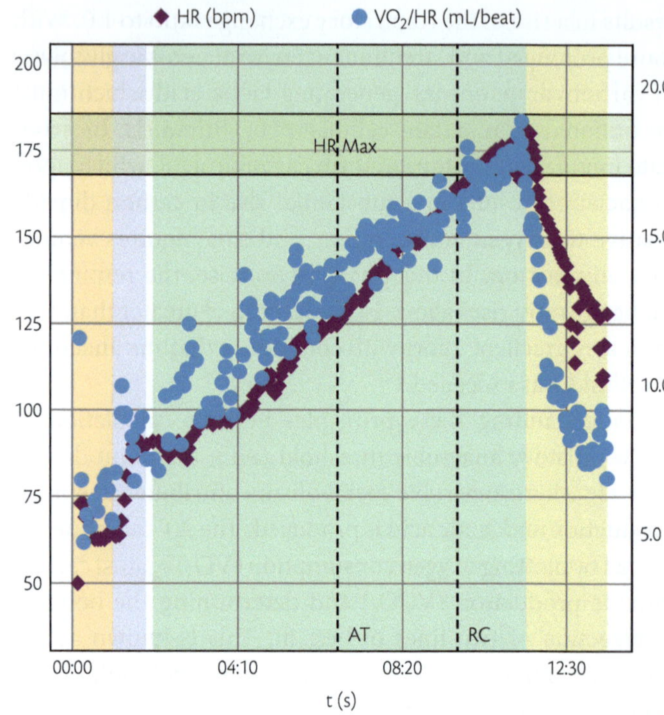

Fig. 1.1.1.2 Heart rate (HR) and oxygen pulse (VO_2/HR) vs time (t). Oxygen pulse, which is a surrogate of stroke volume, rises first and reaches a plateau earlier, followed by heart rate. The vertical dashed lines represent the ventilatory anaerobic threshold (AT) and the respiratory compensation threshold (RC). The normal range of maximal heart rate is indicated (HR Max).

Exercise and the respiratory system

Oxygen is the key to unlocking chemical energy in the cell and regenerating ATP. Ventilation is a crucial factor not only for providing an adequate source of oxygen but also for the excretion of carbon dioxide, which is essential for maintaining acid–base homeostasis. In health, the lungs are easily able to meet the ventilatory requirements for efficient gas exchange, even during maximal exercise when ventilation can increase from approximately 6L/min at rest to over 100L/min. An increase in the depth and rate of ventilation during exercise allows not only replenishment of oxygen but, more importantly, the elimination of carbon dioxide. The control of breathing during exercise is under the influence of many complex integrating neuroanatomical pathways and reflexes.

The accumulation of lactic acid beyond the anaerobic threshold is initially buffered by bicarbonate ions, generating an excess of carbon dioxide. This increase in carbon dioxide level is sensed by chemoreceptors, located in the carotid bodies, which stimulate an increase in ventilation via the medullary respiratory centre. Once the lactic acid buffering capacity of the blood is exceeded during strenuous maximal exercise, the blood pH falls and this is an additional extremely potent trigger for chemoreceptor-mediated stimulation to drive dramatic hyperventilation. The considerable rise in ventilation can be detected on the cardiopulmonary exercise test and is termed either respiratory compensation for acidosis or the ventilatory compensation threshold (➲ Fig. 1.1.1.3(a)).

At low intensity exercise, ventilation increases initially by an increased depth of breathing or tidal volume. After the tidal volume reaches approximately 50–60% of the vital capacity, further increases in ventilation are achieved by increases in respiratory rate. Minute ventilation (V_E) is the product of tidal volume and respiratory rate, which rises continuously throughout exercise approaching the maximum breathing capacity. Gas exchange becomes even more efficient during exercise, through increased pulmonary capillary perfusion and greater recruitment of alveoli, resulting in greater uniformity in ventilation–perfusion matching. The improvement in ventilation–perfusion matching depends not only on increasing the alveolar surface area for gas exchange but also on the adequacy of the circulation, providing sufficient venous return to the right ventricle, good right ventricular function, and responsive pulmonary vasculature.

Although oxygen is consumed at a high rate during strenuous exercise and the arteriovenous oxygen content difference becomes greater, the ability of the lungs to source sufficient oxygen and enrich the blood is not a limiting factor in healthy individuals. Increases in minute ventilation are driven primarily by carbon dioxide production, acidosis, and central command from the brain. Ventilatory efficiency is best represented by the rise in minute ventilation per litre of carbon dioxide output. This relationship is linear below the ventilatory compensation threshold and the normal V_E/VCO_2 slope is approximately 25 (➲ Fig. 1.1.1.3(b)). Any condition that prevents air taken in during a breath from participating in gas exchange increases the physiological dead space in the airways. This may be a pulmonary condition that disturbs alveolar function or a circulatory disorder limiting alveolar perfusion and the delivery of carbon dioxide to the lungs. The result in either case is a steepening of the V_E/VCO_2 slope with high minute ventilation relative to the carbon dioxide output. This manifests clinically as

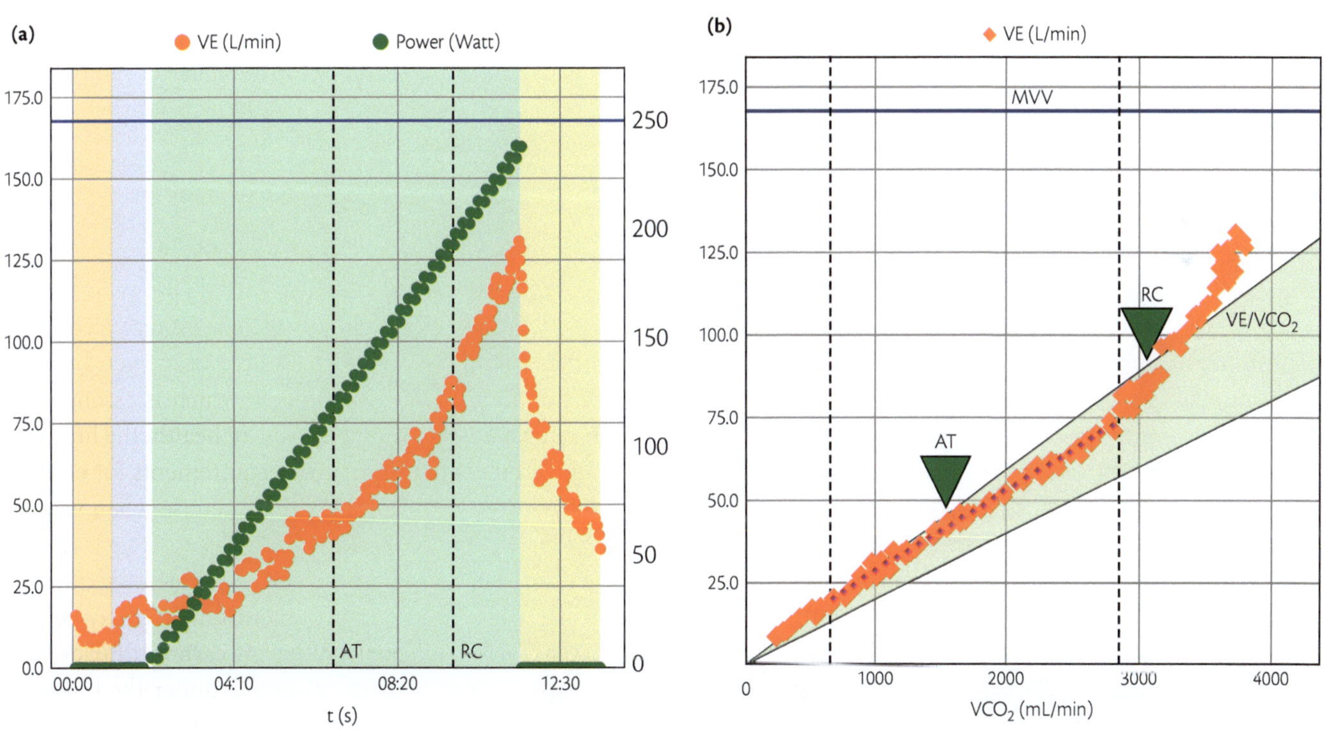

Fig. 1.1.1.3 (a) Minute ventilation (VE) (t) and work (Power) vs time. The vertical dashed lines represent the ventilatory anaerobic threshold (AT) and the respiratory compensation threshold (RC). The horizontal blue line indicates the estimated maximal ventilatory volume (MVV). (b) Minute volume (VE) vs carbon dioxide output (VCO_2). The relationship of this plot is linear until the respiratory compensation threshold is reached. In health the slope is less than 30. The horizontal blue line indicates the estimated maximal ventilatory volume (MVV). The ventilatory anaerobic threshold and respiratory compensation threshold are indicated by AT and RC, respectively. The normal range of vales is indicated (VE/VCO_2).

uncomfortable dyspnoea, which limits functional capacity in disease states.

Alveolar ventilation and pulmonary perfusion both increase during exercise, which results in greater uniformity in ventilation–perfusion matching. End-tidal oxygen levels are relatively stable during early exercise and rise at the ventilatory compensation threshold due to metabolic acidosis-induced hyperventilation. End-tidal carbon dioxide levels increase minimally in the early stages of incremental exercise, resulting from the increase in production from substrate metabolism coupled with the release from the bicarbonate buffering of lactic acid. Once the ventilatory compensation threshold is passed in heavy exercise, acidosis-driven hyperventilation dramatically augments minute ventilation, resulting in a fall in end-tidal carbon dioxide levels.

In summary, exercise reflects the ability of the human body to summon skeletal muscle activity with immediacy and for prolonged periods. From an evolutionary perspective, the ability to fight or flee effectively is a critical determinant of species survival. Physical activity is the culmination of an impeccably orchestrated arrangement incorporating the brain, nervous system, heart, circulation, lungs, adrenal glands, and muscles. Each system has a part to play in energy generation, oxygen uptake, and carbon dioxide elimination, with the ability to respond and modulate outputs akin to fine tuning. It is remarkable how cardiac output and pulmonary ventilation are so precisely adjusted to meet the metabolic demands of exercise until fatigue. The versatility of how chemical energy can be sourced from various substrates, stored, and borrowed permits the necessary transformation from chemical to kinetic energy, harnessing locomotive power. Exercise performance is limited by the role of the cardiovascular system in oxygen transport, although athletes demonstrate considerable functional remodelling of the heart to deliver greater cardiac output and better accommodate the repeated physiological stresses of exercise.

Further reading

Jones NL, Killian KJ. Exercise limitation in health and disease. *N Engl J Med* 2000; 343(9): 632–41.

Laughlin MH. Cardiovascular response to exercise. *Am J Physiol* 1999; 277 (6 Pt 2): S244–59.

Wasserman K, Hansen J, Sue D, et al. *Principles of Exercise Testing and Interpretation* (4th edn) Philadelphia, PA: Lippincott Williams & Wilkins, 2005.

References

1. McArdle W, Catch F, Catch V. Functional capacity of the cardiovascular system. *Exercise Physiology: Nutrition, Energy, and Human Performance* (8th edn), Chapter 17. Baltimore, MD: Wolters Kluwer, 2014 , p. 347.
2. Jones NL, Killian KJ. Exercise limitation in health and disease. *N Engl J Med* 2000; 343(9): 632–41.

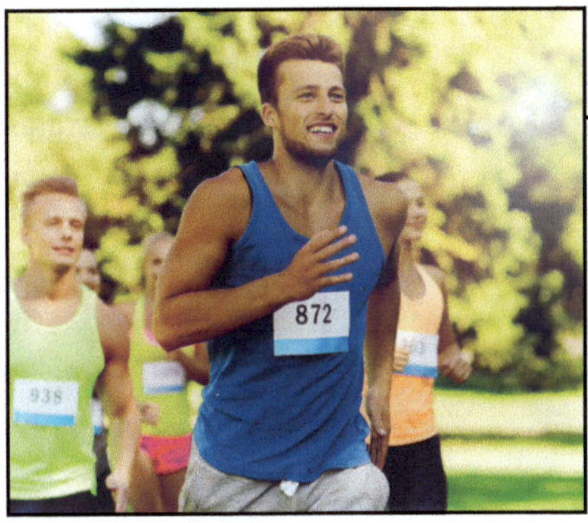

1.2

Long-term adaptation to exercise: athlete's heart and vascular adaptations

Contents

1.2.1 **Structural and functional adaptations in the athlete's heart** Antonio Pelliccia and Stefano Caselli 9
1.2.2 **Impact of sporting discipline, gender, ethnicity, and genetics on the athlete's heart** Nabeel Sheikh 20
1.2.3 **The athlete's heart in children and adolescents** Graham Stuart and Guido E. Pieles 32
1.2.4 **Vascular remodelling** Stephan Gielen, M. Harold Laughlin, and Dirk J. Duncker 41

1.2.1 Structural and functional adaptations in the athlete's heart

Antonio Pelliccia and Stefano Caselli

Historical perspective: from chest percussion to 3D imaging

The human body has an extraordinary ability to respond to environmental changes in a way that guarantees vital function and survival under many circumstances. Sport activity is an example of this impressive adaptation capacity, with a series of integrated changes in structure and function of different organs and systems within the body which allow the accomplishment of greater exercise performance.

The cardiovascular system goes through many adaptations as a consequence of exposure to chronic exercise training, which have been described by scientists for more than a century. Indeed, the first observations regarding cardiac changes associated with high intensity exercise training date back to 1899, when Henshen, from the University of Uppsala, in his publication 'A study in sports medicine; skiing and competitive skiing', stated that 'skiing causes an enlargement of the heart, and this enlarged heart can perform more work than a normal heart. There is, therefore, a physiologic enlargement of the heart due to athletic activity, i.e. the '*Athlete's Heart*' [1]. This accurate definition is impressive considering that the assessment was conducted solely by physical examination consisting of carefully performed chest percussion.

Subsequently, radiological techniques to assess the heart volume in athletes were introduced by the Scandinavian scientists Rohrer and Kahlstorf [2]. Cardiac dimensions were measured using X-rays in athletes participating in the 1928 Olympic Games in Amsterdam, and it was found that cardiac size varied in athletes engaged in different sports, with athletes engaged in endurance disciplines showing the most enlarged cardiac silhouette [3,4]. Subsequently, Reindell and Hollman, using chest X-rays, reported that an increased heart volume was associated with improved physical performance, with athletes with the greatest increase in X-ray cardiac dimension also showing the highest aerobic capacity, as expressed by maximum oxygen uptake [5,6].

Substantial contributions to the clinical issues surrounding the 'athlete's heart' originated in Italy in the 1930s, when Cassinis published *Controllo Medico dello Sport* (Medical Evaluation in Sport) [7], the first manual dedicated to the evaluation of athletes. Subsequently, Venerando and colleagues at the Institute of Sports Medicine in Rome performed a series of radiological and electrocardiographic studies of athletes participating in the 1960 Olympic Games [8]. They made several intriguing observations: a variety of cardiac X-ray silhouettes were described in trained athletes (➲ Fig. 1.2.1.1), in selected cases mimicking those found in patients with valvular or congenital heart disease which raised questions regarding

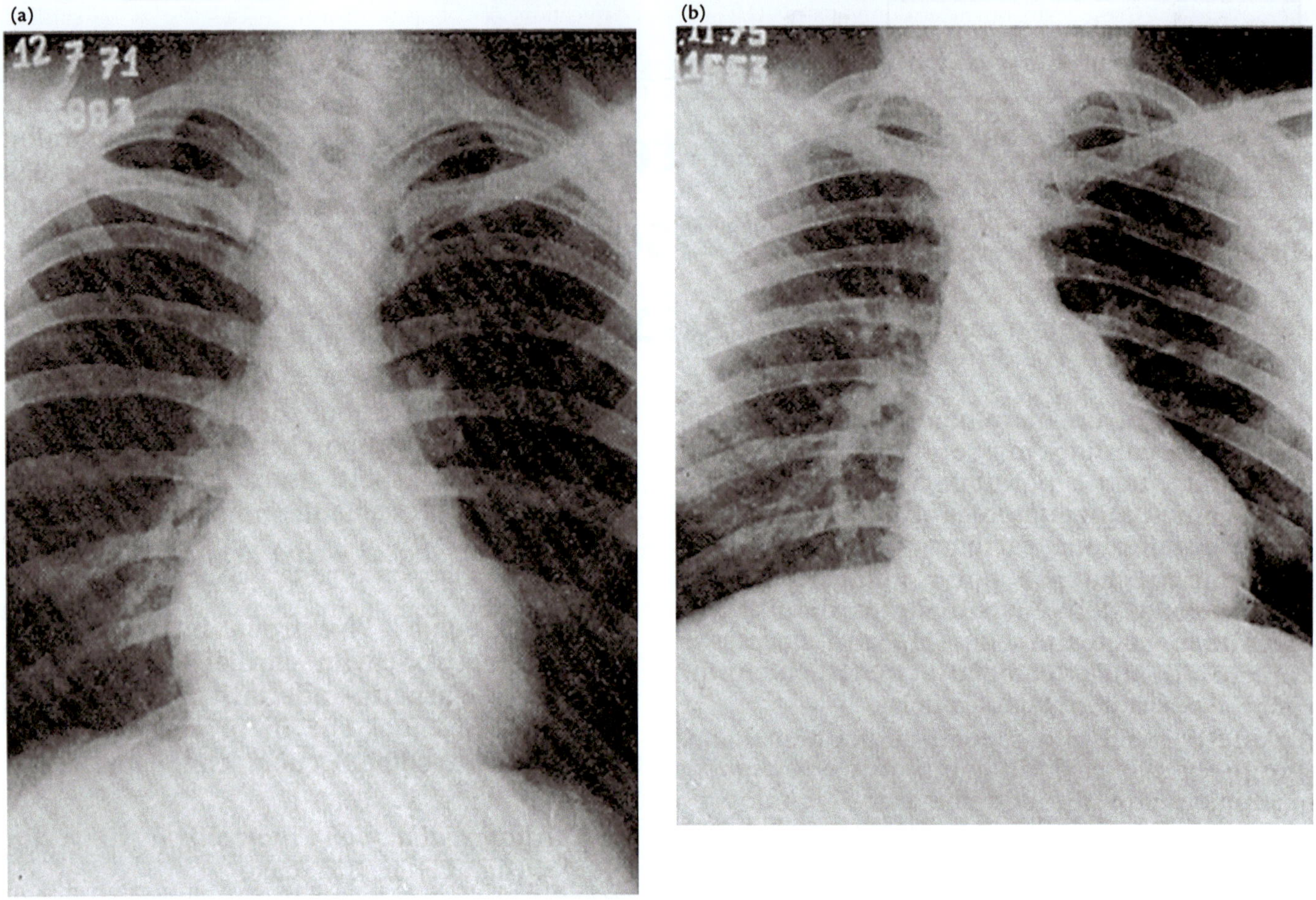

Fig. 1.2.1.1 Chest X-rays from (a) a 27-year-old male professional cyclist, showing a symmetrically enlarged cardiac silhouette, and (b) a 24-year-old male elite water polo player, showing an enlarged cardiac silhouette suggestive of distinctly enlarged LV dimensions. An increased pulmonary vascular tree is also evident in both X-ray images,.

differential diagnosis between cardiac disease and physiological heart adaptation [9].

Echocardiography, introduced in clinical cardiovascular practice at the end of the 1970s, gave a great impulse to investigation of the morphological and functional features of the 'athlete's heart'. In 1975 the first comparative echocardiographic study of athletes engaged in endurance-type and strength-type sports was published by Morganroth et al. in the *Annals of Internal Medicine* [10]. This study compared M-mode echocardiographic measurements of untrained subjects, strength-trained athletes, and endurance-trained athletes. The authors observed that athletes engaged in endurance training showed eccentric left ventricular (LV) remodelling (as a consequence of volume overload), while those in strength training showed concentric hypertrophy (as consequence of pressure overload). Therefore they hypothesized that morphological adaptations in athletes could be related to the type of haemodynamic overload associated with the specific exercise training.

This investigation pioneered a large series of studies assessing the structural changes, upper limits. and clinical correlates of cardiac remodelling in trained athletes. In this context, in 1991 Pelliccia et al. published a pivotal study in the *New England Journal of Medicine* describing the characteristics and upper limits of LV hypertrophy derived from a large athlete cohort from the database of Institute of Sports Medicine and Science [11]. A few years later, in 1995, the largest investigation describing the characteristics of 'athlete's heart' in women appeared in the *Journal of the American Medical Association* [12], and in 1999 a report on the morphological features and clinical correlates of LV dilatation was published in the *Annals of Internal Medicine* [13]. Since then, reports of several subsequent studies have been published describing the determinants of cardiovascular adaptations to exercise training according to age, gender, ethnicity, and the sport participated in [14–17].

In 1976, two episodes of sudden cardiac death in young competitive athletes occurred within 8 weeks of each other, one due to aortic rupture caused by Marfan syndrome and one secondary to hypertrophic cardiomyopathy (HCM). These tragic events attracted the attention of the media and raised the consciousness of the medical community about the potential harm of intense exercise activity in individuals with inherent, often silent, cardiovascular disease [18,19]. These and other detrimental events in subsequent years resulted in a major drive towards the timely identification of cardiac diseases capable of causing sudden cardiac death (SCD) in competitive athletes, and the utility of implementing pre-participation screening programmes to prevent such catastrophes. As a consequence, a large literature has been produced regarding the criteria for identifying the risk of cardiac disease in athletes and the differentiation of physiological cardiac remodelling from cardiac pathology.

Of particular note, a study from the Veneto region of Italy published by Corrado et al. in 2006 [20] demonstrated that, after implementing the mandatory preparticipation screening (including 12-lead ECG), the incidence of SCD in screened athletes progressively declined, mainly due to the ability to identify athletes with underlying cardiomyopathies. Many studies have been performed subsequently in order to emphasize the importance of ECG screening in athletes as a model for identifying pathological conditions at risk of SCD.

In this scenario, cardiac imaging has continuously evolved with substantial advances in cardiac magnetic resonance (CMR) and newer echocardiographic techniques (such as 3D echocardiography (➲ Fig. 1.2.1.2) and speckle tracking imaging). These highly sophisticated techniques have led to further clarification of the geometrical characteristics of cardiac chamber remodelling in athletes and further insight into the physiology of myocardial contraction by making a relevant contribution to the differential diagnosis of physiological cardiac remodelling from cardiovascular disorders, and are part the complete evaluation of athletes in the modern era [21–24].

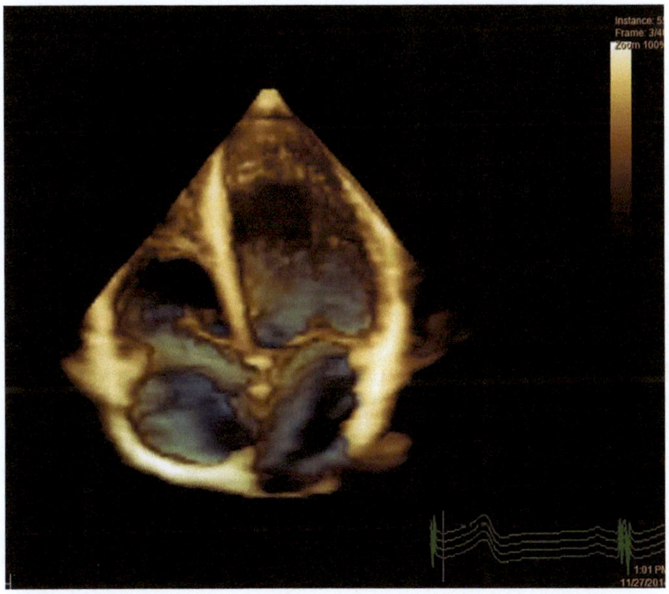

Fig. 1.2.1.2 Three-dimensional echocardiographic evaluation of the athlete's heart. This new technology allows accurate morphological assessment of cardiac structures as well as evaluation of size and function of all cardiac chambers. Notice the global and symmetric enlargement of all cavities, with preserved global left and right cavity shape.

Structural and functional adaptations of cardiac chambers

The cardiovascular system undergoes several modifications as a consequence of exercise training, with acute responses, which occur within few seconds of intensive exercise, and chronic adaptations that include more profound structural remodelling and are a result of long-term conditioning [25,26]

The acute response to exercise training includes substantial increases in heart rate, stroke volume, cardiac output, systolic blood pressure, and maximum oxygen consumption. Chronic cardiovascular adaptations to exercise training determine structural remodelling of the cardiac chambers and vessels which facilitates an increased capacity to deliver oxygen to the working muscles during prolonged bouts of exercise. Expression of cardiac remodelling consists of an increase in left and right ventricular and left atrial cavity size associated with normal (or even improved) diastolic function.

LV wall stress seems to be the most important determinant of LV remodelling, and most changes in LV geometry can be explained by the Laplace law:

$$\text{LV wall stress} = (\text{LV pressure} \times \text{radius})/(2 \times \text{LV wall thickness}).$$

This law describes the factors that determine LV wall stress, which is a major determinant of myocardial hypertrophy. LV wall stress is the force acting against the myocardial cells. This is directly proportional to the ventricular pressure and radius, and inversely proportional to the wall thickness. LV pressure increases in conditions with high afterload, such as systemic hypertension and aortic valve stenosis, while LV radius increases in states of high preload, such as aortic or mitral regurgitation. An increase in LV wall thickness is necessary to normalize wall stress in situations associated with an increase in preload and/or afterload (➲ Fig. 1.2.1.3) [27].

The biomechanical stress induced by the haemodynamic overload stimulates the release of angiotensin II which, in association with other humoral factors and hormones (growth factors, insulin, IGF-1) leads to 'beneficial' adaptive changes in the cardiac myocyte. Experimental models show that exercise training is associated with an over-expression of the isoform α of the myosin heavy chain, which is associated with enhanced cardiac contractility [28]. However, the

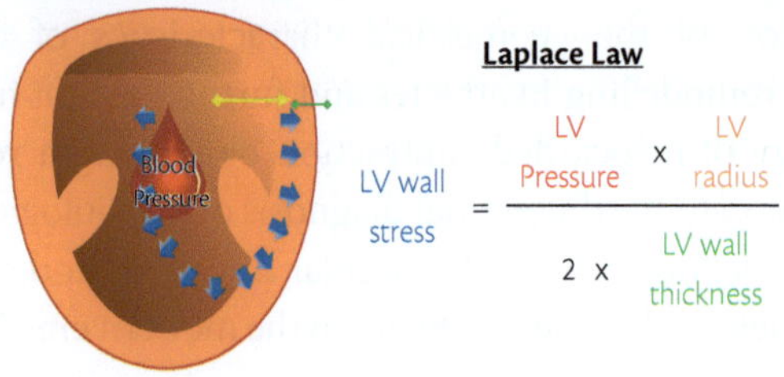

Fig. 1.2.1.3 Cardiac adaptations to athletic training can be explained by the Laplace law: the increase in LV thickness reduces myocardial wall tension that occurs with increased chamber size at a given pressure.

adult cardiomyocyte is a post-mitotic cell without regeneration capacity, and therefore myocardial hypertrophy may occur only through an increase in cellular size [29].

At the molecular level, physiological training is associated with an over-expression of the isoform α of the myosin heavy chain, which enhances cardiac contractility. The expression of mRNA for the α myosin heavy chain is an early event in the adaptation to chronic exercise and occurs before cardiac growth is evident [29,30]. In addition to the hypertrophic growth of contractile fibres, experimental studies suggest that improved LV function in trained animals can be ascribed to an alteration of the Ca^{2+} regulatory systems involved in the excitation–contraction coupling and relaxation processes [31–33].

Consistent with the increase in myocardial mass, adaptations in coronary circulation have been described, including increased vessel size and number and improved endothelial function which ultimately lead to increased coronary flow and myocardial oxygen supply [27,34].

Determinants of cardiac hypertrophy

Macroscopic structural remodelling of the athlete's heart has been extensively studied using echocardiography for almost four decades and this has enabled an appreciation of the determinants and upper limits of the cardiac adaptation in highly trained athletes. It is now well recognized that age, sex, ethnicity, body size, type of sport, and amount of training (with a dose–effect relation) are the main determinants of remodelling, and therefore structural adaptation may vary considerably between one athlete and another. However, the relative contribution of demographic and environmental or genetic determinants of LV remodelling in trained athletes has long been a subject of controversy [35].

Multivariate analysis of data obtained from large athlete populations shows that 75% of variability in LV cavity size is attributable to non-genetic factors, such as body size, type of sport, gender, age, and anthropometric features [12]. The remaining 25% of variability is otherwise unexplained, and is possibly due in part to genetic factors [12,35].

The pattern and magnitude of physiologically increased LV mass varies with respect to the type and intensity of exercise training. The most extreme increases in LV cavity dimension and/or wall thickness are observed in athletes engaged in endurance sports such as rowing, cross-country skiing, cycling, and swimming (➲ Fig. 1.2.1.4). However, other than the sport discipline itself, cardiovascular adaptation may rely on the intrinsic characteristics of training. For instance, the

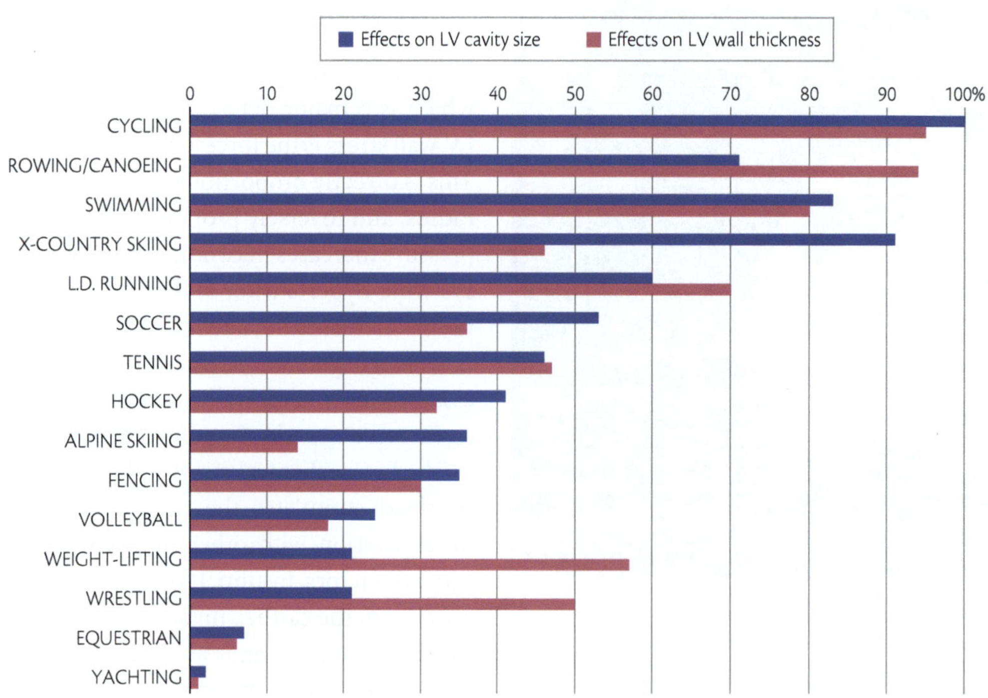

Fig. 1.2.1.4 Impact of different sport disciplines on cardiovascular remodelling in athletes. The relative effect on cavity size and wall thickness is represented.

haemodynamic load may vary even within the same discipline; the paradigm is soccer where the goalkeeper is subject to a different haemodynamic load compared with the striker or midfield players. Indeed, the individual characteristics of the athlete (age, gender, body size, and composition) significantly affect the extent of cardiac remodelling.

For didactic purposes, exercise physiology can be dichotomously divided into isotonic (dynamic) and isometric (static) components [36,37]. Chronic isotonic exercise imparts a volume overload to all cardiac chambers which induces cavity enlargement, whereas isometric exercise is associated with short bursts of a significant increase in afterload. Although the afterload may be very intense, its shorter duration has a lower impact on LV dimensions compared with isotonic exercise [38]. However, this dichotomous classification cannot be applied to the majority of sports disciplines, which may include a varying mixture of components of dynamic and static exercise. Therefore knowledge of the specific exercise training of the athlete is mandatory to improve understanding of the characteristics of cardiac remodelling .

Left heart dimensions and function in athletes

LV wall thickness in athletes varies with regard to sex, ethnicity, and type of sport, but in the vast majority of cases remains within normal limits. The greatest degree of LV hypertrophy is usually seen in male athletes, but values >12mm are observed in less than 2% of Caucasian athletes (➲ Fig. 1.2.1.5). Conversely, in female athletes the degree of hypertrophy is usually milder, with values extending up to 11mm. Interestingly, while white athletes rarely demonstrate an increase in wall thickness in the range overlapping with pathological LV hypertrophy such as HCM, a larger

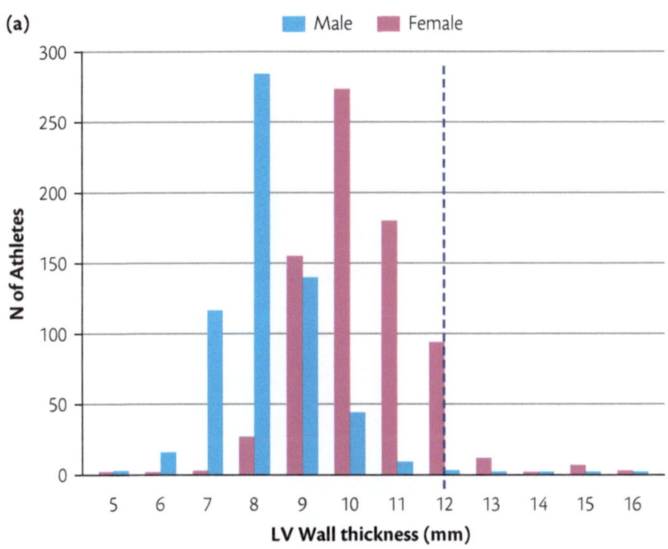

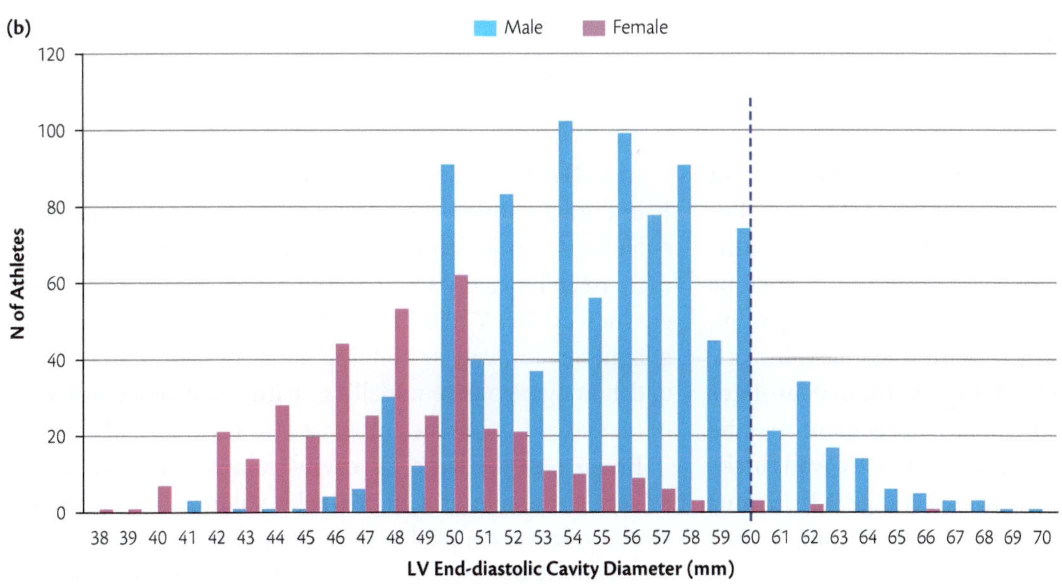

Fig. 1.2.1.5 (a) Distribution of LV wall thickness in a large population of Italian athletes. An increase in wall thickness >12mm (dotted line) is observed in 2% of male and 0% of female athletes. (b) Distribution of LV cavity size in a large population of Italian athletes. Of the overall population, 14% had values >60mm and up to 70mm. (c) Distribution of left atrial dimension in a group of highly trained Italian athletes. The dotted line represents the cut-off of 40mm; approximately 20% of individuals showed an increase in left atrial size, with only 2% showing marked left atrial enlargement >45mm. (d) Distribution of aortic root dimensions in a group of highly trained Italian athletes. The dotted line represents the cut-off of 40mm.

(a) Adapted from *The New England Journal of Medicine*, Antonio Pelliccia, Barry J. Maron, Antonio Spataro, et al. The upper limit of physiologic cardiac hypertrophy in highly trained elite athletes, Volume 324, Issue 5, pp 295–301. Copyright © (1991) Massachusetts Medical Society. Reprinted with permission from Massachusetts Medical Society.

(b) From *Annals of Internal Medicine*, Pelliccia, Antonio; Culasso, Franco. Physiologic left ventricular cavity dilatation in elite athletes, Volume 130, Issue 1, pp. 23–31. Copyright © 1999 American College of Physicians. All Rights Reserved. Reprinted with the permission of American College of Physicians, Inc.

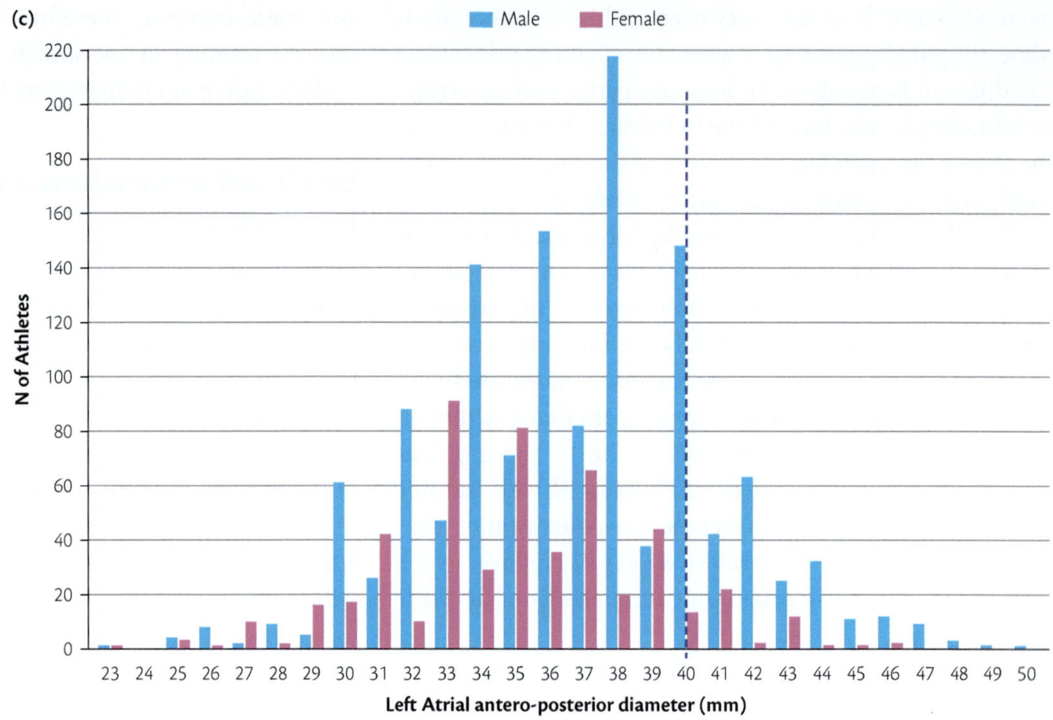

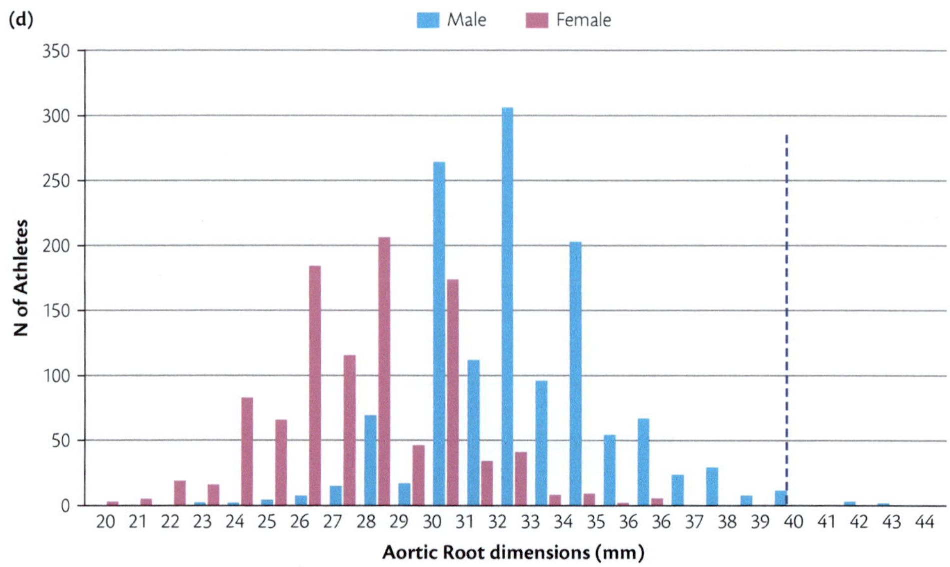

Fig. 1.2.1.5 *(Continued)* (c) Reprinted from *Journal of the American College of Cardiology*, Antonio Pelliccia, Barry J. Maron, Fernando M. Di Paolo, Alessandro Biffi, Filippo M. Quattrini, Cataldo Pisicchio, Alessandra Roselli, Stefano Caselli, Franco Culasso. Prevalence and clinical significance of left atrial remodeling in competitive athletes, Volume 46, edition 4, pp. 690–696. Copyright (2005) with permission from Elsevier. (d) Reproduced with permission from Pelliccia A. et al., Prevalence and clinical significance of aortic root dilation in highly trained competitive athletes, *Circulation*, Volume 122, Issue 7, pp.69–706. Copyright © 2010 Wolters Kluwer Health, Inc.

proportion of black male athletes (up to 18%) may present with LV wall thickness >12mm (➔ Fig. 1.2.1.6) [11,16,39,40].

An increased LV chamber dimension in trained athletes has been well documented. LV cavity dimensions vary widely with respect to type of sport and gender, and may be strikingly enlarged, with end-diastolic values ≥60mm in almost 15% of highly trained athletes [13] (➔ Fig. 1.2.1.5). This chamber enlargement may be accompanied by a small increase in absolute LV wall thickness exceeding upper normal limits (range 13–15mm) when endurance training is associated with components of strength training [11].

In a 3D echocardiography study, LV end-diastolic volume in endurance athletes was on average 50% than in untrained subjects. An interesting and practical observation is that the increase in LV cavity size is always associated with a consistent increase in LV mass, suggesting that in the physiological adaptation to exercise training there is always a balanced and homogeneous remodelling, with consistency in terms of increased LV volume and mass [17] (➔ Fig. 1.2.1.7).

Because of the large LV cavity volume, the heart of an athlete is capable of a high stroke volume. The increased stroke volume, coupled with increased vagal tone, explains why trained athletes usually have low heart rates. The LV

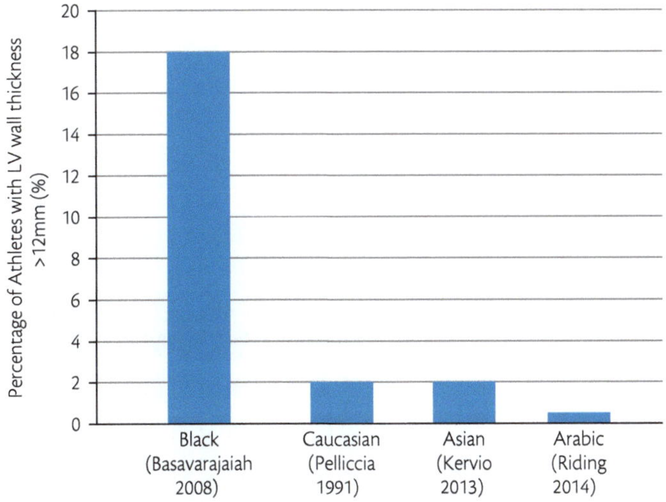

Fig. 1.2.1.6 Proportion of athletes of different ethnicities showing an increase in wall thickness in the range of mild LV hypertrophy (<12mm).
Data from references 11,16, 39, and 40.

ejection fraction is usually unchanged but may be just below normal limits in athletes with large LV dimensions [41]. Several studies and a meta-analysis [42] encompassing 59 studies, including 1451 athletes, confirm that LV function in athletes is no different from that in untrained subjects and (also in our experience) LV ejection fraction is consistently ≥50% (➔ Fig. 1.2.1.8). Therefore detection of a more substantial reduction in systolic function (EF <50%) should not necessarily be considered a benign consequence of athletic training but deserves clinical investigation. Indeed, 2D speckle tracking echocardiography allows better evaluation of the contractile properties of the myocardium by describing the deformation of myocardial fibres during the cardiac cycle. Based on recent observations, the LV deformation pattern of trained athletes is similar to that of untrained individuals, supporting the concept that LV contractile properties are not impaired despite substantial changes in LV wall thickness, cavity size, and mass [22].

Additionally, a 3D echocardiographic study has previously reported that the duration of mechanical systole in athletes is shorter (by an average of 10%) in athletes compared with untrained subjects. This mild shortening of mechanical systole (and a consequent lengthening of diastole), associated with a larger amount of blood ejected, is a demonstration of a more efficient myocardial pumping capacity induced by athletic training [43].

With regard to the impact of cardiac remodelling on diastolic LV function, there is no evidence to suggest a detrimental impact on diastolic function. Commonly, the LV filling in young athletes is characterized by a trans-mitral E/A ratio significantly higher than in untrained subjects, and always >1.0, suggesting that values <1.0 imply a non-physiological condition [44]. The increase in the E/A ratio is mainly due to a decrease in A wave velocity, meaning that the relative contribution of the left atrial (LA) pump, under resting conditions, is lower in athletes compared with untrained controls, and most of the LV filling occurs in early diastole. However, the additional atrial boost becomes important for

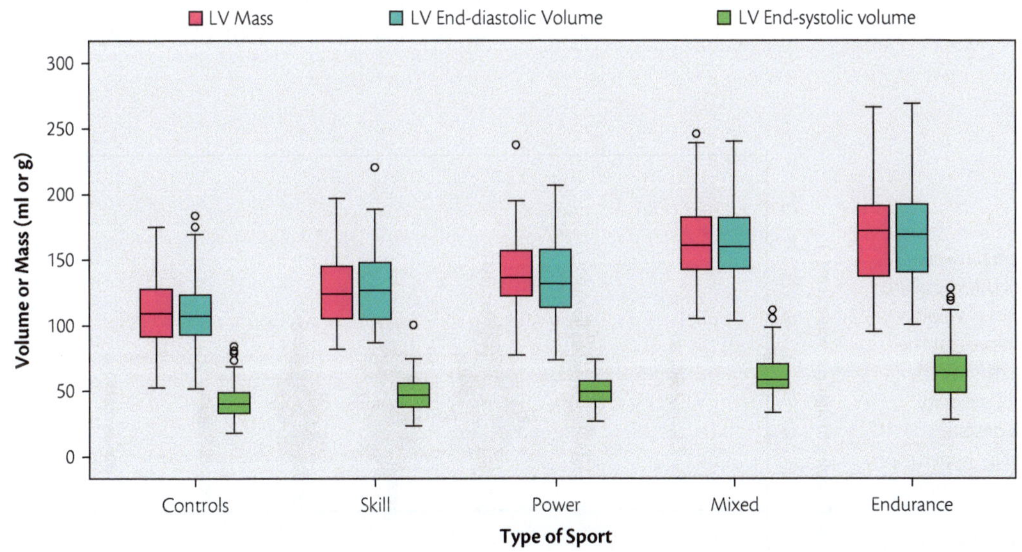

Fig. 1.2.1.7 LV volume and mass measured by 3D echocardiography in elite athletes of different sport disciplines and untrained controls. The increase in LV end-diastolic volume is always associated with a consistent increase in LV mass suggesting that, regardless of the sport discipline, there is always a balanced and homogeneous remodelling.
Reprinted from *The American Journal of Cardiology*, Volume 108, edition 1, Stefano Caselli, Fernando M. Di Paolo, Cataldo Pisicchio, Riccardo Di Pietro, Filippo M. Quattrini, Barbara Di Giacinto, Franco Culasso, Antonio Pelliccia. Three-dimensional echocardiographic characterization of left ventricular remodeling in Olympic athletes, pp. 1-7, Copyright (2011), with permission from Elsevier.

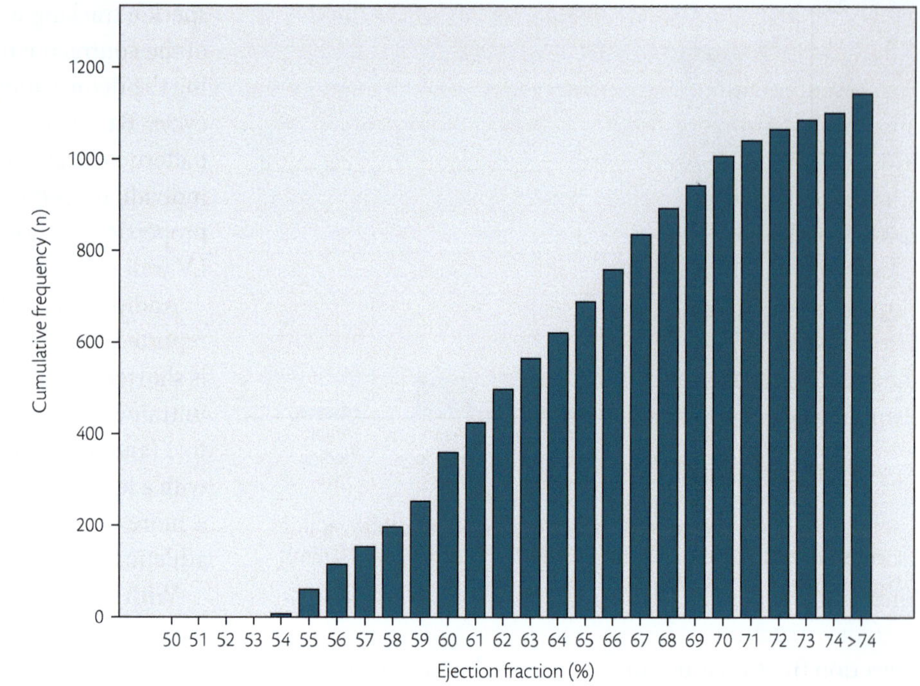

Fig. 1.2.1.8 Ejection fraction, measured by echocardiography using Simpson's rule, in a population of 1159 athletes from the database of the Insitute of Sports Medicine and Science (age 15–45, 65% male, 98% Caucasian). The bars represent the cumulative frequencies of athletes with respect to increasing values of ejection fraction. None of the athletes show values <50%, and only a small minority have values ≤55%.
Reprinted from *Journal of the American Society of Echocardiography*, Volume 28, edition 2, Stefano Caselli, Fernando M. Di Paolo, Cataldo Pisicchio, Natesa G. Pandian, Antonio Pelliccia. Patterns of left ventricular diastolic function in Olympic athletes, pp. 236–44. Copyright (2015), with permission from Elsevier.

increasing output, particularly during peak exercise. In a similar fashion, elite athletes always exhibit a septal e′ velocity >8.0cm/s (assessed by tissue Doppler imaging). This has important clinical implication since lower values have been reported in cases of pathological LV hypertrophy, such as HCM; indeed, even individuals with genotype-positive phenotype-negative HCM may reveal abnormal e′ velocity, emphasizing the principle that abnormal diastolic function may precede the development of pathological LV hypertrophy (➲ Fig. 1.2.1.9) [45–47].

LA remodelling is also recognized in highly trained athletes, most commonly those training for endurance sports, and is largely part of the global increase in cardiac dimensions in response to an increased preload [48]. A transverse LA dimension ≥40mm is present in 20% of young athletes, and is more substantially enlarged (≥45mm) in 2%, overlapping with atrial dimensions observed in patients with cardiac disease such as HCM (➲ Fig. 1.2.1.5). A differential feature peculiar to the physiological atrial enlargement is the direct relationship with LV cavity enlargement, in contrast

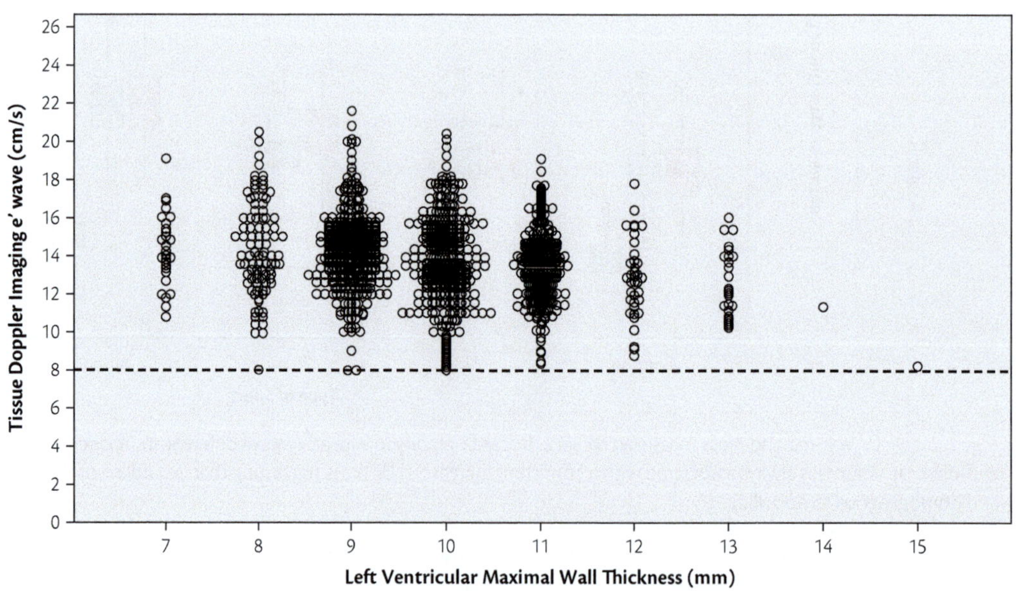

Fig. 1.2.1.9 Relation between the maximal LVl wall thickness and the TDI-derived septal e′ velocity in athletes; dot-line represent the reference value of 8cm/s. All the athletes show septal e′ velocity consistently >8cm/s despite substantial degree of LV hypertrophy (≥13mm) in a small proportion of athletes.
Reprinted from *Journal of the American Society of Echocardiography*, Volume 28, edition 2, Stefano Caselli, Fernando M. Di Paolo, Cataldo Pisicchio, Natesa G. Pandian ,Antonio Pelliccia. Patterns of left ventricular diastolic function in Olympic athletes, pp. 236–44, Copyright (2015), with permission from Elsevier.

with pathological LA enlargement in HCM where the size of the LV cavity is usually normal or reduced.

A recent meta-analysis showed that the LA diameter was on average 4.1mm greater in athletes than in sedentary controls, and that the LA volume index was 7.0ml/m^2 greater in athletes than controls [49]. Moreover, LA remodelling in the context of the athlete's heart is not associated with increased LA stiffness [48,50]. LA enlargement in athletes appears to be clinically benign, and in young healthy athletes is very rarely associated with incident atrial fibrillation (<1%), supporting the view that LA remodelling in athletes is a physiological manifestation of intensive exercise conditioning.

Right heart and aortic remodelling in athletes

Similarly to the left heart, the chambers in the right heart also undergo structural remodelling as a consequence of long-term exercise training, and both the right atrium (RA) and right ventricle (RV) are usually enlarged in athletes [51–58] The RV is subject to a lower pressure overload compared with the left ventricle because the pulmonary resistance is lower than the systemic resistance. However, invasive studies during exercise have revealed that pulmonary artery pressure can reach high values (up to 80mmHg) [51].

Male athletes show significantly larger absolute RV dimensions compared with females, while indexed values are usually larger in female athletes (➔ Fig. 1.2.1.10). With regard to ethnicity, its impact on RV dimensions is minimal, obviating the need for race-specific reference values [56]. The most significant changes in RV size are observed in endurance athletes, while several studies have reported that strength athletes exhibit no significant changes in RV dimensions and systolic function.

Recent studies involving large cohorts of athletes engaged in a broad spectrum of sport disciplines have reported that the greater the duration and intensity of isotonic exercise, the larger the increase in the dimensions of the RV (and RA) chambers [53–58] Interestingly, a large proportion of athletes may present with RV dimensions exceeding normal reference values and compatible with those seen in patients with arrhythmogenic right ventricular cardiomyopathy (ARVC) [56,58]. However, despite these substantial morphological adaptations, RV systolic function is usually unchanged in athletes and no wall motion abnormalities are seen, supporting the physiological nature of RV changes and providing insight into the differential diagnosis between physiological RV remodelling and the pathological RV remodelling occurring in cardiac diseases such as ARVC [56–58]. Another interesting observation is that RV adaptation occurs in synergy with LV remodelling. Therefore a practical clinical insight is the usual finding of a balanced and symmetric enlargement of the RV and LV ventricular cavities, whereas a disproportionate increase in size of either the RV or LV cavity should instinctively suggest non-physiological remodelling.

Aortic remodelling in athletes has also been documented [59–61]. During exercise the aorta is subject to a significant haemodynamic load; both the increased stroke volume and the increase in blood pressure cause increased stress through the aortic wall. As a consequence, athletes usually show a larger aortic root dimension compared with untrained

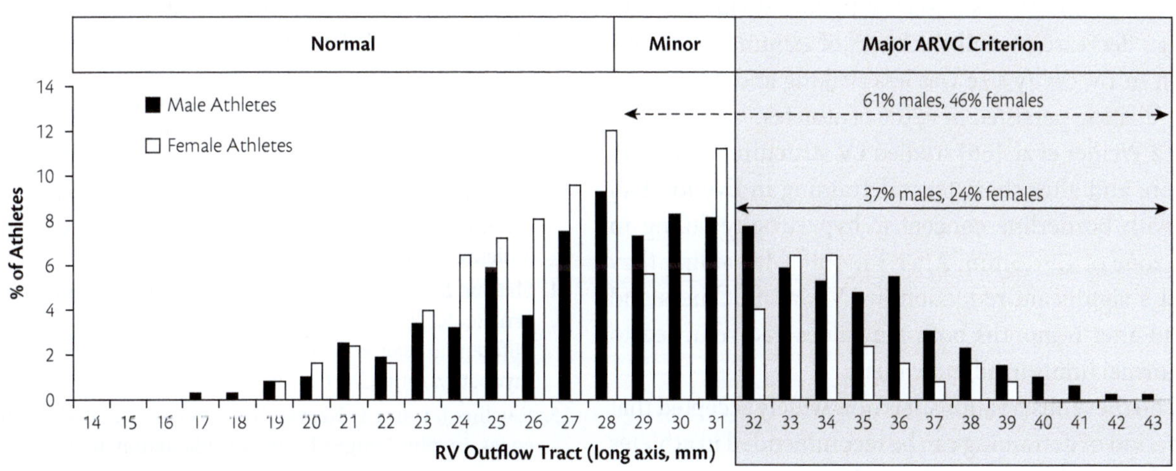

Fig. 1.2.1.10 Distribution of right ventricular outflow tract diameter measured by echocardiography in the parasternal long axis view in 675 athletes. Black bars represent male athletes and white bars represent female athletes. A large proportion of athletes exceed both the minor and major dimensional criteria for arrhythmogenic right ventricular cardiomyopathy.

subjects. However, this change is relatively small; the upper limit of aortic root size in male endurance athletes is 40mm. Finding a larger aortic size should prompt comprehensive evaluation because it may be evidence of a degenerative disease of the aortic wall (➔ Fig. 1.2.1.5) [62,63].

The dynamic nature of cardiac adaptations

The structural remodelling observed in highly trained athletes is dynamic in nature and persists as long as the haemodynamic overload is operating. Interruption of systematic training is associated with reduction in LV mass, and this observation is the basis for a differential diagnosis of physiological LV hypertrophy from the pathological hypertrophy of HCM.

The first observation of reverse remodelling in detrained athletes was reported in 1993, when Maron et al. [64] observed a significant reduction in LV wall thickness in elite endurance athletes after an average 3-month detraining period. The athletes evaluated at peak training (corresponding to the 1988 Seoul Olympic Games) and after detraining showed an average reduction of 3mm in maximal LV wall thickness, confirming the adaptive nature of cardiac LV hypertrophy induced by exercise conditioning.

Some years later Pelliccia et al. [65] studied the effects of long-term deconditioning on a population of 40 Italian elite male athletes who showed marked LV remodelling (i.e. cavity diameter ≥60mm and/or wall thickness ≥13mm). After an average period of 6 years (occasionally extending to 13 years) regression of LV remodelling, including significant reduction in LV cavity size and LV wall thickness, was evident in the athletes. Of particular interest, the resolution of LV hypertrophy (to values of ≤12mm) was observed in all individuals, with an average decrease in wall thickness of ≥2mm; conversely reduction in LV cavity size was less striking and substantial chamber dilation persisted in >20% of athletes.

In 2012 Weiner et al. [66] studied LV structural modification before and after short-term detraining in five football players with borderline concentric hypertrophy falling in the grey zone of 13–15mm. After 3 months detraining they observed a significant reduction in LV wall thickness and mass, and after 6 months both the values had returned to within normal limits in all individuals.

Based on these observations, it is now widely accepted that a short period of detraining can be recommended in athletes with borderline LV hypertrophy to demonstrate regression of the hypertrophy, thus confirming the benign nature of training-induced LV wall thickening. Lack of a reduction in LV hypertrophy is considered to be a non-physiological phenomenon, consistent with a maladaptive process and possible evidence of a pathological condition such as HCM.

Further reading

Caselli S, Di Paolo FM, Pisicchio C, et al. Patterns of left ventricular diastolic function in Olympic athletes. *J Am Soc Echocardiogr* 2015; 28(2): 236–44.

D'Ascenzi F, Pisicchio C, Caselli S, et al. Remodeling in Olympic athletes. *JACC Cardiovasc Imaging* 2017; 10(4): 385–93.

Pelliccia A, Maron BJ, Spataro A, et al. The upper limit of physiologic cardiac hypertrophy in highly trained elite athletes. *N Engl J Med 1991*; 324 295–301.

Sharma S, Merghani A, Mont L. Exercise and the heart: the good, the bad, and the ugly. *Eur Heart J* 2015; 36(23): 1445–53.

References

1. Henschen S. Skilanglauf und Skiwettlauf. Eine medizinische Sportstudie. *Mitt Med Klin Uppsala (Jena) 1899*; 2 15–18.
2. Rohrer F. Volumenbestimmung an Korperhohlen und Organen auf orthodiagraphischem wege. *Fortschr Rontgenstr* 1916; 24 285–9.
3. Deutsch F, Kauf E. *Herz und Sport*. Vienna: Bern, 1924.
4. Buytendijk FJJ, Snapper I. *Ergebnisse sportarztlichen Untersuchungen bei den IX Olympischen Spielen in Amsterdam 1928*. Berlin: Springer, 1929.
5. Reindell H, Klepzig H, Steim H, et al. *Herz-Kreislaufkrankheiten und Sport*. Munich, 1960.
6. Hollman W. Der arbeits und trainingseinfluss auf Kreislauf und Atmung. Darmstadt: Steinkopff, 1959.
7. Cassinis U. *Controllo Medico dello Sport*. Rome: Enzo Pinci, 1934.
8. Venerando A, Rulli V.Frequency, morphology and meaning of the electrocardiographic anomalies found in Olympic marathon runners. *J Sports Med* 1964; 3 135–41.
9. Rossi F, Todaro A, Venerando A. Pulmonary circulation in endurance athletes. *J Sports Med* 1997; 17 269–73
10. Morganroth J, Maron BJ, Henry WL, Epstein SE. Comparative left ventricular dimensions in trained athletes. *Ann Intern Med* 1975; 82: 521–4.
11. Pelliccia A, Maron BJ, Spataro A, et al. The upper limit of physiologic cardiac hypertrophy in highly trained elite athletes. *N Engl J Med* 1991; 324 : 295–301.
12. Pelliccia A.Culasso F, Di Paolo F, Maron BJ. Physiologic left ventricular cavity dilatation in elite athletes. *Ann Intern Med.* 1999; 130 23–31.
13. Pelliccia A, Maron BJ, Culasso F, et al. Athlete's heart in women: echocardiographic characterization of highly trained elite female athletes. *JAMA* 1996; 276 211–15.
14. Sharma S, Maron BJ, Whyte G, et al. Physiologic limits of left ventricular hypertrophy in elite junior athletes: relevance to differential diagnosis of athlete's heart and hypertrophic cardiomyopathy. *J Am Coll Cardiol* 2002; 40(8): 1431–6.
15. Rawlins J, Carré F, Kervio G, Papadakis M, et al. Ethnic differences in physiological cardiac adaptation to intense physical exercise in highly trained female athletes. *Circulation* 2010; 121(9): 1078–85.
16. Basavarajaiah S, Boraita A, Whyte G, et al. Ethnic differences in left ventricular remodeling in highly-trained athletes relevance to differentiating physiologic left ventricular hypertrophy from hypertrophic cardiomyopathy. *J Am Coll Cardiol* 2008; 51(23) : 2256–62.

17. Caselli S, Di Paolo FM, Pisicchio C, et al. Three-dimensional echocardiographic characterization of left ventricular remodeling in Olympic athletes. *Am J Cardiol* 2011; 108(1): 141–7.
18. Maron BJ. Historical perspectives on sudden deaths in young athletes with evolution over 35 years. *Am J Cardiol* 2015; 116(9): 1461–8.
19. Maron BJ, Roberts WC, McAllister HA, et al. Sudden death in young athletes. *Circulation* 1980; 62(2): 218–29.
20. Corrado D, Basso C, Pavei A, et al. Trends in sudden cardiovascular death in young competitive athletes after implementation of a preparticipation screening program. *JAMA* 2006; 296(13): 1593–1601.
21. Scharhag J, Schneider G, Urhausen A, et al. Athlete's heart: right and left ventricular mass and function in male endurance athletes and untrained individuals determined by magnetic resonance imaging. *J Am Coll Cardiol* 2002; 40(10): 1856–63.
22. Caselli S, Montesanti D, Autore C, et al. Patterns of left ventricular longitudinal strain and strain rate in Olympic athletes. *J Am Soc Echocardiogr*; 28(2): 245–53.
23. D'Ascenzi F, Caselli S, Solari M, et al. Novel echocardiographic techniques for the evaluation of athletes' heart: a focus on speckle-tracking echocardiography. *Eur J Prev Cardiol* 2016; 23(4): 437–46.
24. La Gerche A, Baggish AL, Knuuti J, et al. Cardiac imaging and stress testing asymptomatic athletes to identify those at risk of sudden cardiac death. *JACC Cardiovasc Imaging* 2013; 6(9): 993–1007.
25. George K, Whyte GP, Green DJ, et al. The endurance athlete's heart: acute stress and chronic adaptation. *Br J Sports Med* 2012; 46(Suppl 1) : i29–36.
26. Ellison GM, Waring CD, Vicinanza C, Torella D. Physiological cardiac remodelling in response to endurance exercise training: cellular and molecular mechanisms. *Heart* 2012; 98(1): 5–10.
27. Opie LH, Hasenfuss G. Mechanisms of cardiac contraction and relaxation. InBonow RO, Mann DL, Zipes DP, Libby P(eds), *Braunwald's Heart Disease: A Textbook of Cardiology, Volume 1* (9th edn). Philadelphia, PA: Elsevier Saunders, 2012, pp: 459–86.
28. Herron TJ, McDonald KS. Small amounts of alpha-myosin heavy chain isoform expression significantly increase power output of rat cardiac myocyte fragments. *Circ Res* 2002; 90 1150–2.
29. Rafalski K, Abdourahman A, Edwards JG. Early adaptations to training: upregulation of alpha-myosin heavy chain gene expression. *Med Sci Sports Exerc* 2007; 39(1): 75–82.
30. Tardiff JC, Hewett TE, Factor SM, et al. Expression of the beta (slow)-isoform of MHC in the adult mouse heart causes dominant-negative functional effects. *Am J Physiol Heart Circ Physiol* 2000; 278(2): H412–19.
31. Kemi OJ, Ellingsen O, Smith GL, Wisloff U. Exercise-induced changes in calcium handling in left ventricular cardiomyocytes. *Front Biosci* 2008; 13 356–68.
32. Wang S, Ma JZ, Zhu SS, et al. Swimming training can affect intrinsic calcium current characteristics in rat myocardium. *Eur J Appl Physiol* 2008; 104(3): 549–55.
33. Jiao Q, Bai Y, Akaike T, Takeshima H, et al. Sarcalumenin is essential for maintaining cardiac function during endurance exercise training. *Am J Physiol Heart Circ Physiol* 2009; 297(2): H576–82.
34. Pelliccia A, Spataro A, Granata M, et al. Coronary arteries in physiological hypertrophy: echocardiographic evidence of increased proximal size in elite athletes. *Int J Sports Med* 1990; 11(2): 120–6.
35. Pelliccia A, Thompson PD. The genetics of left ventricular remodeling in competitive athletes. *J Cardiovasc Med (Hagerstown)* 2006; 7(4): 267–70.
36. Kovacs R, Baggish AL. Cardiovascular adaptation in athletes. *Trends Cardiovasc Med* 2016; 26(1): 46–52.
37. Baggish AL, Wood MJ. Athlete's heart and cardiovascular care of the athlete: scientific and clinical update. *Circulation*. 2011 Jun 14; 123(23): 2723–35.
38. Pelliccia A, Spataro A, Caselli G, Maron BJ. Absence of left ventricular wall thickening in athletes engaged in intense power training. *Am J Cardiol* 1993; 72(14): 1048–54.
39. Kervio G, Pelliccia A, Nagashima J, et al. Alterations in echocardiographic and electrocardiographic features in Japanese professional soccer players: comparison to African-Caucasian ethnicities. *Eur J Prev Cardiol* 2013; 20(5): 880–8.
40. Riding NR, Salah O, Sharma S, et al. ECG and morphologic adaptations in Arabic athletes: are the European Society of Cardiology's recommendations for the interpretation of the 12-lead ECG appropriate for this ethnicity? *Br J Sports Med* 2014; 48(15): 1138–43.
41. Abergel E, Chatellier G, Hagege AA, et al. Serial left ventricular adaptations in world-class professional cyclists: implications for disease screening and follow-up. *J Am Coll Cardiol* 2004; 44(1): 144–9.
42. Pluim BM, Zwinderman AH, van der Laarse A, van der Wall EE. The athlete's heart: a meta-analysis of cardiac structure and function. *Circulation* 2000; 101(3): 336–44.
43. Caselli S, Di Pietro R, Di Paolo FM, et al. Left ventricular systolic performance is improved in elite athletes. *Eur J Echocardiogr* 2011; 12(7): 514–19.
44. Caselli S, Di Paolo FM, Pisicchio C, et al. Patterns of left ventricular diastolic function in Olympic athletes. *J Am Soc Echocardiogr* 2015; 28(2): 236–44.
45. Ho CY, Sweitzer NK, McDonough B, et al. Assessment of diastolic function with Doppler tissue imaging to predict genotype in preclinical hypertrophic cardiomyopathy. *Circulation* 2002; 105 2992–7.
46. Nagueh SF, Bachinski LL, Meyer D, et al. Tissue Doppler imaging consistently detects myocardial abnormalities in patients with hypertrophic cardiomyopathy and provides a novel means for an early diagnosis before and independently of hypertrophy. *Circulation* 2001; 104 128–30.
47. Cardim N, Perrot A, Ferreira T, et al. Usefulness of Doppler myocardial imaging for identification of mutation carriers of familial hypertrophic cardiomyopathy. *Am J Cardiol* 2002; 90 128–32.
48. Pelliccia A, Maron BJ, DiPaolo FM, et al. Prevalence and clinical significance of left atrial remodeling in competitive athletes. *J Am Coll Cardiol* 2005; 46 690–6.
49. Iskandar A, Mujtaba MT, Thompson PD. Left atrium size in elite athletes. *JACC Cardiovasc Imaging* 2015; 8(7): 753–62.
50. D'Ascenzi F, Pelliccia A, Natali BM, et al. Increased left atrial size is associated with reduced atrial stiffness and preserved reservoir function in athlete's heart. *Int J Cardiovasc Imaging* 2015; 31(4): 699–705.
51. Sharma S, Merghani A, Mont L.Exercise and the heart: the good, the bad, and the ugly. *Eur Heart J* 2015; 36(23): 1445–53.
52. D'Ascenzi F, Pelliccia A, Natali BM, et al. Morphological and functional adaptation of left and right atria induced by training in highly trained female athletes. *Circ Cardiovasc Imaging* 2014; 7(2): 222–9.

53. D'Ascenzi F, Pelliccia A, Corrado D, et al. Right ventricular remodelling induced by exercise training in competitive athletes. *Eur Heart J Cardiovasc Imaging* 2016; 17(3): 301–7.
54. D'Andrea A, La Gerche A, Golia E, et al. Right heart structural and functional remodeling in athletes. *Echocardiography* 2015; 32(Suppl 1): S11–22.
55. D'Andrea A, Riegler L, Morra S, et al. Right ventricular morphology and function in top-level athletes: a three-dimensional echocardiographic study. *J Am Soc Echocardiogr* 2012; 25(12): 1268–76.
56. Zaidi A, Ghani S, Sharma R, et al. Physiological right ventricular adaptation in elite athletes of African and Afro-Caribbean origin. *Circulation* 2013; 127(17): 1783–92.
57. Zaidi A, Sheikh N, Jongman JK, et al. Clinical differentiation between physiological remodeling and arrhythmogenic right ventricular cardiomyopathy in athletes with marked electrocardiographic repolarization anomalies. *J Am Coll Cardiol* 2015; 65(25): 2702–11.
58. D'Ascenzi F, Pisicchio C, Caselli S, et al. RV remodeling in Olympic athletes. *JACC Cardiovasc Imaging* 2017; 10(4): 385–93.
59. Pelliccia A, Di Paolo FM, De Blasiis E, et al. Prevalence and clinical significance of aortic root dilation in highly trained competitive athletes. *Circulation* 2010; 122(7): 698–706.
60. D'Andrea A, Cocchia R, Riegler L, et al. Aortic stiffness and distensibility in top-level athletes. *J Am Soc Echocardiogr* 2012; 25(5): 561–7.
61. Iskandar A, Thompson PD. A meta-analysis of aortic root size in elite athletes. *Circulation* 2013; 127(7): 791–8.
62. Engel DJ, Schwartz A, Homma S. Athletic cardiac remodeling in US professional basketball players. *JAMA Cardiol* 2016; 1(1): 80–7.
63. Boraita A, Heras ME, Morales F, et al. Reference values of aortic root in male and female white elite athletes according to sport. *Circ Cardiovasc Imaging* 2016; 9(10): e005292.
64. Maron BJ, Pelliccia A, Spataro A, Granata M. Reduction in left ventricular wall thickness after deconditioning in highly trained Olympic athletes. *Br Heart J* 1993; 69(2): 125–8.
65. Pelliccia A, Maron BJ, De Luca R, et al. Remodeling of left ventricular hypertrophy in elite athletes after long-term deconditioning. *Circulation* 2002; 105(8): 944–9.
66. Weiner RB, Wang F, Berkstresser B, et al. Regression of 'gray zone' exercise-induced concentric left ventricular hypertrophy during prescribed detraining. *J Am Coll Cardiol* 2012; 59(22): 1992–4.

1.2.2 Impact of sporting discipline, gender, ethnicity, and genetics on the athlete's heart

Nabeel Sheikh

Introduction

Participation in regular intensive exercise requires a five-to-sixfold increase in cardiac output, necessitating a constellation of structural and functional cardiac adaptations collectively termed the 'athlete's heart'. These changes, which include chamber dilatation, ventricular hypertrophy, enhanced diastolic filling, and alterations in autonomic function, are frequently reflected on the resting 12-lead ECG.

Although the electrical and structural manifestations of athlete's heart usually fall well within defined limits of normality for athletic individuals, occasionally a small proportion of athletes may display striking changes which raise suspicion of an underlying cardiac disorder implicated in exercise-related sudden cardiac death (SCD). Such cases can prove challenging for the evaluating physician in differentiating physiology from cardiac pathology [1].

The nature and extent of cardiac remodelling in response to regular bouts of intense exercise are determined by several demographic factors including the gender, sporting discipline, and ethnicity of the athlete. In recent times, the impact of genetic variation on cardiac adaptation to exercise has also emerged. The influence of these variables on the athlete's heart is the topic of this chapter, which will focus on adult athletes aged between 18 and 35 years. Cardiac remodelling in younger cohorts is the subject of Chapter 1.2.3.

The athlete's heart: electrical remodelling

Data from observational studies based on large cardiac screening programmes have established several physiological ECG changes that accompany regular exercise in adult male Caucasian (white) athletes. These changes usually reflect increased vagal tone, changes to the sinoatrial node, and chamber enlargement resulting from exercise training [2–4], and include a resting sinus bradycardia, first-degree and Mobitz type 1 second-degree atrioventricular block, partial right bundle branch block, isolated increases in QRS voltage, and the early repolarization pattern [5]. Numerous studies have demonstrated that these alterations are common, occurring in up to 70% of athletes, and are largely benign [6–9].

In contrast, a minority of adult white athletes (5–17%) may exhibit ECG patterns observed frequently in several cardiac conditions implicated in exercise-related SCD, including the cardiomyopathies [10,11] and ion-channel disorders [12]. These changes, which include pathological Q waves, axis deviation, voltage criteria for atrial enlargement, T-wave inversion, ST-segment depression, and a prolonged corrected QT interval, may result in diagnostic uncertainty between athlete's heart and cardiac pathology. To aid differentiation of benign versus pathological ECG patterns in athletes, the European Society of Cardiology (ESC)

Table 1.2.2.1 Training-related (Group 1) and training-unrelated (Group 2) ECG changed encounter in athletes

Classification of anomalies of the athlete's heart
Group 1: Common and training-related ECG changes
◆ Sinus bradycardia
◆ First-degree atrioventricular block
◆ Incomplete right bundle branch block
◆ Early repolarization
◆ Isolated QRS voltage criteria for LVH
Group 2: Uncommon and training-unrelated ECG changes
◆ T-wave inversion
◆ ST-segment depression
◆ Pathological Q waves
◆ Left atrial enlargement
◆ Left axis deviation/left anterior hemiblock
◆ Right axis deviation/left posterior hemiblock
◆ Ventricular pre-excitation
◆ Complete left or right bundle branch block
◆ Long or short corrected QT interval
◆ Brugada-like early repolarization

Long corrected QT interval: >440 ms (male), >460 ms (female);
Short corrected QT interval: <380 ms.
LVH, left ventricular hypertrophy.

published recommendations in 2010 (➲ Table 1.2.2.1) [5]. These recommendations divided ECG changes in athletes into physiological, training-related 'Group 1' changes which do not require further investigation, and training-unrelated or 'Group 2' changes, for which further evaluation is recommended (➲ Table 1.2.2.1). Although these recommendations have performed well in the detection of cardiac pathology in young athletes, in particular hypertrophic cardiomyopathy (HCM), recent studies have revealed a high burden of false-positive results, particularly in those of African/Afro-Caribbean (black) ethnicity [13–15]. In the light of new evidence on the impact of ethnicity on the athlete's heart and novel research findings regarding the relevance of several isolated ECG patterns currently regarded as abnormal in athletes of all ethnicities [14,16,17], modifications to the ESC recommendations have been proposed [14] and were recently incorporated into international guidelines for ECG interpretation in athletes [18].

The athlete's heart: structural remodelling

The ability of athletes to generate and maintain sizeable cardiac outputs for prolonged periods of time arises largely from an increase in their stroke volume with regular exercise training [19]. There are several mechanisms by which augmentation of stroke volume occurs, including an increase in left ventricular (LV) end-diastolic volume, increase in LV mass, decrease in LV end-systolic volume, and enhanced LV filling.

Evidence that athletes develop quantitatively significant cardiac enlargement first emerged from M-mode echocardiographic studies in the 1970s and 1908s [20,21]. An analysis of 28 such studies demonstrated that, on average, athletic individuals develop a 10% increase in their LV end-diastolic chamber diameter and a 15–20% increase in their LV wall thickness compared with sedentary controls [22]. Since then, the structural cardiac changes accompanying the athlete's heart have been further quantified by cross-sectional studies based on 2D echocardiography in large cohorts of elite athletes. A study of 1309 adult white male Olympian athletes by Pelliccia et al. [23] demonstrated a LV cavity size of >55mm in almost 50%, and extreme LV cavity dilatation of >60mm in 14% (➲ Fig. 1.2.2.1). A second study of 947 white Olympian athletes by same group demonstrated LV wall thicknesses between ≤7mm and 16mm, although only 16 individuals (1.7%) demonstrated values ≥13mm which could be considered in keeping with morphologically mild hypertrophic cardiomyopathy (HCM) [24]. Subsequent work by this group has demonstrated a significant reduction in cavity size and normalization of wall thicknesses after long-term detraining [25].

Based on these studies, the upper limit of normal for LV cavity dimension in adult male white athletes is currently regarded as ≤64mm, and for LV wall thickness ≤12mm (➲ Table 1.2.2.2). However, when interpreting quantitative data, it must be noted that a minority of athletes participating in extreme endurance sports, such as the Tour de France, have been reported to demonstrate LV cavities ≥70mm, with 75% of such individuals demonstrating cavity dimensions of >57mm and 8.7% LV wall thicknesses of >13mm, though almost always <15mm [26].

Owing to the technical challenges of imaging and quantifying the complex and irregular anatomy of the right ventricle using echocardiography, right ventricular (RV) adaptation to exercise has been relatively neglected until recently. Only a few early m-mode echocardiographic studies assessed the right ventricle, reporting transverse diameters up to 25% larger than those seen in sedentary control subjects [27–29]. The practical clinical consequence of RV remodelling is the overlap of increased RV dimensions with the RV morphological criteria for diagnosis of ARVC (Task Force Criteria [11]). Zaidi et al. observed that a large subset of female athletes (14%) showed absolute RV outflow dimensions meeting major Task Force Criteria [35]. To avoid misinterpretation, it appears convenient to refer to RV outflow dimensions indexed to body surface area, which have shown

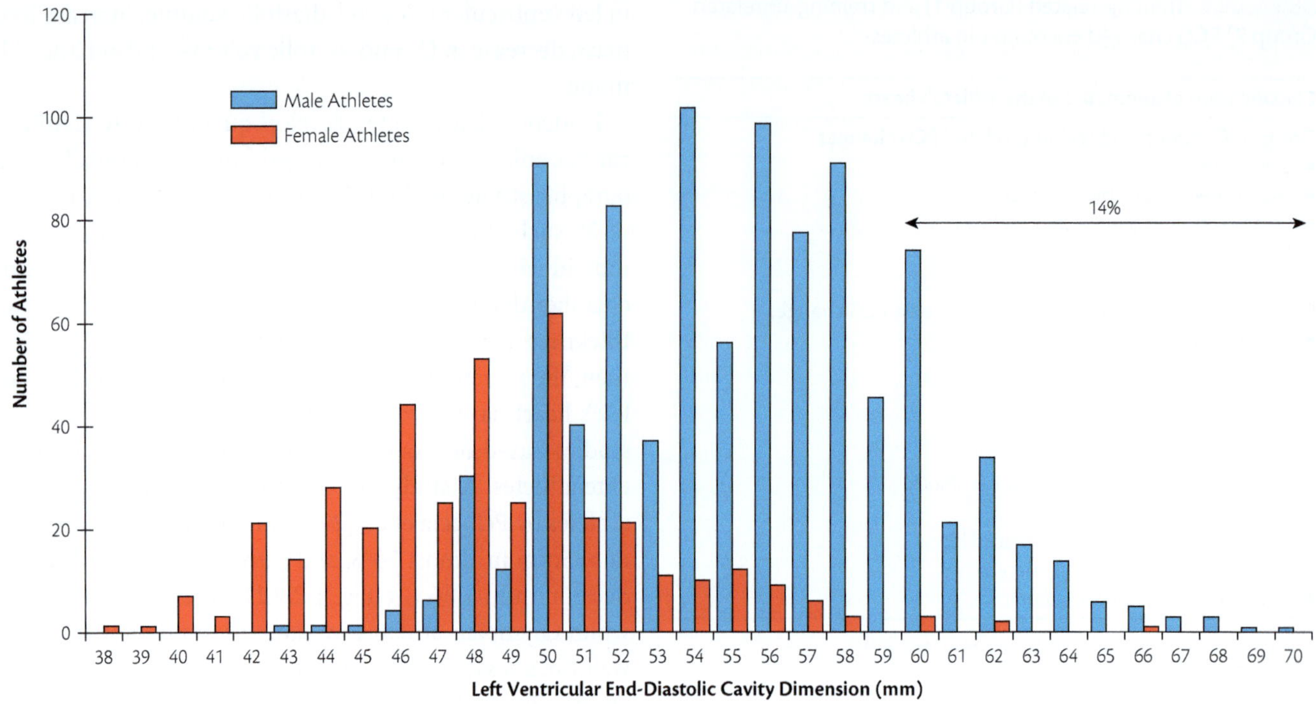

Fig. 1.2.2.1 Distribution of left ventricular end-diastolic cavity dimensions in 1309 highly trained athletes without evidence of structural cardiovascular disease. Fourteen per cent of athletes had markedly enlarged left ventricular cavities ranging in size from 60mm to 70mm.

Table 1.2.2.2 Upper limits of normal for left and right ventricular end-diastolic cavity dimensions and wall thicknesses in adult athletes based on gender and ethnicity

Athlete group	Gender	LV cavity dimension (mm)	LVWT (mm)	RV dimensions (mm)						
				RVOTP	RVOT1	RVOT2	RVD1	RVD2	RVD3	RVWT
Adult white	Male	≤64	≤12	≤40	≤43	≤32	≤55	≤47	≤109	≤6
	Female	≤57	≤11	≤37	≤40	≤29	≤49	≤43	≤100	≤5
Adult black	Male	≤62	≤15	≤40	≤43	≤32	≤55	≤47	≤109	≤6
	Female	≤56	≤12	≤37	≤40	≤29	≤49	≤43	≤100	≤5

LV, left ventricular; LVWT, left ventricular wall thickness; RV, right ventricular; RVOTP, right ventricular outflow tract dimension (parasternal): RVOT1, proximal right ventricular outflow tract dimension; RVOT2, distal right ventricular outflow tract dimension; RVWT, right ventricular free wall thickness; RVD1, right ventricular basal dimension; RVD2, right ventricular mid-ventricular dimension; RVD3, right ventricular longitudinal dimension.
Data from refs 22, 49, 63, and 65.

to drastically reduce the overlap (to 4%) with major Task Force criteria [30]. Indeed, regardless of the extent of morphological remodelling, indices of RV function (TAPSE, % fractional shortening) remain normal in athletes [30]. Newer data from echocardiographic and cardiac magnetic resonance (CMR) imaging studies have confirmed that exercise training induces similar changes in mass, volume, and function in the right ventricle to those in the left, with cardiac remodelling occurring in a 'balanced' fashion [31–36].

Upper limits of normality for RV cavity dimensions in athletes have recently been proposed for adult cohorts, although age- and gender- specific values are currently lacking (➲ Table 1.2.2.2) [32,33,36].

Influence of sporting discipline on the athlete's heart

Although there is a direct relationship between exercise training and development of the athlete's heart, the type of exercise being performed has an important influence on both the nature and extent of cardiac remodelling.

Influence of sporting discipline on electrical remodelling

Exercise results in a resting bradycardia through changes in extrinsic autonomic balance to the heart in addition to intrinsic remodelling within the sinoatrial node itself [3,4]. In comparison with athletes performing static exercise such as weightlifting or wrestling, heart rate is generally lower in athletes engaged in dynamic exercise such as running or cycling [9,37,38]. Some athletes engaged in extreme forms of dynamic exercise may exhibit marked sinus bradycardia of <30bpm, asymptomatic pauses of duration longer than 2 s, and junctional escape rhythms, all of which are overcome by exercise, suggesting a vagal origin [5,39,40].

Sporting discipline also indirectly produces electrical changes on the surface ECG through differential effects on cardiac morphology. Athletes engaged in dynamic exercise reveal a higher prevalence of physiological electrical changes suggestive of chamber enlargement, including partial right bundle branch block and voltage criteria for ventricular hypertrophy [5,9,38]. However, pathological ECG abnormalities are also reported to be commoner in athletes engaged in dynamic exercise than in static exercise. Pelliccia et al. [9] reported that distinctly abnormal ECG patterns were commoner in athletes engaged in cycling, cross-country skiing, rowing, and canoeing than in other sporting disciplines. The majority of individuals revealed absolute increases in cardiac dimensions, including LV end-diastolic dimension and LV wall thickness, suggesting a physiological basis. Only a minority (<10%) were diagnosed with cardiac pathology. Brosnan et al. [38] reported group 2 ECG changes to be twice as common in endurance versus non-endurance athletes (approximately 30% vs 15%), predominately due to ECG findings suggestive of right ventricular remodelling (voltage criteria for RVH and right pre-cordial T-wave inversion). Comprehensive evaluation of these athletes failed to detect any underlying cardiac pathology, although long-term follow-up data from this study were lacking.

Influence of sporting discipline on structural remodelling

The idea that sporting discipline has a direct influence on cardiac structure was first proposed by Morganroth et al. 40 years ago [20]. The 'Morganroth hypothesis' postulated that as dynamic (endurance) exercise places primarily a volume load on the heart, this results in 'eccentric hypertrophy' characterized by an increase in LV mass and a proportional increase in LV end-diastolic volume secondary to chamber enlargement, but little or no increase in LV wall thickness. In contrast, static exercise places mostly a pressure load on the heart, resulting in 'concentric hypertrophy' characterized by an increase in LV mass and wall thickness but with normal LV end-diastolic volume.

The Morganroth hypothesis has been widely accepted in sports cardiology [41] and remained relatively unchallenged for several decades, supported by a few echocardiographic studies which have, in particular, confirmed the concept of eccentric remodelling in endurance athletes [21,42–46]. However, newer data, including that derived from CMR and longitudinal follow-up studies, suggest that the hypothesis is far from absolute [44,47–50]. This probably reflects the fact that training regimes for most sports feature both dynamic and static aspects, resulting in volume and pressure loads on the heart, with a mixed effect [44].

In keeping with studies on the left ventricle, there is now considerable evidence from CMR studies for eccentric RV remodelling in endurance athletes [34,35]. Recent echocardiographic studies have also confirmed these findings, reporting significantly larger right heart measurements in athletes performing dynamic compared with static exercise [32,33]. Specifically, the RV linear and area dimensions show increasing values from athletes engaged in primarily skill activities (golfing, sailing) to endurance sports (cycling, rowing) [29]. A similar trend is observed for RA size. Frequently, particularly in endurance athletes, the RV chamber shape is altered, with a rounded apex and prominent trabecular pattern [30].

Influence of gender on the athlete's heart

Gender influences the athlete's heart independent of age and sporting discipline. In general, changes in female athletes occur to a lesser extent than in male athletes. The exact mechanisms behind these differences remain unclear, although gender variations in body size [51], blood pressure response to exercise [52,53], and the concentration of circulating androgens [54] have all been suggested.

Influence of gender on electrical remodelling

Pelliccia et al. [2] observed a higher prevalence of ECG abnormalities in male compared with female athletes in a large study of 32,652 unselected individuals undergoing pre-participation screening (12.4% vs 9.6%, $p = 0.001$). In another study of 1005 consecutive athletes by the same group [9], significant differences were observed between male and female athletes with respect to both mildly abnormal ECGs (28% male vs 14% female, $p < 0.001$) and distinctly abnormal ECGs (17% male vs 8% female, $p < 0.001$). Compared with male athletes, the majority of female athletes exhibited normal ECGs (78% vs 55%, $p < 0.001$). Although a lower uptake in sports associated with more extensive electrical changes may explain these gender differences, they may also reflect the subtler structural adaptations to exercise demonstrated by females.

Influence of gender on structural remodelling

In their study of 1309 Olympians, Pelliccia et al. [23] reported extremes of LV cavity dilatation (≥60mm) in just 1.7% of female compared with 18.7% of male athletes (➲ Fig, 1.2.2.1).

The same group compared cardiac dimensions in 600 female athletes, 738 male athletes, and 65 sedentary female controls [51]. Female athletes revealed 6% larger LV cavity dimensions and 14% larger LV wall thicknesses compared with control subjects. However, mean LV cavity dimensions were smaller in female compared to male athletes (48.9 ± 3.8cm vs 54.2 ± 4.0cm, $p < 0.001$) and exceeded normal limits (≥55mm) in just 8% of female compared with 47% of male athletes. Only 1% of female athletes ($n = 4$) demonstrated extreme LV cavity dilatation of ≥60mm. Similarly, mean LV wall thicknesses were smaller in female than in male athletes (8.2 ± 0.9cm vs 10.1 ± 1.2cm, $p < 0.001$), and none of the female athletes exceeded the upper limits of normal (>12mm) compared with 2% of the males. Based on these data, the upper limit of normal for LV cavity dimension and LV wall thickness in adult white female athletes is currently regarded as ≤57mm and ≤11mm, respectively (➲ Table 1.2.2.2).

With regard to RV remodelling, available data suggest that female athletes show increased RV cavity dimensions compared with controls, characterized by an enlarged RV inflow (by about 10%), with only mild changes in the outflow tract. In parallel, RV thickness is also increased (by an average of 13%). As with the LV, absolute RV dimensions are lower in female compared to male athletes: RV diastolic area (−23%), RV outflow tract (−8%) [30]. When indexed to body surface area, differences reduce greatly for RV chamber area (<10%) and reverse for RV outflow tract (5% greater in females).

Influence of ethnicity on the athlete's heart

Initial data regarding cardiac adaptation to exercise were derived predominately from white cohorts competing in the USA and Europe. However, the past two to three decades have witnessed a rapid growth in the globalization of professional sport, with the result that athletes from a diverse range of countries now have the opportunity to compete on the world stage and through this undergo routine pre-participation cardiovascular evaluation. The results from such evaluations are informing our understanding of the influence and importance of ethnicity on the athlete's heart. From this perspective, the group most intensely studied has been athletes of African/Afro-Caribbean ethnicity (black athletes), who form an ever growing population competing at the highest level throughout the world and are also reported to be at increased risk of exercise-related SCD [55–59].

Electrical remodelling in athletes of African/Afro-Caribbean ethnicity

The physiological training-related (group 1) ECG changes commonly observed in white athletes are also frequently seen in the black athlete population. In particular, ST-segment elevation, the early repolarization pattern, and voltage criteria for ventricular hypertrophy are highly prevalent in black athlete cohorts [60–62]. However, the most striking feature of electrical remodelling in black athletes is the extent to which they develop ECG changes traditionally regarded as abnormal in white athletes, in particular T-wave inversion.

T-wave inversion in adult male b lack athletes

The high prevalence of training-unrelated ECG changes in black athletes was first observed in professional American football players in the USA. Balady et al. [63] and Choo et al. [60] both reported T-wave inversion to be more common in black compared to white football players. Magalski et al. [61] subsequently reported ECG findings from 1959 elite adult male American football players, noting electrical abnormalities to be twice as common in black compared to white individuals. Of note, T-wave inversion >2mm was 13 times more frequent in black players.

Recently, a landmark European study has corroborated these initial American findings in cohorts of black athletes engaged in other sporting disciplines. Papadakis et al. [62] compared the ECGs of 904 male black athletes with those from 1819 white male athletes, 119 black sedentary controls, and 52 black HCM patients. T-wave inversion was over six times more common in black compared to white athletes (22.8% vs 3.7%, $p < 0.001$) and largely confined to the anterior leads (V1–V4; 12.7%). When confined to V1–V4, T-wave inversion was associated with a characteristic pattern of convex ST-segment elevation in almost two-thirds of cases (➲ Fig. 1.2.2.2). T-wave inversion in the inferior and lateral leads was rarer in black athletes, but nevertheless commoner than in white athletes (6% vs 1.5% and 4.1% vs 0.3%, respectively, $p < 0.001$ in both cases). The prevalence of deep T-wave inversion (≥ −0.2 mV) was also significantly greater in black athletes compared to both white athletes and black controls (12.1% vs 1.0% vs 1.7%, respectively, $p < 0.001$). T-wave inversion was observed less commonly in sedentary black controls than in black athletes (10.1% vs 22.8%, $p < 0.001$), suggesting that exercise modulates repolarization in black athletic individuals.

In contrast, almost all black HCM patients exhibited T-wave inversion (87.2%), particularly in the lateral leads (76.9%). Isolated anterior T-wave inversion and inferior T-wave inversion were comparatively rare in black HCM patients (3.8% and 1.9%, respectively). ST-segment depression was frequently observed in black HCM patients, but was virtually absent in black athletes and controls (50.0% vs 0.4% vs 0.0%, $p < 0.001$).

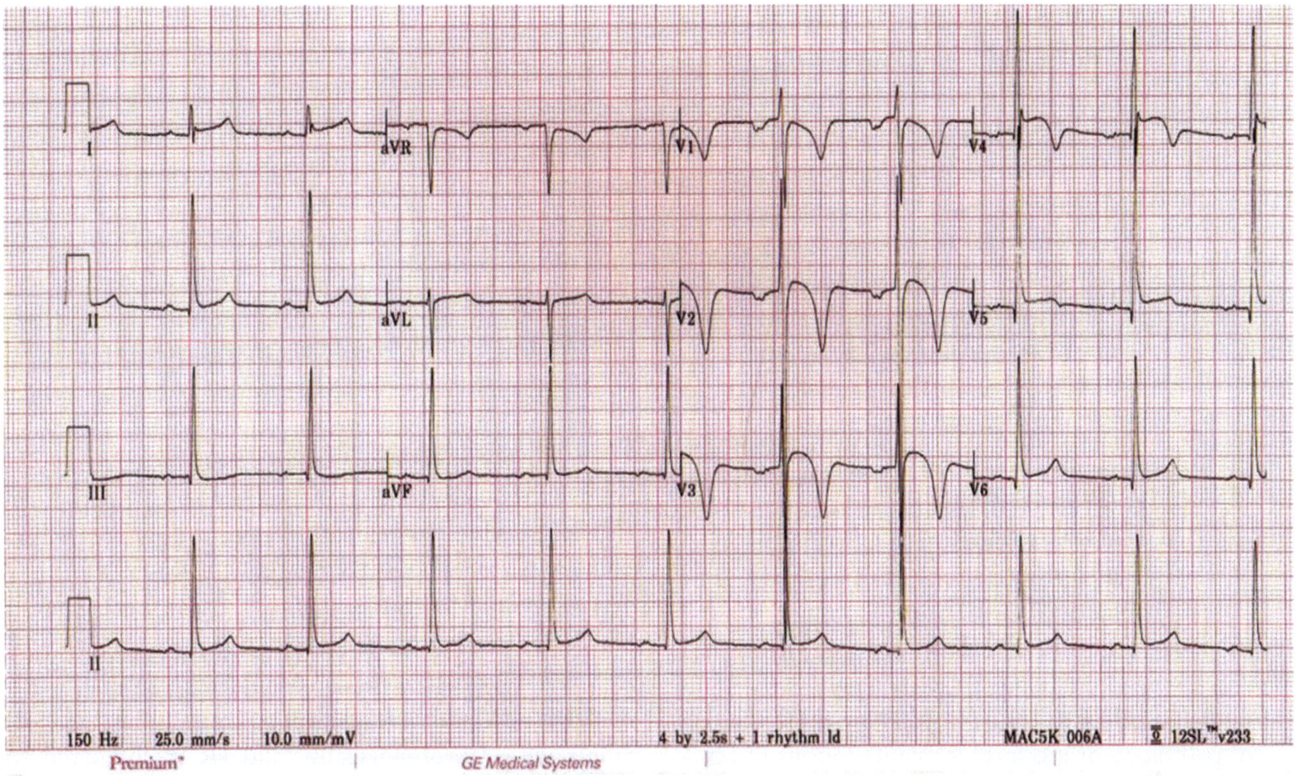

Fig. 1.2.2.2 An ECG from a black athlete demonstrating deep T-wave inversion in leads V1–V4. Note the preceding convex ST-segment elevation and Sokolow–Lyon voltage criteria for left ventricular hypertrophy.

Two-thirds of athletes with T-wave inversion in this study were comprehensively subjected to additional investigations but failed to reveal a definitive diagnosis of cardiomyopathy. However, during long-term follow-up two black athletes and one white athlete were diagnosed with HCM. In keeping with a previous study in white athletes with repolarization abnormalities [64], all three athletes revealed T-wave inversion in the inferior and/or lateral ECG leads. None of the black athletes with isolated anterior T-wave inversion were eventually diagnosed with a cardiomyopathy.

Based on these observations, isolated anterior T-wave inversion preceded by convex ST-segment elevation in black athletes is now considered an ethnic variant of normal. In contrast, T-wave inversion in the lateral leads should be considered abnormal regardless of ethnicity and investigated comprehensively to exclude an underlying cardiomyopathy, with continuing surveillance thereafter.

T-wave inversion in adult female black athletes

Rawlins et al. [65] performed the first and only study to date examining ethnic differences in cardiac adaptation to exercise in a sizeable cohort of adult female black athletes [65]. The ECGs from 240 female black athletes were compared to those from 200 female white athletes. In keeping with observations in male black athletes, female black athletes revealed a higher prevalence of repolarization changes, including ST-segment elevation (11% vs. 1%, p <0.001), T-wave inversion (14% vs. 2%, p <0.001) and deep T-wave inversion (2% vs. 0%, p <0.001). However, in contrast to male black athletes, T-wave inversion was less prevalent and confined exclusively to leads V1–V3. Furthermore, none of the individuals revealed phenotypic features of a cardiomyopathy after comprehensive evaluation. Therefore, as with male black athletes, T-wave inversion in the anterior leads is likely to represent an ethnically mediated variant in female black athletes. The absence of inferior or lateral T-wave inversion suggests that, if observed, these changes should trigger comprehensive evaluation and follow-up in female black athletes.

The prevalence of other ECG changes in black athletes.

Although repolarization abnormalities have commonly been associated with black ethnicity, data from several of the aforementioned studies have also revealed a high prevalence of other ECG patterns traditionally regarded as abnormal in black athletes. For example, in their adult cohort of 904 male black athletes, Papadakis et al.[62] reported a significantly higher prevalence of voltage criteria for right ventricular hypertrophy (RVH) (13.3% vs 2.6%), left atrial enlargement (8.6% vs 2.8%), and right atrial enlargement (6.3% vs 0.3%) compared with white athletes (➲ Fig. 1.2.2.3).

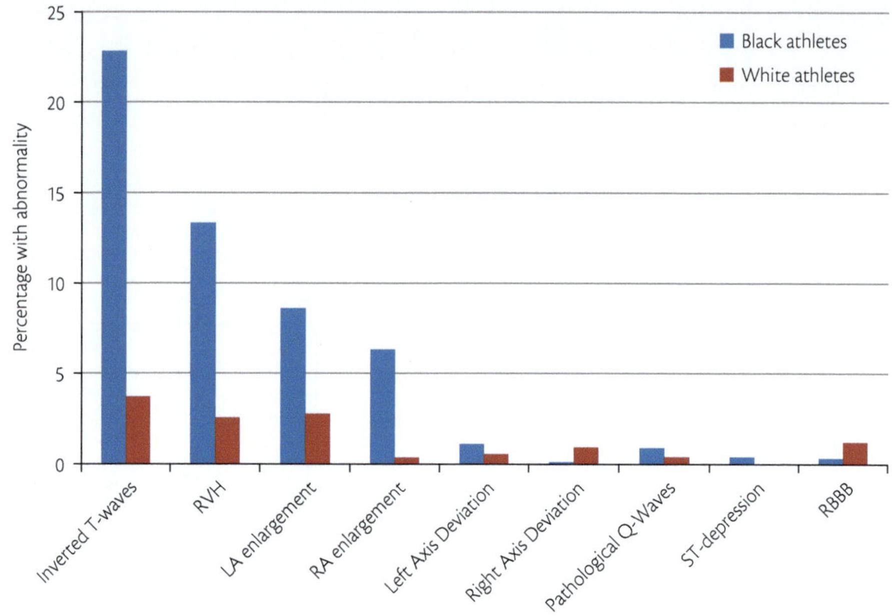

Fig. 1.2.2.3 Bar chart illustrating the prevalence of abnormal ECG patterns other than T-wave inversion in a large cohort of black (n = 904) and white (n = 1819) elite athletes. LA, left atrial; RA, right atrial; RBBB, right bundle branch block; RVH, right ventricular hypertrophy.

Data from Papadakis M, Carré F, Kervio G, Rawlins J, Panoulas VF, Chandra N, et al., The prevalence, distribution, and clinical outcomes of electrocardiographic repolarization patterns in male athletes of African/Afro-Caribbean origin. *European Heart Journal*, Volume 32, Issue 18, pp. 2304–13. Copyright © 2011 Oxford University Press and the European Society of Cardiology (ESC).

The question therefore arises as to whether these changes represent pathology or are further manifestations of black athlete's heart. Recent work has suggested that if found in isolation in an asymptomatic athlete without sinister family history, such changes would probably represent benign training-related variants rather than cardiac pathology in athletes, regardless of ethnicity [16,17].

Structural remodelling in athletes of African/Afro-Caribbean ethnicity

Left ventricular cavity dimensions in black athletes

Black athletes demonstrate similar quantitative changes with respect to LV cavity dimensions as white athletes. Therefore, in general, the upper limits of normal for LV cavity dimensions in white athletes are also applicable to the black athletic population (➔ Table 1.2.2.2).

Left ventricular hypertrophy in male black athletes

In contrast with LV cavity dimensions, several studies have demonstrated an appreciable increase in LV wall thickness and a higher prevalence of LVH on echocardiography in black athletes compared to white athletes. Lewis et al. [66] first noted such changes in a study of 265 predominately (99%) black Howard University collegiate athletes, observing that 11% revealed LV wall thicknesses ≥13mm, mainly 13mm or 14mm (26 out of 29 individuals). Basavarajiah et al. [67] observed a greater mean maximal LV wall thickness (11.3 ± 1.6mm vs 10.0 ± 1.5mm, $p < 0.001$) and higher prevalence of LVH ≥13mm (18% vs 4%, $p < 0.001$) in a UK-based study comparing cardiac dimensions in 300 male black and 300 male white adult athletes. Significantly, 18% of black athletes exhibited a LV wall thickness of >12mm in the range compatible with morphologically mild HCM compared with just 4% of white athletes. Furthermore, 3% of black athletes demonstrated extreme LVH of ≥15mm (➔ Fig. 1.2.2.4). In contrast, LV wall thicknesses did not exceed 14mm in white athletes. None of the athletes revealed LVH exceeding 16mm, irrespective of ethnicity. In athletes with LVH, the pattern of hypertrophy was homogenous and associated with concomitant LV cavity dilatation (55–66mm). Comprehensive evaluation of these athletes failed to reveal the broader phenotypic features of HCM. Papadakis et al. [62] reproduced these findings in a larger cohort of 904 black and 1819 white athletes competing in a wider range of sporting disciplines, demonstrating LV wall thicknesses of >12mm in 12.4% of black athletes compared with just 1.6% of white athletes. Left ventricular wall thicknesses did not exceed 13mm in white athletes and 16mm in black athletes.

Left ventricular hypertrophy in female black athletes

In addition to electrical changes, Rawlins et al. [65] also examined structural cardiac remodelling in adult female black athletes. Although female black athletes demonstrated greater LV wall thicknesses than female white athletes (9.2 ± 1.2 vs 8.6 ± 1.2mm, $p < 0.001$), the magnitude of LVH was significantly smaller than that observed in male athletes. Only 3% of black female athletes revealed a LV wall thickness >11mm and none exhibited a LV wall thickness >13mm. In comparison, none of the female white athletes revealed a LV wall thickness >11mm.

These studies suggest that the upper limit of normal for LV wall thicknesses should be regarded as ≤15mm in adult

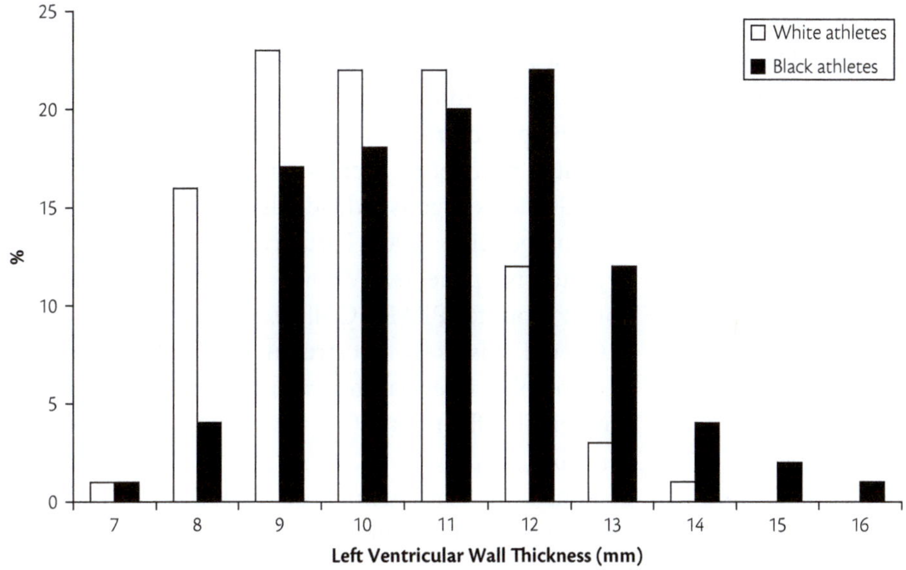

Fig. 1.2.2.4 Distribution of maximal left ventricular wall thicknesses in black and white athletes. Note the greater magnitude of LVH (>12mm) in black athletes, including substantial LVH (≥15mm) in 3%.

Reprinted from *Journal of the American College of Cardiology*, Vol 51, issue 23, Basavarajaiah et al. Ethnic differences in left ventricular remodeling in highly-trained athletes relevance to differentiating physiologic left ventricular hypertrophy from hypertrophic cardiomyopathy, pp. 2256–62. Copyright 2008 with permission from Elsevier.

male black athletes and ≤12mm in adult female black athletes (➔ Table 1.2.2.2).

Right ventricular adaptations in black athletes

The high prevalence of right precordial T-wave inversion observed in the black athletic population invariably raises suspicion of ARVC and underscores the importance of examining RV structural remodelling in black athletes. Zaidi et al. [36] are the only group to have studied the right ventricle in black athletes, comparing data from 300 elite black athletes (predominately male) with that from 375 elite white athletes and 153 sedentary controls (n = 69 black). In keeping with observations from white athletic cohorts, black athletes exhibited significantly greater RV and RV outflow tract dimensions compared with sedentary controls, although marginally smaller dimensions compared with white athletes. Right ventricular outflow tract dilatation compatible with current diagnostic Task Force criteria for ARVC [11] was observed frequently in athletes of both ethnicities. However, 3% of black athletes (n = 9) revealed concomitant anterior T-wave inversion, increasing the diagnostic uncertainty between ARVC and physiological remodelling. Comprehensive evaluation of all nine black athletes failed to reveal firm diagnostic features consistent with ARVC, highlighting the shortcomings of applying diagnostic criteria derived from sedentary diseased cohorts of other ethnicities to black athletic individuals [68].

Athletes of other ethnicities

Data on cardiac remodelling with exercise is now emerging for athletes of Arabic (Middle Eastern), South Asian, and East Asian ethnicity. To date, all such data indicate that the electrical and structural changes associated with athlete's heart in these ethnicities is similar to that observed in white athletic cohorts. Thus ECG and echocardiographic criteria derived from white athletes aiding the differentiation of physiological from pathological changes may also be applied to these ethnic groups. However, further data are awaited in many ethnicities, particularly South and East Asian athletes.

Influence of genetics on the athlete's heart

Although electrical and structural changes in the athlete's heart are now well described, the mechanisms underlying extreme expressions of cardiac remodelling remain poorly understood. In recent years, several studies have pointed towards an important role for genetic factors. In time, these may lead to a better understanding of physiological versus pathological cardiac remodelling in athletes.

Potential candidate genes for electrical and structural remodelling in athletes

Data from work in the 1980s comparing twins or sibling pairs with unrelated individuals demonstrated greater similarity in cardiac dimensions between the former [69,70]. Although this finding was used as evidence for the heritability of cardiac dimensions, it is likely that the observations were a reflection of body size and composition rather than a primary genetic effect [71]. Since then, a number of potential candidate genes have emerged which may directly influence cardiac adaptation to exercise [72–83].

Genes influencing left ventricular remodelling in athletes

Perhaps one of the most studied genetic targets in relation to LV remodelling in athletes has been the angiotensin-converting enzyme (ACE) gene. Montgomery et al. [72] first described associations between LV mass in a group of military recruits and the presence (insertion allele, I) or absence (deletion allele, D) of a 287-base pair marker in the ACE gene, which is known to be associated with increased risk for LVH in the general population [84]. These observations were later confirmed in other studies by different researchers [73–79,82]. In athletes, the DD or DI alleles were associated with a significantly greater increase in LV mass in response to intensive exercise compared with the II allele (72–79,82). ACE activates angiotensin I to angiotensin II which in turn stimulates myocyte growth. Angiotensin II also degrades kinins, which inhibit myocyte growth [85]. Given that exercise training can activate the ACE gene and that the D allele is associated with higher levels of circulating and tissue angiotensin [78], this may be the mechanism by which the DD and DI alleles lead to an increase in LV mass. However, other studies in the general population [86,87], hypertensive patients [88], athletes [80], and policemen [81] have given conflicting results, with no close association observed between the ACE gene D/I alleles and cardiac remodelling.

Changes in LV mass in response to athletic training have also been associated with the presence of polymorphisms in other common allelic variants of the renin–angiotensin system (RAS), such as the angiotensinogen (AGT) and angiotensin II type 1 receptor (AT1R) genes. A methionine-to-threonine substitution at position 235 (M235T) of the AGT gene (T allele) and an adenine-to-cytosine substitution at position 1166 (A1166C) of the AT1R gene have both been linked to an increased risk of hypertension in the general white population [89–92] and of LVH in endurance athletes [73,80]. Furthermore, athletes with both the AGT TT allele and the ACE DD allele reveal the greatest increases in LV mass in response to exercise training [73]. However, as with the ACE gene, results have been conflicting, with some studies reporting no association with the ATR1 gene A116C polymorphism and LVH in athletes [80,82].

More recently, genes other than those comprising the RAS have also been implicated in cardiac remodelling and the development of LVH in humans. The expression of insulin-like growth factor 1 (IGF-1) is increased in both animal models of cardiac hypertrophy and humans with LVH [93–96], implicating the cardiac IGF-1 gene in this process [97]. The mechanism by which this occurs is uncertain, but one possibility is through the effects of IGF-1 on cell signalling via the phosphatidylinsitol 3 kinase–Akt1 pathway [98], which is involved in the regulation of transcription factors and gene product synthesis [99]. Other work has demonstrated that polymorphisms in the peroxisome proliferator-activated receptor (PPARα) are associated with LVH; those individuals homozygous for the C allele of the G/C polymorphism in intron 7 of PPARα gene demonstrated a threefold increase in their LV mass compared with GG homozygous individuals, independent of body size and composition [100]. Furthermore, in a large cohort of hypertensive patients, LVH was commoner in individuals homozygous for PPARα C allele.

Overall, it is likely that structural remodelling in athletes is a complex interplay between multiple genes and environmental influences [101]. Several of the clinical studies described in previous sections and in Chapter 1.2.3 have demonstrated that much of the variability observed in athletic cohorts is accounted for by body size, age, gender, and sporting discipline. Indeed, studies of the ACE I/D polymorphism and AGT M/T polymorphism have revealed that <15% of the variation in left ventricular dimensions and mass is explained by genetic variation in these genes alone [80,100].

Genes influencing electrical remodelling in athletes

In contrast with structural remodelling, there is little data regarding the influence of genetic variability on electrical changes in athletes. The literature has many reports of ethnic variation between black and white individuals in several genes encoding sodium and potassium ion channels involved in the pathogenesis of long QT syndrome and Brugada syndrome, including the KCN family and SCN5A, particularly the Y1102 polymorphism and its association with SCD in the black population [102–107]. Polymorphisms in some of these targets have been show to influence T-wave parameters, including T-wave alternans and repolarization intervals [108]. However, as yet there are no robust reports on potential genetic targets that may specifically influence electrical changes observed in athletic cohorts in response to long-term exercise training.

Summary and conclusion

Structural and electrical remodelling in athletes is a complex phenomenon, influenced by a number of demographic as well as genetic factors. It is clear that gender, sporting discipline, and ethnicity exert a significant impact on the nature and extent of cardiac remodelling in response to exercise. In general, adult male athletes, those of black ethnicity, and those performing dynamic exercise tend to exhibit the largest cardiac dimensions and the most profound electrical alterations (➲ Fig. 1.2.2.5). ➲ Table 1.2.2.2 summarizes

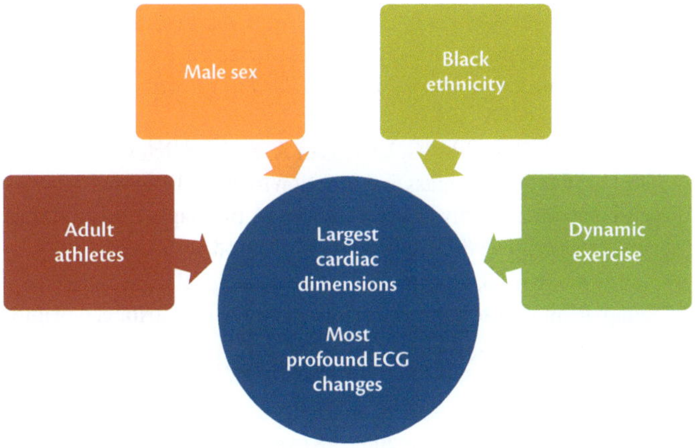

Fig. 1.2.2.5 The impact of age, gender, sporting discipline, and ethnicity on the athlete's heart.

the current upper limits of normality for LV and RV cavity size and wall thicknesses in adult athletes of different gender and ethnicity based on our current knowledge and the clinical studies presented in this chapter. An interaction between environmental influences and the genetic make-up of a particular athlete is likely to explain extreme expressions of athlete's heart and the differences observed between ethnicities. Recognition and complete understanding of the influence of these demographic and genetic factors is crucial for the correct interpretation of an athlete's ECG and echocardiographic data. Future work examining the genetic targets involved may further aid the differentiation of athlete's heart from cardiac pathology.

Further reading

Basavarajaiah S, Boraita A, Whyte G, et al. Ethnic differences in left ventricular remodeling in highly-trained athletes relevance to differentiating physiologic left ventricular hypertrophy from hypertrophic cardiomyopathy. *J Am Coll Cardiol* 2008; 51(23): 2256–62.

Papadakis M, Carré F, Kervio G, et al. The prevalence, distribution, and clinical outcomes of electrocardiographic repolarization patterns in male athletes of African/Afro-Caribbean origin. *Eur Heart J* 2011; 32(18): 2304–13.

Pelliccia A, Thompson PD. The genetics of left ventricular remodeling in competitive athletes. *J Cardiovasc Med (Hagerstown)* 2006; 7(4): 267–70.

Pelliccia A, Maron BJ, Spataro A, et al. The upper limit of physiologic cardiac hypertrophy in highly trained elite athletes. *N Engl J Med* 1991; 324(5): 295–301.

Pelliccia A, Maron BJ, Culasso F, et al. Athlete's heart in women—echocardiographic characterization of highly trained elite female athletes. *JAMA* 1996; 276(3): 211–15.

Pelliccia A, Culasso F, Di Paolo FM, Maron BJ. Physiologic left ventricular cavity dilatation in elite athletes. *Ann Intern Med* 1999; 130(1): 23–31.

Rawlins J, Carré F, Kervio G, et al. Ethnic differences in physiological cardiac adaptation to intense physical exercise in highly trained female athletes. *Circulation* 2010; 121(9): 1078–85.

Sharma S, Drezner J, Baggish A, et al. International consensus standards for electrocardiographic interpretation in athletes. *Eur Heart J* 2017; 69(8).

Sheikh N, Sharma S. Impact of ethnicity on cardiac adaptation to exercise. *Nat Rev Cardiol*; 2014; 11(4): 198–217.

Zaidi A, Ghani S, Sharma R, et al. Physiological right ventricular adaptation in elite athletes of African and Afro-Caribbean origin. *Circulation* 2013; 127(17): 1783–92.

References

1. Chandra N, Bastiaenen R, Papadakis M, Sharma S. Sudden cardiac death in young athletes: practical challenges and diagnostic dilemmas. *J Am Coll Cardiol*; 2013; 61 (10): 1027–40.
2. Pelliccia A, Culasso F, Di Paolo FM, et al. Prevalence of abnormal electrocardiograms in a large, unselected population undergoing pre-participation cardiovascular screening. *Eur Heart J* 2007; 28 (16): 2006–10.
3. Boyett MR, D'Souza A, Zhang H., Viewpoint: Is the resting bradycardia in athletes the result of remodeling of the sinoatrial node rather than high vagal tone? *J Appl Physiol* 2013; 114 (9): 1351–5.
4. Stein R, Medeiros CM, Rosito GA, et al. Intrinsic sinus and atrioventricular node electrophysiologic adaptations in endurance athletes. *J Am Coll Cardiol* 2002; 39 (6): 1033–8.
5. Corrado D, Pelliccia A, Heidbuchel H, et al. Recommendations for interpretation of 12-lead electrocardiogram in the athlete. *Eur Heart J* 2010; 31 (2): 243–59.
6. Oakley DG, Oakley CM. Significance of abnormal electrocardiograms in highly trained athletes. *Am J Cardiol* 1982 Nov; 50 (5): 985–9.
7. Kansal S, Roitman DI, Sheffield LT. A quantitative relationship of electrocardiographic criteria of left ventricular hypertrophy with echocardiographic left ventricular mass: a multivariate approach. *Clin Cardiol* 1983; 6 (9): 456–63.
8. Raskoff WJ, Goldman S, Cohn K. The 'athletic heart': prevalence and physiological significance of left ventricular enlargement in distance runners. *JAMA* 1976; 236 (2): 158–62.
9. Pelliccia A, Maron BJ, Culasso F, et al. Clinical significance of abnormal electrocardiographic patterns in trained athletes. *Circulation* 2000; 102 (3): 278–84.
10. Maron BJ, Wolfson JK, Ciró E, Spirito P. Relation of electrocardiographic abnormalities and patterns of left ventricular hypertrophy identified by 2-dimensional echocardiography in patients with hypertrophic cardiomyopathy. *Am J Cardiol* 1983; 51 (1): 189–94.
11. Marcus FI, McKenna WJ, Sherrill D, et al. Diagnosis of arrhythmogenic right ventricular cardiomyopathy/dysplasia: proposed modification of the task force criteria. *Circulation* 2010; 121 (13): 1533–41.
12. Schwartz P, Moss A, Vincent G, Crampton R. Diagnostic criteria for the long QT syndrome: an update. *Circulation* 1993; 88
13. Brosnan M, La Gerche A, Kalman J, et al. The Seattle Criteria increase the specificity of preparticipation ECG screening among elite athletes. *Br J Sports Med* 2014; 48 (15); 1144–50.

14. Sheikh N, Papadakis M, Ghani S, et al. Comparison of ECG criteria for the detection of cardiac abnormalities in elite black and white athletes. *Circulation* 2014; 129 (16): 1637–49.
15. Riding NR, Sheikh N, Adamuz C, et al. Comparison of three current sets of electrocardiographic interpretation criteria for use in screening athletes. *Heart* 2014; 101 (5): 384–90.
16. Gati S, Sheikh N, Ghani S, et al. Should axis deviation or atrial enlargement be categorised as abnormal in young athletes? The athlete's electrocardiogram: time for re-appraisal of markers of pathology. *Eur Heart J* 2013; 34 (47): 3641–8.
17. Zaidi A, Ghani S, Sheikh N, et al. Clinical significance of electrocardiographic right ventricular hypertrophy in athletes: comparison with arrhythmogenic right ventricular cardiomyopathy and pulmonary hypertension. *Eur Heart J* 2013; 34 (47): 3649–56.
18. Sharma S, Drezner J, Baggish A, et al. International recommendations for electrocardiographic interpretation in athletes. *J Am Coll Cardiol*; 2017; 69 (8): 1057–75.
19. Rowell L. *Human Circulation: Regulation During Physical Stress.* New York: Oxford University Press, 1986.
20. Morganroth J, Maron BJ, Henry WL, Epstein SE. Comparative left ventricular dimensions in trained athletes. *Ann Intern Med* 1975; 82 (4): 521–4.
21. Longhurst JC, Kelly AR, Gonyea WJ, Mitchell JH. Echocardiographic left ventricular masses in distance runners and weight lifters. *J Appl Physiol* 1980; 48 154–62.
22. Maron BJ. Structural features of the athlete heart as defined by echocardiography. *J Am Coll Cardiol* 1986; 7 (1): 190–203.
23. Pelliccia A, Culasso F, Di Paolo FM, Maron BJ. Physiologic left ventricular cavity dilatation in elite athletes. *Ann Intern Med* 1999; 130 (1): 23–31.
24. Pelliccia A, Maron BJ, Spataro A, et al. The upper limit of physiologic cardiac hypertrophy in highly trained elite athletes. *N Engl J Med* 1991; 324 (5): 295–301.
25. Pelliccia A. Remodeling of left ventricular hypertrophy in elite athletes after long-term deconditioning. *Circulation* 2002; 105 (8): 944–9.
26. Abergel E, Chatellier G, Hagege AA, et al. Serial left ventricular adaptations in world-class professional cyclists: implications for disease screening and follow-up. *J Am Coll Cardiol* 2004; 44 (1): 144–9.
27. Roeske WR, Rourke RAO, Klein A, et al. Noninvasive evaluation of ventricular hypertrophy in professional athletes. *Circulation* 1976; 53 (2): 286–91.
28. Wieling W, Borghols EA, Hollander AP, et al. Echocardiographic dimensions and maximal oxygen uptake in oarsmen during training. *Br Heart J* 1981; 46 (2): 190–5.
29. Zoneraich S, Rhee JJ, Zoneraich O, et al. Assessment of cardiac function in marathon runners by graphic noninvasive techniques. *Ann NY Acad Sci* 1977; 301 900–17.
30. D'Ascenzi F, Cataldo P, Caselli S., RV remodelling in Olympic athletes. *JACC Cardiovasc Imaging* 2017; 10 (4): 385–93.
31. Henriksen E, Kangro T, Jonason T, et al. An echocardiographic study of right ventricular adaptation to physical exercise in elite male orienteers. *Clin Physiol* 1998; 18 (6): 498–503.
32. Oxborough D, Sharma S, Shave R, et al. The right ventricle of the endurance athlete: the relationship between morphology and deformation. *J Am Soc Echocardiogr* 2012; 25 (3): 263–71.
33. D'Andrea A, Riegler L, Golia E, et al. Range of right heart measurements in top-level athletes: the training impact. *Int J Cardiol* 2013; 164 (1): 48–57.
34. Prakken NH, Velthuis BK, Teske AJ, et al. Cardiac MRI reference values for athletes and nonathletes corrected for body surface area, training hours/week and sex. *Eur J Cardiovasc Prev Rehabil* 2010; 17 (2): 198–203.
35. Scharhag J, Schneider G, Urhausen A, et al. Athlete's heart: right and left ventricular mass and function in male endurance athletes and untrained individuals determined by magnetic resonance imaging. *J Am Coll Cardiol* 2002; 40 (10): 1856–63.
36. Zaidi A, Ghani S, Sharma R, et al. Physiological right ventricular adaptation in elite athletes of African and Afro-Caribbean origin. *Circulation* 2013; 127 (17): 1783–92.
37. Sztajzel J, Jung M, Sievert K, Bayes De Luna A. Cardiac autonomic profile in different sports disciplines during all-day activity. *J Sports Med Phys Fitness* 2008; 48 (4): 495–501.
38. Brosnan M, La Gerche A, Kalman J, et al. Comparison of frequency of significant electrocardiographic abnormalities in endurance versus nonendurance athletes. *Am J Cardiol* 2014; 113 (9): 1567–73.
39. Baggish AL, Wood MJ. Athlete's heart and cardiovascular care of the athlete: scientific and clinical update. *Circulation* 2011; 123 (23): 2723–35.
40. Viitasalo MT, Kala R, Eisalo A. Ambulatory electrocardiographic recording in endurance athletes. *Br Heart J* 1982; 47 (3): 213–20.
41. Mitchell JH, Haskell WL, Raven PB. Classification of sports. *Med Sci Sports Exerc* 1994; 26 (10 Suppl): S242–5.
42. Baggish AL, Wang F, Weiner RB, et al. Training-specific changes in cardiac structure and function: a prospective and longitudinal assessment of competitive athletes. *J Appl Physiol* 2008; 104 (4): 1121–8.
43. Telford RD, McDonald IG, Ellis LB, et al. Echocardiographic dimensions in trained and untrained 12-year-old boys and girls. *J Sports Sci* 1988; 6 (1): 49–57.
44. Pluim BM, Zwinderman AH, van der Laarse A, van der Wall EE. The athlete's heart: a meta-analysis of cardiac structure and function. *Circulation* 2000; 101 (3): 336–44.
45. George K, Whyte GP, Green DJ, et al. The endurance athletes heart: acute stress and chronic adaptation. *Br J Sports Med* 2012; 46 (2): i29–36.
46. Whyte GP, George K, Nevill A, et al. Left ventricular morphology and function in female athletes: a meta-analysis. *Int J Sports Med* 2004; 25 (5): 380–3.
47. Fagard RH. Impact of different sports and training on cardiac structure and function. *Cardiol Clin* 1997; 15 (3): 397–412.
48. Spence AL, Naylor LH, Carter HH, et al. A prospective randomised longitudinal MRI study of left ventricular adaptation to endurance and resistance exercise training in humans. *J Physiol* 2011; 589 (Pt 22): 5443–52.
49. Utomi V, Oxborough D, Ashley E, et al. Predominance of normal left ventricular geometry in the male 'athlete's heart'. *Heart* 2014; 100 (16): 1264–71.
50. Utomi V, Oxborough D, Whyte GP, et al. Systematic review and meta-analysis of training mode, imaging modality and body size influences on the morphology and function of the male athlete's heart. *Heart* 2013; 99 (23): 1727–33.
51. Pelliccia A, Maron BJ, Culasso F., Athlete's heart in women—echocardiographic characterization of highly trained elite female athletes. *JAMA* 1996; 276 (3): 211–15.
52. Gleim GW, Stachenfeld NS, Coplan NL, Nicholas JA. Gender differences in the systolic blood pressure response to exercise. *Am Heart J* 1991; 121 (2 Pt 1): 524–30.

53. Petrofsky JS, Burse RL, Lind AR. Comparison of physiological responses of women and men to isometric exercise. *J Appl Physiol* 1975; 38 (5): 863–8.
54. McGill HC, Anselmo VC, Buchanan JM, Sheridan PJ. The heart is a target organ for androgen. *Science* 1980; 207 (4432): 775–7.
55. Maron BJ, Doerer JJ, Haas TS, et al. Sudden deaths in young competitive athletes: analysis of 1866 deaths in the United States, 1980–2006. *Circulation* 2009; 119 (8): 1085–92.
56. Maron BJ, Carney KP, Lever HM, et al. Relationship of race to sudden cardiac death in competitive athletes with hypertrophic cardiomyopathy. *J Am Coll Cardiol* 2003; 41 (6): 974–80.
57. Harmon KG, Asif IM, Klossner D, Drezner JA. Incidence of sudden cardiac death in National Collegiate Athletic Association athletes. *Circulation* 2011; 123 (15): 1594–1600.
58. Maron BJ, Haas TS, Murphy CJ, et al. Incidence and causes of sudden death in US college athletes. *J Am Coll Cardiol* 2014; 63 (16): 1636–43.
59. Harmon KG, Asif IM, Maleszewski JJ, et al. Incidence, etiology, and comparative frequency of sudden cardiac death in NCAA athletes: a decade in review. *Circulation* 2015; 132 (1): 10–19.
60. Choo JK, Abernethy WB, Hutter AM. Electrocardiographic observations in professional football players. *Am J Cardiol* 2002; 90 (2): 198–200.
61. Magalski A, Maron BJ, Main ML, et al. Relation of race to electrocardiographic patterns in elite American football players. *J Am Coll Cardiol* 2008; 51 (23): 2250–5.
62. Papadakis M, Carré F, Kervio G, et al. The prevalence, distribution, and clinical outcomes of electrocardiographic repolarization patterns in male athletes of African/Afro-Caribbean origin. *Eur Heart J* 2011; 32 (18): 2304–13.
63. Balady GJ, Cadigan JB, Ryan TJ. Electrocardiogram of the athlete: an analysis of 289 professional football players. *Am J Cardiol* 1984; 53 (9): 1339–43.
64. Pelliccia A, Di Paolo FM, Quattrini FM, et al. Outcomes in athletes with marked ECG repolarization abnormalities. *N Engl J Med* 2008; 358 (2): 152–61.
65. Rawlins J, Carré F, Kervio G, et al. Ethnic differences in physiological cardiac adaptation to intense physical exercise in highly trained female athletes. *Circulation* 2010; 121 (9): 1078–85.
66. Lewis JF, Maron BJ, Diggs JA, et al. Preparticipation echocardiographic screening for cardiovascular disease in a large, predominantly black population of collegiate athletes. *Am J Cardiol* 1989; 64 (16): 1029–33.
67. Basavarajaiah S, Boraita A, Whyte G, et al. Ethnic differences in left ventricular remodeling in highly-trained athletes relevance to differentiating physiologic left ventricular hypertrophy from hypertrophic cardiomyopathy. *J Am Coll Cardiol* 2008; 51 (23): 2256–62.
68. Weinstock J, Estes NA 3rd. The heart of an athlete: black, white, and shades of grey with no gold standard. *Circulation* 2013; 127 (17): 1757–9.
69. Adams T, Yanowitz FG, Fisher AG, et al. Heritability of cardiac size : an echocardiographic and electrocardiographic study of monozygotic and dizygotic twins. *Circulation* 1985; 71 (1): 39–44.
70. Bouchard C, Mailina R. Genetics of physiological fitness and motor performance. *Exerc Sport Sci. Rev* 1983; 11 306–39.
71. Fagard R, Van Den Broeke C, Bielen E, Amery A. Maximum oxygen uptake and cardiac size and function in twins. *Am J Cardiol* 1987; 60 (16): 1362–7.
72. Montgomery HE, Clarkson P, Dollery CM, et al. Association of angiotensin-converting enzyme gene I/D polymorphism with change in left ventricular mass in response to physical training. *Circulation* 1997; 96 (3): 741–7.
73. Diet F, Graf C, Mahnke N, et al. ACE and angiotensinogen gene genotypes and left ventricular mass in athletes. *Eur J Clin Invest* 2001; 31 (10): 836–42.
74. Boraita A, de la Rosa A, Heras ME, et al. Cardiovascular adaptation, functional capacity and angiotensin-converting enzyme I/D polymorphism in elite athletes. *Rev Esp Cardiol* 2010; 63 (7): 810–19.
75. Rizzo M, Gensini F, Fatini C, et al. ACE I/D polymorphism and cardiac adaptations in adolescent athletes. *Med Sci Sports Exerc* 2003; 35 (12): 1986–90.
76. Nagashima J, Musha H, Takada H, et al. Influence of angiotensin-converting enzyme gene polymorphism on development of athlete's heart. *Clin Cardiol* 2002; 23 (1): 621–4.
77. Hernández D, de la Rosa A, Barragán A, et al. The ACE/DD genotype is associated with the extent of exercise-induced left ventricular growth in endurance athletes. *J Am Coll Cardiol* 2003; 42 (3): 527–32.
78. Montgomery H, Brull D, Humphries SE. Analysis of gene-environment interactions by 'stressing-the-genotype' studies: the angiotensin converting enzyme and exercise-induced left ventricular hypertrophy as an example. *Ital Heart J* 2002; 3 (1): 10–14.
79. Mauro M Di, Izzicupo P, Santarelli F, et al. ACE and AGTR1 polymorphisms and left ventricular hypertrophy in endurance athletes. *Med Sci Sport Exerc* 2010; 1 (5): 915–21.
80. Karjalainen J, Kujala UM, Stolt A, et al. Angiotensinogen gene M235T polymorphism predicts left ventricular hypertrophy in endurance athletes. *J Am Coll Cardiol* 1999; 34 (2): 494–9.
81. Alves GB, Oliveira EM, Alves CR, et al. Influence of angiotensinogen and angiotensin-converting enzyme polymorphisms on cardiac hypertrophy and improvement on maximal aerobic capacity caused by exercise training. *Eur J Cardiovasc Prev Rehabil* 2009; 16 (4): 487–92.
82. Fatini C, Guazzelli R, Manetti P, et al. RAS genes influence exercise-induced left ventricular hypertrophy: an elite athletes study. *Med Sci Sports Exerc* 2000; 32 (11): 1868–72.
83. Pelliccia A, Thompson PD. The genetics of left ventricular remodeling in competitive athletes. *J Cardiovasc Med (Hagerstown)* 2006; 7 (4): 267–70.
84. Schunkert H, Hense H, Holmer S, et al. Association between a deletion polymorphism of the angiotensin-converting-enzyme gene and left ventricular hypertrophy. *N Engl J Med* 1994; 330 (23): 1634–8.
85. Brown NJ, Blais C, Gandhi SK, Adam A. ACE insertion/deletion genotype affects bradykinin metabolism. *J Cardiovasc Pharmacol* 1998; 32 (3): 373–7.
86. Lindpaintner K, Lee M, Larson MG, et al. Absence of association or genetic linkage between the angiotensin-converting enzyme gene and left ventricular mass. *N Engl J Med* 1996; 334 (16): 1023–8.
87. Kupari M, Perola M, Koskinen P, et al. Left ventricular size, mass, and function in relation to angiotensin-converting enzyme gene polymorphism in humans. *Am J Physiol* 1994; 267 (3 Pt 2): H1107–11.
88. Gomez-Angelats E, de la Sierra A, Enjuto M, et al. Lack of association between ACE gene polymorphism and left ventricular hypertrophy in essential hypertension. *J Hum Hypertens* 2000; 14 (1): 47–9.

89. Hata A, Namikawa C, Sasaki M, et al. Angiotensinogen as a risk factor for essential hypertension in Japan. *J Clin Invest* 1994; 93 (3): 1285–7.
90. Jeunemaitre X, Soubrier F, Kotelevtsev YV, et al. Molecular basis of human hypertension: role of angiotensinogen. *Cell* 1992; 71 (1): 169–80.
91. Kunz R, Kreutz R, Beige J, et al. Association between the angiotensinogen 235T-variant and essential hypertension in whites: a systematic review and methodological appraisal. *Hypertension* 1997; 30 (6): 1331–7.
92. Bonnardeaux A, Davies E, Jeunemaitre X, et al. Angiotensin II type 1 receptor gene polymorphisms in human essential hypertension. *Hypertension* 1994; 24 (1): 63–9.
93. Ito H, Hiroe M, Hirata Y, et al. Insulin-like growth factor-II induces hypertrophy with increased expression of muscle specific genes in cultured rat cardiomyocytes. *J Mol Cell Cardiol* 1994; 26 (7): 1715–21.
94. Donath MY, Zapf J, Eppenberger-Eberhardt M, et al. Insulin-like growth factor I stimulates myofibril development and decreases smooth muscle alpha-actin of adult cardiomyocytes. *Proc Natl Acad Sci USA* 1994; 91 (5): 1686–90.
95. Decker RS, Cook MG, Behnke-Barclay M, Decker ML. Some growth factors stimulate cultured adult rabbit ventricular myocyte hypertrophy in the absence of mechanical loading. *Circ Res* 1995; 77 (3): 544–55.
96. Reiss K, Cheng W, Kajstura J, et al. Fibroblast proliferation during myocardial development in rats is regulated by IGF-1 receptors. *Am J Physiol* 1995; 269 (3 Pt 2): H943–51.
97. Pauliks LB, Cole KE, Mergner WJ. Increased insulin-like growth factor-1 protein in human left ventricular hypertrophy. *Exp Mol Pathol* 1999; 66 (1): 53–8.
98. DeBosch B, Treskov I, Lupu T. Akt1 is required for physiological cardiac growth. *Circulation* 2006; 113 (117): 2097–104.
99. Schlüter KD, Goldberg Y, Taimor G, et al. Role of phosphatidylinositol 3-kinase activation in the hypertrophic growth of adult ventricular cardiomyocytes. *Cardiovasc Res* 1998; 40 (1): 174–81.
100. Jamshidi Y. Peroxisome proliferator-activated receptor alpha gene regulates left ventricular growth in response to exercise and hypertension. *Circulation* 2002; 105 (8): 950–5.
101. Montgomery HE, Marshall R, Hemingway H, et al. Human gene for physical performance. *Nature* 1998; 393 (6682): 221–2.
102. Ackerman MJ, Splawski I, Makielski JC, et al. Spectrum and prevalence of cardiac sodium channel variants among black, white, Asian, and Hispanic individuals: implications for arrhythmogenic susceptibility and Brugada/long QT syndrome genetic testing. *Heart Rhythm* 2004; 1 (5): 600–7.
103. Killen SA, Kunic J, Wang L, et al. SCN5A allelic expression imbalance in African-Americans heterozygous for the common variant p.Ser1103Tyr. *BMC Med Genet* 2010; 11
104. Van Norstrand DW, Tester DJ, Ackerman MJ. Overrepresentation of the proarrhythmic, sudden death predisposing sodium channel polymorphism S1103Y in a population-based cohort of African-American sudden infant death syndrome. *Heart Rhythm* 2008; 5 (5): 712–15.
105. Ackerman MJ, Tester DJ, Jones GS, et al. Ethnic differences in cardiac potassium channel variants: implications for genetic susceptibility to sudden cardiac death and genetic testing for congenital long QT syndrome. *Mayo Clin Proc* 2003; 78 (12): 1479–87.
106. Plant LD, Bowers PN, Liu Q, et al. A common cardiac sodium channel variant associated with sudden infant death in African Americans, SCN5A S1103Y. *J Clin Invest* 2006; 116 (2): 430–5.
107. Burke A, Creighton W, Mont E, et al. Role of SCN5A Y1102 Polymorphism in sudden cardiac death in blacks. *Circulation* 2005; 112 (6): 798–802.
108. Porthan K, Marjamaa A, Viitasalo M, et al. Relationship of common candidate gene variants to electrocardiographic T-wave peak to T-wave end interval and T-wave morphology parameters. *Heart Rhythm* 2010; 7 (7): 898–903.

1.2.3 The athlete's heart in children and adolescents

Graham Stuart and Guido E. Pieles

Introduction

Healthy children are more active than adults. Public health guidelines recommend that children should minimize sedentary activity and accumulate at least 60 minutes of moderate to vigorous physical activity daily [1]. By 18 years this volume should include at least 150 minutes of moderate intensity exercise per week (➲ Tables 1.2.3.1 and 1.2.3.2). The need for this formal guidance reflects both the overwhelming evidence of health benefit from regular physical exercise and the increasingly sedentary nature of childhood. In 2012 in the UK, 13–15-year-old children spent an average of 4 hours sedentary time including over 2 hours of screen time (television, video, and computer games). Moreover, only 14% of 13–15-year-old boys and 9% of girls achieved recommended physical activity levels—a figure which has fallen from 28% in boys and 14% in girls in 2008 [2].

At the other end of the activity spectrum, there is a subgroup of child and adolescent athletes who compete at an increasingly high level. Many elite competitive child athletes will train for over 20 hours per week—a duration of exercise similar to that of professional adult athletes. Even pre-pubertal club-level swimmers may complete up to 15km swim training weekly, in addition to school sporting activities. Excessive training can have a detrimental effect on the developing musculoskeletal system, leading to overuse injuries [3]. Similarly, the syndrome of overtraining and burnout is now well recognized in elite child athletes [4].

The aim of this chapter is to assess the effect of prolonged exercise on the cardiovascular system of the child and consider whether this can lead to a childhood or adolescent 'athlete's heart' phenotype. In addition, we will address how the sports cardiologist can distinguish adaptive beneficial

Table 1.2.3.1 WHO recommended physical activity levels for health

Age group	Minimum recommended	Alternative strategy	Comments
5–17 years	> 60 min moderate intensity exercise per day	**Additional benefit if more than 60 min*	Most activity should be aerobic. Vigorous PA is recommended at least three times per week and this should include weight-loading activities for muscle and bone health. This should incorporate play, sports, and daily activities
18–65 years	>150 min moderate intensity exercise per week. Aerobic sessions should last >10 min	>75 min of vigorous intensity aerobic PA **or** combination of moderate vigorous intensity PA	Muscle strengthening exercise on >2 days/week **Additional benefit if moderate intensity aerobic PA increased to 300 min/week, or 150 min of vigorous intensity aerobic PA/week, or combination of moderate and vigorous intensity PA*

PA, physical activity

Reprinted from Recommended Levels of Physical Activity for Health. Taken from *Global Recommendations on Physical Activity for Health.* Geneva: World Health Organization; 2010. http://www.who.int/dietphysicalactivity/publications/9789241599979/en/

Table 1.2.3.2 Summary of recommendations for paediatric exercise activity

Guidelines	Year	Key recommendations
Canadian Society for Exercise Physiology (CSEP) (5–17 years)	2012	◆ 60min of moderate to vigorous physical activity daily ◆ Vigorous intensity activities at least 3 days/week ◆ Activities that strengthen muscle and bone at least 3 days/week ◆ Sedentary screen time maximum of 2 hours/day
UK Department of Health (DoH) (5–18 years)	2011	◆ At least 60min of moderate to vigorous physical activity daily ◆ Activities that strengthen muscle and bone at least 3 days/week ◆ Minimize sedentary time
World Health Organization (WHO) (5–17 years)	2011	◆ At least 60min of moderate to vigorous physical activity daily; >60min provides additional health benefits ◆ Most physical activity should be aerobic ◆ Vigorous intensity activities at least 3 days/week ◆ Activities that strengthen muscle and bone at least 3 days/week
US Department of Health and Human Services (HHS) (children and adolescents)	2008	◆ At least 60min of moderate to vigorous physical activity daily ◆ Mostly moderate or vigorous aerobic physical activity ◆ Vigorous intensity activities at least 3 days/week ◆ Activities that strengthen muscle and bone at least 3 days/week
Australian Government Department of Health (5–18 years)	2005	◆ At least 60min of moderate to vigorous physical activity daily ◆ 2 hours/day maximum time using electronic media for entertainment

Reproduced from *Archives of Disease in Childhood*. Guido E Pieles, Richard Horn, Craig A Williams, A Graham Stuart, Vol 99, Issue 4, pp 380–5. Copyright 2014 with permission from BMJ Publishing Group Ltd.

cardiovascular remodelling from underlying pathology such as congenital or inherited cardiovascular disease.

Cardiovascular changes in childhood

The cardiovascular system in the child differs from that in the adult in many ways. These differences vary according to the age and pubertal status of the child.

Infancy

In infancy there is rapid development of both cardiac morphology and electrophysiology. In the first few hours of life, the arterial duct closes and the intra-atrial foramen flap shuts, albeit remaining patent in up to 20% of adults. During the first weeks of life, right ventricular mass decreases and left ventricular mass increases in response to a fall in pulmonary arterial resistance and a rise in systemic blood pressure. There is a similar change in cardiac electrical properties reflected in the electrocardiogram. The newborn infant ECG exhibits right axis deviation and right ventricular hypertrophy but changes rapidly. Thus positive T-waves in V1 are normal on day 1 of life but invert by day 3 and represent a significant abnormality if this has not occurred by day 7. Although these T-wave changes predominantly reflect intracardiac pressures, there are major additional changes in the primary electrophysiological properties of the myocardium over the first 12 months. This can be seen in the propensity for some refractory arrhythmias in the newborn to spontaneously resolve by the first year of life as the electrical properties of the heart stabilize. The specific myocardial properties of infancy are also reflected in significantly lower diastolic relaxation and predominantly late diastolic filling of the left and right ventricles. The infant heart is more vulnerable to load changes and increased output demands are mainly met by an increase in heart rate (HR).

Early childhood and puberty

Children grow rapidly in early childhood. A healthy 3kg neonate may triple in weight to 10kg in the first year of life, but it will be a further 10–12 years before weight triples again to 30kg. Cardiac chambers grow in line with somatic growth and continue growing until somatic growth ends. Maturation of the myocardium leads to normalization of relaxation. Thus diastolic echocardiographic parameters remain relatively stable from 3 years of age. After infancy, systolic function does not change significantly. While most girls stop growing by the late teenage years, some boys continue to grow into their third decade. This variability in cardiac size with somatic growth implies that cardiac chamber size should be referenced to somatic size using *z* scores or relating cardiac dimensions to height or body surface area. Size- and gender-specific paediatric centiles are available for both echocardiographic measurements and cardiac MRI [5–7]. Ideally, cardiac size and physiology should also be related to pubertal stage, but this is seldom carried out because of the practical difficulties and potential embarrassment associated with formally assessing pubertal stage in healthy teenagers. Perhaps one of the most important confounding factors in the assessment of the teenage athlete is this failure to take into account pubertal stage.

At puberty there is a further growth surge. In the early teenage years, the top child athletes are often those who are more physically mature and thus bigger and stronger than their peers. This is recognized in a number of countries; for example, in New Zealand children participating in sports such as rugby are segregated according to weight rather than chronological age. Indeed, it is only after puberty that any prediction can be made regarding potential for adult athletic performance [8].

Puberty is also the stage at which underlying inherited cardiac pathology may present. A genetic predisposition to cardiovascular disease may only manifest when exposed to the rapid growth and hormonal changes that accompany puberty. This is seen in both 'electrical' diseases such as channelopathies and 'structural' diseases such as the cardiomyopathies. Thus, 23% of children with a family history of Brugada syndrome and a negative ajmaline challenge in early childhood will have a positive (diagnostic) ajmaline challenge if repeated after puberty [9]. The effect of puberty is particularly relevant to conditions such as hypertrophic cardiomyopathy. Consequently, at least biennial ECG and echocardiography are recommended for pubertal children with a family history of hypertrophic cardiomyopathy (HCM) [10]. It can sometimes be extremely difficult to distinguish the subtle differences between age-related cardiac maturation, exercise-related remodelling, and the early manifestation of cardiac disease such as cardiomyopathy.

During early childhood the ECG gradually moves from the right dominant infancy pattern to the typical adult appearance at the end of puberty. Typical ECG changes in childhood are shown in ➲ Fig. 1.2.3.1. Normal centiles for the childhood ECG are available [11]. A major issue in the assessment of the ECG of a teenager is the complexity of interpreting the change from pre-pubertal T-wave inversion (TWI) in the right precordial leads to the adult pattern of upright T-waves. Anterior TWI (V1 to V3) in an adult is often abnormal and may suggest pathology such as arrhythmogenic right ventricular cardiomyopathy, but identical T-wave inversion can be normal in a young teenager. In a study of 2765 asymptomatic children undergoing pre-participation athletic screening, Migliore et al. [12] found TWI to be present in 8.4% under 14 years but only in 1.7% over 14 years [12]. The only predictor was incomplete pubertal status. Post-pubertal TWI was regarded as an indication for echocardiography to exclude an underlying cardiomyopathy [12]. Similarly, Calo et al. [13] studied TWI in 2,261 Caucasian soccer players (mean age 12 years, range 8–18 years). TWI was present in 136 (6%) and was virtually always in the anterior leads (>90%). Anterior TWI was associated with mild cardiac disease in 4.8%, but lateral TWI was associated with LH hypertrophy or cardiomyopathy in 60%. Papadakis et al. [14] found TWI in V1–V3 to be common in adolescent Caucasian athletes (<16 years), but only 0.1% had TWI beyond V2 after 16 years.

To conclude, pre-pubertal TWI in the anterior leads (V1,V2) is usually benign and resolves after puberty, while lateral TWI is much less common and should lead to further investigations.

Influence of ethnicity

In adult athletes there are important cardiovascular differences between athletes of Caucasian/white and non-Caucasian/Afro-Caribbean descent [15,16]. Consequently, ethnicity has to be taken into account when assessing the ECG and echocardiographic findings. Very little is known on the effect of ethnicity on the cardiovascular system of the developing child athlete. Sheik et al. [17] have shown that the repolarization changes and left ventricular hypertrophy occurring in black adult athletes are also present in

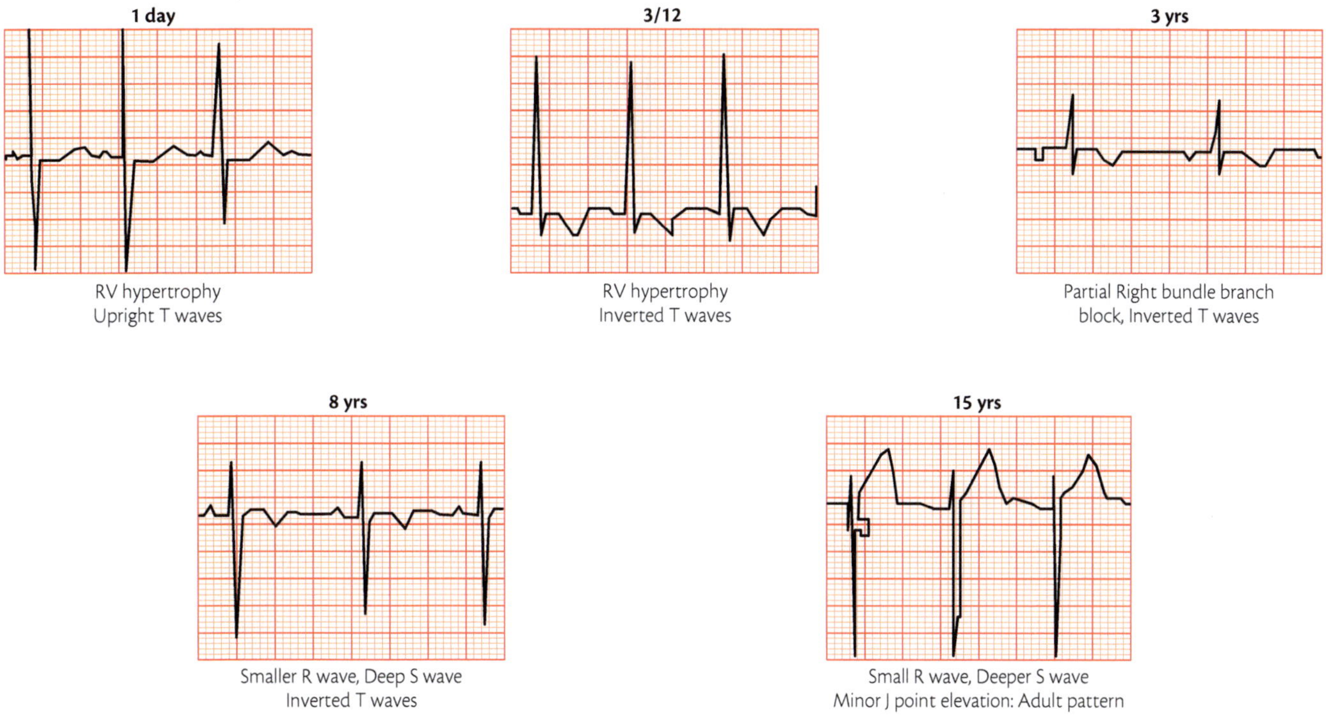

Fig. 1.2.3.1 Age-related changes in the ECG during childhood.

adolescents. Moreover, Pela et al. [18] demonstrated that the concentric LV remodelling that occurs in adolescent footballers of black African origin is much less obvious in their white peers. There is more genetic diversity in Africa than in any other world region, and it is possible that changes in athletes originating from one part of Africa may be a normal variant whereas similar changes in athletes originating from another African region may represent disease. In the multicultural environment of sport and exercise, the influence of ethnicity is a complex confounding variable in the child athlete. It may not be possible to exclude abnormality with confidence. It is important to follow up child athletes in whom a possible ethnically related change has been found, although it is equally important not to label such a change as a definite 'abnormality' without clear evidence.

The effect of exercise training in childhood

General effects

Exercise training has multiple benefits for school age youth. These include improvements in bone strength, kinetic skills, biological maturity, lung and endocrine function, academic performance, and mental health. Many of these are summarized by Strong et al. [19].

Cardiovascular effects and athlete's heart

Prior and La Gerche [20] defined athlete's heart as 'the complex of structural and functional electrical remodelling that accompanies athletic training'. The cardiovascular consequences of vigorous exercise training are well documented in adults but less is known for the developing child athlete [21–23]. As in the adult athlete, exercise training in children leads to significant morphological and functional cardiovascular changes, although studies are sometimes contradictory and show a variable remodelling response. This variation may depend on age, pubertal stage, type of sport, and intensity of exercise training.

Some of the studies reporting training-related cardiovascular changes in peri-pubertal athletes are summarized in ➲ Table 1.2.3.3. Although trained children are able to exercise to a higher level than untrained children (for example, higher VO_2max and heart rates), there is relatively little difference in cardiac chamber size and myocardial mass. This may reflect the different effect of exercise on the immature heart, but it may also be due to the reduced intensity and volume of exercise training participated in by younger children. In intensively trained 11–12-year-old pre-pubertal boys (swim trained for >3 years for >8 hours per week), Ayabakan et al. [24] described a concentric increase in LV wall thickness but no significant change in diastolic diameter in comparison to controls. Interpretation of these studies is made more complex by the lack of formal pubertal assessment. More research is needed to establish the effects of intensive training on cardiac function in children, particularly pre- and peri-pubertal children who may behave differently from adults. Data on the negative impact of

Table 1.2.3.3 Cardiovascular remodelling in peri-pubertal child athletes

Study	Number of athletes/sport	Age range	Evaluation technique	Pubertal status described	Conclusions and effect of exercise
Rowland et al. [41]	14 competitive swimmers; matched active non-trained controls	8.8–13.5 years (mean 11)	ECG/echocardiogram	Yes	Lower resting heart rates and LV volume overload in athletes
Telford et al. [42]	85 trained child athletes (mixed) compared with skeletal age matched controls	11–12 years	Echocardiogram	No	No difference in ventricular dimensions or mass
Rowland et al. [43]	10 male runners, matched with active non-trained controls	11–13 years	ECG/echocardiogram/ metabolic exercise testing	Yes–described as pre-pubertal	No clinically significant differences in ECG or LV mass and wall thickness
Ozer et al. [44]	82 swimmers with mean 32 months swim training; 41 sedentary controls	7–14 years (mean 11.2 years)	Echocardiography	No	Athletes had increased LV dimensions, wall thickness, aortic root size, and LV mass compared with controls
Rowland et al. [45]	7 competitive cyclists compared with control group	11.9 years	Metabolic exercise testing Echocardiography	No	Maximal stroke volume determines VO_2max; lower resting heart rate and higher stroke volume than controls
Obert et al. [46]	29 boys and girls 3 month aerobic training/ detraining for 2 months (26 non-exercised controls)	10–11 years	Echocardiography	No	LV internal dimensions increased (4.6%) and wall thickness decreased (10.7%); returned to normal after detraining Heart rate slowed with training No change in systolic function with training or detraining
Triposkiadis et al. [47]	25 elite swimmers 12–14 hours training per week compared with sedentary controls	11.5 years	Heart rate variability (HRV) Echocardiography	No	Increased vagal dominance LV and LA dimensions increased. No change in wall thickness or HRV
Nottin et al. [48]	12 boy cyclists, 11 untrained controls; 10 adult cyclists and 13 sedentary adults	11–13 years (adults 20-26 years)	Echocardiography	Yes (Tanner stages) Post pubertal boys excluded	Increased LV relaxation in adult and child cyclists but no LV hypertrophy in children
Ayabakan et al. [24]	22 male pubertal swimmers compared with 21 age-matched, sedentary controls. Mean 10 hours training per week.	11 years	Echocardiography including tissue Doppler imaging	Yes (described as pre-pubertal)	No differences in tissue Doppler but increased concentric LV wall thickness in athletes compared with controls No change in diastolic dimensions
Rowland et al. [49]	7 girls, 7 boys trained swimmers (5 h/week) Prone swim simulation Compared with non-trained controls	12 ± 0.5 years	Metabolic exercise testing Exercise Echocardiography	No	No rise in stroke volume during exercise implying peripheral factors (increased filling) and heart rate are main determinants of cardiac output on exercise Minor increase in LV diastolic dimension and mass in trained group.
Zdravkovic [50]	94 highly trained male footballers	12.85 ± 0.84 years	Echocardiography	No	Significant increase in LV dimensions, aortic root and LA size

(Continued)

Study	Number of athletes/sport	Age range	Evaluation technique	Pubertal status described	Conclusions and effect of exercise
Koch et al. [36]	342 elite athletes at sports schools Multiple disciplines	10–15 years	ECG/echocardiogram	No	LV upper limits described Age 11: boys 10mm, girls 9mm Age 13: boys/girls 10 mm Age 15: boys 11mm/girls 10mm. No ECG gender differences
Binnetoglu et al. [51]	140 athletes; six sports Minimum 3h/week for 2 years Sedentary controls	10–16 years	ECG/echocardiogram including strain imaging	No	Normal systolic and diastolic indices in athletes 16% concentric remodelling; 28% eccentric remodelling Strain lower in athletes Myocardial deformation more evident in mixed sports participants
Agrebi et al. [52]	Elite male national handball players; three groups of 12	Mean age 12/16/25 years	ECG/echocardiogram	No	Chamber dilatation occurred in younger athletes but less hypertrophy compared with older athletes.
Calo et al. [13]	2261 male Caucasian soccer players	Mean age 12.4 years	ECG/echocardiogram	No	Anterior T-wave inversion (>2 leads) associated with cardiac disease in 4.8% T-wave inversion (inferolateral leads) associated with disease in 60%

excessive training volume and intensity on the paediatric heart are scarce. However, Komoliatova et al. [25] found that elevation in microvolt T-wave alternans was an insensitive but specific sign of over-training in elite child athletes.

Although many exercise-related cardiovascular changes in children are similar to those in adults, there are important differences in the remodelling process [26]. These are summarized in ➲ Table 1.2.3.4. For example, there is more chamber dilatation and less ventricular hypertrophy than in adults. Nottin et al. [27] showed that 12–13-year-old elite endurance cyclists did not develop LV hypertrophy but demonstrated similar improvements in LV relaxation to adults. In a similar study (720 elite adolescent athletes), Sharma et al. [28] noted that very few had an LV wall thickness greater than 12mm. Moreover, when this was exceeded ventricles were invariably large with end-diastolic measurements >2 SD above the mean. The authors concluded that HCM should be considered in adolescent athletes if LV wall thickness is >12mm (>11mm in girls) and the ventricle is not dilated.

Table 1.2.3.4 Cardiovascular adaption to exercise training in child athletes: comparison with adults

Cardiovascular change in child	Comparison with adult athletes	Comment
Resting heart rate falls	Resting heart rate remains higher than in adult	Age-dependent;younger athletes have higher resting heart rates
Dilatation of left atrium	Similar pattern	Considerable variation between children in the same exercise group and in different studies. Some studies have demonstrated concentric hypertrophy, others predominantly dilatation. If LV dilates above 60 mm in diastole consider pathology.
Left ventricle dilates, mild LV hypertrophy.	Less chamber dilatation and more hypertrophy occurs in adults	
Mild concentric hypertrophy with prolonged vigorous training	Eccentric hypertrophy tends to occur in adults with athlete's heart	
Increased LV relaxation Improved diastolic function	Similar pattern	Occurs in pre- and post-pubertal children
Raised VO_2max compared with untrained	Lower VO_2max relative to body size in comparison with adult athletes	Reflects lower maximal stroke volume and maturity related increase in diastolic filling
Reduced vascular stiffness	Similar pattern	Acute effect known but long-term effects not studied in children
No differences between the sexes	Female athletes have higher resting heart rates, smaller cardiac chambers and less hypertrophy	Pre-pubertal changes present but change to adult pattern post-puberty.

Assessment of the child athlete

Cardiologists may be required to assess child athletes as part of a pre-participation screen or when the athlete presents with possible cardiac symptoms. In both situations, it is important to be aware of the normal cardiac remodelling that occurs with exercise. The most important pathological conditions which mimic these adaptive changes are the cardiomyopathies, in particular hypertrophic cardiomyopathy (HCM).

There are no cardiovascular screening protocols specific to child and adolescent athletes. However, screening protocols for young athletes (teenagers and adults) have been produced [29,30]. These are discussed in detail elsewhere. These guidelines are designed for teenage and young adult athletes, but it is accepted that diagnosis of developing cardiovascular disease can be difficult to predict in the younger age groups [31].

A standardized approach to screening for cardiovascular disease in young people (>12 years old) has been proposed in the USA. This proposal includes a comprehensive history and clinical examination [32].

An approach to the cardiovascular assessment of the child and adolescent athlete is described in ➲ Table 1.2.3.5. This should involve a pre-participation questionnaire, a clinical examination, and an ECG. An echocardiogram is essential for the assessment of athlete's heart.

Screening questionnaire, history, and examination

The pre-participation questionnaire should identify cardiovascular symptoms and any underlying cardiac or inherited condition. When the child is reviewed these questions should be repeated, preferably in the presence of parents, as important facts can be omitted. This should include an exercise participation history. The child who only exercises as part of routine school physical education (<3–4hours/

Table 1.2.3.5 Approach to cardiovascular evaluation of the child and adolescent athlete

	Details	Rationale
Exercise history	Hours of exercise per week Type of exercise (aerobic/isometric). Should include details of training for specific sport *and* any additional exercise such as school sport.	This is to evaluate the likelihood of exercise-related remodelling. Structural changes are unlikely unless there is a significant exercise load.
Medical history	Should include full past medical history (including neonatal history, significant illnesses,/surgery and assessment of current symptoms. Specific attention to be given to exercise-related syncope/near syncope; chest pain; palpitations.	Evaluation of current health status. This aids the interpretation of potential cardiovascular symptoms.
Drug and supplement history	Current medications and supplements including details of origin of supplements if self-administered.	Medications taken inform medical history. Supplements may have cardiovascular consequences if containing illicit anabolic or excessive stimulants.
Family history and ethnicity	Details of sudden death of close relative at young age (<40 years). Details of known inherited cardiac condition in close relative. Ethnicity and family origin (Afro-Caribbean, Arab, etc.) Black.	Identification of inherited familial condition. Ethnicity is important particularly when interpreting ECG (see text).
Physical Examination	Specific emphasis on dysmorphology (e.g. Marfan/Noonan syndrome). Signs of hypertension (including reduced femoral pulses and murmur of coarctation). Pathological murmur suggesting valve dysfunction. Check blood pressure in right arm/both arms. Pubertal status: pre-pubertal/peri-pubertal/post-pubertal	Dysmorphic syndromes can mimic changes of athlete's heart (e.g. Noonan syndrome–ventricular hypertrophy. Marfan syndrome—root and LV dilatation). Pathological murmur may expose cause of left ventricular hypertrophy (e.g. aortic stenosis, coarctation of aorta). Pubertal status has a major influence on manifestation of both inherited cardiac conditions (such as HCM) and athlete's heart.
Electrocardiogram	Use Seattle screening criteria: false-positive rate 1–3%; false negative for HCM, 10%. T-wave inversion in anteroseptal leads is usually normal before puberty but abnormal after puberty. Lateral T-wave inversion is usually abnormal at any age.	Must be supplemented by clinical history and examination.
Echocardiogram	Full congenital and structural assessment using indexed values. The echocardiographic parameters of most child athletes lie within the normal range	See text

week) is unlikely to develop exercise-related cardiac remodelling. A clinical examination is invaluable for identifying syndromes and abnormal physical signs. An assessment of general health and an approximate assessment of pubertal stage should be made.

Electrocardiography

ECG screening in young athletes can be difficult to interpret due to the changes mentioned in previous sections. Thompson et al. [33] found that >50% of 16-year-old elite athletes reached standard criteria for ventricular hypertrophy. However, only 1% had pathological Q waves, TWI, or ST depression compared with 74% of teenagers with HCM. In this study, the Seattle and ESC screening criteria had a false-negative rate of 10% for HCM, but the Seattle criteria had a much lower false-positive rate (1% vs 24%) [29,30,33]. Bessem et al. [34] compared the ESC and Seattle criteria in high level junior soccer players (10–19 years). In this study, 100/188 athletes were under 14 years old. A high rate of abnormalities were detected using the ESC criteria (33%), but this fell to 3% using the Seattle criteria. In a review of electrocardiogram screening in pre-pubertal athletic children, Leger et al. [35] noted that the ECG phenotype of cardiac disease differed significantly from that of adults but concluded that history and physical examination should remain the cornerstone of cardiovascular screening.

Echocardiography screening

In a study of 343 elite athletes (10–15 years old), Koch found that children had fewer abnormal ECGs than adults but, when identifying cardiovascular abnormalities, ECG had a sensitivity of only 38% (specificity 64%) compared with echocardiography. Rowland [26] noted that, although many child athletes have slightly larger and thicker hearts than non-athletes, even the most highly trained are usually within the normal range. Consequently, it is usually feasible to distinguish between exercise-based remodelling and cardiomyopathies. Specific paediatric echocardiography guidelines and normative values for morphology and function are available [37]. The end-diastolic LV diameter, which is reduced in the majority of phenotypic HCM, can be a diagnostic help [38]. As in adults, diastolic tissue Doppler imaging (TDI) parameters are often reduced.

Chamber-size-based echocardiography (e.g. ejection fraction) has limitations in the assessment of ventricular function as it is load dependent and does not measure myocardial performance. Myocardial deformation (strain) imaging by 2D speckle tracking is less load dependent, more sensitive to mild functional impairment, and measures myocardial function. Strain imaging has been validated in children, and normative paediatric values exist although few data for child athletes are available [39]. Recently it has been used successfully as a robust and less load-dependent functional tool in assessing myocardial performance reserve during exercise in adolescents [21]. In addition to functional assessment, echocardiography in the child athlete should include a complete congenital echocardiographic examination as undiagnosed congenital heart disease is encountered more often than in the adult.

Other assessment methods—the cardiomyopathies

In the initial assessment of athlete's heart in the child, it is seldom necessary to use any additional assessment techniques. A cardiopulmonary exercise stress test can be helpful if it is unclear whether hypertrophy is due to exercise remodelling or cardiomyopathy. A normal heart rate and blood pressure response is a reassuring response, but does not exclude cardiomyopathy.

The main differential diagnoses of athlete's heart in the young are HCM and arrhythmogenic right ventricular cardiomyopathy (ARVC). Echocardiography has reduced sensitivity and specificity in detecting inherited myocardial disease, and young adolescents often have minimal symptoms. Cardiac magnetic resonance (CMR) imaging can be of value in assessing the presence of cardiomyopathy. CMR is particularly useful in the context of T-wave changes that may reflect an ethnically related variant or mild hypertrophy that seems disproportionate to the level of exercise participation. The presence of late gadolinium enhancement or diastolic dysfunction supports the presence of underlying cardiomyopathy but does not exclude it. In ARVC, CMR findings such as fatty infiltration and fibrosis are of limited value in children, and the focus is on ventricular function, regional wall motion abnormalities, and *z*-scores of RV and LV dimensions [40].

In the child athlete the developing nature of cardiomyopathies means that a single point assessment does not exclude subsequent manifestation of a genotype-positive, phenotype-negative inherited cardiomyopathy. Serial annual evaluation is paramount.

Future directions

Future work should formulate specific guidelines for the junior athlete population younger than 14 years. The development of normal ranges for the child athlete population should continue, and thought should be given to the use of new diagnostic tools, such as assessment of myocardial performance during exercise stress, in the identification of underlying pathology.

Further reading

Armstrong N, Van Mechelen W. *Paediatric Exercise Science and Medicine* (2nd edn). Oxford: Oxford University Press, 2009.

Koch S, Cassel M, Linne K, et al. ECG and echocardiographic findings in 10–15-year-old elite athletes. *Eur J Prev Cardiol* 2014; 21: 774–81.

Pieles GE, Horn R, Williams CA, Stuart AG. Paediatric exercise training in prevention and treatment. *Arch Dis Child* 2014; 99: 380–5.

Rowland T. Morphologic features of the 'athlete's heart' in children: a contemporary review. *Pediatr Exerc Sci* 2016; 28: 345–52.

References

1. Pieles GE, Horn R, Williams CA, Stuart AG. Paediatric exercise training in prevention and treatment. *Arch Dis Child* 2014; 99: 380–5.
2. Townsend MWK, Williams J, Bhatnagar P, Rayner M. *Physical Activity Statistics 2015*. London: British Heart Foundation, 2015.
3. Brenner JS, American Academy of Pediatrics Council on Sports Medicine and Fitness. Overuse injuries, overtraining, and burnout in child and adolescent athletes. *Pediatrics* 2007; 119: 1242–5.
4. Gustafsson H, Hill AP, Stenling A, Wagnsson S. Profiles of perfectionism, parental climate, and burnout among competitive junior athletes. *Scand J Med Sci Sports* 2016; 26(10): 1256–64.
5 Sarikouch S, Peters B, Gutberlet M, et al. Sex-specific pediatric percentiles for ventricular size and mass as reference values for cardiac MRI: assessment by steady-state free-precession and phase-contrast MRI flow. *Circ Cardiovasc Imaging* 2010; 3: 65–76.
6. Dallaire F, Slorach C, Hui W, et al. 2015. Reference values for pulse wave Doppler and tissue Doppler imaging in pediatric echocardiography. *Circ Cardiovasc Imaging*; 8(2): e002167.
7. Overbeek LI, Kapusta L, Peer PG, et al. New reference values for echocardiographic dimensions of healthy Dutch children. *Eur J Echocardiogr* 2006; 7: 113–21.
8. Costa MJ, Marinho DA, Bragada JA, et al. Stability of elite freestyle performance from childhood to adulthood. *J Sports Sci* 2011; 29: 1183–9.
9. Conte G, De Asmundis C, Ciconte G, et al. Follow-up from childhood to adulthood of individuals with family history of Brugada syndrome and normal electrocardiograms. *JAMA* 2014; 312: 2039–41.
10. Elliott PM, Anastasakis A, Borger MA, et al. 2014 ESC guidelines on diagnosis and management of hypertrophic cardiomyopathy: the Task Force for the Diagnosis and Management of Hypertrophic Cardiomyopathy of the European Society of Cardiology (ESC). *Eur Heart J* 2014; 35: 2733–79.
11. Rijnbeek PR, Witsenburg M, Schrama E, et al. New normal limits for the paediatric electrocardiogram. *Eur Heart J* 2001; 22: 702–11.
12. Migliore F, Zorzi A, Michieli P, et al. Prevalence of cardiomyopathy in Italian asymptomatic children with electrocardiographic T-wave inversion at preparticipation screening. *Circulation* 2012; 125: 529–38.
13. Calo L, Sperandii F, Martino A., et al. Echocardiographic findings in 2261 peri-pubertal athletes with or without inverted T waves at electrocardiogram. *Heart* 2015; 101: 193–200.
14. Papadakis M, Basavarajaiah S, Rawlins J, et al. Prevalence and significance of T-wave inversions in predominantly Caucasian adolescent athletes. *Eur Heart J* 2009; 30: 1728–35.
15. Calore C, Zorzi A, Sheikh N., et al. Electrocardiographic anterior T-wave inversion in athletes of different ethnicities: differential diagnosis between athlete's heart and cardiomyopathy. *Eur Heart J* 2016; 37(32): 2515–27
16. Basavarajaiah S, Boraita A, Whyte G, et al. Ethnic differences in left ventricular remodeling in highly-trained athletes relevance to differentiating physiologic left ventricular hypertrophy from hypertrophic cardiomyopathy. *J Am Coll Cardiol* 2008; 51: 2256–62.
17. Sheikh N, Papadakis M, Carré F, et al. Cardiac adaptation to exercise in adolescent athletes of African ethnicity: an emergent elite athletic population. *Br J Sports Med* 2013; 47: 585–92.
18. Pela G, Li Calzi M, Crocamo A, et al. Ethnicity-related variations of left ventricular remodeling in adolescent amateur football players. *Scand J Med Sci Sports* 2015; 25: 382–9.
19. Strong WB, Malina RM, Blimkie CJ, et al. Evidence based physical activity for school-age youth. *J Pediatr* 2005; 146: 732–7.
20. Prior DL, La Gerche A. The athlete's heart. *Heart* 2012; 98: 947–55.
21. Pieles GE, Gowing L, Forsey J, et al. The relationship between biventricular myocardial performance and metabolic parameters during incremental exercise and recovery in healthy adolescents. *Am J Physiol Heart Circ Physiol* 2015; 309: H2067–76.
22. Weiner RB, Baggish AL. Cardiovascular adaptation and remodeling to rigorous athletic training. *Clin Sports Med* 2015; 34(3): 305–18
23. Gielen S, Schuler G, Adams V. Cardiovascular effects of exercise training: molecular mechanisms. *Circulation* 2010; 122: 1221–38.
24. Ayabakan C, Akalin F, Mengutay S, et al. Athlete's heart in prepubertal male swimmers. *Cardiol Young* 2006; 16: 61–6.
25. Komoliatova VV, Makarov LM, Fedina, NN, Kiseleva II. [Microvolt T-wave alternans in adolescent elite athletes]. *Kardiologiia* 2015; 55: 43–6.
26. Rowland T. Morphologic features of the 'athlete's heart' in children: a contemporary review. *Pediatr Exerc Sci* 2016; 28: 345–52.
27. Nottin S, Nguyen LD, Terbah M, Obert P. Left ventricular function in endurance-trained children by tissue Doppler imaging. *Med Sci Sports Exerc* 2004; 36: 1507–13.
28. Sharma S, Maron BJ, Whyte G, et al. Physiologic limits of left ventricular hypertrophy in elite junior athletes: relevance to differential diagnosis of athlete's heart and hypertrophic cardiomyopathy. *J Am Coll Cardiol* 2002; 40: 1431–6.
29. Drezner JA, Ackerman MJ, Anderson J, et al. Electrocardiographic interpretation in athletes: the 'Seattle criteria'. *Br J Sports Med* 2013; 47: 122–4.
30. Corrado, D., Pelliccia, A., Heidbuchel, H., et al. Recommendations for interpretation of 12-lead electrocardiogram in the athlete. *Eur Heart* 2010; 31: 243–59.
31. Maron BJ, Zipes DP, Kovacs RJ, et al. Eligibility and disqualification recommendations for competitive athletes with cardiovascular abnormalities: preamble, principles, and general considerations. A scientific statement from the American Heart Association and American College of Cardiology. *Circulation* 2015; 132: e256–61.
32. Maron BJ, Friedman RA, Kligfield P, et al. Assessment of the 12-lead electrocardiogram as a screening test for detection of cardiovascular disease in healthy general populations of

young people (12-25 years of age): a scientific statement from the American Heart Association and the American College of Cardiology. *J Am Coll Cardiol* 2014; 64: 1479–1514.
33. Thompson AJ, Cannon BC, Wackel PL, et al. Electrocardiographic abnormalities in elite high school athletes: comparison to adolescent hypertrophic cardiomyopathy. *Br J Sports Med* 2016; 50: 105–10.
34. Bessem B, De Bruijn MC, Nieuwland W. The ECG of high-level junior soccer players: comparing the ESC vs. the Seattle criteria. *Br J Sports Med* 2015; 49: 1000–6.
35. Leger L, Gojanovic B, Sekarski N., et al. The impending dilemma of electrocardiogram screening in athletic children. *Pediatr Cardiol* 2016; 37: 1–13.
36. Koch S, Cassel M, Linne K, et al. ECG and echocardiographic findings in 10–15-year-old elite athletes. *Eur J Prev Cardiol* 2014; 21: 774–81.
37. Lopez L, Colan SD, Frommelt PC., et al. Recommendations for quantification methods during the performance of a pediatric echocardiogram: a report from the Pediatric Measurements Writing Group of the American Society of Echocardiography Pediatric and Congenital Heart Disease Council. *J Am Soc Echocardiogr* 2010; 23: 465–95, quiz 576–7.
38. Lipshultz SE, Orav EJ, Wilkinson JD, et al. Risk stratification at diagnosis for children with hypertrophic cardiomyopathy: an analysis of data from the Pediatric Cardiomyopathy Registry. *Lancet* 2013; 382: 1889–97.
39. Marcus KA, Mavinkurve-Groothuis AM, Barends M, et al. Reference values for myocardial two-dimensional strain echocardiography in a healthy pediatric and young adult cohort. *J Am Soc Echocardiogr* 2011; 24: 625–36.
40. Etoom Y, Govindapillai S, Hamilton R, et al. Importance of CMR within the Task Force Criteria for the diagnosis of ARVC in children and adolescents. *J Am Coll Cardiol* 2015; 65: 987–95.
41. Rowland TW, Delaney BC, Siconolfi SF. 'Athlete's heart" in prepubertal children. *Pediatrics* 1987; 79(5): 800–4.
42. Telford RD, McDonald IG, Ellis LB, et al. Echocardiographic dimensions in trained and untrained 12-year-old boys and girls. *J Sports Sci* 1988; 6: 49–57.
43. Rowland TW, Unnithan VB, MacFarlane NG, et al. Clinical manifestations of the 'athlete's heart' in prepubertal male runners. *Int J Sports Med* 1994; 15: 515–19
44. Ozer, S, Cil E, Baltaci G. et al. Left ventricular structure and function by echocardiography in childhood swimmers Jpn Heart J 1994; 35(3): 295–300.
45. Rowland, T, Wehnert M, Miller K. Cardiac responses to exercise in competitive child cyclists. *Med Sci Sports Exerc* 2000; 32(4): 747–52.
46. Obert P, Mandigout, S, Vinet, A, et al. Effect of aerobic training and detraining on left ventricular dimensions and diastolic function in prepubertal boys and girls. *Int J Sports Med* 2001; 22(2): 90–6.
47. Triposkiadis F, Ghiokas S, Skoulangis I, et al. Cardiac adaptation to intensive training in prepubertal swimmers. *Eur J Clin Invest* 2002; 32: 16–23.
48. Nottin S, Nguyen LD, Terbah M, Obert P. Left ventricular function in endurance-trained children by tissue Doppler imaging. *Med Sci Sports Med* 2004; 36(9); 1507–13.
49. Rowland T, Bougault V, Walther G, et al. Cardiac responses to swim bench exercise in age-group swimmers and non-athletic children. *J Sci Med Sport* 2009;12:266–272
50. Zdravkovic M, Perunicic J, Krotin M, et al. Echocardiographic study of early left ventricular remodeling in highly trained preadolescent footballers. *J Sci Med Sport* 2010; 13: 602–6.
51. Binnetoğlu FK, Babaoğlu K, Altun G, Kayabey Ö. Effects that different types of sports have on the hearts of children and adolescents and the value of two-dimensional strain-strain-rate echocardiography. *Pediatr Cardiol* 2014; 35: 126–39.
52. Agrebi B, Tkatchuk V, Hlila N. Impact of specific training and competition on myocardial structure and function in different age ranges of male handball players. *PLoS One* 2015; 10(12): e0143609.

1.2.4 Vascular remodelling

Stephan Gielen, M. Harold Laughlin, and Dirk J. Duncker

Introduction

Regular exercise training increases whole-body maximal oxygen consumption, which is regarded as an integral measure of exercise capacity. This effect is associated with increased maximal cardiac output and increased maximal arteriovenous oxygen difference [1]. The cardiac output of elite athletes increases to up to 40L/min (e.g. in cross-country skiers) and stroke volume may exceed 200mL [2]. The increase in cardiac output produced by exercise training is accompanied by a corresponding increase in vascular conductance [1,3], which results from functional and structural adaptations in conduit and resistance arteries, and in capillaries in skeletal muscle and myocardium [1,3].

- *Structural adaptations* in cardiac and skeletal muscle vascular beds include angiogenesis (i.e. increased density of capillaries, arterioles, and other microvessels) and vascular remodelling (i.e. increased length, cross-sectional area, and/or diameters of existing arteries and veins).
- *Functional adaptive changes* in the blood flow capacity can result from changes in neurohumoral control, local control systems, and vascular smooth muscle and/or endothelial cells, or from the effects of changes in vascular structure on vascular resistance.

In this chapter we provide a concise overview of the physiological and molecular mechanisms that explain the remarkable vascular adaptations seen in elite athletes. The focus is on changes in the large arterial conductance vessels and the coronary circulation.

Vascular adaptation of the aorta and peripheral circulation

Aorta

Type of exercise and aortic stiffness

High intensity physical activity is associated with recurrent bouts of elevated blood pressure and increased blood flow. The relation between both changes depends on the relation between isometric and isotonic exercise components. The increase in blood pressure and radial circumferential stress is greatest in pure isometric exercise such as weight-lifting. The physiological basis for the differences in aortic wall stiffness seems to be an elevated sympathetic tone in strength training versus resistance training, while endothelium-dependent vasodilation is not different [4]. Additionally, elevated endothelin-1 plasma concentrations have been observed in strength training, and this may contribute to the increased vascular stiffness [5].

Adaptations of the aorta in isometric versus endurance exercise

The increase in blood pressure and radial strain on the aortic wall associated with strength training leads to increases in vascular stiffness and aortic transverse diameter [6]. Endurance athletes, on the other hand, have a lower aortic stiffness index compared with sedentary controls [7]. In strength training the increase in aortic stiffness leads to higher cardiac afterload with consequent concentric LV hypertrophy [8].

In a large meta-analysis of 23 studies with a total of 5580 elite athletes, Iskandar and Thompson [9] compared aortic root dimensions at the aortic valve annulus and the sinus of Valsalva with those of healthy sedentary subjects. The weighted mean aortic root diameter measured at the sinuses of Valsalva was 3.2mm ($p = 0.02$) larger in athletes than in the non-athletic controls, and the aortic root size at the aortic valve annulus was 1.6mm ($p = 0.04$) larger in athletes than in controls. In this meta-analysis, the slightly larger aortic diameters in strength-trained athletes versus controls did not reach statistical significance. The authors conclude that mild aortic enlargement is a normal adaptation to exercise training, but 'large increases in aortic size are unusual in athletes and are therefore consistent with a pathological process' [9]. The relation between physical activity with high isometric strain and aortic dilatation was further corroborated by a Turkish observational study comparing the aortic root diameters of 30 strenuous activity trainers and 30 ordinary activity trainers [10]. They found significantly larger aortic root and ascending aorta diameters in strenuous activity trainers.

Despite these rather reassuring data from the Iskandar meta-analysis [9], a number of cases of acute aortic dissection in weight-lifters—especially those with a history of anabolic steroid use—have been described in the literature (reviewed in [11]). There are no cases of aortic dissections in endurance athletes [11]. These life-threatening complications of high-intensity isometric exercise highlight the risks associated with athletic exercise training and raise the questionof the role of pre-participation screening for aortic diseases in athletes. The general consensus is that patients with genetic syndromes associated with aortopathy should be restricted from vigorous sports participation [12], but the presence of a bicuspid aortic valve with normal aortic dimensions should not influence eligibility to participate in sports competitions.

Conduit arteries

Adaptations of vascular control by exercise

Exercise-training-induced improvement in endothelium-dependent vasodilation has been described in many pathological conditions with reduced baseline endothelial function (e.g. hypertension, old age, diabetes mellitus, hyperlipidaemia). However, if baseline endothelial function is normal—as in young athletes—improvements may not be found. The most common measure of endothelial function in humans is brachial artery flow-mediated dilation (FMD). Shear stress plays a key role in signalling the exercise-training-induced positive adaptation of the endothelium in conduit arteries [13], which is related to changes in eNOS generated NO signalling [13] and is also endothelium independent [1].

In addition to the improvements in endothelium-dependent vasodilation, vasoconstrictive α-adrenergic responsiveness is reduced in large conduit coronary arteries of exercise-trained animals, which may aid in maximizing upstream vessel diameter during bouts of exercise [14,15].

Adaptations in vascular structure by exercise

Changes in arterial luminal diameter

Athletes have larger peripheral arteries (e.g. aorta, carotid, subclavian arteries) relative to matched sedentary controls [16], and many studies have revealed remodelling of conduit arteries with increases in conduit artery lumen diameter after regular exercise, typically in the trained limb [17,18]. Repeated exposure to increased shear stress with exercise is the key stimulus for remodelling. When exploring bilateral brachial artery adaptations to handgrip [19] or cycle [20] exercise, unilateral shear manipulation with sub-diastolic cuff inflation prevented the increases in peak brachial artery diameter observed in the arm exposed to episodic increases in shear. The increase in femoral artery diameter is strongly related to the increase in the regional maximal oxygen uptake ($r = 0.86$) [21] and muscle mass ($r = 0.44$) [22]. It appears that changes in muscle mass along with regional increases in blood flow, tightly coupled with the metabolic demand of the distal muscle, are associated with exercise-induced arterial remodelling and facilitate the ability to perform aerobic work.

Changes in wall thickness of peripheral conduit arteries

Direct comparisons of endurance-trained and sedentary populations often report no significant differences in carotid wall thickness between trained and untrained cohorts [23]. In contrast, cross-sectional and longitudinal training studies both suggest that exercise mediates reductions in the thickness of conduit artery walls supplying the active and non-active areas when adequate intensity and duration of training are employed [18,24,25]. Rowley et al. [26] reported smaller brachial and femoral artery wall thicknesses in subjects who were active, whether they were engaged in lower limb versus upper limb exercise, healthy controls, wheelchair controls, or athletes.

Changes in compliance of peripheral conduit arteries

Arterial wall stiffness can be reliably measured via pulse wave velocity (PWV), which strongly relates to atherosclerotic disease: A 1m/s increase in PWV leads to a 7% increase in the risk for CV events [27]. Both field studies and literature reviews support the notion that PWV is decreased in aerobically trained subjects [28]. The effect on PWV was larger with longer duration training and in subjects with a lower a priori level of arterial stiffness. Furthermore, a larger reduction in PWV after exercise was observed for brachial–ankle PWV compared with carotid–femoral PWV. This observation suggests that exercise training has a larger effect on 'peripheral' conduit artery stiffness than on aortic stiffness [29]. It seems possible that the more muscular, stiffer, peripheral arteries have a potential for larger adaptations of arterial wall properties in response to exercise compared with central arteries.

Skeletal muscle resistance arteries

Consistent with the notion that vascular adaptations need to match supply and demand, multiple studies in athletes confirm that the preferred limb exhibited higher peak vasodilator responses than the non-preferred limbs. Similarly, comparing leg peak blood flow between elite athletes and controls indicates greater peak vasodilator responses in the preferred limb [30]. Higher peak blood flow after exercise training causes remodelling of structure and function/control of resistance arteries, which appears to be focused in the active beds during exercise [24] and to require increases in blood flow [26]. Experiments in animal models also indicate that exercise can increase the size and/or number of resistance arteries/arterioles in skeletal muscle [1].

Studies performed in healthy subjects have reported conflicting results regarding the impact of exercise on resistance artery endothelium-dependent dilation (EDD), with some showing improvement [31], but many reporting no change [32,33]. The majority of longitudinal studies in healthy subjects suggest that exercise training does not increase skeletal muscle resistance artery endothelium-dependent dilation above normal [1,34].

Skeletal muscle capillaries

As early as 1977 quadriceps capillary density was compared between endurance-trained athletes and sedentary age-matched subjects. Brodal et al. [35] described a significant increase in capillaries around each fibre and the numbers of capillaries per mm^2 [35]. The increase in capillary density in skeletal muscle was confirmed in many subsequent studies [1,36,37], and these structural changes are strongly linked to improvements in local and whole-body peak oxygen uptake [38]. Increased capillary density is believed to prolong the capillary transit time of red blood cells, providing increased time for exchange across muscle capillaries [1].

In strength training, capillary density does not seem to increase despite significant muscle hypertrophy—a decrease in capillary density has even been described [39].

Vascular adaptation of the coronary system

Epicardial coronary conduit arteries

Alpha-adrenergic responsiveness is blunted in large conduit coronary arteries of exercise-trained animals, which, together with the lower amount of circulating catecholamines, will translate into lower α-adrenergic influences in trained subjects that may serve to maximize upstream vessel diameter during bouts of exercise [13,14,40].

Exercise training produces a transient increase in endothelium-dependent vasodilation in coronary conduit arteries until outward arterial remodelling reduces shear stress levels to baseline (➲ Fig. 1.2.4.1). This temporarily enhanced responsiveness of the endothelium appears to be principally the result of increased NO bioavailability. As early as 60min after initiation of shear stress, bovine aortic endothelial cells produce 13 times more NO compared with baseline conditions [41] This increase is mediated by both short-term enhancement of endothelial NO synthase (eNOS) activity and activation of eNOS expression. A considerable increase in eNOS expression has been demonstrated in endothelial cell culture experiments after exposure to laminar shear stress, while hydrostatic pressure alone reduces eNOS expression [42]. This is consistent with studies of exercise training in dogs, which documented increased eNOS

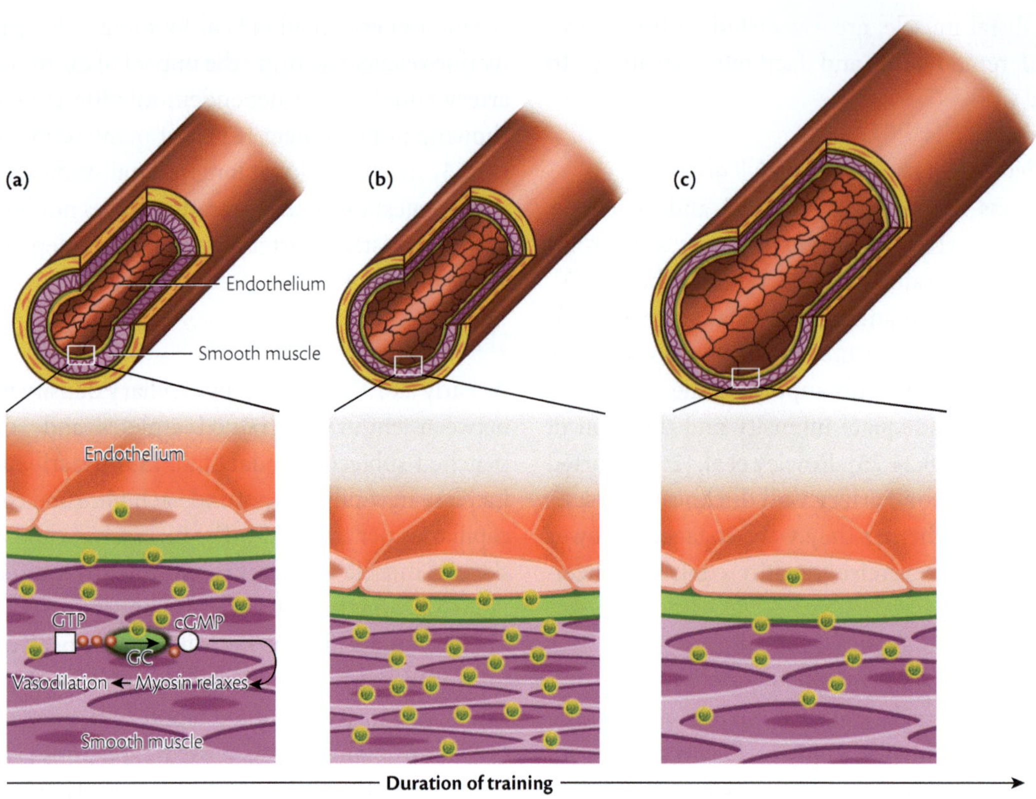

Fig. 1.2.4.1 Hypothesized response of arteries to increased flow and shear stress following varying durations of exercise training. In the vessels of sedentary persons (left panel), basal release of NO causes smooth muscle cell vasodilatation which acts to homeostatically regulate wall shear. In response to medium-term exercise training (middle panel), increase in shear stress during exercise increases endothelial NO production and consecutive vasodilatation. Upregulation of eNOS expression and activity occurs to buffer increased shear stress. Following long-term exercise training (right panel), structural adaptation occurs, possibly in part due to NO-mediated remodelling, resulting in a chronic increase in vessel calibre which 'structurally normalizes' shear stress. NO function returns towards baseline levels.

Adapted with permission from Andrew Maiorana et al. Exercise and the nitric oxide vasodilator system. *Sports Medicine*, Volume 33, Issue 14, pp.1013–35, Copyright © 2003. With permission of Springer.

expression and NO production in coronary conduit vessels [43]. Increases in NO production are caused by: (a) increased eNOS mRNA transcription and eNOS mRNA stabilization mediated by the tyrosine kinase c-Src [44], and (b) eNOS phosphorylation mediated by the serine/threonine protein kinase Akt/PKB [45]. Training-induced eNOS phosphorylation in humans was confirmed by Hambrecht et al. [46] in samples of the left internal thoracic artery obtained from patients scheduled for elective coronary bypass surgery.

However, improvements of endothelium-dependent vasodilatation are not always seen in healthy young individuals. Baseline endothelial function needs to be impaired by one or several cardiovascular risk factors (e.g. physical inactivity, hyperlipidaemia, hypertension, diabetes mellitus, smoking, or old age) to actually measure improved vasodilation after exercise.

Coronary resistance arteries

Exercise training has been shown to increase coronary resistance vessel densities and diameters (➔ Fig. 1.2.4.2) [47,48]. In coronary resistance vessels a sustained augmentation of endothelium-dependent vasodilation is observed, which is mainly due to an increase in NO bioavailability [49].

Available data indicate that in coronary resistance vessels of exercised animals α-adrenergic tone is maintained or slightly increased and β-adrenergic tone is maintained during submaximal exercise. Maintenance of adrenergic tone in the presence of lower circulating catecholamine levels is consistent with the observed increased receptor responsiveness to adrenergic stimulation [50]. There is no evidence for altered parasympathetic control of coronary tone after exercise [50].

Available data also indicate that exercise alters intrinsic vasomotor properties of coronary resistance vessels. Arterioles exhibit increased myogenic tone, which appears specific for stretch-induced contractions, as vasoconstrictor responses to various agonists are not altered [50]. The molecular basis for the increased myogenic tone is probably the result of a calcium-dependent protein kinase C (PKC) signalling mediated alteration in voltage-gated calcium channel activity in response to stretch. It is currently

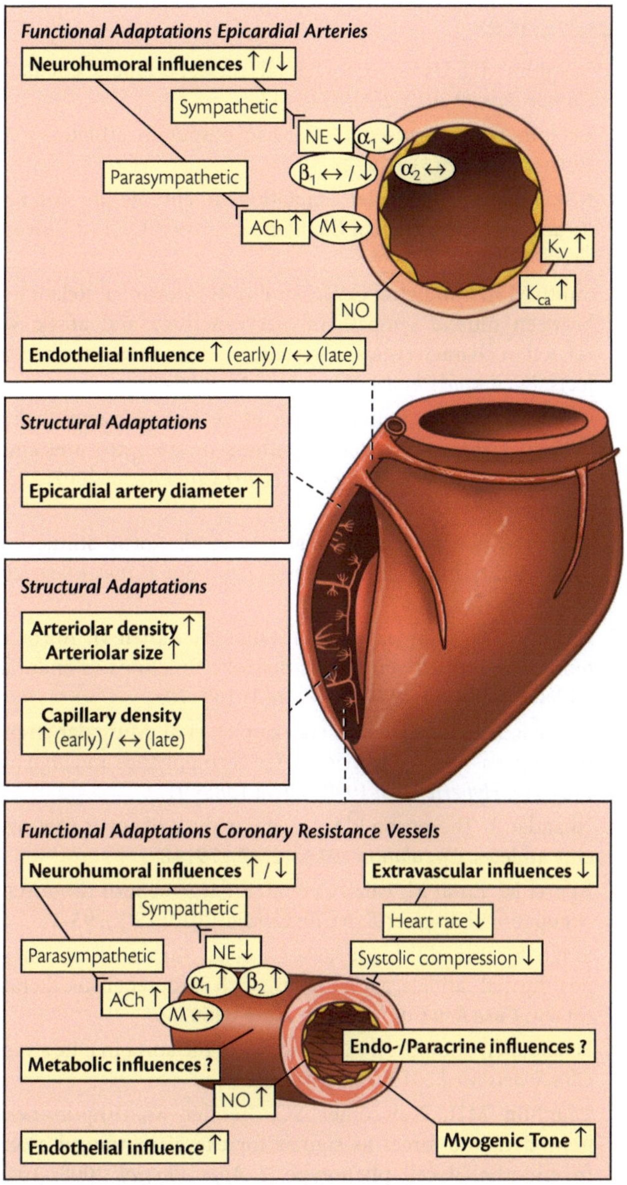

Fig. 1.2.4.2 Summary of the structural and functional coronary adaptations to chronic exercise in normal subjects. Ach, acetylcholine; M, muscarinic receptor; NE, noradrenaline (norepinephrine); α_1, α_1-adrenergic receptor; β_1, β_1-adrenergic receptor; β_2, β_2-adrenergic receptor; K_V voltage-dependent K channel;. K_{Ca}, Ca^{2+}-dependent K channel.

Modified from Laughlin, MH, Bowles DK, Duncker DJ. *AJP Heart* 2012, 47 with permission of the American Physiological Society, and Laughlin MH, Bowles DK, Duncker DJ. The coronary circulation in exercise training. *Am J Physiol Heart Circ Physiol* 2012; 302(1): H10–23.

unclear whether metabolic control mechanisms, including adenosine and K^+-channel activity, are altered in coronary resistance vessels following exercise.

Myocardial capillaries

While there is evidence that exercise increases myocardial capillary density in young rats, larger exercised animals exhibit capillary density matched to cardiac hypertrophy, i.e. capillary density is maintained in the normal range (reviewed in [50] and [51]). This matching of capillary angiogenesis to the degree of myocardial hypertrophy contrasts with pathological forms of myocardial hypertrophy (due to hypertension or aortic stenosis) where capillary rarefaction often occurs [52].

Capillary exchange capacity, measured as the product of permeability and surface area, is determined by capillary permeability and total capillary surface area available for exchange. Although capillary numerical density is not increased by exercise, an increased capillary permeability surface area product could still result from optimization of coronary blood flow (CBF) distribution so that capillaries are fully perfused and their maximal exchange capacity is reached, thus increasing effective capillary surface area. Laughlin and colleagues reported that exercise caused an increase in coronary capillary permeability surface area product in dogs [47,52,53] and miniature swine [54]. When the capillary permeability surface area product and morphometric measurements of capillarization were examined in the same hearts, exercise was found to increase coronary capillary permeability surface area product with no change in capillary density [52,54]. In the maximally vasodilated bed, capillary permeability surface area product is a function of the flow rate, possibly because increased CBF is associated with recruitment of more capillary exchange area [47,52]. As summarized in ➲ Fig 1.2.4.2, exercise training increases capillary diameters and arteriolar densities, two adaptations that act to decrease capillary transit time and could improve matching of capillary blood flow and exchange capacity [55]. Taken together, these studies demonstrate that exercise alters the distribution of coronary vascular resistance, increasing the effective capillary surface area and the capillary permeability surface area product without a change in coronary capillary numerical density. These adaptations probably contribute to the exercise-induced increase in myocardial oxygen extraction capacity [50,56].

Integrative coronary vascular function

Experiments designed to determine the effects of exercise on CBF capacity have reported either no change [40,48,56–59] or an increase in CBF capacity after exercise [54,60–64]. The differing results may be due to several factors, including differences in species, sex, and age of the experimental animals, and the type, intensity and duration of the exercise protocol. Based on our review of the literature we consider the most important factor to be the experimental conditions for assessing CBF capacity, as discussed in detail previously [50,51]. In studies where maximal vasodilation was demonstrated under tightly controlled haemodynamic conditions and the efficacy of the training programme was documented, CBF capacity was consistently reported to be slightly increased following exercise in swine [54,64], dogs [47,52], and rats [61]. Taken together these studies suggest that exercise induces a small increase in maximal CBF per gram of myocardium when the exercise programme is of sufficient intensity to produce a training effect and when CBF capacity is measured under rigorously controlled haemodynamic conditions [50,51].

Summary and conclusions

In summary, vascular adaptations of the coronary and peripheral arteries play a key role in increasing aerobic exercise capacity. The key stimulus for initiating and perpetuating vascular adaptations is a recurrent increase in vascular shear stress. Since shear stress is greatest in muscle regions with the highest workload, improvement in vascular vasodilator response is largest in trained muscle regions.

With continuing endurance training structural adaptations follow the functional adaptations. Large conduit vessels grow in diameter and show greater vascular compliance.

However, strength training does not significantly increase shear stress—rather, the repetitive increases in systolic blood pressure with high peripheral vascular resistance cause increased radial strain. This may lead to aortic dilatation and in rare cases aortic dissection.

In the skeletal muscle, endurance training increases capillary density and improves oxygen exchange, thus adding further functional reserves to aerobic exercise capacity.

Further reading

Ashor AW, Lara J, Siervo M, et al. Effects of exercise modalities on arterial stiffness and wave reflection: a systematic review and meta-analysis of randomized controlled trials. *PloS One* 2014; 9(10): e110034.

Duncker DJ, Bache RJ. Regulation of coronary blood flow during exercise. *Physiol Rev* 2008; 88(3): 1009–86.

Green DJ, Maiorana A, O'Driscoll G, Taylor R. Effect of exercise training on endothelium-derived nitric oxide function in humans. *J Physiol* 2004; 561(Pt 1): 1–25.

Iskandar A, Thompson PD. A meta-analysis of aortic root size in elite athletes. *Circulation* 2013; 127(7): 791–8.

Laughlin MH, Bowles DK, Duncker DJ. The coronary circulation in exercise training. *Am J Physiol Heart Circ Physiol* 2012; 302(1): H10–23.

Montero D, Vinet A, Roberts CK. Effect of combined aerobic and resistance training versus aerobic training on arterial stiffness. *Int J Cardiol* 2015; 178: 69–76.

Spence AL, Carter HH, Naylor LH, Green DJ. A prospective randomized longitudinal study involving 6 months of endurance or resistance exercise: conduit artery adaptation in humans. *J Physiol* 2013; 591(5): 1265–75.

References

1. Laughlin MH, Davis MJ, Secher NH, et al. Peripheral circulation. *Compr Physiol* 2012; 2(1): 321–447.
2. Ekblom B, Hermansen L. Cardiac output in athletes. *J Appl Physiol* 1968; 25(5): 619–25.
3. Rowell L. Cardiovascular adaptations to chronic physical activity and inactivity. *Human Circulation*. Oxford: Oxford University Press; 1986, pp. 257–86.
4. Smith MM, Buffington CAT, Hamlin RL, Devor ST. Relationship between muscle sympathetic nerve activity and aortic wave reflection characteristics in aerobic- and resistance-trained subjects. *Eur J Appl Physiol* 2015; 115(12): 2609–19.
5. Otsuki T, Maeda S, Iemitsu M, et al. Vascular endothelium-derived factors and arterial stiffness in strength- and endurance-trained men. *Am J Physiol Heart Circ Physiol* 2007; 292(2): H786–91.
6. D'Andrea A, Cocchia R, Riegler L, et al. Aortic stiffness and distensibility in top-level athletes. *J Am Soc Echocardiogr* 2012; 25(5): 561–7.
7. Kasikcioglu E, Kayserilioglu A, Oflaz H, Akhan H. Aortic distensibility and left ventricular diastolic functions in endurance athletes. *Int J Sports Med.* 2005;26(3):165–70.
8. Bertovic DA, Waddell TK, Gatzka CD, et al. Muscular strength training is associated with low arterial compliance and high pulse pressure. *Hypertension* 1999; 33(6): 1385–91.
9. Iskandar A, Thompson PD. A meta-analysis of aortic root size in elite athletes. *Circulation* 2013; 127(7): 791–8.
10. Aparci M, Erdal M, Isilak Z, et al. Enlargement of the aorta: an occupational disease? *Exp Clin Cardiol* 2013; 18(2): 93–7.
11. Singh B, Treece JM, Murtaza G, et al. Aortic dissection in a healthy male athlete: a unique case with comprehensive literature review. *Case Rep Cardiol* 2016; 2016: 6460386.
12. Iskandar A, Thompson PD. Diseases of the aorta in elite athletes. *Clin Sports Med* 2015; 34(3): 461–72.
13. Laughlin MH, Newcomer SC, Bender SB. Importance of hemodynamic forces as signals for exercise-induced changes in endothelial cell phenotype. *J Appl Physiol* 2008; 104(3): 588–600.
14. Oltman CL, Parker JL, Adams HR, Laughlin MH. Effects of exercise training on vasomotor reactivity of porcine coronary arteries. *Am J Physiol* 1992; 263(2 Pt 2): H372–82.
15. Rogers PJ, Miller TD, Bauer BA, et al. Exercise training and responsiveness of isolated coronary arteries. *J Appl Physiol* 1991; 71(6): 2346–51.
16. Zeppilli P, Vannicelli R, Santini C, et al. Echocardiographic size of conductance vessels in athletes and sedentary people. *Int J Sports Med* 1995; 16(1): 38–44.
17. Dinenno FA, Tanaka H, Monahan KD, et al. Regular endurance exercise induces expansive arterial remodelling in the trained limbs of healthy men. *J Physiol* 2001; 534(Pt 1): 287–95.
18. Spence AL, Carter HH, Naylor LH, Green DJ. A prospective randomized longitudinal study involving 6 months of endurance or resistance exercise: conduit artery adaptation in humans. *J Physiol* 2013; 591(5): 1265–75.
19. Tinken TM, Thijssen DHJ, Hopkins N, et al. Shear stress mediates endothelial adaptations to exercise training in humans. *Hypertension* 2010; 55(2): 312–18.

20. Birk GK, Dawson EA, Batterham AM, et al. Effects of exercise intensity on flow mediated dilation in healthy humans. *Int J Sports Med.* 2013; 34(5): 409–14.
21. Miyachi M, Tanaka H, Yamamoto K, et al. Effects of one-legged endurance training on femoral arterial and venous size in healthy humans. *J Appl Physiol (1985)* 2001;90(6):2439–44.
22. Zoeller RF, Angelopoulos TJ, Thompson BC, et al. Vascular remodeling in response to 12 wk of upper arm unilateral resistance training. *Med Sci Sports Exerc* 2009; 41(11): 2003–8.
23. Thijssen DHJ, Cable NT, Green DJ. Impact of exercise training on arterial wall thickness in humans. *Clin Sci (Lond)*, 2012; 122(7): 311–22.
24. Rowley NJ, Dawson EA, Birk GK, et al. Exercise and arterial adaptation in humans: uncoupling localized and systemic effects. *J Appl Physiol (1985)* 2011; 110(5): 1190–5.
25. Ranadive SM, Yan H, Lane AD, et al. Aerobic exercise training and arterial changes in African Americans versus Caucasians. *Med Sci Sports Exerc* 2016; 48(1): 90–7.
26. Rowley NJ, Dawson EA, Hopman MTE, et al. Conduit diameter and wall remodeling in elite athletes and spinal cord injury. *Med Sci Sports Exerc* 2012; 44(5): 844–9.
27. Vlachopoulos C, Aznaouridis K, Stefanadis C. Aortic stiffness for cardiovascular risk prediction: just measure it, just do it! *J Am Coll Cardiol* 2014; 63(7): 647–9.
28. Montero D, Vinet A, Roberts CK. Effect of combined aerobic and resistance training versus aerobic training on arterial stiffness. *Int J Cardiol* 2015;178:69–76.
29. Ashor AW, Lara J, Siervo M, et al. Effects of exercise modalities on arterial stiffness and wave reflection: a systematic review and meta-analysis of randomized controlled trials. *PloS One* 2014; 9(10): e110034.
30. Snell PG, Martin WH, Buckey JC, Blomqvist CG. Maximal vascular leg conductance in trained and untrained men. *J Appl Physiol (1985)* 1987; 62(2): 606–10.
31. Montero D, Walther G, Diaz-Cañestro C, et al. Microvascular dilator function in athletes: a systematic review and meta-analysis. *Med Sci Sports Exerc* 2015; 47(7): 1485–94.
32. Maiorana A, O'Driscoll G, Cheetham C, et al. The effect of combined aerobic and resistance exercise training on vascular function in type 2 diabetes. *J Am Coll Cardiol* 2001; 38(3): 860–6.
33. Oudegeest-Sander MH, Olde Rikkert MGM, Smits P, et al. The effect of an advanced glycation end-product crosslink breaker and exercise training on vascular function in older individuals: a randomized factorial design trial. *Exp Gerontol* 2013; 48(12): 1509–17.
34. Green DJ, Maiorana A, O'Driscoll G, Taylor R. Effect of exercise training on endothelium-derived nitric oxide function in humans. *J Physiol* 2004; 561(Pt 1): 1–25.
35. Brodal P, Ingjer F, Hermansen L. Capillary supply of skeletal muscle fibers in untrained and endurance-trained men. *Am J Physiol* 1977; 232(6): H705–12.
36. Andersen P, Henriksson J. Capillary supply of the quadriceps femoris muscle of man: adaptive response to exercise. *J Physiol* 1977; 270(3): 677–90.
37. Hoier B, Hellsten Y. Exercise-induced capillary growth in human skeletal muscle and the dynamics of VEGF. *Microcirculation* 2014; 21(4): 301–14.
38. Duscha BD, Robbins JL, Jones WS, et al. Angiogenesis in skeletal muscle precede improvements in peak oxygen uptake in peripheral artery disease patients. *Arterioscler Thromb Vasc Biol* 2011; 31(11): 2742–8.
39. Tesch PA. Skeletal muscle adaptations consequent to long-term heavy resistance exercise. *Med Sci Sports Exerc* 1988; 20(5 Suppl): S132–4.
40. Yipintsoi T, Rosenkrantz J, Codini MA, Scheuer J. Myocardial blood flow responses to acute hypoxia and volume loading in physically trained rats. *Cardiovasc Res* 1980; 14(1): 50–7.
41. Marsden PA, Heng HHQ, Scherer SWS, et al. Structure and chromosomal localization of the human constitutive endothelial nitric oxide synthase gene. *J Biol Chem* 1993; 268: 17478–88.
42. Malek AM, Izumo S, Alper SL. Modulation by pathophysiological stimuli of the shear stress-induced up-regulation of endothelial nitric oxide synthase expression in endothelial cells. *Neurosurgery* 1999; 45(2): 334–45.
43. Wang J, Wolin MS, Hintze T. Chronic exercise exhances endothelium-mediated dilation of epicardial coronary arteries in conscious dogs. *Circ Res* 1993; 73: 829–38.
44. Davis ME, Cai H, Drummond GR, Harrison DG. Shear stress regulates endothelial nitric oxide synthase expression through c-Src by divergent signaling pathways. *Circ Res* 2001; 89(11): 1073–80.
45. Dimmeler S, Fleming I, Fisslthaler B, et al. Activation of nitric oxide synthase in endothelial cells by Akt-dependent phosphorylation. *Nature* 1999; 399: 601–5.
46. Hambrecht R, Adams V, Erbs S, et al. Regular physical activity improves endothelial function in patients with coronary artery disease by increasing phosphorylation of endothelial nitric oxide synthase. *Circulation* 2003; 107(25): 3152–8.
47. Laughlin MH. Effects of exercise training on coronary transport capacity. *J Appl Physiol* 1985; 58(2): 468–76.
48. Liang IY, Hamra M, Stone HL. Maximum coronary blood flow and minimum coronary resistance in exercise-trained dogs. *J Appl Physiol* 1984; 56(3): 641–7.
49. Muller JM, Myers PR, Laughlin MH. Vasodilator responses of coronary resistance arteries of exercise-trained pigs. *Circulation* 1994; 89: 2308–14.
50. Laughlin MH, Bowles DK, Duncker DJ. The coronary circulation in exercise training. *Am J Physiol Heart Circ Physiol* 2012; 302(1): H10–23.
51. Duncker DJ, Bache RJ. Regulation of coronary blood flow during exercise. *Physiol Rev* 2008; 88(3): 1009–86.
52. Laughlin MH, Tomanek RJ. Myocardial capillarity and maximal capillary diffusion capacity in exercise-trained dogs. *J Appl Physiol (1985)* 1987; 63(4): 1481–6.
53. Laughlin MH, Diana JN. Myocardial transcapillary exchange in the hypertrophied heart of the dog. *Am J Physiol* 1975; 229(3): 838–46.
54. Laughlin MH, Overholser KA, Bhatte MJ. Exercise training increases coronary transport reserve in miniature swine. *J Appl Physiol* 1989; 67: 1140–9.
55. White FC, McKirnan MD, Breisch EA, et al. Adaptation of the left ventricle to exercise-induced hypertrophy. *J Appl Physiol (1985)* 1987; 62(3): 1097–110.
56. Stone HL. Coronary flow, myocardial oxygen consumption, and exercise training in dogs. *J Appl Physiol* 1980; 49(5): 759–68.
57. Barnard RJ, Duncan HW, Baldwin KM, et al. Effects of intensive exercise training on myocardial performance and coronary blood flow. *J Appl Physiol* 1980; 49(3): 444–9.

58. Bove AA, Dewey JD. Proximal coronary vasomotor reactivity after exercise training in dogs. *Circulation* 1985; 71: 620–5.
59. Breisch EA, White FC, Nimmo LE, et al. Exercise-induced cardiac hypertrophy: a correlation of blood flow and microvasculature. *J Appl Physiol(1985)* 1986; 60(4): 1259–67.
60. Baur TS, Brodowicz GR, Lamb DR. Indomethacin suppresses the coronary flow response to hypoxia in exercise trained and sedentary rats. *Cardiovasc Res* 1990; 24(9): 733–6.
61. Buttrick PM, Levite HA, Schaible TF, et al. Early increases in coronary vascular reserve in exercised rats are independent of cardiac hypertrophy. *J Appl Physiol (1985)* 1985; 59(6): 1861–5.
62. DiCarlo SE, Blair RW, Bishop VS, Stone HL. Daily exercise enhances coronary resistance vessel sensitivity to pharmacological activation. *J Appl Physiol (1985)* 1989; 66(1): 421–8.
63. Liang IY, Stone HL. Effect of exercise conditioning on coronary resistance. *J Appl Physiol* 1982; 53(3): 631–6.
64. White FC, Bloor CM, McKirnan MD, Carrol SM. Exercise training in swine promotes growth of arteriolar bed and capillary angiogenesis in heart. *J Appl Physiol* 1998; 85(3): 1160–8.

SECTION 2

Clinical evaluation of the athlete's heart

2.1 History and physical examination *51*

2.1.1 History and physical examination *51*
Maurizio Schiavon, Alessandro Zorzi, and Domenico Corrado

2.2 The electrocardiogram in the athlete *57*

2.2.1 The electrocardiogram in the athlete *57*
Alessandro Zorzi and Domenico Corrado

2.2.2 Common ECG patterns in the athlete's heart *68*
Ricardo Stein and Victor Froelicher

2.2.3 Overlap ECG patterns in the athlete's heart and cardiomyopathies *77*
Harshil Dhutia and Michael Papadakis

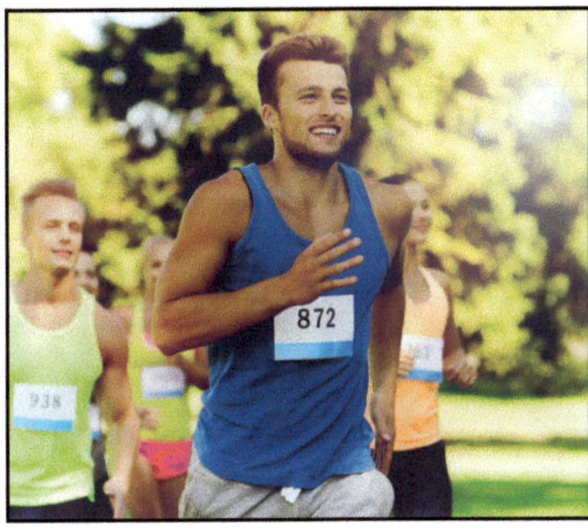

2.1

History and physical examination

Contents

2.1.1 **History and physical examination** Maurizio Schiavon, Alessandro Zorzi, and Domenico Corrado *51*

2.1.1 History and physical examination

Maurizio Schiavon, Alessandro Zorzi, and Domenico Corrado

Introduction

Consensus statements by the American Heart Association (AHA) and the European Society of Cardiology (ESC) agree on the need for cardiovascular evaluation of young competitive athletes before they engage in competitive sports and consider pre-participation screening of athletes to be justifiable and compelling on ethical, legal, and medical grounds [1,2]. Pre-participation screening is also advised by the International Olympic Committee (IOC) [3].

It is well recognized that detailed history and physical examination are the mainstays of cardiovascular screening of young athletes [1–3]. Although personal and family history alone are not adequate for identifying subjects at risk [4], they are an invaluable component in guiding and interpreting subsequent clinical investigations including physical examination and 12-lead electrocardiogram (ECG).

The history and physical examination elements should be assessed in a quiet place (consulting room or similar), preferably using standardized forms [5]. At the discretion of the examiner, a positive response in one or more items concerning personal health may be judged sufficient to trigger second-line cardiovascular tests. To achieve the highest accuracy, screening physicians should be aware of those conditions that confer a predisposition to sudden cardiac death; therefore, education of both physicians and the public (i.e. athlete him/herself and family) is critical for improving the effectiveness of screening by means of history-taking and physical examination. Screening must be carried out at regular time intervals; therefore athletes and their families should be instructed to report new symptoms or new clinical events occurring in family members between screening evaluations.

History

History-taking should focus on possible risk factors that may predict exercise-induced cardiovascular events and is usually carried out using a questionnaire. The short AHA questionnaire is composed of 12 items (➲ Table 2.1.1.1) [1], and the longer questionnaire recommended by the IOC and ESC is composed of 36 items [2,3].

Since 1989 the Italian Cardiological Committee on Sports Eligibility (COCIS) has been editing the *Cardiovascular Guidelines for Competitive Sports Eligibility*, the latest in 2017. These guidelines recommend using a check list of items regarding family and personal history plus additional information about sport history and lifestyle (professional activity, tobacco smoking, alcohol consumption, and use of psychoactive substances) (➲ Table 2.1.1.2) [6,7].

The first important history element that should be collected at the time of pre-participation screening is the type of sport and level of training of the individual athlete. Sport physicians and consultant cardiologists should be able to recognize what organs and functions are involved across the broad spectrum of sports, the physiological and technical requirements of each sport discipline, and the actual or expected

Table 2.1.1.1. Original American Heart Association 12-element screening checklist (2007)

Family history
1. Sudden and unexpected death before the age of 50 years due to heart disease in one or more relatives
2. Disability from heart disease in a close relative less than 50 years old
3. Specific knowledge of certain cardiac conditions in family members: hypertrophic or dilated cardiomyopathy, long QT syndrome or other ion channelopathies, Marfan syndrome, or clinically important arrhythmias
Personal history (parental verification recommended for high school and middle school athletes)
4. Exertional chest pain/discomfort
5. Exertional syncope or near syncope
6. Excessive exertional and unexplained fatigue/fatigue associated with exercise
7. Prior recognition of a heart murmur
8. Elevated systemic blood pressure
Physical examination
9. Heart murmur: examine supine and standing or with the Valsalva manoeuvre, specifically to identify murmurs of dynamic left ventricular outflow tract obstruction
10. Femoral pulses to exclude aortic stenosis
11. Physical stigmata of Marfan syndrome
12. Brachial artery blood pressure (sitting, preferably taken in both arms)

Two new items (prior restriction from participation in sports and prior testing for the heart ordered by a physician) were included in the latest (2015) guidelines update. Reproduced with permission from B.J. Maron, P.D. Thompson, M.J. Ackerman, et al. Recommendations and considerations related to preparticipation screening for cardiovascular abnormalities in competitive athletes: 2007 update. *Circulation*, Volume 115, Issue 12, pp.1013–35. Copyright © 2007 with permission of Wolters Kluwer Health Inc.

Table 2.1.1.2. History-taking checklist (derived from the 2009 Italian guidelines) for pre-participation screening

Questions		Answers	
		No	**Yes**
A. Family history			
Has any family member or relative died of heart problems or had an unexpected or unexplained sudden death before age 50 (including premature myocardial infarction, drowning, unexplained car accident, or sudden infant death syndrome)?		No	Yes
Has anyone in your family:	Had unexplained fainting, seizure, unexplained car accidents, or near-drowning?	No	Yes
	Had a disabling heart problem, or a pacemaker or defibrillator implanted?	No	Yes
	Had cardiac surgery or heart transplantation, or been treated for irregular heart beat (arrhythmia)?	No	Yes
Does anyone in your family	Have hypertrophic cardiomyopathy, dilated cardiomyopathy, Marfan syndrome, arrhythmogenic right ventricular cardiomyopathy, long QT syndrome, short QT syndrome, Brugada syndrome, catecholaminergic polymorphic ventricular tachycardia, or ischaemic heart disease at a young age (<55 in men and <65 in women)?	No	Yes
	Have diabetes, cancer, hypertension (high blood pressure), asthma, allergies, or respiratory, neurological, or haematological disease?	No	Yes

B. Personal history			
Have you ever passed out (fainting/syncope) or nearly passed out (near-fainting/near-syncope)?	During exercise	No	Yes
	After exercise	No	Yes
	Unrelated to exercise	No	Yes
Have you ever had discomfort, pain, tightness, or pressure in your chest?	During exercise	No	Yes
	After exercise	No	Yes
	Unrelated to exercise	No	Yes
Have you ever experienced dizziness or vertigo?	During exercise	No	Yes
	After exercise	No	Yes
	Unrelated to exercise	No	Yes
Do you feel that you are more breathless or more easily tired than your team mates?	During exercise	No	Yes
	After exercise	No	Yes
	Unrelated to exercise	No	Yes

Table 2.1.1.2. History-taking checklist (derived from the 2009 Italian guidelines) for pre-participation screening *(Conitnued)*

Have you ever had respiratory problems (~~difficulty~~ breathing, chest tightness, wheezing, or cough)?	During exercise	No	Yes
	After exercise	No	Yes
	Unrelated to exercise	No	Yes
Have you ever had racing of your heart (palpitations) or skipped heartbeats (irregular heartbeat/premature beat)?	During exercise	No	Yes
	After exercise	No	Yes
	Unrelated to exercise	No	Yes
Has a doctor ever told you that you have any heart problems, high blood pressure, high cholesterol, a heart murmur, a cardiac arrhythmia, or a heart infection (i.e. myocarditis or mononucleosis) within the last month, unexplained seizure, or rheumatic fever?		No	Yes
Has a doctor ever told you that you have asthma, seizure disorders, epilepsy, health conditions that prevent you from exercising, diabetes, obesity, or orthopaedic, neurological, or respiratory problems?		No	Yes
Has a doctor ever ordered a test for your heart (i.e. ECG, Holter monitoring, echocardiography)?		No	Yes
Do you have any allergies (i.e. to pollens, dust mites, medicines, food, insect stings)?		No	Yes
Have you ever had hives, eczema, or skin rashes during or after exercise?		No	Yes
Are you currently taking any prescription or non-prescription (over-the-counter) medications or pills, or using an inhaler?		No	Yes
Have you routinely taken any medication in the past 2 years?		No	Yes

C. Sport history

Type of sport played	Playing position/sport discipline	Starting from age	To age	Training session duration (min)	No. of training sessions per week	No. of competitions per week

D. Additional information

Professional activity

Risk exposure

For how long?

Tobacco smoking

Cigarettes/day

For how long?

Starting from age

Until

Alcohol consumption

Units/day

For how long?

Starting from age

Until

Use of psychoactive substance

Frequency

For how long?

Starting from age

Until

Source data from Corrado D, Biffi A, Schiavon M. Pre-participation cardiovascular screening. *Medicina dello Sport* 2010; 63:15–24.

cardiovascular risk. The classification of sports according to cardiovascular demands (aerobic, anaerobic, or mixed) is based on the evaluation of a few easily detectable variables [8]. It is important to consider that the cardiac involvement can be either constant over time, as is the case in aerobic endurance sports (marathon, cross-country skiing, cycling, swimming, etc.) or alternating, as is the case in team games (aerobic–anaerobic activities). Intense and brief efforts, starting or finishing abruptly, may also be strong arrhythmogenic triggers. Similarly, an abrupt interruption after intense effort may result in haemodynamic and rhythm disturbance. Moreover, sports that entail a moderate increase in hearth rate, but a marked blood pressure elevation, may be dangerous in individuals with cardiovascular disorders. In addition, it is recommended that cardiovascular risk is assessed in special sports activities, so-called intrinsic risk, i.e. the risk related to the specific environment in which the sport takes place (such as scuba diving, climbing, motor sports, etc.).

A family history of unexplained or unexpected sudden cardiac death before the age of 50, sudden infant death syndrome, drowning or near-drowning, or unexplained car accident should raise the suspicion of a genetic arrhythmogenic disorder. It should be noted that close relatives include parents, grandparents, direct aunts/uncles, and siblings.

The occurrence of prodromal symptoms or signs (i.e. exertional chest pain, effort or recurrent syncope or pre-syncope, palpitations or irregular heartbeats, exercise dyspnoea or fatigue disproportionate to the level of exertion, unexplained seizure) should prompt further diagnostic investigations.

Physical examination

Physical examination should be focused on the following items.

- Heart murmur: auscultation should be performed in both supine and standing positions, and with Valsalva manoeuvre. Typical characteristics of innocent murmurs, which are very common in healthy young athletes and do not usually warrant further evaluation, include [9]:
  - (1) low intensity, usually ≤2/6;
  - (2) typically occur during systole, rarely during systole and diastole, and never during diastole alone;
  - (3) often are position dependent as they are produced by normal blood flow, with the intensity usually increasing as the flow increases (e.g. standing after squatting and Valsalva manoeuvre decrease the venous return and the intensity of innocent murmurs; conversely, murmurs that increase with Valsalva manoeuvre or standing suggest dynamic left ventricular outflow tract obstruction, such as in hypertrophic cardiomyopathy);
  - (4) associated with physiological (respiration-dependent) split of the second tone; fixed split of the second tone suggests a shunt such as inter-atrial or inter-ventricular septal defects;
- Pulses: reduced femoral pulses compared with the arms are typical of aortic coarctation, especially if there is an associated infrascapular murmur;
- Physical stigmata of Marfan syndrome, including pectus excavatum or carinatum, thoracolumbar scoliosis, reduced upper-to-lower segment ratio (i.e. the distance from the head to the pubic symphysis divided by the distance of the pubic symphysis to the sole) less than 0.85, positive wrist sign (i.e. the thumb and little finger overlap when encircling the contralateral wrist), positive thumb sign (i.e. the thumb extends beyond the ulnar border of the hand when the digit is held flexed in the palm), flat foot [10].

Accuracy of history and physical examination for screening athletes

Although there is widespread agreement that cardiovascular screening in athletes should be performed, the best screening method is a matter of debate. The ESC, IOC, Fédération Internationale de Football Association (FIFA), and various professional sporting organizations in the USA recommend performing an ECG during an athlete's pre-participation screening [2,3,11]. Conversely, the AHA recommends pre-participation cardiovascular evaluation by means of history (personal and family history) and physical examination alone because of concerns regarding the presumed high false-positive rate of ECG [1,12]. However, supporters of pre-participation ECG screening believe that history and physical examination alone have a low sensitivity for detecting cardiovascular diseases at risk of sudden cardiac death [13].

A recent meta-analysis by Harmon et al. [4] including 15 studies from nine different countries evaluated the sensitivity and specificity of the two pre-participation screening modalities. Overall, more than 47,000 athletes (age ranging from 5 to 39 years) were included. The combined analysis demonstrated that the false-positive rates of history (8%)

and physical examination (10%) were higher than that of ECG (6%). The authors suggest two possible explanations for the lack of specificity of history: (1) the screening history questions that are currently recommended are based on expert opinion and there is little research into the ability of athletes to answer the questions properly; (2) typical history questions enquire about common symptoms that are not specific to cardiac diseases. For this reason, in the case of a positive response to questions a physician review is needed before prescribing further examinations. As far as physical examination is concerned, the most common reason for secondary testing is a murmur, but the accuracy of auscultation to distinguish physiological from pathological murmurs is low [9].

Not only are history and physical examination less specific than 12-lead ECG but, more importantly, they are far less sensitive. The meta-analysis by Harmon et al. [4] suggested that only one out of five athletes with cardiovascular conditions at risk of sudden cardiac death can be identified by history and physical examination alone. In the studies included in the meta-analysis which systematically performed echocardiography [14–16], the sensitivity of ECG (80%) was superior to that of history (50%) and physical examination (33%). This is because the majority of young athletes with potentially lethal cardiovascular conditions are asymptomatic [17,18] and physical examination is usually negative in purely electrical diseases, such as Wolff–Parkinson–White and long QT syndromes, and in many patients with cardiomyopathies. For example, although patients with hypertrophic cardiomyopathy may show a positive family history or a cardiac murmur on physical examination, the spectrum of presentation is broad. Among 22 athletes with hypertrophic cardiomyopathy who were identified by ECG screening (and subsequent testing) at the Centre for Sports Medicine in Padua, only five (23%) would have been suspected on the basis of positive family history, symptoms or abnormal physical findings [2].

Conclusions

In conclusion, history and physical examination are the major components of the pre-participation screening protocol, bearing in mind that (1) the specificity of questionnaires is limited and although the questions may serve as a red flag, the experience of the screening physician is crucial to identify those athletes who needs further investigation, and (2) cardiac murmurs in athletes are usually benign and should not systematically prompt echocardiography. More importantly, the sensitivity of history and physical examination alone are low. Finally, it must be recognized that some cardiovascular diseases at risk of sudden cardiac death in young competitive athletes, such as premature coronary atherosclerosis or anomalous coronary artery, are difficult to detect, regardless of the screening modality [19].

Further reading

Biffi A, Delise P, Zeppilli P, et al. Italian cardiological guidelines for sports eligibility in athletes with heart disease: part 2. *J Cardiovasc Med (Hagerstown)* 2013; 14(7): 500–15.

Biffi A, Delise P, Zeppilli P, et al. Italian cardiological guidelines for sports eligibility in athletes with heart disease: part 1. *J Cardiovasc Med (Hagerstown)* 2013; 14(7): 477–99.

Corrado D, Pelliccia A, Bjornstad HH, et al. Cardiovascular pre-participation screening of young competitive athletes for prevention of sudden death: proposal for a common European protocol. Consensus Statement of the Study Group of Sport Cardiology of the Working Group of Cardiac Rehabilitation and Exercise Physiology and the Working Group of Myocardial and Pericardial Diseases of the European Society of Cardiology. *Eur Heart J* 2005; 26(5): 516–24.

Harmon KG, Zigman M, Drezner JA. The effectiveness of screening history, physical exam, and ECG to detect potentially lethal cardiac disorders in athletes: a systematic review/meta-analysis. *J Electrocardiol* 2015; 48(3): 329–38.

Maron BJ, Levine BD, Washington RL, et al. Eligibility and disqualification recommendations for competitive athletes with cardiovascular abnormalities. Task Force 2: Preparticipation screening for cardiovascular disease in competitive athletes: a scientific statement from the American Heart Association and American College of Cardiology. *Circulation* 2015; 132(22): e267–72.

References

1. Maron BJ, Levine BD, Washington RL, et al. Eligibility and disqualification recommendations for competitive athletes with cardiovascular abnormalities. Task Force 2: Preparticipation screening for cardiovascular disease in competitive athletes: a scientific statement from the American Heart Association and American College of Cardiology. *Circulation* 2015; 132(22): e267–72.
2. Corrado D, Pelliccia A, Bjornstad HH, et al. Cardiovascular pre-participation screening of young competitive athletes for prevention of sudden death: proposal for a common European protocol. Consensus Statement of the Study Group of Sport Cardiology of the Working Group of Cardiac Rehabilitation and Exercise Physiology and the Working Group of Myocardial and Pericardial Diseases of the European Society of Cardiology. *Eur Heart J* 2005; 26(5): 516–24.
3. Ljungqvist A, Jenoure P, Engebretsen L, et al. The International Olympic Committee (IOC) Consensus Statement on periodic health evaluation of elite athletes March 2009. *Br J Sports Med* 2009; 43(9): 631–43.
4. Harmon KG, Zigman M, Drezner JA. The effectiveness of screening history, physical exam, and ECG to detect potentially lethal cardiac disorders in athletes: a systematic review/meta-analysis. *J Electrocardiol* 2015; 48(3): 329–38.

5. Chatard JC, Mujika I, Goiriena JJ, Carré F. Screening young athletes for prevention of sudden cardiac death: practical recommendations for sports physicians. *Scand J Med Sci Sports* 2016; 26(4): 362–74.
6. Biffi A, Delise P, Zeppilli P, et al. Italian cardiological guidelines for sports eligibility in athletes with heart disease: part 2. *J Cardiovasc Med (Hagerstown)* 2013; 14(7): 500–15.
7. Biffi A, Delise P, Zeppilli P, et al. Italian cardiological guidelines for sports eligibility in athletes with heart disease: part 1. *J Cardiovasc Med (Hagerstown)* 2013; 14(7): 477–99.
8. Mitchell JH, Haskell W, Snell P, Van Camp SP. Task Force 8: classification of sports. *J Am Coll Cardiol* 2005; 45(8): 1364–7.
9. Guntheroth WG. Innocent murmurs: a suspect diagnosis in non-pregnant adults. *Am J Cardiol* 2009; 104(5): 735–7.
10. Faivre L, Collod-Beroud G, Ades L, et al. The new Ghent criteria for Marfan syndrome. What do they change? *Clin Genet* 2012; 81(5): 433–42.
11. Dvorak J, Grimm K, Schmied C, Junge A. Development and implementation of a standardized precompetition medical assessment of international elite football players—2006 FIFA World Cup Germany. *Clin J Sport Med* 2009; 19(4): 316–21.
12. Maron BJ, Friedman RA, Kligfield P, et al. Assessment of the 12-lead ECG as a screening test for detection of cardiovascular disease in healthy general populations of young people (12–25 years of age): a scientific statement from the American Heart Association and the American College of Cardiology. *Circulation* 2014; 130(15): 1303–34.
13. Corrado D, McKenna WJ. Appropriate interpretation of the athlete's electrocardiogram saves lives as well as money. *Eur Heart J* 2007; 28(16): 1920–2.
14. Baggish AL, Hutter AM, Jr, Wang F, et al. Cardiovascular screening in college athletes with and without electrocardiography: a cross-sectional study. Ann Intern Med 2010; 152(5): 269–75.
15. Magalski A, McCoy M, Zabel M, et al. Cardiovascular screening with electrocardiography and echocardiography in collegiate athletes. *Am J Med* 2011; 124(6): 511–18.
16. Deligiannis AP, Kouidi EJ, Koutlianos NA, et al. Eighteen years' experience applying old and current strategies in the pre-participation cardiovascular screening of athletes. *Hellenic J Cardiol* 2014; 55(1): 32–41.
17. Maron BJ, Shirani J, Poliac LC, et al. Sudden death in young competitive athletes: clinical, demographic, and pathological profiles. *JAMA* 1996; 276(3): 199–204.
18. Glover DW, Maron BJ. Profile of preparticipation cardiovascular screening for high school athletes. *JAMA* 1998; 279(22): 1817–19.
19. Corrado D, Basso C, Thiene G. Sudden cardiac death in athletes. What is the role of screening? *Curr Opin Cardiol* 2012; 27(1): 41–8.

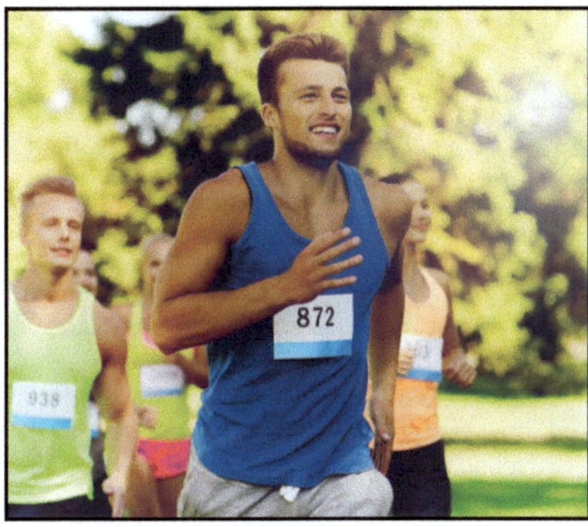

2.2

The electrocardiogram in the athlete

Contents

2.2.1 **The electrocardiogram in the athlete** Alessandro Zorzi and Domenico Corrado 57

2.2.2 **Common ECG patterns in the athlete's heart** Ricardo Stein and Victor Froelicher 68

2.2.3 **Overlap ECG patterns in the athlete's heart and cardiomyopathies** Harshil Dhutia and Michael Papadakis 77

2.2.1 The electrocardiogram in the athlete

Alessandro Zorzi and Domenico Corrado

Introduction

The interpretation of 12-lead electrocardiogram (ECG) abnormalities in the athlete has attracted great interest in recent years, which has resulted in a series of documents aimed at helping sports physicians and cardiologists to interpret the athlete's ECG. The ECGs of trained athletes usually show changes that represent the consequence of the heart's adaptation to physical exercise ('athlete's heart'), such as enlarged cardiac chamber size and increased vagal tone. Such physiological changes must be differentiated from the abnormalities secondary to an underlying cardiovascular disease that can cause sudden cardiac death during exercise [1–4]. Appropriate interpretation of the athlete's ECG should satisfy two different needs: guaranteeing a high sensitivity for cardiovascular disease, and avoiding expensive diagnostic examinations or unnecessary disqualification from competition for abnormalities that fall within the normal range for athletes.

➲ Figure 2.2.1.1 summarizes the historical progression of ECG criteria for evaluation of the athlete's ECG. A modern interpretation of the athlete's ECG was initially provided in 2010 by a consensus document of the European Society of Cardiology (ESC) which aimed to improve the accuracy and cost-effectiveness of the ECG for screening athletes for cardiovascular diseases [5]. The ECG changes in athletes were classified according to prevalence, relation to exercise training, association with an increased risk of cardiovascular disease, and need for further investigations. Two groups were identified: Group 1, including 'common and training-related' ECG changes, and Group 2, including 'uncommon (<5%) and training-unrelated' ECG abnormalities (➲ Fig. 2.2.1.2). According to the ESC recommendations, common ECG changes (Group 1) should be considered as a benign sign of physiological adaptation to exercise and the athlete should be allowed to participate in competitive sports without additional evaluation; on the other hand, further work-up to exclude an underlying cardiac disease should be performed in the case of Group 2 abnormalities, which may be associated with an underlying heart disease at risk of sudden death (➲ Fig. 2.2.1.3). This fundamental document enabled the deveopment of subsequent consensus statements aimed at providing more accurate definitions of ECG parameters such as abnormal Q waves and long/short QT interval, and to further enhance the specificity of interpretation of the athlete's ECG, mostly in sports and ethnic subgroups such as endurance and black athletes [6–12]. Validating studies of different athletic populations proved that this modern approach to ECG interpretation lowers the traditionally high number of false positives and reduces unnecessary and expensive investigations [13]. The present chapter reviews the abnormalities that may be found in an athlete's ECG and proposes criteria

Corrado et al. NEJM 1998 **Screening for HCM**	*Pelliccia et al. Circulation 2000* **Significance of ECG abnormalities**	*Corrado et al. EHJ 2005* **ESC consensus Screening**	*Corrado et al. EHJ 2010* **ECG in the athlete ESC Criteria**	*Drezner et al. Br J Sports Med 2013* **ECG in the athlete Seattle criteria**	*Sheikh et al. Circulation 2014* **ECG in the athlete C.R.Y. criteria.**	*Sharma et al. EHJ 2018* **International criteria**
First presentation of ECG criteria for differentiation between normal and abnormal findings in athletes.	ECG were categorized as normal, mildly abnormal, and abnormal. The three categories were associated with a different prevalence of underlying echo abnormalities.	First consensus document presenting criteria for interpretation of ECG in the athlete in the contest of pre-participation screening.	Formal differentiation between group 1 (common/training related) and group 2 (uncommon/training unrelated) ECG abnormalities in the athlete	Presenting refined quantative definations of various ECG criteria (in particular QT interval and anterior T-wave inversion in black athletes).	Proposed a third group of ECG abnormalities (atrial enlargement, QRS axis deviation, and isolated voltage criteria for right venticular hypertrophy) that should not be considered abnormal if found in isolation.	Updated the Seattle criteria and adopted the classification of the athlete's ECG findings in three groups: normal, abnormal, and borderline.

Fig. 2.2.1.1 The historical progression of ECG criteria for evaluation of the athlete's ECG.

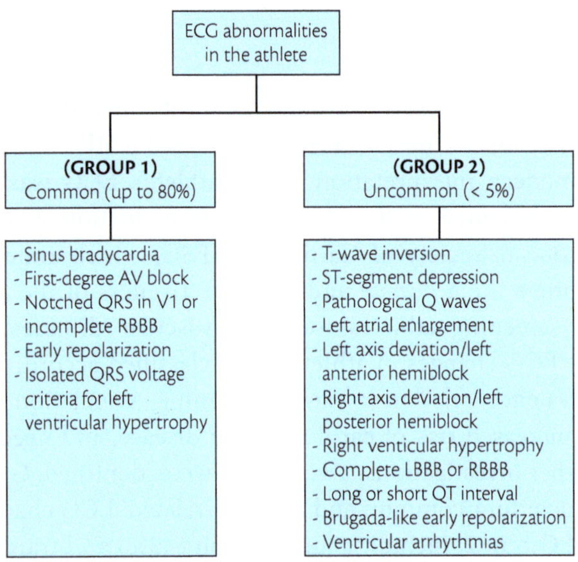

Fig. 2.2.1.2 Classification of ECG abnormalities in the athlete according to the 2010 European Society of Cardiology Recommendations for interpretation of the athlete's ECG. Common ECG abnormalities are the consequence of the physiological cardiovascular adaptation to sustained physical exertion and do not reflect the presence of an underlying cardiovascular disease. Uncommon ECG abnormalities (<5%) are unrelated to athletic conditioning and should be regarded as an expression of possible underlying cardiovascular disorders.

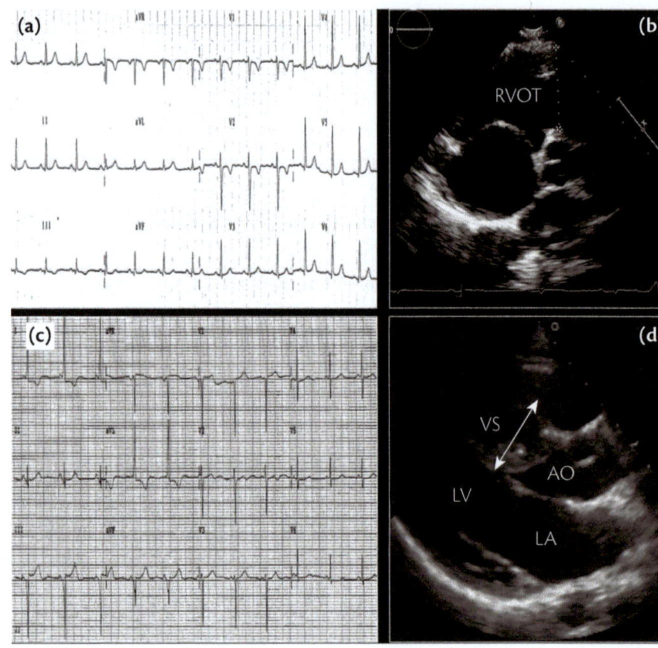

Fig. 2.2.1.3 Uncommon and training-unrelated ECG abnormalities and echocardiographic findings in athletes undergoing pre-participation ECG screening. (a) Electrocardiographic and (b) echocardiographic findings in a 14-year-old male soccer player with arrhythmogenic right ventricular cardiomyopathy. The ECG shows T-wave inversion in right precordial leads (V1–V2) and the echocardiogram reveals right ventricular dilation and dysfunction. (c) Electrocardiographic and (d) echocardiographic findings in a 15-year-old male soccer player with hypertrophic cardiomyopathy. The ECG shows T-wave inversion in the lateral leads (I and aVL) and a pathological Q wave in the inferior leads (III and aVF). The echocardiogram shows an asymmetrical left ventricular hypertrophy with a maximal septal thickness of 31 mm. RVOT, right ventricular outflow tract; VS, ventricular septum; LV, left ventricle; LA, left atrium; AO, aorta.

for interpretation of such changes as normal variants or abnormal findings that need further assessment to exclude an underlying cardiac disease.

Atrial rhythm and atrioventricular conduction abnormalities

Sinus arrhythmia and sinus bradycardia

Sinus arrhythmia and sinus bradycardia are non-pathological conditions commonly associated with aerobic exercise and typical of highly trained endurance athletes [14–16]. Sinus bradycardia is by far the most common bradyarrhythmia in the athlete and can result in heart rates at rest as low as 30–40 bpm. Sinus arrhythmia is also more prevalent in athletes than in the general population. With significant sinus bradycardia, low atrial rhythm (characterized by negative P waves in inferior limb leads II/aVF/III) or junctional rhythm (characterized by narrow QRS not preceded by a P wave) can compete with sinus rhythm.

Atrial enlargement

Left atrial enlargement is diagnosed when the P wave is bifid and has a duration >120 ms in lead II. A biphasic P wave with a prominent terminal negative component is observed in lead V1. Left atrial enlargement can be caused by volume overloading (e.g. mitral regurgitation) or be associated with left ventricular hypertrophy (e.g. hypertrophic cardiomyopathy). It has been proposed that the electrocardiographic pattern of left atrial enlargement is caused by an intra-atrial conduction defect that is often, but not exclusively, associated with left atrial enlargement [18]. Right atrial enlargement (P pulmonale) is characterized by peaked (>2.5 mm) P waves in the inferior leads II/aVF/III. It can be the sign of a right atrial volume overload (e.g. atrial septal defect) as well as pulmonary hypertension. Both left and right atrial enlargement were listed in the 2010 ESC recommendations for interpretation of the ECG of the athlete among the 'uncommon and training-unrelated ECG abnormalities' that should prompt further investigation. This view is supported by a recent study showing that the P-wave morphology is unaffected by physiological training-induced bi-atrial dilatation of the athlete [19]. However, other studies found that right and left atrial enlargements in isolation are relatively common in healthy athletes, while the majority of patients with cardiomyopathy or pulmonary hypertension show atrial enlargement associated with other ECG abnormalities. As a consequence, at present it is proposed that atrial enlargement should be considered benign in the athlete if found in isolation [20,21].

Atrioventricular block

The prevalence of first-degree and Mobitz type I second-degree atrioventricular block (Luciani–Wenckebach) is very high in endurance athletes, whereas Mobitz type II second-degree atrioventricular block and third-degree atrioventricular block are very rare [22–26]. Pathological causes of atrioventricular block in the young athlete include specific forms of infective myocarditis (e.g. Lyme disease and Chagas disease), immune diseases (e.g. cardiac sarcoidosis), and genetic disorders (e.g. Lénègre disease, PRKAG2 syndrome, myotonic dystrophy, and Laminin mutation-related dilated cardiomyopathy). In healthy athletes, first-degree and Luciani–Wenckebach atrioventricular blocks reflect the effect of increased vagal tone on the atrioventricular node and typically disappear with exercise and hyperpnoea (➲ Fig. 2.2.1.4). Persistent forms of atrioventricular block and those unrelated to hypervagotonia contraindicate sports activity. Second-degree atrioventricular Mobitz type 2 advanced or complete atrioventricular block requires careful investigation of the conduction system.

Ventricular depolarization

Depolarization abnormalities include ventricular pre-excitation, pathological Q waves, QRS axis deviation, voltage criteria for ventricular hypertrophy, intraventricular conduction defects. and epsilon waves.

Ventricular pre-excitation

Ventricular pre-excitation (Wolff–Parkinson–White syndrome) reflects the presence of a congenital heart disease characterized by the abnormal persistence of a muscular bundle (accessory atrioventricular pathway) which provides an alternative method of electrical connection between atrial and ventricular myocardium, other than the normal atrioventricular node–His bundle axis. It may be associated with different types of arrhythmia, either benign (atrioventricular re-entrant tachycardia) or malignant (pre-excited atrial fibrillation which can degenerate into ventricular fibrillation). Physical activity may increase the occurrence of arrhythmias in patients with ventricular pre-excitation [27].

Typical ECG features of ventricular pre-excitation include (1) a PR interval <0.12 s, (2) slurring of the initial segment of the QRS complex, known as a delta wave, and (3) QRS complex widening with a total duration >0.12 s. Rare forms of ventricular pre-excitation (e.g. atriofascicular or 'Mahaim' bypass tract) are characterized by the presence of a delta wave and a normal PR interval. The delta wave may be particularly evident in highly trained athletes who exhibit an increased vagal tone and prolonged atrioventricular conduction time. Athletes with ventricular pre-excitation should be referred to a specialist centre for evaluation of appropriate management and sports eligibility.

Q waves

Pathological Q waves are universally recognized as a manifestation of an underlying myocardial disorder (previous myocardial infarction or structural heart disease including cardiomyopathy). Numerous definitions of pathological Q waves have been adopted in the setting of the athlete's ECG interpretation: (1) >4 mm in depth in any lead except III and aVR (ESC recommendations) [5], (2) >3 mm in depth or >40 ms in duration in two or more leads except III and aVR (Seattle criteria) [8], (3) ≥40 ms in duration or ≥25% of the

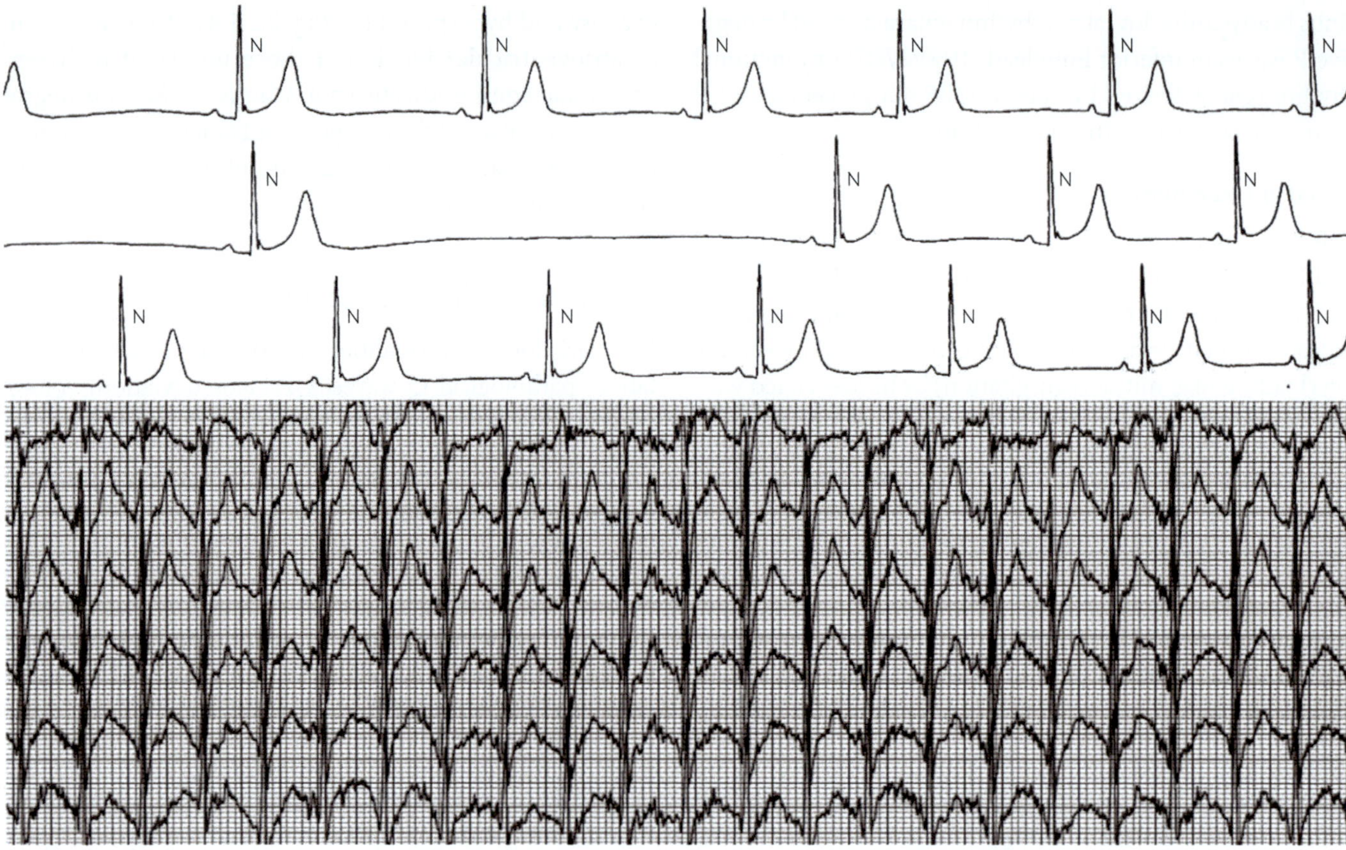

Fig. 2.2.1.4 Luciani–Wenckeback atrioventricular block in an endurance athlete. Top: Second-degree Mobitz I (Luciani–Wenckebach) atrioventricular block during sleep in a 28-year-old runner. Note that sinus bradycardia is also present at the time of block, suggesting the role of increased vagal tone (rather than structural disease of the atrioventricular node) in the aetiopathogenesis of impaired atrioventricular conduction. Bottom: During moderate exercise atrioventricular conduction completely normalizes, confirming the benign (neuro-authonomic) nature of the atrioventricular block.

height of the ensuing R wave in depth (Cardiac Risk in the Young criteria) [11]. According to our personal experience, considering as abnormal a Q wave based on an absolute value of depth is non-specific as a significant proportion of athletes exhibit Q waves >3–4 mm, especially when the QRS voltages are increased. On the other hand, Q waves ≥25% of the following R wave and/or ≥0.04 s are very rare in healthy athletes but are common in patients with previous myocardial infarction or hypertrophic cardiomyopathy.

Intraventricular conduction defects

Incomplete right bundle branch block is a common ECG finding in athletes, with an estimated prevalence of 35–50% compared with 10% in young healthy controls [28–30] (➲ Fig. 2.2.1.5). This ECG pattern is more often noted in athletes engaged in endurance sports, with a striking male preponderance, and should be considered benign in the presence of negative history and physical examination (in particular, a fixed split of the second tone, which may suggest a congenital heart disease with right ventricular volume overloading, should be excluded). It has been suggested that incomplete right bundle branch in the athlete is not caused by slow His–Purkinje system conduction but rather by a conduction delay within the working myocardium secondary to the enlarged RV cavity size and/or increased cardiac mass [30].

Left anterior and posterior fascicular blocks, complete (QRS duration >120 ms) right and left bundle branch block, and non-specific intraventricular conduction defect (QRS >110 ms not satisfying the criteria for either left or right bundle branch block) are rare in athletes, and represent potential markers of a cardiovascular disease requiring accurate clinical investigation [31–34].

Voltage criteria for left and right ventricular hypertrophy

An increase in QRS voltages in the precordial leads (➲ Fig. 2.2.1.6) is one of the most common abnormalities in the athlete's ECG [5], but it can be also a sign of pathological left ventricular hypertrophy as in the case of

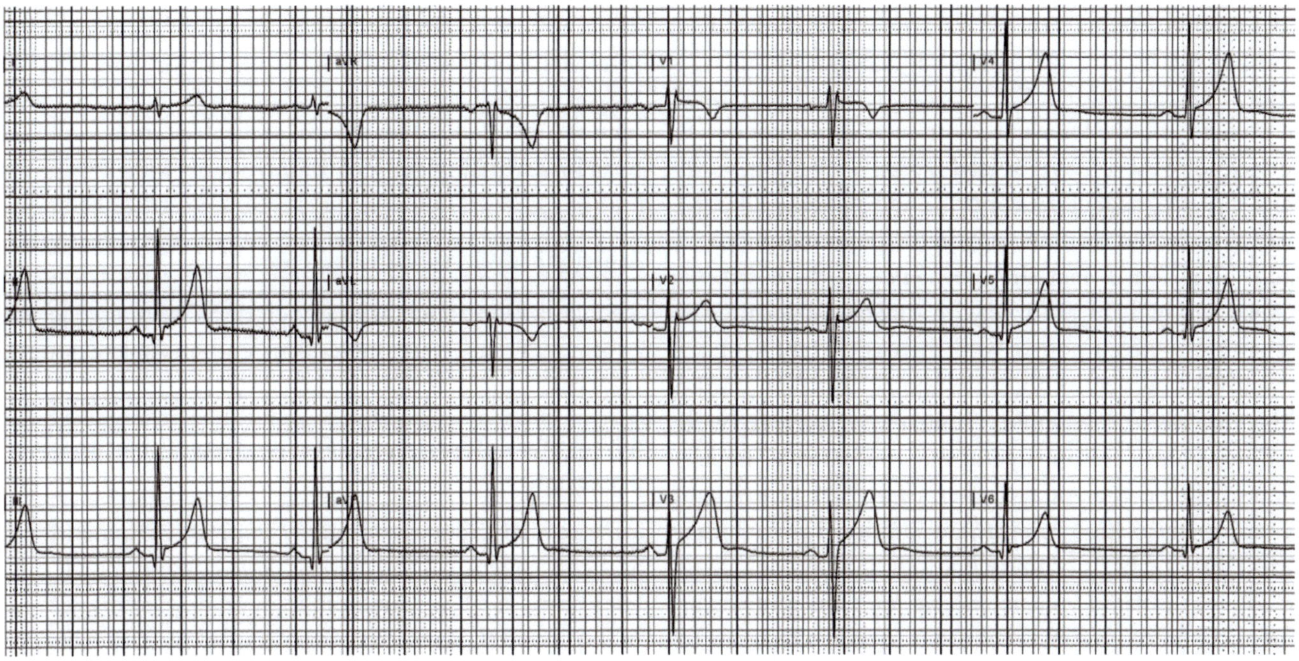

Fig. 2.2.1.5 Voltage criteria for left ventricular hypertrophy and early repolarization in a highly trained athlete. A 12-lead electrocardiogram of a 21-year-old runner showing pure voltage criteria (Sokolow–Lyon) for left ventricular hypertrophy and diffuse early repolarization (J-point elevation).

hypertrophic cardiomyopathy (HCM) [35]. Recent studies have demonstrated that isolated Sokolow–Lyon voltage criteria for left ventricular hypertrophy (S wave in V1 + R wave in V5 >35 mm) in the absence of other depolarization–repolarization abnormalities are very common in the athletes but rare (~2%) in isolation in HCM patients, who usually exhibit associated other ECG abnormalities such as ST-segment depression and/or T-wave inversion, left atrial enlargement, and abnormal Q waves [11,36,37]. These findings support current ESC recommendations

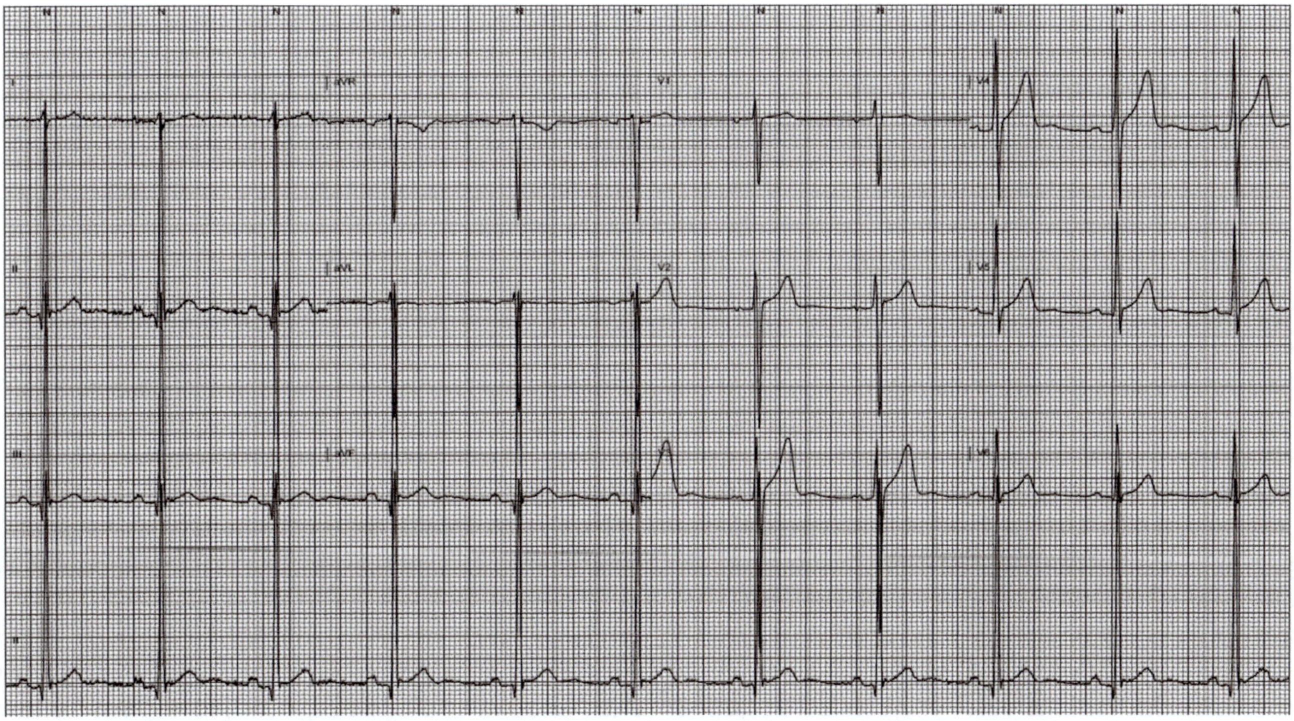

Fig. 2.2.1.6 Incomplete bundle branch block and early repolarization in an endurance athlete. A 12-lead ECG in a 37-year-old cyclist showing incomplete right bundle branch block and diffuse early repolarization (J-point elevation). This pattern is common and benign in athletes.

which consider isolated voltage criteria for left ventricular hypertrophy to be normal in athletes.

Zaidi et al. [20] studied the prevalence of the Sokolow–Lyon voltage criteria for right ventricular hypertrophy (R wave in lead V1 + S wave in lead V5 or V6 >1.05mV) in normal athletes, sedentary controls, and patients affected by arrhythmogenic cardiomyopathy or pulmonary hypertension. They found that the prevalence of these criteria was relatively high in both healthy subjects and patients, and that it correlated poorly with increased right ventricular wall thickness on echocardiography. However, unlike healthy athletes and sedentary controls, no patients with arrhythmogenic cardiomyopathy or pulmonary hypertension exhibited the voltage criteria for right ventricular hypertrophy in isolation (i.e. without additional ECG abnormalities). On the basis of these findings, it is reasonable to conclude that isolated voltage criteria for right ventricular hypertrophy are representative of the normal spectrum of physiological cardiac adaptations resulting from regular exercise training, similarly to isolated voltage criteria for left ventricular hypertrophy.

Left and right axis deviation

Left axis deviation (QRS axis in limb leads <–30°) and right axis deviation (QRS axis in limb leads >90°) were listed among the 'uncommon and training-unrelated ECG changes' by the 2010 ESC recommendations for interpretation of the athlete's ECG. In patients with cardiovascular diseases, left and right axis deviations are usually associated with other ECG abnormalities. Left and right axis deviation in isolation are found in about 2% of healthy athletes [20,21,36,38]. As a consequence, it is proposed that, as for atrial enlargement, axis deviation in isolation should be considered to be benign in the athlete [20,21].

Epsilon wave

The epsilon wave is defined as a 'reproducible low-amplitude signal between the end of the QRS complex to the onset of the T wave in the right precordial leads V1 to V3' and is a major criteria for the diagnosis of arrhythmogenic cardiomyopathy[39]. This ECG abnormality reflects a delayed and fragmented propagation of ventricular depolarization in the right ventricle, and is usually observed in advanced disease stage in association with other ECG abnormalities such as T-wave inversion. It should be differentiated from an incomplete right bundle branch block pattern with a slurred R′ wave, which can be found in healthy athletes. A recent study demonstrated that the inter-observer agreement in epsilon wave definition is low even among experienced physicians, and that finding an epsilon wave as an isolated abnormal ECG finding is highly unlikely. The authors conclude that physicians should be cautious in the assessment of epsilon waves, especially in individuals undergoing ECG screening who do not satisfy other clinical or electrocardiographic criteria for arrhythmogenic cardiomyopathy [40].

Ventricular repolarization

Repolarization abnormalities include ST-segment elevation or depression, T-wave inversion, and short and long QT interval.

ST-segment elevation: early repolarization vs Brugada syndrome

Early repolarization is commonly observed in trained athletes as a consequence of intensive athletic conditioning (i.e. athlete's heart) [5]. It is characterized by an upward displacement of the J point (QRS–ST junction) ≥0.1 mV. Slurring or notching of the terminal part of the QRS complex (J wave) may be observed in the inferolateral leads (➲ Figs 2.2.1.5 and 2.2.1.6).

The most common pattern of early repolarization in anterior leads V1–V4 is characterized by J-point and ST-segment elevation followed by a peaked and tall positive T wave. Another variant of anterior early repolarization exists, consisting of an elevated and convex ST segment preceding a negative T wave. This variant is particularly common in Afro-Caribbean athletes and has many similarities with the type 1 ('coved-type') ECG of Brugada syndrome [41]. The 2010 ESC criteria proposed that the two conditions can be differentiated based on the ST-segment configuration: a down-sloping ST-segment elevation is typical of Brugada syndrome whereas an upsloping ST-segment elevation is characteristic of early repolarization. These criteria have recently been validated by a study showing that an upsloping ST-segment configuration (ST-segment elevation at J point/ST-segment elevation at 80 ms after J point <1) had a diagnostic accuracy of 99% for differentiating between athlete's heart and Brugada syndrome [42] (➲ Fig. 2.2.1.7). The type 2/3 Brugada ECG, characterized by J-point elevation ≥0.2 mV in V1–V2 and a positive T wave, overlaps with early repolarization and does not require further testing in asymptomatic athletes with negative family history [43].

In the last decade there have been several reports of patients with idiopathic ventricular fibrillation (ventricular fibrillation in the absence of overt heart diseases) showing prominent early repolarization (J-point elevation ≥2mm) particularly in the inferolateral leads and associated with a flat or down-sloping ST segment [44–48]. An increased prevalence of early repolarization was also found among athletes who had been resuscitated from idiopathic ventricular

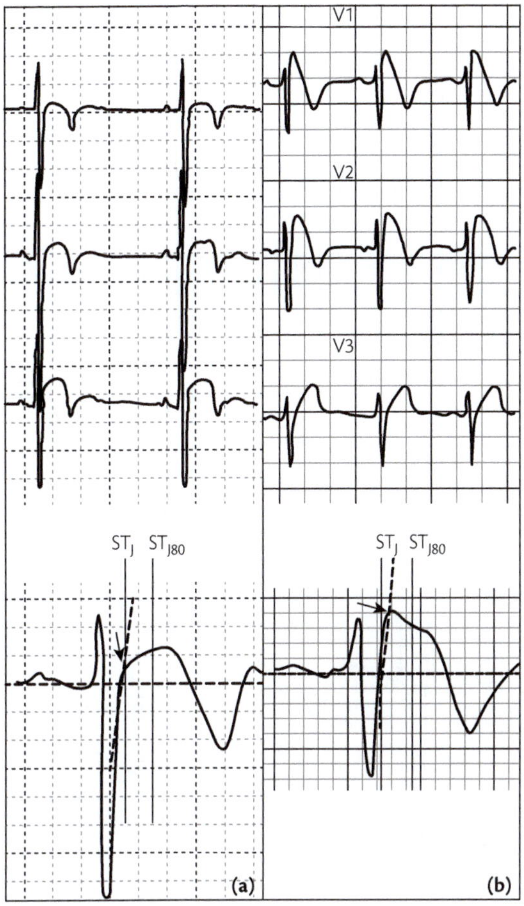

Fig. 2.2.1.7 Differential diagnosis between 'domed-type' early repolarization of athlete's heart and a coved-type Brugada electrocardiogram. (a) the athlete's 'domed-type' early repolarization is characterized by an upsloping ST-segment elevation ($ST_J/ST_{j+80ms} < 1$), while (b) the patient with Brugada syndrome shows a downsloping ST segment ($ST_J/ST_{j+80ms} > 1$).

Reprinted from *The American Journal of Cardiology*, Vol 115, issue 4, Alessandro Zorzi et al. Differential diagnosis between early repolarization of athlete's heart and coved-type Brugada electrocardiogram, pp. 529–32, © 2105 with permission from Elsevier.

fibrillation or who died suddenly without evidence of structural heart disease [49]. However, to put these studies into clinical perspective, it must be kept in mind that idiopathic ventricular fibrillation is an extremely rare condition, while early repolarization is very common in highly trained athletes. Using the Bayes formula, it has been calculated that finding a J wave and/or QRS slurring in an athlete increases the probability of experiencing idiopathic ventricular fibrillation from 2 in 1,000,000 to 3.5 in 1,000,000 [49]. Given the above considerations, in asymptomatic athletes early repolarization should still be considered to be a physiological ECG pattern reflecting cardiac adaptation to exercise [5,50,51]. However, in athletes with a history of cardiac arrest with no evidence of structural heart disease, an ECG pattern of early repolarization should raise the suspicion of an idiopathic ventricular fibrillation [5,52].

ST-segment depression

ST-segment depression at rest, particularly if associated with T-wave inversion, is a typical electrocardiographic sign of pathological left ventricular hypertrophy. This finding is rarely observed in healthy athletes, and demonstration of ST-segment depression on resting ECG, either isolated or associated with T-wave inversion, should prompt further investigations to exclude heart disease [5].

T-wave inversion

T-wave inversion ≥1 mm in two or more contiguous leads (excluding V1, III, and aVR) should be interpreted differently according to the regional distribution on the 12 ECG leads.

Anterior (V1–V4) T-wave inversion is a possible sign of an underlying cardiac disease [5,6,9]. Anterior T-wave inversion is rarely (2–4%) observed in patients with hypertrophic cardiomyopathy, who more often show T-wave inversion in inferolateral leads [51], but it may be present in as many as 80% of patients with arrhythmogenic cardiomyopathy [38,53–55]. However, anterior T-wave inversion is very common in children ('juvenile pattern of repolarization') and may also be observed on the ECG of healthy athletes, with a reported prevalence of up to 25% in athletes of Afro-Caribbean descent [51,56,57]. As a consequence, anterior T-wave inversion is one of the most common causes of false-positive ECG findings [13]. However, findings of recent studies may help to interpret the clinical meaning of anterior T-wave inversion in an athlete.

Negative T waves in right precordial leads are typically observed in children ('juvenile pattern of repolarization'), so they are traditionally considered a normal finding in athletes aged less than 14 years. However, it is difficult to provide a precise age cut-off to differentiate between the benign 'juvenile pattern of repolarization' and anterior repolarization abnormalities which may represent the sign of an underlying cardiomyopathy. Migliore et al. [38] found a 4.7% prevalence of T-wave inversion in V1–V2/V3 among young Caucasian athletes (aged 9–19 years) and demonstrated a decreasing prevalence of T-wave inversion with increasing age (8.4% in athletes younger than 14 years vs 1.7% in those older than 14 years). Multivariate analysis showed that pubertal development rather than age was independently associated with right precordial T-wave inversion. The clinical meaning of this ECG feature also depended more on the development stage than on the actual age: no cardiac disease was found among pre-pubertal children with right-precordial T-wave inversions, whereas 11% of post-pubertal individuals with persistent negative T waves in V1–V2/V3 were diagnosed with definite or borderline arrhythmogenic cardiomyopathy.

According to this study, right-precordial T-wave inversion should be regarded in the context of pubertal development, and further investigation should be performed only if the ECG abnormality persists beyond puberty.

In view of the very high prevalence of the early repolarization variant characterized by ST-segment elevation and negative T-waves in anterior leads in black athletes [51], the 2018 International criteria recommended that anterior T-wave inversion preceded by a convex ST-segment elevation in black athletes should not require further assessment to exclude a cardiomyopathy in the absence of symptoms, positive family history, or abnormal physical examination findings [11]. According to a recent study comparing healthy athletes of both white and black ethnicity with anterior T-wave inversion and patients with arrhythmogenic cardiomyopathy or hypertrophic cardiomyopathy who also exhibited anterior T-wave inversion, J-point elevation >1 mm in at least one anterior lead exhibiting an inverted T-wave is much more specific than ST-segment elevation in differentiating between benign and possibly malignant anterior T-wave inversion (➲ Fig. 2.2.1.8). The study concluded that T-wave inversion can be considered as a normal ECG sign in the athlete when it is (1) limited to V1–V4, (2) preceded by J-point elevation in at least one lead exhibiting T-wave inversion, and (3) not associated with concomitant pathological ECG abnormalities. These combined criteria provide excellent accuracy for differentiating between anterior T-wave inversion secondary to early repolarization and possibly due to a cardiomyopathy, thus reducing the number of healthy athletes with such an ECG pattern who are subjected to further unnecessary and expensive clinical investigation [12].

T-wave inversion in leads other than V1–V4 is rare in athletes and is a potential marker for an underlying cardiac disease that should prompt further investigation. A normal echocardiography may not be sensitive enough to exclude a pathological myocardial substrate in athletes with inferolateral repolarization abnormalities, and contrast-enhanced cardiac magnetic resonance should be performed to exclude apical variants of hypertrophic cardiomyopathy [58] or myocardial scars that typically involve the subepicardial/midmyocardial layers of the lateral left ventricular wall. Myocardial scar in athletes, irrespective of the aetiology (healed myocarditis, 'left-dominant' arrhythmogenic cardiomyopathy, etc.) may act as a substrate for life-threatening ventricular arrhythmias [59,60]. Regular follow-up with cardiac imaging is necessary for athletes with inferolateral T-wave inversion and normal initial evaluation as repolarization abnormalities may precede the development of an overt cardiomyopathy phenotype [56,61].

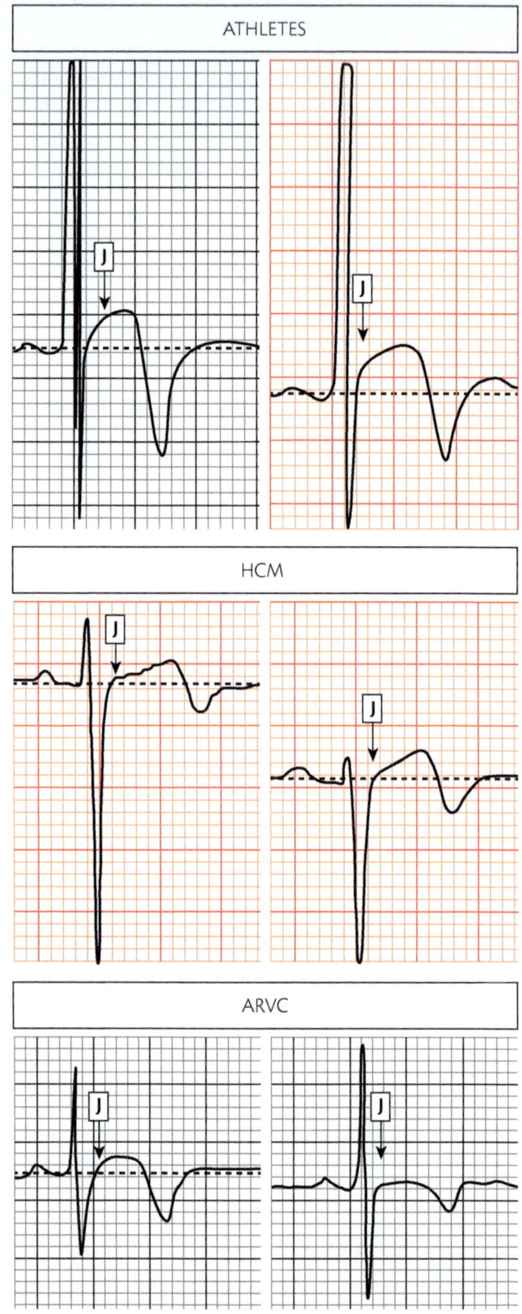

Fig. 2.2.1.8 Patterns of anterior T-wave inversion in healthy athletes and athletes with cardiomyopathy. Note that athletes typically demonstrate J-point elevation preceding the negative T wave so that this J-point elevation–T-wave inversion pattern can be considered an early repolarization variant and further investigations can be avoided if T-wave inversion is confined to leads V1–V4. However, in patients with hypertrophic cardiomyopathy (HCM) or arrhythmogenic right ventricular cardiomyopathy (ARVC) and anterior T-wave inversion, there is no J-point elevation. Anterior T-wave inversion with no J-point elevation or extending beyond V4 or to the limb leads should prompt additional investigations to exclude an underlying structural heart disease.

QT interval

The QT interval is defined as the interval between the beginning of the QRS complex and the end of the T wave, measured in II and V5 (whichever is the longest) and corrected to heart rate according to the Bazett formula (QTc = QT ms/square root of the previous RR in seconds), remembering that the formula is less accurate at slow heart rates and can underestimate the QTc at heart rates <50–60 bpm. If the heart rate is variable, multiple measurements should be performed and an averaged value should be considered. The main difficulty in QT measurement lies in correct identification of the end of the T wave when the T and U waves are close together. When the T wave is followed by a distinct U wave, the T-wave offset is identified when the descending limb of the T wave returns to the baseline before the onset of the U wave. When the T wave and the U wave are fused, the end of the T wave is calculated as the point of intersection between a straight line tangent to the downslope of the T wave and the isoelectric line ('teach the tangent' method). It is important to differentiate the U wave (lower amplitude compared with the T wave) from a notched T wave (the second portion of the T wave following the notch which is higher than the first portion). Manual confirmation should be performed if the computer-derived QT interval is outside normal values.

According to the ESC recommendation for interpretation of the athlete's ECG, a long QT is defined as a QTc ≥440 ms in men and ≥460 ms in women, but the recent International criteria have suggested higher cut-offs (above 470 ms in male and 480 ms in female athletes) to account for the longer QTc values in athletes [5,11]. If QTc slightly exceeds normal values (470/480–500 ms) in the absence of family or personal history, a second ECG should be obtained, ideally on a different day, to confirm the diagnosis. If an abnormal QT is confirmed or if QTc exceeds 500 ms, the athlete should be referred for consultation to a referral centre. A definite diagnosis of long QT syndrome may require molecular genetics analysis, which has a sensitivity of approximately 70% [62].

Short QT syndrome is a recently identified genetic disorder which is characterized by QTc <320 ms, often associated with a tall and peaked T wave. Short QT syndrome has been associated with paroxysmal atrial fibrillation and ventricular fibrillation. Although data are still limited, adrenergic stress has been linked to the development of premature atrial fibrillation and life-threatening ventricular arrhythmias [62]. Eligibility for competitive sport in athletes who are diagnosed with short QT syndrome is controversial [5,17], but it has to be emphasized that a recent study of a large cohort of asymptomatic individuals and athletes found a prevalence of QTc <320 ms of 0.1% and that no subject with short QT suffered any adverse event during follow-up [63]. Therefore great caution should be used in diagnosing short QT syndrome in athletes with no suggestive family or personal history.

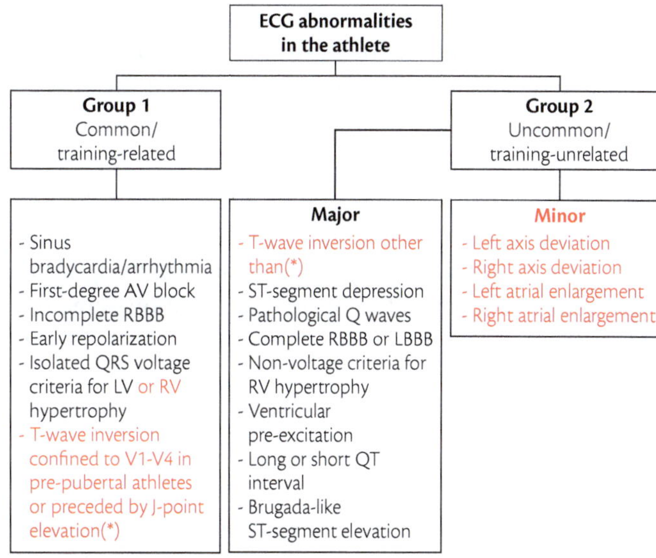

Fig. 2.2.1.9 Proposed modification of the 2010 European Society of Cardiology classification of ECG abnormalities in the athlete. Compared with the original classification (Fig. 2.2.1.2), isolated voltage criteria for right ventricular (RV) hypertrophy and T-wave inversion confined to V1–V4 in prepubertal athletes or preceded by J-point elevation are now included among common ECG abnormalities. Group 2 ECG abnormalities comprising uncommon and training-unrelated abnormalities are further divided into 'major', i.e. those that are uncommon in athlete's heart but frequent in cardiomyopathy (e.g. T-wave inversion beyond leads V1–V4) and 'minor', i.e. those that are infrequent in both athletes and patients with cardiomyopathy (atrial enlargement or axis deviation). AV, atrioventricular, LBBB, left bundle branch block, LV, left ventricular, RBBB, right bundle branch block.
Adapted with permission from Corrado D, Calore C, Zorzi A, Migliore F. Improving the interpretation of the athlete's electrocardiogram. *European Heart Journal*, Volume 34, Issue 47, pp. 3606–9. Copyright © 2013 Oxford University Press and the European Society of Cardiology (ESC).

Modern interpretation of the athlete's electrocardiogram

➔ Figure 2.2.1.9 shows a possible revision of the original classification (➔ Fig. 2.2.1.2) of ECG abnormalities in the athlete based on the results of recent studies. At variance with the 2010 ESC guidelines for interpretation of the athlete's ECG, two more ECG findings that are much more common in the athlete's heart than in cardiomyopathies are now included in the training-related ECG abnormalities (group 1): (1) isolated voltage criteria for right ventricular hypertrophy and (2) anterior T-wave inversion confined to leads V1–V4 in pre-pubertal athletes or preceded by J-point elevation.

Group 2 ECG abnormalities comprising those that are uncommon and training unrelated are further divided into 'major', i.e. those that are uncommon in athletes but frequent in cardiomyopathies (e.g. T-wave inversion beyond leads V1–V4), and 'minor', i.e. those that are infrequent in both athletes and patients with cardiomyopathies (atrial enlargement or axis deviation). Recommendations for management of athletes showing the new subset of 'minor' Group 2 ECG changes are open to debate. While some authors suggest excluding these patterns from the abnormal category of ECG changes [20,21], it should be emphasized that ignoring such 'minor' abnormalities at pre-participation screening increases the specificity of the screening ECG by 2–4%, but decreases the sensitivity for identification of a potentially lethal cardiomyopathy by a similar figure (2–3%).

Further reading

Corrado D, McKenna WJ. Appropriate interpretation of the athlete's electrocardiogram saves lives as well as money. *Eur Heart J* 2007; 28: 1920–2.

Corrado D, Pelliccia A, Heidbuchel H, et al. Recommendations for interpretation of 12-lead electrocardiogram in the athlete. *Eur Heart J* 2010; 31: 243–59.

Drezner JA, Ackerman MJ, Cannon BC, et al. Abnormal electrocardiographic findings in athletes: recognising changes suggestive of primary electrical disease. *Br J Sports Med* 2013; 47: 153–67.

Drezner JA, Ashley E, Baggish AL, et al. Abnormal electrocardiographic findings in athletes: recognising changes suggestive of cardiomyopathy. *Br J Sports Med* 2013; 47: 137–52.

Drezner JA, Fischbach P, Froelicher V, et al. Normal electrocardiographic findings: recognising physiological adaptations in athletes. *Br J Sports Med* 2013; 47: 125–36.

Drezner J, Sharma S, Baggish A, et al. International criteria for electrocardiographic interpretation in athletes: Consensus standards. *Br J Sports Med* 2017; 51(9): 704–31.

Maron BJ, Friedman RA, Kligfield P, et al. Assessment of the 12-lead ECG as a screening test for detection of cardiovascular disease in healthy general populations of young people (12-25 years of age): a scientific statement from the American Heart Association and the American College of Cardiology. *Circulation* 2014; 130: 1303–34.

Zorzi A, ElMaghawry M, Corrado D. Evolving interpretation of the athlete's electrocardiogram: from European Society of Cardiology and Stanford criteria, to Seattle criteria and beyond. *J Electrocardiol* 2015; 48: 283–91.

References

1. Pelliccia A, Di Paolo FM, Maron BJ. The athlete's heart: remodeling, electrocardiogram and preparticipation screening. *Cardiol Rev* 2002; 10(2): 85–90.
2. Corrado D, McKenna WJ. Appropriate interpretation of the athlete's electrocardiogram saves lives as well as money. *Eur Heart J* 2007; 28(16): 1920–2.
3. Maron BJ, Pelliccia A. The heart of trained athletes: cardiac remodeling and the risks of sports, including sudden death. *Circulation* 2006; 114(15): 1633–44.
4. Maron BJ, Friedman RA, Kligfield P, et al. Assessment of the 12-lead ECG as a screening test for detection of cardiovascular disease in healthy general populations of young people (12–25 years of age): a scientific statement from the American Heart Association and the American College of Cardiology. *Circulation* 2014; 130(15): 1303–34.
5. Corrado D, Pelliccia A, Heidbuchel H, et al. Recommendations for interpretation of 12-lead electrocardiogram in the athlete. *Eur Heart J* 2010; 31(2): 243–59.
6. Uberoi A, Stein R, Perez MV, et al. Interpretation of the electrocardiogram of young athletes. *Circulation* 2011; 124(6): 746–57.
7. Drezner JA, Ackerman MJ, Cannon BC, et al. Abnormal electrocardiographic findings in athletes: recognising changes suggestive of primary electrical disease. *Br J Sports Med* 2013; 47(3): 153–67.
8. Drezner JA, Ashley E, Baggish AL, et al. Abnormal electrocardiographic findings in athletes: recognising changes suggestive of cardiomyopathy. *Br J Sports Med* 2013; 47(3): 137–52.
9. Drezner JA, Fischbach P, Froelicher V, et al. Normal electrocardiographic findings: recognising physiological adaptations in athletes. *Br J Sports Med* 2013; 47(3): 125–36.
10. Sheikh N, Papadakis M, Ghani S, et al. Comparison of electrocardiographic criteria for the detection of cardiac abnormalities in elite black and white athletes. *Circulation* 2014; 129(16): 1637–49.
11. Sharma S, Drezner JA, Baggish A, et al. International recommendations for electrocardiographic interpretation in athletes. *Eur Heart J* 2018; 39(16):1466–80.
12. Calore C, Zorzi A, Sheikh N, et al. Electrocardiographic anterior T-wave inversion in athletes of different ethnicities: differential diagnosis between athlete's heart and cardiomyopathy. *Eur Heart J* 2016; 37(32): 2515–27.
13. Zorzi A, ElMaghawry M, Corrado D. Evolving interpretation of the athlete's electrocardiogram: from European Society of Cardiology and Stanford criteria, to Seattle criteria and beyond. *J Electrocardiol* 2015; 48(3): 283–91.
14. Chapman JH. Profound sinus bradycardia in the athletic heart syndrome. *J Sports Med Phys Fitness* 1982; 22(1): 45–8.
15. Hanne-Paparo N, Kellermann JJ. Long-term Holter ECG monitoring of athletes. *Med Sci Sports Exerc* 1981; 13(5): 294–8.
16. Zehender M, Meinertz T, Keul J, Just H. ECG variants and cardiac arrhythmias in athletes: clinical relevance and prognostic importance. *Am Heart J* 1990; 119(6): 1378–91.
17. Corrado D, Pelliccia A, Bjornstad HH, et al. Cardiovascular pre-participation screening of young competitive athletes for prevention of sudden death: proposal for a common European protocol. Consensus Statement of the Study Group of Sport Cardiology of the Working Group of Cardiac Rehabilitation and Exercise Physiology and the Working Group of Myocardial and Pericardial Diseases of the European Society of Cardiology. *Eur Heart J* 2005; 26(5): 516–24.
18. Bayes de Luna A, Platonov P, Cosio FG, et al. Interatrial blocks. A separate entity from left atrial enlargement: a consensus report. *J Electrocardiol* 2012; 45(5): 445–51.
19. D'Ascenzi F, Solari M, Biagi M, et al. P-wave morphology is unaffected by training-induced biatrial dilatation: a prospective, longitudinal study in healthy athletes. *Int J Cardiovasc Imaging* 2016; 32(3): 407–15.
20. Zaidi A, Ghani S, Sheikh N, et al. Clinical significance of electrocardiographic right ventricular hypertrophy in athletes: comparison with arrhythmogenic right ventricular cardiomyopathy and pulmonary hypertension. *Eur Heart J* 2013; 34(47): 3649–56.

21. Gati S, Sheikh N, Ghani S, et al. Should axis deviation or atrial enlargement be categorised as abnormal in young athletes? The athlete's electrocardiogram: time for re-appraisal of markers of pathology. *Eur Heart J* 2013; 34(47): 3641–8.
22. Palatini P, Maraglino G, Sperti G, et al. Prevalence and possible mechanisms of ventricular arrhythmias in athletes. *Am Heart J* 1985; 110(3): 560–7.
23. Talan DA, Bauernfeind RA, Ashley WW, et al. Twenty-four hour continuous ECG recordings in long-distance runners. *Chest* 1982; 82(1): 19–24.
24. Viitasalo MT, Kala R, Eisalo A. Ambulatory electrocardiographic recording in endurance athletes. *Br Heart J* 1982; 47(3): 213–20.
25. Meytes I, Kaplinsky E, Yahini JH, et al. Wenckebach A-V block: a frequent feature following heavy physical training. *Am Heart J* 1975 Oct; 90(4):426–30.
26. Zeppilli P, Fenici R, Sassara M, Pirrami MM, Caselli G. Wenckebach second-degree A-V block in top-ranking athletes: an old problem revisited. *Am Heart J* 1980; 100(3): 281–94.
27. Di Mambro C, Drago F, Milioni M, et al. Sports eligibility after risk assessment and treatment in children with asymptomatic ventricular pre-excitation. *Sports Med* 2016; 46(8): 1183–90.
28. Pelliccia A, Maron BJ, Culasso F, et al. Clinical significance of abnormal electrocardiographic patterns in trained athletes. *Circulation* 2000; 102(3): 278–84.
29. Sharma S, Whyte G, Elliott P, et al. Electrocardiographic changes in 1000 highly trained junior elite athletes. *Br J Sports Med* 1999; 33(5): 319–24.
30. Langdeau JB, Blier L, Turcotte H, et al. Electrocardiographic findings in athletes: the prevalence of left ventricular hypertrophy and conduction defects. *Can J Cardiol* 2001; 17(6): 655–9.
31. Kreger BE, Anderson KM, Kannel WB. Prevalence of intraventricular block in the general population: the Framingham Study. *Am Heart J* 1989; 117(4): 903–10.
32. Agarwal AK, Venugopalan P. Right bundle branch block: varying electrocardiographic patterns. Aetiological correlation, mechanisms and electrophysiology. *Int J Cardiol* 1999; 71(1): 33–9.
33. Hardarson T, Arnason A, Eliasson GJ, et al. Left bundle branch block: prevalence, incidence, follow-up and outcome. *Eur Heart J* 1987; 8(10): 1075–9.
34. Elizari MV, Acunzo RS, Ferreiro M. Hemiblocks revisited. *Circulation* 2007; 115(9): 1154–63.
35. Maron BJ. Hypertrophic cardiomyopathy and other causes of sudden cardiac death in young competitive athletes, with considerations for preparticipation screening and criteria for disqualification. *Cardiol Clin* 2007; 25(3): 399–414.
36. Calore C, Melacini P, Pelliccia A, et al. Prevalence and clinical meaning of isolated increase of QRS voltages in hypertrophic cardiomyopathy versus athlete's heart: relevance to athletic screening. *Int J Cardiol* 2013; 168(4): 4494–7.
37. Corrado D, Basso C, Schiavon M, Thiene G. Screening for hypertrophic cardiomyopathy in young athletes. *N Engl J Med* 1998; 339(6): 364–9.
38. Migliore F, Zorzi A, Michieli P, et al. Prevalence of cardiomyopathy in Italian asymptomatic children with electrocardiographic T-wave inversion at preparticipation screening. *Circulation* 2012; 125(3): 529–38.
39. Marcus FI, McKenna WJ, Sherrill D, et al. Diagnosis of arrhythmogenic right ventricular cardiomyopathy/dysplasia: proposed modification of the task force criteria. *Circulation* 2010; 121(13): 1533–41.
40. Platonov PG, Calkins H, Hauer RN, et al. High interobserver variability in the assessment of epsilon waves: implications for diagnosis of arrhythmogenic right ventricular cardiomyopathy/dysplasia. *Heart Rhythm* 2016; 13(1): 208–16.
41. Zorzi A, ElMaghawry M, Corrado D. ST-segment elevation and sudden death in the athlete. *Card Electrophysiol Clin* 2013; 5: 73–84.
42. Zorzi A, Leoni L, Di Paolo FM, et al. Differential diagnosis between early repolarization of athlete's heart and coved-type Brugada electrocardiogram. Am J Cardiol. 2015; 115(4): 529–32.
43. Zorzi A, Migliore F, Marras E, et al. Should all individuals with a nondiagnostic Brugada-electrocardiogram undergo sodium-channel blocker test? *Heart Rhythm* 2012; 9(6): 909–16.
44. Riera AR, Ferreira C, Schapachnik E, et al. Brugada syndrome with atypical ECG: downsloping ST-segment elevation in inferior leads. *J Electrocardiol* 2004; 37(2): 101–4.
45. Sahara M, Sagara K, Yamashita T, et al. J wave and ST segment elevation in the inferior leads: a latent type of variant Brugada syndrome? *Jpn Heart J* 2002; 43(1): 55–60.
46. Sugao M, Fujiki A, Nishida K, et al. Repolarization dynamics in patients with idiopathic ventricular fibrillation: pharmacological therapy with bepridil and disopyramide. J *Cardiovasc Pharmacol* 2005; 45(6): 545–9.
47. Tsunoda Y, Takeishi Y, Nozaki N, et al. Presence of intermittent J waves in multiple leads in relation to episode of atrial and ventricular fibrillation. *J Electrocardiol* 2004; 37(4): 311–14.
48. Komiya N, Imanishi R, Kawano H, et al. Ventricular fibrillation in a patient with prominent J wave in the inferior and lateral electrocardiographic leads after gastrostomy. *Pacing Clin Electrophysiol* 2006; 29(9): 1022–4.
49. Cappato R, Furlanello F, Giovinazzo V, et al. J wave, QRS slurring, and ST elevation in athletes with cardiac arrest in the absence of heart disease: marker of risk or innocent bystander? *Circ Arrhythm Electrophysiol* 2010; 3(4): 305–11.
50. Rosso R, Adler A, Halkin A, Viskin S. Risk of sudden death among young individuals with J waves and early repolarization: putting the evidence into perspective. *Heart Rhythm* 2011; 8(6): 923–9.
51. Papadakis M, Carré F, Kervio G, et al. The prevalence, distribution, and clinical outcomes of electrocardiographic repolarization patterns in male athletes of African/Afro-Caribbean origin. *Eur Heart J* 2011; 32(18): 2304–13.
52. Rosso R, Glikson E, Belhassen B, et al. Distinguishing 'benign' from 'malignant early repolarization': the value of the ST-segment morphology. *Heart Rhythm* 2012; 9(2): 225–9.
53. Bhonsale A, James CA, Tichnell C, et al. Risk stratification in arrhythmogenic right ventricular dysplasia/cardiomyopathy-associated desmosomal mutation carriers. *Circ Arrhythm Electrophysiol* 2013; 6(3): 569–78.
54. Steriotis AK, Bauce B, Daliento L, et al. Electrocardiographic pattern in arrhythmogenic right ventricular cardiomyopathy. *Am J Cardiol* 2009; 103(9): 1302–8.
55. Zorzi A, Migliore F, ElMaghawry M, et al. Electrocardiographic predictors of electroanatomic scar size in arrhythmogenic right ventricular cardiomyopathy: implications for arrhythmic risk stratification. *J Cardiovasc Electrophysiol* 2013; 24(12): 1321–7.

56. Pelliccia A, Di Paolo FM, Quattrini FM, et al. Outcomes in athletes with marked ECG repolarization abnormalities. *N Engl J Med* 2008; 358(2): 152–61.
57. Basavarajaiah S, Boraita A, White G, et al. Ethinic differences in left ventricular remodeling in highly-trained athletes: relevance to differentiating physiologic left ventricular hypertrophy from hypertrophic cardiomyopathy. *J Am Coll Cardiol* 2008; 51(23): 2256–62.
58. Moon JC, Fisher NG, McKenna WJ, Pennell DJ. Detection of apical hypertrophic cardiomyopathy by cardiovascular magnetic resonance in patients with non-diagnostic echocardiography. *Heart* 2004; 90(6): 645–9.
59. Zorzi A, Perazzolo Marra M, Rigato I, et al. Nonischemic left ventricular scar as a substrate of life-threatening ventricular arrhythmias and sudden cardiac death in competitive athletes. *Circ Arrhythm Electrophysiol* 2016; 9(7): e004229.
60. Schnell F, Claessen G, La Gerche A, et al. Subepicardial delayed gadolinium enhancement in asymptomatic athletes: let sleeping dogs lie? *Br J Sports Med* 2016; 50(2): 111–17.
61. Schnell F, Riding N, O'Hanlon R, et al. Recognition and significance of pathological T-wave inversions in athletes. *Circulation* 2015; 131(2): 165–73.
62. Priori SG, Blomstrom-Lundqvist C, Mazzanti A, et al. 2015 ESC Guidelines for the management of patients with ventricular arrhythmias and the prevention of sudden cardiac death: The Task Force for the Management of Patients with Ventricular Arrhythmias and the Prevention of Sudden Cardiac Death of the European Society of Cardiology (ESC). Endorsed by: Association for European Paediatric and Congenital Cardiology (AEPC). *Eur Heart J* 2015; 36(41): 2793–867.
63. Dhutia H, Malhotra A, Parpia S, et al. The prevalence and significance of a short QT interval in 18,825 low-risk individuals including athletes. *Br J Sports Med* 2016; 50(2): 124–9.

2.2.2 Common ECG patterns in the athlete's heart

Ricardo Stein and Victor Froelicher

Key Points

1. High intensity dynamic endurance sports are associated with electrocardiographic rhythm and conduction alterations as well as with waveform amplitude increases. The former are due to lower intrinsic heart rate and changes in parasympathetic and sympathetic tone, and the latter are due to physiological myocardial remodelling.
2. Sinus bradycardia is by far the most common bradyarrhythmia in the athlete and is a benign finding unless associated with symptoms or with other arrhythmias.
3. Repolarization abnormalities can result from structural changes and autonomic adaptations to exercise training.
4. Several ECG findings can mimic cardiac disease.

Box 2.2.2.1 ECG findings associated with low heart rate in athletes

Very common

Sinus bradycardia
Sinus arrhythmia
Sinus pauses

Common

Junctional escape beats
First-degree AV block
Type I second-degree AV block (Wenckebach phenomenon)

Introduction

The electrocardiogram (ECG) of the endurance athlete may show certain distinguishing features that are similar to those seen in patients with phenotypic expressions which can cause sudden cardiac death. In this scenario it is important to make a distinction between what is considered a normal adaptation to regular intense exercise that does not require further evaluation and the electrocardiographic expression of a serious pathological process.

More than 70% of athletes demonstrate ECG changes [1,2] such as rhythm disturbances, atrioventricular (AV) block, morphological alterations, and repolarization abnormalities (➲ Box 2.2.2.1) [3]. Sinus bradycardia may be found in the great majority of endurance athletes, and first-degree AV block may be observed in up to a third of long-distance runners [4]. These changes have been related to sinus automaticity and AV node conduction alterations that are linked to intrinsic physiology [5] as well as to higher parasympathetic activity (➲ Box 2.2.2.2) [1].

Isolated voltage criteria for left ventricular hypertrophy are common, and repolarization anomalies comprising J-point and ST-segment elevation and high amplitude T waves are also frequent, particularly in black athletes (African/Afro-Caribbean) [6]. T-wave inversion in leads V1–V4 can be normal in all athletes aged <15 years,

Box 2.2.2.2 Hints for evaluating the athlete's ECG

Further evaluation for sinus bradycardia as low as 30bpm is not recommended.

A prolonged PR interval up to 300ms should not prompt further work-up, but longer intervals should be resolved with an exercise test (the PR interval should shorten as vagal tone is withdrawn).

Wenckebach phenomenon in isolation does not require further evaluation, but an exercise test could be reassuring.

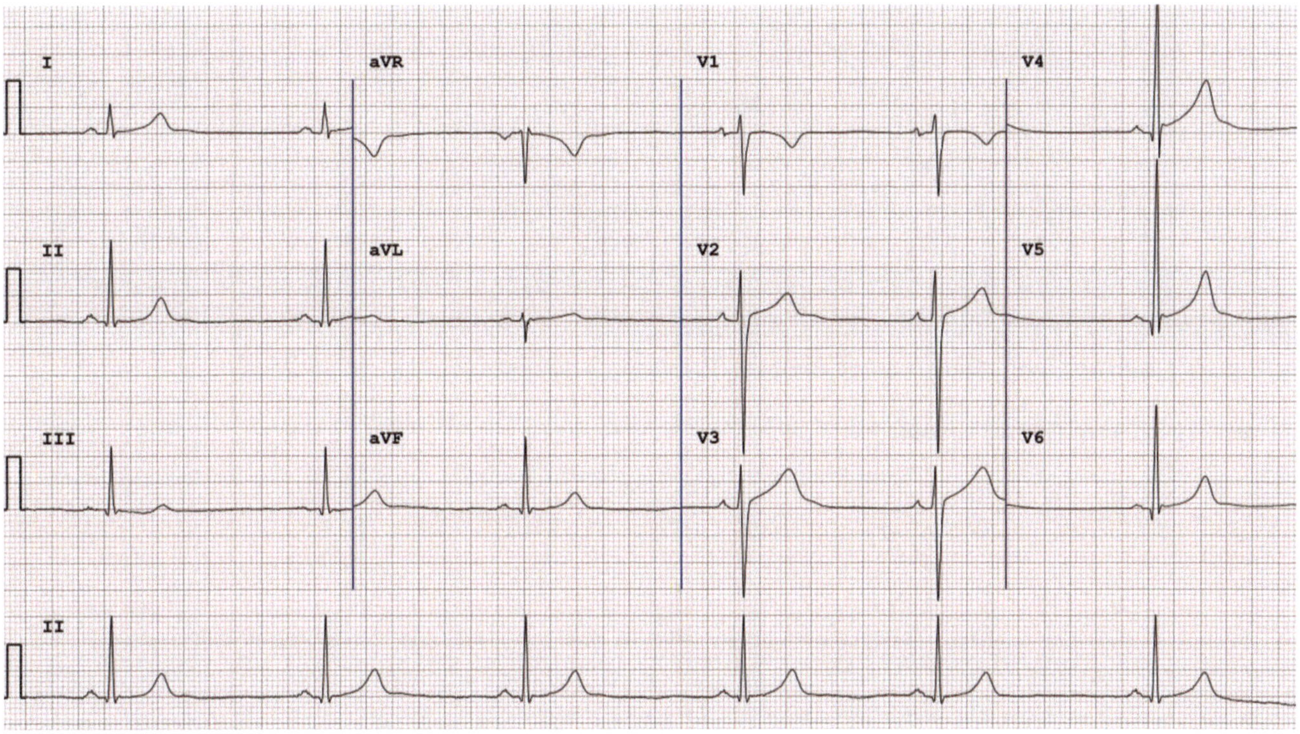

Fig. 2.2.2.1 Sinus bradycardia.

and in black athletes in particular if there is J-point and ST elevation in these leads [6].

It is important to point out that, in addition to ethnicity and age, ECG changes also depend on the athlete's gender, sporting discipline, and level of training and competition [7–9.

The effects of increasing age may modify some of the physiological adaptations at the sinus node level. In this context, resting bradycardia is more pronounced in the older athlete whose maximum heart rate is also less. This may account in part for the drop off in performance that occurs with age [4].

Sinus bradycardia

Sinus bradycardia is defined as a heart rate <60bpm and is present in up to 80% of highly trained athletes [9,10] (➔ Fig. 2.2.2.1). Resting sinus bradycardia is particularly prevalent in endurance athletes and is mainly mediated by intrinsic electrophysiological adaptations in the sinus node (decrease in sinus automaticity) and by the increased parasympathetic and reduced sympathetic input during the resting state [5].

Resting bradycardia is related to training level and may predispose to increased atrial or ventricular ectopic activity and rarely atrial fibrillation. However, sinus bradycardia is considered a normal finding in the athlete unless symptoms such as fatigue, dizziness, or syncope are present. Even heart rates ≥30bpm are considered normal in the asymptomatic athlete. Interestingly, in some cases of severe sinus bradycardia, the sinus rhythm competes with the nodal rhythm and an isorhythmic atrioventricular dissociation can be seen. However, ventricular escape rhythm is a rare finding.

Sinus arrhythmia

Sinus arrhythmia (➔ Fig. 2.2.2.2) is mediated by the pulmonary centre in the brainstem which blocks vagal activity in the lungs during inspiration in order to cause bronchodilation and facilitate breathing. There is cross-talk with the cardiac centre resulting in an increase in heart rate during inspiration [11]. Atrial stretch receptors, which respond to increased and decreased venous return during inspiration and expiration by speeding or slowing heart rate, respectively, may also be involved.

A more pronounced sinus bradycardia is typically associated with more obvious sinus arrhythmia. It is common in children and young adults. Importantly, it has been estimated that over half of well-trained endurance athletes have sinus arrhythmia [9,12]. In fact, sinus arrhythmia is a marker of a healthy well-functioning heart.

It should not be confused with sinus node dysfunction (sick sinus syndrome). In sinus arrhythmia, the P-wave axis remains normal and the fluctuation in heart rate should resolve with

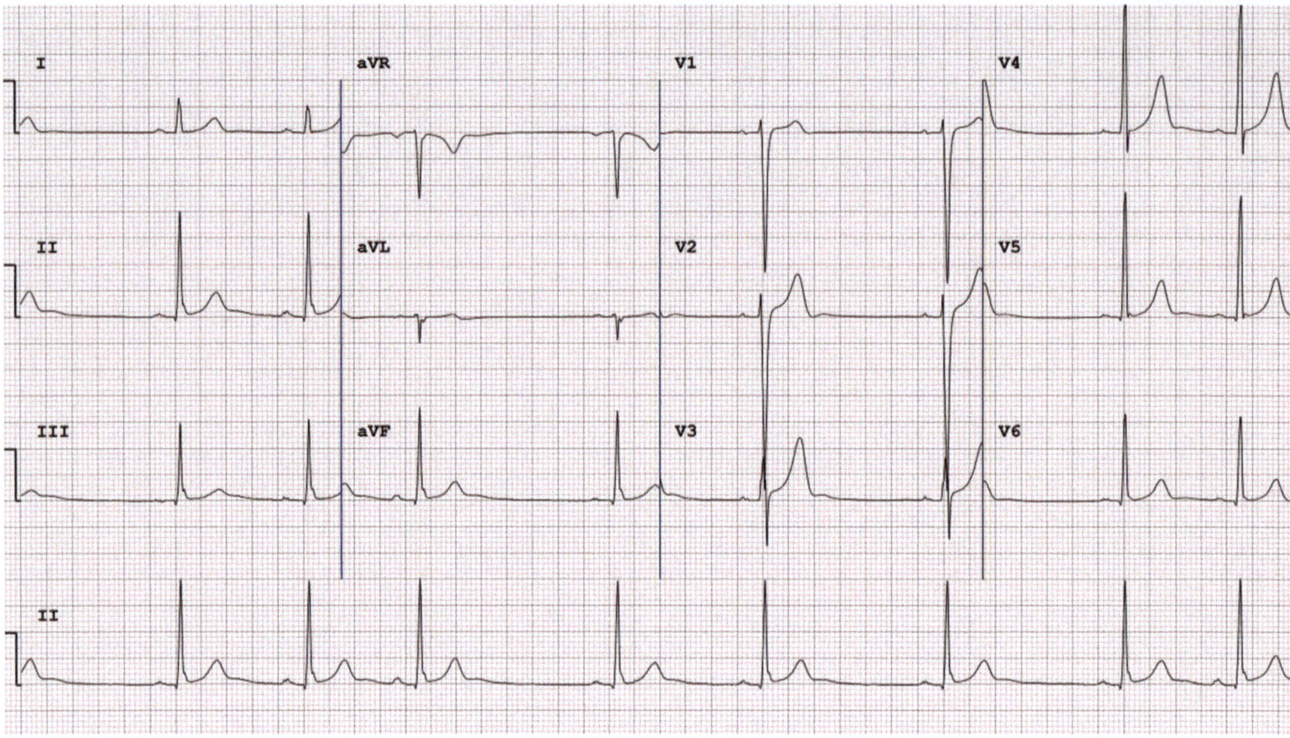

Fig. 2.2.2.2 Sinus arrhythmia.

the onset of exercise. Since sinus arrhythmia is a normal finding, it does not require any special treatment, precautions, or restrictions, and is a normal finding in an athlete. Only profound sinus bradycardia and/or marked sinus arrhythmia (heart rate less than 30bpm and/or pauses of 3s during waking hours) need to be distinguished from sinus node disease.

Sinus pauses

Sinus pauses are very frequent among athletes, with almost a third of subjects presenting pauses greater than 2s [4] (➲ Fig. 2.2.2.3). Holter monitoring captures sinus pauses in up to 25% of highly trained endurance athletes during rest. Vitasalo et al. [12] reported sinus pauses in over a third of 35 young athletes. Impressive pauses can also occur as a result of intense bursts of vagal activity. These typically occur during REM sleep, and can result in prolonged sinus node arrest (>6s) in some cases. These phenomena may occur in athletically trained individuals with slow resting heart rates. Invasive electrophysiological studies typically demonstrate normal sinus node and AV node function and normal sinus rhythm appears during exercise.

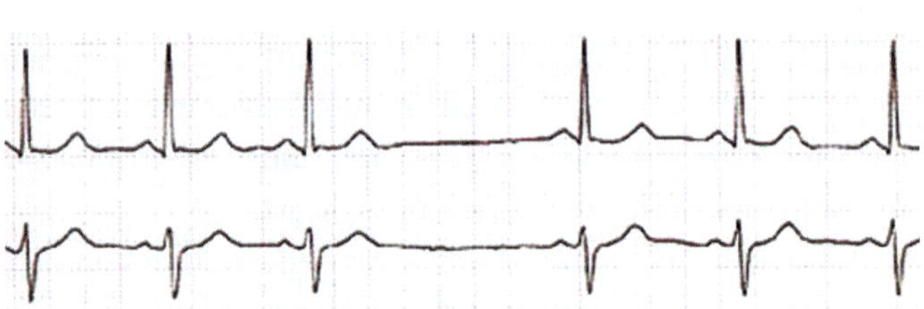

Fig. 2.2.2.3 Sinus pause.

Junctional escape rhythm

A junctional escape (nodal) rhythm occurs when the QRS rate is faster than the resting P-wave or sinus rate. It is typically slower in athletes owing to intrinsic electrophysiological adaptation and/or increased vagal tone (➲ Fig. 2.2.2.4). The R–R interval is regular in a junctional escape rhythm, and the QRS rate is usually less than 100bpm with a narrow complex (<120ms) unless the baseline QRS has a bundle branch block. A junctional escape rhythm or wandering atrial pacemaker is observed in up to 8% of all athletes under resting conditions [13]. Sinus rhythm should resume with the onset of physical activity.

Ectopic atrial rhythm

These should be considered when P waves are of different morphology from sinus P waves and their rates are typically ≤100bpm. Ectopic P waves are most easily seen when the P waves are negative in the inferior leads, i.e. a coronary sinus rhythm (➲ Fig. 2.2.2.5). Ectopic atrial rhythms occur because of a slowed resting sinus rate from intrinsic

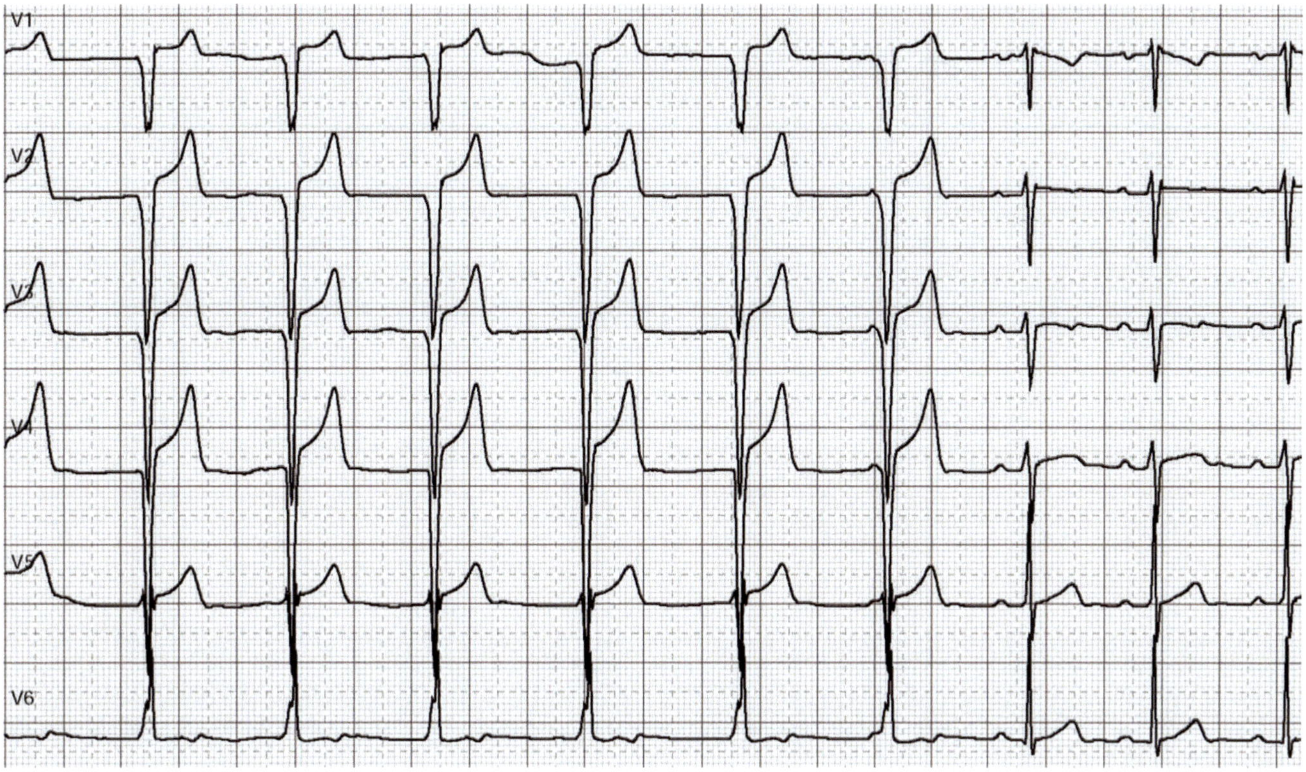

Fig. 2.2.2.4 Junctional escape rhythm.

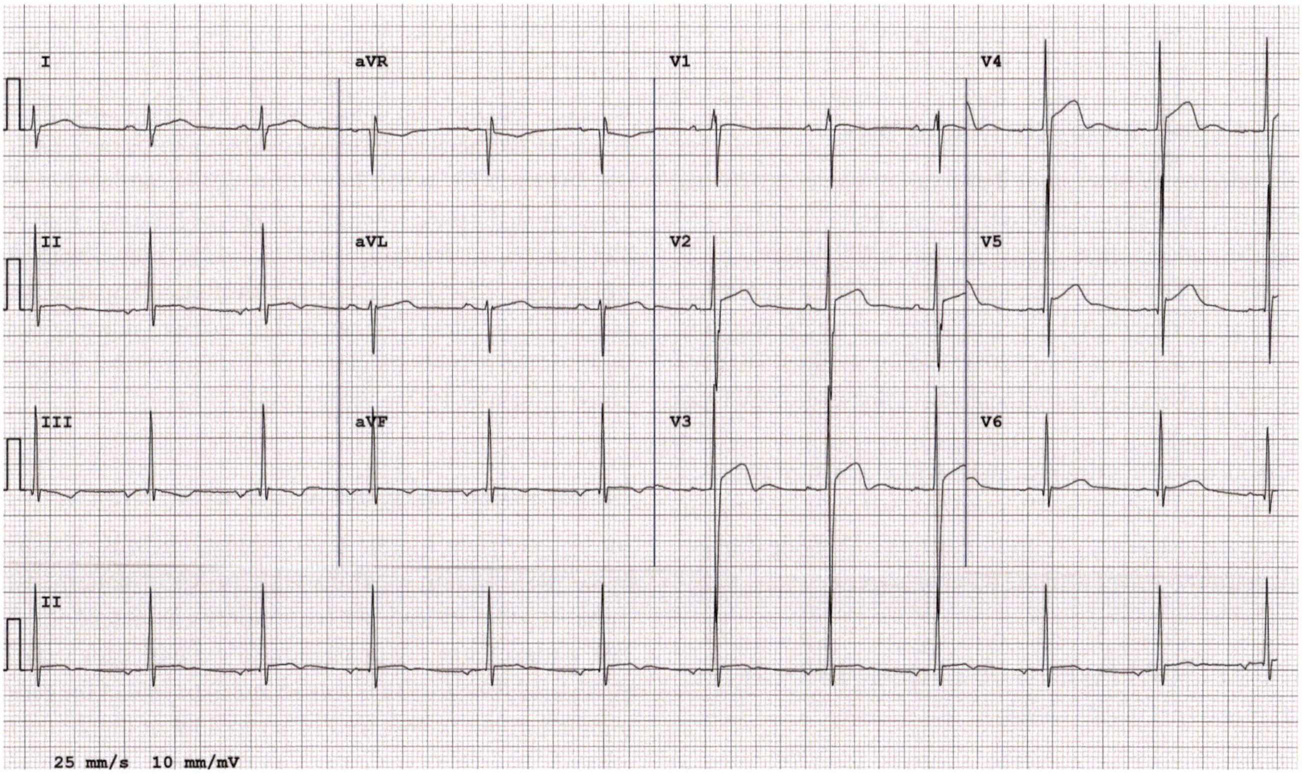

Fig. 2.2.2.5 Ectopic atrial rhythm.

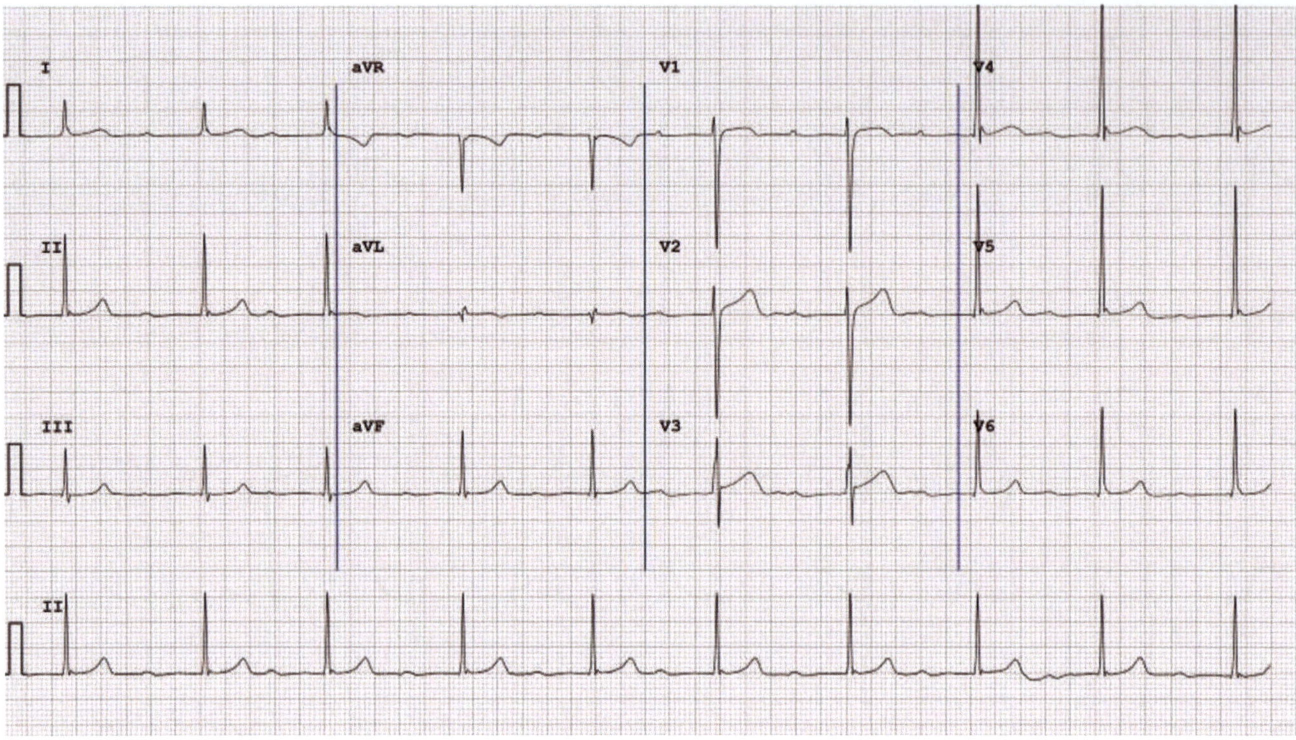

Fig. 2.2.2.6. First-degree AV block

electrophysiological adaptation and/or increased vagal tone in athletes [1,5]. The detection of more than two types of P-wave morphology on an ECG is described as a wandering atrial pacemaker, and this also occurs in athletes as a result of increased vagal tone. Normal P-wave morphology should resume with the onset of physical activity.

First-degree atrioventricular block

In first-degree AV block, the PR interval is prolonged (>200ms) but it presents the same duration on every beat (➔ Fig. 2.2.2.6). Mild to moderate first-degree AV block (PR interval up to 399ms) may be present in athletes as a result of intrinsic adaptations and/or increased parasympathetic drive. In a seminal paper analysing more than 120,000 young aviators, Hiss and Lamb [14] observed that the incidence of first-degree AV block was approximately 0.65%. In competitive endurance athletes the frequency of this finding can be as high as a third [9,13,15]. This represents a delay in AV nodal conduction in athletes due to increased vagal activity and/or intrinsic AV node changes, and typically resolves with the onset of exercise.

Mobitz type I (Wenckebach) second-degree atrioventricular block

In Mobitz type I second-degree AV block the PR interval progressively lengthens from beat to beat until there is a non-conducted P wave with no QRS complex (➔ Fig. 2.2.2.7). The first PR interval after the dropped beat is shorter than the last conducted. Even if the PR interval can be augmented by increased vagal tone, the occurrence of AV blocks depends mostly on individual susceptibility.

Mobitz type I second-degree AV block occurred in 10% of a sample of 25 Japanese marathon runners, and the finding was clearly dependent on training conditions and occurred only at rest [15]. On the other hand, Meytes et al. [16] found the incidence in another 126 endurance athletes to be only 2.4% on the resting ECG. When long-term ECG examinations were performed, the prevalence of Mobitz type I second-degree AV block increased, ranging from 15% to 22% (non-athletes control group = 2.5–6%) [11,17,18]. However, in a Spanish study of Spanish athletes (128 men and 41 women) utilizing Holter monitoring, a lower incidence of this type of AV block was noted (10.1% and 9.7%, respectively).

Incomplete right bundle branch block

Incomplete right bundle branch block (IRBBB) is defined by a QRS duration <120 ms with an RBBB pattern: a terminal R wave in lead V1 (commonly characterized as an rSR′ pattern) and a wide terminal S wave in leads I and V6 (➔ Fig. 2.2.2.8). IRBBB is seen in less than 10% of the general population but is observed in up to 40% of highly trained athletes. It occurs particularly in those engaged in endurance training and mixed sport disciplines that include both aerobic and anaerobic components [3,20,21]. IRBBB may be

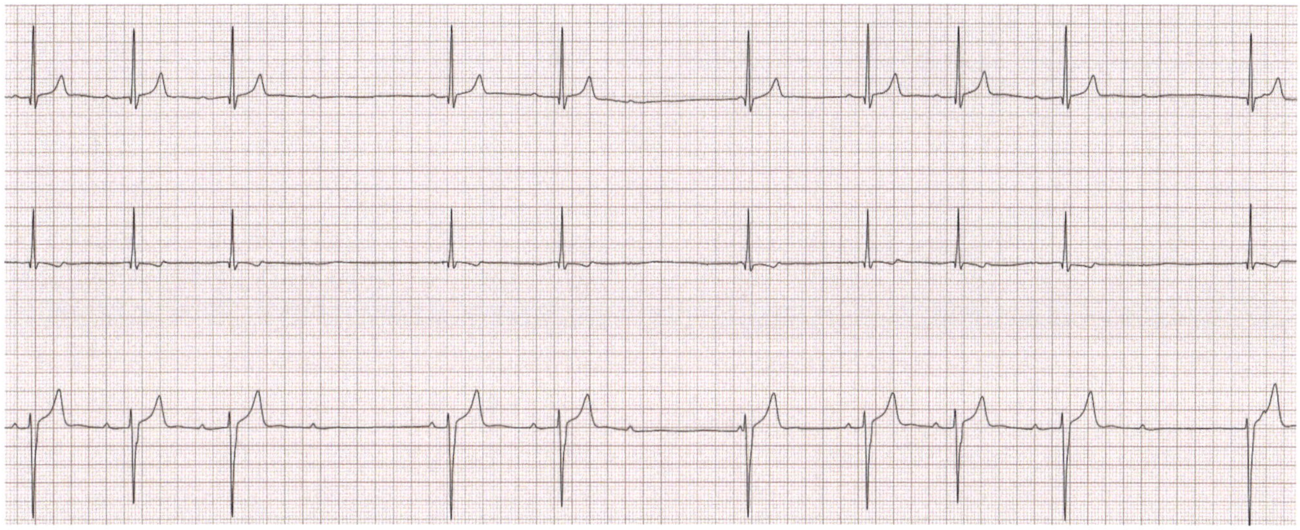

Fig. 2.2.2.7 Second-degree atrioventricular block.

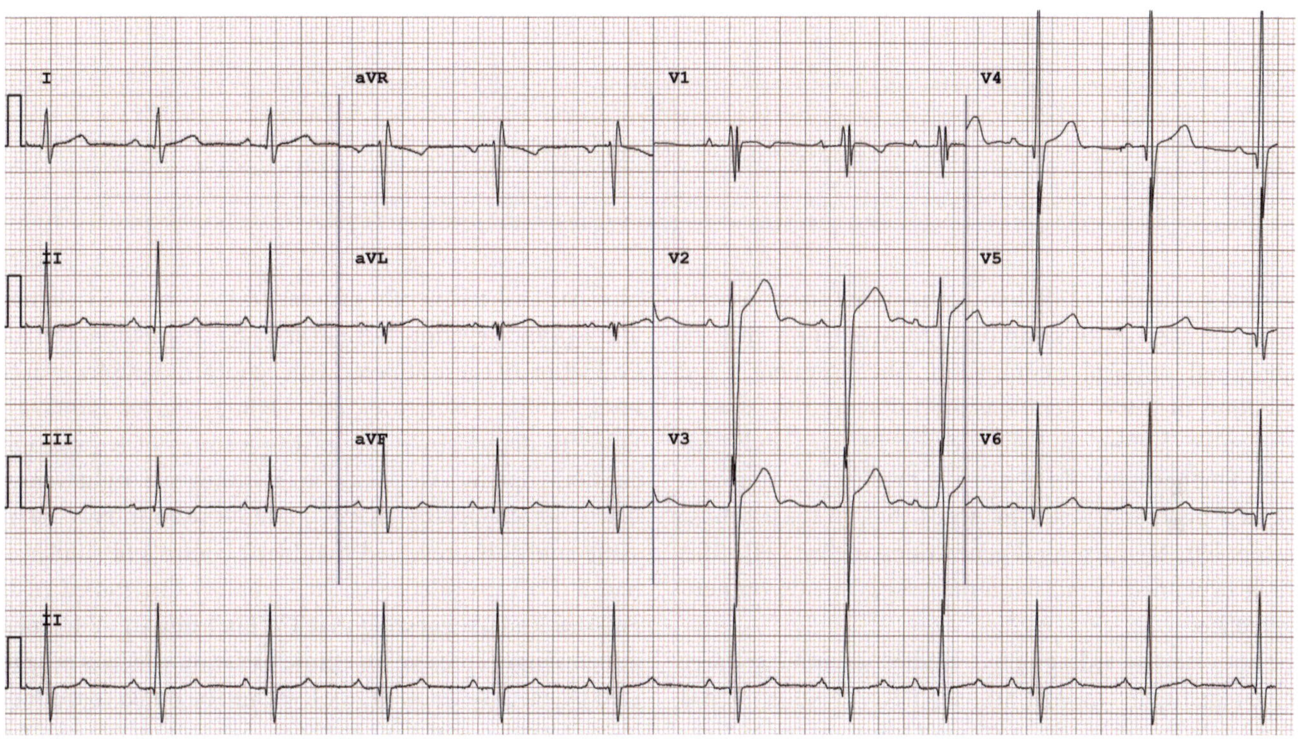

Fig. 2.2.2.8 Incomplete right bundle branch block and first-degree AV block.

related to the structural and physiological cardiac remodelling triad (right ventricle dilation, a relative reduction in the right ventricle systolic function at rest, and interventricular dyssynchrony) rather than to an intrinsic delay within the His–Purkinje system [22]. The occurrence of IRBBB in an asymptomatic athlete with a negative family history and physical examination does not require further evaluation. In the absence of other ECG abnormalities, symptoms, or a cardiac murmur suggestive of an intracardiac shunt, no further investigation is required.

Convex ST-segment elevation combined with T-wave inversion in leads V1–V4 in black/African athletes

Participation in regular intensive exercise can be associated with repolarization changes affecting the ST-segment and T-wave morphology. It is suggested that T-wave inversion (TWI) preceded by convex ST-segment elevation in leads V1–V4 (➲ Fig. 2.2.2.9) is a common phenomenon in Black/African athletes and, according to the most recent published

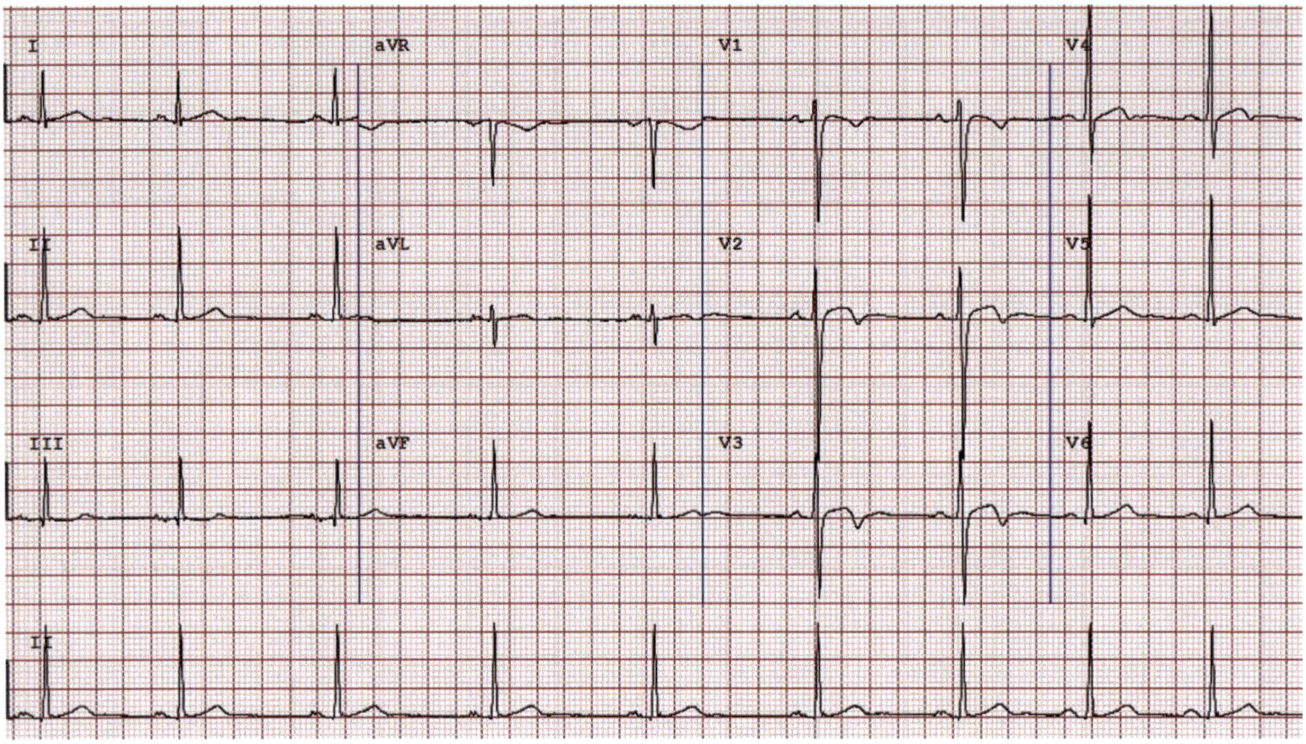

Fig. 2.2.2.9 Convex ST-segment elevation (domed) combined with T-wave inversion in leads V1–V4.

consensus guidelines [23], does not require further assessment in the absence of symptoms, positive family history, or abnormal physical examination. The prevalence and distribution of these alterations are influenced by several demographic factors including ethnicity, age, and gender [7]. Furthermore, the pattern is much more common in athletes born and raised in Africa than in those whose ancestors left Africa several generations earlier [24]. This could be explained by racial intermarriages or environmental influence.

Specific electrocardiographic studies examining large numbers of highly trained athletes have demonstrated a TWI prevalence up to 4% in young Caucasian individuals [13]. We have seen the pattern in white twin athletes with a black great-grandparent who came directly from Africa; the pattern disappeared with detraining. In contrast, 12% or more of black athletes born and raised in Africa can demonstrate a repolarization variant consisting of convex ST-segment elevation in the anterior leads (V1–V4) followed by TWI (dome-shaped) [6,9].

Examination of 904 black athletes and 1819 white athletes aged 14–35 years participating in 22 different sporting disciplines revealed that the presence of TWI in up to 25% of the athletes, half of whom exhibited deep TWI (-0.2 mV)[6]. TWI in leads V1–V4 was usually asymmetric or biphasic and frequently proceeded by convex ST-segment and J-point elevation, but never by ST depression. Detailed evaluation of these athletes with echocardiography, exercise tests, cardiac resonance, and 24 hour Holter monitoring failed to demonstrate any of the features of hypertrophic cardiomyopathy (HCM) or arrhythmogenic right ventricular cardiomyopathy (ARVC) after 7 years follow-up. The same study also revealed that black controls of similar age had a TWI prevalence of 10%, mainly distributed in the anterior leads, suggesting that TWI in leads V1–V4 in black athletes may represent an ethnic variation which is exaggerated by exercise training [6]. It should be noted that a much lower prevalence of TWI has been seen in American athletes of all ethnicities [25,26] This leaves the possibility that TWI in athletes in other countries than those considered by our UK colleagues may be due to cardiomyopathies rather than being a 'normal' finding.

Isolated QRS voltage criteria for left ventricular hypertrophy

ECGs with increased QRS amplitudes considered to be consistent with left ventricular hypertrophy (LVH) are very prevalent. This pattern is present in up to 45% of athletes (particularly endurance runners) and 25% of sedentary

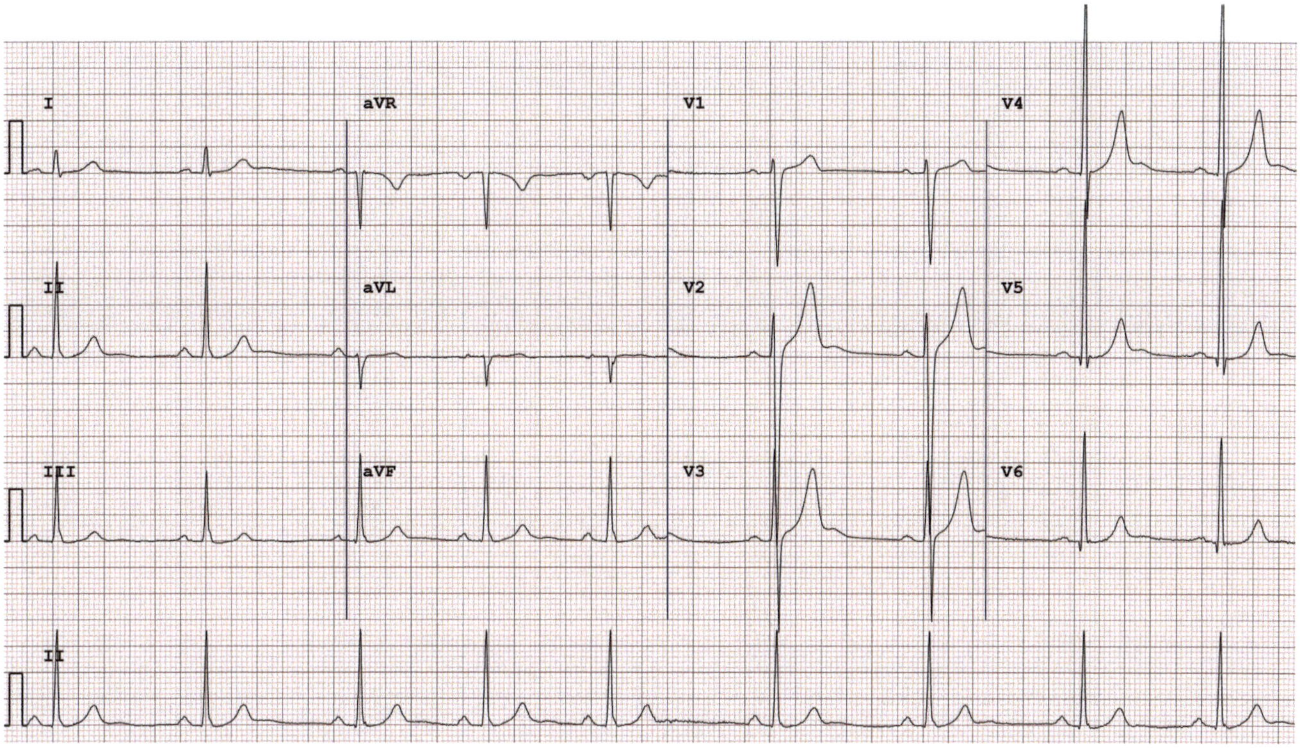

Fig. 2.2.2.10 Voltage criteria for LVH in a cross-country runner with a normal echocardiogram.

young adults [3,13]. In fact, these changes constitute physiological LVH in trained athletes and usually manifest as an isolated increase in QRS amplitude. Pathological ECG LVH always exhibits other abnormalities such as ST depression, pathological Q waves, left axis deviation, left atrial abnormality, and/or TWI [27].

Several studies have evaluated athletes and young individuals with isolated increased QRS voltage using echocardiography or cardiac MRI, and none have reported any subjects with HCM [6,9,28]. Furthermore, increased QRS voltage in the absence of other ECG abnormalities is uncommon in HCM patients.

The ECG in ➲ Fig. 2.2.2.10 shows, in addition to sinus arrhythmias, an S wave in V2 (3.2mV) and an R wave in V5 (3.0mV) exceeding the 3.5mV criteria. This 20-year-old white male cross-country runner had a normal echocardiogram.

Early repolarization

Early repolarization is common in athletes (➲ Fig. 2.2.2.11), whether the classical definition using ST elevation or the more recent definition considering QRS terminal slurs and/or J waves is used [29]. Although it was proposed that the latter pattern with slurs/J waves in the inferior leads is associated with arrhythmic risk, this was not substantiated in a large clinical population [30]. The classical definition using ST elevation could result in a phenotype confused with pericarditis or acute ischaemia. The more recent definition using terminal QRS findings was also noted in patients with a very rare cause of SCD. Certain morphological features differentiate the early repolarization pattern common in athletes from that observed in patients at risk of ventricular fibrillation, including the association with other peculiarities of the athlete's ECG such as increased QRS voltages (in 76%), ST-segment elevation (in 84%), predominance in males engaged in endurance sport disciplines, and larger LV remodelling [31]. Indeed, recent reports have shown that in a medium-term follow-up period the early repolarization pattern in athletes does not convey any risk for adverse cardiac events, including sudden death or ventricular tachyarrhythmias [31].

Further reading

Corrado D, Pelliccia A, Heidbuchel H, et al. Recommendations for interpretation of 12-lead electrocardiogram in the athlete. *Eur Heart J* 2010; 31: 243–59.

Drezner JA, Ackerman MJ, Anderson J, et al. Electrocardiographic interpretation in athletes: the 'Seattle criteria'. *Br J Sports Med* 2013; 47: 122–4.

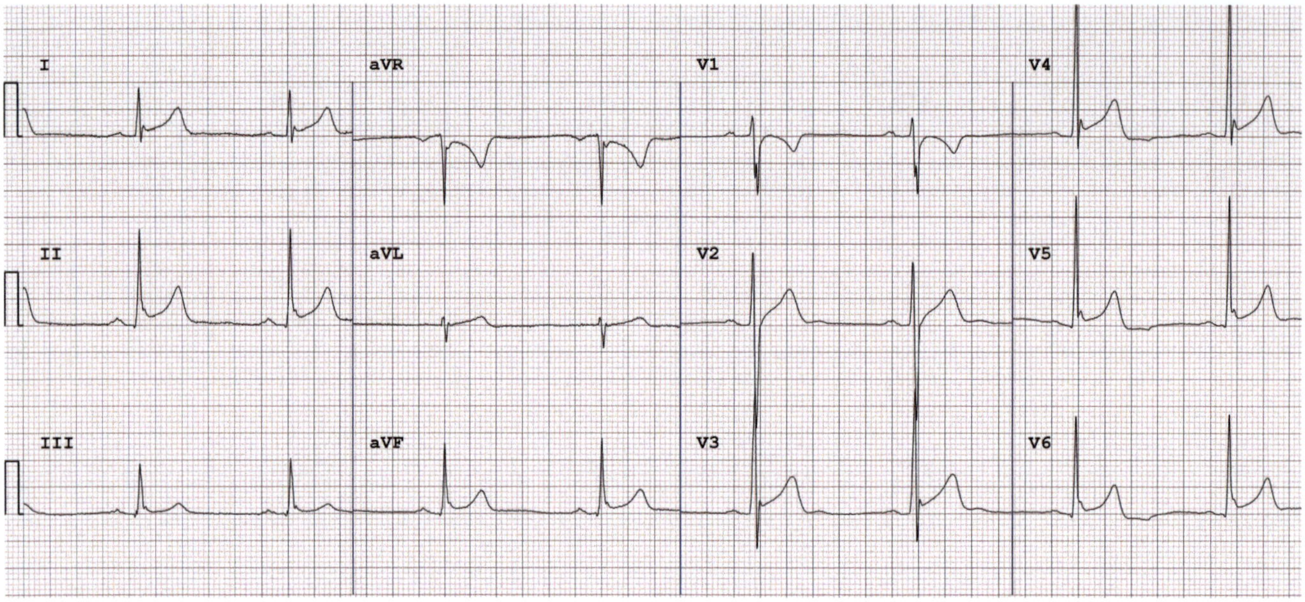

Fig. 2.2.2.11 Early repolarization.

Drezner JA, Fischbach P, Froelicher V, et al. Normal electrocardiographic findings: recognizing physiological adaptations in athletes. *Br J Sports Med* 2013;47:125–36.

Drezner JA, Sharma S, Baggish A, et al. International criteria for electrocardiographic interpretation in athletes. Consensus statement. *Br J Sports Med* 2017; 51(9): 704–31.

Froelicher V, Wagner G. The ECG and the pre-participation examination of young athletes. *J Electrocardiol* 2015; 48: 281–2.

Perez M, Fonda H, Le VV, et al. Adding an electrocardiogram to the pre-participation examination in competitive athletes: a systematic review. *Curr Probl Cardiol* 2009; 34: 586–662.

Uberoi A, Stein R, Perez MV, et al. Interpretation of the electrocardiogram of young athletes. *Circulation* 2011; 124: 746–57.

References

1. Huston TP, Puffer JC, Rodney WM. The athletic heart syndrome. *N Engl J Med* 1985; 313: 24–32.
2. Holly RG, Shaffrath JD, Amsterdam EA. Electrocardiographic alterations associated with the hearts of athletes. *Sports Med* 1998; 25: 139–48.
3. Pelliccia A, Culasso F, Di Paolo FM, et al. Prevalence of abnormal electrocardiograms in a large, unselected population undergoing pre-participation cardiovascular screening. *Eur Heart J* 2007; 28: 2006–10.
4. Zehender M, Meinertz T, Keul J, Just H. ECG variants and cardiac arrhythmias in athletes: clinical relevance and prognostic importance. *Am Heart J* 1990; 6: 1378–90.
5. Stein R, Medeiros CM, Rosito GA, et al. Intrinsic sinus and atrioventricular node electrophysiologic adaptations in endurance athletes. *J Am Coll Cardiol* 2002; 39: 1033–8.
6. Papadakis M, Carré F, Kervio G, et al. The prevalence, distribution, and clinical outcomes of electrocardiographic repolarization patterns in male athletes of African/Afro-Caribbean origin. *Eur Heart J* 2011; 32: 2304–13.
7. Sharma S. Athlete's heart: effect of age, sex, ethnicity and sporting discipline. *Exp Physiol* 2003; 88: 665–9.
8. Wilson MG, Chatard JC, Carré F, et al. Prevalence of electrocardiographic abnormalities in West-Asian and African male athletes. *Br J Sports Med* 2011;46:341–7.
9. Sharma S, Whyte G, Elliott P, et al. Electrocardiographic changes in 1000 highly trained junior elite athletes. *Br J Sports Med* 1999; 33: 319–24.
10. Hammond HK, Froelicher VF. Normal and abnormal heart rate responses to exercise. *Prog Cardiovasc Dis* 1985; 27: 271–96.
11. Freeman JV, Dewey FE, Hadley DM, et al. Autonomic nervous system interaction with the cardiovascular system during exercise. *Prog Cardiovasc Dis* 2006; 48: 342–62.
12. Vitasalo MT, Kala R, Eisalo A. Ambulatory electrocardiographic findings in young athletes between 14 and 16 years of age. *Eur Heart J* 1984; 5: 2–6.
13. Papadakis M, Basavarajaiah S, Rawlins J, et al. Prevalence and significance of T-wave inversions in predominantly Caucasian adolescent athletes. *Eur Heart J* 2009; 30: 1728–35.
14. Hiss RG, Lamb LE. Electrocardiographic findings in 122,043 individuals. *Circulation* 1962; 25: 947–61.
15. Nakamoto K. Electrocardiograms of 25 marathon runners before and after 100 meter dash. *Jpn Circ J* 1969; 33: 105–28.
16. Meytes I, Kaplinsky E, Yahini JH, et al. Wenckebach A-V block: a frequent feature following heavy physical training. *Am Heart J* 1975; 90: 426–30.
17. Hanne-Paparo N, Kellermann JJ. Long-term Holter ECG monitoring of athletes. *Med Sci Sports Exerc* 1981; 13: 294–8.
18. Talan DA, Bauernfeind RA, Ashley WW et al. Twenty-four hour continuous ECG recordings in long distance runners. *Chest* 1982; 19: 24–32.

19. Boraita A, Serratosa L, Antón P, et al. Las arritmias del deportista. *Rev Lat Cardiol* 1996; 17: 124–31.
20. Moore EN, Boineau JP, Patterson DF. Incomplete right bundle-branch block: an electrocardiographic enigma and possible misnomer. *Circulation* 1971; 44: 678–87.
21. Fagard R, Aubert A, Lysens R, et al. Noninvasive assessment of seasonal variations in cardiac structure and function in cyclists. *Circulation* 1983; 67: 896–901.
22. Kim JH, Noseworthy PA, McCarty D, et al. Significance of electrocardiographic right bundle branch block in trained athletes. *Am J Cardiol* 2011; 107: 1083–9.
23. Drezner JA, Ackerman MJ, Anderson J, et al. Electrocardiographic interpretation in athletes: the 'Seattle criteria'. *Br J Sports Med* 2013; 47: 122–4.
24. Stein R, Garcia M, Araújo CGS, et al. Do T wave inversions in athletes of African ancestry disappear over generations after migration? *Arq Bras Cardiol* 2012; 99(Suppl 1): 166.
25. Magalski A, Maron BJ, Main ML, et al. Relation of race to electrocardiographic patterns in elite American football players. *J Am Coll Cardiol* 2008; 51: 2250–55.
26. Pickham D, Zarafshar S, Sani D, et al. Comparison of three ECG criteria for athlete pre-participation screening. *J Electrocardiol* 2014; 47: 769–74.
27. Singla V, Jindal A, Pargaonkar V, et al. Examining QRS amplitude criteria for electrocardiographic left ventricular hypertrophy in recommendations for screening criteria in athletes. *J Electrocardiol* 2015; 48: 368–72.
28. Weiner RB, Hutter AM, Wang F, et al. Performance of the 2010 European Society of Cardiology criteria for ECG interpretation in the athlete. *Heart* 2011; 97: 1573–7.
29. Muramoto D, Yong CM, Singh N, et al. Patterns and prognosis of all components of the J-wave pattern in multiethnic athletes and ambulatory patients. *Am Heart J* 2014; 167: 259–66.
30. Pargaonkar VS, Perez MV, Jinda A, et al. Long-term prognosis of early repolarization with J-wave and QRS slur patterns on the resting electrocardiogram: a cohort study. *Ann Intern Med* 2015; 163: 747–55.
31. Quattrini FM, Pelliccia A, Assorgi R, et al. Benign clinical significance of J-wave pattern (early repolarization) in highly trained athletes. *Heart Rhythm* 2014; 11(11): 1974–82.

2.2.3 Overlap ECG patterns in the athlete's heart and cardiomyopathies

Harshil Dhutia and Michael Papadakis

Introduction

Individuals who engage in regular intensive exercise develop a constellation of physiological alterations in autonomic tone, cardiac structure, and cardiac function, collectively referred as 'the athlete's heart'. Fundamental to the interpretation of an athlete's electrocardiogram (ECG) is a clear understanding of the phenotypes that reflect cardiac adaptation to exercise and those which are likely to indicate quiescent cardiac pathology. Occasionally, however, ECG changes in athletes overlap with those considered characteristic of cardiomyopathies, one of the leading causes of exercise-related sudden cardiac death (SCD) in young athletes. In such cases, multimodal algorithms including cardiac imaging, exercise testing, prolonged ECG monitoring, reassessment after a period of detraining, familial evaluation, and genetic testing may be useful in facilitating the differentiation between cardiac physiology and pathology.

This chapter outlines the ECG phenotypes that are likely to cause a diagnostic conundrum in clinical practice, attempts to delineate the size of the problem for individual cardiomyopathies, and provides practical algorithms relating to which ECG abnormalities should prompt comprehensive evaluation (➲ Fig. 2.2.3.1).

T-wave inversions

T-wave inversions (TWIs) are the hallmark of primary cardiomyopathies with certain patterns being indicative of specific conditions. However, it is not uncommon to see TWIs in athletes. Differentiating physiological TWIs from those suggestive of pathology may be challenging, especially in the context of concomitant left or right ventricular dilatation, left ventricular hypertrophy, or left ventricular trabeculations which are commonly present in athletes. The interpretation of such ECG phenotypes should be guided by the distribution of the TWIs, concurrent ECG changes, and the demographic characteristics of the athlete.

Anterior T-wave inversions

Anterior TWIs are detected in 2–4% of patients with hypertrophic cardiomyopathy (HCM), but may be present in as many as 80% of patients with arrhythmogenic right ventricular cardiomyopathy (ARVC) and constitute a major diagnostic criterion for ARVC [1–4]. However, anterior TWIs are also observed on the ECGs of healthy athletes and can be a marker of physiological adaptation to exercise (➲ Fig. 2.2.3.2). TWIs in leads V1–V4 are considered part of the 'black athlete's heart' and should not result in further investigations in the absence of other clinical or ECG features of cardiomyopathy. Papadakis et al. [1] demonstrated that up to 13% of male black athletes exhibited isolated TWI in leads V1–V4, commonly preceded by convex ST-segment elevation

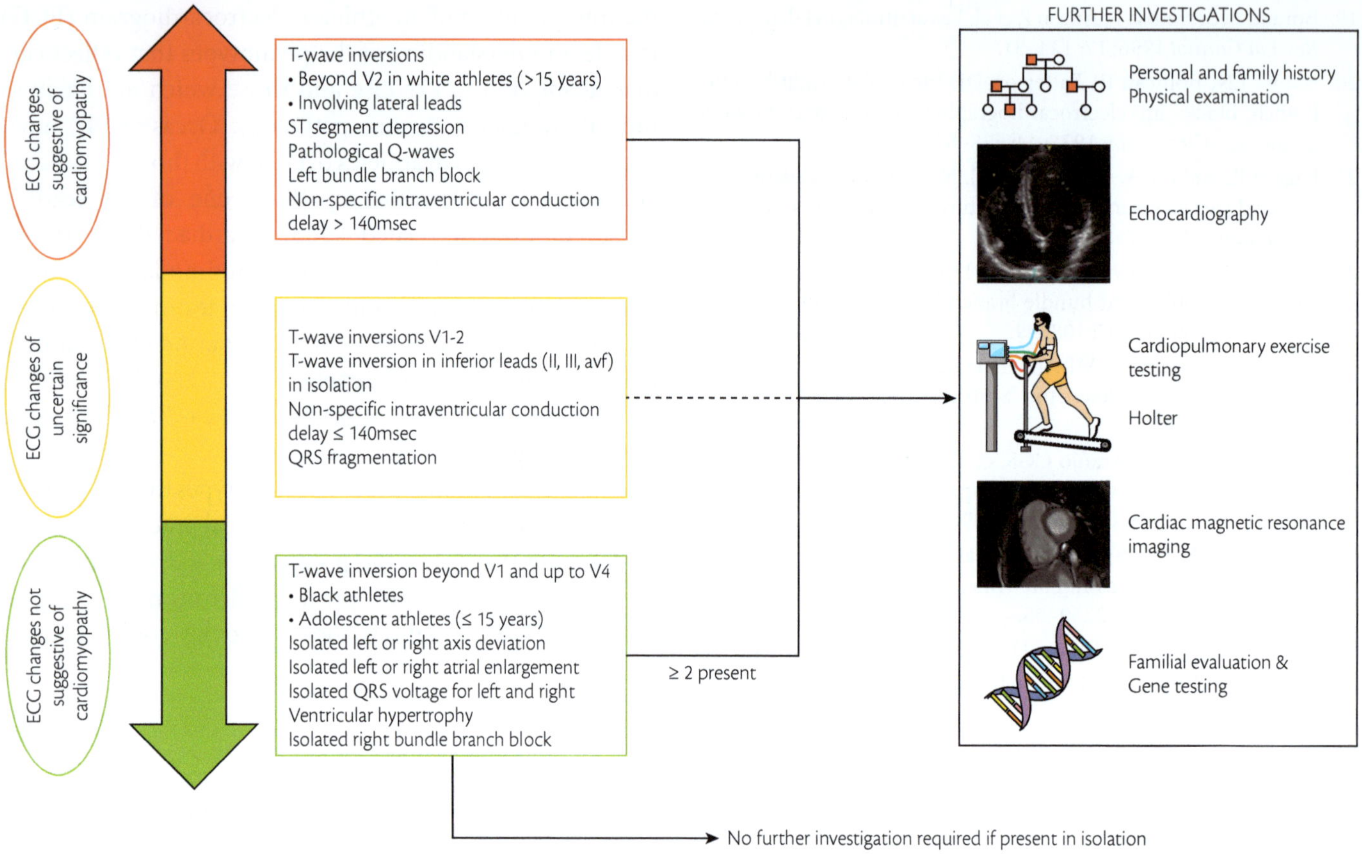

Fig. 2.2.3.1 Algorithm for differentiating ECG changes that are physiological and do not warrant further investigation from those that are indicative of cardiomyopathy and always warrant further investigation. The armamentarium of investigations includes transthoracic echocardiogram, cardiac magnetic resonance imaging, cardiopulmonary exercise testing, prolonged ECG monitoring (Holter), familial evaluation, genetic testing, and detraining.

Fig. 2.2.3.2 Schematic representation of the ECG overlap zone between athletes and ARVC in individuals with anterior TWIs. The figure demonstrates the ECG and other features that would point towards a diagnosis of physiology or pathology, respectively [1,13,14]. BA, black athlete; ETT, exercise tolerance test; LGE, late gadolinium enhancement; LVEDD, left ventricular end diastolic diameter; LVEDV, left ventricular end diastolic volume; LVH, left ventricular hypertrophy; NSVT, non-sustained ventricular tachycardia; RVD1, right ventricle basal diameter; RVEDV, right ventricular end diastolic volume; RVFAC, right ventricular fractional area change; RVH, right ventricular hypertrophy; RV RWMA, right ventricular regional wall motion abnormalities; SAECG, signal average ECG; TWI, T-wave inversion; VE, ventricular ectopy; VT, ventricular tachycardia; WA, white athlete.

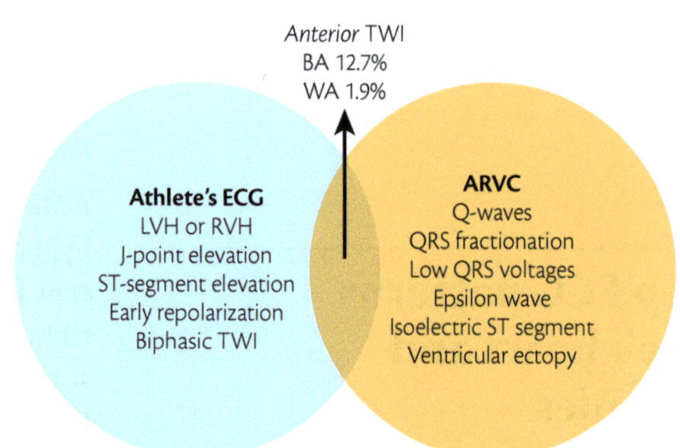

Clinical history	Asymptomatic, No family history	Symptoms, Positive family history
Echocardiography	Symmetrical chamber dilatation RVD1/LVEDD ≤0.9	RVFAC ≤ 30%
Exercise testing	-	ETT <12 minutes Increase in VE during ETT
24 hour ECG	-	>1000 VE's, NSVT/VT
Cardiac MRI	RVEDV/LVEDV ≤1.2	RVEF ≤45%, RV RWMA, LGE
Other	-	3 abnormal SAECG parameters, +ve gene test

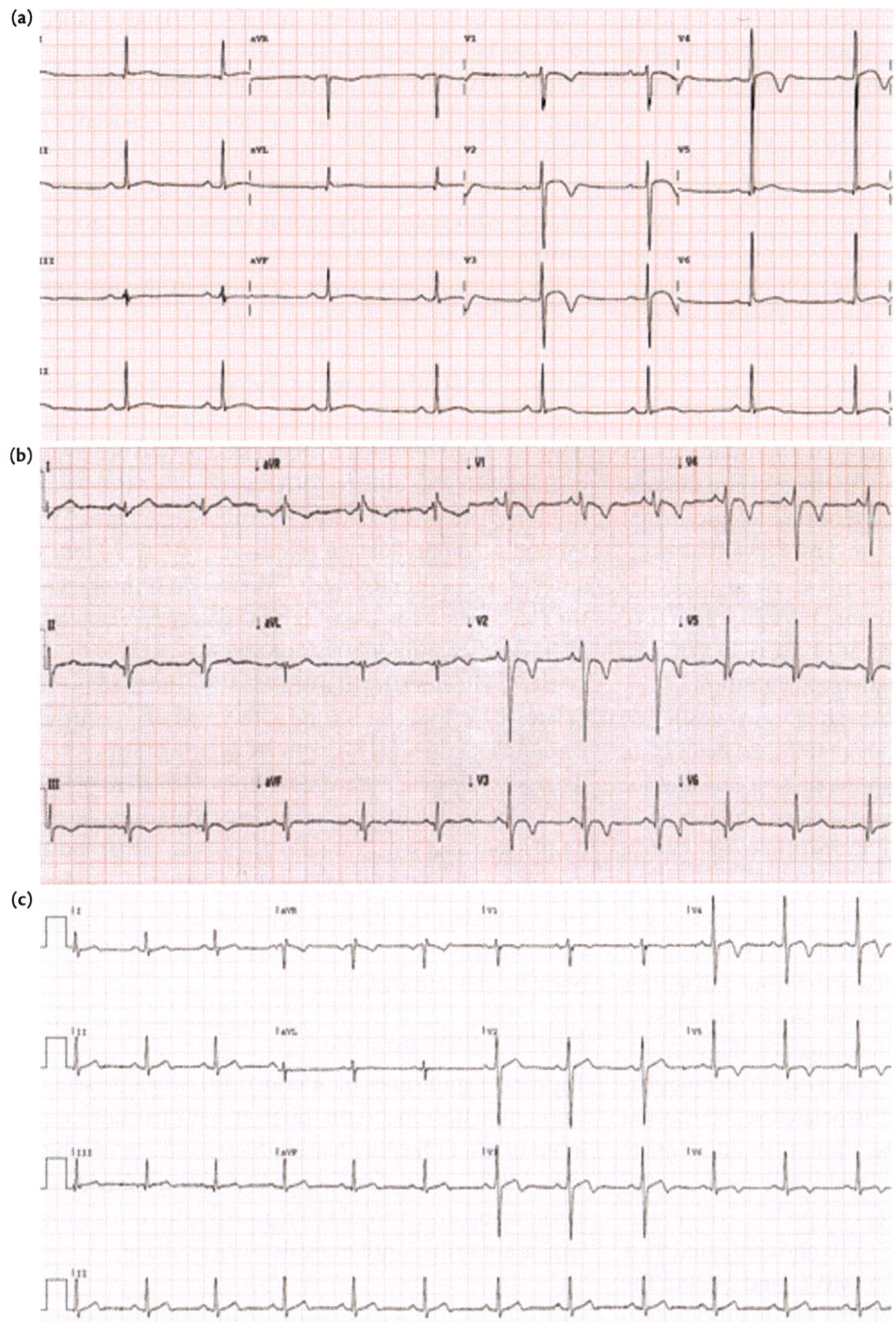

Fig. 2.2.3.3 Comparison of the distribution of TWIs and associated ECG features. (a) A healthy black athlete demonstrating TWI in leads V1–V4 preceded by J-point elevation and convex ST-segment elevation. (b) A young white athlete with ARVC demonstrating TWIs in leads V1–V4 with isoelectric J point and ST segment. There is associated right axis deviation and suspicion of epsilon wave in lead V1. (c) A young white athlete with HCM demonstrating TWIs in the anterior leads extending to the lateral leads.

(➔ Fig. 2.2.3.3(a)). None of these athletes showed symptoms or signs of cardiomyopathy despite comprehensive evaluation and a 5-year follow-up period. Similar findings have been described in female and adolescent black athletes [5,6].

Anterior TWIs have also been reported in healthy adolescent athletes [2,7]. Anterior TWIs are a normal variant in children, and gradually resolve and eventually disappear as the child goes through puberty. In the absence of symptoms, signs, or a family history of cardiac disease, TWI beyond V1 in adolescents who have yet to reach physical maturity is often termed the 'juvenile' ECG pattern. This ECG pattern is present in 2.5–4.7% of young adolescent Caucasian athletes aged <16 years and is not associated with cardiomyopathy

[2,7]. However, TWI beyond V2 is uncommon in Caucasian athletes aged ≥16 years (0.2%) or younger athletes who have reached physical maturity, and should raise suspicion of ARVC [2,7].

The significance of TWI in V1–V2 in post-pubertal Caucasian athletes is less clear. The paucity of evidence is reflected in the difference of opinion in existing recommendations [8,9]. The 2010 European Society of Cardiology (ESC) guidelines recommend investigation of post-pubertal Caucasian athletes with TWIs beyond V1. However, in the Seattle criteria TWIs in leads V1–V2 are considered a normal variant for all athletes and do not warrant further investigation. TWIs in V1-V2 are highly prevalent (14–28%) in athletes competing in high endurance sports [10,11]. These changes in endurance athletes were thought to possibly reflect the higher degree of physiological right ventricular remodelling. However, in a recent cardiac magnetic resonance (CMR) study of healthy endurance athletes the increased prevalence of anterior TWI in endurance athletes reflected lateral displacement of the right ventricle rather than right ventricular dilatation or hypertrophy [12].

At present, anterior TWIs remain a major diagnostic criterion for ARVC in the general population [4]. Zaidi et al. [13] demonstrated that, in athletes, the presence of anterior TWIs alone did not discriminate between patients with ARVC and healthy athletes with TWIs. They reported as ECG markers of physiology the presence of J-point elevation, early repolarization, biphasic TWIs, and the presence of voltage criteria for left or right ventricular hypertrophy. On the contrary, ECG features more likely to favour a diagnosis ARVC included TWIs preceded by an isoelectric ST segment and the presence of low QRS voltages (➲ Figs 2.2.3.2, 2.2.3.3(a), and 2.2.3.3(b)). Calore et al. [14] further emphasized the importance of assessing associated repolarization parameters, and in particular the J point, to differentiate between physiological adaptation and cardiomyopathy in the presence of anterior TWIs. They comprehensively evaluated healthy athletes with anterior TWIs and compared their ECGs with those of patients with ARVC and HCM. The study demonstrated that the correlation of J-point elevation with TWIs limited to the anterior leads accurately differentiated athletes from patients with cardiomyopathy. Although both studies are a useful addition to our understanding of the athlete's ECG, the results should be interpreted with caution, as most patients with pathology were sedentary.

Lateral T-wave inversions

Irrespective of the demographics of the athlete, there are certain TWI patterns that should always raise suspicion of underlying cardiomyopathy and prompt comprehensive evaluation. Such patterns include TWIs that affect two or more lateral leads (I, aVL, V5, V6) (➲ Fig. 2.2.3.3(c)). Lateral TWIs in individuals with cardiomyopathy commonly extend to the inferior territory and are deep (≥2mm). However, minor TWI (<2mm) should also be treated with suspicion, as there is no compelling evidence to suggest that athletes with minor TWI are at lower risk of harbouring a cardiomyopathy.

Even if pathology is not identified in the first instance, subsequent surveillance is prudent with repeat evaluation annually, or sooner if the athlete becomes symptomatic. In a study of 12,550 athletes referred for pre-participation screening, Pelliccia et al. [15] evaluated 81 athletes with widespread deep TWI and followed them up for a period of 12 years. All of the 29 (0.2%) athletes diagnosed with cardiomyopathy exhibited lateral TWI. More recently, Schnell et al. [16] performed a comprehensive evaluation of 155 asymptomatic athletes who exhibited deep TWI in two or more leads. Of the 155 athletes, 137 (88%) exhibited deep TWI affecting the lateral leads, commonly ($n = 100$; 65%) present in the inferolateral territories (II, III, aVF, V5, V6). The high prevalence of lateral TWI was associated with a high diagnostic yield of cardiomyopathies (41%), with HCM being the predominant diagnosis. Despite echocardiography identifying pathology in more than half of these cases (36 of 63 cardiomyopathies), CMR identified an additional 21 cases of athletes with disease where ECHO was reported as normal or inconclusive. On this basis, the authors recommended that CMR must be considered as routine in athletes presenting with TWIs with normal echocardiography.

Inferior T-wave inversions

The exact significance of inferior TWI, when present in isolation, remains uncertain. Inferior TWI has been reported in up to 6% of healthy black athletes and 2% of white athletes, but is also occasionally observed in individuals with cardiomyopathy. It would be reasonable to consider this pattern as abnormal until more data are available.

ST-segment changes

Assessment of the ST segment is also useful when assessing an athlete's ECG, especially when they precede TWIs. ST-segment elevation is not a good discriminator between physiology and pathology as it is present in the great majority (83%) of healthy athletes with TWIs [14] and 64% of athletes with HCM [17]. On the contrary, ST-segment depression is commonly observed in athletes with cardiomyopathy [17], but is rarely seen in healthy athletes and should always warrant investigation irrespective of the demographic of the athlete [1].

Pathological Q waves

Q waves are a normal component of the ECG. However, pathological Q waves are frequently present in individuals with cardiomyopathy, and in athletes are generally considered an abnormal finding warranting further evaluation [13,17–19]. The overlap between physiology and pathology stems from the lack of consensus relating to the definition of a pathological Q wave. Most criteria examine the depth and the duration of Q waves and require their presence in two or more contiguous leads, excluding aVR. A Q-wave duration ≥40ms is always pathological [17–20]. An absolute depth of >3mm is considered pathological by some [9,20], whereas others [17] recommend an amplitude ≥25% of the ensuing R wave. Although both criteria are associated with a high specificity, the latter is associated with a higher positive predictive value and therefore a lower false-positive rate. Therefore the ≥25% of the ensuing R wave rule is likely to result in a smaller number of athletes falsely identified as being at potential risk of harbouring a cardiomyopathy, resulting in a reduction of unnecessary investigations and significant cost savings [21].

Voltage criteria for ventricular hypertrophy

The ECGs of trained athletes often exhibit isolated voltage criteria for left ventricular hypertrophy (LVH) such as the Sokolow–Lyon and the Cornell criteria. Such ECG patterns are thought to reflect increased left ventricular remodelling, although they correlate poorly with left ventricular mass in young athletes. Conversely, the presence of an *isolated* QRS voltage criterion for LVH is unusual in HCM patients (<2%) in whom pathological LVH is commonly associated with additional ECG features including TWIs and ST-segment depression [22]. QRS voltage criteria for LVH are also uncommon in individuals with ARVC [13]. Therefore the presence of high QRS voltages in the absence of other ECG or clinical markers suggestive of pathology are considered part of normal and training-related ECG changes in athletes and do not require further evaluation.

The voltage criterion for RVH is also common in athletes; it is observed in 12% of healthy athletes, and is twice as common in athletes as in sedentary individuals [23]. Similar to LVH, correlation between the presence of ECG criteria for RVH and increased right ventricular wall thickness/cavity size on echocardiography is poor. Furthermore, an investigation of electrocardiographic changes in 35 patients with ARVC reported that none of the individuals demonstrated a voltage criterion for RVH in isolation [13]. Based on these reports, it is reasonable to conclude that isolated QRS voltage RVH represents part of the normal spectrum of physiological cardiac adaptations to exercise and, in the absence of other ECG or clinical markers of pathology, does not require further investigation [24].

Voltage criteria for QRS axis deviation and atrial enlargement

Left axis deviation (LAD) and left atrial enlargement (LAE) are considered by the ESC and Seattle criteria as ECG phenotypes that should prompt further comprehensive evaluation of athletes [8,9]. These recommendations are based on the fact that both LAD and LAE are a common finding in cardiomyopathies, being present in up to 12% and 44% of HCM patients, respectively. The recommendations for right axis deviation (RAD) and right atrial enlargement (RAE) are less clear. The ESC recommendations and Seattle criteria discuss these phenotypes within the context of underlying cardiac disease and suggest further evaluation. RAD can be a feature of ARVC, whilst RAE has been reported in nearly a fifth of patients with HCM. Both may be present in pulmonary hypertension.

There is, however, concern regarding the significance of these ECG anomalies in isolation in presumed healthy young athletes and the subsequent contribution to the high false-positive ECG rates in athletes. Gati et al. [25] investigated whether non-specific anomalies such as axis deviation and atrial enlargement in isolation require further assessment in highly trained young athletes. In a study of more than 2500 athletes and nearly 10,000 controls, they reported that these ECG changes in isolation failed to identify any major structural or functional cardiac abnormalities. Similarly, studies of athletes from diverse ethnic backgrounds [24,26] have demonstrated that these ECG anomalies in isolation do not correlate with quiescent cardiomyopathy and their exclusion improves the specificity of ECG as a screening tool without compromising the sensitivity to detect athletes at risk of sudden cardiac death. Based on the available evidence, the presence of voltage criteria for LAD, RAD, LAE or RAE *in isolation* should not prompt further investigations of asymptomatic athletes with no family history of cardiac disease or sudden cardiac death [24].

Interventricular conduction abnormalities and QRS fragmentation

Right bundle branch block

Association of a right bundle branch block (RBBB) pattern with a QRS duration <120ms is termed incomplete or partial RBBB. Incomplete RBBB is recognized as a training-related

ECG anomaly, and is commonly seen in healthy young athletes with a reported prevalence of 7–20% [1,27,28]. Complete RBBB is far less common, with a reported incidence ranging from 0.2% to 3% of athletes [27,29–31]. Although its clinical significance in young athletes has not yet been elucidated, Kim et al. [31] observed a positive correlation between increasing QRS duration in athletes with the RBBB pattern and increasing RV size and LV mass. They concluded that complete RBBB might be an ECG phenotype of cardiac adaptation to exercise and, in the absence of other features suggestive of disease, does not require further evaluation. However, RBBB in the presence of repolarization abnormalities (e.g. Brugada type 1 pattern, anterior TWI, and epsilon waves) should not be interpreted as a benign ECG finding and should prompt further evaluation.

Left bundle branch block

The detection of left bundle branch block (LBBB) in asymptomatic athletes is rare, with an estimated prevalence ranging between 0.1% and 0.8% [32]. On the contrary, LBBB is commonly observed in cardiomyopathies, particularly DCM, and has important prognostic implications [9,33]. In a series of 608 patients with DCM, LBBB was present in a third of the cohort (31%) at baseline ECG [33]. Another 11.2% of the same cohort developed LBBB during follow-up, and new-onset LBBB was a predictor of all-cause mortality. Based on existing literature, all individuals with LBBB should be investigated comprehensively and, even if no cardiovascular pathology is identified in the first instance, should be followed up on a long-term basis.

Non-specific intraventricular conduction delay

Non-specific intraventricular conduction delay is defined as a QRS duration of >110ms without the specific patterns of LBBB or RBBB. Its exact significance is unknown, and it can be observed in cardiomyopathies and occasionally in healthy populations and athletes. The ESC recommends further evaluation of all athletes with QRS prolongation, while the Seattle group places emphasis on athletes where the QRS duration is severely prolonged (>140ms).

QRS fragmentation

QRS fragmentation is considered to represent distortion of signal conduction and a depolarization process within ventricles associated with myocardial scar and myocardial fibrosis. QRS fragmentation in the right precordial leads (V1–V3) is very prevalent in ARVC cases and has a high diagnostic value. Peters et al. [34] analysed the ECGs of 360 ARVC patients and compared them with 52 controls. Fragmented QRS complexes were present in 85% of the patients compared with only 4% of the controls. Therefore the presence of fragmented QRS complexes in the right precordial leads may be a useful screening tool for cases highly suspicious for ARVC. The prevalence and significance of isolated QRS fragmentation in an asymptomatic athlete without a relevant family history or cardiovascular risk factors is unknown. In the presence of QRS prolongation (>110ms) further evaluation is considered prudent, while a narrow QRS complex is not deemed to warrant investigation.

Ventricular ectopy

Ventricular ectopy is occasionally seen amongst healthy athletes and is due to increased vagal tone and resting bradycardia. Biffi et al [35] reported that 2.2% of athletes had three or more ventricular premature beats (VPBs) on a standard 10s ECG. The same group also followed up 70 athletes with ventricular arrhythmias (defined as 2000 or more VPBs and/or at least one burst of non-sustained ventricular tachycardia over 24 hours) who had undergone deconditioning [36]. Sixteen of these demonstrated complete reversibility with no VPBs on follow-up ECG monitoring, and 54 demonstrated only partial or no reversibility. None of the athletes with complete resolution demonstrated evidence of cardiovascular pathology on further investigations and follow-up of 8 years. In contrast, 20 of the 54 athletes (37%) in whom arrhythmias persisted exhibited evidence of cardiac disease, namely cardiomyopathy in ten, mitral valve prolapse in six, and myocarditis in four [36]. Additionally, there is emerging evidence that genetically susceptible athletes competing in high endurance events may be prone to right ventricular arrhythmias due to exercise-induced right ventricular dysfunction [37,38]. The majority of 46 endurance athletes with complex RV arrhythmias exhibited RV structural abnormalities following RV angiography or MRI, and ~90% satisfied the diagnostic criteria for ARVC. These athletes had a perilous clinical course, with nearly 40% going on to experience a major arrhythmic event (see also Chapter 5.2)

When the clinician is faced with an athlete with ventricular ectopy, the morphology of the VPBs may provide clues relating to their aetiology. VPBs with LBBB morphology and an inferior axis (positive QRS complex in leads II, III, and aVF) indicate a right ventricular outflow tract origin consistent with idiopathic right ventricular outflow tract arrhythmia, which is a benign condition. Conversely, VPBs with an LBBB morphology and superior axis (negative QRS in leads II, III, and aVF) indicate a right ventricular free wall or apex origin and are more suggestive of ARVC. Given the overlap, it is recommended that athletes with more than one

VPB on a resting 12-lead ECG should undergo further evaluation. This includes an assessment of cardiac structure and function with an echocardiogram, and an assessment of the ectopy burden over 24-hour Holter monitoring.

Conclusion

The overlap between physiological adaptation to exercise and cardiomyopathies remains substantial, and there are still a number of unanswered questions relating to the significance of certain ECG phenotypes in young athletes. In the era of preparticipation screening, understanding which ECG patterns require further investigation is crucial to avoid unnecessary additional investigations and, more importantly, to detect athletes harbouring potentially sinister disease.

Further reading

Chandra N, Bastiaenen R, Papadakis M, Sharma S. Sudden cardiac death in young athletes: practical challenges and diagnostic dilemmas. *J Am Coll Cardiol* 2013; 61:1027–40.

Sheikh N, Sharma S. Impact of ethnicity on cardiac adaptation to exercise. Nat Rev Cardiol. 2014; 11:198–217.

References

1. Papadakis M, Carré F, Kervio G, et al. The prevalence, distribution, and clinical outcomes of electrocardiographic repolarization patterns in male athletes of African/Afro-Caribbean origin. *Eur Heart J* 2011; 32(18): 2304–13.
2. Migliore F, Zorzi A, Michieli P, et al. Prevalence of cardiomyopathy in Italian asymptomatic children with electrocardiographic T-wave inversion at preparticipation screening. *Circulation* 2012; 125: 529–38.
3. Steriotis AK, Bauce B, Daliento L, et al. Electrocardiographic pattern in arrhythmogenic right ventricular cardiomyopathy. *Am J Cardiol* 2009; 103: 1302–8.
4. Marcus FI, McKenna WJ, Sherrill D, et al. Diagnosis of arrhythmogenic right ventricular cardiomyopathy/dysplasia: proposed modification of the Task Force Criteria. *Circulation* 2010; 121: 1533–41.
5. Rawlins J, Carré F, Kervio G, et al. Ethnic differences in physiological cardiac adaptation to intense physical exercise in highly trained female athletes. *Circulation* 2010; 121: 1078–85.
6. Sheikh N, Papadakis M, Carré F, et al. Cardiac adaptation to exercise in adolescent athletes of African ethnicity: an emergent elite athletic population. *J Sports Med* 2013; 47: 585–92.
7. Papadakis M, Basavarajaiah S, Rawlins J, et al. Prevalence and significance of T-wave inversions in predominantly Caucasian adolescent athletes. *Eur Heart J* 2009; 30: 1728–35.
8. Corrado D, Pelliccia A, Heidbuchel H, et al. Recommendations for interpretation of 12-lead electrocardiogram in the athlete. *Eur Heart J* 2010; 31: 243–59.
9. Drezner JA, Ackerman MJ, Anderson J, et al. Electrocardiographic interpretation in athletes: the 'Seattle criteria'. *Br J Sports Med* 2013; 47(3): 1 22–4.
10. Wasfy MM, DeLuca J, Wang F, et al. ECG findings in competitive rowers: normative data and the prevalence of abnormalities using contemporary screening recommendations. *Br J Sports Med* 2015; 49: 200–6.
11. Brosnan M, La Gerche A, Kalman J, et al. Comparison of frequency of significant electrocardiographic abnormalities in endurance versus nonendurance athletes. *Am J Cardiol* 2014; 113(9): 1567–73.
12. Brosnan MJ, Claessen G, Heidbuchel H, et al. Right precordial T-wave inversion in healthy endurance athletes can be explained by lateral displacement of the cardiac apex. *JACC Clin Electrophysiol* 2015; 1: 84–91.
13. Zaidi A, Sheikh N, Jongman JK, et al. Clinical differentiation between physiological remodeling and arrhythmogenic right ventricular cardiomyopathy in athletes with marked electrocardiographic repolarization anomalies. *J Am Coll Cardiol* 2015; 65: 2702–11.
14. Calore C, Zorzi A, Sheikh N, et al. Electrocardiographic anterior T-wave inversion in athletes of different ethnicities: differential diagnosis between athlete's heart and cardiomyopathy. *Eur Heart J* 2016; 37: 2515–27.
15. Pelliccia A, Di Paolo FM, Quattrini FM, et al. Outcomes in athletes with marked ECG repolarization abnormalities. *N Engl J Med* 2008; 358: 152–61.
16. Schnell F, Riding N, O'Hanlon R, et al. Recognition and significance of pathological T-wave inversions in athletes. *Circulation* 2015; 131: 165–73.
17. Sheikh N, Papadakis M, Schnell F, et al. Clinical profile of athletes with hypertrophic cardiomyopathy. *Circ Cardiovasc Imaging* 2015; 8: e003454.
18. Bent RE, Wheeler MT, Hadley D, et al. Computerized Q wave dimensions in athletes and hypertrophic cardiomyopathy patients. *J Electrocardiol* 2015; 48: 362–7.
19. Thompson AJ, Cannon BC, Wackel PL, et al. Electrocardiographic abnormalities in elite high school athletes: comparison to adolescent hypertrophic cardiomyopathy. *Br J Sports Med* 2016; 50: 105–10.
20. Konno T, Shimizu M, Ino H, et al. Diagnostic value of abnormal Q waves for identification of preclinical carriers of hypertrophic cardiomyopathy based on a molecular genetic diagnosis. *Eur Heart J* 2004; 25: 246–51.
21. Prakash K, Malhotra A, Dhutia H, et al. When is a pathological Q wave truly pathological? *Circulation* 2015; 132(Suppl 3):A17015.
22. Lakdawala NK, Thune JJ, Maron BJ, et al. Electrocardiographic features of sarcomere mutation carriers with and without clinically overt hypertrophic cardiomyopathy. *Am J Cardiol* 2011; 108: 1606–13.
23. Zaidi A, Ghani S, Sheikh N, et al. Clinical significance of electrocardiographic right ventricular hypertrophy in athletes: comparison with arrhythmogenic right ventricular cardiomyopathy and pulmonary hypertension. *Eur Heart J* 2013; 34: 3649 56.
24. Sheikh N, Papadakis M, Ghani S, et al. Comparison of electrocardiographic criteria for the detection of cardiac abnormalities in elite black and white athletes. *Circulation* 2014; 129: 1637–49.
25. Gati S, Sheikh N, Ghani S, et al. Should axis deviation or atrial enlargement be categorised as abnormal in young athletes? The athlete's electrocardiogram: time for re-appraisal of markers of pathology. *Eur Heart J* 2013; 34: 3641–8.

26. Riding NR, Sheikh N, Adamuz C, et al. Comparison of three current sets of electrocardiographic interpretation criteria for use in screening athletes. *Heart* 2014; 101: 384–90.
27. Chandra N, Bastiaenen R, Papadakis M, et al. Prevalence of electrocardiographic anomalies in young individuals: relevance to a nationwide cardiac screening program. *J Am Coll Cardiol* 2014; 63: 2028–34.
28. Pelliccia A, Culasso F, Di Paolo FM, et al. Prevalence of abnormal electrocardiograms in a large, unselected population undergoing pre-participation cardiovascular screening. *Eur Heart J* 2007; 28: 2006–10.
29. Pelliccia A, Maron BJ, Culasso F, et al. Clinical significance of abnormal electrocardiographic patterns in trained athletes. *Circulation* 2000; 102: 278–84.
30. Baggish AL, Hutter AM Jr, Wang F, et al. Cardiovascular screening in college athletes with and without electrocardiography: a cross-sectional study. *Ann Intern Med* 2010; 152: 269–75.
31. Kim JH, Noseworthy PA, McCarty D, et al. Significance of electrocardiographic right bundle branch block in trained athletes. *Am J Cardiol* 2011; 107: 1083–9.
32. Kim JH, Baggish AL. Electrocardiographic right and left bundle branch block patterns in athletes: prevalence, pathology, and clinical significance. *J Electrocardiol* 2015; 48: 380–4.
33. Aleksova A, Carriere C, Zecchin M, et al. New-onset left bundle branch block independently predicts long-term mortality in patients with idiopathic dilated cardiomyopathy: data from the Trieste Heart Muscle Disease Registry. *Europace* 2014; 16: 1450–9.
34. Peters S, Trümmel M, Koehler B. QRS fragmentation in standard ECG as a diagnostic marker of arrhythmogenic right ventricular dysplasia–cardiomyopathy. *Heart Rhythm* 2008; 5: 1417–21.
35. Biffi A, Pelliccia A, Verdile L, et al. Long-term clinical significance of frequent and complex ventricular tachyarrhythmias in trained athletes. *J Am Coll Cardiol* 2002; 40: 446–52.
36. Biffi A, Maron BJ, Verdile L, et al. Impact of physical deconditioning on ventricular tachyarrhythmias in trained athletes. *J Am Coll Cardiol* 2004; 44: 1053–8.
37. Heidbüchel H, Hoogsteen J, Fagard R, et al. High prevalence of right ventricular involvement in endurance athletes with ventricular arrhythmias: role of an electrophysiologic study in risk stratification. *Eur Heart J* 2003; 24: 1473–80.
38. Heidbüchel H, Prior DL, Gerche AL. Ventricular arrhythmias associated with long-term endurance sports: what is the evidence? *Br J Sports Med* 2012; 46(Suppl 1): i44–50.

SECTION 3

Additional testing in the evaluation of the athlete's heart

3.1 Exercise testing *87*

3.1.1 Protocols of exercise testing in athletes and cardiopulmonary testing: assessment of fitness *87*
Marco Guazzi and Paolo Emilio Adami

3.1.2 Evaluation of ischaemia, blood pressure, QT interval, and arrhythmias *98*
Frédéric Schnell and François Carré

3.2 Arrhythmia registration *107*

3.2.1 Ambulatory (24-hour Holter monitoring, event recorders) and signal-averaged ECG for arrhythmia registration in the athlete's heart *107*
Mahdi Sareban and Josef Niebauer

3.2.2 Class 1 anti-arrhythmic drug provocation test *114*
Matthias Antz

3.2.3 Electrophysiological study *116*
Matthias Antz

3.3 Imaging the athlete's heart: anatomical and functional *120*

3.3.1 Echocardiogram: morphological and functional evaluation including new echocardiographic techniques *120*
Stefano Caselli and Flavio D'Ascenzi

3.3.2 Cardiac magnetic resonance imaging *140*
Guido Claessen and André La Gerche

3.3.3 Coronary computed tomography *153*
Stefan Möhlenkamp

3.3.4 Nuclear imaging *159*
Stefan Möhlenkamp

3.3.5 Coronary angiography *162*
Stefan Möhlenkamp

3.4 Genotyping *166*

3.4.1 Indications for genetic testing in athletes and its application in daily practice *166*
Andrea Mazzanti, Katherine Underwood, and Silvia G. Priori

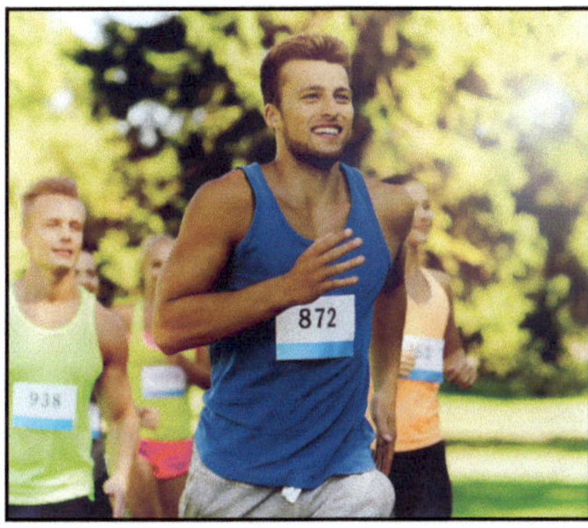

3.1

Exercise testing

Contents

3.1.1 **Protocols of exercise testing in athletes and cardiopulmonary testing: assessment of fitness** Marco Guazzi and Paolo Emilio Adami 87

3.1.2 **Evaluation of ischaemia, blood pressure, QT interval, and arrhythmias** Frédéric Schnell and François Carré 98

3.1.1 Protocols of exercise testing in athletes and cardiopulmonary testing: assessment of fitness

Marco Guazzi and Paolo Emilio Adami

Introduction

The relationship between fitness and longevity, hypothesized over 150 years ago [1], has been demonstrated by large cohort studies in recent years. In particular, these studies show the remarkable ability of fitness and physical activity to reduce cardiovascular risk factors and overall mortality from cardiovascular causes [2,3].

Physical fitness is defined as a set of attributes enabling an individual to perform physical activity which are determined by anthropometric features, such as genetics, sex, age, body composition, medical status, and by regular physical activity [4]. These features are divided into health-related and skill-related components of physical fitness. The health-related components are cardiorespiratory endurance, body composition (the relative amount of muscle mass, bone, and fat), muscular strength, muscular endurance, and flexibility. The skill-related components are agility, coordination, balance, power, reaction time, and speed [5]. Cardiorespiratory endurance is the ability of the circulatory and respiratory systems to supply oxygen during sustained physical activity and can be assessed by measurement of peak oxygen uptake (VO_{2peak}). VO_2 can be measured directly using the cardiopulmonary exercise test (CPET) [6].

CPET is not always feasible because of the associated costs of equipment, space, and staff required. Therefore a variety of maximal and submaximal exercise test outcomes can be used as surrogate markers of fitness. Exercise testing uses electrocardiography (ECG) to establish the presence of exercise-induced cardiovascular diseases, and CPET addresses a large number of issues involving the physiology and pathophysiology of exercise in addition to cardiac function (➔ Fig. 3.1.1.1) [7,8]. The choice of the test modalities and protocol depends on the indications for testing, the characteristics of the subject, and the equipment available.

Indications for exercise testing

Exercise testing can be used for diagnostic, prognostic, or functional evaluation purposes, and it can also be adopted using various ergometers depending on the objective protocols of the test. An exercise test conducted for diagnostic purposes investigates the presence of abnormal or pathological responses to exercise, whereas a prognostic exercise test evaluates the severity of a disease which has already been diagnosed. Exercise tests conducted to evaluate the subject's functional capacity provide important information with respect to disability evaluation, progress of rehabilitation, assessment of preoperative risk, physical activity counselling, and assessment of ability to return to work or training.

Diagnostic exercise testing

Exercise testing is an important tool to differentiate diagnosis of conditions which limit exercise. Depending on the

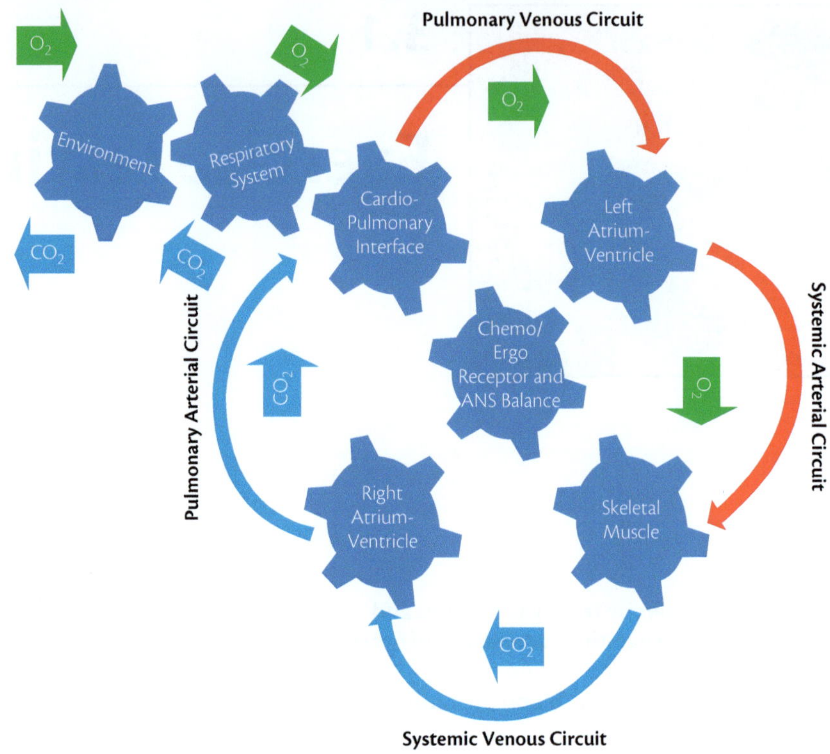

Fig. 3.1.1.1. Schematic diagram of the multiple organ systems involved in O_2 transfer from air to tissues and CO_2 elimination.
Reprinted from *Current Problems in Cardiology*, Vol 40, issue 8, Jonathan Myers, Ross Arena, Lawrence P. Cahalin, Valentina Labate, Marco Guazzi. Cardiopulmonary exercise testing in heart failure, pp. 322–72. Copyright 2015, with permission from Elsevier.

characteristics (age, sex and symptomatology) of the population being examined, some conditions may be more probable than others. For instance, exercise testing can be particularly useful in young or athletic subjects, to reveal the occurrence of exercise-induced arrhythmias, while in individuals aged >35 years it contributes to investigations on the presence of a silent ischaemic cardiovascular disease through specific alterations in the ECG. ST-segment depression, failure to reach 85% of the predicted maximal heart rate (HR_{max}), reduced exercise capacity at peak exercise, exercise-induced arrhythmias, or the occurrence of symptoms are clear examples of signs defining a positive exercise test. A diagnostic exercise test may also be advisable for subjects without risk factors who want to start an intense training programme, those with risk factors/symptoms receiving an exercise prescription, and those involved in occupations in which an acute cardiac event could compromise public safety.

Prognostic exercise testing

Exercise testing plays a key role in the evaluation of individuals with known cardiovascular disease (CVD). The response to exercise is an important indicator of disease severity. In subjects with coronary artery disease the magnitude of ischaemia is directly proportional to the degree and duration of ST-segment depression and the number of ECG leads involved, and is inversely proportional to ST slope, the rate pressure product (RPP) at which ST-segment depression occurs, the maximal heart rate (HR_{max}), systolic blood pressure (SBP), and the metabolic equivalents (METs) achieved.

The prognostic value of exercise testing appears to be high, regardless of the individual's health status, in particular when there is a progressively diminished aerobic capacity which is a warning of prognosis deterioration [9]. In this context CPET provides even more important prognostic information, in particular in patients with cardiac heart failure [8,10] and hypertrophic cardiomyopathy [11].

Functional exercise testing

Exercise testing provides important information for the assessment of functional capacity, and is helpful in disability evaluation, rehabilitation progress, performance improvement, physical activity counselling, and exercise prescription. Integrative CPET provides valuable and comprehensive information when assessing functional capacity in athletes [12], sedentary healthy subjects at risk of CVD [13], and in patients, by measuring VO_{2peak}. Response to functional exercise testing can be evaluated based on percentile ranking [14], and exercise capacity can be expressed as expected METs percentage for age and gender using nomograms [15]. Normal values of exercise capacity for age and gender, based on directly measured oxygen consumption, are available [16].

Exercise test modalities

Exercise tests can be performed on all ergometers, depending on the objective of the test, the subject's characteristics, and the equipment and personnel available. The most commonly used ergometers are the treadmill, the cycle ergometer, and the arm ergometer. Exercise tests can also be conducted in the field, evaluating the subjects while performing their own specific activity.

- A motor-driven treadmill can be used for both maximal and sub-maximal testing. Providing a familiar form of exercise, it is suitable for all types of subject, from the least fit to highly trained athletes. In subjects with balance or gait problems it may be advisable to use a cycle ergometer. Other problems frequently associated with treadmill use are ECG artefacts caused by movement and the size and cost of the device. Treadmills should have handrails for balance and stability, but their use might affect metabolic work output and VO_2 measurement. Therefore use of handrails should be discouraged or minimized when possible.
- Cycle ergometers can be mechanically or electronically braked. Electronically braked cycles have more sensitive incremental work rates that can be maintained over a wide range of pedal rates. Cycle ergometers are less expensive and require less space than treadmills, and can easily be transported. As this is a non-weight-bearing exercise it might be the most appropriate modality for obese subjects or those with orthopaedic, neurological, or vascular limitations. Since less body movement is required during cycling, it is easier to obtain high quality ECG recordings and blood pressure measurements. However, cycling is highly dependent on patient motivation, and so the test might end prematurely, due to localized leg fatigue, before reaching the maximal or submaximal endpoints. VO_{2peak} values are usually 5–15% lower than those achieved on the treadmill, depending on the subject's physical conditioning, leg strength, and motivation.
- Arm ergometry is an alternative testing modality for subjects who cannot perform lower-limb exercise (e.g. subjects with lower-body impairments or spinal cord injury) [17,18] or those whose regular sport activity involves mostly the upper body (e.g. kayakers, sailors) [19,20]. Because a smaller muscle mass is used during arm cranking, VO_{2peak} is usually 20–25% lower than the values obtained with the treadmill. Difficulties might also arise with ECG monitoring, which can be jeopardized by movement of the thoracic muscular mass, or blood pressure monitoring which cannot be performed during the arm cranking exercise.
- Other ergometers based on the specific discipline practised (e.g. rowing ergometers, kayaking ergometers, cross-country skiing ergometers) can be used if available. These testing modalities provide important information for trainers, coaches, and athletes regarding sport performance and response to the specific athletic capacity, but may not be suitable for diagnostic, prognostic, or functional evaluation purposes.

Exercise testing protocols

A number of protocols for evaluating different types of discipline have been proposed, most of which are classified as either *ramp* or *graded* protocols. For the specific study of VO_2 on kinetics, a constant workload protocol at variable load is indicated. ➲ Figure 3.1.1.2 shows three different protocols: graded, ramp, and constant workload.

Ramp protocol

The ramp protocol is physiologically more appropriate since it allows assessment of the physiological linear increment in VO_2 vs work rate well identified as 10 mlO_2/min/kg (➲ Fig. 3.1.1.2(a)). Ramp-like incremental running/cycling tests to exhaustion are performed on the track, on a treadmill, or using an ergometer. On the track, the Track Test protocol proposed by the University of Montreal (UM-TT [21]) is most commonly used with athletes [22,23], although interest in the Vam-Eval protocol, which only differs from the UM-TT in its smaller speed increments and shorter distances between inner cones, is increasing as it is easier to administer in young populations and/or subjects who are not specialists in distance running [24,25]. The final peak incremental test speed/power reached at the end of these tests ($V/p_{Inc\cdot Test}$) is only an approximation of velocity/power associated with maximal oxygen uptake (V/pVO_{2max}) because the 'true' V/pVO_{2max} attained during incremental tests requires VO_2 measures to determine the lowest speed/power that stimulates VO_{2max} (generally defined as a plateau in VO_2 or an increase less than 2.1ml/min/kg despite an increase in running speed of 1km/h [26]). The value of $V/p_{Inc\cdot Test}$ can be 5–10% greater than V/pVO_{2max}, with individuals having greater anaerobic reserves generally presenting a greater difference between V/pVO_{2max} and $V/p_{Inc\cdot Test}$. This is very useful in the field because it is largely correlated with distance running performance and match running capacity in team sports (but only for some positions [25,27]). For training prescription, $V_{Inc\cdot Test}$, as determined in the field by the UM-TT or the Vam-Eval protocol, is probably the preferred method considering that, in addition to not requiring sophisticated apparatus, the tests account for the anaerobic

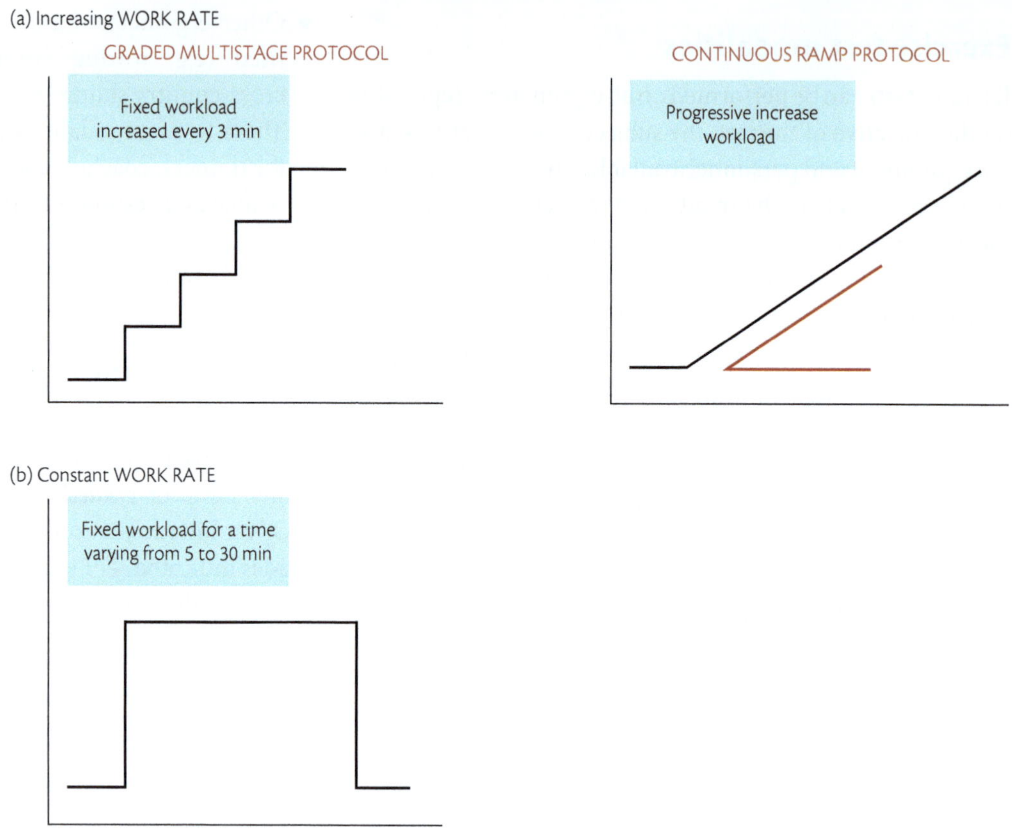

Fig. 3.1.1.2. Diagrammatic representation of exercise protocol modalities using (a) increasing work rate and (b) constant work rate.

contribution necessary to stimulate VVO_{2max} [28]. The use of velocity at maximal oxygen uptake VVO_{2max} or $V_{Inc\text{-}Test}$ as the reference running speed is particularly suitable for long intervals (2–6min) run at around VVO_{2max} (90–105%).

Another protocol in common use is the *step test protocol*, as used, for example, in the study by Zinner et al. [29]. The participants performed a step protocol to physical exhaustion on a motorized running treadmill, starting at 2.4m/s and increasing by 0.4m/s every 5min. Gas exchange data were collected with an open breath-by-breath spirometry using standard algorithms to dynamically account for the time delay between gas consumption and the volume signal. The respiratory variables were averaged every 30s, and the highest 30s value of VO_2 during the test was assumed to be VO_{2peak}. The heart rate of each participant was determined every 5s using short-range telemetry (Polar S 810, Kempele, Finland). All respiratory and heart rate data were averaged every 30s and used for further analyses. Immediately after each step and the termination of the test, a blood sample (20 µl) was collected from the right ear lobe. All samples were analysed using an amperometric enzymatic biosensor. The running economy (RE) was calculated using the average oxygen uptake of the final 30s at 3.2m/s. This velocity was below 85% of VO_{2peak} for all subjects and is required to assess RE [30]. The first significant elevation of blood lactate above baseline levels (at 2 mmol^{-1}) was taken as the velocity at the lactate threshold (V_{LT}) [31].

Graded exercise test

The graded exercise test is used less frequently than the ramp test (➔ Fig. 3.1.1.2(a)). For example, in a large population study by Zinner et al. [29] (491 athletes, 250 males and 241 females), graded exercise testing was performed to voluntary maximal exertion. Several sub-maximal and maximal physiological variables were measured, enabling assessment of the cardiopulmonary capacity, explanation of the possible mechanisms of non-optimal exercise tolerance, and comparison of inter- and intra-individual differences among various disciplines, ages, and genders.

Parameters measured during exercise testing and CPET

Blood pressure

Blood pressure (BP) can be measured by auscultation during exercise by skilled technicians or physicians, but assessing the fourth and fifth Korotkoff phase diastolic pressure and may be challenging because of the background noise of the ergometer. An American Heart Association statement [32] addressed the problems related to the measurement of blood pressure by sphygmomanometry, although the gold standard remains invasive evaluation. Intra-arterial pressures can be accurately and continuously measured by means of a pressure transducer attached to an indwelling arterial catheter whenever arterial blood specimens are not being drawn through the catheter. Accurate intra-arterial blood pressure values are more difficult to obtain during treadmill ergometry because of movement artefacts. When the subject is using the cycle, the hand on the handlebar stabilizes the arm and transducer, but tight gripping should be avoided to minimize the hypertensive effect of isometric exercise. Although resting pressures are higher in older men, the mean maximum exercise systolic and diastolic pressures are similar in both groups. Note that the true mean arterial pressure closely approximates the diastolic pressure plus half the pulse pressure, rather than one-third the pulse pressure during exercise when using a cuff [33].

Heart rate

The maximum or peak heart rate (HR) achieved declines with age in all studies, and consistent differences have been found between men and women or among the types of exercise used (e.g. leg cycling, stepping, inclined treadmill, walking, running) [34]. The two most common formulas for predicting peak HR are as follows [35]:

220 – age (years)

210 – 0.65 × age (years).

The standard deviation for each formula is 10bpm. As reported by Sheffield et al. [36] and Astrand and Rodahl [37], the peak HRs derived from fit individuals approximate either formula reasonably well. The concept of heart rate reserve (HRR), determined from the change in HR from rest to peak exercise divided by the difference between the resting HR and the age-predicted maximal heart rate (APMHR) can be useful for estimating the relative stress of the cardiovascular system during exercise, but it should be used with caution. The mean predicted peak HR may not be reached because of normal population variability, poor motivation, temporary use of medications such as β-adrenergic blockers, or heart, peripheral vascular, lung, endocrine, or musculoskeletal diseases.

Stroke volume

Stroke volume is a main determinant of the increase in oxygen delivery to working muscles. Unlike athletes, deconditioned people are cardiac limited due to chronotropic incompetence and insufficient stroke volume increase. The oxygen pulse is defined as the ratio of VO_2 to HR, and its value reflects the stroke volume assuming fixed

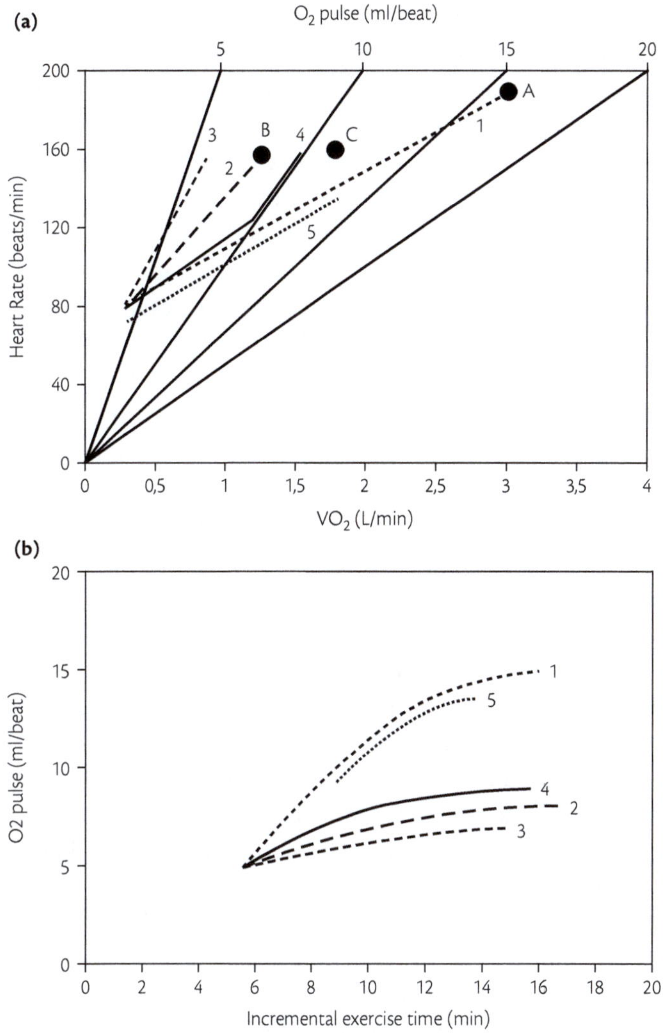

Fig. 3.1.1.3. Examples of HR vs VO_2 responses and the oxygen pulse for different cases. (see text for explanation).

Reproduced with permission from Wasserman et al., *Principles of Exercise Testing and Interpretation: Including Pathophysiology and Clinical Applications*, Fifth Edition. Lippincott Williams & Wilkins, Baltimore, Copyright © 2012.

arteriovenous oxygen extraction. The arteriovenous oxygen difference changes depending on the availability of haemoglobin, arterial blood oxygenation in the lung, and net peripheral oxygen extraction. Examples of normal and abnormal VO_2 vs HR responses and oxygen pulse responses are shown in ➲ Fig. 3.1.1.3. The linearity of the normal relationship between VO_2 and HR (subjects 1 and 2) is maintained over a wide range with a positive intercept on the HR axis. Both have normal responses, even though sedentary subjects 1 and 2 differ considerably in their predicted peak values (because they differ in age, gender, or size). An exercise response with a higher VO_2 and HR than predicted indicates better than average cardiorespiratory function, whereas a response with a lower VO_2 and HR indicates poorer than average cardiorespiratory function (subject 3).

Generally, the rate of increase in oxygen pulse declines gradually as it approaches maximum values. This is a necessary consequence of a linear VO_2 vs HR response with a positive intercept on the HR axis. The curvilinear response of the O_2 pulse during incremental exercise is clearly demonstrated in ➲ Fig. 3.1.1.3(b). The predicted peak O_2 pulse at any given work rate is strongly dependent on body size, gender, age, degree of fitness, and haemoglobin concentration. Normal values for the predicted peak O_2 pulse on the cycle ergometer range from approximately 5 ml/beat in a 7-year-old child to 8 ml/beat in a 70-year-old woman of height 150 cm, or 17 ml/beat in 30-year-old man of height 190 cm. The actual peak oxygen pulse may be considerably higher than predicted in the cardiovascularly fit person. Beta-adrenergic blocking drugs may also increase the oxygen pulse.

VO_2 and blood lactate

Five major variables have been described to explain the inter-individual variation in aerobic endurance performance [38]. VO_2peak is one of the most important parameters for endurance performance and has been extensively assessed in individuals of different ages, genders, and performance levels. VO_2peak is directly influenced by maximal cardiac output and arteriovenous oxygen difference, and therefore has become a standard in CPET evaluation [39]. Some variables, such as the level of blood lactate, demonstrate intensity-dependent benchmarks during graded exercise testing, and this has led to the development of numerous lactate threshold (LT) concepts [40]. Previous studies of endurance athletes have demonstrated that the velocity at the lactate threshold (V_{LT}) is closely linked to endurance performance [38,39]. Consequently, V_{LT} and fractional utilization of VO_2 at V_{LT} (% VO_2peak) are regarded as good indicators of endurance performance in individuals of different ages, genders, and disciplines [38,41]. Running economy (RE), defined as the steady state VO_2 expressed in ml/kg/min at a standard velocity [42] or as the energy cost of running per metre (ml/min'm) [43], differentiates among athletes with different performance levels [44]. Finally, peak treadmill running velocity (V_{peak}) has been described as a good predictor of endurance performance [45]. It can be assumed that $\%VO_{2peak}$, V_{LT}, RE, and V_{peak} are important for comparison of endurance performance amongst well-trained individuals, and the characteristics of these variables are of particular interest for elite athletes of different ages, genders, and performance levels. In practice, information about the determinants of endurance performance may aid in distinguishing individual differences in cardiopulmonary fitness, as well as for designing appropriate conditioning programmes for athletes of different ages, genders, and disciplines.

Minute ventilation (VE)

Minute ventilation is the volume of air moving into and out of the lungs expressed in litres per minute, body temperature and pressure saturated (BTPS). VE is determined by the product of respiratory rate and the volume of air exhaled with each breath (the tidal volume). As O_2 (the difference between inspired and expired oxygen content) differs a little among individuals, even in those with widely varying fitness levels, VE is usually a major determinant of VO_2max. However, fit individuals with high maximal VE and high VO_2max values must be able to increase cardiac output so that the increase in ventilation corresponds to the increase in cardiac output in the lung. The ratio of alveolar ventilation to alveolar capillary blood flow (the ventilation–perfusion ratio) is approximately 0.0 at rest. During exercise, VE and alveolar blood flow increase and this ratio may reach 5.0. In patients with congestive heart failure and pulmonary disease an abnormal VE is an important characteristic, in part because of a mismatching of the ratio of ventilation to perfusion. The ventilatory response to exercise can be important in identifying these conditions and evaluating patient's response to therapy.

Carbon dioxide production (VCO_2)

CO_2 (expressed in litres per minute, STPD) is produced by the body during exercise, and is generated from two sources. The first source is metabolic CO_2which is produced by the oxidative metabolism: 75% of the oxygen consumed by the body is converted to CO_2, which is returned to the right side of the heart by the venous blood, enters the lungs, and is exhaled as VCO_2. The second source is non-metabolic CO_2 which results from buffering of lactate at higher levels of exercise. Thus VCO_2 closely matches VE during exercise, except at higher levels of exercise (final hyperventilation), and the body keeps a relatively normal pH under most conditions. VO_2 increases in parallel with VE and VCO_2 during exercise levels of up to 50–70% of VO_2max.

Respiratory exchange ratio (RER)

RER is defined as the amount of CO_2 produced divided by the amount of oxygen consumed. Generally, about 75% of oxygen consumed is converted to CO_2. Hence RER at rest usually ranges from 0.70 to 0.85. RER depends on the type of fuel used by the cells, so it can provide an index of carbohydrate or fat metabolism. At high levels of exercise, CO_2 production exceeds oxygen uptake, so an RER exceeding 1.1–1.2 is often used to indicate that the subject is exerting maximal effort. RER values generally vary greatly and they are not a precise criterion for maximal exercise.

Ventilatory equivalents for oxygen and carbon dioxide (VE/VO_2 and VE/VCO_2)

These are calculated by dividing VE (L/min, BPTS) by VO_2 or VCO_2 (L/min, STPD), respectively. A great deal of VE (25–40 L) is required to consume a single litre of O_2; thus VE/VO_2 is often 30–40 at rest. A decrease in VE/VO_2 is normally observed on going from rest to submaximal exercise, followed by a rapid increase at higher levels of exercise when VE increases in response to the need to buffer lactate. VE/VO_2 is an index of ventilatory efficiency as it reflects ventilatory requirement for any given oxygen uptake. VE/VCO_2 represents the ventilatory requirement to eliminate a given amount of CO_2 produced by the metabolizing tissues. After a drop early in exercise, VE/VCO_2 does not normally increase significantly during submaximal exercise.

Ratio of ventilatory dead space to tidal volume (Vd/Vt)

Vd/Vt determined by gas exchange is an evaluation of the fraction of tidal volume that represents physiological dead space, i.e. the difference between minute ventilation and alveolar ventilation. Vd/Vt is another measure of ventilatory efficiency and represents the degree to which ventilation matches perfusion in the lung. Vd/Vt is high when there is significant ventilation–perfusion mismatching. The additional measurement of arterial CO_2 pressure directly from the blood is necessary to quantify Vd/Vt accurately. In normal conditions, Vd/Vt falls from roughly a third to between a tenth and a fifth at peak exercise. However, in the presence of pulmonary disease or heart failure, Vd/Vt is elevated and remains relatively unchanged throughout exercise. Ventilation–perfusion mismatching, and thus a high Vd/Vt, accounts in large part for the abnormally high ventilation observed in cardiopulmonary diseases.

Breathing reserve

Breathing reserve is calculated as the ratio of maximal voluntary ventilation (MVV) at rest to maximal exercise ventilation. Thus, breathing reserve is commonly used to help differentiate pulmonary from cardiovascular limitations to exercise.

Interestingly, in a study by Blaber et al. [46] the main purpose was to determine the changes of pulmonary function and autonomic cardiovascular control and their relation to performance after an ultramarathon in seven males and one female out of a field of 19 registered entrants in the Canadian Championship 100km running race. Pulmonary function and 30s maximum voluntary ventilation (MVV 30s) tests were conducted one day before the race and within 5min of race completion. MVV-Vt was used to examine the relationship between pulmonary function, ventilatory power, and cardiovascular race performance. It was found that MVV 30s and MVV 30s tidal volumes were lower post-race ($p < 0.001$). Pre-race supine total harmonic variation ($p < 0.01$) and pre-race MVV values (10–30 s) ($p < 0.05$) were correlated with race finish time. Thus it was concluded that maximal sustainable ventilator power and dynamic autonomic cardiovascular control are important factors in determining overall performance in an ultramarathon.

Ventilatory threshold

A sudden rise in the blood lactate level during exercise has long been associated with muscle anaerobiosis and therefore has been termed the anaerobic threshold [47], defined as the highest VO_2 during exercise above which a sustained lactic acidosis occurs. When this level of exercise is reached, excess H^+ ions of lactate must be buffered to maintain physiological pH. Moreover, VE is stimulated because bicarbonate buffering produces an additional CO_2 source. This point of non-linear increase is used to detect the anaerobic threshold non-invasively and is often termed the gas exchange anaerobic ventilatory threshold (VT). Changes in VO_2 at the VT, used clinically during pharmacological and other interventions, imply that there has been a change in oxygen supply to the working muscle. Connett et al. [48] studied dog gracilis muscle, which is a pure red fibre containing only type I and type IIA fibres, and observed lactate accumulation during fully aerobic mild (10% VO_2max) conditions. These investigators also observed that lactate accumulation was not altered by changes in blood flow, and that the accumulation occurred even though no anoxic areas were present in the muscle. This suggests that there is no relationship between lactate production and muscle hypoxia. Many studies, using tracer technology, now suggest that lactate production occurs at all times, even in resting conditions. Moreover, the turnover rate of lactate is linearly related to oxygen uptake during exercise, and this relation is possible because studies have demonstrated that lactate is shuttled from fibres where it is produced (presumably the fast-twitch fibres) to those where it is used as an energy source (the heart and slow-twitch fibres). Identification of the lactate shuttle led to the concept that production, transport, and use of lactate represent an important source of energy from carbohydrates during exercise [49]. Some studies have concluded that the anaerobic threshold is not strictly related to muscle anaerobiosis, but instead reflects an imbalance between lactate appearance and lactate disappearance. The term *ventilatory threshold* has been suggested as preferable to *anaerobic threshold*, as it does not imply the onset of anaerobiosis. Lactate accumulates in the blood during exercise, ventilation must respond to maintain physiological pH, a breakpoint in ventilation does appear to occur reproducibly, and this point is related to various measures of cardiopulmonary performance in both normal subjects [50–54] and patients with heart disease [55–62]. The use of VT, as a submaximal parameter, is better associated with the patient's everyday activities than maximal exercise, so using VT avoids the increased risk and discomfort of maximal exercise testing. Methods used for estimating VT are the V-slope and the ventilatory equivalent methods. The V-slope concept is calculated based on the relationship between VCO_2 and VO_2 which is composed of two apparently linear components, the lower of which has a slope of slightly less than 1, whereas the upper one has a slope steeper than 1. The intercept is the VT as measured by gas exchange. The ventilatory equivalent methods rely on the following features:

- the point at which a systematic increase in the ventilatory equivalent for oxygen (VE/VO_2) occurs without an increase in the ventilatory equivalent for carbon dioxide (VE/VCO_2)
- the point at which a systematic rise in end-tidal carbon dioxide pressure ($P_{ET}CO_2$) occurs.

Implications for high intensity training (HIT)

The simplicity (no need to monitor HR) and versatility of rating of perceived exertion (RPE) are very attractive. Coaches normally prescribe independent variables such as the duration or distance of work and relief intervals [63]. Consequently, the athlete can self-regulate the intensity, which is typically the maximal intensity of exercise perceived as sustainable and is based on athlete's experience, the session goal, and external considerations related to training periodization. RPE responses may be a reflection of how hard, heavy, and effortful exercise is, correlated with the physiological, biomechanical, and psychological [64] stress/fatigue imposed on the body during exercise [65]. RPE responses are gender independent [66] and comparable during free versus constant-pace exercise [67]. RPE is used for assessing HIT programme results with advantages and some limitations. The advantage of RPE-guided HIT sessions is that they do not require any knowledge of the athlete's fitness level (no test results necessary). Finally, we can state that it is a universal 'exercise regulator', irrespective of locomotor mode and variations in environmental conditions. Since RPE does not allow for the precise manipulation of the physiological response to a given HIT session, it still has some limitations. In fact, this could limit the ability to

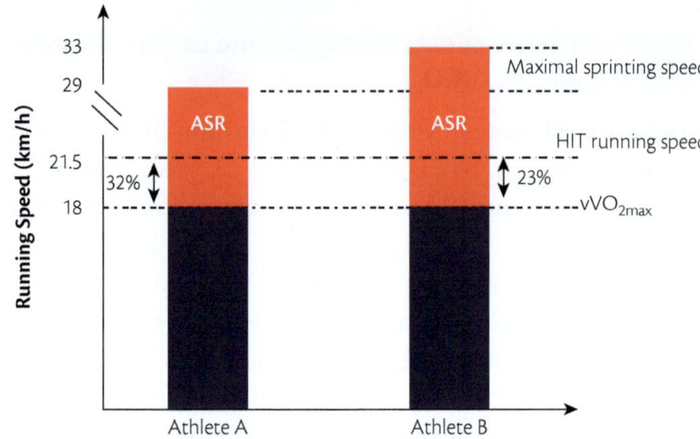

Fig. 3.1.1.4. Illustration of the importance of anaerobic speed reserve (ASR) for two athletes processing similar running speeds associated with VO_2max, but different maximal sprinting speeds. During an HIT session, athlete B with a greater ASR will work at a lower percentage of his ASR and will achieve a lower exercise load compared with athlete A. HIT training: vVO_2max, minimal running speeds associated with maximal VO_2.
Reproduced from *Sports Medicine*, High-intensity interval training, solutions to the programming puzzle. Vol. 43, issue 10, 2013, pp. 927–54, Martin Buchheit. With permission of Springer.

target a specific adaptation (➲ Fig. 3.1.1.4) [68] and could cause difficulties in a team sport setting. There is some evidence to suggest that the ability to evaluate exercise intensity by relying on RPE may be dependent on age, fitness, exercise intensity, and pleasure.

Gas exchange analysis assessment of repeated sprint sequences (RSSs)

An RSS is generally defined as a repetition of more than two short (≤10s) all-out sprints interspersed with a short recovery period (<60s). Early in the 1990s, Balsom et al. [69] showed that RSSs were aerobically demanding (i.e. >65% VO_2max). Moreover, Dupont et al. [70] have demonstrated that footballers can reach VO_2max during repeated sprinting. However, time at maximal oxygen consumption (T@VO_2max) during RSSs was not reported, so data from other studies [71–74] were reanalysed to provide T@VO_{2max} values for several forms of RSS (➲ Fig. 3.1.1.5) [69,70,72,73,75]. VO_2max was frequently reached and sustained for 10–40% of the entire RSS duration (i.e. 10–60s). When RSS is repeated two or three times per session, as is usually the case, athletes may spend up to 2–3min at VO_2max during repeated sprints. It seems that sprints should last at least 4s to increase T@VO_{2max} during an RSS, and that the recovery period should be less than 20s. However, with very short passive recovery periods, some athletes can reach VO_2max by repeating 3s sprint only (15 m). In addition, some athletes

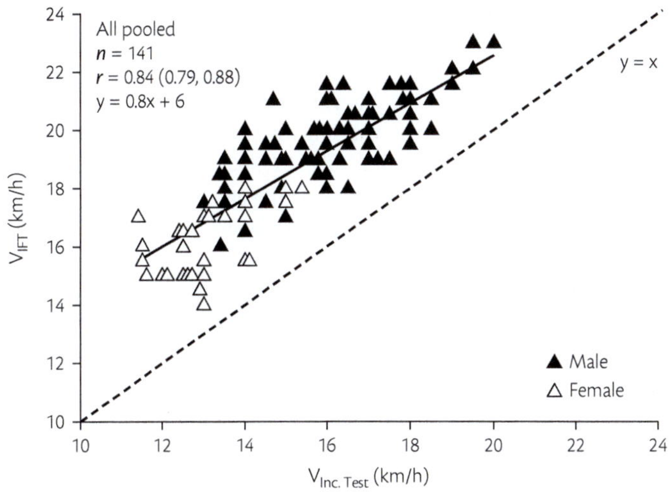

Fig. 3.1.1.5. Relationship (90% confidence limits) between the V_{IFT} and $V_{Inc\text{-}Test}$. V_{IFT}, speed reached at the end of the 30–15 IFT.
Reproduced from *Sports Medicine*, High-intensity interval training, solutions to the programming puzzle. Vol. 43, issue 10, 2013, pp. 927–54, Martin Buchheit. With permission of Springer.

may not reach VO_2max and T@VO_2max. When considering four different forms of RSS performed by the same group of 13 athletes [71,74], it was observed that six (45%) of them reached VO_2max on four occasions, one (8%) on three occasions, and four (31%) on two occasions, with two (15%) never reaching VO_2max during any of the RSSs. Thus, using RSSs to increase T@VO_2max may be questionable in some athletes, especially those with high fitness levels [68].

Metabolic equivalents (METs)

Metabolic equivalents are an index of energy expenditure. The MET unit represents the rate of energy expenditure while sitting at rest and was derived from the average resting VO_2 for a 40-year-old man weighing 70kg. Conventionally, 1 MET is equal to an oxygen uptake of 3.5ml/kg/min. The adoption of METs to establish VO_2 is an estimation that assumes a fixed relationship between the ergometer work rate and VO_2. This is inaccurate and does not take into account several factors that impair the linearity of this relationship, such as the presence of cardiovascular disease, pulmonary disease, or obesity [28]. METs may be adopted to obtain a rough estimate of the VO_2 in non-laboratory settings, such as fitness centres or training venues. In order to estimate the VO_2 per kilogram from the MET value it is necessary to multiply it by 3.5. The MET value can easily be calculated from the peak VO_2 by dividing the VO_2 per kilogram of body weight by 3.5. For convenience and ease of use, daily living activities, physical activities and sports have been classified in detail by their average MET expenditure.

Summary

Assessment of physical performance in athletes is a composite task that requires skill and a fundamental physiological background. Irrespective of testing modalities, a knowledge of VO_2max and a careful analysis of its cardiac and non-cardiac determinants (i.e. ventilation, muscular oxygen diffusion and extraction) is preparatory to training programmes and physical fitness improvement. CPET plays a major role in this respect by helping to differentiate a normal expected response from the typical abnormalities encountered in patients affected by coronary artery disease, heart failure, and cardiopulmonary disorders in general. Information derived from CPET provides the exercise physiologist and clinicians with pathophysiological and prognostic insights.

Further reading

Ainsworth BE, Haskell WL, Herrmann SD, Meckes N, Bassett DR Jr, Tudor-Locke C, Greer JL, Vezina J, Whitt-Glover MC, Leon AS. 2011 Compendium of Physical Activities: a second update of codes and MET values. Med Sci Sports Exerc. 2011 Aug;43(8): 1575–81. doi: 10.1249/MSS.0b013e31821ece12

Balady GJ, Arena R, Sietsema K, Myers J, Coke L, Fletcher GF, Forman D, Franklin B, Guazzi M, Gulati M, Keteyian SJ, Lavie CJ, Macko R, Mancini D, Milani RV, American Heart Association Exercise CR, Prevention Committee of the Council on Clinical C, Council on E, Prevention, Council on Peripheral Vascular D, Interdisciplinary Council on Quality of C, Outcomes R. Clinician's guide to cardiopulmonary exercise testing in adults: A scientific statement from the american heart association. Circulation. 2010;122:191–225

Balsom PD, Seger JY, Sjodin B, Ekblom B. Physiological responses to maximal intensity intermittent exercise. Eur J Appl Physiol Occup Physiol. 1992;65:144–149

Myers J, Prakash M, Froelicher V, Do D, Partington S, Atwood JE. Exercise capacity and mortality among men referred for exercise testing. N Engl J Med. 2002;346:793–801

Zinner C, Sperlich B, Wahl P, Mester J. Classification of selected cardiopulmonary variables of elite athletes of different age, gender, and disciplines during incremental exercise testing. Springerplus. 2015;4:544

References

1. Darwin C. On the Origin of Species by Means of Natural Selection, Or The Preservation of Favoured Races in the Struggle for Life. London: John Murray, 1859. Reprinted as Darwin C. The Origin of Species. New York: Random House, 1993.
2. Kodama S, Saito K, Tanaka S, et al. Cardiorespiratory fitness as a quantitative predictor of all-cause mortality and cardiovascular events in healthy men and women: a meta-analysis. *JAMA* 2009; 301: 2024–35
3. Myers J, Prakash M, Froelicher V, et al. Exercise capacity and mortality among men referred for exercise testing. *N Engl J Med* 2002; 346: 793–801

4. US Department of Health and Human Services. *PhysicalActivity and Health: A Report of the Surgeon General.* Atlanta, GA: Centers for Disease Control and Prevention, 1996
5. Physical Activity Guidelines Advisory Committee. *Physical Activity Guidelines for Americans.* Washington, DC: US Department of Health and Human Services, 2008.
6. Guazzi M, Arena R, Halle M, et al. 2016 focused update: clinical recommendations for cardiopulmonary exercise testing data assessment in specific patient populations. *Eur Heart J* 2018; 39: 1149–61.
7. Balady GJ, Arena R, Sietsema K, et al. Clinician's guide to cardiopulmonary exercise testing in adults: a scientific statement from the American Heart Association. *Circulation* 2010; 122: 191–225.
8. Myers J, Arena R, Cahalin LP, et al. Cardiopulmonary exercise testing in heart failure. *Curr Probl Cardiol* 2015; 40: 322–72.
9. Arena R, Myers J, Guazzi M. The future of aerobic exercise testing in clinical practice. Is it the ultimate vital sign? *Future Cardiol* 2010; 6: 325–42
10. Corra U, Agostoni P, Giordano A, et al. The metabolic exercise test data combined with cardiac and kidney indexes (mecki) score and prognosis in heart failure: a validation study. *Int J Cardiol* 2016; 203: 1067–72.
11. Magri D, Limongelli G, Re F, et al. Cardiopulmonary exercise test and sudden cardiac death risk in hypertrophic cardiomyopathy. *Heart* 2016; 102(8), 602–9.
12. Bernardi M, Carucci S, Faiola F, et al. Physical fitness evaluation of paralympic winter sports sitting athletes. *Clin J Sport Med* 2012; 22: 26–30.
13. Guazzi M, Arena R, Pellegrino M, et al. Prevalence and characterization of exercise oscillatory ventilation in apparently healthy individuals at variable risk for cardiovascular disease: A subanalysis of the Euro-Ex trial. *Eur J Prev Cardiol* 2016; 23: 328–34.
14. Cooper Institute. *Physical Fitness Assessments and Norms for Adults and Law Enforcement.* Dallas, TX: Cooper Institute,.
15. Gibbons RJ, Balady GJ, Bricker JT, Chaitman. ACC/AHA 2002 guideline update for exercise testing: summary article. A Report of the American College of Cardiology/American Heart Association Task Force on Practice Guidelines (committee to update the 1997 exercise testing guidelines). *J Am Coll Cardiol* 2002; 40: 1531–40.
16. Wasserman K Hansen JE, Sue DY, et al. Normal values. *Principles of Exercise Testing and Interpretation: Including Pathophysiology and Clinical Applications* (5th edn). Baltimore, MD: Lippincott Williams & Wilkins, 2011, pp. 154–80.
17. Drory Y, Ohry A, Brooks ME, et al. Arm crank ergometry in chronic spinal cord injured patients. *Arch Phys Med Rehabil* 1990; 71: 389–92.
18. Ordonez FJ, Rosety MA, Camacho A, et al. Arm-cranking exercise reduced oxidative damage in adults with chronic spinal cord injury. *Arch Phys Med Rehabil* 2013; 94: 2336–41.
19. Adami PE, Delussu AS, Rodio A, et al. Upper limb aerobic training improves aerobic fitness and all-out performance of America's Cup grinders. *Eur J Sport Sci* 2015; 15: 235–41.
20. Forbes SC, Chilibeck PD. Comparison of a kayaking ergometer protocol with an arm crank protocol for evaluating peak oxygen consumption. *J Strength Cond Res* 2007; 21: 1282–5.
21. Leger L, Boucher R. An indirect continuous running multistage field test: the Université de Montreal track test. *Can J Appl Sport Sci* 1980; 5: 77–84.
22. Buchheit M. The 30–15 intermittent fitness test: accuracy for individualizing interval training of young intermittent sport players. *J Strength Cond Res.* 2008; 22: 365–74.
23. Dupont G, Akakpo K, Berthoin S. The effect of in-season, high-intensity interval training in soccer players. *J Strength Cond Res* 2004; 18: 584–89.
24. Mendez-Villanueva A, Buchheit M, Kuitunen S, et al. Is the relationship between sprinting and maximal aerobic speeds in young soccer players affected by maturation? *Pediatr Exerc Sci* 2010; 22: 497–510.
25. Buchheit M, Mendez-Villanueva A, Simpson BM, Bourdon PC. Match running performance and fitness in youth soccer. *Int J Sports Med* 2010; 31: 818–25.
26. Billat V, Renoux JC, Pinoteau J, et al. Reproducibility of running time to exhaustion at VO_2max in subelite runners. *Med Sci Sports Exerc* 1994; 26: 254–7.
27. Rampinini E, Bishop D, Marcora SM, et al. Validity of simple field tests as indicators of match-related physical performance in top-level professional soccer players. *Int J Sports Med* 2007; 28: 228–35.
28. Berthon P, Fellmann N. General review of maximal aerobic velocity measurement at laboratory. Proposition of a new simplified protocol for maximal aerobic velocity assessment. *J Sports Med Phys Fitness* 2002; 42: 257–66.
29. Zinner C, Sperlich B, Wahl P, Mester J. Classification of selected cardiopulmonary variables of elite athletes of different age, gender, and disciplines during incremental exercise testing. *SpringerPlus* 2015; 4: 544.
30. Saunders PU, Pyne DB, Telford RD, Hawley JA. Factors affecting running economy in trained distance runners. *Sports Med* 2004; 34: 465–85.
31. Skinner JS, McLellan TM. The transition from aerobic to anaerobic metabolism. *Res Q Exerc Sport* 1980; 51: 234–48.
32. American Heart Association. Human blood pressure determination by sphygmomanometry. *Circulation* 1993; 88: 2460–70.
33. Robinson TE, Sue DY, Huszczuk A, et al. Intra-arterial and cuff blood pressure responses during incremental cycle ergometry. *Med Sci Sports Exerc* 1988; 20: 142–9.
34. Wasserman K Hansen JE, Sue DY, et al. *Principles of Exercise Testing and Interpretation: Including Pathophysiology and Clinical Applications* (5th edn). Baltimore, MD: Lippincott Williams & Wilkins, 2011.
35. Jones NL, Summers E, Killian KJ. Influence of age and stature on exercise capacity during incremental cycle ergometry in men and women. *Am Rev Respir Dis* 1989; 140: 1373–80.
36. Sheffield LT, Maloof JA, Sawyer JA, Roitman D. Maximal heart rate and treadmill performance of healthy women in relation to age. *Circulation* 1978; 57: 79–84.
37. Astrand I. Aerobic work capacity in men and women with special reference to age. *Acta Physiol Scand Suppl* 1960; 49: 1–92.
38. Midgley AW, McNaughton LR, Jones AM. Training to enhance the physiological determinants of long-distance running performance. Can valid recommendations be given to runners and

coaches based on current scientific knowledge? *Sports Med* 2007; 37: 857–80.
39. Bassett DR, Jr, Howley ET. Limiting factors for maximum oxygen uptake and determinants of endurance performance. *Med Sci Sports Exerc* 2000; 32: 70–84.
40. Faude O, Kindermann W, Meyer T. Lactate threshold concepts. How valid are they? *Sports Med* 2009; 39: 469–90.
41. Ziogas GG, Patras KN, Stergiou N, Georgoulis AD. Velocity at lactate threshold and running economy must also be considered along with maximal oxygen uptake when testing elite soccer players during preseason. *J Strength Cond Res* 2011; 25: 414–19.
42. Costill DL, Thomason H, Roberts E. Fractional utilization of the aerobic capacity during distance running. *Med Sci Sports* 1973; 5: 248–52.
43. di Prampero PE. The energy cost of human locomotion on land and in water. *Int J Sports Med* 1986; 7: 55–72.
44. Conley DL, Krahenbuhl GS. Running economy and distance running performance of highly trained athletes. *Med Sci Sports Exerc* 1980; 12: 357–60.
45. Noakes TD, Myburgh KH, Schall R. Peak treadmill running velocity during the VO_2max test predicts running performance. *J Sports Sci* 1990; 8: 35–45.
46. Blaber AP, Walsh ML, Carter JB, et al. Cardiopulmonary physiology and responses of ultramarathon athletes to prolonged exercise. *Can J Appl Physiol* 2004; 29: 544–63.
47. Wasserman K, McIlroy MB. Detecting the threshold of anaerobic metabolism in cardiac patients during exercise. *Am J Cardiol* 1964; 14: 844–52.
48. Connett RJ, Gayeski TE, Honig CR. Lactate accumulation in fully aerobic, working, dog gracilis muscle. *Am J Physiol* 1984; 246: H120–8.
49. Brooks GA. Mammalian fuel utilization during sustained exercise. *Comp Biochem Physiol B Biochem Mol Biol* 1998; 120: 89–107.
50. Davis JA, Frank MH, Whipp BJ, Wasserman K. Anaerobic threshold alterations caused by endurance training in middle-aged men. *J Appl Physiol Respir Environ Exerc Physiol* 1979; 46: 1039–46.
51. Niess AM, Fehrenbach E, Strobel G, et al. Evaluation of stress responses to interval training at low and moderate altitudes. *Med Sci Sports Exerc* 2003; 35: 263–9.
52. Ready AE, Quinney HA. Alterations in anaerobic threshold as the result of endurance training and detraining. *Med Sci Sports Exerc* 1982; 14: 292–6.
53. Tanaka K, Watanabe H, Konishi Y, et al. Longitudinal associations between anaerobic threshold and distance running performance. *Eur J Appl Physiol Occup Physiol* 1986; 55: 248–52.
54. Millett PJ, Allen MJ, Bostrom MP. Effects of alendronate on particle-induced osteolysis in a rat model. *J Bone Joint Surg Am* 2002; 84A: 236–49.
55. Brubaker PH, Marburger CT, Morgan TM, et al. Exercise responses of elderly patients with diastolic versus systolic heart failure. *Med Sci Sports Exerc* 2003; 35: 1477–85.
56. Guazzi M, Tumminello G, Matturri M, Guazzi MD. Insulin ameliorates exercise ventilatory efficiency and oxygen uptake in patients with heart failure-type 2 diabetes comorbidity. *J Am Coll Cardiol* 2003; 42: 1044–50.
57. Matsumura N, Nishijima H, Kojima S, et al. Determination of anaerobic threshold for assessment of functional state in patients with chronic heart failure. *Circulation* 1983; 68: 360–7.
58. Myers J, Atwood JE, Sullivan M, et al. Perceived exertion and gas exchange after calcium and beta-blockade in atrial fibrillation. *J Appl Physiol (1985)* 1987; 63: 97–104.
59. Sullivan M, Atwood JE, Myers J, et al. Increased exercise capacity after digoxin administration in patients with heart failure. *J Am Coll Cardiol.* 1989; 13: 1138–43.
60. Sullivan MJ, Cobb FR. The anaerobic threshold in chronic heart failure: relation to blood lactate, ventilatory basis, reproducibility, and response to exercise training. *Circulation* 1990; 81: II47–58.
61. Weber KT, Kinasewitz GT, Janicki JS, Fishman AP. Oxygen utilization and ventilation during exercise in patients with chronic cardiac failure. *Circulation* 1982; 65: 1213–23.
62. Auricchio A, Stellbrink C, Butter C, et al. Clinical efficacy of cardiac resynchronization therapy using left ventricular pacing in heart failure patients stratified by severity of ventricular conduction delay. *J Am Coll Cardiol* 2003; 42: 2109–16.
63. Seiler S, Sjursen JE. Effect of work duration on physiological and rating scale of perceived exertion responses during self-paced interval training. *Scand J Med Sci Sports* 2004; 14: 318–25.
64. Marcora SM, Staiano W, Manning V. Mental fatigue impairs physical performance in humans. *J Appl Physiol (1985)* 2009; 106: 857–64.
65. Ulmer HV. Concept of an extracellular regulation of muscular metabolic rate during heavy exercise in humans by psychophysiological feedback. *Experientia* 1996; 52: 416–20.
66. Garcin M, Fleury A, Mille-Hamard L, Billat V. Sex-related differences in ratings of perceived exertion and estimated time limit. *Int J Sports Med* 2005; 26: 675–81.
67. Garcin M, Danel M, Billat V. Perceptual responses in free vs. constant pace exercise. *Int J Sports Med* 2008; 29: 453–9.
68. Buchheit M, Laursen PB. High-intensity interval training, solutions to the programming puzzle. Part II: Anaerobic energy, neuromuscular load and practical applications. *Sports Med* 2013; 43: 927–54.
69. Balsom PD, Seger JY, Sjodin B, Ekblom B. Maximal-intensity intermittent exercise: effect of recovery duration. *Int J Sports Med* 1992; 13: 528–33.
70. Dupont G, Millet GP, Guinhouya C, Berthoin S. Relationship between oxygen uptake kinetics and performance in repeated running sprints. *Eur J Appl Physiol* 2005; 95: 27–34.
71. Buchheit M. Performance and physiological responses to repeated-sprint and jump sequences. *Eur J Appl Physiol* 2010; 110: 1007–18
72. Buchheit M, Cormie P, Abbiss CR, et al. Muscle deoxygenation during repeated sprint running: effect of active vs passive recovery. *Int J Sports Med* 2009; 30: 418–25.
73. Buchheit M, Laursen PB, Ahmaidi S. Parasympathetic reactivation after repeated sprint exercise. *Am J Physiol Heart Circ Physiol* 2007; 293: H133–41.
74. Buchheit M, Bishop D, Haydar B, et al. Physiological responses to shuttle repeated-sprint running. *Int J Sports Med* 2010; 31: 402–9.
75. Balsom PD, Seger JY, Sjodin B, Ekblom B. Physiological responses to maximal intensity intermittent exercise. *Eur J Appl Physiol Occup Physiol* 1992; 65: 144–9.

3.1.2 Evaluation of ischaemia, blood pressure, QT interval, and arrhythmias

Frédéric Schnell and François Carré

Interest and limits of exercise testing

Exercise testing has two main applications in athletes: it enables performance evaluation to guide individual training regimes and can identify exercise-induced cardiovascular (CV) disorders. In this chapter we will only consider the second application. As the indications for exercise testing have been described in Chapter 3.1.1, we will focus on the evaluation of ischaemia, blood pressure, QT interval, and arrhythmias using exercise tests (➲ Fig. 3.1.2.1).

First, it must be emphasized that exercise testing has some major limitations, which should be considered by the physician and clearly explained to the athlete. A 'normal' exercise test does not mean that there is no CV risk during intense exercise. The rate of false-negative exercise tests is high, as is false-positive detection of asymptomatic coronary artery disease (CAD) and arrhythmia. Moreover, because of the low pre-test probability due to the low CV risk level in athletes, the rate of false-positive exercise tests for CAD is higher in athletes than in sedentary subjects [1,2]. Therefore in order to avoid unnecessary complementary examinations, exercise test results should be interpreted with caution.

Evaluation of ischaemia

Positive or false positive test?

In asymptomatic athletes with a high risk factor profile for CAD, the detection of ischaemia may be indicated, especially prior to initiating a vigorous exercise programme (see Chapters 6.5 and 6.6) [3]. In athletes, exercise testing is better accepted than pharmacological tests. The usual interpretation criteria (i.e. ECG change, clinical parameters, and haemodynamic parameters) are the same in athletes as in the general population. An asymptomatic upsloping ST-segment depression with normalization in the early (<1min) phase of recovery should not be considered pathological (➲ Fig. 3.1.2.2) [4]. However, a horizontal or downsloping ST-segment depression ≥1mm, or an ascending elevation of the ST segment ≥1.5mm detected 60ms after the J point are criteria for coronary disease. Persistent (>1min) or aggravated ST-segment abnormality during recovery, adrenergic premature ventricular contractions (PVCs), abnormally slow heart rate (HR) recovery [5], and/or chronotropic [3] insufficiency are further indications of CAD. The performance achieved during exercise testing is also of major value; it should be greater than 10 metabolic equivalents (METs), and must be correlated with the training load [6].

In this context, criteria derived from cardiopulmonary exercise testing (CPET) may add valuable information; a decrease in the VO_2/W ratio and a decrease in oxygen pulse (VO_2/HR) indicate a CAD [7–10]. Indeed, abnormalities of left ventricular function during exercise invariably precede ST-segment depression and angina in patients with stable CAD. Thus, VO_2 kinetics may be delayed, reflecting

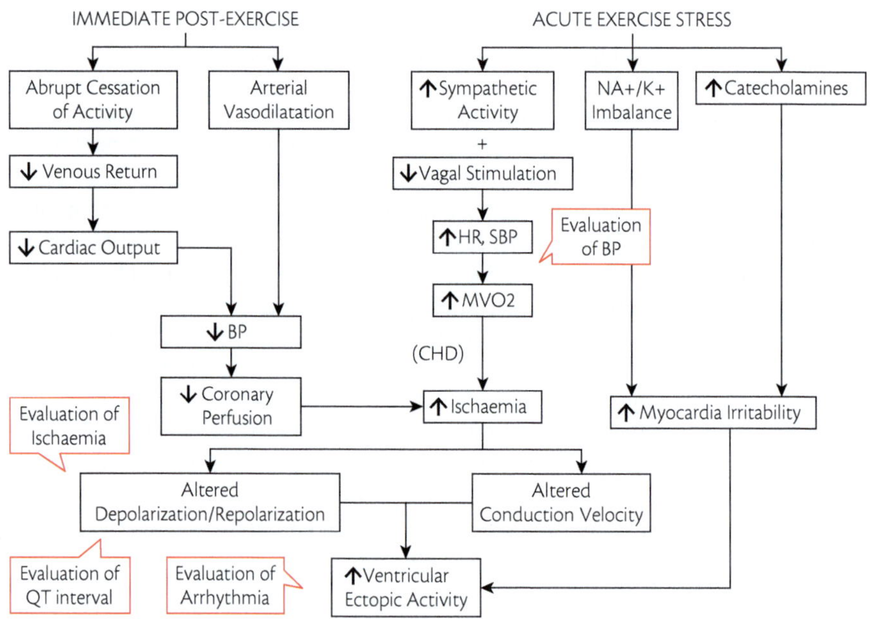

Fig. 3.1.2.1 Physiopathology of ECG changes and arrhythmic disorders during an exercise test. BP, blood pressure; HR, heart rate; MVO_2, myocardial oxygen uptake.

Adapted from *British Journal of Sports Medicine*, J. Freeman, V. Froelicher, E. Ashley, Volume 43, issue 9. Copyright 2009 with permission from BMJ Publishing Group Ltd.

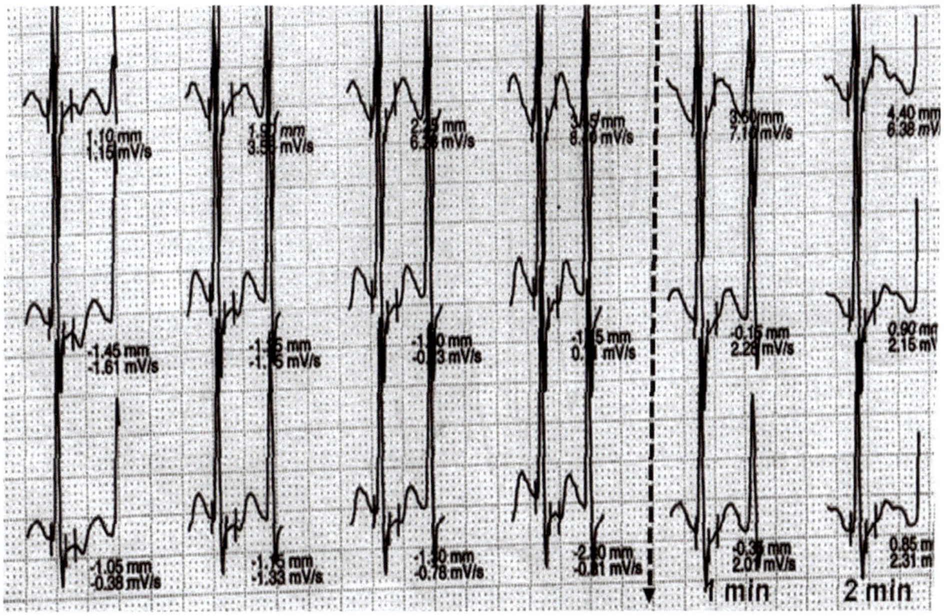

Fig. 3.1.2.2 Example of a false-positive exercise test. Exercise test performed on an asymptomatic cyclist aged 42 years. Notice the downsloping ST-segment depression in leads V4–V6, but with a fast normalization in <1min. The good exercise capacity is shown by the high workload achieved. Dotted arrow, end of the exercise phase.

exercise-induced myocardial dysfunction, and CPET abnormalities may be evident earlier than ECG changes and clinical signs. This hypothesis is suggested by the correlation of both O_2 pulse flattening or decreasing kinetics and a $\Delta VO_2/\Delta WR$ decrease with the degree of contractile dysfunction expressed by the systolic wall-thickening score index at peak exercise as assessed by SPECT [7].

All these parameters must be taken into account to avoid false-positive results, which are more frequent (10–15%) in athletes, especially those over 35 years of age [11,12]. The physiopathology of these false-positive tests is not well known, but it has been proposed that they might be related to left ventricular hypertrophy and/or an abnormality in the coronary microcirculation [2,12].

It should be remembered that exercise tests can detect angina and significant stenosis (≥70%) which impairs the coronary blood flow during exercise, but cannot detect non-significant unstable vulnerable atherosclerotic plaques which might lead to thrombotic occlusion [3].

Indications for complementary tests

If the exercise test results are abnormal or doubtful, further tests are needed before medical clearance for competitive sport participation can be given. Exercise-imaging techniques are more sensitive and specific than exercise tests; indeed ECG ST-segment changes are more delayed than regional myocardial dysfunction due to perfusion abnormalities [13]. Exercise echocardiography is non-invasive, physiological, and easy to perform in athletes. NMR imaging is also well validated, but it exposes the patient to radiation. Anatomical tests may also be helpful, especially CT angiography [14].

Conclusions

Detection of ischaemia is generally indicated for veteran athletes with a high risk factor profile for CAD, but there is high rate of false-positive tests in this healthy population. However, it should be remembered that a normal exercise test does not exclude the occurrence of a coronary syndrome due to an acute vessel occlusion.

Evaluation of arrhythmia

Which arrhythmia or conduction disorder should we assess with exercise tests?

Because of the well-described training-induced electrical remodelling, athletes present more frequent innocent arrhythmias, such as marked sinus bradycardia, slowing of atrioventricular nodal conduction, and ectopic supraventricular rhythms [15].

In athletes without heart disease, asymptomatic frequent premature ventricular contractions (PVCs) which do not worsen following acute exercise are reported to have a long-term benign prognostic significance [15], especially when they are reduced by physical deconditioning [16].

Atrial fibrillation (AF) is the most common arrhythmia in the general population, and recent studies have demonstrated that long-term endurance exercise may increase the incidence of AF in this population [17–19]. In athletes with AF, it is essential to assess the ventricular rate and haemodynamic impairment during recurrent paroxysms of AF or during permanent AF in order to resume sports activity. Exercise testing can help to assess the tolerance of AF in this specific population [20,21].

Moderate sinus bradycardia and first- or second-degree AV block Mobitz type 1 are common findings in athletes [22], and do not require systematic exercise testing if they are asymptomatic. Nevertheless, when an exercise test is performed, chronotropic adaptation and the conductance disturbances should resolve quickly during exercise [22]. In the case of second-degree AV block Mobitz type 2 or third-degree AV block, a more comprehensive diagnostic evaluation is warranted to exclude underlying structural heart disease which is more often present in these patients. Moreover, exercise tests should be performed in order to assess the tolerance of the conduction disorder and to identify associated ventricular tachyarrhythmia [20].

In patients without heart disease and a pacemaker, competitive or recreational sports participation is allowed in sports with minor to moderate cardiovascular demand [23]. Exercise testing will help to exclude significant arrhythmias and to programme an appropriate pacing rate responsiveness during exercise [24]. In a recreational athlete with implantable cardiac defibrillator, exercise testing is warranted to optimize its adjustment during exercise and prevent the occurrence of an inappropriate shock.

Exercise testing can be used for risk assessment of an asymptomatic pre-excitation discovered in an athlete; indeed, a beat-to-beat disappearance of pre-excitation during exercise testing is classically a good prognosis (see also Chapter 5.4) [25,26]. Nevertheless, even if the sensitivity of exercise testing for fast anterograde conduction is good, its specificity is low [26], meaning that approximately half the patients will need a subsequent electrophysiological study to rule out an increased risk of sudden death. Therefore, an electrophysiological study should be performed in competitive athletes with pre-excitation.

Specific protocols in the evaluation of arrhythmia

Because classical exercise testing is not really adapted to studying arrhythmias, some specific exercise test protocols might be proposed for symptomatic athletes. An 'abrupt' exercise test on cyclo-ergometer can be used. After a short warm-up phase, the subject has to cycle as fast and as long as possible against at least the peak load achieved during a previous standard exercise test. The cessation of exercise should also be abrupt in order to make the test even more arrhythmogenic. Sometimes an exercise test that simulates high intensity interval training performed on the field can be used to cause abnormal tachycardia.

Conclusions

Symptomatic arrhythmia and/or adrenergic PVCs that increase in frequency with repetitive forms during exercise testing need further evaluation. Search for a morphological substrate is usually the primary goal [20]. It determines both the prognosis and the recommendations for participation in sport. Echocardiography is the first-line imaging examination, and in selected cases cardiac magnetic resonance might be performed. A 24-hour ECG monitor is also mandatory. It must include an intense training session. Exercise testing in the laboratory does not completely reflect the effort performed in the field which includes dehydration and environmental (heat, cold) constraints. If necessary, an electrophysiological study could also be performed [23]. There should be no doubt associated with medical clearance for participation in competitive sports.

Evaluation of blood pressure during exercise

Limits of blood pressure evaluation during exercise

The responses of systolic and diastolic blood pressure (BP) induced by a dynamic progressive and maximal exercise have been described in Chapter 1.2.1. Briefly, systolic BP increases linearly with exercise intensity throughout exercise, while diastolic BP varies only slightly.

However, it must be remembered that the classical exercise test used in cardiology is designed to diagnose an abnormal response of coronary circulation and not to detect an inadequate BP response. First, this protocol with short step duration does not take into account the peripheral resistance inertia, which is the main peripheral parameter involved in the BP response. Secondly, because of its marked limitations the automatic method of measuring BP during exercise has not been validated. Thus the manual method is more reliable method, even though its true accuracy for diastolic and maximal systolic values is questionable [27]. Finally, BP responses depend on the main component of the exercise (dynamic, static or mixed), which vary greatly depending on the different sport practices. Thus, it is difficult to extrapolate BP values observed during a classical maximal exercise test to BP evolution in an athlete on the field [28,29].

Clinical interest of blood pressure values recorded during exercise testing

A decrease or small elevation in systolic BP during exercise is always pathological and should always alert the physician. Conversely, an exaggerated BP response to exercise suggests an impaired individual capacity for exercise-induced vasodilation, but its clinical interest is more questionable. Indeed, the diagnosis of hypertension is solely based on resting systolic and diastolic BP values higher than 140/90mmHg; exercise BP values themselves are not used for the diagnosis. this is mainly because the cut-off value of abnormal maximal exercise BP is still under debate, partly because of differences between study populations, testing procedures, and definitions used for abnormal BP response to exercise.

Several upper limits have been proposed for exercise systolic BP, but none have been generally accepted. Ageing alters BP responses to exercise [27], and so observational studies based on general populations have identified different upper limits on peak systolic BP according to age. On cyclo-ergometer tests, systolic BP should not exceed 300mmHg before age 40 years, 280mmHg from 40 to 50 years, 260mmHg from 51 to 60 years, and 250mmHg after 60 years [30,31]. These values should be considered as abnormal.

One of the major interests in exaggerated systolic exercise BP is the detection of 'masked' hypertension [32]. Even if its real predictive value is debated [27,33,34], positive correlations between high systolic BP and occurrence of hypertension, cardiovascular events, and early mortality have been reported in a number of studies. The most frequently cited cut-off values for peak systolic exercise BP used to predict incident hypertension in healthy untrained women and men are 190mmHg and 210mmHg, respectively, in the cyclo-ergometer test [35]. On the treadmill, the peak and relative (i.e. the difference between peak and resting BP) systolic BP values proposed for predicting future hypertension in the general population are 181mmHg and 52mmHg, respectively [36].

With regard to diastolic BP, an exaggerated response to exercise (≥110mmHg) could be predictive of risk for new-onset hypertension in normotensive men and women [37]. Observation of a peak diastolic BP value >130mmHg is very rare, and should be treated with caution [27].

Some studies have proposed a limit of 200/100mmHg on submaximal BP values recorded during prolonged exercise on cyclo-ergometer (100W over 6min) for subjects aged between 20 and 50 years [38,39], whereas another study proposed a lower cut-off value of 160mmHg for systolic BP [35].

Finally, an inadequate decrease in BP during the recovery phase, such as a 3min recovery (systolic BP/peak systolic BP) ratio >0.9, or a delayed decrease in BP with a value above 140/90mmHg after 5min or above the basal value after more than 6min recovery, has also been proposed as a predictive marker of cardiovascular events [27,38].

Specificities of blood pressure responses to exercise in athletes

During exercise, BP increases in a similar manner in athletes and sedentary subjects with no significant difference at the same relative workloads (ratio of power/maximal power).

With regard to the maximal BP values observed during exercise, diastolic BP limits proposed in the general population are consistent in athletes. In one study of young normotensive elite athletes the upper reference values reported during a maximal bicycle exercise test were 200mmHg and 220 mmHg for systolic BP, and 80mmHg and 85mmHg diastolic BP for female and male athletes, respectively[40]. It must be emphasized that, in athletes, it is not uncommon for the fifth Korotkoff sound to be heard all the way to zero [27].

The interpretation of maximal systolic BP may be difficult, and the clinical relevance and true prognostic value of this parameter in normotensive athletes is still under debate. First, both resting and exercise BP values in athletes depend on their training period [41] as the arterial stiffness involved in maximal exercise systolic BP increases after high volume training [42]. Secondly, it has been proved that, apart from gender and age, functional capacity markedly influences the response of systolic BP to exercise [43]. There is a linear relation between maximal power and peak systolic BP. Therefore it is recommended to correct exercise systolic BP response with working capacity expressed in metabolic equivalents (METs). For example, an upper limit of 11.3mmHg/MET has been proposed for exercise on a treadmill [44]. Thus, in athletes, Rost's formula is usually adopted to evaluate peak systolic pressure responses on the cyclo-ergometer [45]:

$$\text{systolic BP (mmHg)} = 147 + 0.334 \times \text{maximal power (W)} + 0.31 \times \text{age (years)}.$$

This has recently been confirmed in young endurance athletes (10–18 years old) using the formulas

$$\text{systolic BP (mmHg)} = 120.84 + 0.55 \times \text{workload (W)} - 1.92 \times \text{age (years)}$$
$$\text{systolic BP (mmHg)} = 111.22 + 0.48 \times \text{workload (W)} - 0.88 \times \text{age (years)}$$

for boys and girls, respectively [46].

Finally, physical training does not induce hypertension; in fact the prevalence of hypertension in athletes is lower than that in a sedentary population [47]. It is well known that physical training in hypertensive patients is associated with a slower rise and a lower peak of systolic BP during exercise testing [48]. Moreover, in the general population excessive systolic BP values during exercise are mainly observed in less trained subjects with a lower physical capacity. These subjects present with a high arterial stiffness linked to ageing and other classical cardiovascular risk factors, mainly metabolic syndrome [49]. Aerobic physical training attenuates their BP elevation during physical exertion and daytime activities, as assessed by ambulatory BP monitoring [50].

Few studies have investigated exercise hypertension in athletic populations, and all concerned only systolic BP responses. One study demonstrated that in athletes with abnormal systolic BP response to exercise the risk of developing hypertension was increased by a factor of 10 [51] and that they had higher systolic BP values on 24-hour ambulatory BP monitoring, although remaining within normal values [52].

A positive correlation between maximal exercise systolic BP and left ventricular (LV) mass has been reported in the general population [53]. In endurance athletes, the LV mass is related to maximal exercise loads ($r = 0.65$ for mass and 0.58 for indexed mass, $p = 0.001$) [54]. It was found that BP values at the anaerobic threshold in male athletes with higher LV mass (>220g) and a concentric echocardiographic myocardial remodelling pattern was obtained [55]. However, these athletes also recorded the best maximal power and VO_2max values. Because exercise capacity is decreased in hypertensive subjects, whether they are trained or not [56], it is difficult to be sure whether the features reported for these triathletes were really deleterious.

Middle-aged amateur marathon runners presenting with exaggerated systolic BP response to exercise showed lower VO_2max and higher LV mass index as LV diastolic dysfunction than runners with normal exercise BP responses [57]. Moreover, their increases in cTnI, NT-proBNP, endothelin-1, and hs-CRP after a marathon were higher than in normal runners [58].

Finally, the merit of assessing blood pressure during exercise in hypertensive athletes who are well equilibrated with pharmacological therapy is not proved. However, exercise testing should be performed in this population in order to detect disorders of the coronary circulation and/or adrenergic arrhythmias [23].

Conclusions

The current diagnosis of hypertension in athletes, as in the general population, is based only on resting BP values measured according to standard recommendations [59]. In view of the limits discussed in the preceding sections, until further data are validated by large studies, we propose the following approach to exercise BP responses in athletes. In asymptomatic normotensive athletes with physical performance adapted to level training, it is more appropriate to analyse the global kinetics of BP changes during exercise rather than checking only the peak BP. However, if there is a marked increase in systolic BP, adjusted for age and maximal power, ambulatory BP monitoring to detect 'masked' hypertension is recommended. Competitive athletes with marked abnormal response of BP to exercise testing should have an annual cardiological evaluation. Exercise testing is valuable for detecting coronary or rhythm abnormalities in hypertensive athletes, but its use for assessing the pharmacological quality of BP control is questionable.

Evaluation of QT interval adaptations during exercise

Normal QT interval adaptation during exercise

Because of its implications for the practice of sports in competition, a diagnosis of pathological long QT (LQT) should be confirmed in the athlete. As in the general population, LQT diagnosis in athletes is based on a set of criteria; therefore analysis of QT adaptation during ET is an integral part of the score determined for LQT diagnosis [60].

The QT duration on the ECG reflects the time elapsed from the depolarization of the first ventricular cell to the repolarization of the last one. The ventricular myocardium is comprised of three main electrophysiologically and functionally distinct cell types: epicardial, M, and endocardial cells. Under most QT conditions, epicardial cells are the earliest and M cells are often the last to repolarize. Repolarization of the epicardial action potential coincides with the peak of the T wave (Tp), and repolarization of the M cells coincides with the end of the T wave (Te). Thus, the Tp–Te interval provides an index of transmural dispersion of repolarization, which may be of prognostic value [61].

The QT duration depends on many factors, among which the autonomic nervous system (ANS), heart rate (RR interval duration), and gender have a major impact. The autonomic control of the QT is complex, with rate-dependent mechanisms such as membrane ion potentials, intracellular calcium handling, and electrotonic effects. When HR increases, QT duration decreases and vice versa. During exercise in healthy untrained subjects, QT shortens and T waves become more symmetric and increase in amplitude. The major determinant of QT shortening concerns the Te component of the T wave. Under steady-state conditions (e.g. at rest), the QT interval correlates well with the previous RR interval and responds to temporary deviations in instantaneous HR. However, the QT interval at a given HR during exercise is longer than that during recovery [62]. This physiological phenomenon, which is called QT–RR hysteresis, seems to be mainly mediated by differential ANS effects during exercise and recovery [63,64]. During the recovery period a small variation in QTc, within normal limits, is described in normal subjects.

Because of the QT–RR relation, several formulas have been proposed for calculating the corrected QT (QTc).

However, they can only be used over a narrow window of resting heart rates [65]. During exercise the QTc is non-linearly related to HR, and the QTc interval is related to the peak workload achieved. Thus, ideally (even occasionally used in studies) an individual linear QT–HR relation

$$QT = \alpha + \beta \times HR$$

where α is the intercept and β is the slope of the relation, is adopted [65–67]. At baseline the QTc interval is longer in females than in males [60], and QT–RR hysteresis is more marked in women than in men with a greater QT prolongation during decelerating heart rates in recovery [66,68].

Abnormal QT interval adaptation during exercise

LQT is characterized by a disorder of the dynamic adaptations of QT duration to abrupt RR variations. Thus an abnormal adaptation of the QT interval, with a marked increase in its duration, after a rapid transition from the supine to the standing position has been reported (lasting for 2–7min) [69]. LQT patients show several anomalies in QT adaptation to exercise and recovery. Because almost 40% of patients with long QT syndrome may have a non-diagnosis of QTc at rest, treadmill and cycle exercise testing are used in the diagnostic evaluation of LQT [70].

The QT adaptation features occurring during exercise can also help to characterize the specific LQT genotype [71]. For example, during exercise the QT interval shortens less in LQT1 than in LQT2 and LQT3 patients [70,72,73]. In LQT1 and LQT3 patients this abnormal adaptation is progressive and persists at higher HR. In LQT2 patients, the smaller shortening is observed at submaximal HR (50% of predicted maximum HR). The TPe duration is unchanged in LQT1 patients, but decreases in LQT2 and LQT3 patients and is longest in LQT2 carriers at the end of the recovery phase [70,73]. The HR response to exercise is frequently impaired in LQT1 patients [72]. These observations seem to be independent of age, gender, or exercise type [74].

The recovery phase must be abruptly passive, and it is recommended that a long period (at least 5–9min) is recorded in children [70,71,74]. Typically, there are two stages of QT adaptation during recovery. LQT1 patients present the most prolonged QT interval with an initial abrupt exaggerated lengthening, described as QT overshoot, followed by a decrease in QT duration [73,75,76]. Conversely, LQT2 patients begin recovery ($\leq$1min) with their lowest QTc value which then increases during the second part of recovery [70]. The following cut-off values have been proposed: a QTc duration $\geq$460 ms at the start of recovery identifies 80% of LQT1 and 92% of LQT2 patients, and a QTc duration $\geq$445 ms identifies 92% of LQT patients from controls [70,75]. Finally, LQT1 patients are also identified by a paradoxical increase in QTc, i.e. a difference of $\geq$30 ms between QTc recovery and QTc baseline [70]. QT hysteresis is more pronounced in LQT2 patients than in LQT1 patients and normal subjects.

A burst cyclo-ergometer protocol has been proposed for detecting latent long QT (LQT patients with normal resting QTc value). It consists of a sudden maximal exertion against a fixed workload (200W) for 1min, with 5min of recovery. During exercise, QTc increases to a greater extent in latent long LQT patients (98 $\pm$ 36ms) than in controls (65 $\pm$ 19ms). A ΔQTc value >85ms has a sensitivity of 85% and a specificity of 86% for LQTS [77]. Beta-blockers do not blunt these abnormal repolarization exercise profiles, but reduce QT hysteresis in patients with LQT syndrome [70,78]. This improved QT adaptation to HR changes may explain the clinical benefit of beta-blockers [78].

The exercise adaptation of ECG interventricular dispersion of repolarization, evaluated by the difference in QT intervals between left and right ventricle type leads, has also been studied. An increased interventricular dispersion of repolarization is observed in LQT1 patients, but there is almost no variation in normal subjects [76].

Short QT syndrome is a rare arrhythmogenic inherited heart disease and its diagnosis can be challenging in subjects with slightly shortened QT interval [79]. The possibility of using exercise testing for diagnosis has recently been suggested. Patients with short QT show a reduced adaptation of the QT interval to HR, with a shallower slope (<–0.90ms/beat/min) of the QT–HR linear relationship than in normal subjects [80].

QT interval adaptation to exercise in athletes

Regular intense training may modify repolarization with bizarre T-wave shapes and prolonged QT duration. The upper QTc limits proposed for athletes are 470ms and 480ms for males and females, respectively [81].

There have been very few studies of the specific adaptation of QT parameters during exercise in athletes. To our knowledge, no study has compared athletes with LQT patients. Nevertheless, it is considered that the abnormal QT adaptations described for LQT patients should help in the diagnosis of athletes with prolonged resting QT duration.

QT interval prolongation is observed both at rest and during exercise in pathological left ventricular hypertrophy [82]. Conversely, training-induced left ventricular hypertrophy does not affect the relation between QT parameters and the RR interval during exercise testing [82,83]. The slopes of individual QT–RR relations in athletes and untrained controls seem to be similar, but QT hysteresis is less marked and return to the basal value of the QT duration during recovery is faster in athletes [82].

Conclusions

Currently, the diagnosis scheme proposed for confirming LQT in athletes is the same as that in untrained subjects. The place of exercise testing is interesting. Because of the lack of specific studies of athletes, interpretation of QT responses to exercise validated in the general population must be used in athletes.

Further reading

Biffi A, Maron BJ, Culasso F, et al. Patterns of ventricular tachyarrhythmia associated with training, deconditioning and retraining in elite athletes without cardiovascular abnormalities. *Am J Cardiol* 2011; 107: 697–703.

Freeman J, Froelicher V, Ashley E. The ageing athlete: screening prior to vigorous exertion in asymptomatic adults without known cardiovascular disease. *Br J Sports Med* 2009; 43: 696–701.

Schwartz PJ, Ackerman MJ. The long QT syndrome: a transatlantic clinical approach to diagnosis and therapy. *Eur Heart J* 2013; 34: 3109–16.

Turmel J, Bougault V, Boulet L-P, Poirier P. Exaggerated blood pressure response to exercise in athletes: dysmetabolism or altered autonomic nervous system modulation? *Blood Press Monit* 2012; 17: 184–92.

van de Sande DAJP, Breuer MAW, Kemps HMC. Utility of exercise electrocardiography in pre-participation screening in asymptomatic athletes: a systematic review. *Sports Med* 2016

References

1. van de Sande DAJP, Hoogeveen A, Hoogsteen J, Kemps HMC. The diagnostic accuracy of exercise electrocardiography in asymptomatic recreational and competitive athletes. *Scand J Med Sci Sports* 2015; 26: 214–20.
2. van de Sande DAJP, Breuer MAW, Kemps HMC. Utility of exercise electrocardiography in pre-participation screening in asymptomatic athletes: a systematic review. *Sports Med* 2016; 46: 1155–64.
3. Freeman J, Froelicher V, Ashley E. The ageing athlete: screening prior to vigorous exertion in asymptomatic adults without known cardiovascular disease. *Br J Sports Med* 2009; 43: 696–701.
4. Desai MY, Crugnale S, Mondeau J, et al. Slow upsloping ST-segment depression during exercise: does it really signify a positive stress test? *Am Heart J* 2002; 143: 482–7.
5. Cole CR, Blackstone EH, Pashkow FJ, et al. Heart-rate recovery immediately after exercise as a predictor of mortality. *N Engl J Med* 1999; 341: 1351–7.
6. La Gerche A, Baggish AL, Knuuti J, et al. Cardiac imaging and stress testing asymptomatic athletes to identify those at risk of sudden cardiac death. *JACC Cardiovasc Imaging* 2013; 6:993–1007.
7. Belardinelli R, Lacalaprice F, Carle F, et al. Exercise-induced myocardial ischaemia detected by cardiopulmonary exercise testing. *Eur Heart J* 2003; 24: 1304–13.
8. Chaudhry S, Arena RA, Hansen JE, et al. The utility of cardiopulmonary exercise testing to detect and track early-stage ischemic heart disease. *Mayo Clin Proc* 2010; 85: 928–32.
9. Chaudhry S, Arena R, Wasserman K, et al. Exercise-induced myocardial ischemia detected by cardiopulmonary exercise testing. *Am J Cardiol* 2009; 103: 615–19.
10. Chaudhry S, Arena R, Wasserman K, et al. The utility of cardiopulmonary exercise testing in the assessment of suspected microvascular ischemia. *Int J Cardiol* 2011; 148: e7–9.
11. Katzel LI, Fleg JL, Busby-Whitehead MJ, et al. Exercise-induced silent myocardial ischemia in master athletes. *Am J Cardiol* 1998; 81: 261–5.
12. Spirito P, Maron BJ, Bonow RO, Epstein SE. Prevalence and significance of an abnormal S-T segment response to exercise in a young athletic population. *Am J Cardiol* 1983; 51: 1663–6.
13. Jengo JA, Oren V, Conant R, et al. Effects of maximal exercise stress on left ventricular function in patients with coronary artery disease using first pass radionuclide angiocardiography: a rapid, noninvasive technique for determining ejection fraction and segmental wall motion. *Circulation* 1979; 59: 60–5.
14. Ermolao A, Roman F, Gasperetti A, et al. Coronary CT angiography in asymptomatic middle-aged athletes with ST segment anomalies during maximal exercise test. *Scand J Med Sci Sports* 2015; 26: 57–63.
15. Delise P, Sitta N, Lanari E, et al. Long-term effect of continuing sports activity in competitive athletes with frequent ventricular premature complexes and apparently normal heart. *Am J Cardiol* 2013; 112: 1396–1402.
16. Biffi A, Maron BJ, Culasso F, et al. Patterns of ventricular tachyarrhythmia associated with training, deconditioning and retraining in elite athletes without cardiovascular abnormalities. *Am J Cardiol* 2011; 107: 697–703.
17. Calvo N, Brugada J, Sitges M, Mont L. Atrial fibrillation and atrial flutter in athletes. *Br J Sports Med* 2012; 46: 37–43.
18. Turagam MK, Velagapudi P, Kocheril AG. Atrial fibrillation in athletes. *Am J Cardiol* 2012; 109: 296–302.
19. Claessen G, Colyn E, La Gerche A, et al. Long-term endurance sport is a risk factor for development of lone atrial flutter. *Heart* 2011; 97: 918–22.
20. Heidbuchel H, Panhuyzen-Goedkoop N, Corrado D, et al. Recommendations for participation in leisure-time physical activity and competitive sports in patients with arrhythmias and potentially arrhythmogenic conditions. Part I: Supraventricular arrhythmias and pacemakers. *Eur J Cardiovasc Prev Rehabil* 2006; 13: 475–84.
21. Camm AJ, Kirchhof P, Lip GYH, et al. Guidelines for the management of atrial fibrillation: the Task Force for the Management of Atrial Fibrillation of the European Society of Cardiology (ESC). *Eur Heart J* 2010; 31: 2369–429.
22. Zeppilli P, Fenici R, Sassara M, et al. Wenckebach second-degree A-V block in top-ranking athletes: an old problem revisited. *Am Heart J* 1980; 100: 281–94.
23. Pelliccia A, Fagard R, Bjørnstad HH, et al. Recommendations for competitive sports participation in athletes with cardiovascular disease: a consensus document from the Study Group of Sports Cardiology of the Working Group of Cardiac Rehabilitation and Exercise Physiology and the Working Group of Myocardial and Pericardial Diseases of the European Society of Cardiology. *Eur Heart J* 2005; 26: 1422–45.

24. Bennekers JH, van Mechelen R, Meijer A. Pacemaker safety and long-distance running. *Neth Heart J* 2004; 12: 450–4.
25. Wellens HJ, Rodriguez LM, Timmermans C, Smeets JP. The asymptomatic patient with the Wolff–Parkinson–White electrocardiogram. *Pacing Clin Electrophysiol* 1997; 20: 2082–6.
26. Gaita F, Giustetto C, Riccardi R, et al. Stress and pharmacologic tests as methods to identify patients with Wolff–Parkinson–White syndrome at risk of sudden death. *Am J Cardiol* 1989; 64: 487–90.
27. Le VV, Mitiku T, Sungar G, et al. The blood pressure response to dynamic exercise testing: a systematic review. *Prog Cardiovasc Dis* 2008; 51: 135–60.
28. Palatini P. Exercise haemodynamics: field activities versus laboratory tests. *Blood Press Monit* 1997; 2: 133–7.
29. Palatini P. Exaggerated blood pressure response to exercise: pathophysiologic mechanisms and clinical relevance. *J Sports Med Phys Fitness* 1998; 38: 1–9.
30. Douard H, Vuillemin C, Bordier P, et al. Normal blood pressure profiles during exercise according to age, sex and protocols. *Arch Mal Coeur Vaiss* 1994; 87: 311–18.
31. Palatini P. Blood pressure behaviour during physical activity. *Sports Med* 1988; 5: 353–74.
32. Peacock J, Diaz KM, Viera AJ, et al. Unmasking masked hypertension: prevalence, clinical implications, diagnosis, correlates and future directions. *J Hum Hypertens* 2014; 28: 521–8.
33. Schultz MG, Sharman JE. Exercise hypertension. *Pulse* 2013; 1: 161–76.
34. Smith RG, Rubin SA, Ellestad MH. Exercise hypertension: an adverse prognosis? *J Am Soc Hypertension* 2009; 3: 366–73.
35. Lorbeer R, Ittermann T, Völzke H, et al. Assessing cutoff values for increased exercise blood pressure to predict incident hypertension in a general population. *J Hypertens* 2015;33:1386–93
36. Jae SY, Franklin BA, Choo J, Choi Y-H, Fernhall B. Exaggerated exercise blood pressure response during treadmill testing as a predictor of future hypertension in men: a longitudinal study. *Am J Hypertens* 2015; 28: 1362–7.
37. Singh JP, Larson MG, Manolio TA, et al. Blood pressure response during treadmill testing as a risk factor for new-onset hypertension. The Framingham Heart Study. *Circulation* 1999; 99: 1831–3.
38. Franz IW. Blood pressure measurement during ergometric stress testing. *Z Kardiol* 1996; 85(Suppl 3): 71–5.
39. Kjeldsen SE, Mundal R, Sandvik L,. Supine and exercise systolic blood pressure predict cardiovascular death in middle-aged men. *J Hypertens* 2001; 19: 1343–8.
40. Caselli S, Vaquer Segui A, Quattrini F, et al. Upper normal values of blood pressure response to exercise in Olympic athletes. *Am Heart J* 2016; 177: 120–8.
41. Turmel J, Bougault V, Boulet L-P, Poirier P. Exaggerated blood pressure response to exercise in athletes: dysmetabolism or altered autonomic nervous system modulation? *Blood Press Monit* 2012; 17: 184–92.
42. Tomoto T, Sugawara J, Hirasawa A, et al. Impact of short-term training camp on arterial stiffness in endurance runners. *J Physiol Sci* 2015; 65: 445–9.
43. Leiba A, Baur DM, Kales SN. Exercise-induced hypertension among healthy firefighters: a comparison between two different definitions. *J Am Soc Hypertens* 2013; 7: 40–5.
44. Zanettini JO, Fuchs FD, Zanettini MT, Zanettini JP. Is hypertensive response in treadmill testing better identified with correction for working capacity? A study with clinical, echocardiographic and ambulatory blood pressure correlates. *Blood Press* 2004; 13: 225–9.
45. Rost R, Heck H. Exercise hypertension: significance from the viewpoint of sports. *Herz* 1987; 12: 125–33.
46. Szmigielska K, Szmigielska-Kapłon A, Jegier A. Blood pressure response to exercise in young athletes aged 10 to 18 years. *Appl Physiol Nutr Metab* 2016; 41: 41–8.
47. Hernelahti M, Kujala UM, Kaprio J, et al. Hypertension in master endurance athletes. *J Hypertens* 1998; 16: 1573–7.
48. Carnethon MR, Evans NS, Church TS, et al. Joint associations of physical activity and aerobic fitness on the development of incident hypertension: coronary artery risk development in young adults. *Hypertension* 2010; 56: 49–55.
49. Thanassoulis G, Lyass A, Benjamin EJ, et al. Relations of exercise blood pressure response to cardiovascular risk factors and vascular function in the Framingham Heart Study. *Circulation* 2012; 125: 2836–43.
50. Miyai N, Arita M, Miyashita K, et al. Antihypertensive effects of aerobic exercise in middle-aged normotensive men with exaggerated blood pressure response to exercise. *Hypertens Res* 2002; 25: 507–14.
51. Dlin RA, Dotan R, Inbar O, et al. Exaggerated systolic blood pressure response to exercise in a water polo team. *Med Sci Sports Exerc* 1984; 16: 294–8.
52. Turmel J, Poirier P, Bougault V, et al. Cardiorespiratory screening in elite endurance sports athletes: the Quebec study. *Phys Sportsmed* 2012; 40: 55–65.
53. Lauer MS, Levy D, Anderson KM, Plehn JF. Is there a relationship between exercise systolic blood pressure response and left ventricular mass? The Framingham Heart Study. *Ann Intern Med* 1992; 116: 203–10.
54. Karjalainen J, Mäntysaari M, Viitasalo M, Kujala U. Left ventricular mass, geometry, and filling in endurance athletes: association with exercise blood pressure. *J Appl Physiol* 1997; 82: 531–7.
55. Leischik R, Spelsberg N, Niggemann H, et al. Exercise-induced arterial hypertension: an independent factor for hypertrophy and a ticking clock for cardiac fatigue or atrial fibrillation in athletes? *F1000 Res* 2014; 3: 105
56. Mazic S, Lazic JS, Dekleva M, et al. The impact of elevated blood pressure on exercise capacity in elite athletes. *Int J Cardiol* 2015; 180: 171–7.
57. Kim YJ, Goh CW, Byun YS, et al. Left ventricular hypertrophy, diastolic dysfunction, pulse pressure, and plasma ET-1 in marathon runners with exaggerated blood pressure response. *Int Heart J* 2013; 54: 82–7.
58. Kim YJ, Ahn JK, Shin KA, et al. Correlation of cardiac markers and biomarkers with blood pressure of middle-aged marathon runners. *J Clin Hypertens* 2015; 17: 868–73.
59. Mancia G, Fagard R, Narkiewicz K, et al. 2013 ESH/ESC guidelines for the management of arterial hypertension: the Task Force for the Management of Arterial Hypertension of the European Society of Hypertension (ESH) and of the European Society of Cardiology (ESC). *Eur Heart J* 2013; 34: 2159–219.

60. Schwartz PJ, Ackerman MJ. The long QT syndrome: a transatlantic clinical approach to diagnosis and therapy. *Eur Heart J* 2013; 34: 3109–16.
61. Antzelevitch C. Drug-induced spatial dispersion of repolarization. *Cardiol J* 2008; 15: 100–21.
62. Zhang Y, Bao M, Dai M, et al. QT hysteresis index improves the power of treadmill exercise test in the screening of coronary artery disease. *Circ J* 2014; 78: 2942–9.
63. Kannankeril PJ, Harris PA, Norris KJ, et al. Rate-independent QT shortening during exercise in healthy subjects: terminal repolarization does not shorten with exercise. *J Cardiovasc Electrophysiol* 2008; 19: 1284–8.
64. Pelchovitz DJ, Ng J, Chicos AB, et al. QT-RR hysteresis is caused by differential autonomic states during exercise and recovery. *Am J Physiol Heart Circ Physiol* 2012; 302: H2567–73.
65. Malik M, Färbom P, Batchvarov V, et al. Relation between QT and RR intervals is highly individual among healthy subjects: implications for heart rate correction of the QT interval. *Heart* 2002; 87: 220–8.
66. Kligfield P, Lax KG, Okin PM. QT interval-heart rate relation during exercise in normal men and women: definition by linear regression analysis. *J Am Coll Cardiol* 1996; 28: 1547–55.
67. Rabkin SW, Cheng XJ. Newer QT correction formulae to correct QT for heart rate changes during exercise. *Am J Med Sci* 2016; 351: 133–9.
68. Chauhan VS, Krahn AD, Walker BD, et al. Sex differences in QTc interval and QT dispersion: dynamics during exercise and recovery in healthy subjects. *Am Heart J* 2002; 144: 858–64.
69. Adler A, van der Werf C, Postema PG, et al. The phenomenon of 'QT stunning': the abnormal QT prolongation provoked by standing persists even as the heart rate returns to normal in patients with long QT syndrome. *Heart Rhythm* 2012; 9: 901–8.
70. Horner JM, Horner MM, Ackerman MJ. The diagnostic utility of recovery phase QTc during treadmill exercise stress testing in the evaluation of long QT syndrome. *Heart Rhythm* 2011; 8: 1698–704.
71. Wong JA, Gula LJ, Klein GJ, et al. Utility of treadmill testing in identification and genotype prediction in long-QT syndrome. *Circ Arrhythm Electrophysiol* 2010; 3: 120–5.
72. Swan H, Viitasalo M, Piippo K, et al. Sinus node function and ventricular repolarization during exercise stress test in long QT syndrome patients with KvLQT1 and HERG potassium channel defects. *J Am Coll Cardiol* 1999; 34: 823–9
73. Hekkala AM, Viitasalo M, Vaananen H, et al. Abnormal repolarization dynamics revealed in exercise test in long QT syndrome mutation carriers with normal resting QT interval. *Europace* 2010; 12: 1296–1301.
74. Sy RW, Chattha IS, Klein GJ, et al. Repolarization dynamics during exercise discriminate between LQT1 and LQT2 genotypes. *J Cardiovasc Electrophysiol* 2010; 21: 1242–6.
75. Chattha IS, Sy RW, Yee R, et al. Utility of the recovery electrocardiogram after exercise: a novel indicator for the diagnosis and genotyping of long QT syndrome? *Heart Rhythm* 2010; 7: 906–11
76. Haapalahti P, Viitasalo M, Perhonen M, et al. Ventricular repolarization and heart rate responses during cardiovascular autonomic function testing in LQT1 subtype of long QT syndrome. *Pacing Clin Electrophysiol* 2006; 29: 1122–9.
77. Walker BD, Krahn AD, Klein GJ, et al. Burst bicycle exercise facilitates diagnosis of latent long QT syndrome. *Am Heart J* 2005; 150: 1059–63.
78. Krahn AD, Yee R, Chauhan V, et al. Beta blockers normalize QT hysteresis in long QT syndrome. *Am Heart J* 2002; 143: 528–34.
79. Gaita F. Short QT syndrome: a familial cause of sudden death. *Circulation* 2003; 108: 965–70.
80. Giustetto C, Scrocco C, Schimpf R, et al. Usefulness of exercise test in the diagnosis of short QT syndrome. *Europace* 2015; 17: 628–34.
81. Sheikh N, Papadakis M, Ghani S, et al. Comparison of ECG criteria for the detection of cardiac abnormalities in elite black and white athletes. *Circulation* 2014; 129: 1637–49.
82. Rajappan K, O'Connell C, Sheridan DJ. Changes in QT interval with exercise in elite male rowers and controls. *Int J Cardiol* 2003; 87: 217–22.
83. Braschi A, Francavilla VC, Abrignani MG, et al. Behavior of repolarization variables during exercise test in the athlete's heart. *Ann Noninvasive Electrocardiol* 2012; 17: 95–100.

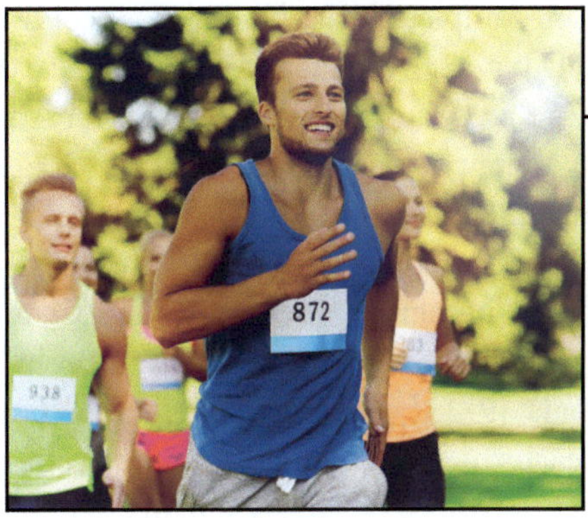

3.2

Arrhythmia registration

Contents

3.2.1 **Ambulatory (24-hour Holter monitoring, event recorders) and signal-averaged ECG for arrhythmia registration in the athlete's heart** Mahdi Sareban and Josef Niebauer *107*
3.2.2 **Class 1 anti-arrhythmic drug provocation test** Matthias Antz *114*
3.2.3 **Electrophysiological study** Matthias Antz *116*

3.2.1 Ambulatory (24-hour Holter monitoring, event recorders) and signal-averaged ECG for arrhythmia registration in the athlete's heart

Mahdi Sareban and Josef Niebauer

Ambulatory ECG

Introduction

The evolution of telemetry as an electronic tool in the biological sciences started with an aim stated by Norman J. Holter in 1947 [1]: '... trying to broadcast by radio the more obvious electrophysiological phenomena occurring in humans so that they could be free to do something besides lie quietly on a couch'. A few years later Holter accomplished this when a 34kg portable unit, kept in a backpack, permitted single-lead ECG recording for several hours [2]. In recognition of this seminal contribution the conventional ambulatory ECG-monitor was named, and is commonly known as, the 'Holter monitor'.

Athlete's heart syndrome exhibits a broad range of heart rhythm variations commonly seen in the resting ECG of asymptomatic athletes, but also present in the ECGs of patients with underlying cardiac disease. If such an athlete consults a doctor for unspecific symptoms, such as chest discomfort, palpitations, or light-headedness, a resting ECG which exhibits ambiguous ECG characteristics might make the medical work-up both challenging and possibly unnecessarily complicated. On the other hand, a normal resting ECG in such an athlete does not necessarily exclude an arrhythmic cause of the symptoms. Ambulatory Holter monitoring plays a critical role in the diagnostic work-up of these athletes. However, progress in science and technology has led to the development of numerous devices for assessing cardiac arrhythmias in an ambulatory setting. Cardiac rhythm can now be recorded continuously or intermittently, devices can be worn externally or implanted subcutaneously, and many are capable of automatically transmitting recordings to a monitoring station for real-time evaluation. In addition, some common heart rate monitors regularly used for controlling training intensity in endurance sports provide precise data on RR intervals from which information about occurrence, frequency, onset and termination, regularity of the rhythm, and duration of arrhythmias in athletes can be derived. However, in view of the lack of information about the morphology of the QRS complex, no precise differentiation between supraventricular and ventricular arrhythmias can be made. Data on heart rate monitors for ambulatory arrhythmia registration are scarce, but the increasing trend to monitor human physiological function in the athletic environment and progress in technology may open up new diagnostic opportunities.

In the next section we highlight the relevance of 24-hour Holter monitoring and event recorders in documenting three clinically relevant arrhythmias related to athlete's heart syndrome: bradyarrhythmias, premature ventricular contractions/non-sustained ventricular tachycardia, and atrial fibrillation (AF).

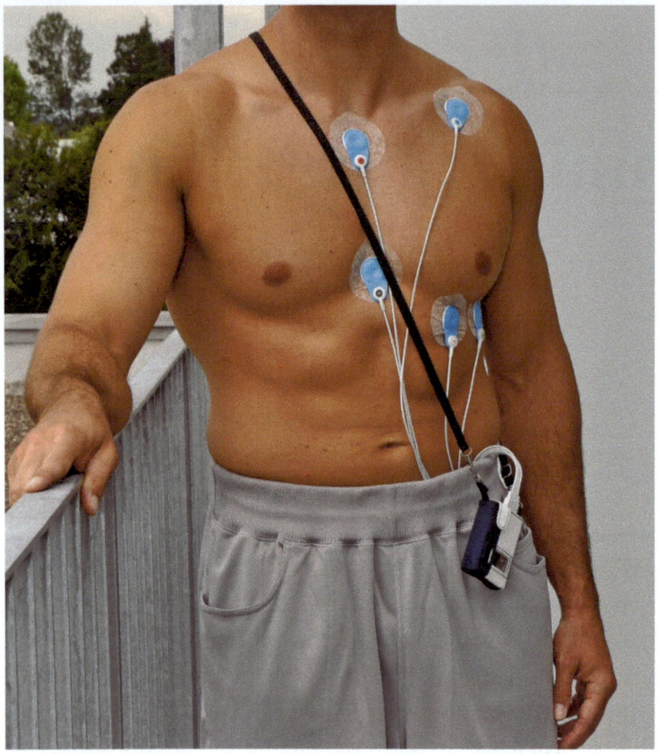

Fig. 3.2.1.1 Holter monitor using five electrodes for a three-lead recording. Used with the permission of Schiller AG, Baar. © 2016, Schiller AG, Baar.

Holter monitoring

Holter monitoring is a non-invasive diagnostic tool which is inexpensive to set up. Monitoring is usually performed for 24 hours, and involves continuous recording in up to 12 leads (➔ Fig. 3.2.1.1). Holter monitoring is the first choice for additional work-up in detecting and quantifying suspected arrhythmias that occur at least once a day in athletes presenting with clinical symptoms and cardiac manifestations suggestive of athlete's heart syndrome or cardiac diseases [3].

According to the current literature, resting bradyarrhythmias, such as sinus bradycardia (≤30 bpm), junctional bradycardia, sinus exit block, and sinus pauses (>3s), are frequently seen in trained athletes. They are attributed to enhanced vagal tone caused by systematic conditioning and thus represent normal ECG findings resulting from physiological adaptation [4–6]. However, when these arrythmias are documented during exercise or accompanied by relevant symptoms, a 24-hour Holter ECG should be obtained [7]. First-degree atrioventricular (AV) block (PR interval >200 ms), and second-degree AV block Mobitz type 1 (Wenckebach) are also commonly seen and taken as normal in athletes [4,6]. If the QRS complex is abnormal, or the PR interval is excessively prolonged (≥0.3s) or documented during exercise, Holter monitoring is warranted because these athletes could be at increased risk for progression to higher-degree AV or complete heart block [7]. Second-degree AV block Mobitz type 2 (Mobitz) and complete heart block are not exercise-related and are generally considered an indication for permanent pacemaker implantation [7].

The most common ventricular arrhythmias seen in athletes are premature ventricular contractions (PVCs) [8]. However, it is debatable whether the incidence of PVCs is increased in highly trained athletes compared with healthy non-athletic individuals [9–11] and thus whether PVCs are part of athlete's heart syndrome. In addition,the occurrence of PVCs has been shown to be largely independent of training-related physiological left ventricular remodelling indices [12], but is sensitive to brief periods of deconditioning in trained athletes [13]. According to the Seattle Criteria for interpretation of athletes' ECGs, two or more PVCs per 10s tracing, ventricular couplets, triplets, and non-sustained ventricular tachycardia are abnormal findings in athletes and prompt further evaluation [6]. In addition to a 12-lead ECG, exercise stress test, and echocardiography, a 24-hour ambulatory monitor may be helpful in determining the frequency, response to exercise, and pattern of the arrhythmias. PVCs recorded at a frequency of >2000 per 24 hours have a higher likelihood of association with underlying cardiac disease [14] and require further evaluation [7,15]. Even when structural heart disease is excluded, annual cardiological evaluation with ambulatory Holter monitoring is recommended [7,14]. Likewise, PVCs that become more frequent or convert to runs of non-sustained ventricular tachycardia (NSVT) during exercise prompt further evaluation [7]. PVCs generally have an inferior axis, indicating an origin in the right ventricular outflow tract which is recognized as a benign entity. However, according to the latest recommendations, multiform/multifocal single PVCs may be equivalent to uniform/unifocal PVCs in terms of risk assessment [7]. In all borderline cases, deconditioning-induced reduction of PVC burden during follow-up Holter monitoring is indicative of a benign condition, which is important for further risk stratification [13].

NSVT, defined as three or more consecutive PVCs up to a maximum duration of 30s, is occasionally detected in trained athletes by Holter monitoring. It is unclear whether this represents another expression of athlete's heart syndrome [14], albeit that NSVT has a higher probability of reflecting an underlying disorder than single PVCs [15]. If NSVTs detected at rest disappear with exercise, this indicates a probable benign condition [7]. Thus, it is of great importance that Holter monitoring is also performed during training and that an accurate diary of the activities is kept in order to relate arrhythmia burden to exercise. Rarely, longitudinal follow-up studies in athletes with NSVT have documented sustained ventricular tachycardia defined by a duration of ≥30s. In addition, sustained ventricular tachyarrhythmias were not inducible during electrophysiological studies of these athletes, and thus are unlikely to be an expression of athlete's heart syndrome [14].

Atrial remodelling and an increased vagal tone are not only characteristics of athlete's heart syndrome but are also the substrate and trigger for promoting re-entry mechanisms in the atrium [16]. Thus athletes undergoing systematic, high volume, and prolonged endurance training appear to be particularly prone to AF, and there is an increasing body of evidence suggesting a correlation between long-term endurance training, ageing, and risk for AF [17–19]. AF has recently been stigmatized as the Achilles tendon of the ageing master athlete [20]. Symptomatic paroxysmal AF, defined as any documented episode of AF with spontaneous conversion to sinus rhythm within 7 days [21], is the most common type of AF presentation in athletes. The majority of AFs in athletes are vagally induced, and so usually occur at night [22]. The diagnosis of AF requires ECG documentation and, because of the intermittent nature of paroxysmal AF, Holter monitoring should be considered for its early detection [21]. As mentioned previously, during Holter monitoring athletes should perform at their usual level of exercise with the monitor in place and keep an accurate diary of their activities in order to be able to relate symptoms to the presence of arrhythmias.

Event recorders

External event recorders are generally devices attached to the individual by chest electrodes during electrophysiological studies of these athletes and they record data either when activated by the patient or when an automatic trigger recognizes an arrhythmia. In *continuous looping event recorders* or *external loop recorders (ELRs)* data are stored for a programmable fixed amount of time before the activation (looping memory) and a period of time after the activation. Other devices are not worn continuously but instead are applied to the chest once a symptom develops. Because of the missing looping feature, these devices are commonly referred to as *post-event non-looping event recorders* (➲ Fig. 3.2.1.2). In these devices the initiation of the arrhythmia that may provide a clue to the arrhythmic mechanism and short arrhythmias that terminate before the device is activated will not be recorded. The major advantage of these devices compared with traditional Holter monitors is that they are small, allow ECG monitoring for longer time periods, and can provide nearly real-time data analysis when the patient transmits a recording in proximity to the symptomatic event. However, asymptomatic arrhythmias cannot be diagnosed and the patient has to be awake to activate the device unless the unit offers automatic activation if arrhythmias occur. *Real-time continuous event recorders* (mobile cardiac telemetry (MCT)) overcome these limitations, and do not require any intervention to capture ECG data as they record continuously for hours a day.

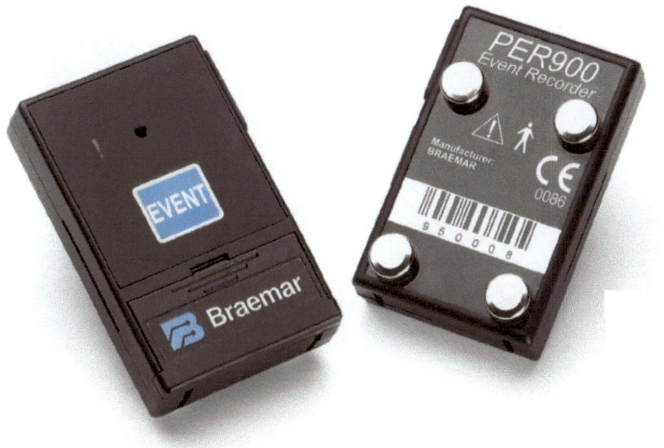

Fig. 3.2.1.2 Post-event non-looping event monitors (PER900).
Courtesy of Braemar. The PER device is CE marked, but the 900L is not and cannot be sold in European CE Mark countries at this time.

Several studies have demonstrated a better diagnostic yield for patient-activated event recorders compared with 24-hour Holter monitoring in the detection of arrhythmias in patients with paroxysmal palpitation or dizziness suggestive of cardiac arrhythmias without underlying structural heart disease [23]. All three external event recorder types can send ECG data wirelessly to a transmitter of the size of a mobile phone which has to be within the radius of radio reception. Data are then relayed through a SIM-card-enabled cellular network to an ECG monitoring centre (the company's monitoring facility or the patient's personal physician) and thus can be analysed in real time. The ECG study duration of all event recorder systems is typically up to 30 days, but can be extended in special cases. If the patient is away away from home the device communicates continuously with the monitoring centre and thus offers real-time ECG analysis even in case of travel.

Limitations on both external event recorders and Holter monitors for use in athletes are skin irritation if electrodes are regularly used and the poor skin contact with the electrodes during exercise, both of which cause artefacts. Some suppliers offer chest patches (➲ Fig. 3.2.1.3) or straps for single-lead ECG recording, which can be sequentially extended to 12-lead recording in some systems. However, the 12-lead results obtained from single-lead systems are sequential, unlike the results obtained with most standard 12-lead systems which are simultaneous. Thus, 12-lead ECG recordings cannot be made continuously during exercise, as with Holter

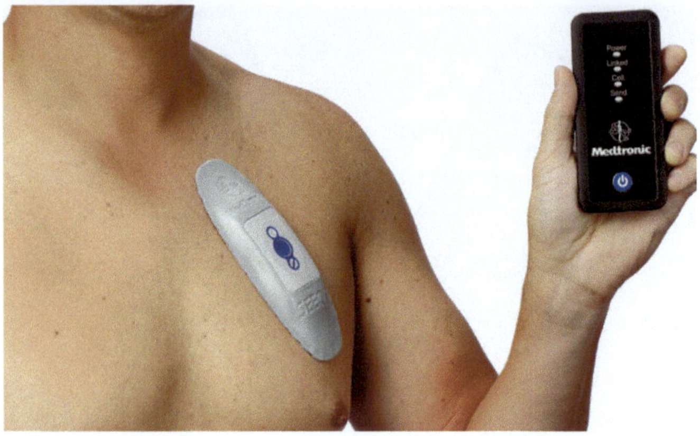

Fig. 3.2.1.3 External real-time continuous event recorder patch (SEEQ Mobile Cardiac Telemetry system). A distance of less than 9m from the transmitter is needed for successful data transmission. The transmitter remains charged for up to 12 hours. Data are sent via global satellite cellular signals with built-in cellular technology.
Used with the permission of Medtronic, Inc. © 2016 Medtronic, Inc. Material not commercially available in Europe (mid-2016).

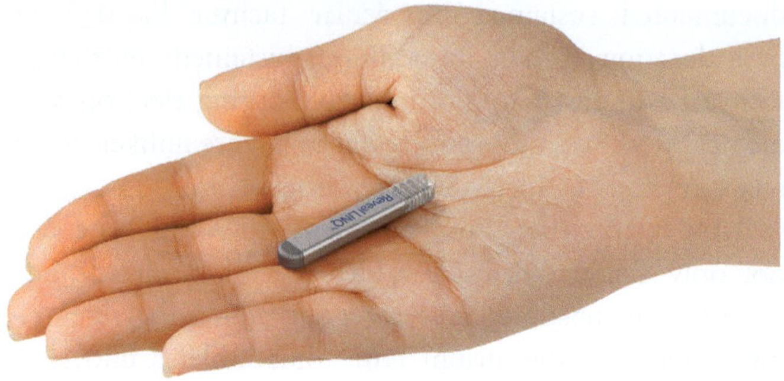

Fig. 3.2.1.4 Implantable loop recorder (Reveal LINQ). Distance of less than 2 meters from the transmitter is needed for successful data transmission.
Used with the permission of Medtronic, Inc. © 2016 Medtronic, Inc. Material not commercially available in Europe (mid-2016).

units or standard stress-testing equipment, because of artefacts induced by muscle activation. Instead, rapid recordings must be made during brief interruptions of exercise.

Implantable event recorders are the next diagnostic step for documenting arrhythmias in symptomatic athletes in cases where Holter monitors and external event recorders have been unsuccessful, for example because of the rare frequency of symptoms or missed arrhythmias when using a non-looping device. New generation implantable devices are becoming smaller (➲ Fig. 3.2.1.4), can be inserted with a syringe, are safe for use in MRIs, and continuously record a single-lead ECG for up to 3 years. Nevertheless, they are still invasive and are associated with considerable costs, and therefore they should be used with great caution, especially in athletes participating in body contact sports. ➲ Table 3.2.1.1 gives an overview of different types of event recorder.

Table 3.2.1.1 Overview of different types of event recorder

	Allows complete monitoring and storage of data (24 h/d)	**Remote monitoring capability**	**Usual duration of monitoring**	**Technical cost**	**Examples for use in arrhythmias and symptoms seen in athletes**	**Relevant specifications from illustrated devices**
Post-event non-looping event monitors (Fig. 3.2.1.2)	No	Yes	up to 1 month	€200	Atrial fibrillation	Single-channel recording; max. no. of events, 30; max. recording time, 30min; max. event time, 60s, dimensions, 84 × 54 × 18 mm
Continuous looping event monitor/external loop recorder (ELR)	No	Yes	Up to 1 month	€300	Symptomatic premature ventricle contractions/ non-sustained ventricular tachycardia, atrial fibrillation	1–3-channel recording; programmable max. pre/ post-event and total recording time
Real-time continuous event recorder (Fig. 3.2.1.3)	Yes	Yes	Up to 1 month	€500	Recurrent presyncope/ syncope, palpitations	Wearable water-resistant sensor; single-channel recording; max. recording time, 7.5 days; weight, 50 g; dimensions, 160 × 60 × 15mm
Implantable loop recorder (Fig. 3.2.1.4)	Yes	Yes	Up to 3 years	€3500	Otherwise unexplained infrequent syncope	Single-channel recording; weight, 2.5 g; dimensions, 45 × 7 × 4mm

Adapted with permission from Peter Zimetbaum, Alena Goldman. Ambulatory arrhythmia monitoring. *Circulation*, Volume 122, Issue 16, pp. 1629–36. Copyright © 2010 Wolters Kluwer Health, Inc.

The role of event recorders in the evaluation of the athlete's heart starts with continuing clinical suspicion of relevant arrhythmias after Holter monitoring has failed to document any abnormalities. The choice of event recorder is based on the presenting symptoms, symptom frequency, and degree of suspicion of a life-threatening arrhythmia, and should be individualized to the athlete.

Since most bradyarrhythmias in athlete's heart are training-induced adaptations to which the athlete is accustomed, dizziness or unexplained syncope should always raise suspicion and prompt further evaluation [7]. Syncope, defined as transient loss of consciousness caused by transient global cerebral hypoperfusion and spontaneous complete recovery [24], in athletes has a neurally-mediated origin in most cases, is not related to exercise, and has a low recurrence rate [25]. Syncope during exercise has a higher probability of being caused by serious underlying cardiovascular disease, and athletes with exercise-induced syncope should be restricted from all competitive sport until evaluated by a qualified medical professional [7]. Holter monitoring is of low diagnostic value in detecting underlying arrhythmias during an episode because of the low recurrence rates of syncopes in athletes. If further evaluation is considered, a real-time continuous event recorder is the device of choice. Because of poor compliance with an intensive monitoring protocol due to skin irritation and the inconvenience associated with performing activities [26], an implantable loop recorder should be considered in unexplained and infrequent syncopal episodes.

Although reassuring data have been published regarding the benign nature of PVC and NSVT in athletes without structural heart disease [12,14,27], athletes may still present with intimidating palpitations which may lead to considerable psychological strain, reduced performance, and reduction of sporting activities or even abandonment of an active lifestyle. Athletes may be particularly sensitive to PVCs, presuming they are sensitive to their body, and often perceive abnormalities with greater intensity. After exclusion of structural heart disease, failed documentation, or a clear association between symptoms and PVC/NSVT during Holter monitoring, use of an external event recorder should be discussed with the athlete noting that documentation as well as reassurance might help them to deal with benign alterations. In asymptomatic cases with a high pre-test probability for underlying cardiomyopathy, an event recorder should be considered for further risk stratification.

In symptomatic athletes with a high pre-test probability for AF, although none occur during Holter monitoring, further ambulatory monitoring approaches should be considered. Presuming that paroxysmal AF episodes in athletes are accompanied by symptoms and usually last for at least several minutes, external loop recorders or post-event non-looping recorders are reasonable choices. The lower the AF burden and the shorter the duration of the paroxysm, the greater is the chance of catching an episode on a continuous looping recorder. Implantable event recorders have a high diagnostic yield for detecting the presence of AF [28,29], but given the invasive nature of the device implantation should only be considered if asymptomatic AF is presumed and establishing a diagnosis has clinical consequences.

Signal-averaged ECG

Introduction

Since the early 1960s, signal averaging has been increasingly used to improve the signal-to-noise ratio of highly amplified bioelectric signals [30]. Signal averaging has even been used for differentiating ECG signals recorded during exercise from movement artefacts [31]. In the 1970s scientists looked for non-invasive ECG techniques which provided direct information about the electrical activity of the conducting system, and Berbari et al. [32] attempted to record His bundle deflection by signal-averaged ECG (SAECG). The next step in signal averaging was the non-invasive detection of late potentials on the surface ECG as a surrogate for risk of sudden cardiac death (SCD) in patients with myocardial ischaemia. Late potentials were described as low amplitude, high frequency ECG signals which occur at the end of the QRS complex and/or the ST segment and were conceptualized as reflecting slow and inhomogeneous conduction in scarred myocardium. It was already known that slow conduction was a prerequisite for re-entrant ventricular arrhythmias. In the 1980s several important technical contributions for both recording and analysing late potentials [33] were made by introducing bidirectional Butterworth filter and a combination of bipolar X, Y, and Z leads. Algorithms were developed to determine the end of the filtered signal-averaged vector magnitude, and this was referred to as 'time-domain analysis'. The testing protocol and the time-domain analysis of SAECG is still used in clinical routine. In short, SAECG recordings are performed with special high-resolution recording devices. Silver chloride electrodes are placed in an orthogonal manner using Frank bipolar X, Y, and Z leads after careful skin preparation to eliminate artefacts. Subsequently, patients lie still and supine for 10 min to minimize noise from muscle movements while recording is performed. The signals derived are then amplified, digitized, averaged, and filtered between 1 and 300Hz.

Although the most recent guidelines for the management of patients with ventricular arrhythmias [3] no longer recommend SAECG for risk stratification for SCD after myocardial infarction, it is a class I recommendation for improving the diagnosis of arrhythmogenic right ventricular dysplasia/cardiomyopathy (ARVD/C) [3]. In addition, SAECG should be performed on all first-degree relatives of patients diagnosed with ARVD/C. In view of these recommendations, the relevance of late potentials derived from SAECG in sports cardiology practice will be discussed in more detail and the role of signal averaging of the P wave as a surrogate to identify endurance athletes at risk of AF will be outlined.

Signal-averaged ECG in sports cardiology

ARVD/C is an inherited cardiomyopathy and an important contributor to SCDs in young athletes [34].An international Task Force of experts included several ECG features in the modified Task Force Criteria for the diagnosis ARVD/C [35]. A combination of criteria from different diagnostic modalities is needed for the clinical diagnosis of ARVC and, referring to the modified Task Force criteria, SAECG is regarded as a minor diagnostic criterion for ARVD/C, if one out of the following three time-domain parameters (➲ Fig. 3.2.1.5) is abnormal in the absence of a QRS duration of ≥110 ms on the standard ECG:

(1) filtered QRS duration (fQRS) ≥114 msl

(2) low amplitude signal duration ≥38 ms

(3) root mean square voltage of terminal 40ms ≤20μV.

Previously, the SAECG was classified as positive if two of the above three parameters were abnormal, but according to the modified criteria any one of the three parameters obtained was proposed as a criterion for this modality.

However, these criteria were derived from patients in the North American ARVC Registry [36] and have limited diagnostic power for athletes. Thus they may give rise to exercise-induced cardiovascular changes. Jongman et al. [37] have recently demonstrated that all elite athletes and the majority of amateur athletes participating in high dynamic and high static sports reveal a prolonged fQRS duration on SAECG, and these athletes would satisfy minor ARVD/C criteria. Adding to the diagnostic dilemma of differentiating the athlete's heart from ARVD/C, in the study conducted by Jongman et al. [37], the extent of fQRS prolongation was positively correlated with the right ventricular dimension and a majority of athletes demonstrated at least one major echocardiographic criterion for ARVD/C. The number of athletes exhibiting two or three abnormal SAECG parameters was comparable to the prevalence of 8.5% of late potentials reported in the literature [38]. In summary, the present cut-off values for the diagnosis of ARVD/C are of limited use in the athletic population, especially elite athletes

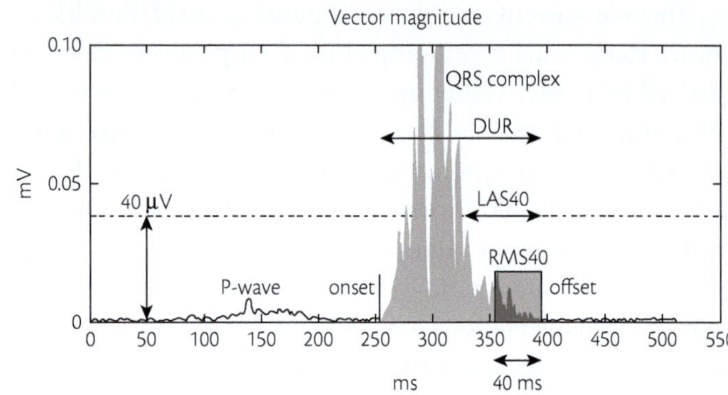

Fig. 3.2.1.5: Time-domain parameters in a signal-averaged ECG. Onset and offset represent the limits of the ventricular activation and are automatically detected. Parameters calculated from the vector magnitude: (1) duration of the signal-averaged filtered QRS complex (DUR, ms); (2) duration in the terminal region of ventricular activation with a magnitude <40μV (LAS40, ms); (3) root mean square (RMS) value of the potentials in the 40ms terminal of the filtered QRS (RMS40, μV).

Reproduced from Marocolo, et al. The effect of an aerobic training program on the electrical remodeling of the heart: high-frequency components of the signal-averaged electrocardiogram are predictors of the maximal aerobic power. *Brazilian Journal of Medical and Biological Research*, Volume 40, issue 2, pp. 199–208. 2007. Reproduced under the Creative Commons Attribution Licence.

participating in high dynamic and high static sports where cardiovascular adaptation is most pronounced [39] and probably represents physiological cardiac adaptation resulting from regular physical exercise.

The signal-averaging technique has also been used as a surrogate risk index for AF using the same lead positions (bipolar X, Y, Z leads) and the same filter settings as in the detection of late potentials [40]. In a study conducted by Wilhelm et al. [40], 60 non-elite middle-aged male endurance athletes were stratified according to their lifetime training hours into low (<1500 hours), medium (1500–4500 hours), and high (>4500 hours). The signal-averaging P-wave duration increased from low to high training groups and the study concluded that signal averaging of the P wave may reflect conduction delay within the left atrium or the pulmonary veins. In view of the increasing evidence of adverse atrial remodelling due to prolonged and intense endurance training, further research is needed to establish the diagnostic value of signal-average analysis of the P wave in the early detection of athletes at risk of AF.

New technologies

Some lead-less ambulatory heart rate monitors regularly used for controlling training intensity in endurance sport provide precise data on RR intervals from which basic information about arrhythmias in athletes can be derived [41,42]. Smartphone-based ECG devices can create single-lead ECG tracings and have already shown their utility in the detection of AF [43]. In addition, the field of wearable electronics, i.e. integration of small electronic devices into textile fabrics, is rapidly emerging. Single-lead ECG derived from a biomedical shirt which captures a medical-quality ECG signal via textile electrodes with wireless transmission of the signal to a platform for further analysis has already achieved high diagnostic accuracy [44,45] and will serve as a new alternative for cardiac monitoring and the detection of arrhythmias in athletes.

Conclusions

Ambulatory ECG registration is an invaluable diagnostic tool for differentiating benign arrhythmias commonly seen in the athlete's heart syndrome and life-threatening arrhythmias caused by cardiac pathologies. However, considering the vast number of existing devices and software applications as well as possible misinterpretations, the need for appropriate training of the team in charge of the management of athletes presenting with arrhythmias should be emphasized. Furthermore, longitudinal ambulatory ECG studies are needed in order to improve characterization of the athlete's heart syndrome.

Further reading

Abdulla J, Nielsen JR. Is the risk of atrial fibrillation higher in athletes than in the general population? A systematic review and meta-analysis. *Europace* 2009; 11:1156–9.

Baggish AL, Wood MJ. Athlete's heart and cardiovascular care of the athlete: scientific and clinical update. *Circulation* 2011; 123: 2723–35.

Lampert R. Evaluation and management of arrhythmia in the athletic patient. Prog Cardiovasc Dis 2012;54: 423–31.

Priori SG, Blomström-Lundqvist C, Mazzanti A, et al. 2015 ESC Guidelines for the management of patients with ventricular arrhythmias and the prevention of sudden cardiac death: the Task Force for the Management of Patients with Ventricular Arrhythmias and the Prevention of Sudden Cardiac Death of the European Society of Cardiology (ESC): endorsed by Association for European Paediatric and Congenital Cardiology (AEPC). *Europace* 2015; 17: 1601–87.

Zimetbaum P, Goldman A. Ambulatory arrhythmia monitoring: choosing the right device. *Circulation* 2010; 122: 1629–36.

References

1. Roberts WC, Silver MA. Norman Jefferis Holter and ambulatory ECG monitoring. *Am J Cardiol* 1983; 52: 903–6.
2. Zimetbaum P, Goldman A. Ambulatory arrhythmia monitoring: choosing the right device. *Circulation* 2010; 122: 1629–36.
3. Priori SG, Blomström-Lundqvist C, Mazzanti A, et al. 2015 ESC Guidelines for the management of patients with ventricular arrhythmias and the prevention of sudden cardiac death: the Task Force for the Management of Patients with Ventricular Arrhythmias and the Prevention of Sudden Cardiac Death of the European Society of Cardiology (ESC): endorsed by Association for European Paediatric and Congenital Cardiology (AEPC). *Europace* 2015; 17: 1601–87.
4. Ector H, Bourgois J, Verlinden M, Hermans L, Vanden Eynde E, Fagard R, et al. Bradycardia, ventricular pauses, syncope, and sports. Lancet. 1984 Sep;2(8403):591–4.
5. Holly RG, Shaffrath JD, Amsterdam EA. Electrocardiographic alterations associated with the hearts of athletes. Sports Med. 1998 Mar;25(3):139–48.
6. Drezner JA, Ackerman MJ, Anderson J, Ashley E, Asplund CA, Baggish AL, et al. Electrocardiographic interpretation in athletes: the 'Seattle criteria'. Br J Sports Med. 2013 Feb;47(3):122–4.
7. Zipes DP, Link MS, Ackerman MJ, Kovacs RJ, Myerburg RJ, Estes NA, et al. Eligibility and Disqualification Recommendations for Competitive Athletes With Cardiovascular Abnormalities: Task Force 9: Arrhythmias and Conduction Defects: A Scientific Statement From the American Heart Association and American College of Cardiology. Circulation. 2015 Dec;132(22):e315–25.
8. Huston TP, Puffer JC, Rodney WM. The athletic heart syndrome. N Engl J Med. 1985 Jul;313(1):24–32.
9. Lampert R. Evaluation and management of arrhythmia in the athletic patient. Prog Cardiovasc Dis. 2012 Mar-Apr;54(5):423–31.
10. Bjørnstad H, Storstein L, Meen HD, Hals O. Ambulatory electrocardiographic findings in top athletes, athletic students and control subjects. Cardiology. 1994;84(1):42–50.
11. Palatini P, Maraglino G, Sperti G, Calzavara A, Libardoni M, Pessina AC, et al. Prevalence and possible mechanisms of ventricular arrhythmias in athletes. Am Heart J. 1985 Sep;110(3):560–7.
12. Biffi A, Maron BJ, Di Giacinto B, Porcacchia P, Verdile L, Fernando F, et al. Relation between training-induced left ventricular hypertrophy and risk for ventricular tachyarrhythmias in elite athletes. *Am J Cardiol* 2008 Jun;101(12):1792–5.
13. Biffi A, Maron BJ, Verdile L, Fernando F, Spataro A, Marcello G, et al. Impact of physical deconditioning on ventricular tachyarrhythmias in trained athletes. J Am Coll Cardiol. 2004 Sep;44(5):1053–8.
14. Biffi A, Pelliccia A, Verdile L, Fernando F, Spataro A, Caselli S, et al. Long-term clinical significance of frequent and complex ventricular tachyarrhythmias in trained athletes. J Am Coll Cardiol. 2002 Aug;40(3):446–52.
15. Heidbüchel H, Corrado D, Biffi A, Hoffmann E, Panhuyzen-Goedkoop N, Hoogsteen J, et al. Recommendations for participation in leisure-time physical activity and competitive sports of patients with arrhythmias and potentially arrhythmogenic conditions. Part II: ventricular arrhythmias, channelopathies and implantable defibrillators. Eur J Cardiovasc Prev Rehabil. 2006 Oct;13(5):676–86.
16. Chen PS, Tan AY. Autonomic nerve activity and atrial fibrillation. Heart Rhythm. 2007 Mar;4(3 Suppl):S61–4.
17. Abdulla J, Nielsen JR. Is the risk of atrial fibrillation higher in athletes than in the general population? A systematic review and meta-analysis. Europace. 2009 Sep;11(9):1156–9.
18. Andersen K, Farahmand B, Ahlbom A, Held C, Ljunghall S, Michaëlsson K, et al. Risk of arrhythmias in 52 755 long-distance cross-country skiers: a cohort study. Eur Heart J. 2013 Dec;34(47):3624–31.
19. Mont L, Elosua R, Brugada J. Endurance sport practice as a risk factor for atrial fibrillation and atrial flutter. Europace. 2009 Jan;11(1):11–7.

20. Baggish AL. Athletic Left Atrial Dilation: Size Matters? JACC Cardiovasc Imaging. 2015 Jul;8(7):763–5.
21. Camm AJ, Kirchhof P, Lip GY, Schotten U, Savelieva I, Ernst S, et al. Guidelines for the management of atrial fibrillation: the Task Force for the Management of Atrial Fibrillation of the European Society of Cardiology (ESC). Eur Heart J. 2010 Oct;31(19):2369–429.
22. Hoogsteen J, Schep G, Van Hemel NM, Van Der Wall EE. Paroxysmal atrial fibrillation in male endurance athletes. A 9-year follow up. Europace. 2004 May;6(3):222–8.
23. de Asmundis C, Conte G, Sieira J, Chierchia GB, Rodriguez-Manero M, Di Giovanni G, et al. Comparison of the patient-activated event recording system vs. traditional 24 h Holter electrocardiography in individuals with paroxysmal palpitations or dizziness. Europace. 2014 Aug;16(8):1231–5.
24. Moya A, Sutton R, Ammirati F, Blanc JJ, Brignole M, Dahm JB, et al. Guidelines for the diagnosis and management of syncope (version 2009). Eur Heart J. 2009 Nov;30(21):2631–71.
25. Colivicchi F, Ammirati F, Santini M. Epidemiology and prognostic implications of syncope in young competing athletes. Eur Heart J. 2004 Oct;25(19):1749–53.
26. Vasamreddy CR, Dalal D, Dong J, Cheng A, Spragg D, Lamiy SZ, et al. Symptomatic and asymptomatic atrial fibrillation in patients undergoing radiofrequency catheter ablation. J Cardiovasc Electrophysiol. 2006 Feb;17(2):134–9.
27. Baldesberger S, Bauersfeld U, Candinas R, Seifert B, Zuber M, Ritter M, et al. Sinus node disease and arrhythmias in the long-term follow-up of former professional cyclists. Eur Heart J. 2008 Jan;29(1):71–8.
28. Pürerfellner H, Pokushalov E, Sarkar S, Koehler J, Zhou R, Urban L, et al. P-wave evidence as a method for improving algorithm to detect atrial fibrillation in insertable cardiac monitors. Heart Rhythm. 2014 Sep;11(9):1575–83.
29. Pürerfellner H, Sanders P, Pokushalov E, Di Bacco M, Bergemann T, Dekker LR, et al. Miniaturized Reveal LINQ insertable cardiac monitoring system: First-in-human experience. Heart Rhythm. 2015 Jun;12(6):1113–9.
30. Gomes JA. Signal Averaged Electrocardiography: Concepts, Methods and Applications: Springer Science; 1993.
31. Pryor TA, Ridges JD. A computer program for stress test data processing. Comput Biomed Res. 1974 Aug;7(4):360–8.
32. Berbari EJ, Lazzara R, Samet P, Scherlag BJ. Noninvasive technique for detection of electrical activity during the P-R segment. Circulation. 1973 Nov;48(5):1005–13.
33. Simson MB. Use of signals in the terminal QRS complex to identify patients with ventricular tachycardia after myocardial infarction. Circulation. 1981 Aug;64(2):235–42.
34. Corrado D, Basso C, Pavei A, Michieli P, Schiavon M, Thiene G. Trends in sudden cardiovascular death in young competitive athletes after implementation of a preparticipation screening program. JAMA. 2006 Oct;296(13):1593–601.
35. Marcus FI, McKenna WJ, Sherrill D, Basso C, Bauce B, Bluemke DA, et al. Diagnosis of arrhythmogenic right ventricular cardiomyopathy/dysplasia: proposed modification of the Task Force Criteria. Eur Heart J. 2010 Apr;31(7):806–14.
36. Marcus FI, Zareba W, Calkins H, Towbin JA, Basso C, Bluemke DA, et al. Arrhythmogenic right ventricular cardiomyopathy/dysplasia clinical presentation and diagnostic evaluation: results from the North American Multidisciplinary Study. Heart Rhythm. 2009 Jul;6(7):984–92.
37. Jongman JK, Zaidi A, Muggenthaler M, Sharma S. Relationship between echocardiographic right-ventricular dimensions and signal-averaged electrocardiogram abnormalities in endurance athletes. Europace. 2015 Sep;17(9):1441–8.
38. Moroe K, Kimoto K, Inoue T, Annoura M, Oku K, Arakawa K, et al. Evaluation of abnormal signal-averaged electrocardiograms in young athletes. Jpn Circ J. 1995 May;59(5):247–56.
39. Luijkx T, Cramer MJ, Prakken NH, Buckens CF, Mosterd A, Rienks R, et al. Sport category is an important determinant of cardiac adaptation: an MRI study. Br J Sports Med. 2012 Dec;46(16):1119–24.
40. Wilhelm M, Roten L, Tanner H, Wilhelm I, Schmid JP, Saner H. Atrial remodeling, autonomic tone, and lifetime training hours in nonelite athletes. Am J Cardiol 2011 Aug;108(4):580–5.
41. Müssigbrodt A, Richter S, Wetzel U, Van Belle Y, Bollmann A, Hindricks G. Diagnosis of arrhythmias in athletes using leadless, ambulatory HR monitors. Med Sci Sports Exerc. 2013 Aug;45(8):1431–5.
42. Weippert M, Kumar M, Kreuzfeld S, Arndt D, Rieger A, Stoll R. Comparison of three mobile devices for measuring R-R intervals and heart rate variability: Polar S810i, Suunto t6 and an ambulatory ECG system. Eur J Appl Physiol. 2010 Jul;109(4):779–86.
43. Chung EH, Guise KD. QTC intervals can be assessed with the AliveCor heart monitor in patients on dofetilide for atrial fibrillation. J Electrocardiol. 2015 2015 Jan-Feb;48(1):8–9.
44. Despang HG, Netz S, Heinig A, Holland HJ, Fischer WJ. Wireless long-term ECG integrated into clothing. Biomed Tech (Berl). 2008 Dec;53(6):270–8.
45. Perez de Isla L, Lennie V, Quezada M, Guinea J, Arce C, Abad P, et al. New generation dynamic, wireless and remote cardiac monitorization platform: a feasibility study. Int J Cardiol. 2011 Nov;153(1):83–5.

3.2.2 Class 1 anti-arrhythmic drug provocation test

Matthias Antz

The Brugada syndrome is associated with potentially lethal arrhythmias and sudden cardiac death [1,2]. The diagnosis of Brugada syndrome is made from the surface ECG showing a coved type ST-segment elevation ≥0.2 mV (Brugada type 1 ECG) in one or more right precordial leads (V1 and/or V2) positioned in the second, third, or fourth intercostal space [1,2]. These diagnostic ECG characteristics occur either spontaneously or can be provoked by intravenous administration of class 1 anti-arrhythmic drugs (i.e. sodium channel blocking agents such as ajmaline, flecainide, or procainamide). The latter is frequently performed in suspicious but not diagnostic ECGs (incomplete or complete bundle branch block pattern, saddle-type ECG with ST-segment elevation less than 0.2mV; class I level C recommendation) [2].

In most centres the drug of choice for the class 1 antiarrhythmic provocation test is ajmaline because of its high sensitivity and specificity as well as its short half-life (➔ Fig. 3.2.2.1) [3]. Ajmaline is injected intravenously at a rate of 10mg every 2min up to a total dose of 1mg/kg body weight [4]. Ajmaline administration should be stopped if the QRS increases by more than 30%, premature ventricular ectopy appears, or a diagnostic Brugada type I ECG is visible [4]. The provocation test should be performed by experienced physicians and nurses in a room in which advanced life support is readily available, because the sodium channel blocker may provoke life-threatening ventricular arrhythmias in 1% of tests (any ventricular arrhythmia in 2.4%, non-sustained ventricular tachycardia (VT) in 0.34%, and sustained VT in 0.59%) [4,5]. These ventricular arrhythmias can usually be managed by defibrillator shocks, isoproterenol and (as a last resort), an extra-corporeal membrane oxygenator [5].

Predictors of induced ventricular arrhythmias are younger age and conduction disturbance in the baseline ECG (longer QRS interval, macroscopic T-wave alternans, high ST-segment elevation in V2, longer QTc interval, sinus node dysfunction) [5]. Survivors of these induced arrhythmias did not have a worse prognosis [5]. However, the class 1 antiarrhythmic drug provocation test is only useful for diagnosing a Brugada syndrome, and not for establishing the indication for an implantable cardioverter defibrillator (ICD). For further risk stratification and management, see Chapter 5.1.

References

1. Ackerman MJ, Priori SG, Willems S, et al. HRS/EHRA expert consensus statement on the state of genetic testing for the channelopathies and cardiomyopathies. Heart Rhythm 2011; 8(8): 1308–35.
2. Priori SG, Blomström-Lundqvist C, Mazzanti A, et al. 2015 ESC guidelines for the management of patients with ventricular arrhythmias and the prevention of sudden cardiac death. Eur Heart J 2015; 36: 2793–867.
3. Arbelo E, Brugada J. Risk stratification and treatment of Brugada syndrome. Curr Cardiol Rep 2014; 16: 508–18.
4. Rolf S, Bruns HJ, Wichter T, et al. The ajmaline challenge in Brugada syndrome: diagnostic impact, safety, and recommended protocol. Eur Heart J 2003; 24: 1104–12.
5. Dobbels B, De Cleen D, Ector J. Ventricular arrhythmia during ajmaline challenge for the Brugada syndrome. Europace 2016; 18: 1501–6.

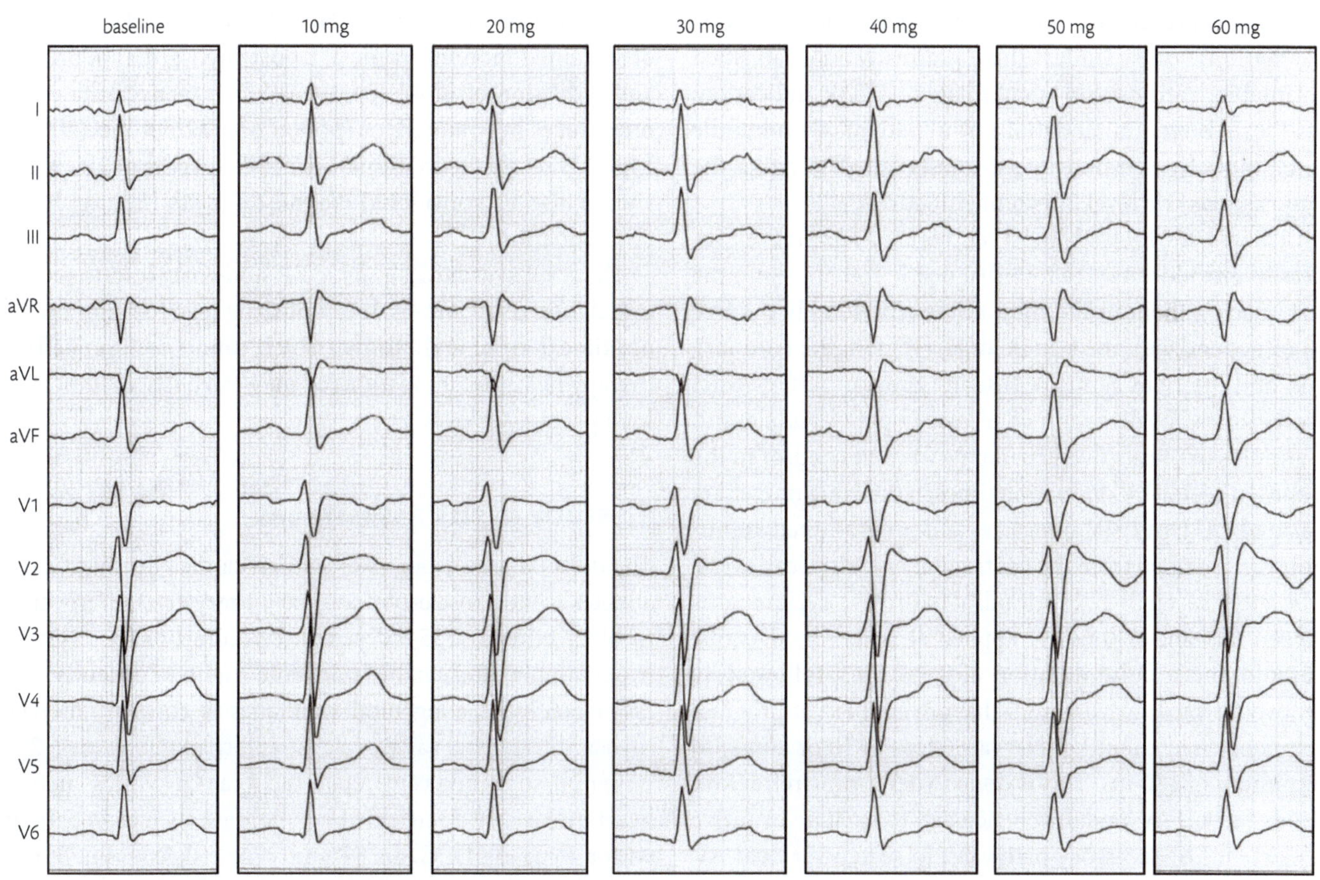

Figure 3.2.2.1 Ajmaline test in a patient with suspected Brugada syndrome. The baseline 12-lead ECG is almost normal with a slightly elevated J point in V2. After administration of 30mg ajmaline the J point in V2 is elevated by 3mm with a saddle-back type ST-segment elevation of 2mm resembling a type 2 Brugada ECG. After injection of 60mg ajmaline the J point is elevated by 3mm in V1 and by 6 mm in in V2 with a coved-type ST-segment elevation followed by a negative T wave, which is consistent with a diagnostic type 1 Brugada ECG.

3.2.3 Electrophysiological study

Matthias Antz

Introduction

An electrophysiological (EP) study can be performed for diagnostic reasons (athletes with palpitations or documented arrhythmias of unclear origin), for risk assessment (non-sustained ventricular tachycardia, structural heart disease, or electrical abnormalities such as the Brugada syndrome) and for therapy of arrhythmias (ablation of ectopic beats, supraventricular or ventricular tachycardia, atrial fibrillation).

Diagnostic EP study

In athletes with documented narrow or broad complex tachycardias, syncope, or palpitations a diagnostic EP study can be performed for further evaluation. According to the 2009 guidelines of the European Society of Cardiology [1] an EP study is especially recommended in syncope patients with ischaemic heart disease when initial evaluation suggests an arrhythmic cause (unless there is already an established implantable cardioverter defibrillator (ICD) indication; class I level B recommendation) or in patients with bundle branch block (when non-invasive tests failed to make the diagnosis; class IIa level B recommendation).

In a diagnostic EP study most centres use a femoral venous access to introduce two to four diagnostic catheters into the heart, placing them in the right atrium (preferably the free wall or appendage), the bundle of His region, the coronary sinus, and the right ventricle (usually apex or outflow tract or sometimes, for detection of accessory pathways, close to the annulus of the atrioventricular (AV) valves and/or in the parahisian region). Conduction times in the His catheter are measured (AH and HV intervals) and programmed stimulation is performed from the ventricular and atrial catheters. In the latter, seven or eight stimuli at base drive cycle lengths between 600 and 400ms are applied at twice the diastolic threshold and a pulse duration of 0.5–2.0ms, followed by one, two, or three extrastimuli that are coupled at progressively shortened coupling intervals (steps of 10 or 20ms) to a minimum of 180 ms. This is done to determine refractory periods (atrial, AV nodal, ventricular), to exclude or prove the existence of accessory pathways, to search for dual AV nodal conduction properties, and to induce arrhythmias (especially re-entry tachycardias) as shown in ➲ Fig. 3.2.3.1. To further elucidate AV conduction properties continuous atrial and ventricular stimulation is performed and the cycle length is progressively shortened to determine the antegrade and retrograde Wenckebach cycle length ('ramp pacing'). Brief pacing at short constant cycle lengths ('burst pacing') can be used for arrhythmia induction. All pacing manoeuvres can be repeated during isoproterenol infusion or after atropine administration. To assess sinus nodal function the atrium is stimulated at a constant cycle length for 30–60s and the time between the last atrial stimulus and the first sinus beat is determined (sinus nodal recovery time). This interval is usually corrected for the heart rate during sinus rhythm before stimulation is started (corrected sinus nodal recovery time). Drug testing can also be performed to investigate whether intravenous administration of an anti-arrhythmic agent can successfully terminate or suppress induction (or spontaneous occurrence) of a symptomatic arrhythmia not amenable to catheter ablation.

For the general population the 2009 guidelines of the European Society of Cardiology [1] consider an EP study diagnostic in syncope patients with sinus bradycardia and a prolonged corrected sinus nodal recovery time >525ms (however, this criterion may not be valid for athletes), bundle branch block and either a baseline HV interval ≥100ms or second- or third-degree His–Purkinje block, induction of sustained monomorphic VT post-myocardial infarction, and induction of rapid supraventricular tachycardia which reproduces hypotensive or spontaneous symptoms (all class I level B recommendations). An HV interval of 70–100ms should also be considered diagnostic (class IIa level B recommendation) [1].

The results of the diagnostic EP study may lead to recommendation of an anti-arrhythmic drug (e.g. in symptomatic multifocal atrial arrhythmia which cannot be mapped) or therapy by catheter ablation, or may establish an indication for a pacemaker or ICD.

EP study of risk assessment

The most common causes of sudden cardiac death (SCD) in athletes are atherosclerotic coronary artery disease (especially in older athletes >35–40 years), cardiomyopathies (mainly hypertrophic and arrhythmogenic right ventricular cardiomyopathies), congenital anomalies of coronary arteries, myocarditis, mitral valve prolapse and channelopathies [2].

In non-sustained ventricular tachycardia (VT), structural heart disease, or electrical abnormalities, such as in patients with a Brugada ECG, an EP study for risk assessment may be indicated. However, the induction of polymorphic VT or ventricular fibrillation (VF), especially with aggressive stimulation, is not specific [2].

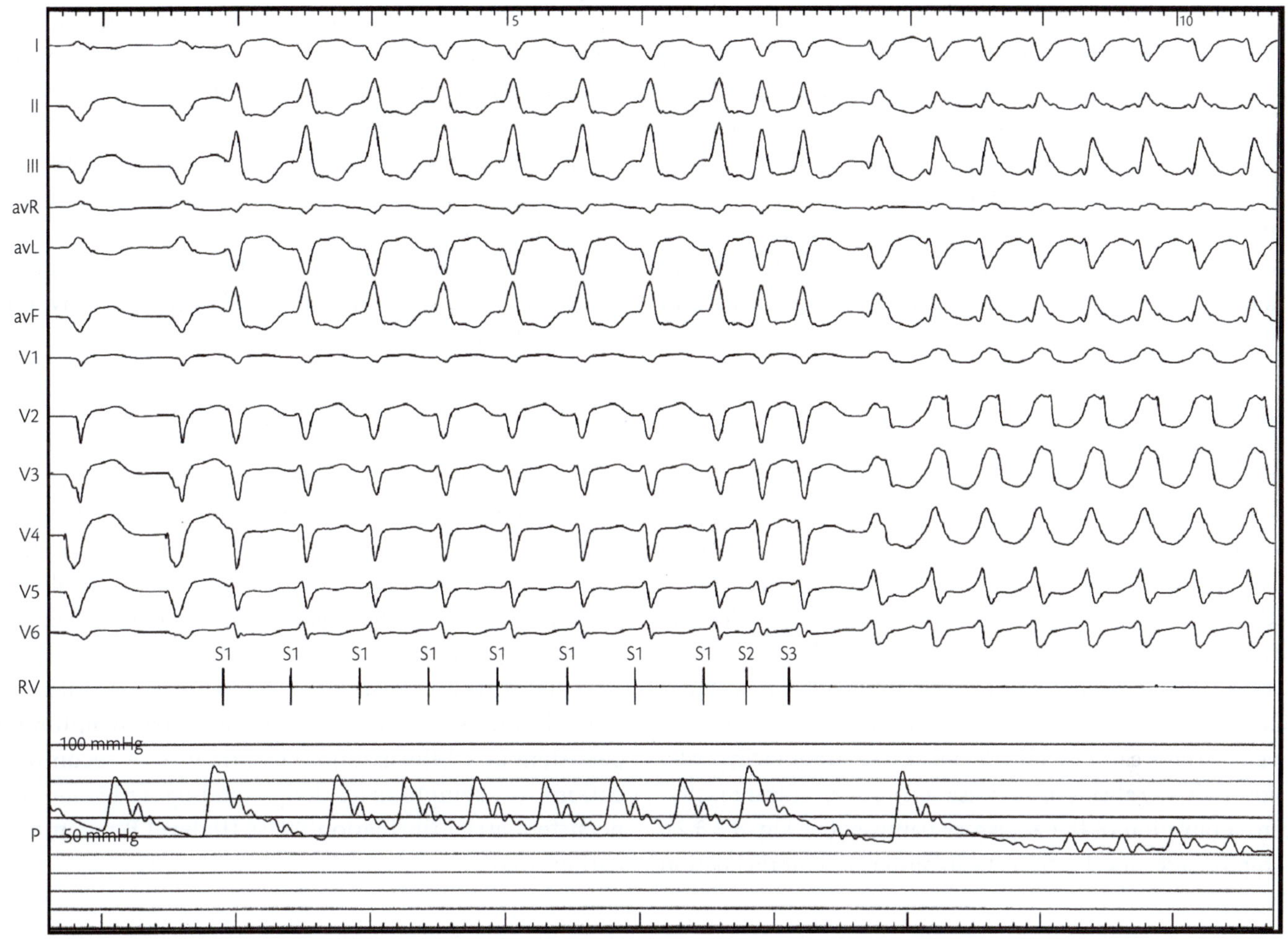

Fig. 3.2.3.1 Programmed ventricular stimulation in a patient with syncope, coronary artery disease, reduced left ventricular function, and a pacemaker with a single ventricular lead. The pacemaker is stimulating the ventricle at a rate of 80/min (two left QRS complexes). With eight stimuli (S1) from the right ventricle (RV) at a base drive cycle length of 510ms followed by two extrastimuli (S2 = 320ms, S3 = 320ms) a monomorphic ventricular re-entrant tachycardia (heart rate 150bpm) is induced that is not haemodynamically tolerated as indicated by the marked drop in the invasively measured blood pressure (P).

If ventricular arrhythmias are suspected or known, an EP study is especially helpful for stratification of SCD risk in patients with left ventricular dysfunction after myocardial infarction, and may be considered in arrhythmogenic right ventricular cardiomyopathy (class IIb level C recommendation), dilated cardiomyopathy (class IIb level B recommendation), and the Brugada syndrome (class IIb level C recommendation) [2]. In the latter, however, there is conflicting evidence whether or not the induction of VF during an EP study with two or three extrastimuli from two different sites should lead to ICD implantation [2]. Although a recent pooled analysis of eight studies (1312 patients) found an increased risk for sudden cardiac death in Brugada syndrome mainly when a polymorphic VT or VF is inducible with one or two extrastimuli (rather than more aggressive protocols), the authors point out that clinical risk stratification remains most important (such as spontaneous type 1 ECG pattern and syncope) and that non-inducibility should not be considered as indicative of a low risk of cardiac events [3].

In athletes with asymptomatic pre-excitation who engage in moderate or high level competitive sports, an EP study for risk assessment is considered reasonable (class IIa level B recommendation) [4]. Signs in an EP study for an increased risk of developing malignant arrhythmias in the future are as follows: (1) an R–R interval of <250ms between two pre-excited complexes during induced atrial fibrillation; (2) the presence of multiple accessory pathways; (3) the ability to induce sustained AV re-entrant tachycardias; (4) the finding that an AV re-entrant tachycardia leads to pre-excited atrial fibrillation; (5) a short accessory pathway refractory period of <240ms [4]. If the EP study reveals one of these risk factors, catheter ablation of the accessory pathway is considered reasonable (see also Chapter 5.4).

An EP study for risk assessment by programmed ventricular stimulation is usually not indicated in the absence of structural heart disease or patients with a normal ECG, or in most channelopathies (long QT syndrome, short QT syndrome, and catecholaminergic polymorphic ventricular tachycardia) and hypertrophic cardiomyopathy [2]. In the latter case, the European Society of Cardiology recommends using the HCM Risk-SCD calculator to estimate the 5-year sudden cardiac death risk. However, this cannot be used in elite athletes [2].

EP study for arrhythmia therapy

Ablation of ectopic beats, supraventricular or ventricular tachycardia, and atrial fibrillation may be warranted, in particular for athletes in order to avoid anti-arrhythmic drugs that may be pro-arrhythmogenic, not well tolerated, or forbidden in certain competitive sports (such as beta-blockers in archery or shooting). The 2015 ACC/AHA/HRS Guideline for the Management of Adult Patients with Supraventricular Tachycardia considers catheter ablation as a class I alternative to drug treatment for AV nodal re-entrant tachycardia (slow pathway ablation/modification), AV re-entrant tachycardia (ablation of the accessory pathway (➔ Fig. 3.2.3.2), symptomatic focal atrial tachycardia (recommendation level B), cavotricuspid isthmus dependent atrial flutter, and symptomatic recurrent non-cavotricuspid isthmus dependent atrial flutter after failure of at least one anti-arrhythmic agent) [4]. In contrast, anti-arrhythmic drug treatment is the preferred first-line treatment in inappropriate sinus tachycardia, multifocal atrial tachycardia, and junctional tachycardia [4].

Paroxysmal and persistent atrial fibrillation is common in athletes (autonomically mediated or triggered by other supraventricular tachycardia), and contributing conditions (hypertension, coronary artery disease) should be considered [5,6]. Radiofrequency catheter ablation can be considered as first-line therapy in athletes with paroxysmal atrial fibrillation (class IIa level C recommendation) [5,6]. The success rates of paroxysmal atrial fibrillation ablation in athletes appear to be similar to those in non-athletes [7,8]. However, in persistent atrial fibrillation treatment with catheter ablation is considered a second-line therapy and therefore can be considered in patients who are refractory or intolerant to at least one class I or class III anti-arrhythmic drug if they have symptomatic persistent atrial fibrillation (class IIa level A recommendation) or symptomatic long-standing (>12 months) persistent atrial fibrillation (class IIb level B recommendation) [5,6].

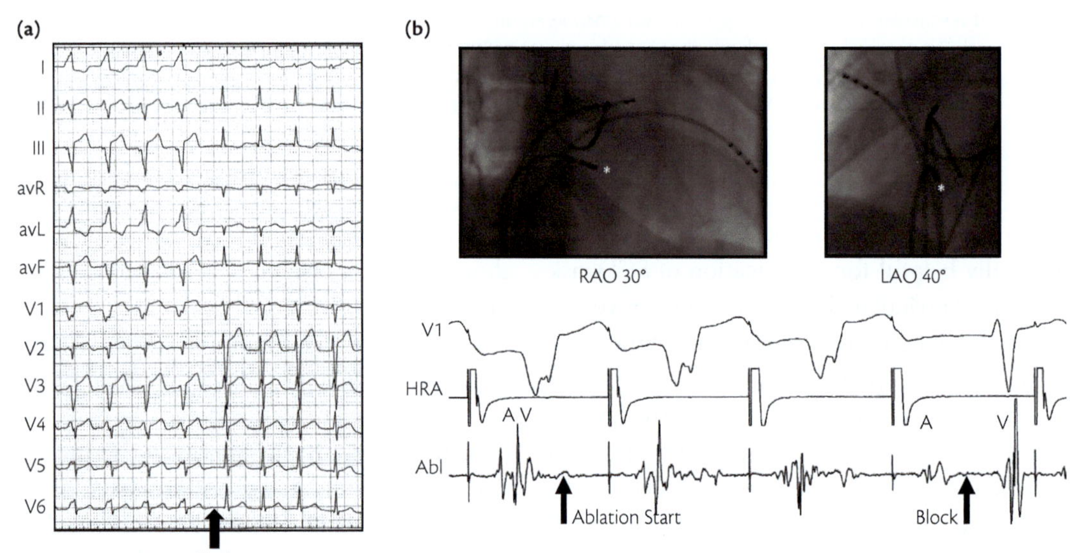

Fig. 3.2.3.2 (a) Ablation of a right posteroseptal accessory pathway during atrial stimulation. Note the disappearance of the delta wave in the 12-lead surface ECG (arrow) when the accessory pathway is blocked by radiofrequency ablation. (b) Upper panel: Location of the ablation catheter at the successful right posteroseptal ablation site (asterisk) in a RAO 30° and LAO 40° X-ray projection. The other catheters are located in the high right atrium, at the His, inside the coronary sinus, and in the right ventricular apex. Lower panel: The surface lead V1 and intracardiac recordings from the pacing catheter located in the high right atrium (HRA) and the ablation catheter (Abl). During atrial stimulation radiofrequency current is delivered from the ablation catheter, resulting in successful blockade of the accessory pathway (Block), indicated by the disappearance of the delta wave and sudden separation of the local ventricular activation (V) from the local atrial activation (A).

Ablation of ventricular arrhythmias in patients with structurally normal hearts is considered a first-line therapy in idiopathic left ventricular VT (class I level B recommendation), and an alternative to anti-arrhythmic drugs for premature ventricular contractions (PVCs) or VT originating in the right ventricular outflow tract (class I level B recommendation) or left ventricular outflow tract, aortic cusp, or epicardially (class IIa level B recommendation) as well as in patients with idiopathic VF in whom PVCs are triggering an electrical storm or VF (class I level B recommendation) [2]. In patients with structural heart disease ablation is indicated in patients with ischaemic heart disease presenting with incessant VT, electrical storm, or recurrent ICD shocks (class I level B recommendation) and possibly after the first episode of sustained VT in ICD patients (class IIa level B recommendation) [2]. Ablation is the first-line therapy in bundle branch re-entrant tachycardia (class I level C recommendation) [2]. Catheter ablation is considered as an alternative to amiodarone therapy in patients with PVCs or non-sustained VT and left ventricular dysfunction, (class IIa level B recommendation), and this is also the case for patients with arrhythmogenic right ventricular cardiomyopathy (class IIa level B recommendation) [2]. Catheter ablation could also be an option (class IIb level C recommendation) in dilated cardiomyopathy and drug refractory ventricular arrhythmia [2].

For channelopathies, catheter ablation is a possible option in Brugada syndrome patients presenting with electrical storms or repeated appropriate ICD shocks (class IIb level C recommendation) [2]. Preliminary data suggests that in these patients epicardial catheter ablation over the anterior right ventricular outflow tract may prevent electrical storm recurrences [9].

Mapping and ablation of arrhythmias can be performed conventionally or by utilizing 3D mapping systems. Radiofrequency current is most frequently used (irrigated or non-irrigated electrodes) for ablation of supraventricular und ventricular tachyarrhythmias, whereas other energy sources (cryo, laser, ultrasound) are also utilized in ablation of atrial fibrillation.

Further reading

Calvo N, Mont L, Tamberero D, et al. Efficacy of circumferential pulmonary vein ablation of atrial fibrillation in endurance athletes. *Europace* 2010; 12: 30–6.

Camm AJ, Kirchhoff G, Lip GY, et al. Guidelines for the management of atrial fibrillation. *Europace* 2010; 12: 1360–1420.

January CT, Wann LS, Alpert JS, et al. 2014 AHA/ACC/HRS Guideline for the management of patients with atrial fibrillation. *J Am Coll Cardiol* 2014; 64: e1–76.

Koopmann P, Nuyens D, Garweg C, et al. Efficacy of radiofrequency catheter ablation in athletes with atrial fibrillation. *Europace* 2011; 13: 1386–93.

Moya A, Sutton R, Ammirati F, et al. Guidelines for the diagnosis and management of syncope (version 2009). *Eur Heart J* 2009; 30: 2631–71.

Nademanee K, Veerakul G, Chandanamattha P, et al. Prevention of ventricular fibrillation episodes in Brugada syndrome by catheter ablation over the right ventricular outflow tract epicardium. *Circulation* 2011; 123: 1270–9.

Page RL, Joglar JA, Caldwell MA, et al. 2015 ACC/AHA/HRS Guideline for the management of adult patients with supraventricular tachycardia. *Heart Rhythm* 2016; 13: e 136–221.

Priori SG, Blomström-Lundqvist C, Mazzanti A, et al. 2015 ESC Guidelines for the management of patients with ventricular arrhythmias and the prevention of sudden cardiac death. *Eur Heart J* 2015; 36: 2793–867.

Sroubek J, Probst V, Mazzanti A, et al. Programmed ventricular stimulation for risk stratification in the Brugada syndrome: a pooled Analysis. *Circulation* 2016; 133: 622–30.

References

1. Moya A, Sutton R, Ammirati F, et al. Guidelines for the diagnosis and management of syncope (version 2009). *Eur Heart J* 2009; 30: 2631–71.
2. Priori SG, Blomström-Lundqvist C, Mazzanti A, et al. 2015 ESC Guidelines for the management of patients with ventricular arrhythmias and the prevention of sudden cardiac death. *Eur Heart J* 2015; 36: 2793–867.
3. Sroubek J, Probst V, Mazzanti A, et al. Programmed ventricular stimulation for risk stratification in the Brugada syndrome: a pooled analysis. *Circulation* 2016; 133: 622–30.
4. Page RL, Joglar JA, Caldwell MA, et al. 2015 ACC/AHA/HRS Guideline for the management of adult patients with supraventricular tachycardia. *Heart Rhythm* 2016; 13: e136–221.
5. January CT, Wann LS, Alpert JS, et al. 2014 AHA/ACC/HRS Guideline for the management of patients with atrial fibrillation. *J Am Coll Cardiol* 2014; 64: e1–76.
6. Camm AJ, Kirchhoff G, Lip GY, et al. Guidelines for the management of atrial fibrillation. *Europace* 2010; 12: 1360–1420.
7. Calvo N, Mont L, Tamberero D, et al. Efficacy of circumferential pulmonary vein ablation of atrial fibrillation in endurance athletes. *Europace* 2010; 12: 30–6.
8. Koopmann P, Nuyens D, Garweg C, et al. Efficacy of radiofrequency catheter ablation in athletes with atrial fibrillation. *Europace* 2011; 13: 1386–93.
9. Nademanee K, Veerakul G, Chandanamattha P, et al. Prevention of ventricular fibrillation episodes in Brugada syndrome by catheter ablation over the right ventricular outflow tract epicardium. *Circulation* 2011; 123: 1270–9.

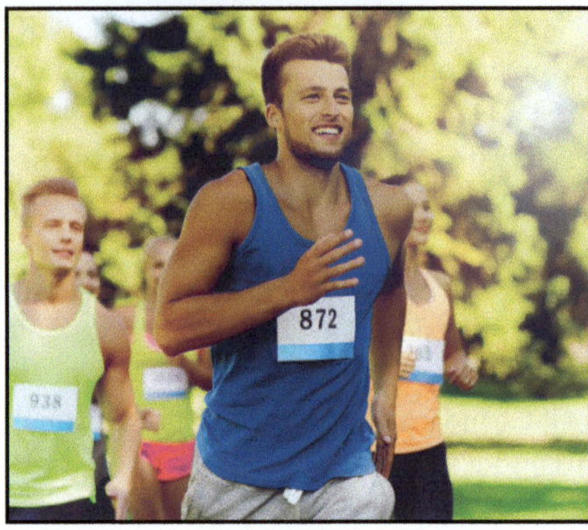

3.3

Imaging the athlete's heart: anatomical and functional

Contents

3.3.1 **Echocardiogram: morphological and functional evaluation including new echocardiographic techniques** Stefano Caselli and Flavio D'Ascenzi *120*
3.3.2 **Cardiac magnetic resonance imaging** Guido Claessen and André La Gerche *140*
3.3.3 **Coronary computed tomography** Stefan Möhlenkamp *153*
3.3.4 **Nuclear imaging** Stefan Möhlenkamp *159*
3.3.5 **Coronary angiography** Stefan Möhlenkamp *162*

3.3.1 Echocardiogram: morphological and functional evaluation including new echocardiographic techniques

Stefano Caselli and Flavio D'Ascenzi

Introduction

Echocardiography is the cardiovascular imaging method of choice in the athletic population by virtue of its widespread availability, relatively low cost, and safety. Indeed, echocardiography has the unique ability to provide complementary information on cardiac morphology, functional properties, and haemodynamics, playing an important role in the diagnosis and clinical management of a broad spectrum of cardiovascular conditions [1].

Over the last three or four decades advances in ultrasound and computer technology have resulted in the evolution of this technique from the simple and relatively limited M-mode to two-dimensional imaging, Doppler assessment of intracardiac flows and pressures, three-dimensional anatomical imaging, and two- and three-dimensional analysis of myocardial deformation. In parallel with this technological evolution a large amount of data on the cardiovascular adaptation of athletes has been assembled, improving our understanding of the physiology of cardiac contraction and morphological adaptations to increased haemodynamic load [2–5].

Compared with untrained individuals of the same age and body size, athletes show an increase in cardiac mass and a global and harmonious enlargement of all chambers which makes it possible to achieve very high cardiac output during exercise, guaranteeing oxygen supply to working muscles [1,3,4].

From a pathophysiological point of view, cardiac adaptations in athletes are closely correlated with the characteristics, intensity, and cumulative duration of training protocols, showing a 'dose–effect' relation with different cardiac remodelling associated with the practice of different sport disciplines [2–4,6–8] (see Chapter 1.2.1 for details).

Since these changes in cardiac structure depend on the persistent haemodynamic overload, several investigations have reported that the degree of hypertrophy changes with the status of fitness and is reversible after discontinuation of training [9]. In this scenario echocardiography, by virtue of its easy availability, is the ideal technique for following up athletes and allows dynamic evaluation of morpho-functional changes related to the intensity of training [10].

In recent years, morphological cardiac adaptations with respect to age, gender, and ethnicity have also been extensively reported. While the interest has been limited to the left ventricle in the past, attention has recently been directed to other structures such as the right ventricle, the atria, and the aorta [5,8,11–13]. Training-induced morphological remodelling of the athlete's heart is rarely extreme, although in some cases there may be a dimensional overlap with pathological conditions, raising the dilemma of differential diagnosis and eligibility for participation in sport. For example, the left ventricle may show an increase in chamber size with a potential overlap with dilated cardiomyopathy in 12% of cases, and an increase in wall thickness which, in 2% of cases, requires differential diagnosis from mild hypertrophic cardiomyopathy (HCM). Similarly, increased trabeculations which resemble left ventricular non-compaction are evident in 8% of athletes, and a dilated right ventricle potentially overlaps with arrhythmogenic cardiomyopathy in 0.3–3.4% cases [14]. Differential diagnosis is of utmost importance because these cardiomyopathies represent a pathological substrate on which different stimuli related to intense training and competitions may trigger malignant tachyarrhythmias, eventually culminating in sudden cardiac death (SCD). Therefore many studies have reported echocardiographic criteria for appropriate differential diagnosis in the setting of overlap with cardiomyopathies [15].

Beyond cardiomyopathies, which are the most important causes of SCD related to sports, in expert hands echocardiography is able to identify other diseases which, if not promptly recognized, may worsen or evolve to adverse outcomes such as anomalous origin of the coronary arteries, myocarditis and pericarditis, valvular heart disease, and aortic root pathologies [16].

Box 3.3.1.1 Indications for performing an echocardiographic examination.

Clinical history

Sudden cardiac death in the family
Known genetic/familiar cardiovascular disorder or cardiomyopathy in a first-degree relative
Palpitations
Syncope/pre-syncope (particularly during effort)

Physical examination

Pathological murmurs
Abnormal heart sounds

12-lead electrocardiogram

T-wave inversion beyond V1 in white athletes and beyond V4 in black athletes
ST-segment depression
Pathological Q waves
Ventricular pre-excitation
Complete right or left bundle branch block
Atrial or ventricular arrhythmias
Left or right axis deviation
Right ventricular hypertrophy
Left or right atrial enlargement

Exercise testing

Exercise-induced atrial and/or ventricular arrhythmias
ST-segment or T-wave abnormalities at peak exercise

Indications for echocardiographic examination

Echocardiography is particularly useful in the athletic population, and the low acoustic impedance of the chest makes it possible to obtain high quality images and assess all the cardiac structures. In the majority of cases echocardiography is a second-level examination, preceded by physical examination and/or a 12-lead electrocardiogram [17,18]. ➲ Box 3.3.1.1 shows the most common indications for echocardiographic examination which may originate from clinical history, physical examination, or 12-lead ECG. Abnormalities identified at 12-lead resting ECG and requiring an echocardiographic examination are derived from the current recommendations [17–21].

Standard examination protocol

Echocardiographic examination should follow a standardized protocol, which may be modified, on an individual basis, in order to allow the recognition of specific conditions. Before starting the examination it is important to record some individual characteristics such as height, weight, race, body surface, sporting discipline, training volume and intensity, previous years of training, and period of the active season, as all these features may affect the interpretation of the examination. The echocardiographic examination should be performed under resting condition before training (or an exercise test) in order to avoid tachycardia or dehydration, which may alter cardiac volumes and flows. Subjects should lie in a comfortable position in the left lateral decubitus and a continuous ECG tracing should be obtained (three electrodes are placed on the right shoulder, right hip, and left hip, respectively) with proper adjustment of gain in order to visualize the QRS complex and allow correct image trigger. Images should be stored digitally and properly archived in order to allow review of examination and off-line analysis.

Several reference values with regard to age, gender, ethnicity, and sport disciplines have been published in literature, and therefore there are no universally accepted cut-offs for basic echocardiographic measurements. ➲ Table 3.3.1.1 shows reference values that can be used for routine echocardiographic examination. However, they should be used with caution and interpreted on the basis of all the clinical and demographic variables.

Table 3.3.1.1 Reference values from a population of 2000 healthy consecutive athletes (age 15–45), members of the Italian Olympic Team

	Female (*n*=700)	Male (*n*=1300)
LV end-diastolic diameter (mm)	43–54	48–61
LV end-diastolic diameter index (mm/m²)	25–33	23–32
LV end-systolic diameter (mm)	25–37	28–41
Septal wall thickness (mm)	7–10	9–12
LV posterior wall (mm)	7–10	8–11
LV mass (g)	96–203	140–295
LV mass index (g/m²)	60–112	75–144
Relative wall thickness	0.31–0.39	0.33–0.41
Aortic root (mm)	23–32	26–37
LA antero-posterior diameter (mm)	26–38	29–42
LV ejection fraction (%)	56–75	56–75
RVOT long axis diameter (mm)	20-32	22–34
RVOT long axis diameter index (mm/m²)	12–19	11–18
RVOT short axis diameter (mm)	21-34	23–36
RVOT short axis diameter index (mm/m²)	12–21	12–19
RV basal diameter (mm)	27–44	33–49
RV fractional area change (%)	38–66	39–65
TAPSE (mm)	19–30	19–31
Doppler parameters		
Transmitral E/A ratio	1.3–2.8	1.3–2.8
Tissue Doppler E′ velocity (septal) (cm/s)	11–17	10–17
Tissue Doppler S velocity (septal) (cm/s)	7–11	7–11
E/e′ ratio	4.8–8.7	4.6–8.5
Pulmonary artery systolic pressure (mmHg)	16–29	17-30

Athletes were of Caucasian origin and covered the broad spectrum of all Olympic disciplines. The reference values were calculated as the gender-specific 5th–95th percentile.LV, left ventricle; LA, left atrium; RVOT, right ventricular outflow tract; RV, right ventricle; TAPSE, tricuspid annular plane systolic excursion.
Data from the Institute of Sports Medicine and Science. Italian National Olympic Committee, Rome, Italy.

Parasternal long axis

This view is obtained with the probe in the third or fourth intercostal space proximal to the left border of the sternum (➲ Fig. 3.3.1.1). It is usually the first echocardiographic view of the examination and provides a good general overview of the main cardiac structures. The scan is usually started at a high depth (18–20cm) in order to allow visualization of structures in proximity, such as the descending aorta and pericardium, and then is reduced to 15–16cm in order to obtain better definition of cardiac chambers and valves. The aortic root, sino-tubular junction, and proximal ascending aorta can be accurately assessed and measured. The aortic root is measured at end-diastole at the sinuses of Valsalva using the leading-edge method (➲ Fig. 3.3.1.2) [22]. The right and non-coronary cusps of the aortic root and their mobility are then evaluated. Colour Doppler is particularly useful for identifying aortic or mitral valve regurgitation. Anterior and posterior mitral valve leaflets can be accurately assessed by tilting the probe and allowing assessment of all the scallops. The image is frozen in end-diastole (corresponding to the onset of QRS on the ECG tracing) in order to measure the septal and posterior left ventricular (LV) wall thickness, the LV end-diastolic diameter, the LV outflow tract, and the diameter of the right ventricular outflow tract (RVOT) (➲ Fig. 3.3.1.3). The LV end-systolic diameter and the left atrial antero-posterior diameter are measured in the same cardiac cycle, in end systole (corresponding to the end of T wave on ECG tracing) [22].

Right ventricular inflow

This view is obtained by tilting the tail of the transducer towards the right shoulder. The tricuspid valve is well

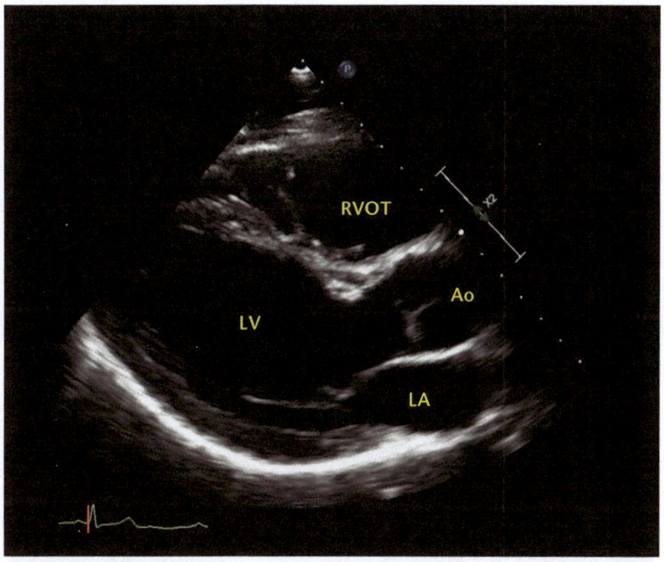

Fig. 3.3.1.1 Parasternal long-axis view. LV, left ventricle; LA, left atrium; Ao, aortic root; RVOT, right ventricular outflow tract.

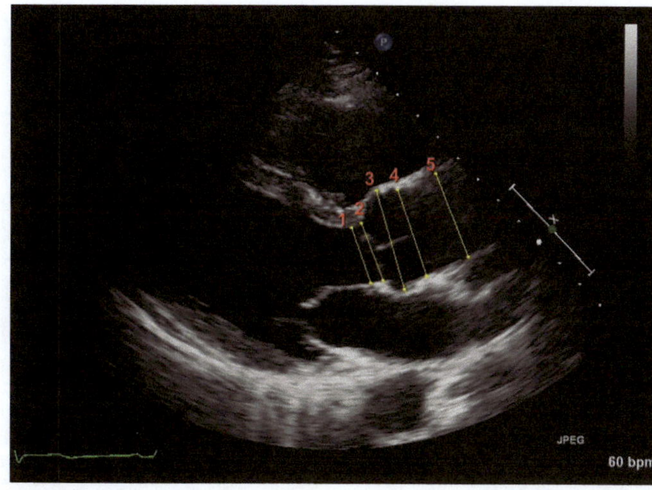

Fig. 3.3.1.2 Parasternal long-axis view in end-diastole. The measurements of left ventricular outflow tract (1), aortic annulus (2), aortic root at sinuses of Valsalva (3), sinotubular junction (4) and ascending aorta (5) are reported.

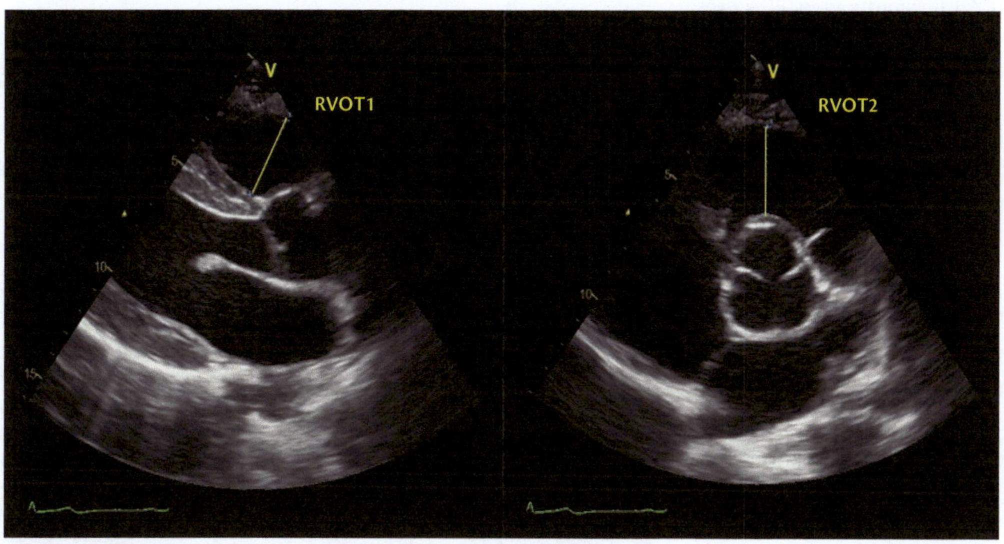

Fig. 3.3.1.3 Right ventricular outflow tract assessment from parasternal long axis (left panel, RVOT1) and parasternal short-axis view (right panel, RVOT2).

characterized, allowing assessment of the morphology and mobility of the anterior and posterior leaflets. Colour and CW Doppler is used here to assess the tricuspid regurgitation and estimate the pulmonary artery systolic pressure. RV morphology and function may also be assessed. This view is particularly useful for identifying possible RV wall motion abnormalities if there is suspicion of ARVC.

Parasternal short axis

Rotating the probe clockwise by 90° from the parasternal long axis, a transverse view of the cardiac structures is obtained. Starting from an upper position, which allows assessment of the great vessels, the probe is subsequently tilted downwards in order to obtain a series of tomographic views of the heart. At the level of the great vessels the aortic valve is seen in the middle. The number and morphology of the cusps is analysed with special attention to identifying the bicuspid aortic valve and the presence and position of a raphe. The origin of the coronary artery must be sought in all individuals in order to exclude any potential abnormality, especially in (but not limited to) those athletes with ECG abnormalities on exercise testing (➲ Fig. 3.3.1.4). The pulmonic valve and the pulmonary artery are then visualized with Doppler, and specific attention is paid to excluding a patent ductus arteriosus when a murmur is indicated by the examination. Special attention should be paid to the assessment of RVOT, since pathological enlargement and saccular dilatations may be identified in individuals with ARVC.

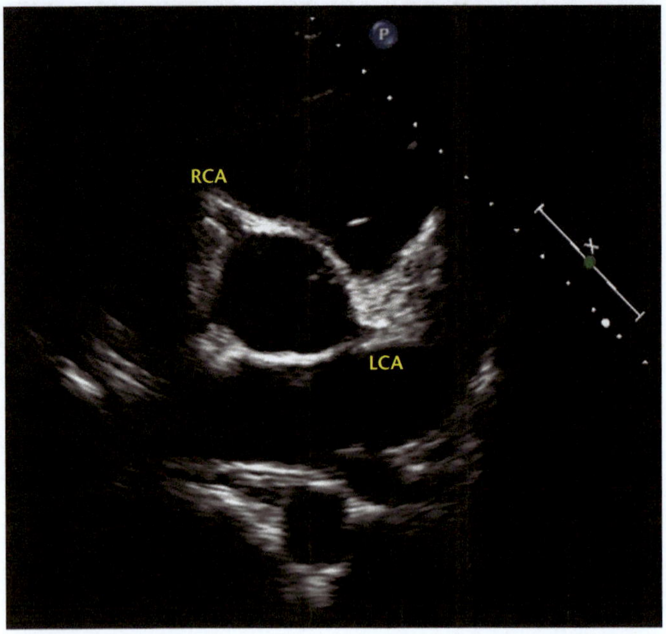

Fig. 3.3.1.4 Parasternal short-axis view at the level of sinuses of Valsalva showing the origin of coronary arteries: LCA, left coronary artery; RCA, right coronary artery.

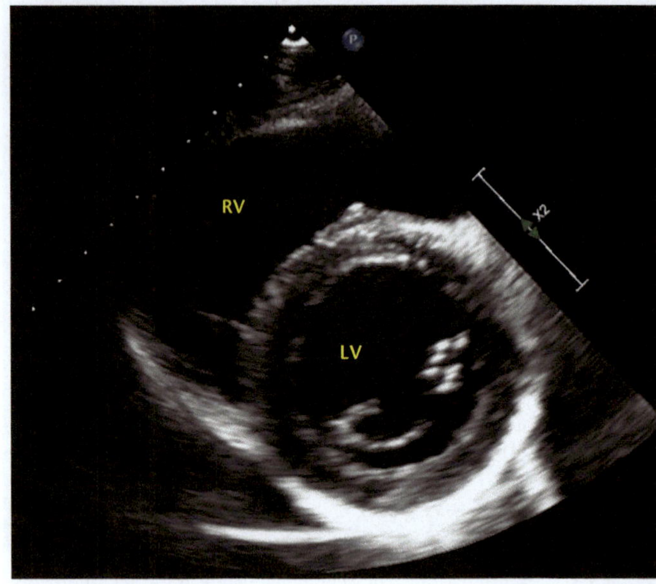

Fig. 3.3.1.5 Parasternal short-axis view at the basal level: LV, left ventricle; RV, right ventricle.

On tilting the probe slightly downwards the mitral valve is well visualized, allowing correct morphological and functional evaluation of the leaflets, chordae, and number and position of papillary muscles.

The LV can be accurately evaluated in all segments by tiliting the probe from the mitral valve through the apex (➲ Fig. 3.3.1.5). The wall motion of all segments should be carefully evaluated and the presence and location of focal areas of hypertrophy should be described. The presence and characteristics of excessive trabeculations should be described, and the number of trabeculations, and thickness of compact and non-compact layer in systole and diastole should be measured when there is a suspicion of LV non-compaction (LVNC).

Apical four-chamber view

The apical four-chamber is visualized by placing the transducer directly at the level of cardiac apex and provides a good overview of atrioventricular valves, chamber size, and morphology (➲ Fig. 3.3.1.6). Particular attention should be paid to obtaining a correct imaging plane, avoiding foreshortened views which may affect the accuracy of measurements. The LV usually appears as a truncated ellipse and the volumes are assessed by the Simpson method of discs, tracing the endocardial border from the mitral annulus plane through the apex in diastole and systole. The wall motion of the inferoseptum and anterolateral wall can be evaluated. Left atrial volume is assessed in end-systole, ensuring

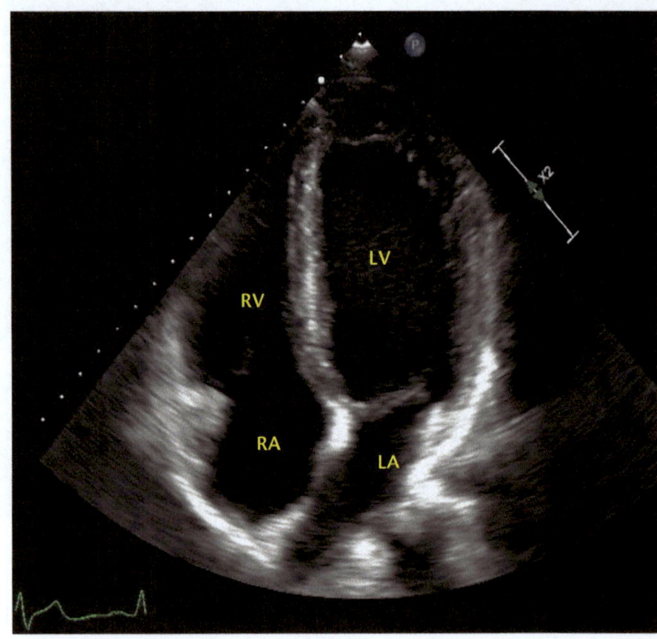

Fig. 3.3.1.6 Apical four-chamber view: LV, left ventricle; RV, right ventricle; LA, left atrium; RA, right atrium.

that the pulmonary veins and left appendage are excluded from the tracing. LV inflow velocities are recorded by pulse wave (PW) Doppler with a small sample volume positioned at the tip of the mitral leaflets and the ultrasound beam aligned parallel to the flow, allowing measurements of peak early filling, deceleration time, and late diastolic filling (A) at end-expiration during breath-holding (➲ Fig. 3.3.1.7). Isovolumic relaxation time (IVRT) is measured by means of CW Doppler, placing the ultrasound beam in the LV outflow

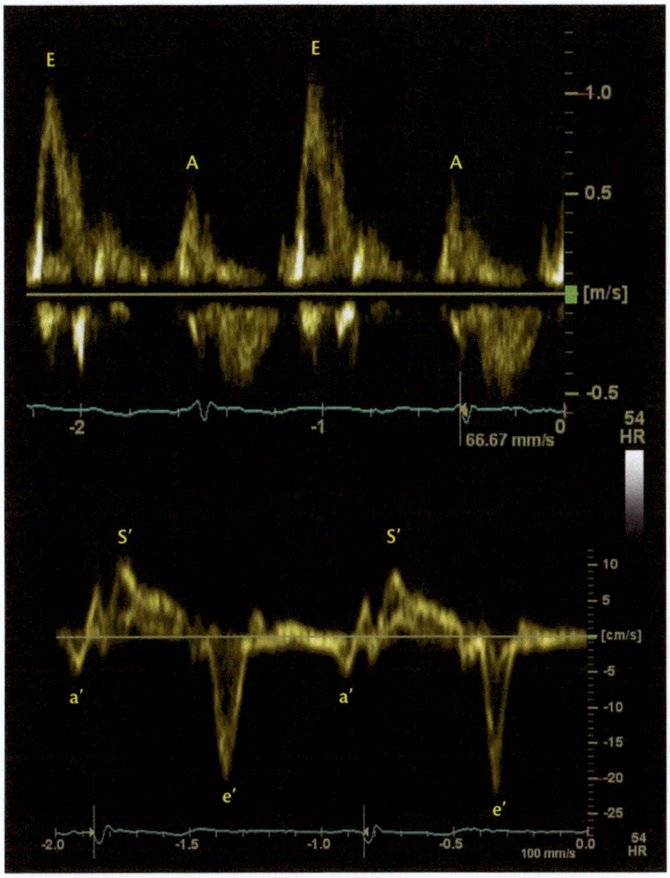

Fig. 3.3.1.7. Evaluation of diastolic function from the apical four-chamber view. The upper panel shows trans-mitral pulse-wave Doppler analysis (E, early filling; A, atrial contraction): the lower panel shows tissue Doppler imaging from the lateral annulus of the mitral valve (e′, early left ventricular (LV) filling; a′, late LV filling; s′, LV contraction).

tract in order to calculate the time from the end of aortic ejection to the onset of mitral inflow. Myocardial tissue Doppler imaging (TDI) signals can be recorded using PW Doppler with a 5mm sample volume positioned at the septal and lateral aspect of the mitral annulus (➲ Fig. 3.3.1.7). Early (e′) and late (a′) diastolic peak velocities are measured at end-expiration.

The mitral valve and subvalvular apparatus are morphologically assessed by tilting the probe in order to visualize all the scallops. If a regurgitation is found by colour Doppler, spectral analysis is performed using CW Doppler.

Mapping of the LV outflow tract with PW Doppler is usually performed in order to exclude any pathological flow acceleration. Flows across the aortic valve are then analysed by colour and CW Doppler. Colour Doppler is then placed on the inter-atrial and inter-ventricular septum in order to exclude any intra-cardiac shunt.

RV measurements including basal, middle, and longitudinal diameters, and end-diastolic and end-systolic areas are performed in this view (➲ Fig. 3.3.1.8). RV function can be assessed using TAPSE, fractional area change, and/or TDI of the tricuspid annulus. The right atrial area can be measured in systole. Tricuspid regurgitation can be identified in order to allow estimation of systolic pulmonary artery pressure (sPAP).

Apical two- and three-chamber views

These views are obtained from the apical position by rotating the transducer counterclockwise by 90° and 120° (➲ Fig. 3.3.1.9). They allow further assessment of regional wall motion of the left ventricle. LV volumes can also be calculated from the two-chamber view, allowing a more precise estimate using the biplane Simpson rule. The mitral valve is further evaluated by colour Doppler in order to look for regurgitation. Further analysis of the LV outflow tract and aortic valve is performed in the three-chamber view.

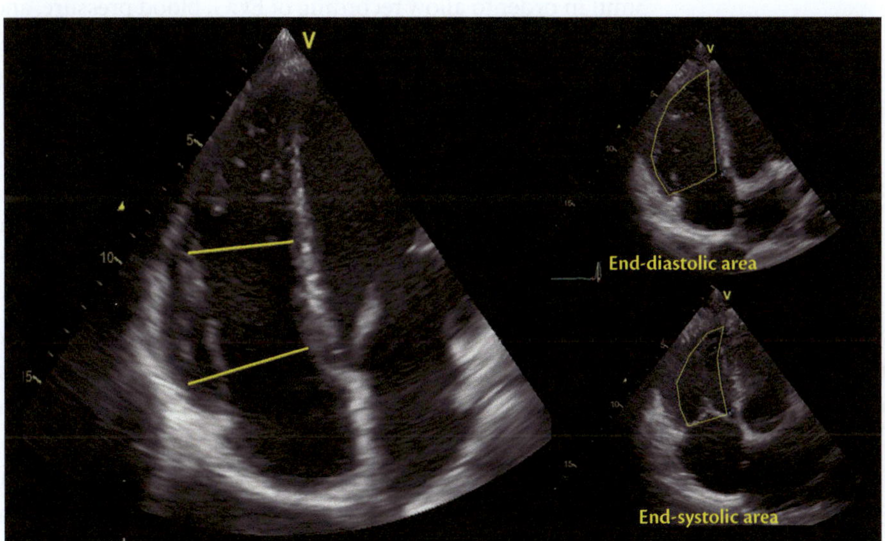

Fig. 3.3.1.8. Evaluation of right ventricular (RV) size from the apical four-chamber view. The left panel shows mid-cavity and basal RV diameters; the right panel shows RV end-diastolic and end-systolic areas for the assessment of RV fractional area change.

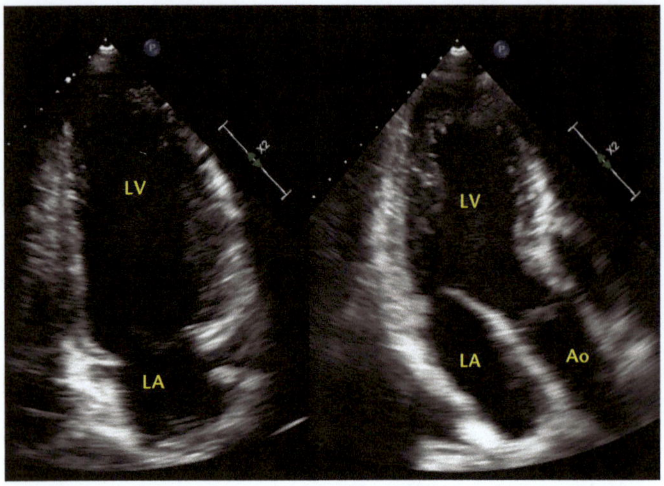

Fig. 3.3.1.9 Apical two- and three-chamber view: LV, left ventricle; LA; left atrium; Ao, aorta.

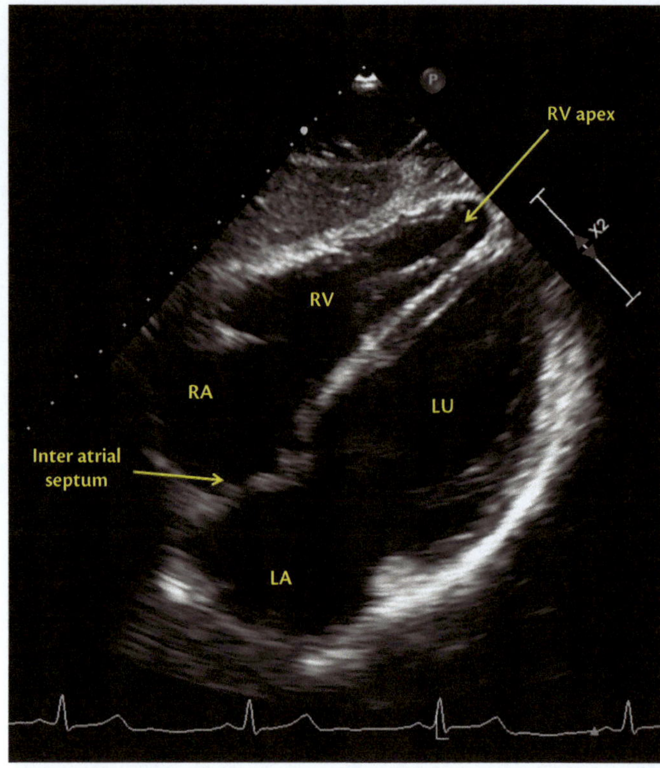

Fig. 3.3.1.10 Subcostal view: LV, left ventricle; LA, left atrium; RV, right ventricle; RA, right atrium.

Subcostal view

The subcostal view is obtained placing the transducer in the subxyphoid region (➔ Fig. 3.3.1.10). The RV free wall and its contractile function can be assessed in detail, and RV inflow and outflow regions can be clearly characterized in this acoustic view. Colour flow Doppler is usually positioned over the inter-atrial and inter-ventricular septum in order to look for pathological shunts.

The presence and location of pericardial effusion is described. The diameter and collapse of the inferior vena cava is finally assessed.

Suprasternal view

This is the last part of the echocardiographic examination. The probe is positioned in the suprasternal notch to assess the great vessels. The aortic arch is measured and flow in the descending aorta is evaluated in order to exclude aortic coarctation.

Stress echocardiography

Stress echocardiography allows dynamic evaluation of cardiac function during exercise and is useful for identifying pathological conditions that may not be present at rest. In the general population it is usually performed to detect myocardial ischaemia but in young competitive athletes it may have additional applications, most commonly the dynamic assessment of a valvular lesion and of sPAP or the evaluation of systolic function if there is suspicion of dilated cardiomyopathy (DCM) [23,24].

Pharmacological stress is generally not indicated in athletes and an exercise test is usually performed. Echocardiographic examination can be performed soon after exercise on a treadmill or upright bicycle, but in athletes it is preferable to perform the examination during exercise because they usually have a brisk recovery phase and in some cases they may already have returned to baseline heart rate and blood pressure a minute after exercise.

Therefore, use of a special supine bicycle ergometer, which allows image acquisition by echocardiography, is recommended. The exercise protocol is the same as that of a normal exercise test with an incremental increase in workload every 3min in order to allow recording of ECG, blood pressure, and echocardiographic imaging planes. Echocardiographic images are acquired under resting conditions and at submaximal exercise, peak exercise, and during the recovery phase in order to obtain an overview of dynamic changes during exercise.

Since the time for image acquisition is limited, the echocardiographic protocol is usually tailored to the clinical indication. When there is a suspicion of coronary artery disease short-axis planes, apical four-chamber and two-chamber planes, and long-axis planes are obtained to allow accurate assessment of regional wall motion abnormalities. When there is a suspicion of DCM good apical windows are needed in order to measure LV volumes and ejection fraction accurately. In cases of valvular heart disease attention is directed towards LV function and aortic or mitral valve flows and assessment of sPAP.

New echo modalities

The development and rapid dissemination of 2D echocardiography has led to a comprehensive understanding of cardiac adaptation to exercise conditioning. However, advanced echocardiographic techniques have recently begun to clarify significant functional adaptations of the myocardium that accompany previously reported morphological features of athlete's heart. In particular, speckle-tracking echocardiography (STE) and 3D echocardiography have recently provided further insights into the characterization of the myocardial properties of athletes.

These very advanced echocardiographic techniques are not used in routine echocardiographic examinations, but may be required, under specific circumstances, to allow a deeper investigation of cardiac structure and function. ➲ Box 3.3.1.2 summarizes the main indications to perform speckle tracking and three-dimensional echocardiography in athletes.

Speckle-tracking echocardiography

STE is a relatively new non-invasive imaging technique, which is largely independent of angle, that allows an objective and quantitative evaluation of global and regional myocardial function. Myocardial strain is a dimensionless parameter expressed as the percentage of myocardial deformation; negative values indicate shortening or compression, and positive values indicate lengthening or stretching. Depending on the spatial resolution, selective analysis of epicardial, mid-wall, and endocardial function may be possible, allowing longitudinal, radial, and circumferential strain to be obtained [25–27]. In addition, STE permits evaluation of the occurrence, velocity, and direction of LV rotation (➲ Fig. 3.3.1.11) [28]. STE can be applied to both ventricles and atria. However, while all LV segments can be analysed successfully in most patients, signal quality may be suboptimal for the atria and the right ventricle because of their thin walls [29]. It should be noted that, although feasibility is best for longitudinal and circumferential strain, it is more challenging for radial strain [29]. The main limitation of STE is that it relies on good imaging quality, and there are still differences among manufacturers because STE analysis is performed on data stored in a proprietary scan line format which cannot be analysed by software from another manufacturer. This lack of standardization of different speckle-tracking algorithms makes it difficult to establish normal values and to compare data generated in different centres.

Left ventricle

The main echocardiographic studies of athlete's heart performed using 2D STE are summarized in ➲ Table 3.3.1.2. These studies demonstrate that a reduction in LV global longitudinal strain is an uncommon feature in athlete's heart and cannot be considered a physiological adaptation to training. Indeed, when STE was used to differentiate between physiological (adaptive) and pathological (maladaptive) LV hypertrophy, i.e. between athletes and patients with essential hypertension or non-obstructive hypertrophic cardiomyopathy, a reduction in longitudinal strain was found in patients but not in the athletic population, suggesting that it is an early sign of LV dysfunction [30–34]. This finding can be explained by the fact that the subendocardium is the first layer to be involved in many cardiac diseases (e.g. ischaemic, hypertensive, diabetic, and valvular heart diseases), and longitudinal strain, primarily related to the myocardial

Box 3.3.1.2 Usefulness of speckle-tracking and/or 3D echocardiography when evaluating the athlete's heart

Speckle-tracking echocardiography

- Identification of regional wall motion abnormalities
- Pre-clinical impairment of LV function in individuals with early DCM
- Pre-clinical anomalies useful for differentiating between athlete's heart and early HCM
- Improved ability to recognize RV functional abnormalities suggestive for ARVC

3D echocardiography

- Assessment of LV function (i.e. LV ejection fraction)
- Assessment of cavity size
- Assessment of LV mass
- Improvement of the characterization of LV hypertrabeculation

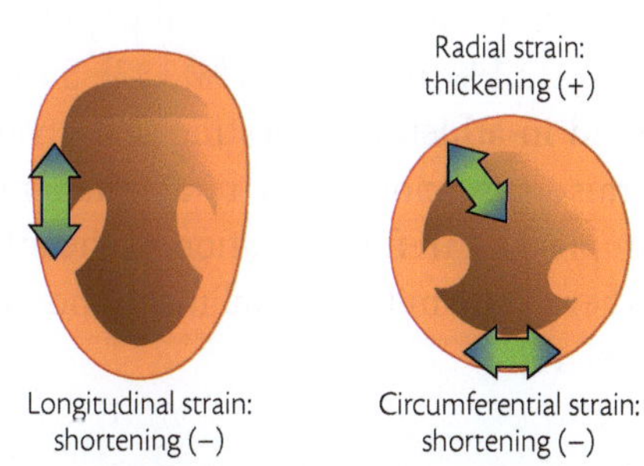

Fig. 3.3.1.11. Schematic representation of the three major components of myocardial deformation. Longitudinal strain is evaluated from apical views and has a negative value, indicating shortening of myocardial fibres. Radial and circumferential strain are evaluated from the short-axis view and reflect myocardial thickening (radial strain) and shortening (circumferential strain) of the left ventricle.

Table 3.3.1.2 Main echocardiographic studies using two-dimensional speckle tracking echocardiography for the assessment of left and right ventricles.

Reference	Year	Sport discipline	*n*	Longitudinal strain (%)
Left ventricle				
Caselli et al. [32]	2015	Olympic athletes	200	−18.1±2.2
Nottin et al. [37]	2008	Elite cyclists	16	−19.2±1.9
Cappelli et al. [30]	2010	Endurance athletes	50	−18.4±3.0
Galderisi et al. [31]	2010	Top-level rowers	22	−22.2±2.7
Simsek et al. [39]	2013	Marathon runners	22	−22.3±2.2 (global)
Simsek et al. [39]	2013	Wrestlers	24	−21.8±1.7 (global)
Weiner et al. [38] (longitudinal study)	2010	University rowers	15	−16.8±2.1 (pre-training) −18.3±2.8 (post–training)
Right ventricle				
Oxborough et al. [41]	2012	Endurance athletes	102	−27.0±6.0 (range: −18 to −41)
Teske et al. [40]	2009	Endurance athletes (group I)/Olympic endurance athletes (Group II)	58/63	−28.5±2.9/−7.6±3.1
Pagourelias et al. [42]	2013	Endurance/strength athletes	108 (80/28)	−23.1±3.7/−25.1±3.2 (septal+++free wall segments)
Esposito et al. [43]	2013	Top-level rowers	40	−26.3±3.6 (global) −29.1±4.1 (free wall)

deformation of subendocardial fibres, is expected to be impaired in the early stages of the cardiac disease.

In view of the increasing application of 2D STE to the integrated imaging-based diagnosis of cardiomyopathies, it is extremely important to know whether exercise modifies LV strain. Recent longitudinal studies suggest that, despite an exercise-induced increase in LV size, changes in LV strain cannot be found in either top-level athletes or in untrained subjects assigned to a training protocol [35,36].

Because the definition of a normal range is constrained by inherent variability due to age, haemodynamic conditions, disciplines, and differences between manufacturers, the current normal value for the general population varies from −15.9% to −22.1% (mean −19.7%) [37]. Similar values have been found in athletes, suggesting that a value below 15% should raise suspicion of an underlying myocardial disease and implies a careful evaluation of the athlete, particularly if other concomitant subclinical anomalies exist [30,31,34,35,38–41].

Right ventricle

Although athletic training results in remodelling of all cardiac cavities, morphological and functional adaptations of the right ventricle have been given considerably less attention than those of the left ventricle and atrium. The formal assessment of the right ventricle has often been neglected, primarily because of the absence of simple and reliable methods of estimating RV function. However, STE is able to overcome some of the major limitations on RV quantification. STE has recently been applied to the investigation of the RV in athletes, and has provided new insights into the investigation of its physiological remodelling (➲ Fig. 3.3.1.12) and the assessment of possible detrimental effects of strenuous chronic exercise training on RV function, particularly in endurance athletes [42–50]. Strain and strain rate imaging, which are able to objectively quantify regional RV dysfunction, have demonstrated an improved ability to diagnose ARVC and to distinguish between physiology and pathology [42]. Studies in which STE was used to evaluate RV function in the context of athlete's heart are summarized in ➲ Table 3.3.1.2. However, to date, the evidences remain limited and it is crucial to qualify the normal reference values for strain imaging of each RV regional segment in the athletic population and to know whether significant changes do occur during the season, before deciding whether such findings should provoke further evaluation.

Left and right atrium

Increased atrial size in competitive athletes is a component of athlete's heart [50]. Since atrial size alone is insufficient to provide mechanistic information about the atrium itself, STE has been applied to left and right atrium, demonstrating

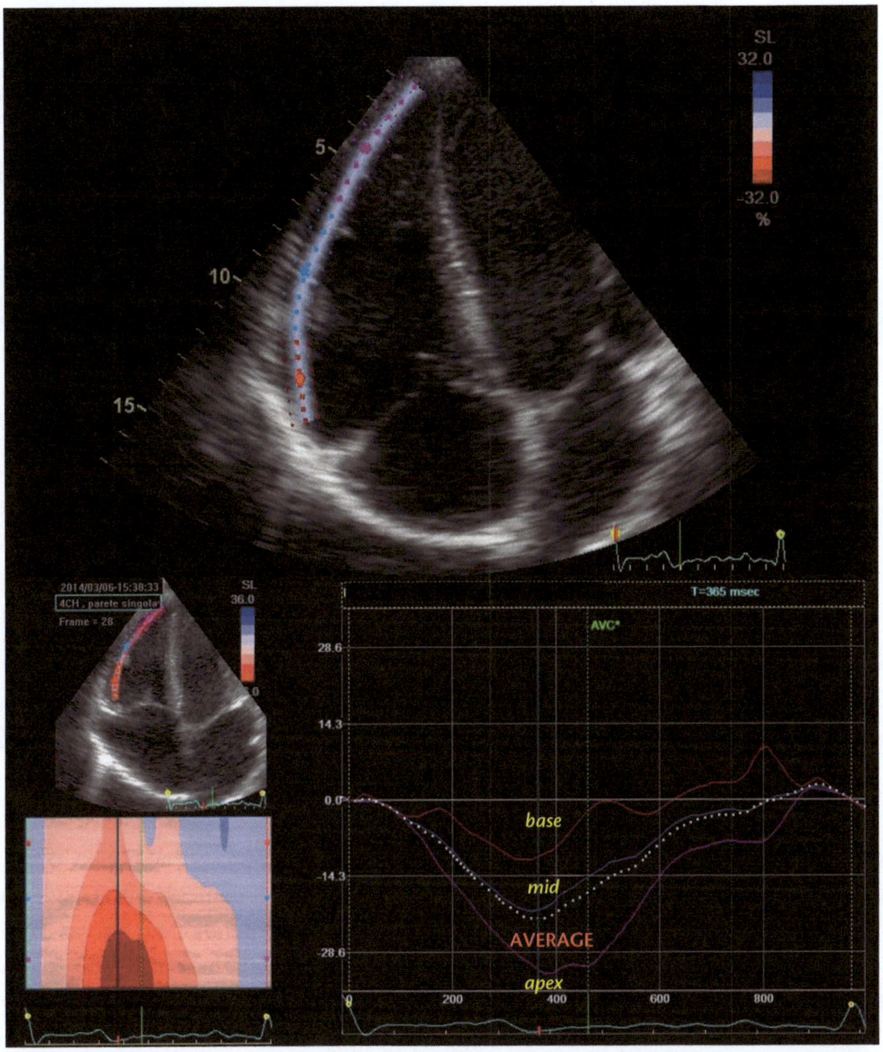

Fig. 3.3.1.12 Application of two-dimensional speckle-tracking echocardiography to the right ventricle from modified apical four-chamber view. The curves represent the right ventricular (RV) myocardial deformation during the cardiac cycle. Regional function is also provided by the assessment of basal, mid, and apical strain. Dot line represents the average values of RV strain.

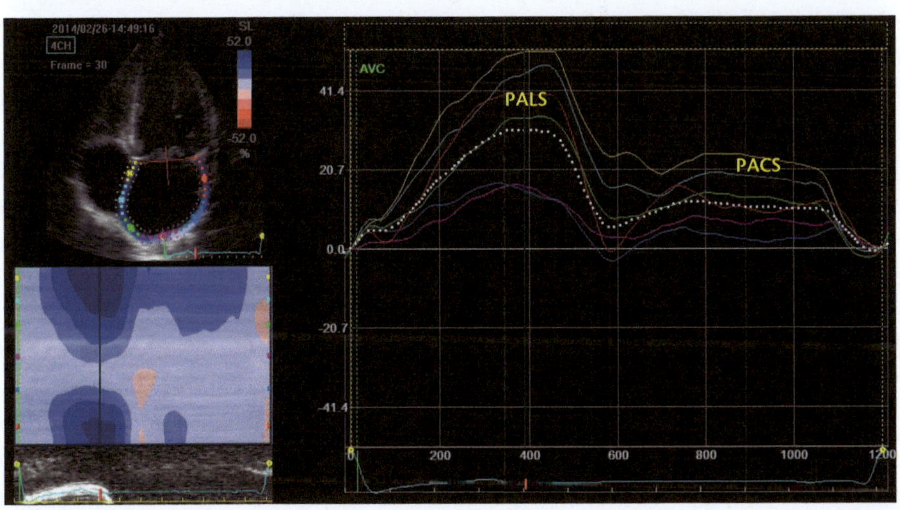

Fig. 3.3.1.13 Application of two-dimensional speckle-tracking echocardiography to the left atrium. The coloured lines represent regional strain values and the dotted line represents the average value. Peak atrial longitudinal strain (PALS) is an estimate of left atrial reservoir function; peak atrial contraction strain (PACS) is an estimate of left atrial contractile function. The ratio of endocavity filling pressure (estimated by the ratio E/e′) to atrial PALS (i.e. (E/e′ ratio)/PALS) can be used to estimate atrial stiffness.

that strain imaging is able to identify specific adaptation of biatrial myocardial deformation to exercise conditioning in competitive athletes [42,51–54] (➲ Fig. 3.3.1.13). This functional remodelling, in both male and female athletes, is dynamic in nature and is accompanied by normal, or even reduced, atrial stiffness and, despite a marked dilatation, does not have a significant impact on biatrial function [53–55].

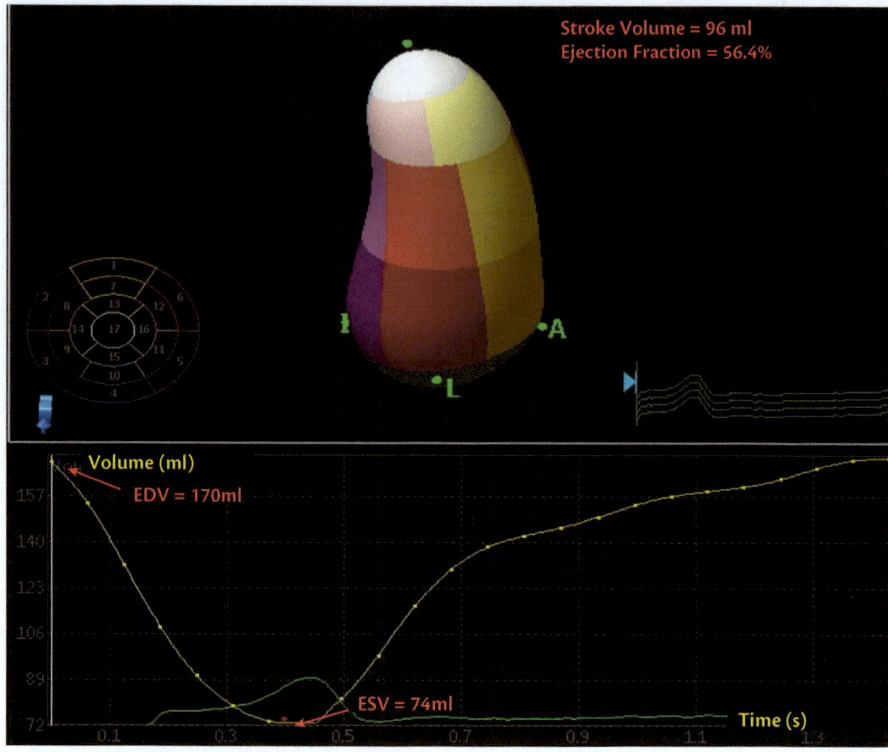

Fig. 3.3.1.14 Analysis of left ventricular function by three-dimensional echocardiography (QLab, Philips). The graph represents left ventricular volume over time and allows the dynamic assessment of left ventricular emptying and filling. EDV, end-diastolic volume; ESV, end-systolic volume.

The application of STE to the atria of competitive athletes has demonstrated a functional adaptation that goes beyond mere cavity enlargement, suggesting a possible future use of this technique as a new parameter for distinguishing between athlete's heart and cardiomyopathies.

Three-dimensional echocardiography

Three-dimensional echocardiography has been developed to overcome the limits of 2D echocardiography, not only the dependence on geometric assumptions for deriving volumetric parameters, but also the high inter-observer variability and probe positioning bias [56–59]. Real-time 3D echocardiography is a widely available, accurate, and reproducible technique. It has been employed successfully in different clinical settings and has been recently used in sports cardiology to evaluate training-induced LV remodelling through the assessment of more precise LV volume, LV ejection fraction, and LV mass [8,60–62] (➲ Fig. 3.3.1.14). Three-dimensional echocardiography has confirmed that athletes have greater LV volume and LV mass compared to sedentary controls, with the largest values observed in endurance athletes [8].

De Castro et al. [61] proposed a new parameter called the LV remodelling index (LVRI), which is calculated as the ratio of LV mass to LV end-diastolic volume. It has been shown that LVRI does not significantly differ between athletes and controls, with values around unity regardless of body surface area, age, sex, or type of sport engaged in. Healthy controls have a balanced ratio between volume and mass that is also found in the healthy athletic population. Thus, despite the high level of conditioning and the development of an increased LV mass and LV end-diastolic volume, the ratio remains constant, demonstrating that remodelling induced by training is balanced and appropriate. LVRI is also able to discriminate between physiological and pathological adaptation of the left ventricle, such as in dilated cardiomyopathy or HCM where low and high values were respectively observed [61].

Using 3D echocardiography, Caselli et al. [60] described the regional distribution of LV mass using a 12-segment model. They calculated a mass dispersion index (MDI) as the standard deviation among these values and found that this parameter could efficiently identify HCM patients from those with other forms of LV hypertrophy, such as athletes and hypertensive patients [60].

Although 3D echocardiography has been used together with 2D strain imaging to provide a comprehensive assessment of biventricular morphology and function and of aortic stiffness, a novel application field is represented by the evaluation of athlete's heart by 3D speckle-tracking imaging [62,63]. However, further data derived from 3D echocardiography are needed to understand the potential clinical utility of this novel imaging technique which also has the potential to be useful in challenging scenarios, such as the differential diagnosis between exercise-induced LV hypertrabeculation and LVNC.

Specific abnormalities

Hypertrophic cardiomyopathy

The differential diagnosis between left ventricular hypertrophy induced by training and that secondary to hypertrophic cardiomyopathy is one of the most challenging and most studied issues in sports cardiology [64–66]. Echocardiography plays an important role in this scenario and several parameters have been proposed to solve the clinical dilemma of an athlete presenting with borderline hypertrophy of 12–15mm which defines the so-called 'grey zone' [65]. However, it is important to emphasize that no single parameter can be definitely diagnostic, and that the final judgement always requires the integration of all clinical data and information derived from cardiac imaging.

HCM is defined as the presence of a hypertrophied and non-dilated left ventricle in the absence of cardiac or systemic diseases capable of producing the same magnitude of LV hypertrophy [67]. In the athlete population the highest degree in terms of increase in wall thickness has been observed in sport disciplines with high intensity static and dynamic components, which are characterized by pressure and volume overload of the left ventricle [3]. The left ventricle adapts to this haemodynamic overload by an increase in both wall thickness and cavity size with an eccentric hypertrophy. Therefore one of the most useful parameters for differential diagnosis is the left ventricular cavity size, which in normal athletes is consistently ≥54mm (➲ Fig. 3.3.1.15). Similarly, the ratio of cavity size to wall thickness (relative wall thickness equals the sum of interventricular septum thickness and posterior wall thickness divided by left ventricular end-diastolic diameter) is usually <0.45 suggesting an eccentric geometry [68].

Other features that may suggest a physiological adaptation are the homogeneous distribution of left ventricular mass without areas of focal hypertrophy (differences between contiguous segments usually ≤2mm) and absence of mitral leaflet elongation, systolic anterior motion of the mitral valve, and LV outflow tract obstruction, which in turn are hallmarks of HCM [68–70].

Diastolic function is usually normal in athletes and characterized by low velocity of the A wave. Consequently, the E/A ratio on transmitral filling is consistently >1.0, meaning that the atrial contribution to LV filling under resting condition is usually mild. Similarly, regardless of the magnitude of LV hypertrophy, it has been reported that in athletes the e′ velocity on TDI is consistently above 8cm/s. Therefore finding an inversion of the E/A ratio or reduced e′ velocity may imply a non-physiological condition and expression of altered relaxation, which often occur in HCM [68,71].

The ejection fraction is normal, or sometimes higher, in HCM patients and cannot be used to differentiate from physiological hypertrophy. Speckle-tracking echocardiography studies have reported that HCM may show a subclinical impairment on myocardial strain, with values of global longitudinal strain (GLS) <15 potentially useful for the differential diagnosis [32,72].

Finally, since all myocardial adaptations are dynamic in nature, short-term detraining may be useful for demonstrating regression of dimensional/functional cardiac changes. Failure to reduce myocardial thickness after discontinuation of training is suggestive of hypertrophic cardiomyopathy [9,10].

Dilated cardiomyopathy

DCM is a common phenotype of different causes. The main features are LV dilatation, systolic and diastolic dysfunction,

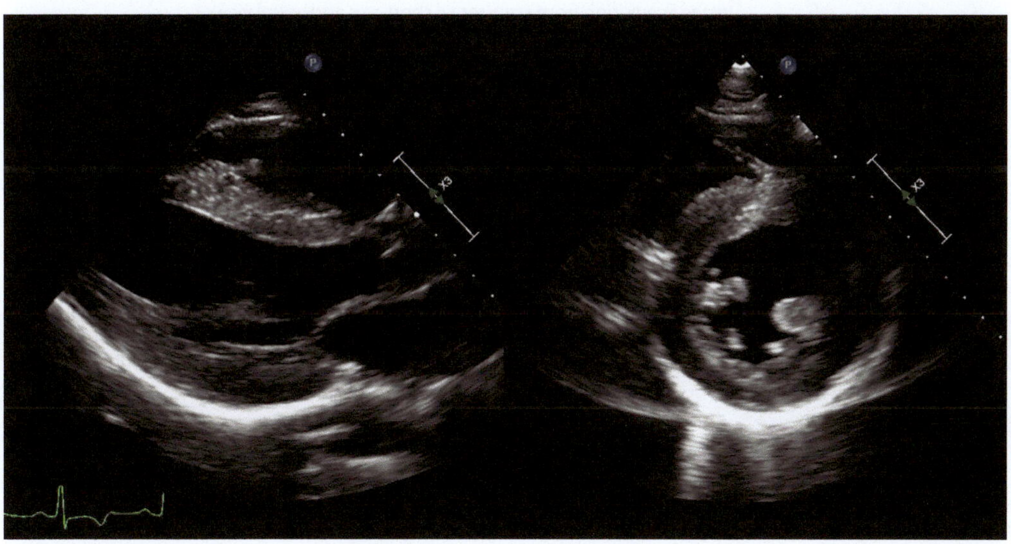

Fig. 3.3.1.15 Parasternal long-axis (left panel) and short-axis (right panel) views of a young basketball player with hypertrophic cardiomyopathy. The images clearly show a hypertrophic and non-dilated left ventricle with maximal wall thickness of 15mm and end-diastolic diameter of 52mm.

myocyte death, and myocardial fibrosis. DCM is sometimes inherited with other phenotypes, both cardiac (e.g. conduction disorder) and non-cardiac (e.g. sensorineural hearing loss) [73]. Although it has been observed that some disciplines may cause an exercise-induced dilatation of the LV, in DCM the dilatation of the cardiac chamber is typically accompanied by a certain degree of systo-diastolic dysfunction, as opposite to the main features of athlete's heart which is rarely associated with a mild loss of function. In an assessment of the LV dimensions in 1309 elite athletes from different sports disciplines, Pelliccia et al. [4] found that LV cavity enlargement varied widely in top-level athletes, but a degree compatible with primary DCM was found in almost 15% of participants. These athletes had normal global LV systolic function and no regional wall-motion abnormalities. The major determinants of cavity dimension were greater body surface area and participation in certain endurance sports (cycling, cross-country skiing, and canoeing) [4]. In the absence of systolic dysfunction, this cavity dilatation was interpreted as an extreme physiological adaptation to intensive athletic conditioning. Although cardiac adaptation also occurs in women, absolute LV cavity size exceeding normal limits is found in only a minority (8%) of women athletes and is rarely (1% of athletes) within the range of DCM [5]. The ejection fraction in athletes is within the normal range (≥55%) and almost never falls below the cut-off of <50% [8,32]. Therefore exercise echocardiography may be helpful in cases with an enlarged left ventricle and borderline reduction in EF. Indeed, athletes show a significant improvement in systolic function even at low exercise intensity, and therefore the lack of the ability to increase ejection fraction during exercise (by an average 20%) could suggest a pathological condition [23,24].

Novel echocardiographic techniques, particularly 2D STE, have demonstrated that in DCM the amplitude of the peak LV systolic twist angle is impaired in proportion to the global LV function [29]. This reduction in LV twist angle is accounted for by the marked attenuation of LV apical rotation, whereas basal rotation may be spared. A delay in the time to peak untwisting can also be found in DCM [29]. Finally, in borderline cases, loss of the decrease in LV dilatation with detraining, confirmation of LV dysfunction using 3D echocardiography, low TDI velocities, reduced LV strain, and identification of late gadolium enhancement by cardiac magnetic resonance allow the identification of the pathological substrate.

Left ventricular non-compaction

Determination of appropriate criteria for the identification of LVNC in athletes has become a novel challenge for sport physicians and cardiologists, who are required to solve this question in the setting of pre-participation cardiovascular screening [74–76].

Echocardiography is the imaging modality of first choice to establish a diagnosis, and several criteria have been proposed (➲ Table 3.3.1.3). Three major echocardiographic criteria are generally used, i.e. those initially proposed by Chin et al. [77], Jenni et al. [78]. and Stollberger et al. [79] However,

Table 3.3.1.3 Proposed diagnostic criteria for left ventricular non-compaction by echocardiography

Reference	Technique	Phase	Cut-off	Description
Chin et al. [76]	2D echo	Diastole	X/Y <0.5	X = compact layerY = non-compacted layer Image acquisition from parasternal short-axis and apical views
Jenni et al. [77]	2D echo	Systole	NC/C >2	Thickened myocardium with a bilayered structure NC, non compacted C, compacted Evidence by colour Doppler of inter-trabecular recesses filled from LV cavity Image acquisition from parasternal short-axis view
Stollberger et al. [78]	2D echo	Diastole	More than three trabeculae	Qualitative evaluation. Four or more trabeculations with the same echogenicity of the myocardium Perfusion of the inter-trabecular spaces from the LV cavity Image acquisition from the apical view Trabeculations should be identified apically to the papillary muscles
Gebhard et al. [79]	2D echo	Systole	Compacta <8mm	Reduced compacta thickness measured in systole in addition to the Jenni criterion
Caselli et al. [84]	3D echo	Diastole	TLV>13%	TLV calculated as the difference between LV end-diastolic volume obtained including and excluding the trabeculae in the cavity contour and normalized by the LV end-diastolic volume (TLV%)

2D, Two-dimensional; 3D, three-dimensional; NC/C, non-compacted/compacted; LV, left ventricle; TLV, trabeculated left ventricular volume.

despite the reasonable accuracy of each diagnostic criterion, they seem to lack specificity with low agreement between the three and high inter-observer variability. Therefore additional parameters have been developed. Gebhard et al. [80] demonstrated that a reduced compacta layer (<8mm in systole) in association with Jenni criteria helped the differentiation from normal hearts and proved to be accurate for LVNC diagnosis. Another study [81] reported that in 22 asymptomatic athletes with LV hypertrabeculation reduced thickness of the compacta layer (<5mm in diastole) was able to identify subjects with decreased LV systolic function, potentially affected by LVNC. More recently, evaluation by speckle-tracking echocardiography showed that patients with LVNC present a twisting pattern characterized by rotation at the basal and apical level predominantly in the same direction, which is also known as 'rigid body rotation'. This pattern is different from the normal LV twisting, characterized by counterclockwise basal and clockwise apical rotation followed by end-systolic clockwise basal and counterclockwise apical rotation [82,83].

Finally, an interesting insight has been derived from 3D echocardiography. Comparing LVNC patients, athletes, and control subjects, Caselli et al. [84] introduced the concept of the trabeculated left ventricular volume (TLV%), calculated as the LV end-diastolic volume obtained including and excluding the trabeculae in the cavity contour, and normalized by the LV end-diastolic volume. In this analysis, LVNC patients had approximately 24% of LV cavity occupied by trabeculae, i.e. a fourfold increase compared with other groups. The larger extent of trabeculations in patients corresponded to a higher degree of systolic dysfunction and LV chamber sphericity.

However, an increased trabecular pattern incidentally observed in an otherwise normal heart should not be considered sufficient per se to support the final diagnosis of LVNC, and the echocardiographic findings should always be interpreted on the basis of family history and all available clinical data [74,75] (➲ Fig. 3.3.1.16). The absence of LV systolic or diastolic dysfunction, positive family history, ECG abnormalities, or ventricular tachyarrhythmias may support the diagnosis of a clinically benign adaptation of the left ventricle, and the athlete should be reassured without any unwarranted restriction for sport participation but advised to have a clinical follow-up.

Aortic root dilation

An increase in aortic root size has been reported as part of cardiovascular adaptation in athletes. Indeed, intense and prolonged physical activity is associated with haemodynamic overload, which increases the wall tension through

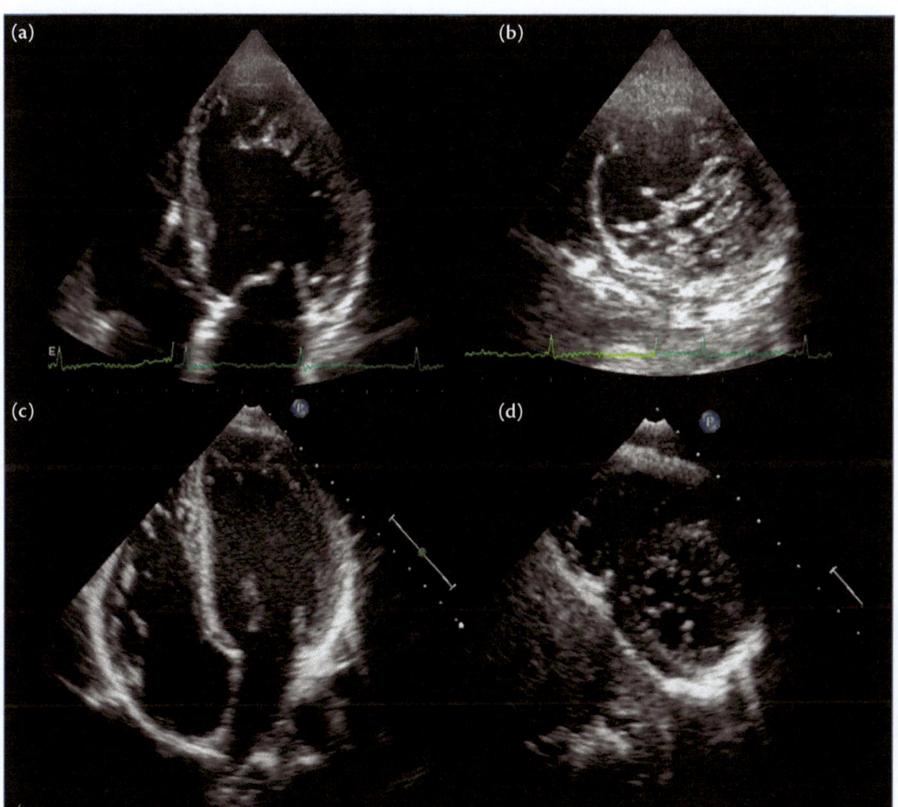

Fig. 3.3.1.16 Echocardiographic images of a patient with left ventricular non-compaction ((a), b)) and an athlete with prominent trabeculation ((c), (d)). The patient with LVNC was characterized by a more spherical shape of the left ventricle, a depressed systolic function, and impaired diastolic function. The athlete had preserved shape of the left ventricle and normal indexes of systolic and diastolic function.

the aortic walls causing an increase in aortic dimension [85,86]. However, the absolute increase in aortic root diameter is usually mild and falls within the universally accepted limits for untrained controls. A recently published meta-analysis of 5580 athletes and 727 controls reported that the aortic root size was larger in athletes with an average increase of 3mm [87].

A study by Pelliccia et al. [85] showed that the upper reference values, corresponding to the 99th percentile for the aortic root diameter were 40mm and 34mm for male and female athletes, respectively. An increase in aortic root diameter to ≥40mm was present only in a small minority of male athletes (1.7% of the population) [85]. Long-term follow-up of these athletes showed that aortic root size continued to increase, approaching or reaching 50mm in some cases (3/17).

This finding substantiates the concept that a marked increase in aortic root diameter may be an initial sign of aorthopathy, especially if associated with other features such as a bicuspid aortic valve or clinical findings suggesting Marfan syndrome.

The universally accepted technique is to measure the aortic root diameter at end-diastole at the sinuses of Valsalva using the leading-edge method, even if this may lead to a small over-estimate compared with other imaging techniques [22] (see ➲ Fig. 3.3.1.2).

Mitral valve prolapse

Mitral valve prolapse (MVP) is the most common valve disease, with an estimated prevalence of 2–3% in the general population [88]. Although MVP is generally regarded as a benign condition, the outcome is widely heterogeneous, and complications such as mitral regurgitation, atrial fibrillation, congestive heart failure, endocarditis, and stroke are well known; ventricular arrhythmias and sudden cardiac death (SCD) have also been reported [89–92]. The estimated rate of SCD in MVP ranges from 0.2% to 0.4% per year in prospective follow-up studies [91]. LV dysfunction resulting from severe mitral regurgitation identifies a patient subgroup at high risk of SCD [93]. However, life-threatening ventricular arrhythmias also occur in patients with MVP with trivial or absent mitral regurgitation, and recent evidence suggest that MVP is an underestimated cause of arrhythmic SCD, mostly in young adult women [94,95].

MVP is defined as abnormal systolic displacement of one or both leaflets into the left atrium below the mitral annulus due to structural enlargement or abnormal distensibility of the mitral valve. Two forms of MVP have been described: classic and non-classic. In classic MVP the displacement exceeds 2mm and the maximal thickness is at least 5mm; in non-classic MVP the displacement exceeds 2mm but the maximal thickness is less than 5mm [91,96,97]. Borderline degrees of displacement (≤2 mm) are not associated with increased leaflet thickness, mitral regurgitation, left atrial enlargement, valve-related complications, or progression over a period of 10 years, and are not usually included in the definition of MVP [96,97] (➲ Fig. 3.3.1.17). Levine et al. [96] demonstrated that leaflet displacement limited to the apical four-chamber view is a normal geometric finding without associated evidence of pathological significance, suggesting that, with 2D echocardiography, the diagnosis of MVP should be made in the parasternal or eventually the apical long-axis view, but not in the apical four-chamber view because the saddle-shaped mitral annulus may lead to a false-positive diagnosis [96,98].

Bicuspid aortic valve

Bicuspid aortic valve (BAV) is a common congenital heart abnormality affecting 0.5–2% of the population. It is a very heterogeneous disease, which may also be associated with aortopathy caused by a common pathogenic mechanisms [99–101].

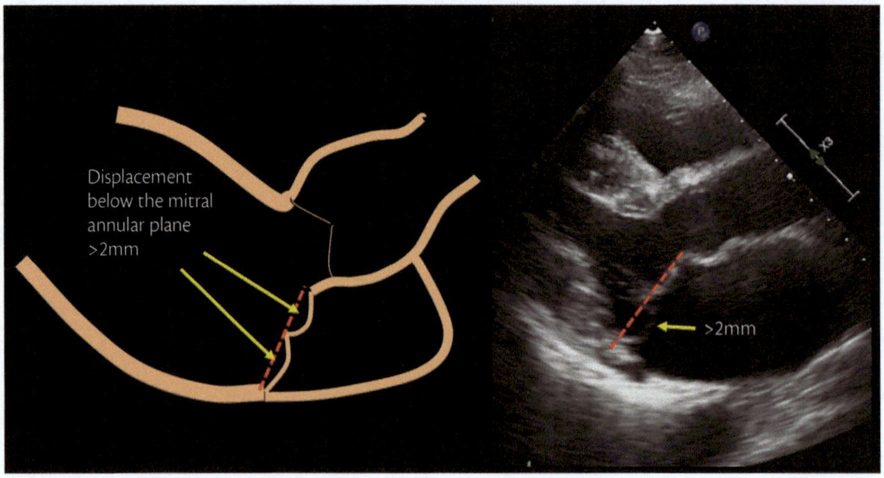

Fig. 3.3.1.17 Mitral valve prolapse is defined as an abnormal systolic displacement of one or both leaflets into the left atrium below the mitral annulus. In the classic form the displacement exceeds 2mm and the maximal thickness of the leaflets is at least 5mm; in the non-classic form the displacement exceeds 2mm but the maximal thickness of leaflets is less than 5mm.

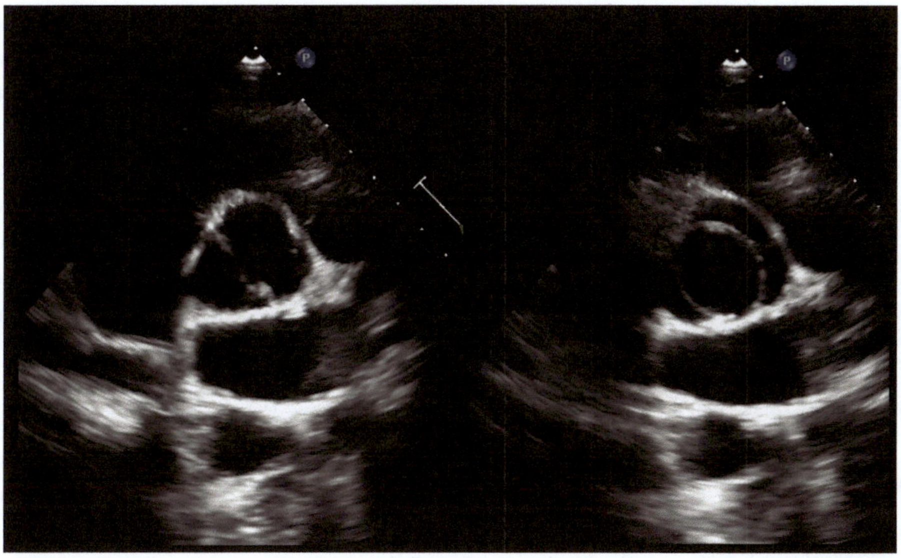

Fig. 3.3.1.18 Short bicuspid valve results from the fusion of right and left coronary cusps.

The variable morphology of BAV is due to different cusp fusion patterns [102]. The two most common patterns are fusion of the left and right coronary cusps, which occurs in 70–85% of BAV cases, and fusion of the right and non-coronary cusps, which is less common and occurs in the remaining 15–30% of cases [103] (➲ Fig. 3.3.1.18). Rarely, there is fusion of the left and non-coronary cusps. A raphe is present on the right and anterior cusps, respectively, and this can make the valve appear tricuspid on echocardiography [104].

The mainstay of diagnosis is echocardiography (transthoracic or trans-oesophageal), which can provide a definitive diagnosis in the majority of patients with 92% sensitivity and 96% specificity when images are adequate. The echocardiographic report should adequately evaluate aortic valve morphology and measure the severity of any stenosis or regurgitation [104,105]. The functional characterization of the aortic valve is extremely important because of the possible progression to aortic valve stenosis, especially in men, or to aortic regurgitation, finally requiring aortic valve replacement [106–108].

In cases of BAV the echocardiographic examination should also include aortic measurements at the aortic annulus, sinuses, sinotubular junction, mid-ascending aorta, and aortic arch. Notably, different cusp fusion patterns in BAV are associated with specific dilatation patterns of the aorta. BAV patients with right–left cusp fusion have a significantly larger aortic root diameter with normal aortic shape compared with patients with right–non-coronary cusp fusion, and the histological changes in the ascending aortic wall are more pronounced in the former [109]. Conversely, fusion of right–non-coronary cusps is associated with larger distal ascending aorta and aortic arch diameters [110]. In addition, evaluation of aortic coarctation using Doppler interrogation of the proximal descending aorta should be performed [111].

Atrial and ventricular septal defects

Atrial septal defects

An atrial septal defect (ASD) is a persistent inter-atrial communication. It is distinct from a patent foramen ovale in which there is a flap with intermittent communication. ASD types strictly include ostium secundum (~75% of cases), ostium primum (15–20%), and sinus venosus (5–10%), and rare coronary sinus defects are closely related [112,113]. Secundum ASDs are positioned by the fossa ovalis, primum ASDs inferiorly as part of the spectrum of endocardial cushion defects, and sinus venosus ASDs near the superior or inferior vena caval entry [112]. An ASD is diagnosed by echocardiography demonstrating shunting across the inter-atrial septum, with evaluation of the right heart and for associated abnormalities [112]. Clues to an ASD on 2D trans-thoracic echocardiography include a hypermobile inter-atrial septum, abrupt septal irregularity, right atrial and ventricular volume overload, and pulmonary artery dilatation. If a satisfactory subcostal view can be obtained, this is the preferred window because the inter-atrial septum is approximately perpendicular to the echo signal. The apical four-chamber view can also be particularly useful in evaluation of the right heart. However, the parallel orientation of the atrial septum to the echo signal in this view can be misleading. Applying colour flow Doppler can confirm the ASD diagnosis, show directionality of flow, and help to appreciate the ASD size better; a larger width of the colour flow jet across the inter-atrial septum indicates a larger ASD and

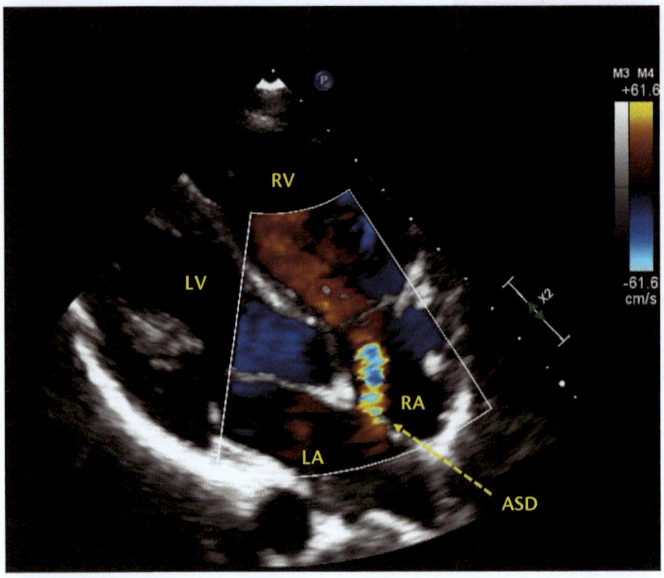

Fig. 3.3.1.19 Atrial septum defect. This is an off-axis view clearly showing an ostium secundum atrial septal defect with left atrium to right atrium shunt demonstrated by colour Doppler: LV, left ventricle; RV, right ventricle; LA, left atrium; RA, right atrium; ASD, atrial septal defect.

predicts a higher shunt ratio (➔ Fig. 3.3.1.19). Pulse wave Doppler allows assessment of lower velocity flows across the inter-atrial septum and can be useful for estimating the ratio of pulmonary to systemic flow. The Qp/Qs ratio (i.e. the pulmonary–systemic shunt ratio) can be estimated in patients who have intra-cardiac shunts by using 2D echocardiography and spectral Doppler measurements. This ratio describes the magnitude of an intra-cardiac shunt; normally, it is 1:1 while in left-to-right shunts it is >1 and in right-to-left shunts it is <1. The Qp/Qs ratio is usually greater than 1.5:1 in haemodynamically relevant left-to-right shunts [112].

In patients diagnosed with an ASD, the right heart should be carefully assessed on an echocardiogram. Right ventricular enlargement and inter-ventricular septal flattening during diastole indicate a state of volume overload. Accompanying right atrial and pulmonary artery enlargement may be present. This evaluation is particularly complicated in an athlete where exercise-induced right heart enlargement may mimic a negative haemodynamic impact of an ASD on the RV, and where training-induced changes in volume and pressure overload may represent a challenge for the RV [113]. However, the presence of pulmonary hypertension in the athlete's heart is uncommon and should raise suspicion of a pathological substrate.

Ventricular septal defects

Ventricular septal defects (VSDs) are openings in the ventricular septum and are classified according to their location, i.e. the membranous septum or the muscular septum. The membranous septum is small and is located at the base of the heart between the inlet and outlet components of the muscular septum and below the right and non-coronary cusps of the aortic valve. The muscular septum is a non-planar structure that can be divided into inlet, trabecular, and infundibular components. All defects should be assessed for location, size, and multiplicity. The relationship of the defect to the atrioventricular valves, infundibular septum, and great arteries should be noted.

Two-dimensional echocardiography accurately delineates the morphology and associated defects of VSDs. A thorough echocardiographic examination is best achieved by imaging the intra-ventricular septum in multiple planes using colour flow and spectral Doppler echocardiography. Echocardiography is most sensitive for defects >5mm that are located in the membranous, inlet, or outlet portion of the septum. It is least sensitive for apical muscular defects.

Echocardiography can confidently identify the morphological features of the defect, including its size and borders and associated defects [114]. It also provides an accurate haemodynamic assessment of the shunt, severity, volume overload, subpulmonic (double-chambered right ventricle) or pulmonic stenosis, and pulmonary hypertension [115]. In addition, echocardiography can assess the degree of aortic valve distortion and prolapse (right and non-coronary cusp) in patients with subarterial VSD, and evaluate the severity of aortic regurgitation and right ventricular outflow tract obstruction caused by the prolapsing coronary cusp [116].

Further reading

Lang RM, Badano LP, Mor-Avi V, et al. Recommendations for cardiac chamber quantification by echocardiography in adults: an update from the American Society of Echocardiography and the European Association of Cardiovascular Imaging. *Eur Heart J Cardiovasc Imaging* 2015; 16(3): 233–70.

Maron BJ, Pelliccia A. The heart of trained athletes: cardiac remodelling and the risks of sports, including sudden death. *Circulation* 2006; 114: 1633–44.

Mor-Avi V, Lang RM, Badano LP, et al. Current and evolving echocardiographic techniques for the quantitative evaluation of cardiac mechanics: ASE/EAE consensus statement on methodology and indications endorsed by the Japanese Society of Echocardiography. *Eur J Echocardiogr* 2011; 12: 167–205.

Pelliccia A, Di Paolo FM, De Blasiis E, et al. Prevalence and clinical significance of aortic root dilation in highly trained competitive athletes. *Circulation* 2010;1 22: 698–706.

Wasfy MM, Weiner RB, Wang F, et al. Endurance exercise-induced cardiac remodeling: not all sports are created equal. *J Am Soc Echocardiogr* 2015; 28: 1434–40.

References

1. Sharma S, Merghani A, Mont L. Exercise and the heart: the good, the bad, and the ugly. *Eur Heart J* 2015; 36: 1445–53.
2. Morganroth J, Maron BJ, Henry WL, Epstein SE. Comparative left ventricular dimensions in trained athletes. *Ann Intern Med* 1975; 82: 521–4.
3. Pelliccia A, Maron BJ, Spataro A, et al. The upper limit of physiologic cardiac hypertrophy in highly trained elite athletes. *N Engl J Med* 1991; 324: 295–301.
4. Pelliccia A. Culasso F, Di Paolo F, Maron BJ. Physiologic left ventricular cavity dilatation in elite athletes. *Ann Intern Med* 1999; 130: 23–31.
5. Pelliccia A, Maron BJ, Culasso F, et al. Athlete's heart in women: echocardiographic characterization of highly trained elite female athletes. *JAMA* 1996; 276: 211–15.
6. Pelliccia A, Spataro A, Caselli G, Maron BJ. Absence of left ventricular wall thickening in athletes engaged in intense power training. *Am J Cardiol* 1993; 72: 1048–54.
7. Wasfy MM, Weiner RB, Wang F, et al. Endurance exercise-induced cardiac remodeling: not all sports are created equal. *J Am Soc Echocardiogr* 2015; 28: 1434–40.
8. Caselli S, Di Paolo FM, Pisicchio C, et al. Three-dimensional echocardiographic characterization of left ventricular remodeling in Olympic athletes. *Am J Cardiol* 2011; 108: 141–7.
9. Pelliccia A, Maron BJ, De Luca R, et al. Remodeling of left ventricular hypertrophy in elite athletes after long-term deconditioning. *Circulation* 2002; 105: 944–9.
10. Weiner RB, Wang F, Berkstresser B, et al. Regression of 'gray zone' exercise-induced concentric left ventricular hypertrophy during prescribed detraining. *J Am Coll Cardiol* 2012; 59: 1992–4.
11. Sharma S, Maron BJ, Whyte G, et al. Physiologic limits of left ventricular hypertrophy in elite junior athletes: relevance to differential diagnosis of athlete's heart and hypertrophic cardiomyopathy. *J Am Coll Cardiol* 2002; 40: 1431–6.
12. Rawlins J, Carré F, Kervio G, et al. Ethnic differences in physiological cardiac adaptation to intense physical exercise in highly trained female athletes. *Circulation* 2010; 121: 1078–85.
13. Basavarajaiah S, Boraita A, Whyte G, et al. Ethnic differences in left ventricular remodeling in highly-trained athletes relevance to differentiating physiologic left ventricular hypertrophy from hypertrophic cardiomyopathy. *J Am Coll Cardiol* 2008; 51(23): 2256–62.
14. Merghani A, Malhotra A, Sharma S. The U-shaped relationship between exercise and cardiac morbidity. *Trends Cardiovasc Med* 2016; 26: 232–40.
15. Heidbuchel H, Carré F. Exercise and competitive sports in patients with an implantable cardioverter-defibrillator. *Eur Heart J* 2014; 35: 3097–102.
16. Corrado D, Basso C, Rizzoli G, et al. Does sports activity enhance the risk of sudden death in adolescents and young adults? *J Am Coll Cardiol* 2003; 42: 1959–63.
17. Corrado D, Pelliccia A, Bjørnstad HH, et al. Cardiovascular pre-participation screening of young competitive athletes for prevention of sudden death: proposal for a common European protocol. Consensus Statement of the Study Group of Sport Cardiology of the Working Group of Cardiac Rehabilitation and Exercise Physiology and the Working Group of Myocardial and Pericardial Diseases of the European Society of Cardiology. *Eur Heart J* 2005; 26: 516–24.
18. Pelliccia A, Fagard R, Bjørnstad HH, et al. Recommendations for competitive sports participation in athletes with cardiovascular disease: a consensus document from the Study Group of Sports Cardiology of the Working Group of Cardiac Rehabilitation and Exercise Physiology and the Working Group of Myocardial and Pericardial Diseases of the European Society of Cardiology. *Eur Heart J* 2005; 26: 1422–45.
19. Drezner JA, Fischbach P, Froelicher V, et al. Normal electrocardiographic findings: recognising physiological adaptations in athletes. *Br J Sports Med* 2013; 47: 125–36.
20. Corrado D, Pelliccia A, Heidbuchel H, et al. Recommendations for interpretation of 12-lead electrocardiogram in the athlete. *Eur Heart J* 2010; 31: 243–59.
21. Drezner JA, Ashley E, Baggish AL, et al. Abnormal electrocardiographic findings in athletes: recognising changes suggestive of cardiomyopathy. *Br J Sports Med* 2013; 47(3): 137–52.
22. Lang RM, Badano LP, Mor-Avi V, et al. Recommendations for cardiac chamber quantification by echocardiography in adults: an update from the American Society of Echocardiography and the European Association of Cardiovascular Imaging. *Eur Heart J Cardiovasc Imaging* 2015; 16: 233–70.
23. Picano E, Pellikka PA. Stress echo applications beyond coronary artery disease. *Eur Heart J* 2014; 35(16): 1033–40.
24. Galderisi M, Cardim N, D'Andrea A, et al. The multi-modality cardiac imaging approach to the athlete's heart: an expert consensus of the European Association of Cardiovascular Imaging. *Eur Heart J Cardiovasc Imaging* 2015 Apr;16(4):353.
25. Alharthi MS, Jiamsripong P, Calleja A, et al. Selective echocardiographic analysis of epicardial and endocardial left ventricular rotational mechanics in an animal model of pericardial adhesions. Eur J Echocardiogr. 2009; 10: 357–62.
26. Jiamsripong P, Alharthi MS, Calleja AM, et al. Quantification of left ventricular twisting mechanics by velocity vector imaging in an animal model of pericardial adhesions. Ultrasound Med Biol. 2009; 35: 1963–72.
27. Kim DH, Kim HK, Kim MK, et al. Velocity vector imaging in the measurement of left ventricular twist mechanics: head-to-head one way comparison between speckle tracking echocardiography and velocity vector imaging. *J Am Soc Echocardiogr* 2009; 22: 1344–52.
28. Teske AJ, De Boeck BW, Melman PG, et al. Echocardiographic quantification of myocardial function using tissue deformation imaging: a guide to image acquisition and analysis using tissue Doppler and speckle tracking. *Cardiovasc Ultrasound* 2007; 5: 27.
29. Mor-Avi V, Lang RM, Badano LP, et al. Current and evolving echocardiographic techniques for the quantitative evaluation of cardiac mechanics: ASE/EAE consensus statement on methodology and indications endorsed by the Japanese Society of Echocardiography. *Eur J Echocardiogr* 2011; 12: 167–205.
30. Cappelli F, Toncelli L, Cappelli B, et al. Adaptative or maladaptative hypertrophy, different spatial distribution of myocardial contraction. *Clin Physiol Funct Imaging* 2010; 30: 6–12.
31. Galderisi M, Lomoriello VS, Santoro A, et al. Differences of myocardial systolic deformation and correlates of diastolic function in competitive rowers and young hypertensives: a speckle-tracking echocardiography study. *J Am Soc Echocardiogr* 2010; 23: 1190–8.

32. Caselli S, Montesanti D, Autore C, et al. Patterns of left ventricular longitudinal strain and strain rate in Olympic athletes. *J Am Soc Echocardiogr* 2015; 28(2): 245–53.
33. Soullier C, Obert P, Doucende G, et al. Exercise response in hypertrophic cardiomyopathy: blunted left ventricular deformational and twisting reserve with altered systolic-diastolic coupling. *Circ Cardiovasc Imaging* 2012; 5: 324–32.
34. D'Ascenzi F, Pelliccia A, Alvino F, et al. Effects of training on LV strain in competitive athletes. *Heart* 2015; 101: 1834–39
35. Spence AL, Naylor LH, Carter HH, et al. A prospective randomised longitudinal MRI study of left ventricular adaptation to endurance and resistance exercise training in humans. *J Physiol* 2011; 589: 5443–52.
36. Yingchoncharoen T, Agarwal S, Popović ZB, Marwick TH. Normal ranges of left ventricular strain: a meta-analysis. *J Am Soc Echocardiogr* 2013; 26: 185–91.
37. Nottin S, Doucende G, Schuster-Beck I, et al. Alteration in left ventricular normal and shear strains evaluated by 2D-strain echocardiography in the athlete's heart. *J Physiol* 2008; 586: 4721–33.
38. Weiner RB, Hutter AM, Jr, Wang F, et al. The impact of endurance exercise training on left ventricular torsion. *JACC Cardiovasc Imaging* 2010; 3: 1001–9.
39. Simsek Z, Hakan Tas M, Degirmenci H, et al. Speckle tracking echocardiographic analysis of left ventricular systolic and diastolic functions of young elite athletes with eccentric and concentric type of cardiac remodeling. *Echocardiography* 2013; 30: 1202–8.
40. Teske AJ, Cox MG, De Boeck BW, et al. Echocardiographic tissue deformation imaging quantifies abnormal regional right ventricular function in arrhythmogenic right ventricular dysplasia/cardiomyopathy. *J Am Soc Echocardiogr* 2009; 22: 920–7.
41. Oxborough D, Sharma S, Shave R, et al. The right ventricle of the endurance athlete: the relationship between morphology and deformation. *J Am Soc Echocardiogr* 2012; 25: 263–71.
42. Pagourelias ED, Kouidi E, Efthimiadis GK, et al. Right atrial and ventricular adaptations to training in male Caucasian athletes: an echocardiographic study. *J Am Soc Echocardiogr* 2013; 26: 1344–52.
43. Esposito R, Galderisi M, Schiano-Lomoriello V, et al. Nonsymmetric myocardial contribution to supranormal right ventricular function in the athlete's heart: combined assessment by speckle tracking and real time three-dimensional echocardiography. *Echocardiography* 2014; 31: 996–1004.
44. D'Ascenzi F, Pelliccia A, Corrado D, et al. Right ventricular remodelling induced by exercise training in competitive athletes. *Eur Heart J Cardiovasc Imaging* 2016; 17(3):301–7
45. La Gerche A, Burns AT, D'Hooge J, et al. Exercise strain rate imaging demonstrates normal right ventricular contractile reserve and clarifies ambiguous resting measures in endurance athletes. *J Am Soc Echocardiogr* 2012; 25: 253–62 e1.
46. Heidbuchel H, La Gerche A. The right heart in athletes: evidence for exercise-induced arrhythmogenic right ventricular cardiomyopathy. *Herzschrittmacherther Elektrophysiol* 2012; 23: 82–6.
47. La Gerche A, Burns AT, Mooney DJ, et al. Exercise-induced right ventricular dysfunction and structural remodelling in endurance athletes. *Eur Heart J* 2012; 33: 998–1006.
48. Oxborough D, Shave R, Warburton D, et al. Dilatation and dysfunction of the right ventricle immediately after ultraendurance exercise: exploratory insights from conventional two-dimensional and speckle tracking echocardiography. *Circ Cardiovasc Imaging* 2011; 4: 253–63.
49. Teske AJ, Cox MG, Te Riele AS, et al. Early detection of regional functional abnormalities in asymptomatic ARVD/C gene carriers. *J Am Soc Echocardiogr* 2012; 25: 997–1006.
50. Iskandar A, Mujtaba MT, Thompson PD. Left atrium size in elite athletes. *JACC Cardiovasc Imaging* 2015; 8: 753–62.
51. D'Ascenzi F, Cameli M, Zaca V, et al. Supernormal diastolic function and role of left atrial myocardial deformation analysis by 2D speckle tracking echocardiography in elite soccer players. *Echocardiography* 2011; 28: 320–6.
52. D'Ascenzi F, Cameli M, Padeletti M, et al. Characterization of right atrial function and dimension in top-level athletes: a speckle tracking study. *Int J Cardiovasc Imaging* 2013; 29: 87–94.
53. D'Ascenzi F, Pelliccia A, Natali BM, et al. Morphological and functional adaptation of left and right atria induced by training in highly trained female athletes. *Circ Cardiovasc Imaging* 2014; 7: 222–9.
54. D'Ascenzi F, Pelliccia A, Natali BM, et al. Increased left atrial size is associated with reduced atrial stiffness and preserved reservoir function in athlete's heart. *Int J Cardiovasc Imaging* 2015; 31: 699–705.
55. Gjerdalen GF, Hisdal J, Solberg EE, et al. Atrial size and function in athletes. *Int J Sports Med* 2015; 36: 1170–6.
56. Dorosz JL, Lezotte DC, Weitzenkamp DA, et al. Performance of 3-dimensional echocardiography in measuring left ventricular volumes and ejection fraction: a systematic review and meta-analysis. *J Am Coll Cardiol* 2012; 59: 1799–1808.
57. Jenkins C, Moir S, Chan J, et al. Left ventricular volume measurement with echocardiography: a comparison of left ventricular opacification, three-dimensional echocardiography, or both with magnetic resonance imaging. *Eur Heart J* 2009; 30: 98–106.
58. Mor-Avi V, Sugeng L, Lang RM. Real-time 3-dimensional echocardiography: an integral component of the routine echocardiographic examination in adult patients? *Circulation* 2009; 119: 314–29.
59. Jenkins C, Bricknell K, Hanekom L, et al. Reproducibility and accuracy of echocardiographic measurements of left ventricular parameters using real-time three-dimensional echocardiography. *J Am Coll Cardiol* 2004; 44: 878–86.
60. Caselli S, Pelliccia A, Maron M, et al. Differentiation of hypertrophic cardiomyopathy from other forms of left ventricular hypertrophy by means of three-dimensional echocardiography. *Am J Cardiol* 2008; 102: 616–20.
61. De Castro S, Caselli S, Maron M, et al. Left ventricular remodelling index (LVRI) in various pathophysiological conditions: a real-time three-dimensional echocardiographic study. *Heart* 2007; 93: 205–9.
62. Vitarelli A, Capotosto L, Placanica G, et al. Comprehensive assessment of biventricular function and aortic stiffness in athletes with different forms of training by three-dimensional echocardiography and strain imaging. *Eur Heart J Cardiovasc Imaging* 2013; 14: 1010–20.

63. Monte IP, Mangiafico S, Buccheri S, et al. Myocardial deformational adaptations to different forms of training: a real-time three-dimensional speckle tracking echocardiographic study. *Heart Vessels*. 2015; 30: 386–95.
64. Maron BJ. Sudden death in young athletes. *N Engl J Med* 2003; 349: 1064–75.
65. Maron BJ, Pelliccia A, Spirito P. Cardiac disease in young trained athletes: insights into methods for distinguishing athlete's heart from structural heart disease, with particular emphasis on hypertrophic cardiomyopathy. *Circulation* 1995; 91: 1596–1601.
66. Maron BJ, Pelliccia A. The heart of trained athletes: cardiac remodelling and the risks of sports, including sudden death. *Circulation* 2006 10; 114: 1633–44.
67. Elliott PM, Anastasakis A, Borger MA, et al. 2014 ESC Guidelines on diagnosis and management of hypertrophic cardiomyopathy: the Task Force for the Diagnosis and Management of Hypertrophic Cardiomyopathy of the European Society of Cardiology (ESC). *Eur Heart J* 2014; 35: 2733–79.
68. Caselli S, Maron MS, Urbano-Moral JA, et al. Differentiating left ventricular hypertrophy in athletes from that in patients with hypertrophic cardiomyopathy. *Am J Cardiol* 2014; 114: 1383–9.
69. Sheikh N, Papadakis M, Schnell F, et al. Clinical profile of athletes with hypertrophic cardiomyopathy. *Circ Cardiovasc Imaging* 2015; 8: e003454.
70. Maron MS, Olivotto I, Harrigan C, et al. Mitral valve abnormalities identified by cardiovascular magnetic resonance represent a primary phenotypic expression of hypertrophic cardiomyopathy. *Circulation* 2011; 124: 40–7.
71. Caselli S, Di Paolo FM, Pisicchio C, et al. Patterns of left ventricular diastolic function in Olympic athletes. *J Am Soc Echocardiogr* 2015; 28: 236–44.
72. Kansal MM, Lester SJ, Surapaneni P, et al. Usefulness of two-dimensional and speckle tracking echocardiography in 'Gray Zone' left ventricular hypertrophy to differentiate professional football player's heart from hypertrophic cardiomyopathy. *Am J Cardiol* 2011; 108: 1322–26.
73. Watkins H, Ashrafian H, Redwood C. Inherited cardiomyopathies. *N Engl J Med* 2011; 364: 1643–56.
74. Caselli S, Attenhofer Jost CH, et al. Left ventricular noncompaction diagnosis and management relevant to pre-participation screening of athletes. *Am J Cardiol* 2015; 116: 801–8.
75. Gati S, Chandra N, Bennett RL, et al. Increased left ventricular trabeculation in highly trained athletes: do we need more stringent criteria for the diagnosis of left ventricular non-compaction in athletes? *Heart* 2013; 99: 401–8.
76. D'Ascenzi F, Pelliccia A, Natali BM, et al. Exercise-induced left ventricular hypertrabeculation in athlete's heart. *Int J Cardiol* 2015; 181: 320–2.
77. Chin TK, Perloff JK, Williams RG, et al. Isolated noncompaction of left ventricular myocardium. A study of eight cases. *Circulation* 1990; 82: 507–13.
78. Jenni R, Oechslin E, Schneider J, et al. Echocardiographic and pathoanatomical characteristics of isolated left ventricular non-compaction: a step towards classification as a distinct cardiomyopathy. *Heart* 2001; 86: 666–71.
79. Stollberger C, Finsterer J, Blazek G. Left ventricular hypertrabeculation/noncompaction and association with additional cardiac abnormalities and neuromuscular disorders. *Am J Cardiol* 2002; 90: 899–902.
80. Gebhard C, Stahli BE, Greutmann M, et al. Reduced left ventricular compacta thickness: a novel echocardiographic criterion for non-compaction cardiomyopathy. *J Am Soc Echocardiogr* 2012; 25: 1050–57.
81. Poscolieri B, Bianco M, Vessella T, et al. Identification of benign form of ventricular non-compaction in competitive athletes by multiparametric evaluation. *Int J Cardiol* 2014; 176: 1134–36.
82. Peters F, Khandheria BK, Libhaber E, et al. Left ventricular twist in left ventricular noncompaction. *Eur Heart J Cardiovasc Imaging* 2014; 15: 48–55.
83. van Dalen BM, Caliskan K, Soliman OI, et al. Diagnostic value of rigid body rotation in noncompaction cardiomyopathy. *J Am Soc Echocardiogr* 2011; 24: 548–55.
84. Caselli S, Autore C, Serdoz A, et al. Three-dimensional echocardiographic characterization of patients with left ventricular noncompaction. *J Am Soc Echocardiogr* 2012; 25: 203–9.
85. Pelliccia A, Di Paolo FM, De Blasiis E, et al. Prevalence and clinical significance of aortic root dilation in highly trained competitive athletes. *Circulation* 2010; 122: 698–706.
86. D'Andrea A1, Cocchia R, Riegler L, et al. Aortic root dimensions in elite athletes. *Am J Cardiol* 2010; 105: 1629–34.
87. Iskandar A, Thompson PD. A meta-analysis of aortic root size in elite athletes. *Circulation* 2013; 127: 791–8.
88. Dellin FN, Vasan RS. Epidemiology and pathophysiology of mitral valve prolapse: new insights into disease progression, genetics, and molecular basis. *Circulation* 2014; 129: 2158–70.
89. Freed LA, Levy D, Levine RA, et al. Prevalence and clinical outcome of mitral-valve prolapse. *N Engl J Med* 1999; 341: 1–7.
90. Freed LA, Benjamin EJ, Levy D, et al. Mitral valve prolapse in the general population: the benign nature of echocardiographic features in the Framingham Heart Study. *J Am Coll Cardiol* 2002; 40(7): 1298–1304.
91. Nishimura RA, McGoon MD, Shub C, et al. Echocardiographically documented mitral-valve prolapse: long-term follow-up of 237 patients. *N Engl J Med* 1985; 313: 1305–9.
92. Düren DR, Becker AE, Dunning AJ. Long-term follow-up of idiopathic mitral valve prolapse in 300 patients: a prospective study. *J Am Coll Cardiol* 1988; 11: 42–7.
93. Kligfield P, Levy D, Devereux RB, Savage DD. Arrhythmias and sudden death in mitral valve prolapse. *Am Heart J* 1987; 113: 1298–1307.
94. Vohra J, Sathe S, Warren R, et al. Malignant ventricular arrhythmias in patients with mitral valve prolapse and mild mitral regurgitation. *Pacing Clin Electrophysiol* 1993; 16: 387–93.
95. Basso C, Perazzolo Marra M, Rizzo S, et al. Arrhythmic mitral valve prolapse and sudden cardiac death. *Circulation* 2015; 132:556–66.
96. Levine RA, Stathogiannis E, Newell JB, et al. Reconsideration of echocardiographic standards for mitral valve prolapse: lack of association between leaflet displacement isolated to the apical four chamber view and independent echocardiographic evidence of abnormality. *J Am Coll Cardiol* 1988; 11: 1010–19.
97. Perloff JK, Child JS. Mitral valve prolapse: evolution and refinement of diagnostic techniques. *Circulation* 1989; 80: 710–1.
98. Lancellotti P, Moura L, Pierard LA, et al. European Association of Echocardiography recommendations for the assessment of valvular regurgitation. Part 2: mitral and tricuspid regurgitation (native valve disease). *Eur J Echocardiogr* 2010; 11: 307–32.
99. Roberts WC. The congenitally bicuspid aortic valve: a study of 85 autopsy cases. *Am J Cardiol* 1970; 26: 72–83.

100. Larson EW, Edwards WD. Risk factors for aortic dissection: a necropsy study of 161 cases. *Am J Cardiol* 1984; 53: 849–55.
101. Steinberger J, Moller JH, Berry JM, Sinaiko AR. Echocardiographic diagnosis of heart disease in apparently healthy adolescents. Pediatrics 2000; 105(4 Pt 1):815–8.
102. Cotrufo M, Della Corte A. The association of bicuspid aortic valve disease with asymmetric dilatation of the tubular ascending aorta: identification of a definite syndrome. *J Cardiovasc Med* 2009; 10: 291–7.
103. Schaefer BM, Lewin MB, Stout KK, et al. The bicuspid aortic valve: an integrated phenotypic classification of leaflet morphology and aortic root shape. *Heart* 2008; 94: 1634–8.
104. Sabet HY, Edwards WD, Tazelaar HD, Daly RC. Congenitally bicuspid aortic valves: a surgical pathology study of 542 cases (1991 through 1996) and a literature review of 2715 additional cases. *Mayo Clin Proc* 1999; 74: 14–26.
105. Schaefer BM, Lewin MB, Stout KK, et al. The bicuspid aortic valve: an integrated phenotypic classification of leaflet morphology and aortic root shape. *Heart* 2008; 94: 1634–8.
106. Subramanian R, Olson LJ, Edwards WD. Surgical pathology of pure aortic stenosis: a study of 374 cases. *Mayo Clin Proc* 1984; 59: 683–90.
107. Roberts WC, Ko JM. Frequency by decades of unicuspid, bicuspid, and tricuspid aortic valves in adults having isolated aortic valve replacement for aortic stenosis, with or without associated aortic regurgitation. *Circulation* 2005; 111: 920–5
108. Kang JW, Song HG, Yang DH, et al. Association between bicuspid aortic valve phenotype and patterns of valvular dysfunction and bicuspid aortopathy: comprehensive evaluation using MDCT and echocardiography. *JACC Cardiovasc Imaging* 2013; 6: 150–61.
109. Roberts WC, Morrow AG, McIntosh CL, et al. Congenitally bicuspid aortic valve causing severe, pure aortic regurgitation without superimposed infective endocarditis: analysis of 13 patients requiring aortic valve replacement. *Am J Cardiol* 1981; 47: 206–9.
110. Russo CF, Cannata A, Lanfranconi M, et al. Is aortic wall degeneration related to bicuspid aortic valve anatomy in patients with valvular disease? *J Thorac Cardiovasc Surg* 2008; 136; 937–42.
111. Schaefer B, Lewin M, Stout K, et al. Usefulness of bicuspid aortic valve phenotype to predict elastic properties of the ascending aorta. *Am J Cardiol* 2007; 99: 686–90.
112. Warnes CA, Williams RG, Bashore TM, et al. ACC/AHA 2008 guidelines for the management of adults with congenital heart disease: a report of the American College of Cardiology/American Heart Association Task Force on Practice Guidelines (Writing Committee to Develop Guidelines on the Management of Adults With Congenital Heart Disease). Developed in Collaboration With the American Society of Echocardiography, Heart Rhythm Society, International Society for Adult Congenital Heart Disease, Society for Cardiovascular Angiography and Interventions, and Society of Thoracic Surgeons. *J Am Coll Cardiol* 2008; 52: e143–263.
113. D'Ascenzi F, Malandrino M, Bonifazi M, Mondillo S. Atrial septal defect and training-induced changes in loading conditions: clinical management and implications for competitive athletes. *BMJ Case Rep* 2015; doi: 10.1136/bcr-2015-211119.
114. Pieroni DR, Nishimura RA, Bierman FZ, et al. Second natural history study of congenital heart defects. Ventricular septal defect: echocardiography. *Circulation* 1993; 87Suppl): I80–8.
115. Kurokawa S, Takahashi M, Katoh Y, et al. Noninvasive evaluation of the ratio of pulmonary to systemic flow in ventricular septal defect by means of Doppler two-dimensional echocardiography. *Am Heart J* 1988; 116(4): 1033–44.
116. Schmidt KG, Cassidy SC, Silverman NH, Stanger P. Doubly committed subarterial ventricular septal defects: echocardiographic features and surgical implications. *J Am Coll Cardiol* 1988; 12: 1538–46.

3.3.2 Cardiac magnetic resonance imaging

Guido Claessen and André La Gerche

Introduction

Cardiac magnetic resonance imaging (CMR) is an extremely useful tool in the clinical evaluation of athletes. It is a gold standard for the assessment of cardiac structure (dimensions, volume, and mass) and provides a volumetric assessment of cardiac function. Perhaps of greatest incremental benefit is that CMR can be used to identify oedema, inflammation, and fibrosis within the myocardium.

Where does CMR fit in the clinical evaluation of athletes?

In most circumstances, CMR remains a tertiary tool for the evaluation of athletes. As depicted in ➲ Fig. 3.3.2.1, significant symptoms, abnormal examination findings, and abnormalities identified on 12-lead electrocardiography should first be evaluated using echocardiography. Echocardiography is a cost-effective investigational tool that is widely available and is sufficient for addressing many clinical questions. Furthermore, far more experience is available in the evaluation of athletes with echocardiography, and as a result our understanding of the range of measures that we would consider as normal in athletes is more extensive than with CMR. On the other hand, it is clear that CMR is more sensitive in identifying some abnormalities, particularly in potential echocardiographic 'blind-spots' such as the cardiac apex and right ventricle (RV). Thus the two main roles of CMR in the evaluation of athletes are (1) to complement and clarify abnormalities identified on echocardiography, and (2) as an additional evaluation even when the echocardiographic study appears normal but significant clinical suspicion persists. A third clinical indication is when echocardiographic images are not diagnostic because of obesity or incompatible body habitus, but this is rarely a major issue in athletes.

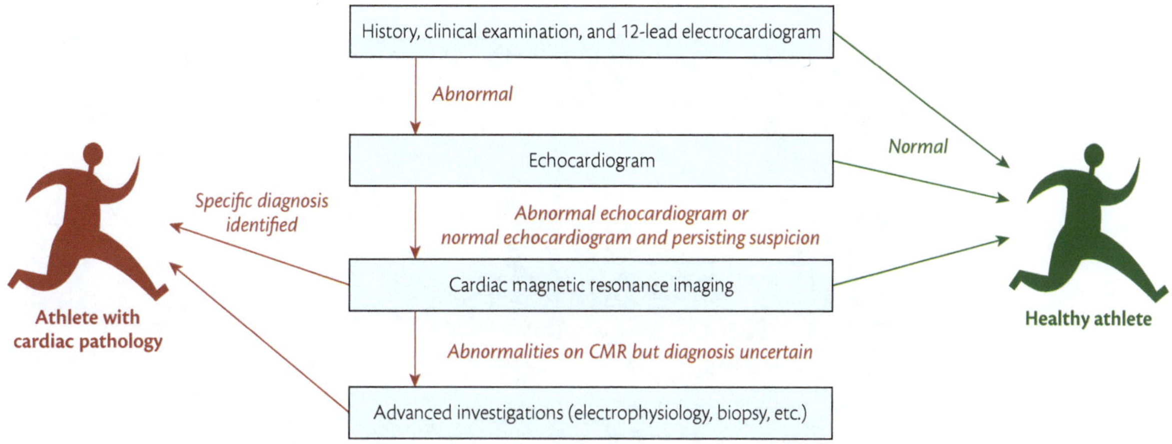

Fig. 3.3.2.1 Clinical scheme for incorporating CMR into the evaluation of an athlete.

It is not always possible to form a conclusive diagnosis at first presentation, and an additional value of CMR is that it serves as an excellent baseline investigation against which future evaluations can be compared. There is no risk of cumulative radiation and, moreover, the extremely high reproducibility and ability to compare similarly acquired images directly makes CMR the ideal modality for serial comparisons. Furthermore, in the recent era in which familial cardiomyopathies are being diagnosed using cascade screening of affected family members, it is increasingly recognized that CMR is a more sensitive diagnostic tool. Compared with ECG and echocardiography, CMR including delayed gadolinium enhancement (DGE) assessment can identify cardiac abnormalities when the ECG and echocardiogram are normal [1]. Thus CMR should be considered the most comprehensive imaging modality for the exclusion of pathology, making it extremely valuable for assessing athletes with concerning symptoms. However, the relative expense and limited availability of CMR make it less suitable for broad-based screening, and the specificity of CMR testing in athletes with little pre-test probability for disease is not sufficiently high to preclude a significant burden of false-positive results.

CMR imaging sequences: acquisition and post-processing

In clinical CMR, several imaging sequences are used to assess cardiac morphology, function, and viability. These sequences include spin echo imaging, gradient echo imaging, phase-contrast velocity encoding, and contrast-enhanced inversion-recovery imaging. Historically, spin echo sequences were the first available to study cardiac anatomy. Because of the moving spins in the blood, it appears dark (hence the name 'black blood imaging'), whereas stationary tissues such as myocardium are bright [2,3]. Spin echo black blood sequences provide high resolution imaging with accurate delineation between the dark blood pool and the myocardium. Therefore these sequences are mainly used to assess cardiac anatomy and for identifying fatty infiltration in arrhythmogenic right ventricular cardiomyopathy (ARVC) [4].

In contrast with spin echo sequences, in gradient echo imaging blood appears bright and myocardium black. The most commonly used gradient echo sequence is balanced steady state free precession (bSSFP). In bSSFP residual transverse magnetization is maintained using a balanced gradient scheme, such that remnant magnetization is superimposed on subsequent read-outs, improving the signal-to-noise ratio. bSSFP provides bright blood images, with excellent contrast between myocardium and blood pool, and high temporal resolution. Thus, bSSFP is ideally suited for the study of cardiac dynamics and detailed evaluation of cardiac anatomy, and has become the standard for cardiac cine imaging [5].

CMR cine imaging is generally considered the gold standard for measurement of biventricular volumes and mass [6]. Rather than depending on single-image slices and multiple geometrical assumptions, the entire heart can be sampled without limitations in acoustic windows. Typically, cine imaging requires electrocardiographic gating and multiple breath-holds. For each phase in the cardiac cycle, an image is acquired over several heart beats. All acquired images are then displayed as a cine loop with optimal spatial and temporal resolution. To measure ventricular volumes, a stack of short-axis slices covering both ventricles from base to apex is acquired. Each slice contains a cine loop of image frames throughout the cardiac

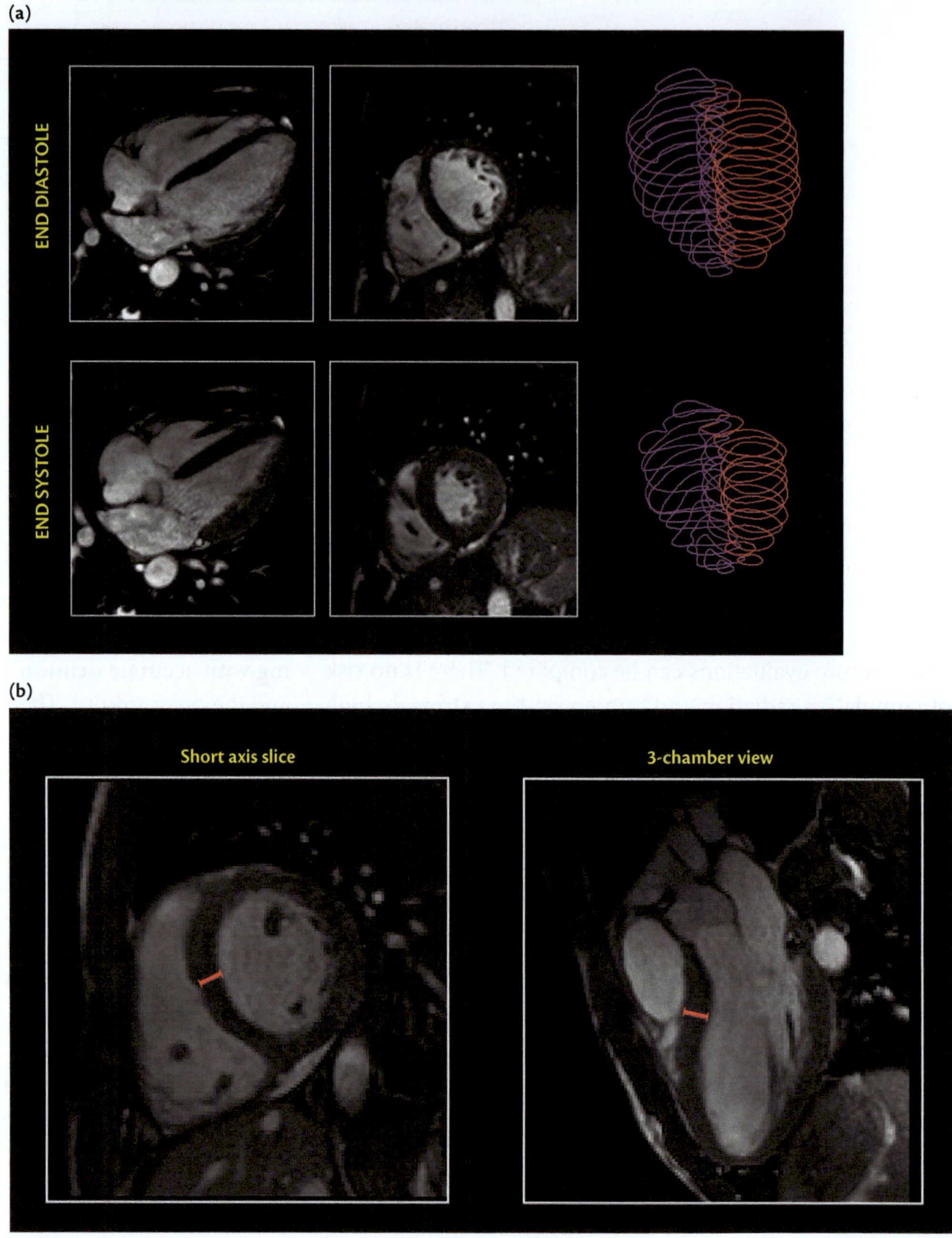

Fig. 3.3.2.2 Assessment of biventricular volumes and left ventricular wall thickness by CMR. (a) A stack of short-axis slices covering both ventricles from base to apex is acquired. Endocardial and epicardial (not shown) borders from end-diastolic and end-systolic frames can be contoured in a manual or automated manner for both the LV (red traces) and the RV (purple traces). Volume and mass for both ventricles can then be calculated using the slice summation method. (b) Wall thickness is measured on a basal short-axis slice or on a three-chamber view. The latter is similar to the parasternal long-axis view by echocardiography.

cycle. Endocardial and epicardial borders from end-diastolic and end-systolic frames can be contoured in a manual or automated manner. Then, volumes and mass for both ventricles can be calculated using the slice summation method (➲ Fig. 3.3.2.2). The acquisition of a complete set of cine CMR images can be performed in 5–10 breath-hold periods of 6–12s each. In addition to ventricular mass and volumes, feature tracking techniques have recently been developed to derive myocardial strain and strain rate from routine SSFP cine CMR images [7]. This technique promises easy and fast quantitative wall motion assessment without the need for tagged images.

CMR phase-contrast velocity encoding is used for velocity measurements and is based on the accumulated phase of moving protons. In this technique bipolar magnetic field gradients are applied to encode the velocity of the moving blood. Stationary objects have a net phase of zero because all phase induced by the first lobe of the gradient is reversed by the second lobe. However, moving objects gain a net phase depending on the direction of blood flow and proportional to the velocity of the blood [8]. This net phase is then displayed as a phase map with differences in signal intensity representing different velocities. CMR phase-contrast velocity encoding is used to quantify the severity of valvular regurgitation and stenosis. In addition, velocity maps can be used to determine flow volume throughout the cardiac cycle, enabling the assessment of forward and regurgitant volumes from which stroke volume can be calculated [9].

Another important feature of CMR is its ability to provide tissue characterization using techniques such as DGE imaging and T1 mapping. DGE imaging exploits the fact that gadolinium-based contrast agents accumulate in areas of extracellular expansion in comparison with normal myocardium, and this can be detected in the late washout phase [10]. The expanded extracellular space in the myocardium can be caused by fibrosis, but also by oedema or protein infiltration, depending on the clinical context. The increased gadolinium concentration in areas of myocardial fibrosis causes shortening of T1 time, thereby appearing as bright signal intensity in the CMR image (T1-weighted imaging). The pattern of DGE enhancement can be used to distinguish myocardial damage due to ischaemia from non-ischaemic causes of fibrosis [11,12] as well as to differentiate non-ischaemic aetiologies.

As the DGE signal intensity typically depends on differences between fibrotic and normal myocardium, DGE imaging is of limited use for the detection of diffuse myocardial pathology when large signal intensity differences are lacking. More recently, T1 mapping techniques have been developed, which enable assessment of diffuse myocardial fibrosis either using native T1 values or by quantification of the extracellular volume (ECV) from pre- and post-contrast T1 mapping [13]. T1 mapping techniques work by measuring absolute myocardial T1 relaxation time (and whole blood T1) on a pixel-wise basis. Any abnormality on T1 mapping is determined by comparison with reference values expressed in units of time, rather than by just assessing regional differences, thereby enabling the detection of both focal and diffuse disease processes. The emergence of T1 and ECV mapping techniques may have the potential to aid in earlier diagnosis and risk stratification, detecting subclinical changes prior to the onset of replacement fibrosis.

CMR in the evaluation of cardiac pathology

The dominant clinical indication for CMR in the evaluation of athletes is symptoms or abnormal findings on clinical examination, ECG, or echocardiography that raise suspicion of cardiac pathology.

CMR is not ideally suited to evaluation of valvular heart disease, and there is rarely an indication to progress beyond echocardiography for issues related to valvular morphology or function. On the other hand, CMR is ideally suited to evaluating structural heart disease including congenital anomalies, inherited cardiomyopathies, and acquired pathologies. Of particular importance are those pathologies associated with sudden cardiac death (SCD) in which specific management and appropriate sports restriction may be important preventative strategies.

The most common inherited or congenital pathologies associated with SCD in athletes are hypertrophic cardiomyopathy (HCM) (prevalence ~0.05–0.2%) [14–16], anomalous coronary arteries (prevalence ~0.2%) [17], ARVC (prevalence ~0.1%) [18], and ion-channel disorders (prevalence ~0.007–0.2%) [16,19]. Ion-channel disorders and channelopathies are not associated with structural changes and cannot be identified with cardiac imaging. The role of CMR in each of the relevant pathologies will be discussed in the following sections.

Hypertrophic cardiomyopathy

HCM is the most common cause of sudden cardiac death amongst young competitive athletes in most series [20,21]. It is an inherited autosomal dominant condition, defined clinically by the presence of unexplained LV hypertrophy. Although the traditional form of asymmetric septal hypertrophy is most common, it has become increasingly clear that many atypical patterns occur, with focal hypertrophy at various sites within the LV or even hypertrophy isolated to the RV. These atypical patterns are common amongst athletic cohorts. In particular, apical HCM (defined by hypertrophy isolated only to the LV apex) is encountered frequently, perhaps due to the fact that it is frequently associated with profound ECG changes and because it may have less impact upon cardiac function and exercise performance, thereby being seen during ECG screening of ostensibly healthy athletes [22]. The characteristic histopathological appearance of HCM consists of myocyte disarray, expansion of the extracellular compartment, and areas of replacement fibrosis and intramural small vessel coronary artery disease [23]. Given its widespread availability, low cost, and reliability in quantifying dynamic outflow tract gradients [24], echocardiography, in conjunction with an electrocardiogram, has been the first-line imaging modality for the diagnosis of HCM for decades. However, CMR has emerged as an important complementary technique, mainly because of its superior visualization of specific areas of the LV such as the apex (➲ Fig. 3.3.2.3) and the anterolateral free wall (➲ Fig. 3.3.2.4) [25,26], and the ability to perform tissue characterization (i.e. DGE imaging) [27]. The additive value of CMR for the diagnosis of HCM was elegantly shown in a recent study by Schnell et al. [28] who evaluated 6372 athletes referred for pre-participation screening, of which 155 presented with pathological T-wave inversion.

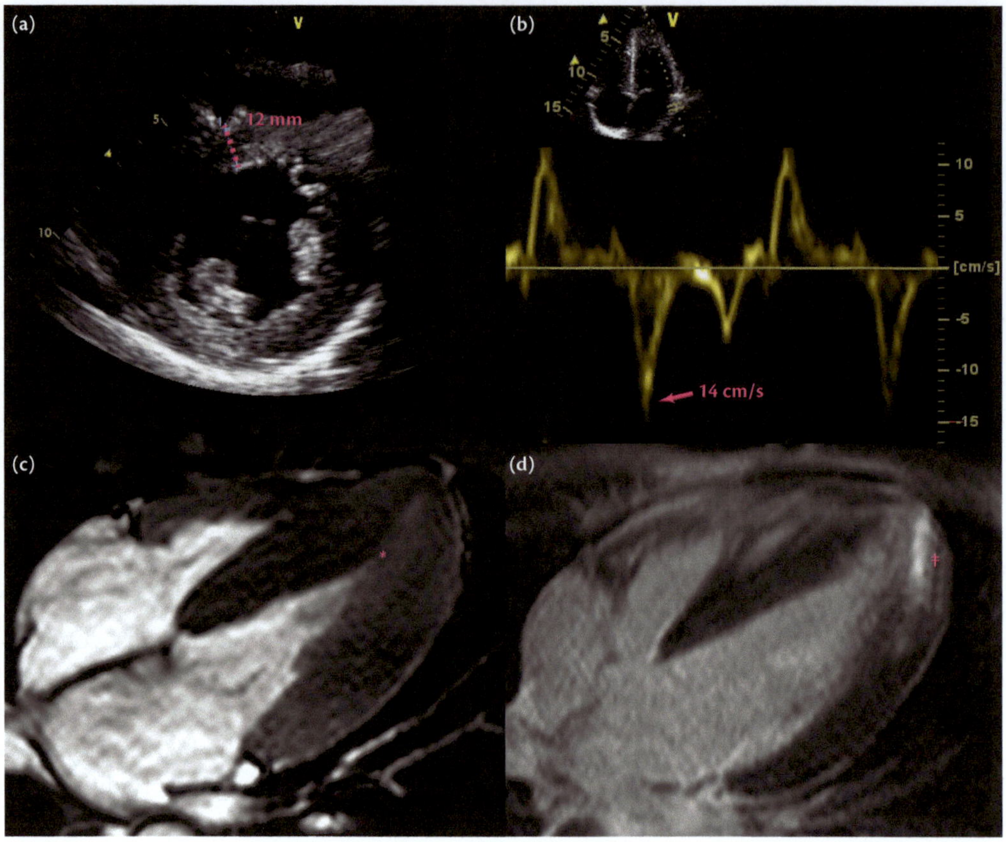

Fig. 3.3.2.3 This triathlete survived a VF arrest during a triathlon race. His left ventricular wall thickness on echocardiography was at the upper limits of normal (a) and his diastolic myocardial velocities were normal (b). CMR revealed mid-cavity obstruction during systole (c, indicated by *) and apical gadolinium enhancement (d, indicated by‡) suggestive of hypertrophic cardiomyopathy.

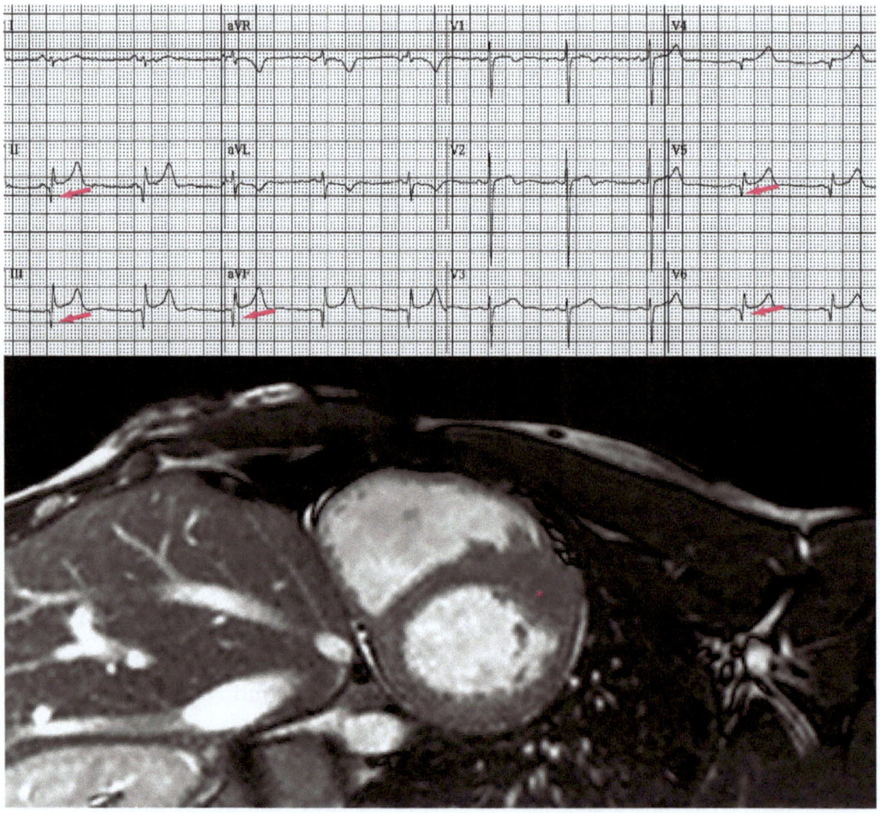

Fig. 3.3.2.4 An Olympic skier with abnormal inferolateral Q waves (pink arrows). Despite an echocardiogram that was reported as normal, a CMR study was performed given the unexplained ECG changes. The focal thickening of the LV anteroseptal wall (indicated by *) was very suggestive of HCM and the diagnosis was confirmed in first-degree family members.

Echocardiography provided a diagnosis of HCM in 31 subjects. CMR significantly increased the diagnostic capability, as evidenced by diagnosis of a further 20 cases with HCM [28]. As suggested in ➲ Fig. 3.3.2.1, we recommend that CMR is performed in all athletes in whom there is reasonable suspicion of HCM even if the echocardiogram appears normal.

As mentioned above, a clinical diagnosis of HCM is suspected by the presence of unexplained LV hypertrophy. Although CMR has become the investigation of choice for the assessment of ventricular mass, the majority of data on LV mass and wall thickness in athletes are derived from studies using echocardiography. To enable differentiation of pathology from normal athletic remodelling, a comprehensive definition of what constitutes physiological cardiac remodelling is required. The largest investigation describing the normal range of cardiac morphology and function is provided by Velthuis and colleagues [29], who compared biventricular volumes, masses, and dimensions in 222 endurance athletes (79 elite and 143 recreational, 42% female) with 114 age- and sex-matched non-athletes. They have also described morphological differences in cardiac adaptation according to training and sport-type in a manner similar to the experience with echocardiography [30,31]. Furthermore, they reported the only direct comparison between CMR and echocardiography in the assessment of athletes' cardiac morphology in which, similar to non-athletic findings, measures of cardiac volumes are consistently larger and wall thickness and mass are lower when measured by CMR [32]. In total, this constitutes an impressive body of work, although the application of this single-centre experience to clinical decision-making may be confounded by operator-specific differences in image acquisition and analysis techniques. For example, considerable differences between ventricular volumes determined from axial compared with short-axis acquisitions have been observed even when analysed at a single institution using the same software [33,34]. Thus, a broader and larger experience of CMR values for healthy athletes is required before being able to use these to accurately identify athletes who have cardiac dimensions which may be considered abnormal.

It is important to note that the heart undergoes profound structural and functional changes in response to systematic athletic training, including increased LV wall thickness and mass. The increase in wall thickness in response to exercise also depends on several other factors, including ethnicity, type of sport, age, and gender. Amongst 947 white Olympic athletes, LV wall thickness assessed by echocardiography ranged from ≤7mm to 16mm. Only 16 individuals had LV wall thickness >13mm, all of whom were males participating in endurance sports with concomitant LV dilation >54mm [35]. The thickest LV wall observed in females was 12mm [36]. Based on these observations, values of ≤12mm and ≤11mm for white male and female athletes, respectively, are currently regarded as the upper limits of normal beyond which further evaluation to exclude HCM is recommended. Compared with white athletes, black athletes exhibit an appreciable increase in LV wall thickness in response to exercise [37]. In a study of 300 black and 300 white athletes, the prevalence of LV hypertrophy ≥13mm assessed by echocardiography was 18% in black athletes versus only 4% in white athletes. Moreover, 3% of black athletes had LV wall thickness >15mm compared with none of the white athletes [37]. These data highlight the difficulty of using wall-thickness measurements in isolation to distinguish between physiological remodelling and HCM.

To better distinguish between physiological and pathological LV remodelling, Petersen et al.[38] evaluated CMR-derived LV volume parameters and geometric indices in patients with HCM and compared them with athletes. They found that the diastolic wall-to-volume ratio was the best parameter for discriminating athlete's heart from HCM. A cut-off value of <0.15mm/m^2/ml was found to have 80% sensitivity and 99% specificity for differentiating physiological LV hypertrophy from HCM. Another feature suggesting HCM is the presence of myocardial fibrosis. A recent meta-analysis demonstrated that myocardial scarring visualized by DGE imaging occurs in approximately 60% of patients with HCM [39], most commonly in those LV segments with the greatest wall thickening [40,41]. The presence of scarring has been shown to be a predictor of arrhythmias [42] and is associated with cardiovascular death, heart failure death, and all-cause mortality in HCM [27,39]. Recently, T1 mapping has emerged as a promising tool for discriminating normal from diffusely diseased myocardium in the context of HCM [43]. As there is some evidence that the development of overt LV hypertrophy is preceded by a low-grade or more diffuse pro-fibrotic state without fibrosis visible on CMR [44], T1 mapping may hold promise for identifying subjects at an earlier stage of the disease process. However, this warrants further investigation.

Arrhythmogenic cardiomyopathy

In the athlete with disproportionate enlargement of the right ventricle, a diagnosis of arrhythmogenic right ventricular cardiomyopathy (ARVC) should be considered. This condition is also referred to as arrhythmogenic cardiomyopathy, reflecting the fact that the LV is also frequently involved and the tendency for arrhythmias to be an early manifestation. Original or revised Task Force criteria should be applied, and although CMR may be useful for a more detailed assessment of both right and left ventricular volume and structure, imaging may only provide one major criterion for diagnosis and is not sufficient by itself. Careful examination of the ECG, a detailed family history, and in some cases endomyocardial biopsy may be required for a definitive diagnosis. The majority of ventricular arrhythmias in athletes originate from the RV. ARVC is a condition characterized by structural and functional abnormalities of the RV due to inflammation, fibrosis, or fibro-fatty replacement of the myocardium. The differentiation between RV changes due to ARVC and those due to physiological remodelling is crucial, given the adverse effects of strenuous exercise on the progression of the disease [45] and the propensity of subjects with ARVC to develop life-threatening arrhythmias [46,47]. However, this can be a challenging task, particularly in endurance athletes, as endurance training induces more prominent remodelling of the RV compared with the LV [48,49]. This is probably due to the greater haemodynamic impact on the RV during exercise [48,50] Therefore endurance athletes typically develop a more dilated RV with slightly reduced resting systolic function, thereby making it difficult to distinguish these from early-stage ARVC when abnormalities are often relatively subtle.

Imaging criteria form an important part of the international diagnostic framework for ARVC, as defined in the modified Task Force criteria that were proposed in 2010 [51]. The ARVC Task Force criteria rely on the presence of both qualitative findings (RV regional akinesia, dyskinesia, or dyssynchronous contraction) and quantitative metrics (decreased RV ejection fraction or increased indexed RV end-diastolic volume (EDV)). However, it should be noted that the criteria are based on comparing ARVC patients with normal controls, not with healthy athletes. This is important because up to 30% of athletes have RV dimensions that would qualify as a 'major criterion' [52]. Few data are available comparing dimensions in normal athletes with ARVC athletes, and those that are available have shown considerable overlap, especially when considering endurance athletes who have the largest RV [53,54]. Therefore RV dimensions alone are an unreliable criterion for distinguishing physiological from pathological RV dilatation, and currently there are no cut-offs to guide clinical practice [55]. In contrast, the size of the RV relative to that of the LV as an indicator of asymmetrical remodelling may be a more accurate means of distinguishing patients with ARVC. A ratio of RVEDV to LVEDV >1.2 has demonstrated a high specificity for ARVC [54].

Functional measures may be more useful than pure dimensions in athletes. RV ejection fraction ≤40–45%, as a measure of global RV dysfunction, has been shown to be a good discriminator between athlete's heart and ARVC [54]. Similarly, regional wall abnormalities limited to the RV are highly specific to the disease and occur in more than 50–94% of patients with ARVC [54.56], most commonly in the subtricuspid region (➔ Fig. 3.3.2.5). The demonstration of functional abnormalities may be too

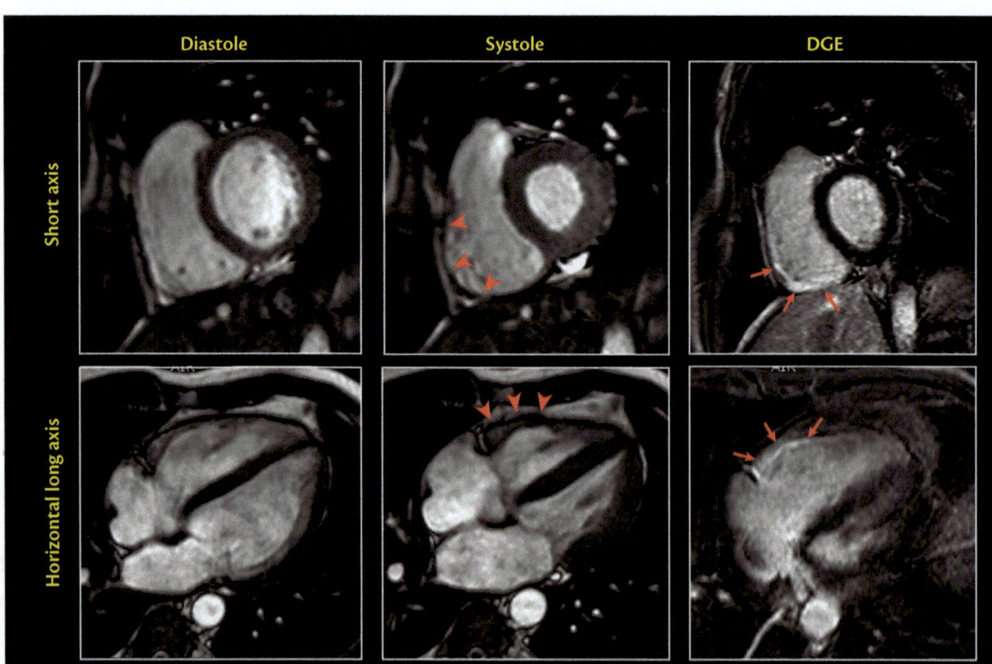

Fig. 3.3.2.5 This triathlete presented with sustained ventricular tachycardia. On CMR there was akinesis of the basal lateral RV free wall (indicated by arrowheads) corresponding to areas of delayed gadolinium enhancement (DGE, indicated by arrows) consistent with localized scarring suggestive of ARVC.

cumbersome for identifying subjects with ARVC who are engaged in endurance training. Hence, amongst endurance athletes presenting with complex ventricular arrhythmias of RV origin, functional abnormalities (both regional and global) are often relatively modest at rest and not distinguishable from athletic RV remodelling [53,57]. New data indicate that morphological and functional evaluation during exercise (i.e. not at rest) can be of help in the differential diagnosis of pathological RV remodelling in these cases [53]. Experimental technology for CMR imaging during uninterrupted exercise has been developed, allowing evaluation of classical volumetric measures (such as end-diastolic volume, end-systolic volume, and ejection fraction) during different stages of exercise [53,58]

CMR tissue characterization may be very useful in the evaluation of ARVC. DGE has been observed in the RV in up to 88% of ARVC patients [59,60] and correlates with histopathology and inducibility of ventricular arrhythmias in electrophysiological study [59]. Furthermore, detection of DGE in the LV may provide important clues for the diagnosis of early and/or predominant LV involvement. This is important because LV-dominant ARVC often occurs in the absence of wall motion abnormalities [61]. Although an ongoing contention, it is important to recognize that DGE is not part of the current Task Force criteria because of several limitations. Firstly, detection of DGE in the RV is hampered by the thin wall of the RV, which is particularly pronounced in ARVC patients [62]. In addition, LV DGE is non-specific and occurs in other conditions affecting the LV such as sarcoidosis, myocarditis, amyloidosis, and dilated cardiomyopathy (DCM).

Dilated cardiomyopathy and left ventricular non-compaction

Myocarditis and DCM have been implicated in a minority of SCD cases [20,63,64] In an asymptomatic population with extremely high levels of fitness, the accurate identification of segmental or global ventricular dilation and hypokinesis is extremely challenging. Abergel et al. [65] assessed 424 cyclists competing in the Tour de France and found that 51.4% exhibited significant LV dilation and 11.6% had an LV ejection fraction <53%, which could be compatible with a diagnosis of DCM. Furthermore, Gati et al. [66] recently reported that 8.1% athletes satisfied conventional criteria for LV non-compaction syndrome but only a very small minority of these had any other features suspicious of an underlying cardiomyopathy. Exercise testing may prove a useful discriminator in these settings. Using echocardiography, Plehn et al. [67] reported that exercise caused a reduction in end-systolic volumes amongst healthy controls but not in patients with HCM or DCM. The recent descriptions of using exercise CMR in the assessment of athletes offers promise in the evaluation of subtle cardiomyopathies [58,68], the hypothesis being that cardiomyopathies are characterized by myocardial contractile impairment that is likely to be more apparent under the haemodynamic and metabolic stress of exercise.

Considerable interest has recently been generated by a number of studies in which DGE has been observed within the LV myocardium of ostensibly healthy athletes [69–71]. It has been hypothesized that these small patches of DGE found in 12–50% of extensively trained veteran athletes may represent fibrosis resulting from extreme physical training [70,71]. However, there is still very limited data on which to assess causality, and a number of studies, albeit in younger, less trained cohorts, have reported that DGE is not a feature of athlete's heart [72–74]. The fact that DGE has been observed in healthy athletic cohorts suggests that it is of limited clinical significance, and we have no long-term clinical data to suggest otherwise. Recently, Trivax and McCullough [75] described the case of a middle-aged runner in whom aborted SCD was attributed to proarrhythmic myocardial fibrosis, as evidenced by a small patch of DGE (➲ Fig. 3.3.2.6). However, if these changes can be identified in approximately 12% of asymptomatic 'healthy' athletes, then it may be presumptive to cite this as the probable cause of cardiac arrest.

Finally, the finding of focal DGE is somewhat surprising given that the haemodyamic load of exercise is imposed on the whole myocyte mass in all cardiac chambers, and thus we would expect any remodelling process, including any potential for fibrosis, to be generalized. New CMR techniques have evolved that use the principle that inversion recovery times are shorter in tissues with fibrosis, and therefore mapping of inversion recovery times may enable diffuse fibrosis to be quantified [76]. These techniques can be performed with or without gadolinium contrast. Mordi et al. [77] recently used these techniques to compare athletes with early DCM patients and again noted small patches of DGE in 10% of the athletes, but found no evidence of diffuse fibrosis. The native T1 times ('native' refers to without gadolinium contrast, and in this case longer T1 times suggest greater fibrosis) were similar for athletes and controls, but both were significantly shorter than in the patients with cardiomyopathy. One clear issue with these techniques is that although they are capable of separating groups in research studies, the standard deviations are high and there is very significant cross-over between groups, making these currently unsuitable for clinical use in diagnosing or excluding pathology in a single individual.

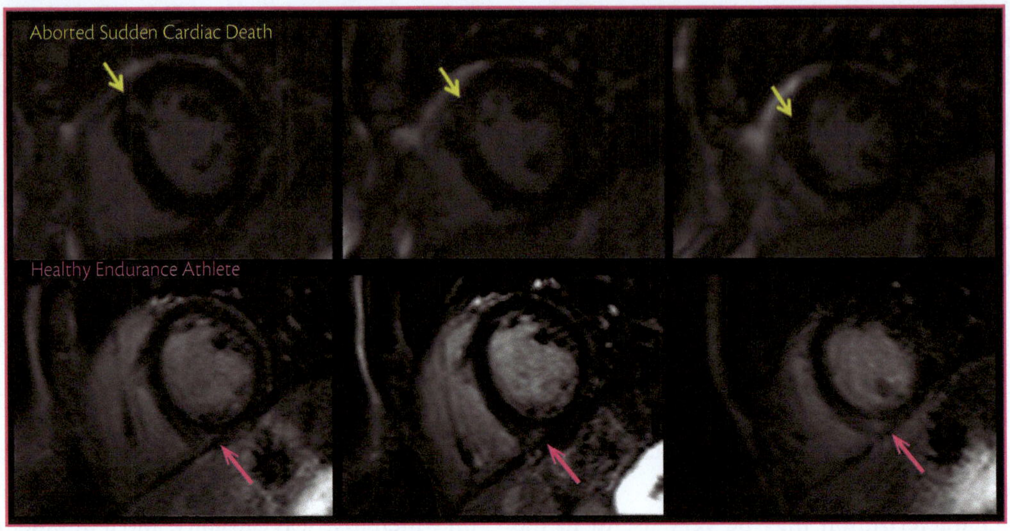

Fig. 3.3.2.6 Delayed gadolinium enhancement (DGE) in two competitive runners with very different clinical outcomes. Cardiac magnetic resonance images of consecutive short-axis slices following gadolinium contrast are shown. The three upper images are taken from a case report of an athlete who survived SCD. The authors speculated that the patch of DGE in the anteroseptal wall of the LV (yellow arrows) may represent pro-arrhythmic myocardial fibrosis resulting from extreme exercise training [75]. However, there have been similar findings in 12–50% of well-trained endurance athletes [69–71]. The three lower images are from an apparently healthy 36-year-old marathon runner undergoing a CMR for research purposes, There is a similar small patch of DGE in the postero-septum of the LV. Given the uncertainty of the significance of these findings, identification of small patches of DGE on screening may be of limited clinical value in older endurance athletes.

Myocarditis

Myocarditis is a pathological entity that has serious potential consequences for competitive athletes. It commonly presents with disproportionate dyspnoea on exertion, chest pain, and arrhythmias. However, it can also present with sudden death without antecedent symptoms or macroscopic cardiovascular abnormalities [78,79]. A definite diagnosis of myocarditis requires confirmation with endomyocardial biopsy. However, given the invasive nature of this technique, the work-up of a suspected myocarditis is generally based on cardiac imaging modalities. CMR has become a vital tool for non-invasive assessment of suspected myocarditis because of its ability to visualize tissue changes, including oedema, hyperaemia, and capillary leak (myocardial early gadolinium enhancement), and myocardial fibrosis (DGE) [80]. Regional oedema can be visualized using T2-weighted images in up to 36% of patients with histologically active myocarditis [81]. Contrast-enhanced T1-weighted imaging can be used to assess regional hyperaemia and capillary leakage [82]. DGE typically involves the subepicardial regions of the LV with variable extension through the ventricular wall. The DGE may be localized in inferolateral and, less frequently, anteroseptal segments, but it can also be multifocal or diffuse in distribution [80]. Usually, this pattern can be distinguished from ischaemic injury because the subendocardium is relatively less affected. The distinction from other conditions such as LV-dominant ARVC or dilated cardiomyopathy is more difficult. A myocarditis-like DGE pattern (➲ Fig. 3.3.2.7) has been described in asymptomatic athletes presenting with abnormalities on their pre-participation screening evaluation, and was associated with progressive LV dysfunction and arrhythmias [83]. Although the possibility of underlying LV-dominant ARVC cannot be excluded, it was suggested that this subepicardial DGE pattern may have resulted from an underlying myocarditis with subsequent negative remodelling through repeated bouts of intensive exercise. Further prospective studies in a larger group of athletes are required to better characterize the prevalence and outcome of asymptomatic athletes with manifest subepicardial DGE.

Coronary artery disease and coronary anomalies

Coronary artery disease accounts for a significant proportion of cases of SCD. In younger athletes, a coronary artery arising from the incorrect coronary sinus and having a proximal course passing between the aorta and the pulmonary artery is a risk for SCD due to obstruction of coronary flow with the distension of the major vessels during exercise. In middle-aged and older athletes, atherosclerotic coronary disease is the major cause of sudden death during exercise. In athletes of all ages, a less common but potentially overlooked cause of myocardial ischaemia is coronary artery dissection (➲ Fig. 3.3.2.8). The risk of dissection increases with exercise, and some authors have

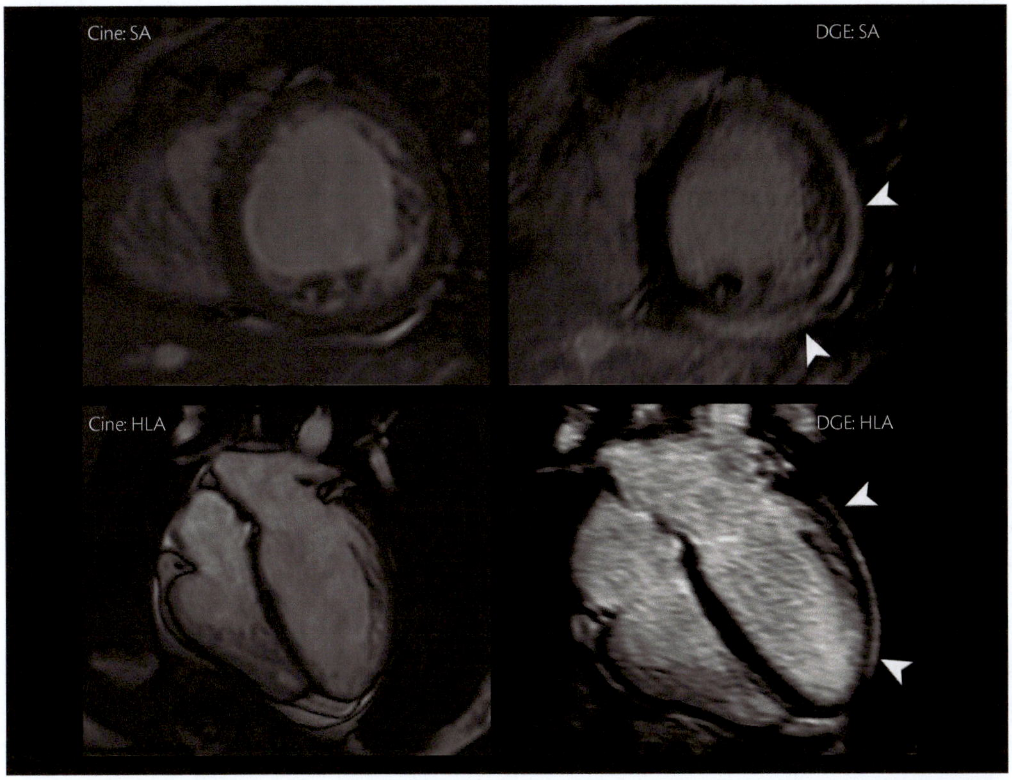

Fig. 3.3.2.7 Myocarditis-like pattern in an asymptomatic athlete presenting with abnormalities during pre-participation screening evaluation. Arrowheads denote areas of delayed gadolinium enhancement (DGE). SA, short-axis view, HLA, horizontal long-axis view in cine and the corresponding DGE images.
Reproduced from *British Journal of Sports Medicine*. Subepicardial delayed gadolinium enhancement in asymptomatic athletes: let sleeping dogs lie? Frédéric Schnell et al., Volume 50, Issue 2, copyright 2016 with permission from BMJ Publishing Group Ltd.

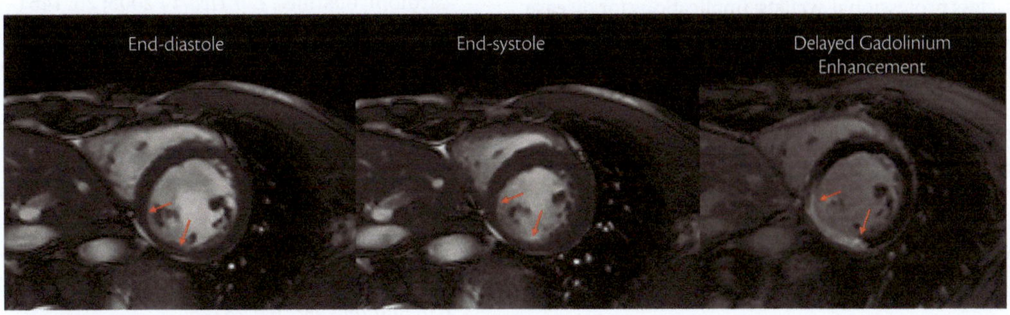

Fig. 3.3.2.8 A triathlete experienced chest pain and nausea 1 hour into an ultra-endurance triathlon. He finished the event but still felt lethargic and unwell a week later. An abnormal ECG and an elevated troponin prompted a coronary angiogram that showed a large dissection of the distal right coronary artery. A subsequent CMR showed inferoseptal thinning, akinesis (left and middle panels highlighted by red arrows) and full-thickness DGE in the same region (right panel).

suggested that this is not as uncommon as previously thought [84].

CMR is the ideal modality for investigating the possibility of previous infarction. It is an excellent tool for assessing wall motion abnormalities that can be combined with the assessment of DGE. The classical pattern of DGE in ischaemic damage is from the 'inside out.' That is, damage starts first in the endocardium and then mid-wall and epicardium. Sub-endocardial enhancement is relatively specific for ischaemic myocardial damage.

However, CMR is not the best modality for assessing the risk of *future* ischaemic damage. It is not as good as computed tomography (CT) for assessing the presence and burden of atherosclerosis. Stress perfusion CMR can be performed, but in most centres other tests (exercise echocardiography or nuclear testing) are preferred. When anomalous coronary circulation is suspected, CT is again the test of choice although Prakken et al. [85] reported that 3D CMR coronary angiography can be added to standard CMR imaging and enables assessment of the coronary ostia in more than 90% of patients. This is not standard practice in most centres, and it cannot be assumed that coronary anomalies have been excluded in a CMR scan unless it has specifically been assessed and reported.

Conclusions

CMR is an extremely useful modality for the investigation of athletes with symptoms or abnormalities on simple investigations that require further characterization. CMR has greater sensitivity than echocardiography for identifying cardiomyopathies and myocarditis, and thus should be included in the assessment of athletes in whom suspicion persists even if the echocardiogram fails to identify an abnormality. On the other hand, there is much that we have yet to learn regarding the application of CMR in athletes. The normal ranges are not as well established as for echocardiography, and the sensitivity for identifying subtle abnormalities is high. As a result, CMR needs to be used carefully. It is not appropriate for screening and careful consideration should also be given to findings that are unexpected or unrelated to the clinical question being addressed. Despite this, CMR has enormous potential for both clarifying difficult clinical questions and advancing our understanding of the athlete's heart.

Further reading

Abergel E, Chatellier G, Hagege AA, et al. Serial left ventricular adaptations in world-class professional cyclists: implications for disease screening and follow-up. *J Am Coll Cardiol* 2004;44:144–9.

La Gerche A, Claessen G, Dymarkowski S, et al. Exercise-induced right ventricular dysfunction is associated with ventricular arrhythmias in endurance athletes. *Eur Heart J* 2015; 36: 1998–2010.

Maron MS, Maron BJ, Harrigan C, et al. Hypertrophic cardiomyopathy phenotype revisited after 50 years with cardiovascular magnetic resonance. *J Am Coll Cardiol* 2009; 54: 220–8.

Schnell F, Riding N, O'Hanlon R, et al. Recognition and significance of pathological T-wave inversions in athletes. *Circulation* 2015; 131: 165–73.

Zaidi A, Sheikh N, Jongman JK, et al. Clinical differentiation between physiological remodeling and arrhythmogenic right ventricular cardiomyopathy in athletes with marked electrocardiographic repolarization anomalies. *J Am Coll Cardiol* 2015; 65: 2702–11.

References

1. Rowin EJ, Maron BJ, Appelbaum E, et al. Significance of false negative electrocardiograms in preparticipation screening of athletes for hypertrophic cardiomyopathy. *Am J Cardiol* 2012; 110: 1027–32.
2. Hawkes RC, Holland GN, Moore WS, et al. Nuclear magnetic resonance (NMR) tomography of the normal heart. *J Comput Assist Tomogr* 1981; 5: 605–12.
3. Higgins CB, Lanzer P, Stark D, et al. Assessment of cardiac anatomy using nuclear magnetic resonance imaging. *J Am Coll Cardiol* 1985; 5: 77S–81S.
4. Menghetti L, Basso C, Nava A, et al. Spin-echo nuclear magnetic resonance for tissue characterisation in arrhythmogenic right ventricular cardiomyopathy. *Heart* 1996; 76: 467–70.
5. Carr JC, Simonetti O, Bundy J, et al. Cine MR angiography of the heart with segmented true fast imaging with steady-state precession. *Radiology* 2001; 219: 828–34.
6. Semelka RC, Tomei E, Wagner S, et al. Interstudy reproducibility of dimensional and functional measurements between cine magnetic resonance studies in the morphologically abnormal left ventricle. *Am Heart J* 1990; 119: 1367–73.
7. Hor KN, Gottliebson WM, Carson C, et al. Comparison of magnetic resonance feature tracking for strain calculation with harmonic phase imaging analysis. *JACC Cardiovasc Imaging* 2010; 3: 144–51.
8. Cawley PJ, Maki JH, Otto CM. Cardiovascular magnetic resonance imaging for valvular heart disease: technique and validation. *Circulation* 2009; 119: 468–78.
9. Hundley WG, Li HF, Hillis LD, et al. Quantitation of cardiac output with velocity-encoded, phase-difference magnetic resonance imaging. *Am J Cardiol* 1995; 75: 1250–5.
10. Kim RJ, Chen EL, Lima JA, Judd RM. Myocardial Gd-DTPA kinetics determine MRI contrast enhancement and reflect the extent and severity of myocardial injury after acute reperfused infarction. *Circulation* 1996; 94: 3318–26.
11. McCrohon JA, Moon JC, Prasad SK, et al. Differentiation of heart failure related to dilated cardiomyopathy and coronary artery disease using gadolinium-enhanced cardiovascular magnetic resonance. *Circulation* 2003; 108: 54–9.
12. Mahrholdt H, Wagner A, Judd RM, et al. Delayed enhancement cardiovascular magnetic resonance assessment of non-ischaemic cardiomyopathies. *Eur Heart J* 2005; 26: 1461–74.
13. Moon JC, Messroghli DR, Kellman P, et al. Myocardial T1 mapping and extracellular volume quantification: a Society for Cardiovascular Magnetic Resonance (SCMR) and CMR Working Group of the European Society of Cardiology consensus statement. *J Cardiovasc Magn Reson* 2013; 15: 92.
14. Maron BJ, Gardin JM, Flack JM, et al. Prevalence of hypertrophic cardiomyopathy in a general population of young adults. Echocardiographic analysis of 4111 subjects in the CARDIA Study: Coronary Artery Risk Development in (Young) Adults. *Circulation* 1995; 92: 785–9.
15. Maron BJ, Mathenge R, Casey SA, et al. Clinical profile of hypertrophic cardiomyopathy identified *de novo* in rural communities. *J Am Coll Cardiol* 1999; 33: 1590–5.
16. Rodday AM, Triedman JK, Alexander ME, et al. Electrocardiogram screening for disorders that cause sudden cardiac death in asymptomatic children: a meta-analysis. *Pediatrics* 2012; 129: e999–1010.
17. Davis JA, Cecchin F, Jones TK, Portman MA. Major coronary artery anomalies in a pediatric population: incidence and clinical importance. *J Am Coll Cardiol* 2001; 37: 593–7.
18. Gemayel C, Pelliccia A, Thompson PD. Arrhythmogenic right ventricular cardiomyopathy. *J Am Coll Cardiol* 2001; 38: 1773–81.
19. Cerrone M, Napolitano C, Priori SG. Genetics of ion-channel disorders. *Curr Opin Cardiol* 2012; 27: 242–52.
20. Maron BJ, Doerer JJ, Haas TS, et al. Sudden deaths in young competitive athletes: analysis of 1866 deaths in the United States, 1980–2006. *Circulation* 2009; 119: 1085–92.
21. Maron BJ. Sudden death in young athletes. *N Engl J Med* 2003; 349: 1064–75.

22. Sheikh N, Papadakis M, Schnell F, et al. Clinical profile of athletes with hypertrophic cardiomyopathy. *Circ Cardiovasc Imaging* 2015; 8: e003454.
23. Elliott P, McKenna WJ. Hypertrophic cardiomyopathy. *Lancet* 2004; 363: 1881–91.
24. Klues HG, Schiffers A, Maron BJ. Phenotypic spectrum and patterns of left ventricular hypertrophy in hypertrophic cardiomyopathy: morphologic observations and significance as assessed by two-dimensional echocardiography in 600 patients. *J Am Coll Cardiol* 1995; 26: 1699–1708.
25. Rickers C, Wilke NM, Jerosch-Herold M, et al. Utility of cardiac magnetic resonance imaging in the diagnosis of hypertrophic cardiomyopathy. *Circulation* 2005; 112: 855–61.
26. Maron MS, Maron BJ, Harrigan C, et al. Hypertrophic cardiomyopathy phenotype revisited after 50 years with cardiovascular magnetic resonance. *J Am Coll Cardiol* 2009; 54: 220–8.
27. Chan RH, Maron BJ, Olivotto I, et al. Prognostic value of quantitative contrast-enhanced cardiovascular magnetic resonance for the evaluation of sudden death risk in patients with hypertrophic cardiomyopathy. *Circulation* 2014; 130: 484–95.
28. Schnell F, Riding N, O'Hanlon R, et al. Recognition and significance of pathological T-wave inversions in athletes. *Circulation* 2015; 131: 165–73.
29. Prakken NH, Velthuis BK, Teske AJ, et al. Cardiac MRI reference values for athletes and nonathletes corrected for body surface area, training hours/week and sex. *Eur J Cardiovasc Prev Rehabil* 2010; 17: 198–203.
30. Luijkx T, Velthuis BK, Backx FJ, et al. Anabolic androgenic steroid use is associated with ventricular dysfunction on cardiac MRI in strength trained athletes. Int J Cardiol 2012.
31. Luijkx T, Cramer MJ, Prakken NH, et al. Sport category is an important determinant of cardiac adaptation: an MRI study. Br J Sports Med 2012; 46: 119–24.
32. Prakken NH, Teske AJ, Cramer MJ, et al. Head-to-head comparison between echocardiography and cardiac MRI in the evaluation of the athlete's heart. *Br J Sports Med* 2012; 46: 348–54.
33. Fratz S, Schuhbaeck A, Buchner C, et al. Comparison of accuracy of axial slices versus short-axis slices for measuring ventricular volumes by cardiac magnetic resonance in patients with corrected tetralogy of Fallot. *Am J Cardiol* 2009; 103: 1764–9.
34. Alfakih K, Plein S, Bloomer T, et al. Comparison of right ventricular volume measurements between axial and short axis orientation using steady-state free precession magnetic resonance imaging. *J Magn Reson Imaging* 2003; 18: 25–32.
35. Pelliccia A, Maron BJ, Spataro A, et al. The upper limit of physiologic cardiac hypertrophy in highly trained elite athletes. *N Engl J Med* 1991; 324: 295–301.
36. Pelliccia A, Maron BJ, Culasso F, et al. Athlete's heart in women: echocardiographic characterization of highly trained elite female athletes. *JAMA* 1996; 276: 211–15.
37. Basavarajaiah S, Boraita A, Whyte G, et al. Ethnic differences in left ventricular remodeling in highly-trained athletes relevance to differentiating physiologic left ventricular hypertrophy from hypertrophic cardiomyopathy. *J Am Coll Cardiol* 2008; 51: 2256–62.
38. Petersen SE, Selvanayagam JB, Francis JM, et al. Differentiation of athlete's heart from pathological forms of cardiac hypertrophy by means of geometric indices derived from cardiovascular magnetic resonance. *J Cardiovasc Magn Reson* 2005; 7: 551–8.
39. Green JJ, Berger JS, Kramer CM, Salerno M. Prognostic value of late gadolinium enhancement in clinical outcomes for hypertrophic cardiomyopathy. *JACC Cardiovasc Imaging* 2012; 5: 370–7.
40. Choudhury L, Mahrholdt H, Wagner A, et al. Myocardial scarring in asymptomatic or mildly symptomatic patients with hypertrophic cardiomyopathy. *J Am Coll Cardiol* 2002; 40: 2156–64.
41. Moon JC, McKenna WJ, McCrohon JA, et al. Toward clinical risk assessment in hypertrophic cardiomyopathy with gadolinium cardiovascular magnetic resonance. *J Am Coll Cardiol* 2003; 41: 1561–7.
42. Fluechter S, Kuschyk J, Wolpert C, et al. Extent of late gadolinium enhancement detected by cardiovascular magnetic resonance correlates with the inducibility of ventricular tachyarrhythmia in hypertrophic cardiomyopathy. *J Cardiovasc Magn Reson* 2010; 12: 30.
43. Puntmann VO, Voigt T, Chen Z, et al. Native T1 mapping in differentiation of normal myocardium from diffuse disease in hypertrophic and dilated cardiomyopathy. *JACC Cardiovasc Imaging* 2013; 6: 475–84.
44. Ho CY, Lopez B, Coelho-Filho OR, et al. Myocardial fibrosis as an early manifestation of hypertrophic cardiomyopathy. *N Engl J Med* 2010; 363: 552–63.
45. James CA, Bhonsale A, Tichnell C, et al. Exercise increases age-related penetrance and arrhythmic risk in arrhythmogenic right ventricular dysplasia/cardiomyopathy-associated desmosomal mutation carriers. *J Am Coll Cardiol* 2013; 62: 1290–7.
46. Corrado D, Basso C, Schiavon M, Thiene G. Screening for hypertrophic cardiomyopathy in young athletes. *N Engl J Med* 1998; 339: 364–9.
47. Tabib A, Loire R, Chalabreysse L, et al. Circumstances of death and gross and microscopic observations in a series of 200 cases of sudden death associated with arrhythmogenic right ventricular cardiomyopathy and/or dysplasia. *Circulation* 2003; 108: 3000–5.
48. La Gerche A, Heidbuchel H, Burns AT, et al. Disproportionate exercise load and remodeling of the athlete's right ventricle. *Med Sci Sports Exerc* 2011; 43: 974–81.
49. Arbab-Zadeh A, Perhonen M, Howden E, et al. Cardiac remodeling in response to 1 year of intensive endurance training. *Circulation* 2014; 130: 2152–61.
50. La Gerche A, MacIsaac AI, Burns AT, et al. Pulmonary transit of agitated contrast is associated with enhanced pulmonary vascular reserve and right ventricular function during exercise. *J Appl Physiol (1985)* 2010; 109: 1307–17.
51. Marcus FI, McKenna WJ, Sherrill D, et al. Diagnosis of arrhythmogenic right ventricular cardiomyopathy/dysplasia: proposed modification of the Task Force Criteria. *Eur Heart J* 2010; 31: 806–14.
52. Oxborough D, Sharma S, Shave R, et al. The right ventricle of the endurance athlete: the relationship between morphology and deformation. *J Am Soc Echocardiogr* 2012; 25: 263–71.
53. La Gerche A, Claessen G, Dymarkowski S, et al. Exercise-induced right ventricular dysfunction is associated with ventricular arrhythmias in endurance athletes. *Eur Heart J* 2015; 36: 1998–2010.

54. Zaidi A, Sheikh N, Jongman JK, et al. Clinical differentiation between physiological remodeling and arrhythmogenic right ventricular cardiomyopathy in athletes with marked electrocardiographic repolarization anomalies. *J Am Coll Cardiol* 2015; 65: 2702–11.
55. Luijkx T, Velthuis BK, Prakken NH, et al. Impact of revised Task Force Criteria: distinguishing the athlete's heart from ARVC/D using cardiac magnetic resonance imaging. *Eur J Prev Cardiol* 2012; 19: 885–91.
56. Te Riele AS, James CA, Philips B, et al. Mutation-positive arrhythmogenic right ventricular dysplasia/cardiomyopathy: the triangle of dysplasia displaced. *J Cardiovasc Electrophysiol* 2013; 24: 1311–20.
57. Ector J, Ganame J, van der Merwe N, et al. Reduced right ventricular ejection fraction in endurance athletes presenting with ventricular arrhythmias: a quantitative angiographic assessment. *Eur Heart J* 2007; 28: 345–53.
58. La Gerche A, Claessen G, van de Bruaene A, et al. Cardiac MRI: a new gold standard for ventricular volume quantification during high-intensity exercise. *Circ Cardiovasc Imaging* 2013; 6: 329–38.
59. Tandri H, Saranathan M, Rodriguez ER, et al. Noninvasive detection of myocardial fibrosis in arrhythmogenic right ventricular cardiomyopathy using delayed-enhancement magnetic resonance imaging. *J Am Coll Cardiol* 2005; 45: 98–103.
60. Santangeli P, Pieroni M, Dello Russo A, et al. Noninvasive diagnosis of electroanatomic abnormalities in arrhythmogenic right ventricular cardiomyopathy. *Circ Arrhythm Electrophysiol* 2010; 3: 632–8.
61. Sen-Chowdhry S, Syrris P, Prasad SK, et al. Left-dominant arrhythmogenic cardiomyopathy: an under-recognized clinical entity. *J Am Coll Cardiol* 2008; 52: 2175–87.
62. Tandri H, Calkins H, Nasir K, et al. Magnetic resonance imaging findings in patients meeting task force criteria for arrhythmogenic right ventricular dysplasia. *J Cardiovasc Electrophysiol* 2003; 14: 476–82.
63. Corrado D, Basso C, Rizzoli G, et al. Does sports activity enhance the risk of sudden death in adolescents and young adults? *J Am Coll Cardiol* 2003; 42: 1959–63.
64. de Noronha SV, Sharma S, Papadakis M, et al. Aetiology of sudden cardiac death in athletes in the United Kingdom: a pathological study. *Heart* 2009; 95: 1409–14.
65. Abergel E, Chatellier G, Hagege AA, et al. Serial left ventricular adaptations in world-class professional cyclists: implications for disease screening and follow-up. *J Am Coll Cardiol* 2004; 44: 144–9.
66. Gati S, Chandra N, Bennett RL, et al. Increased left ventricular trabeculation in highly trained athletes. Do we need more stringent criteria for the diagnosis of left ventricular non-compaction in athletes? *Heart* 2013; 99: 401–8.
67. Plehn G, Vormbrock J, Perings S, et al. Comparison of right ventricular functional response to exercise in hypertrophic versus idiopathic dilated cardiomyopathy. *Am J Cardiol* 2010; 105: 116–21.
68. La Gerche A, Claessen G, Dymarkowski S, et al. Exercise-induced right ventricular dysfunction is associated with ventricular arrhythmias in endurance athletes. *Eur Heart J* 2015; 36: 1998–2010.
69. Mohlenkamp S, Lehmann N, Breuckmann F, et al. Running: the risk of coronary events: prevalence and prognostic relevance of coronary atherosclerosis in marathon runners. *Eur Heart J* 2008; 29: 1903–10.
70. La Gerche A, Burns AT, Mooney DJ, et al. Exercise-induced right ventricular dysfunction and structural remodelling in endurance athletes. *Eur Heart J* 2012; 33: 998–1006.
71. Wilson M, O'Hanlon R, Prasad S, et al. Diverse patterns of myocardial fibrosis in lifelong, veteran endurance athletes. *J Appl Physiol* 2011; 110: 1622–6.
72. O'Hanlon R, Wilson M, Wage R, et al. Troponin release following endurance exercise: is inflammation the cause? A cardiovascular magnetic resonance study. *J Cardiovasc Magn Reson* 2010;12:38.
73. Trivax JE, Franklin BA, Goldstein JA, et al. Acute cardiac effects of marathon running. *J Appl Physiol* 2010; 108: 1148–53.
74. Mousavi N, Czarnecki A, Kumar K, et al. Relation of biomarkers and cardiac magnetic resonance imaging after marathon running. *Am J Cardiol* 2009; 103: 1467–72.
75. Trivax JE, McCullough PA. Phidippides cardiomyopathy: a review and case illustration. *Clin Cardiol* 2012; 35: 69–73.
76. Jellis C, Martin J, Narula J, Marwick TH. Assessment of nonischemic myocardial fibrosis. *J Am Coll Cardiol* 2010; 56: 89–97.
77. Mordi I, Carrick D, Bezerra H, Tzemos N. T1 and T2 mapping for early diagnosis of dilated non-ischaemic cardiomyopathy in middle-aged patients and differentiation from normal physiological adaptation. *Eur Heart J Cardiovasc Imaging* 2016; 17: 797–803.
78. Weber MA, Ashworth MT, Risdon RA, et al. Clinicopathological features of paediatric deaths due to myocarditis: an autopsy series. *Arch Dis Child* 2008; 93: 594–8.
79. Corrado D, Basso C, Thiene G. Sudden cardiac death in young people with apparently normal heart. *Cardiovasc Res* 2001; 50: 399–408.
80. Friedrich MG, Sechtem U, Schulz-Menger J, et al. Cardiovascular magnetic resonance in myocarditis: a JACC White Paper. *J Am Coll Cardiol* 2009; 53: 1475–87.
81. De Cobelli F, Pieroni M, Esposito A, et al. Delayed gadolinium-enhanced cardiac magnetic resonance in patients with chronic myocarditis presenting with heart failure or recurrent arrhythmias. *J Am Coll Cardiol* 2006; 47: 1649–54.
82. Friedrich MG, Strohm O, Schulz-Menger J, et al. Contrast media-enhanced magnetic resonance imaging visualizes myocardial changes in the course of viral myocarditis. *Circulation* 1998; 97: 1802–9.
83. Schnell F, Claessen G, La Gerche A, et al. Subepicardial delayed gadolinium enhancement in asymptomatic athletes: let sleeping dogs lie? *Br J Sports Med* 2016; 50: 111–17.
84. Tweet MS, Hayes SN, Pitta SR, et al. Clinical features, management, and prognosis of spontaneous coronary artery dissection. *Circulation* 2012; 126: 579–88.
85. Prakken NH, Cramer MJ, Olimulder MA, et al. Screening for proximal coronary artery anomalies with 3-dimensional MR coronary angiography. *Int J Cardiovasc Imaging* 2010; 26: 701–10.

3.3.3 Coronary computed tomography

Stefan Möhlenkamp

General considerations

Coronary computed tomography (CCT) allows high resolution imaging of coronary atherosclerosis and other coronary pathologies, such as abnormal origin of coronary arteries or myocardial bridging. It is widely accepted for quantifying obstructive and non-obstructive coronary artery disease (CAD) with therapeutic and prognostic implications in asymptomatic and symptomatic individuals [1–4]. While invasive coronary angiography quantifies vessel lumen diameter, CCT allows additional visualization and quantification of vessel wall morphology, including plaque imaging.

For appropriate use of CCT in sports cardiology, it is important to be aware of the epidemiological aspects and specific cardiac adaptations in response to regular exercise (see Section 1). The risk of cardiovascular disease (CVD) in physically active people and athletes depends on age. Risk in younger athletes (<35 years) is frequently attributable to channelopathies, cardiomyopathies, or myocarditis, whereas CAD is the main underlying cause of CVD in older athletes, (>35 years) [5]. Therefore CCT is paricularly useful in older athletes with symptoms suggestive of CAD, and in asymptomatic individuals with CVD risk factors.

Current recommendations usually focus on competitive athletes, who are characterized by regular participation in organized sport competitions and systematic training [6]. However, individually organized non-supervised leisure-time recreational sport may also include high intensity activity, such as marathons or triathlons, and the number of people participating in such activities has increased markedly over recent decades. The rationale for the use of coronary imaging in general, and CCT in particular, in sports cardiology is not confined to athletes, but also applies to individuals participating in regular recreational leisure-time physical activity.

Identification of athletes who are candidates for CCT imaging

The clinical work-up of *symptomatic* athletes is essentially identical to that in non-athletes. Depending on the local availability of a CT scanner and local expertise in the use of the technology, CCT angiography can be useful in older athletes with risk factors, symptoms, and exercise stress test results that raise suspicion of CAD [1]. In younger athletes with symptoms suggestive of CAD and/or if origins of coronary arteries cannot be identified on echocardiography, coronary variants and anomalies should be considered. In such cases CCT angiography is the method of choice [7–9].

In *asymptomatic* athletes and physically active individuals, who constitute the vast majority of sport participants, the purpose of advanced imaging, as in other individuals, is improved risk stratification beyond traditional risk assessment. CT-based coronary artery imaging, by virtue of quantifying coronary artery calcium, can improve cardiovascular risk stratification, particularly in asymptomatic adults at intermediate risk (10–20% 10-year risk) (Class IIa B) and, with less certainty, individuals at low to intermediate risk (6–10% 10-year risk) (Class IIb B) [2]. If and to what degree the data from the general population can be applied to athletes, if and how athletes can be identified as candidates for CT imaging, and how the findings of CCT imaging can guide therapeutic decision-making, and thus improve cardiovascular health and prognosis in physically active individuals, is a matter of debate [5,10,11].

Coronary artery calcium

Coronary artery calcium (CAC) is a non-invasive measure of the presence, localization, and extent of coronary atherosclerosis. Although it is not a marker of rupture-prone plaque or coronary artery stenosis at the site of CAC, several studies have demonstrated that the presence and extent of the calcified plaque burden is closely linked to future CAD and CVD events [12–14].

Long-term physical activity has been shown to be inversely related to CAC burden [15]. The prevalence of an advanced CAC burden (>75th percentile) in a high activity group was 38% lower than that in a sedentary group ($p<0.05$), and this remained significant after adjusting for established risk factors [15]. In contrast, a study of the prevalence and predictive role of CAC in recreational marathon runners aged >50 years demonstrated a much higher than expected CAC burden compared with age-matched controls from the general population (➲ Fig. 3.3.3.1), even though the Framingham risk was only half that in the controls (7.0±3.6 vs 14.3±8.2% in 10 years, $p<0.0001$) [16]. In this study, 108 marathon runners aged >50 years with no history of CAD, diabetes, or cardiovascular symptoms, who had completed five full-distance marathons during the previous 3 years, were thoroughly phenotyped and followed prospectively [16,17]. Runners were more often free from atherosclerosis than age-matched controls (➲ Fig. 3.3.3.1). However, marathon runners had higher CAC scores than

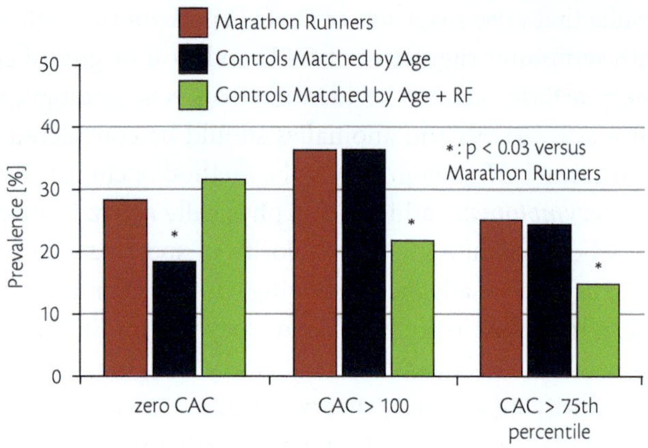

Fig. 3.3.3.1 Calcified coronary plaque burden (CAC) measured by CCT in athletes. Marathon runners were more likely to have no CAC compared with age-matched controls, but similar prevalences of advanced CAC as determined by clinically established thresholds of CAC >100 and CAC >75th percentile. However, controls matched by age and risk factors (i.e. those who presumably have had a beneficial risk factor profile throughout their lives) had less CAC than athletes.

Reproduced with permission from Möhlenkamp, Stefan; Lehmann, Nils. Running: the risk of coronary events: Prevalence and prognostic relevance of coronary atherosclerosis in marathon runners. *European Heart Journal*, Volume 29, Issue 15, pp.1903–10, Copyright © 2008 Oxford University Press and the European Society of Cardiology.

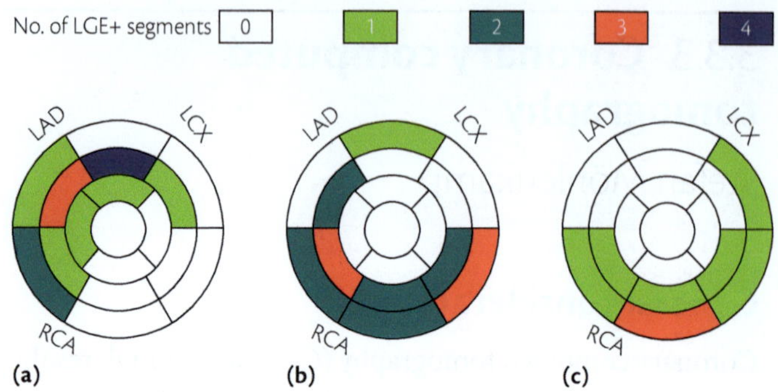

Fig. 3.3.3.2 Bull's eye plots demonstrating the number of runners with MRI-based positive late gadolinium enhancement (LGE) in each particular segment in (a) marathon runners with a CAD pattern of LGE ($n = 5$), (b) marathon runners with a non-CAD-pattern of LGE ($n = 7$), and (c) controls ($n = 4$ of 102 age-matched individuals without exceptional endurance sports activity and without a known history of cardiac disease who were taken from a large population-based MRI screening study). Note that more than one segment could be affected. The LAD territory was more frequently affected in runners with a CAD pattern of LGE than in runners with a non-CAD pattern of LGE and controls, which may indicate a difference in aetiology in the different patterns of LGE.

Reproduced with permission from Breuckmann F, Möhlenkamp S, Nassenstein K, et al., Myocardial late gadolinium enhancement: Prevalence, pattern, and prognostic relevance in marathon runners. *Radiology*, Volume 251, Issue 1, pp.50-57. Copyright © 2009 Radiological Society of North America (RSNA®.)

controls matched for age and risk factors, i.e. individuals who can be assumed to have had a beneficial risk factor profile throughout their lives (➲ Fig. 3.3.3.1). A CAC score >100, a threshold that has been proposed to raise risk awareness [18], was observed in 36% of the runners, and a CAC score <15, a threshold considered safe for high intensity physical activity [18], was present in only 43% of the runners. These findings are in line with observations from the Twin Cities Marathon in Minneapolis–St.Paul [19]. Fifty men aged 59 ± 7 years, who had completed at least one marathon a year for 25 consecutive years, underwent CVD risk assessment including CCT imaging. Compared with 23 sedentary controls, runners had increased calcified plaque volume (84 vs 44mm^3, p <0.0001) [19].

Data from these two studies suggest that the burden of atherosclerosis may be underestimated in older athletes. The mismatch between a presumably healthy CVD risk factor profile and an unexpectedly high burden of subclinical coronary atherosclerosis may be explained by a higher exposure to risk factors earlier in life. This is supported by the fact that 52% of the runners had smoked at some time during their lives [16]. It appears that lifestyle conversion may reduce, but not eliminate, the risk arising from prior long-term risk factor exposure. This has also been observed in other studies of carotid atherosclerosis in marathon runners [20,21]. These findings emphasize the importance of taking a thorough history including past CVD risk factor exposure. CCT imaging may then be appropriate as a second-line test in athletes with a 10-year risk >5% [22].

The presence and burden of coronary plaque also has implications for eligibility and disqualification recommendations in athletes. Athletes with subclinical atherosclerosis by virtue of identification of calcified or non-calcified plaque in CCT should undergo LV function assessment and ischaemia testing (see Chapter 3.3.5), and aggressive lipid-lowering medication should be considered to stabilize potentially rupture-prone plaque [23]. This cautious strategy also appears appropriate in light of the association between CAC and myocardial fibrosis: CAC scores have been found to be predictive of myocardial fibrosis [16]. The distribution of myocardial fibrosis in runners and controls is shown in ➲ Fig. 3.3.3.2 [24]. Runners with myocardial fibrosis had higher increases in high sensitive cardiac troponin I (➲ Fig. 3.3.3.3) and a higher rate of coronary events than runners without myocardial fibrosis [25,26]. However, there was no association between CAC and hs-TnI.

Long-term follow-up data further suggest that an increased coronary plaque burden, as measured by CCT, is also associated with worse outcome in athletes (➲ Fig. 3.3.3.4). Marathon runners had a similar coronary event rate for every given category of CAC as controls matched for age or for age and risk factors [25]. Of note,

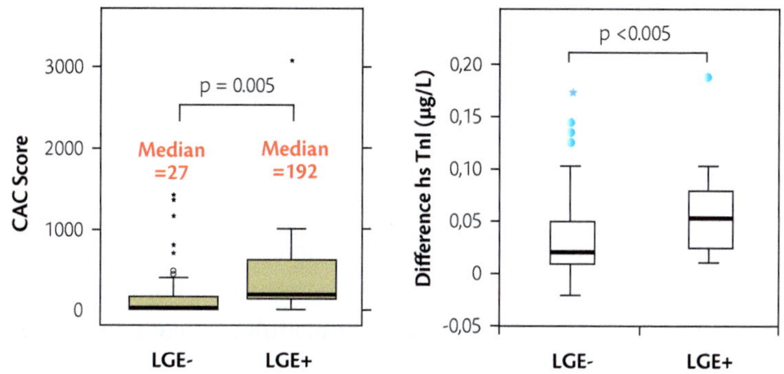

Fig. 3.3.3.3 CAC scores (left) and increase in cardiac troponin values during a marathon (right) by presence or absence of late gadolinium enhancement (LGE) indicating myocardial fibrosis on MRI in marathon runners.

Reproduced with permission from S. Möhlenkamp, G. Heusch, R. Erbel., Cardiovascular risks of strenuous physical exercise, *Aktuelle Kardiologie*, Volume 3, Issue 6, pp. 355-360, Copyright © 2014 Thieme.

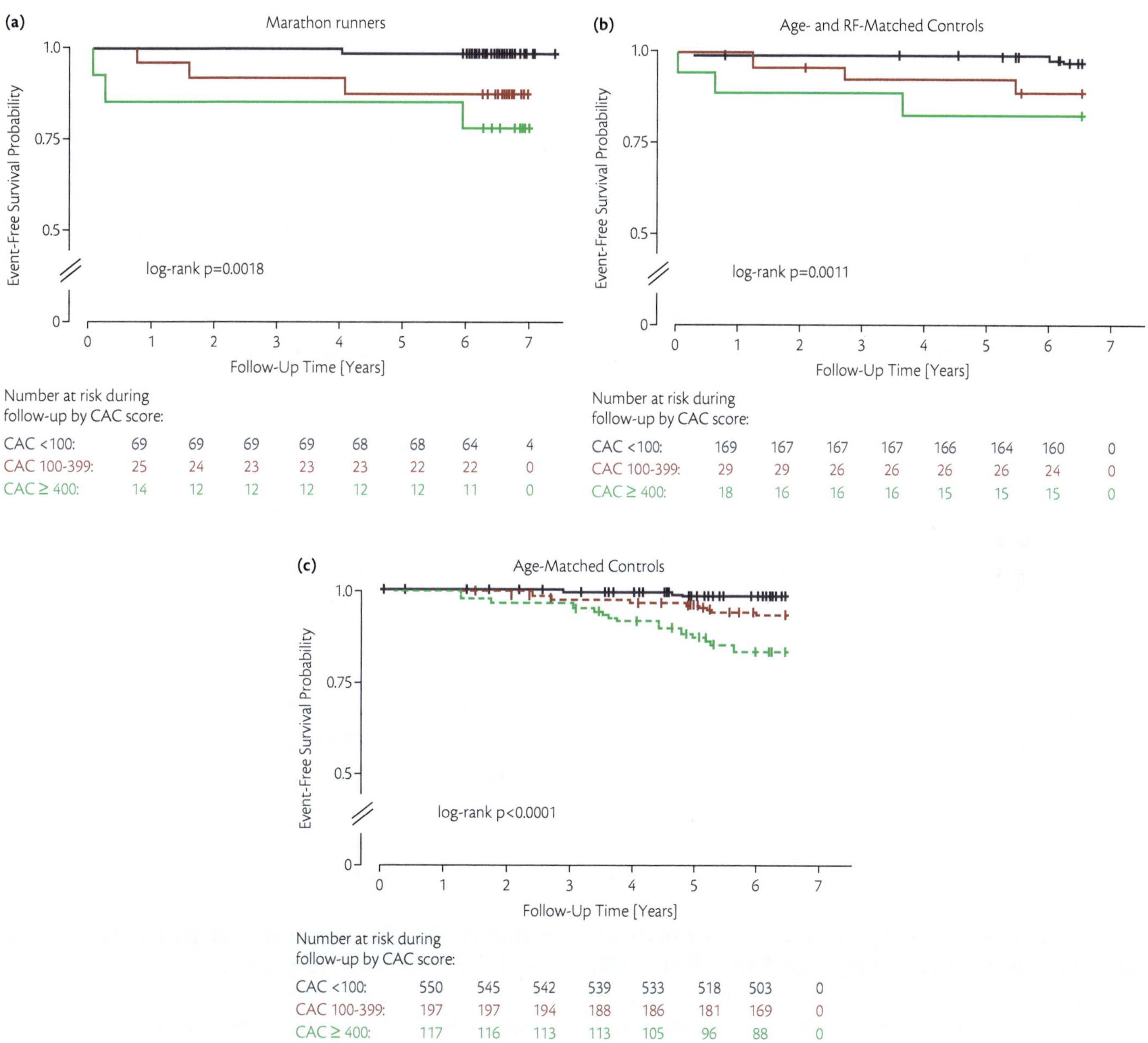

Fig. 3.3.3.4 Kaplan–Meier event-free survival curves in (a) marathon runners, (b) age- and risk-factor-matched controls, and (c) age-matched controls.

Reproduced from *Basic Research in Cardiology*. Coronary atherosclerosis burden, but not transient troponin elevation, predicts long-term outcome in recreational marathon runners. Volume 109, Issue 1, 2013, pp 391–402, Stefan Möhlenkamp. With permission of Springer.

none of the coronary events in that study occurred during a marathon, but in four of seven runners the events were precipitated by some degree of physical activity. Two events were revascularizations unrelated to acute coronary syndrome in runners with few symptoms. In line with clinical data, athletes with elevated CAC scores should be advised on symptoms and on risk factor modification, including aspirin and statins, and should be considered for ischaemia testing and/or CCT angiography.

Coronary computed tomography angiography

To date, few studies have systematically addressed the prevalence of calcified and non-calcified plaque using contrast-enhanced CCT angiography (CCTA) in athletes. In a single-centre observational study, Schwartz et al. [19] assessed 50 men that had participated in at least one marathon every year for 25 consecutive years and compared the findings with controls ($n = 23$) from a contemporary database. Male athletes ($n = 50$) had increased total plaque volume (200 vs 126mm^3, $p < 0.01$), calcified plaque volume (84 vs 44mm^3, $p < 0.0001$), and non-calcified plaque volume (116 vs 82 mm^3, $p = 0.04$), even though age and HDL cholesterol were higher in runners than in controls, while heart rate, body mass index, and rates of hypertension, hyperlipidaemia, and diabetes were much lower. Lesion area, diameter stenosis, and length differences were similar in the two groups. Unfortunately, lumen reduction, remodelling, and follow-up data were not reported.

Tsiflikas et al. [27] invited 50 male runners aged >45 years (mean, 53 ± 6 years) to undergo CCTA, standard risk assessment, and pre-participation screening. The runners had completed a mean of 13.8 marathons (range, 1–72). PROCAM risk scores were very low (1.9% in 10 years,range 0.39–8.5%). However, half the runners (48%) had some degree of atherosclerosis, and five runners (10%) had a CAC score >100. One participant (2%) had significant CAD (>75% lumen reduction), three (6%) had moderate CAD (>50% lumen reduction), and 20 (40%) had mild plaque burden (<50% lumen narrowing). Athletes with CAD on CCTA were 3.5 years older, and had slightly higher blood pressures, PROCAM-scores, and individual best finishing times [27]. A control cohort and follow-up data were not reported. Karlstedt et al. [28] recruited 25 elite marathon athletes (21 males aged 55 ± 4 years), who had run at least three marathons during the preceding two years. Participants had to be free from hypertension, dyslipidaemia, and diabetes, and never been smokers. Two runners (8%) had myocardial fibrosis at the subendocardium in the anterior wall of the left ventricle, and these runners had >70% stenosis on CCTA. Even though absolute numbers were low, these prevalence rates are consistent with findings by Breuckmann et al. [24] in their marathon cohort.

Ermolao et al. [29] recently used CCTA as a second-line test in pre-participation screening of athletes. In a prospective cross-sectional all-comers study, they included 940 asymptomatic athletes (aged 45 ± 7 years, range 30–60 years, 84% men) and performed treadmill or bicycle stress testing prior to high intensity (mostly competitive) sports activities. Only those athletes with pathological or equivocal ST-segment or repolarization changes ($n = 46$ (4.9%)) underwent CCTA. Of those, two were not studied, 23/44 (52%) did not have evidence of CAD, and 14/44 (32%) had CAD on CCTA. Those with CAD were 10 years older (not significant), were more hypertensive, and had a higher risk score. Coronary anomalies were detected in five athletes (11.4%). Six athletes (14%) had significant (>50%) proximal stenosis.

High risk plaque features have recently been characterized using high resolution CCTA. They included low attenuation plaques (0–30 HU) suggestive of lipid-rich plaque, positive remodelling (>110%), reflecting the Glagov phenomenon, and spotty calcification/napkin ring sign which has been associated with thin-cap fibroatheroma (TCFA) and increased coronary event rates [30,31]. Measurement of fractional flow reserve (FFR) using cardiac CT imaging (FFR_{CT}) has been proposed as a non-invasive tool for assessing the functional consequences of epicardial stenoses on CT images [32]. Whether these additional morphological and functional CT-derived parameters help to provide a better diagnosis, guide therapy, and improve outcomes in athletes remains to be shown.

Pathophysiological and prognostic implications of coronary CT imaging in athletes

The presence and extent of asymptomatic coronary atherosclerosis (with potential plaque erosion or plaque rupture and micro-embolization) clearly has a role in CAD events in athletes [25]. Increased coronary plaque burden with endothelial dysfunction may alter coronary microvascular integrity and increase myocardial susceptibility to injury. Repetitive bouts of exhaustive exercise may be one cause of such an injury, as reflected by increases in serum troponin concentrations related to high intensity sport, and eventually lead to myocardial fibrosis. This is supported by a link between the number of completed athletic events and myocardial fibrosis [16,33]. Such fibrosis, in states of increased catecholamine concentrations, may trigger and sustain arrhythmic events [34,35]. It appears that the burden of vessel wall atherosclerosis and/or the presence of myocardial fibrosis, and not the history of how the alteration has arisen, determine prognosis. The types of CVD event occurring in athletes seems as heterogeneous as the mechanisms that cause these events, including plaque rupture with epicardial thrombotic occlusion, sudden death due to VT/VF, or progression from subclinical to overtly symptomatic CAD [26,36,37].

Importantly, there is currently no evidence that long-term endurance exercise is a cause of the unexpectedly high coronary plaque burden in some athletes. Longitudinal studies on coronary atherosclerosis progression in athletes are lacking. Others have argued that the findings of the studies discussed in this chapter are largely attributable to past risk factor exposure [38], a late start in athletic activity [39], or recruitment bias [40]. Indeed, younger athletes are at very low risk of CVD and CAD. However, Kim et al. [36] showed that incidence rates of CVD events in male marathon runners have increased during the past decade, which 'is troubling and may indicate that long-distance racing has recently been attracting more high-risk men with occult cardiac disease who seek the health benefits of routine physical exercise'. The existing CCT studies show that a considerable number of athletes at older age can be identified as carrying a higher than anticipated CAD risk.

Additional considerations of CCT

The aim of advanced imaging is to avoid CVD events at appropriately low side-effects and costs. CT imaging exposes the athlete to radiation (<1mSv for CAC scoring, and <1 to ~10mSv for CCT angiography, with low values for lean athletes with low heart rates) [41,42]. Coronary CT angiography requires administration of ~100cm^3 of contrast agent, and necessitates normal thyroid and (near-)normal kidney function. Finally, like nuclear imaging and MRI, the costs and availability of CT imaging as well as expertise in its use in athletes can vary considerably and must be weighed against the expected improvement in prognosis. To date, no studies have analysed the cost-effectiveness of CT imaging in athletes. Initial data from clinical cohorts suggest that coronary CT imaging may be cost-effective under limited conditions [43–45]. Thus, it is not recommended as a broad screening tool in low-risk cohorts, but should be considered as a second-line technique in athletes.

Further reading

Breuckmann F, Möhlenkamp S, Nassenstein K, et al. Myocardial late gadolinium enhancement: prevalence, pattern, and prognostic relevance in marathon runners. *Radiology* 2009; 251: 50–7

Chugh SS, Weiss JB. Sudden cardiac death in the older athlete. *J Am Coll Cardiol* 2015; 65: 493–502

Kim JH, Malhotra R, Chiampas G, et al. Cardiac arrest during long-distance running races. *N Engl J Med* 2012; 366: 130–40.

La Gerche A, Baggish AL, Knuuti J, et al. Cardiac imaging and stress testing asymptomatic athletes to identify those at risk of sudden cardiac death. *JACC Cardiovasc Imaging* 2013; 6: 993–1007.

La Gerche A, Heidbuchel H. Can intensive exercise harm the heart? You can get too much of a good thing. *Circulation* 2014; 130: 992–1002

Lauer MS. Elements of danger: the case of medical imaging. *N Engl J Med* 2009; 361: 841–3.

Möhlenkamp S, Lehmann N, Breuckmann F, et al. Running the risk of coronary events: prevalence and prognostic relevance of coronary atherosclerosis in marathon runners. *Eur Heart J* 2008; 29: 1903–10

Möhlenkamp S, Leineweber K, Lehmann N, et al. Coronary atherosclerosis burden, but not transient troponin elevation, predicts long-term outcome in recreational marathon runners. *Basic Res Cardiol* 2014; 109: 391–402

Schwartz R, Merkel-Kraus S, Schwartz JG, et al. Increased coronary artery plaque volume among male marathon runners. *Mo Med* 2014; 111: 85–90

Thompson PD, Myerburg RJ, Levine BD, et al. Eligibility and Disqualification Recommendations for Competitive Athletes With Cardiovascular Abnormalities: Task Force 8: Coronary Artery Disease: A Scientific Statement from the American Heart Association and American College of Cardiology. *J Am Coll Cardiol* 2015; 66: 2406–11.

References

1. Montalescot G, Sechtem U, Achenbach S, et al. 2013 ESC guidelines on the management of stable coronary artery disease. *Eur Heart J* 2013; 34, 2949–3003.
2. Greenland P, Alpert JS, Beller GA, et al. 2010 ACCF/AHA guideline for assessment of cardiovascular risk in asymptomatic adults: a report of the ACC Foundation/AHA Task Force on Practice Guidelines. *J Am Coll Cardiol* 2010; 56: e50–103.
3. Möhlenkamp S, Lehmann N, Moebus S, et al. Quantification of coronary atherosclerosis and inflammation to predict coronary events and all-cause mortality. *J Am Coll Cardiol* 2011; 57(13): 1455–64.
4. Cho I, Chang HJ, O'Hartaigh B, et al. Incremental prognostic utility of coronary CT angiography for asymptomatic patients based upon extent and severity of coronary artery calcium: results from the COronary CT Angiography EvaluatioN For Clinical Outcomes InteRnational Multicenter (CONFIRM) study. *Eur Heart J* 2015; 36: 501–8.
5. La Gerche A, Baggish AL, Knuuti J, et al. Cardiac imaging and stress testing asymptomatic athletes to identify those at risk of sudden cardiac death. *JACC Cardiovasc Imaging* 2013; 6: 993–1007.
6. Maron BJ, Zipes DP, Kovacs RJ. Eligibility and disqualification recommendations for competitive athletes with cardiovascular abnormalities: preamble, principles, and general considerations. *J Am Coll Cardiol* 2015; 66: 2343–9.

7. Van Hare GF, Ackerman MJ, Evangelista JA, et al. Eligibility and Disqualification Recommendations for Competitive Athletes With Cardiovascular Abnormalities: Task Force 4: Congenital Heart Disease. *J Am Coll Cardiol.* 2015; 66: 2372–84.
8. Achenbach S, Barkhausen J, Beer M, et al. Consensus recommendations of the German Radiology Society (DRG), the German Cardiac Society (DGK) and the German Society for Pediatric Cardiology (DGPK) on the use of cardiac imaging with CT and MRI. *Rofo* 2012; 184: 345–68.
9. Attili A, Hensley AK, Jones FD, et al. Echocardiography and coronary CT angiography imaging of variations in coronary anatomy and coronary abnormalities in athletic children: detection of coronary abnormalities that create a risk for sudden death. *Echocardiography* 2013; 30(2): 225–33
10. Plicht B, Erbel R, Möhlenkamp S. Is there a preventive value in non-invasive cardiac imaging? Debate on the case of a marathon runner. *Dtsch Med Wochenschr* 2009; 134: e1–5, 1990–4.
11. Lauer MS. Elements of danger: the case of medical imaging. *N Engl J Med* 2009; 361: 841–3.
12. Erbel R, Möhlenkamp S, Moebus S, et al. Coronary risk stratification, discrimination, and reclassification improvement based on quantification of subclinical coronary atherosclerosis: the Heinz Nixdorf Recall study. *J Am Coll Cardiol.* 2010; 56: 1397–1406.
13. Yeboah J, McClelland RL, Polonsky TS, et al. Comparison of novel risk markers for improvement in cardiovascular risk assessment in intermediate-risk individuals. *JAMA* 2012; 308: 788–95.
14. Detrano R, Guerci AD, Carr JJ, et al. Coronary calcium as a predictor of coronary events in four racial or ethnic groups. *N Engl J Med* 2008; 358: 1336–45.
15. Desai MY, Nasir K, Rumberger JA, et al. Relation of degree of physical activity to CAC score in asymptomatic individuals with multiple metabolic risk factors. *Am J Cardiol* 2004; 94: 729–32.
16. Möhlenkamp S, Lehmann N, Breuckmann F, et al. Running: the risk of coronary events: prevalence and prognostic relevance of coronary atherosclerosis in marathon runners. *Eur Heart J* 2008; 29: 1903–10.
17. Möhlenkamp S, Schmermund A, Kröger K, et al. Coronary atherosclerosis and cardiovascular risk in master male marathon runners: rationale and design of the 'Marathon Study'. *Herz* 2006; 31: 575–85
18. Thompson PD, Balady GJ, Chaitman BR, et al. Eligibility recommendations for competitive athletes with cardiovascular abnormalities. Task Force 6: Coronary Artery Disease. *J Am Coll Cardiol* 2005; 45: 1348–53.
19. Schwartz R, Merkel-Kraus S, Schwartz JG, et al. Increased coronary artery plaque volume among male marathon runners. *Mo Med* 2014; 111: 85–90.
20. Taylor BA, Zaleski AL, Capizzi JA, et al. Influence of chronic exercise on carotid atherosclerosis in marathon runners. *BMJ Open* 2014; 4: e004498.
21. Kröger K, Lehmann N, Rappaport L, et al. Carotid and peripheral atherosclerosis in male marathon runners. *Med Sci Sports Exerc* 2011; 43: 1142–7.
22. Chugh SS, Weiss JB. Sudden cardiac death in the older athlete. *J Am Coll Cardiol* 2015; 65: 493–502.
23. Thompson PD, Myerburg RJ, Levine BD, et al. Eligibility and Disqualification Recommendations for Competitive Athletes With Cardiovascular Abnormalities: Task Force 8: Coronary Artery Disease: A Scientific Statement from the American Heart Association and American College of Cardiology. *J Am Coll Cardiol.* 2015; 66: 2406–11.
24. Breuckmann F, Möhlenkamp S, Nassenstein K, et al. Myocardial late gadolinium enhancement: prevalence, pattern, and prognostic relevance in marathon runners. *Radiology* 2009; 251: 50–7.
25. Möhlenkamp S, Leineweber K, Lehmann N, et al. Coronary atherosclerosis burden, but not transient troponin elevation, predicts long-term outcome in recreational marathon runners. *Basic Res Cardiol* 2014; 109: 391–402.
26. Möhlenkamp S, Heusch G, Erbel R. Cardiovascular risks of strenuous physical exercise. *Aktuel Kardiol* 2014; 3: 355–60.
27. Tsiflikas I, Thomas C, Fallmann C, et al. Prevalence of subclinical coronary artery disease in middle-aged, male marathon runners detected by cardiac CT. *Rofo* 2015; 187: 561–8.
28. Karlstedt E, Chelvanathan A, Da Silva M, et al. The impact of repeated marathon running on cardiovascular function in the aging population. *J Cardiovasc Magn Reson* 2012; 14: 58–64.
29. Ermolao A, Roman F, Gasperetti A, et al. Coronary CT angiography in asymptomatic middle-aged athletes with ST segment anomalies during maximal exercise test. *Scand J Med Sci Sports* 2016: 26: 57–63.
30. Hecht HS, Achenbach S, Kondo T, Narula J. High-risk plaque features on coronary CT angiography. *JACC Cardiovasc Imaging* 2015; 8: 1336–9.
31. Otsuka K, Fukuda S, Tanaka A, et al. Napkin-ring sign on coronary CT angiography for the prediction of acute coronary syndrome. *JACC Cardiovasc Imaging* 2013; 6: 448–57.
32. Douglas PS, Pontone G, Hlatky MA, et al. Clinical outcomes of fractional flow reserve by computed tomographic angiography-guided diagnostic strategies vs. usual care in patients with suspected coronary artery disease: the prospective longitudinal trial of FFR-CT: outcome and resource impacts study. *Eur Heart J* 2015; 36: 3359–67.
33. Wilson M, O'Hanlon R, Prasad S, et al. Diverse patterns of myocardial fibrosis in lifelong, veteran endurance athletes. *J Appl Physiol* 2011; 110: 1622–6.
34. La Gerche A, Heidbuchel H. Can intensive exercise harm the heart? You can get too much of a good thing. *Circulation* 2014; 130: 992–1002.
35. Möhlenkamp S, Heusch G, Erbel R. Can intensive exercise harm the heart? *Circulation* 2015; 131: e524.
36. Kim JH, Malhotra R, Chiampas G, et al. Cardiac arrest during long-distance running races. *N Engl J Med* 2012; 366: 130–40.
37. Albano AJ, Thompson PD, Kapur NK. Acute coronary thrombosis in Boston marathon runners. *N Engl J Med* 2012; 366: 184–5.
38. Levine BD. Response to the letters regarding article, 'can intensive exercise harm the heart? The benefits of competitive endurance training for cardiovascular structure and function'. *Circulation* 2015; 131: e525.
39. La Gerche A, Heidbuchel H. Response to letters regarding article, 'Can intensive exercise harm the heart? You can get too much of a good thing'. *Circulation* 2015; 131: e526.
40. Yared K, Wood MJ. Is marathon running hazardous to your cardiovascular health? The jury is still out. *Radiology* 2009; 251: 3–5.
41. Mahabadi AA, Achenbach S, Burgstahler C, et al. Safety, efficacy, and indications of beta-adrenergic receptor blockade to reduce heart rate prior to coronary CT angiography. *Radiology* 2010; 257: 614–23.
42. Meinel FG, Nance JW Jr, Harris BS, et al. Radiation risks from cardiovascular imaging tests. *Circulation* 2014; 130: 442–5.

43. Galper BZ, Wang YC, Einstein AJ. Strategies for primary prevention of coronary heart disease based on risk stratification by the ACC/AHA Lipid Guidelines, ATP III Guidelines, Coronary Calcium Scoring, and C-Reactive Protein, and a Global Treat-All Strategy: a comparative–effectiveness modelling study. *PLoS One* 2015; 10: e0138092.
44. Pletcher MJ, Pignone M, Earnshaw S, et al. Using the coronary artery calcium score to guide statin therapy: a cost-effectiveness analysis. *Circ Cardiovasc Qual Outcomes* 2014; 7: 276–84.
45. Roberts ET, Horne A, Martin SS, et al. Cost-effectiveness of coronary artery calcium testing for coronary heart and cardiovascular disease risk prediction to guide statin allocation: the Multi-Ethnic Study of Atherosclerosis (MESA). *PLoS One* 2015; 10: e0116377.

3.3.4 Nuclear imaging

Stefan Möhlenkamp

Nuclear imaging

Myocardial perfusion imaging by means of scintigraphy is an established non-invasive method for detecting coronary artery disease (CAD) [1] and is a powerful prognostic indicator in patients with known or suspected CAD [2]. In addition, it improves risk stratification in individuals without known CAD [3] and in patients with high exercise tolerance, i.e. about 12 METs on the Bruce treadmill protocol [4]. Overall, a normal nuclear stress test is associated with an excellent prognosis for CAD or CVD events.

Like CT imaging and invasive angiography, it is not a first-line diagnostic test because of costs and radiation exposure (~3–10mSv) [5]. A few small-scale studies have addressed the role of SPECT imaging specifically in athletes [6]. In 18 young male elite athletes, myocardial perfusion defects were associated with left ventricular hypertrophy, resulting in low specificity in athletes with chest pain [7], which is in line with the results of another study [8]. Because of several unexpected cardiac deaths in Swedish orienteers in the 1980s, Andersson et al. [9] used thallium-201 perfusion imaging at rest to search for evidence of myocardial fibrosis. Perfusion defects were associated with left ventricular mass and body weight in orienteers and athlete controls, but were unrelated to wall motion abnormalities on echocardiography. Others have used nuclear imaging techniques such as [^{18}F]-FDG positron emission tomography (PET) or [^{123}I]-MIBG scintigraphy in athletes, especially in research settings, but the clinical role of these imaging modalities is uncertain, particularly in asymptomatic athletes [6]. Siegel et al. [10,11] used myocardial scintigraphy to exclude relevant myocardial cell necrosis in marathon runners with elevated post-race CK-MB or cardiac troponin levels. However, in larger studies nuclear imaging has not been shown to allow identification of coronary or myocardial disease in symptomatic or asymptomatic athletes.

Single-case studies suggest a mismatch between advanced coronary atherosclerosis burden and comparatively small myocardial perfusion defects in athletes. A 64-year-old marathon runner with an asymptomatic increase in heart rate during training had unexpected signs of ischaemia on treadmill exercise testing, which required further work-up. Coronary CT angiography (CCTA) revealed severe coronary atherosclerosis with >50% stenosis (➲ Fig. 3.3.4.1(a)). Consistent with lack of exertional angina, an additional myocardial perfusion scintigraphy demonstrated no evidence of ischaemia (➲ Fig. 3.3.4.1(b)). There was no late enhancement in the MRI study. Invasive coronary angiography was not performed in this case, but the runner received aggressive lipid-lowering medication and aspirin [12]. Nonetheless, the runner underwent right coronary artery stenting two years later at a different clinic.

Another runner, a 57-year-old asymptomatic and otherwise healthy participant in the Essen Marathon study, had an initial coronary artery calcium (CAC) score of 210 (77th percentile). His risk factor profile was as follows: high blood pressure, 160/110mmHg; LDL-cholesterol, 107mg/dL; HDL cholesterol, 60mg/dL; Lp(a), 58mg/dL; body mass index, 23.5 kg/m^2; Framingham score, 14%/10 years. At that time, he had mild late gadolinium enhancement on MRI. He received blood pressure lowering medication. Four years later he returned with atypical chest pain radiating to his left shoulder during running (but not during high intensity cycling). During these episodes he reported dyspnoea and felt 'like a lame duck'. His CAC score had increased to 416 (79th percentile). A bicycle stress test (peak exercise 175W; max. heart rate, 135bpm) was stopped because of a peak blood pressure of 250/130mmHg. He had no angina and no ST-segment changes. On 99mTc-MIBI scintigraphy he had very mild reversible ischaemia (6–10%) (➲ Fig. 3.3.4.2(a)). Long-term follow-up data from scintigraphic trials suggest that prognosis with <10% of ischaemic myocardium benefits more from lifestyle changes and aggressive risk factor medication than from revascularization [13]. However, because of severe LAD stenosis and myocardial bridging of the LAD on CCTA (not shown), he underwent invasive angiography which confirmed several significant (>75%) stenoses of LAD and LCX and additional myocardial bridging of the mid-LAD (➲ Fig. 3.3.4.2(b)) [14]. This runner refused coronary artery bypass grafting; he was not revascularized, but received aggressive blood pressure and lipid-lowering medication.

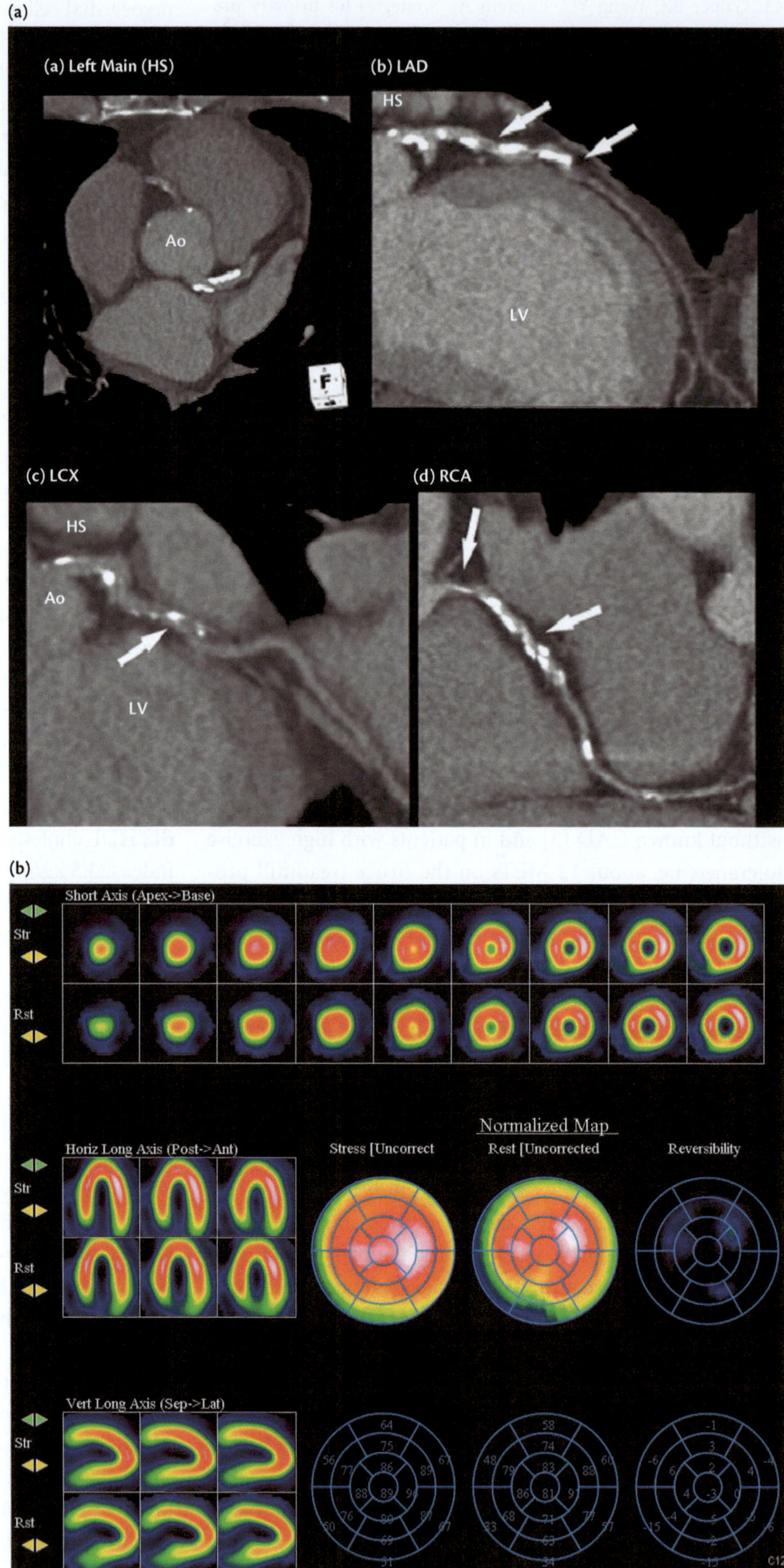

Fig. 3.3.4.1 (a) Multi-slice CT angiography with multiplanar reconstruction of all coronary arteries showing severe calcification, especially in the proximal segments including the left main (LM = Hauptstamm (HS)). A detailed analysis showed no left main obstruction, but high suspicion of significant stenoses in several segments (white arrows). Ao, aortic root, LV, left ventricle. (b) Myocardial scintigraphy during bicycle stress testing up to 225W showing no evidence of stress-induced reversible perfusion deficit.

Reproduced with permission from B. Plicht, R. Erbel, S. Möhlenkamp. Is there a preventive value in non-invasive cardiac imaging? *DMW - Deutsche Medizinische Wochenschrift*, Volume 134, Issue 40, pp.1990–4. Copyright © 2009 Thieme.

(a) (b)

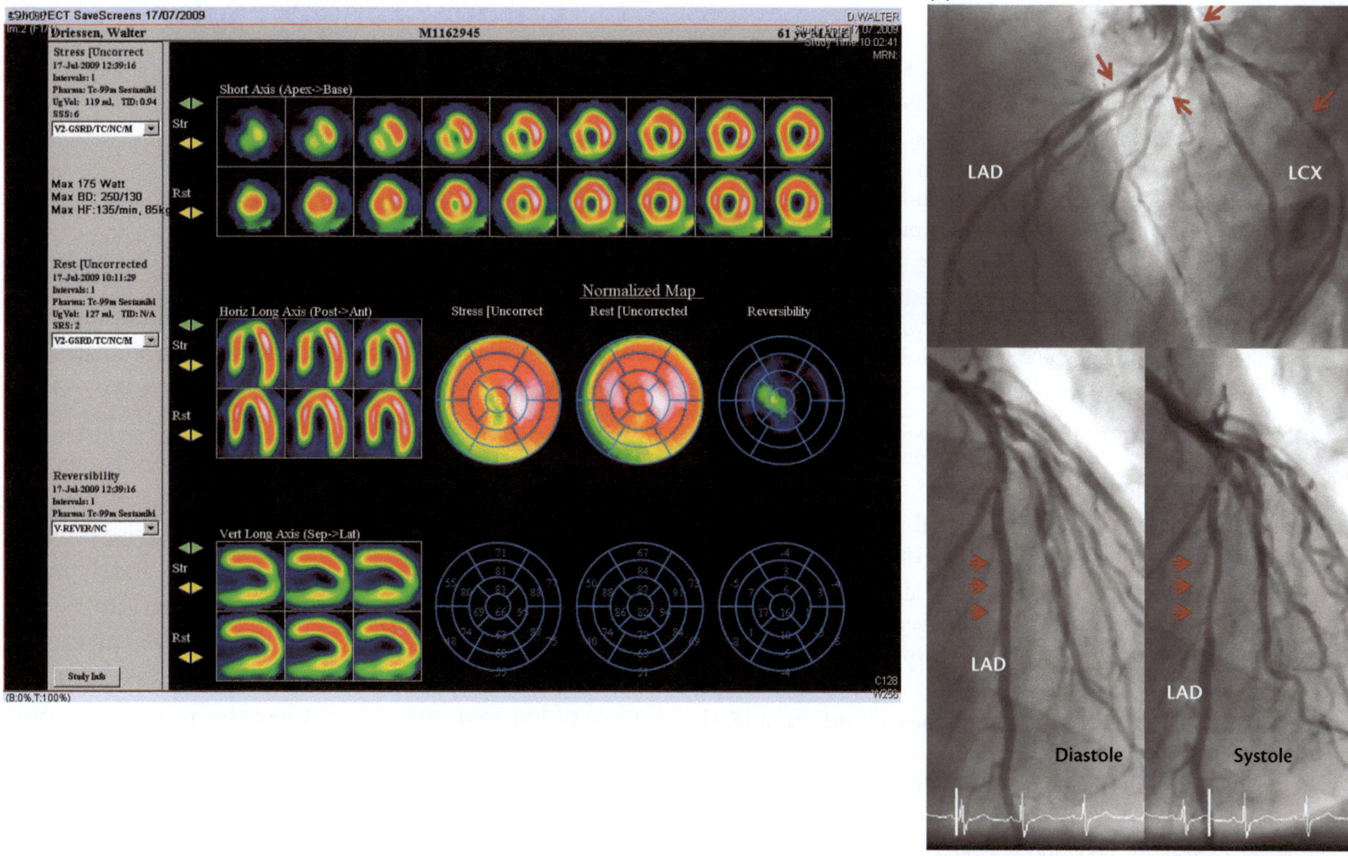

Fig. 3.3.4.2 (a) Myocardial perfusion scintigraphy in a runner with exertional fatigue, mild late gadolinium enhancement on MRI, and high coronary artery calcium (CAC) scores. A small ischaemic array at the apex and the apico-septal segment suggests that modification of lifestyle and risk factor may be sufficient in this runner (see text for details). (b) This runner underwent invasive angiography showing several severe stenoses (>75%, red arrows top) and a long myocardial bridge of the LAD (red arrows, bottom). He did not receive PTCA/stents or coronary artery bypass grafts.

These cases indicate a discrepancy of no or minimal findings on nuclear perfusion imaging in the presence of advanced coronary artery disease. Others have observed the opposite, i.e. relevant ischaemia in the absence of coronary atherosclerosis or other pathology ('athlete's syndrome X') [15]. A well-trained 55-year-old male athlete complained of reduced exercise capacity. He had an episode of infectious mononucleosis at age 23, and a second-degree relative with myocardial infarction at age 50. During myocardial perfusion scintigraphy he had frequency-dependent left bundle branch block and ischaemia in the anteroseptal and inferior regions of four of the 18 segments. Coronary angiography showed no coronary atherosclerosis. He was treated with a calcium-channel blocker and statins. Seven years later, this athlete was admitted with exercise-induced aborted sudden death. Cardiac MRI showed normal right and left ventricular dimensions, normal ventricular wall thickness, normal ventricular function, and no signs of cardiomyopathy or myocardial fibrosis as evidenced by lack of delayed enhancement. He received an automated external defibrillator. The mechanism of the clinical course in this athlete is not clear. Evidence of a channelopathy or Brugada syndrome were not reported.

The findings imply that normal or near-normal myocardial perfusion on nuclear rest and stress imaging studies does not exclude even severe coronary artery disease in athletes. Equally, exercise-related cardiovascular symptoms in athletes requires thorough evaluation. Evidence of ischaemia on nuclear imaging studies deserves careful clinical work-up and monitoring of athletes, even in the absence of CAD or cardiomyopathy.

Further reading

1. Hachamovitch R, Hayes SW, Friedman JD, et al. Comparison of the short-term survival benefit associated with revascularization compared with medical therapy in patients with no prior CAD undergoing stress myocardial perfusion SPECT. *Circulation* 2003; 107: 2900–7.

References

1. Maddahi J, Kiat H, Van Train KF, et al. Myocardial perfusion imaging with technetium-99m sestamibi SPECT in the evaluation of CAD. *Am J Cardiol* 1990; 66: 55E–62E.
2. Berman DS, Hachamovitch R, Kiat H, et al. Incremental value of prognostic testing in patients with known or suspected ischemic heart disease: a basis for optimal utilization of exercise technetium-99m sestamibi myocardial perfusion SPECT. *J Am Coll Cardiol* 1995; 26: 639–47.
3. Hachamovitch R, Berman DS, Kiat H, et al. Exercise myocardial perfusion SPECT in patients without known coronary artery disease: incremental prognostic value and use in risk stratification. *Circulation* 1996; 93: 905–14.
4. Chatziioannou SN, Moore WH, Ford PV, et al. Prognostic value of myocardial perfusion imaging in patients with high exercise tolerance. *Circulation* 1999; 99: 867–72.
5. Meinel FG, Nance JW Jr, Harris BS, et al. Radiation risks from cardiovascular imaging tests. *Circulation* 2014; 130: 442–5.
6. Galderisi M, Cardim N, D'Andrea A, et al. The multi-modality cardiac imaging approach to the athlete's heart: an expert consensus of the European Association of Cardiovascular Imaging. *Eur Heart J Cardiovasc Imaging* 2015; 16: 353
7. Bartram P, Toft J, Hanel B, et al. False-positive defects in technetium-99m sestamibi myocardial single-photon emission tomography in healthy athletes with left ventricular hypertrophy. *Eur J Nucl Med* 1998; 25: 1308–12.
8. Bouvier F, Nejat M, Berglund B, et al. High incidence of scintigraphic myocardial uptake defects at rest and during exercise in male elite runners. *Heart* 1997; 77: 252–5.
9. Andersson LG, Henriksen E, Damm S, et al. Thallium-201 myocardial imaging at rest in male orienteers and other endurance athletes. *Ups J Med Sci* 2001; 106: 59–66.
10. Siegel AJ, Silverman LM, Holman BL. Normal results of post-race thallium-201 myocardial perfusion imaging in marathon runners with elevated serum MB creatinine kinase levels. *Am J Med* 1985; 79: 431–4.
11. Siegel AJ, Lewandrowski KB, Strauss HW, et al. Normal post-race antimyosin myocardial scintigraphy in asymptomatic marathon runners with elevated serum creatine kinase MB isoenzyme and troponin T levels: evidence against silent myocardial cell necrosis. *Cardiology* 1995; 86: 451–6.
12. Plicht B, Erbel R, Möhlenkamp S. Is there a preventive value in non-invasive cardiac imaging? Debate on the case of a marathon runner. *Dtsch Med Wochenschr* 2009; 134: e1–5, 1990–4.
13. Hachamovitch R, Hayes SW, Friedman JD, et al. Comparison of the short-term survival benefit associated with revascularization compared with medical therapy in patients with no prior CAD undergoing stress myocardial perfusion SPECT. *Circulation* 2003; 107: 2900–7.
14. Wilson M, O'Hanlon R, Prasad S, et al. Diverse patterns of myocardial fibrosis in lifelong, veteran endurance athletes. *J Appl Physiol* 2011; 110: 1622–6.
15. van de Sande DAJP, Hoogsteen J, Liem IH, Kemps HMC. Athlete's syndrome X. *Int J Cardiol* 2014; 177: e49–50

3.3.5 Coronary angiography

Stefan Möhlenkamp

Coronary angiography

Because of its its invasive nature, radiation exposure (~2–7mSv) [1], and the need for contrast agent (~50–70cm^3), coronary angiography is not a first-line imaging modality for clinical evaluation of asymptomatic or symptomatic athletes with suspected heart disease. It is used in sports-related acute coronary syndromes and myocardial infarction [2–7], mostly demonstrating plaque rupture, plaque erosion, coronary vasospasm, thrombosis, or a combination of these. These can be explained by an exercise-induced prothrombotic–fibrinolytic imbalance [8,9] and burst of inflammation [8,10] in the presence of coronary artery disease (CAD). Traumatic coronary artery dissection may be demonstrated by coronary angiography but is rare [11,12]. Causes of hypercoagulation that have been linked to coronary thrombus formation in athletes and visualized by coronary angiography include high altitude [7], epinephrine abuse [13], antithrombin III deficiency [14], and left main coronary artery aneurysm [15].

A finding on coronary angiography that remains incompletely understood in athletes and others is Tako–Tsubo cardiomyopathy, characterized by chest pain, apical ballooning, and troponin elevation, but normal non-obstructed coronary arteries. Several cases have been reported in association with exercise testing [16–20]. Tako–Tsubo cardiomyopathy is usually associated with physical or emotional stress, and has been reported in swimmers and divers and in relation to anabolic steroid abuse [21–24]. Therefore it is surprising that there have been few reports of Tako–Tsubo cardiomyopathy in athletes during or after vigorous physical activity.

A number of case reports and case series describe coronary events associated with coronary anomalies in athletes, the majority of which have been confirmed using coronary angiography [25–29]. The most frequent coronary anomaly in the general population (prevalence of up to 30%), and hence also in athletes, is myocardial bridging (see Chapter 4.1.5). On coronary angiography, it is characterized by systolic compression of the tunnelled segment. It is described in less than 5% of coronary angiographies as vessel compression is usually mild, but it can be observed in up to 40% of coronary angiograms for patients with chest pain without atherosclerotic CAD [30]. Because of intra-coronary pressure changes and the subsequent alterations in the vessel wall, severe systolic coronary compression can be viewed as an anatomical risk factor for myocardial infarction [31,32]. However, it has a benign prognosis in the majority of those affected, including athletes [30,33]. Individuals with asymptomatic myocardial bridging and no evidence of myocardial ischaemia need not generally be restricted from vigorous activity [33]. However, athletes with a myocardial bridge as the only explanation for chest pain, who intend to engage in vigorous sports activities, require careful counselling and medication, and may even need surgery for definitive treatment [30].

Additional intra-coronary artery imaging helps to improve understanding of the coronary microvascular adaptations to exercise [34–36] (see Chapter 1.2). Advanced intra-coronary imaging allows detailed assessment of high risk plaque features and functional evaluation of epicardial stenosis and its myocardial sequelae. In the case of an asymptomatic runner in whom significant coronary artery stenosis was detected in a research setting (➲ Fig. 3.3.5.1(a) [37], intravascular ultrasound-based virtual histology (IVUS-VH) revealed high-risk plaque features, i.e. TCFA lesions (➲ Fig. 3.3.5.1(b)), which are associated with higher

(a)

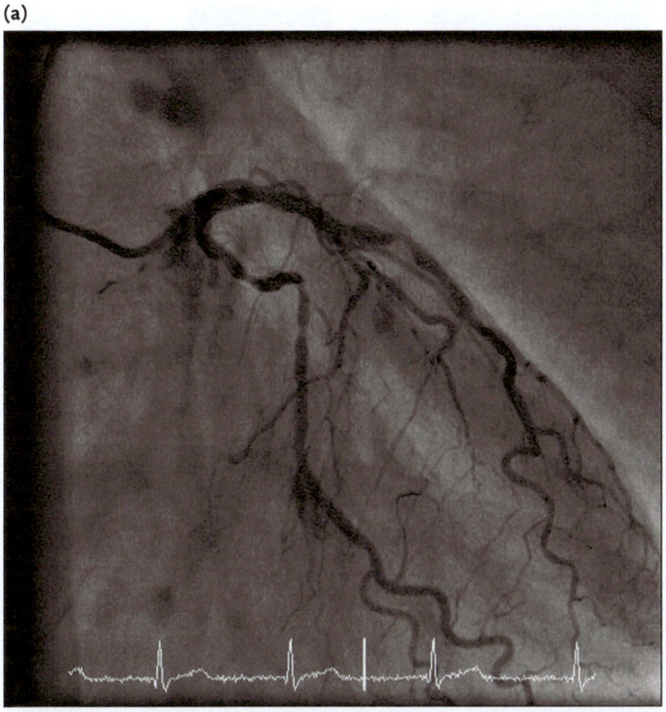

(b)

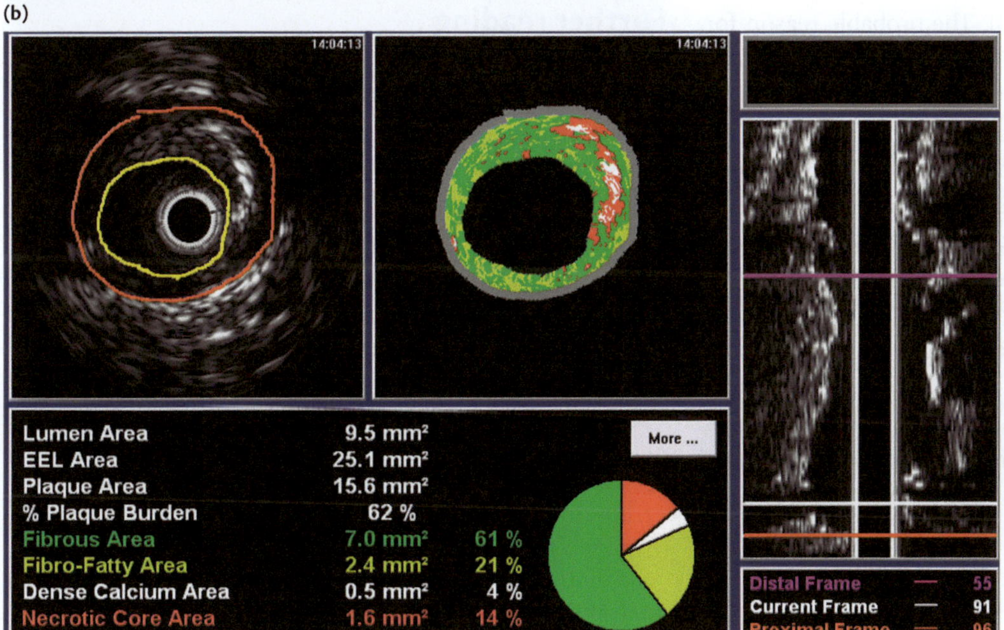

Fig. 3.3.5.1 (a) Coronary angiography demonstrating lumen reduction in the mid-LAD and mid-LCX. The RCA showed no stenosis (not shown). (b) Intravascular ultrasound (IVUS) image of the LAD using a 2.9F, 20MHz catheter (Eagle-Eye©, Volcano, USA). Automated pullback was performed at 0.5mm/s beginning in the distal LAD. Radiofrequency data analysis of the IVUS signal was used for virtual histology (IVUS-VH) assessment. This technique allows in vivo characterization and quantification of different coronary plaque components, i.e. fibrous, fibro-fatty, lipidic–necrotic, and calcium. The IVUS-VH study in this runner demonstrates a high amount of necrotic core plaque component (14%, red). Fibrous tissue is marked in dark green (61%), fibro-fatty tissue (21%) in light green, and calcified plaque in white (4%). The plaque area at this non-culprit lesion site is 62%.

(c)

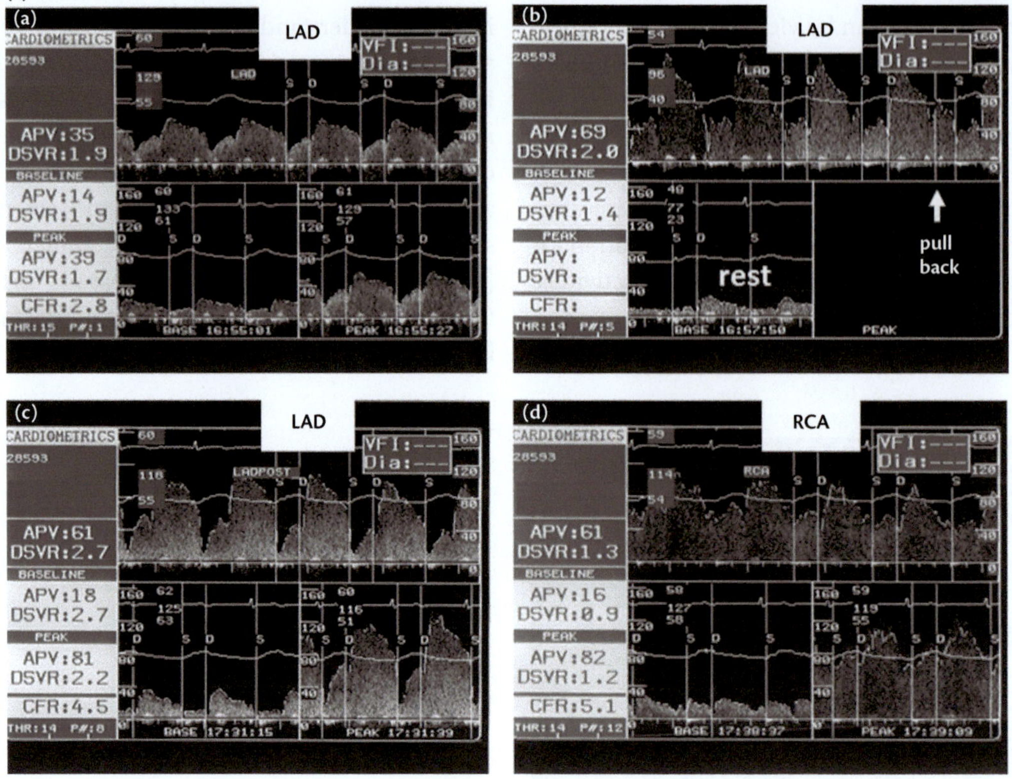

Fig. 3.3.5.1 (*Continued*) (c) Intra-coronary Doppler ultrasound (ICD) in the distal LAD and during pull-back. Doppler flow velocity spectra are measured at the tip of the Doppler wire. The FloMap or FloMod system (Endosonics) was used to automatically detect maximum coronary blood flow (CBF) and calculate absolute coronary flow reserve (CFR) as the ratio of average peak velocity (APV) during maximum adenosine-induced hyperaemia divided by baseline APV. Coronary blood flow (CBF) increased from 14 to 39cm/s, i.e. a near-normal CFR of 2.8 (a, top left). During pull-back, CBF increased 5.75-fold at the lesion site (b, top right). After stenting, maximum average peak velocity (APV) during adenosine doubled to 81 cm/s (c, bottom left). In comparison, CFR in the right coronary artery was 5.1, i.e. an increase in APV from 16 to 82cm/s (d, bottom right). CFR >5 and flow >80cm/s have been observed in <1% of subjects in a series of patients with normal coronary arteries [39], indicating improved microvascular function in this marathon runner, consistent with observations from others [36].

rates of adverse CAD events [38]. The probable reason for this runner being asymptomatic even during exertional exercise is the above-normal microvascular function, as seen in the unobstructed RCA, and a near-normal coronary flow reserve (CFR) of 2.8 in the LAD (➲ Fig. 3.3.5.1(c)) [36,39]. Many mechanisms, including epicardial flow mediated vasodilation, arteriogenesis, angiogenesis, and reduced arterial stiffness contribute to these findings [34,35].

Invasive coronary angiography is used in symptomatic athletes with clinical suspicion of CAD which presumably requires interventional therapy, i.e. mainly in acute coronary syndrome and myocardial infarction. If the cause of chest pain cannot readily be identified on coronary angiography, advanced intra-coronary artery imaging, including intravascular ultrasound (IVUS) and intra-coronary Doppler ultrasound (ICD), can help in understanding the epicardial and intra-myocardial microvascular causes of the symptoms.

Further reading

Möhlenkamp S, Hort W, Ge J, Erbel R. Update on myocardial bridging. *Circulation* 2002; 106(20): 2616–22.

Möhlenkamp S, Leineweber K, Lehmann N, et al. Coronary atherosclerosis burden, but not transient troponin elevation, predicts long-term outcome in recreational marathon runners. *Basic Res Cardiol* 2014; 109: 391–402.

Schuler G, Adams V, Goto Y. Role of exercise in the prevention of cardiovascular disease: results, mechanisms, and new perspectives. *Eur Heart J* 2013; 34: 1790–9.

References

1. Meinel FG, Nance JW Jr, Harris BS, et al. Radiation risks from cardiovascular imaging tests. *Circulation* 2014; 130: 442–5.
2. Albano AJ, Thompson PD, Kapur NK. Acute coronary thrombosis in Boston marathon runners. *N Engl J Med* 2012; 366: 184–5.
3. Ciampricotti R, el Gamal MI, Bonnier JJ, Relik TH. Myocardial infarction and sudden death after sport: acute coronary angiographic findings. *Cathet Cardiovasc Diagn* 1989; 17: 193–7.

4. Ciampricotti R, el-Gamal M, Relik T, et al. Clinical characteristics and coronary angiographic findings of patients with unstable angina, acute myocardial infarction, and survivors of sudden ischemic death occurring during and after sport. *Am Heart J* 1990; 120: 1267–78.
5. Halna du Fretay X, Akoudad H, Nejjari M, Benamer H. Myocardial infarction related to sport. Acute clinical and coronary angiographic characteristics in 16 cases. *Ann Cardiol Angeiol (Paris)* 2013; 62: 398–403.
6. Cuneo A, Oeckinghaus R, Tebbe U. Leisure sport activity as a trigger for acute coronary events in men without known CAD: a single-center case study. *Herz* 2011; 36: 637–42.
7. Indermuehle A, Cook S, Marty H. A young mountaineer surviving sudden cardiac arrest at high altitude. *BMJ Case Rep* 2010; doi:10.1136/bcr.07.2009.2130
8. Siegel AJ, Stec JJ, Lipinska I, et al. Effect of marathon running on inflammatory and hemostatic markers. *Am J Cardiol* 2001; 88: 918–20.
9. Bartsch P. Platelet activation with exercise and risk of cardiac events. *Lancet* 1999; 354: 1747–8.
10. Suzuki K, Nakaji S, Yamada M, et al. Impact of a competitive marathon race on systemic cytokine and neutrophil responses. *Med Sci Sports Exerc* 2003; 35: 348–55.
11. van Mieghem NM, van Weenen S, Nollen G, et al. Traumatic coronary artery dissection: potential cause of sudden death in soccer. *Circulation* 2013; 127: e280–2.
12. Kalaga RV, Malik A, Thompson PD. Exercise-related spontaneous coronary artery dissection: case report and literature review. *Med Sci Sports Exerc* 2007; 39: 1218–20.
13. Kranjec I, Cerne A, Noc M. Ephedrine-induced acute myocardial infarction in a young athlete: a case of thrombus management. *Angiology* 2009; 60: 254–8.
14. Peovska I, Maksimovic J, Kalpak O, et al. Recurrent myocardial infarction in a young football player with antithrombin III deficiency. *Cardiol J* 2008; 15: 463–6.
15. Park SH, Kim SE, Ryu SK. Left main coronary artery aneurysm with chronic total occlusion of both left coronary arteries in a young athlete. *Heart* 2001; 85: E1.
16. Dorfman T, Aqel R, Allred J, et al. Takotsubo cardiomyopathy induced by treadmill exercise testing: an insight into the pathophysiology of transient left ventricular apical (or midventricular) ballooning in the absence of obstructive coronary artery disease. *J Am Coll Cardiol* 2007; 49: 1223–5.
17. Vasconcelos Filho FJ, Gomes CA, Queiroz OA, Barreto JE. Dobutamine stress echocardiography-induced broken heart syndrome (Takotsubo syndrome). *Arq Bras Cardiol* 2009; 93: e5–7.
18. Dhoble A, Abdelmoneim SS, Bernier M, et al. Transient left ventricular apical ballooning and exercise induced hypertension during treadmill exercise testing: is there a common hypersympathetic mechanism? *Cardiovasc Ultrasound* 2008; 18;6: 37.
19. Vértesaljai M, Szoke S, Szonyi T, et al. Transient left ventricular apical akinesis with systolic dysfunction after physical exercise: a form of Tako-Tsubo syndrome. *Orv Hetil* 2008; 149: 687–90.
20. Digne F, Paillole C, Pillière R, et al. Tako-Tsubo syndrome after an exercise echocardiography. *Int J Cardiol* 2008; 127: 420–2.
21. De Gennaro L, Brunetti ND, Ruggiero M, et al. Adrift: Takotsubo cardiomyopathy in an old woman in distress while taking a swim off coast. *Int J Cardiol* 2014; 177: e161–2.
22. Chenaitia H, Coullange M, Benhamou L, Gerbeaux P. Takotsubo cardiomyopathy associated with diving. *Eur J Emerg Med* 2010; 17: 103–6.
23. Madias JE. Adrift while swimming and Takotsubo syndrome: the vagotonia connection. *Int J Cardiol* 2014; 177: 123.
24. Placci A, Sella G, Bellanti G, Margheri M. Anabolic androgenic steroid-induced Takotsubo cardiomyopathy. *BMJ Case Rep* 2015; doi:10.1136/bcr.2014-209089.
25. 2Attili A, Hensley AK, Jones FD, et al. Echocardiography and coronary CT angiography imaging of variations in coronary anatomy and coronary abnormalities in athletic children: detection of coronary abnormalities that create a risk for sudden death. *Echocardiography* 2013; 30: 225–33.
26. Vogt S, Koenig D, Prettin S, et al. Unusual cause of exercise-induced ventricular fibrillation in a well-trained adult endurance athlete: a case report. *J Med Case Rep* 2008; 2: 120.
27. Basso C, Maron BJ, Corrado D, Thiene G. Clinical profile of congenital coronary artery anomalies with origin from the wrong aortic sinus leading to sudden death in young competitive athletes. *J Am Coll Cardiol* 2000; 35: 1493–1501.
28. Maron BJ. Sudden death in young athletes. *N Engl J Med* 2003; 349: 1064–75.
29. Joggerst S, Monge J, Uribe C, et al. Sudden cardiac arrest at the finish line: in coronary ectopia, the cause of ischemia is from intramural course, not ostial location. *Tex Heart Inst J* 2014; 41: 212–16.
30. Möhlenkamp S, Hort W, Ge J, Erbel R. Update on myocardial bridging. *Circulation* 2002; 106: 2616–22.
31. Erbel R, Ge J, Möhlenkamp S. Myocardial bridging: a congenital variant as an anatomic risk factor for myocardial infarction? *Circulation* 2009; 120: 357–9.
32. Kurt IH. A case of muscular bridge resulting in myocardial infraction following heavy effort: a case report. *Cases J* 2009; 2: 135
33. Gowd BM, Thompson PD. Isolated myocardial bridging and exercise-related cardiac events. *Int J Sports Med* 2014; 35: 1145–50.
34. Schuler G, Adams V, Goto Y. Role of exercise in the prevention of cardiovascular disease: results, mechanisms, and new perspectives. *Eur Heart J* 2013; 34: 1790–9.
35. Kojda G, Hambrecht R. Molechular mechanisms of vascular adaptations to exercise. Physical activity as an effective antioxidant therapy? *Cardiovasc Res* 2005; 67: 187–97.
36. Windecker S, Allemann Y, Billinger M, et al. Effect of endurance training on coronary artery size and function in healthy men: an invasive follow-up study. *Am J Physiol Heart Circ Physiol* 2002; 282: H2216–23.
37. Möhlenkamp S, Böse D, Mahabadi AA, et al. On the paradox of exercise: coronary atherosclerosis in an apparently healthy marathon runner. *Nature Clin Pract Cardiovasc Med* 2007; 4: 396–401.
38. Stone GW, Maehara A, Lansky AJ, et al. A prospective natural-history study of coronary atherosclerosis. *N Engl J Med* 2011; 364: 226–35.
39. Wieneke H, Haude M, Ge J, et al. Corrected coronary flow velocity reserve: a new concept for assessing coronary perfusion. *J Am Coll Cardiol* 2000; 35: 1713–20.

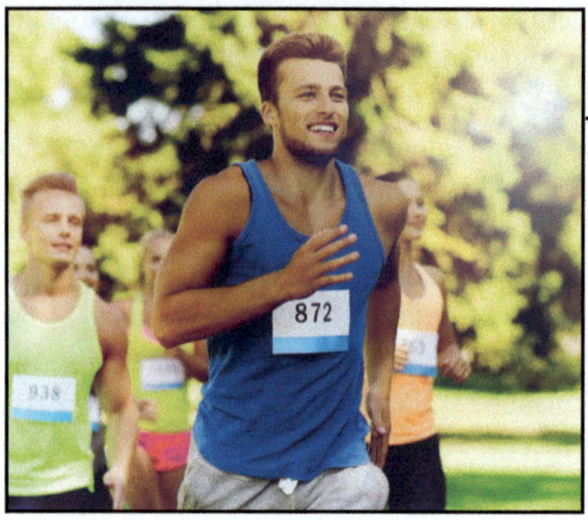

3.4

Genotyping

Contents

3.4.1 **Indications for genetic testing in athletes and its application in daily practice** Andrea Mazzanti, Katherine Underwood, and Silvia G. Priori *166*

3.4.1 Indications for genetic testing in athletes and its application in daily practice

Andrea Mazzanti, Katherine Underwood, and Silvia G. Priori

Introduction

Owing to the tremendous advances in the field of DNA sequencing that have dramatically reduced both the cost and throughput time of genetic analysis, molecular testing for a variety of conditions is offered today by commercial companies all over the world. Specifically, in the field of sports medicine, direct to consumer genetic screening is now available 'to evaluate an athlete's potential to excel in a particular sport or to assess if athletes are predisposed to particular health risks, including arrhythmia, slow recovery from concussions and hypertrophic cardiomyopathy' [1].

The ability to mine this massive amount of genetic material is appealing, but, as is the case with any powerful tool, there is also a great burden of responsibility. Genetic information is undoubtedly vital in the management of patients with primary arrhythmia syndromes (see Section 5) and cardiomyopathies (see Section 4), both of which increase the risk of sudden cardiac death (SCD) [2], and even more so for athletes, whose hearts are exposed to intense stress over the years.

The decision to undergo genetic testing should be justified on a clinical basis and handled by professionals who are capable of framing the results in the correct perspectives [3]. Otherwise, if used as a shortcut to bypass standard clinical evaluation, genetic information may instead serve to increase uncertainty in doctors and anxiety in their patients.

In this chapter we will answer the following questions:

1. When should genetic testing be performed in athletes?
2. Which genetic tests should be requested for athletes?
3. What impact should a positive genetic result have on sports eligibility?

Inherited arrhythmogenic disorders have a special interest for sports cardiology

It is universally acknowledged that a moderate and regular physical exercise regimen contributes to a healthier life, affecting both physical and mental well-being in numerous positive ways [4]. Nevertheless, several lines of evidence suggest that extreme exercise may have detrimental effects on the heart in the long term, prompting some authors to elaborate on the existence of 'exercise-induced' cardiomyopathies [5].

The potential harmful effects of strenuous exercise are especially evident in patients with inherited cardiovascular diseases [6] which predispose them to the development of life-threatening arrhythmias [2]:

(1) primary arrhythmia syndromes, also called channelopathies (long QT syndrome (LQTS), short QT syndrome (SQTS), catecholaminergic polymorphic ventricular tachycardia (CPVT), and Brugada syndrome (BrS));

(2) cardiomyopathies (hypertrophic cardiomyopathy (HCM), dilated cardiomyopathy (DCM), and arrhythmogenic right ventricular cardiomyopathy (ARVC)).

Taken as a whole, this group of inherited arrhythmogenic disorders shares some characteristics.

- They are rare diseases, but globally they might affect up to 1 in 1000 individuals.
- They are familial diseases, transmitted across generations most frequently as autosomal dominant traits.
- They are monogenic disorders, characterized by incomplete penetrance and variable expressivity, so that a molecular diagnosis is often possible.
- They are phenotypically heterogeneous entities and their clinical manifestations range, sometimes even within the same family, from asymptomatic cases to cases manifesting with palpitations, syncope, and SCD, which may be the first presentation of disease in apparently healthy individuals;
- They are generally recognized as the leading cause of SCD in the young athlete. In an examination of 1866 SCDs in young athletes, the most common cause was HCM (up to 53%), followed by other inherited diseases: ARVC (4%), LQTS (4%), aortic rupture (3%), and DCM (2%) [7]. Importantly, inherited arrhythmias are considered to be under-reported, as this diagnosis is usually missed by autopsy. However, ion channel diseases can be identified through post-mortem genetic analyses in up to 10–30% of cases with a normal conventional autopsy including histological and toxicological assessment [8–12].

With all these considerations, it should be evident that molecular testing can play a pivotal role in establishing a clinical diagnosis and in the management of patients affected by inherited cardiovascular diseases.

Athlete's heart or inherited arrhythmogenic disorder?

As outlined in Section 1, intense and prolonged exercise may induce physiological changes in cardiac structure and electrophysiological properties that can be globally collected under the term 'exercise-induced cardiac remodelling' [13] or, more informally, 'athlete's heart' [14].

From a structural standpoint, cardiac remodelling associated with systematic training mainly includes increased ventricular and atrial volumes. Up to 15% of trained athletes will have substantial enlargement of the left ventricular cavity, with end-diastolic dimensions of up to 70mm in men and 66mm in women [15,16]. The chamber enlargement may occasionally be accompanied by a relatively mild increase in left ventricular wall thickness that exceeds the upper normal limits (range of 13–15mm) [14].

Increased cavity size can produce a higher stroke volume, and thus the ejection fraction at rest may be in the low normal range. The ejection fraction in trained athletes has been shown to be as low as 50% [15].

Additionally, a wide spectrum of electrocardiographic alterations have been reported in up to 40% of trained athletes, twice as common in men as in women [17]. The most common electrocardiographic (ECG) alterations in athletes are sinus bradycardia, first-degree AV block, increased QRS voltages, incomplete right bundle branch block, early repolarization pattern, and prolonged QTc interval (in up to 0.4% of elite adult athletes) [18].

The majority of these mild structural and ECG alterations represent the extremes of physiological effects on the athlete's heart, but sometimes the same changes can also serve to define a grey zone of overlap with inherited heart conditions, particularly with the milder phenotypes of HCM [19] and LQTS [18].

The distinction between physiological adaptation to exercise and pathology is crucial, since both cardiomyopathies and channelopathies are well-recognized causes of SCD in athletes. In most cases, such as CPVT, the adrenergic drive brought on by intense exercise acts as an arrhythmic trigger [20–22]. In other cases, including ARVC, intense exercise not only increases the risk of ventricular arrhythmia, but may also enhance and accelerate the phenotypic expression of the underlying disease (➔ Fig. 3.4.1.1). In 2006 Kirchhof et al. [23] demonstrated that endurance training accelerated the development of right ventricular dysfunction and arrhythmias in a mouse model of ARVC. In humans, Saberniak et al. [24] investigated the impact of exercise on myocardial function in 37 ARVC subjects (either clinically affected patients or mutation-positive family members) who participated in at least 4 hours/week of vigorous training for six years or more, compared with 73 non-athletes with similar clinical characteristics. The study found that the systolic function of both ventricles was significantly reduced in athletes compared with non-athletes; interestingly, the amount and intensity of exercise was also correlated with impaired ventricular function. To further validate this finding, James et al. [6] found that carriers of an ARVC-causing mutation who participate in strenuous exercise develop clinically evident ARVC on average 10 years earlier than sedentary patients.

Cardiac structural and electrical remodelling processes related to exercise are dynamic in nature, may develop relatively rapidly after the initiation of vigorous conditioning, and are usually reversible with cessation of training [18,25]; in contrast, abnormalities attributed to true pathological conditions will persist despite abstinence from sports.

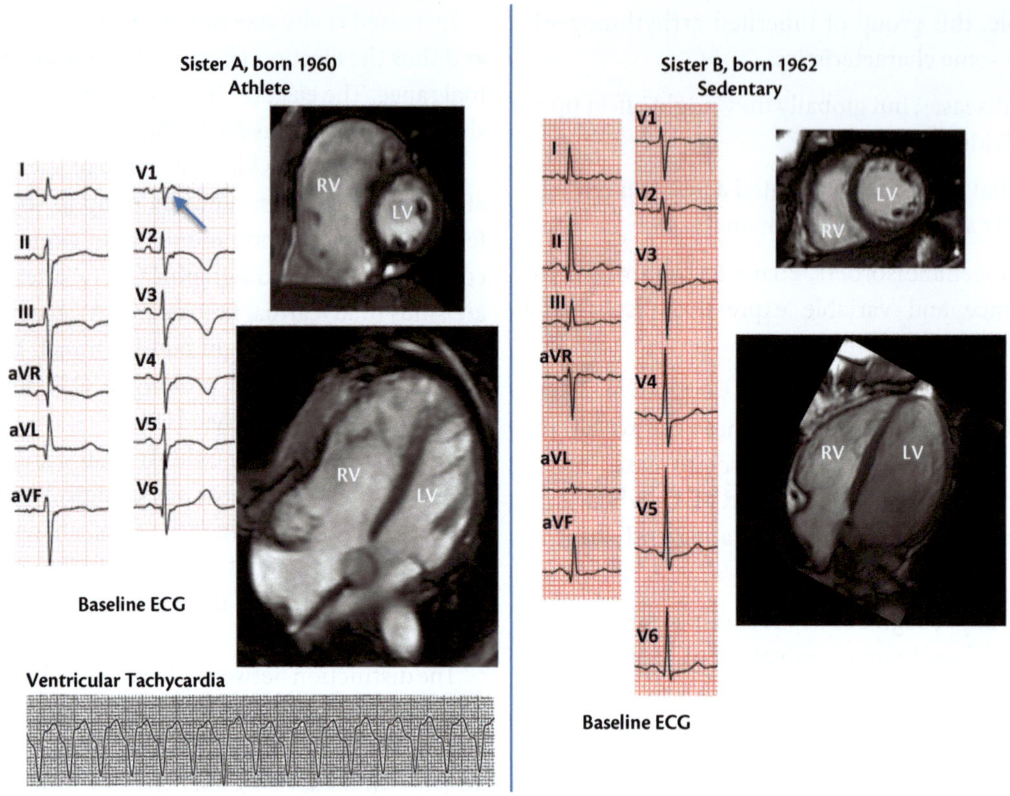

Fig. 3.4.1.1 Strenuous exercise and development of phenotype in arrhythmogenic right ventricular cardiomyopathy (ARVC). The figure shows the effect of the prolonged practice of vigorous physical activity on the development of electrocardiographic, arrhythmic, and structural alterations in patients with ARVC. The images refer to two sisters who are carriers of a non-sense mutation on the plakophillin-2 (PKP-2) gene and no other variants on the main desmosomal genes. **Sister A**, born in 1960, has been practising endurance sport (running) from early adulthood, training 12 hours per week for over 30 years and participating in several marathons. Her basal 12-lead ECG presents the typical changes of ARVC (epsilon wave, indicated by the arrow, and negative T waves on precordial derivations V1–V4). Cardiac magnetic resonance showed a marked dilation and severe contractile dysfunction of the right ventricle (RV) compared with the left ventricle (LV). She also presented with one episode of sustained monomorphic ventricular tachycardia (left bundle branch block morphology and superior axis) with a heart rate of 170 bpm that she tolerated well (she continued working). She is currently being evaluated for a potential heart transplant. **Sister B**, born in 1962, has never practised intense sports and shows almost normal ECG and cardiac magnetic resonance. She is currently asymptomatic and has never experienced arrhythmic episodes.

In cases where there is still doubt of pathological structural alterations persisting after a complete clinical and familial evaluation and a period of detraining, molecular screening may help to clarify the picture [3].

When should genetic testing for inherited heart diseases be performed in athletes?

Generally speaking, the indications for genetic testing are the same for athletes and non-athletes. However, it may have additional utility in athletes by contributing to the early detection of genetic cardiac conditions that may increase the risk of experiencing life-threatening arrhythmias and SCD [3].

The indications for genetic testing cannot be summarized in a 'one size fits all' manner; instead physicians must tailor them on an individual patient basis. Therefore in the following sections we will explore the indications for genetic testing in four different groups of individuals, referring to the consensus document released by the Heart Rhythm Society/European Heart Rhythm Association on the appropriate use of genetic testing in inherited cardiovascular diseases [3]:

Athletes with an established clinical diagnosis of an inherited cardiovascular disease

These individuals should be screened for mutations in the genes related to the phenotype observed [3], taking into account that the likelihood of finding a disease-causing mutation responsible for a diagnosis varies by disease. For example, a patient with a clinical diagnosis of LQTS or HCM has up to an 60–80% chance of testing positive for a disease-causing mutation, whereas someone with BrS or SQTS only has about a 20–30% chance of carrying an identifiable mutation [3]. Importantly, the pre-test probability of a positive genetic result is maximal only if it is considered in the context of an established clinical diagnosis, whereas it decreases when the clinical phenotype is less evident [26].

Even though the diagnosis for primary arrhythmia syndromes and cardiomyopathies is generally based on clinical parameters, it should be noted that in ARVC (see Chapter 4.1.2) genetic screening may also have diagnostic value; in fact, genetic results constitute one of the parameters used for diagnosis, along with electrocardiographic features, structural alterations assessed by imaging techniques/histology, and arrhythmias [27].

Finally, there are some situations in which the results of genetic testing can be used to modify medical management. In patients with LQTS, for instance, genetic testing can determine the subtype of the disease, helping to identify (and avoid) triggering events and stratify the risk of life-threatening arrhythmias [28,29]. Similarly, genetic testing can differentiate between isolated cardiomyopathies and systemic diseases with cardiac involvement. For example, mutations in the *LMNA* gene are associated with familial DCM, which has a high risk of conductive defects and arrhythmias, so pacemakers and ICD placement may be indicated earlier than for traditional DCM patients [2].

Athletes with a suspected diagnosis of an inherited cardiovascular disease

Genetic testing may help to establish a diagnosis when the clinical picture is unclear or in the presence of structural/electrocardiographic features suggestive of an overlap between different disorders, such as exercise-induced cardiac remodelling or mild pathological features [13]. For example, an elite basketball player with borderline left ventricular hypertrophy who undergoes genetic testing and is found to carry an established disease-causing variant in a sarcomere protein gene will have a high level of suspicion for HCM [30]. Similarly, a competitive swimmer with borderline QT prolongation who tests positive for a definitive potassium-channel gene variant will receive the diagnosis of LQTS [2,31].

This is particularly important when an early diagnosis can factor into decisions that may be life-saving, such as abstinence from competitive performances in a patient with CPVT (Section 5) or reduced exercise in a patient with an initial/hidden form of ARVC (Section 4). The yield of any genetic screening should be expected to decrease when the clinical picture is less clear, but it is important to emphasize that a clinical diagnosis cannot be excluded solely on the basis of a negative result of molecular screening.

Athletes who are first-degree relatives of a patient with an inherited cardiovascular disease and an identified disease-causing mutation

The identification of a clearly disease-causing mutation in an index case is the gold standard for the diagnosis of inherited cardiovascular disease, as it promotes further assessment of relatives. According to current recommendations, genetic testing conducted in a cascade fashion is useful in families with any of the diseases described in this chapter to identify at-risk family members, determine their likelihood of disease manifestations, and help them to adopt therapy, protective measures, or lifestyle adaptations [2,32,33]. In the case of a negative genetic result for the mutation that causes an inherited cardiovascular disease in his/her family, an individual may be dismissed from cardiology. However, in the case of a positive genetic result in a relative without clinical evidence for the disease (i.e. genotype positive/phenotype negative (GP/PN)), a series of prophylactic measures and scheduled follow-ups might be appropriately planned [34].

When applied to the field of sports medicine, the possible consequences of a positive genetic result need to be discussed before performing the test, particularly since the presence of a pathogenic variant might warrant disqualification from competitive sport, even in GP/PN cases [35]. The age at which genetic testing should be offered to asymptomatic relatives varies with the disease and should also be carefully discussed with the families [3]. For diseases such as LQTS and CPVT, in which preventive measures and prophylactic therapies are advised for the GP/PN individual, experts recommend that mutation-specific genetic testing should be performed as early as infancy [3]. In contrast, in the case of cardiomyopathies experts consider it reasonable to discuss monitoring for onset of clinical signs of the disease, rather than testing for pathogenic mutations that may never manifest until later in life, if at all [3]. While it is true that no data actually exist on the occurrence of life-threatening arrhythmias in the population of GP/PN patients with HCM [36], we have also seen that GP/PN ARVC individuals who participate in strenuous exercise may develop more severe manifestations of the disease at an earlier age [6]. Moreover, evidence is now emerging from the autopsies on athletes who died suddenly that SCD may be the first manifestation of ARVC in individuals with absent/mild signs of the disease during life [37]. For this reason, we consider it appropriate to screen children in families with a clearly identified pathogenic ARVC genetic variant before any clinical manifestations first arise.

An entirely different situation presents itself when genetic testing has identified a genetic variant in an index case that does not yet have an established pathological correlation and is not directly actionable (the so-called 'variant of unknown significance'). In this case, cascade screening in family members should not be performed routinely because of the potential for generating unnecessary stress in the family [3]. It appears reasonable in these instances to advise patients to seek expert consultation at a referral centre.

Athletes who experience SCD

According to the guidelines for the prevention of SCD released by the European Society of Cardiology, an autopsy is recommended for all victims of sudden unexpected death [2]. In these cases the heart should be analysed by expert pathologists, and when a cardiomyopathy is determined to be the cause of death or when the heart is normal in the absence of any clear cause of tdeath, blood or tissue should be collected to allow for potential genetic testing and DNA banking for future genetic investigations. According to recent data, genetic testing performed on a victim of a sudden and unexplained death has a diagnostic yield of up to 44% [38]. If a mutation is identified in the deceased athlete, then cascade screening can be performed in the surviving relatives to determine who is at risk.

Although several scientific societies around the world have supported the preservation of biological samples of victims of sudden unexplained death to allow for molecular autopsy, it is becoming increasingly difficult in many countries to collect samples from young victims of sudden death, since reimbursement for these investigations is often not covered by insurance plans.

The contribution of family history to defining the diagnosis of inherited cardiovascular diseases may be valid for all four of clinical scenarios discussed above [39]. Because of the genetic components underlying many cases of inherited arrhythmias and cardiomyopathies, a careful analysis of family history can be instrumental in establishing a diagnosis. According to Gimeno et al. [40], when a diagnosis of an inherited cardiovascular disease is made in a patient, it is possible to identify other affected individuals among the first-degree family members in up to 47% of cases for cardiomyopathies and up to 30% of cases for channelopathies. Most of these diseases are autosomal dominant, but recessive, X-linked, or mitochondrial modes of inheritance may also be observed for syndromic diseases or for paediatric patients in particular.

When the clinical picture is unclear for an athlete, screening of their family members may provide valuable information. If the blood relatives have obvious disease or a history of sudden death, this may suggest that the athlete is in the early stages of disease. On the other hand, absence of evidence of disease in any first-degree consanguineous relative can provide some reassurance, although it is important to remember that in situations where the inheritance pattern is not easily recognized within a family, the possibility of either incomplete penetrance or a sporadic case should be considered.

Is there a role for genetic screening to predict athletic performance?

Several lines of animal and human studies have suggested the there is a genetic component to individual cardiorespiratory fitness and response to exercise training [41,42].

The first attempts to identify genetic markers for sports performance date to the 1968 Mexico and 1976 Montreal Olympic Games. They were based on common blood genetic markers and were ultimately unsuccessful [43]. Since then, many studies have been published focusing on the difference in allele frequencies between athletes and non-athlete controls, mainly investigating angiotensin I converting enzyme (*ACE*) and α-actinin-3 (*ACTN3*) polymorphisms [44,45]. Several positive findings have been reported over the years, but most results were based on small sample sizes or derived from post hoc subgroup analyses [46].

Finally, genome-wide approaches have been attempted in the search for common DNA variants associated with physical performance [47]. The most recent example of this came from the international GAMES consortium, which was established to compare the genetic profile of 1520 elite endurance athletes and 2760 ethnicity-matched controls. Despite a sample size larger than any previous study in the field and a solid methodology, this study still did not have the power to identify alleles with small effect sizes and therefore failed to form a group of genomic variants common to the elite endurance athlete group [46].

Nevertheless, even with this lack of evidence, a market of unregulated direct to consumer tests, mainly targeted towards coaches and parents, has begun to emerge in recent years [44]. A large number of private companies claim to be able to predict future athletic potential in children through the screening of large panels of genetic variants, including the *ACTN3* and *ACE* polymorphism alleles. The consensus among internationally recognized sport and exercise genetics researchers [44] is that while large-scale collaborative projects may help to develop a stronger scientific foundation on these issues in the future [48], currently genetic testing has no role to play in talent prediction or individualized training regimens to maximize performance.

What genetic testing should be requested in athletes?

According to current practice, there are no indications for 'non-clinical' genetic testing, as outlined in the previous section. Genetic testing should instead be considered as a diagnostic tool for use when there is clinical suspicion of a specific inherited heart disease [3]. If the clinical diagnosis is in question, it may be prudent first to refer the patient to a centre that specializes in the particular disease rather than proceeding directly with genetic testing [3].

Over a hundred distinct channelopathy/cardiomyopathy-associated genes with thousands of discrete mutations have been described, but only a minority of them are known to be responsible for a significant proportion of each given disease. According to the recommendations of the principal heart rhythm societies, only genes that cause ≥5% of any channelopathy or cardiomyopathy should be routinely screened for clinical purposes (➲ Table 3.4.1.1) [3].

Current expert recommendations state that genetic screening should not include large panels directed towards a wide range of cardiomyopathies and channelopathies all at once, since this may increase the number of identified 'variants of unknown significance'. The potential for false-positive results rises significantly when genetic testing is pursued in settings in which the phenotype is ambiguous or absent, as it is in broad screening.

'Minor' genes may be studied for research, but the 'non-conventional' nature of these investigations and the lesser degree of certainty of the results should be clearly explained to patients before starting the screening.

What impact should a positive genetic result have on sports eligibility?

When genetic testing has identified one or more variants related to the presence of an inherited arrhythmogenic disorder, this information may impact several aspects of a patient's life, including the possibility of participating in competitive sport. The European approach [35] to sport eligibility (which is discussed in detail in Section 7) has traditionally been more cautious on this point, attributing a relatively high importance to genetic information, whereas the American guidelines [49] have conventionally been more permissive in selected circumstances. Indeed,

Table 3.4.1.1 Prevalence, associated genes, contribution, and yield of genetic testing in primary arrhythmia syndromes and cardiomyopathies

	Prevalence	Yield of genetic screening	Genes associated with >5% of disease		Current contribution of genetic testing?		
					Diagnosis	Prognosis	Therapy
LQTS	1:2000	75–80%	*KCNQ1*	30–35%	+++	+++	++
			KCNH2	25–40%			
			SCN5A	5–10%			
SQTS	Unknown	20% ?	*KCNH2*	<5%	+/–	–	–
			KCNQ1	<5%			
			KCNJ2	<5%			
CPVT	1:10,000	60–70%	*RYR2*	60%	+++	+	–
BrS	1:1000	20–30%	*SCN5A*	20–30%	+	+	–
HCM	1:500		*MyBPC3*	20–45%	+++	++	+
			MYH7	15–20%			
			TNNT2	1–7%			
			TNNI3	1–7%			
ARVC	1:2000		*PKP2*	25–40%	++	+/–	–
			DSG2	5–10%			
			DSP	2–12%			
			DSC2	2–7%			
DCM	1:2500		None		+/–	–	–

Adapted with permission from Ackerman, Michael J.; Priori, Silvia G., HRS/EHRA Expert Consensus Statement on the State of Genetic Testing for the Channelopathies and Cardiomyopathies: This document was developed as a partnership between the Heart Rhythm Society (HRS) and the European Heart Rhythm Association (EHRA). *Europace*, Volume 13, Issue 8, pp.1077–1109. Copyright © 2011 Oxford University Press.

the weight of genetic information may vary when the clinical manifestations in the individual patient are taken into account, as is outlined below.

Importantly, both the European and the American guidelines regulate sport eligibility in competitive athletes, defined as those who 'participate in an organized team or individual sport that requires regular competition against others as a central component, places a high premium on excellence and achievement, and requires some form of systematic (and usually intense) training' [49]. Both the European and American recommendations agree that non-competitive and leisure activities should be allowed for all patients, based on individual interests and patient characteristics [50].

Athletes with an established diagnosis of a primary arrhythmia syndrome or a cardiomyopathy should follow recommendations for sport eligibility independent of genetic results. According to current guidelines, no genotype-specific recommendations exist for these individuals, with the exception of the avoidance of swimming for symptomatic patients with LQTS Type 1 [49]. In the field of cardiomyopathies, the specific sarcomere mutation is expressly not considered as a factor with regard to exercise restriction for HCM patients [49].

This very conservative approach reflects the lack of satisfactory genotype–phenotype data for all cardiomyopathies/channelopathies, with the possible exception of LQTS. When more data are available, hopefully the new findings will also be applied to the field of sports medicine.

Athletes with the suspected diagnosis of a primary arrhythmia syndrome or a cardiomyopathy who receive a positive result in genetic testing with an identified pathogenic mutation should be treated as those described above, as the diagnosis is now confirmed.

If targeted genetic testing fails to identify a mutation, athletes with abnormal ECG and/or structural findings should still be followed up clinically, since the current sensitivity of genetic testing for inherited cardiovascular diseases is not 100% [3] (➲ Table 3.4.1.1) and a negative result can never rule out the disorder. In this regard, ECG abnormalities are particularly important as potential 'red flags' to raise the concern for an initial form of cardiomyopathy. For example, Pelliccia et al. [51] collected a database of 12,550 trained athletes, from which they identified 81 (0.6%) with marked ECG repolarization abnormalities (diffusely and deeply inverted T waves) who had no apparent cardiac disease and were followed up for 9 ± 7 years. Of the 81 athletes with abnormal ECGs, five (6%) ultimately proved to have cardiomyopathies: three developed HCM (one of them had an aborted cardiac arrest), one died suddenly at the age of 24 years from clinically undetected ARVC, and the third demonstrated DCM after 9 years of follow-up.

Athletes without a phenotype but who are carriers of a pathogenic mutation that may cause a primary arrhythmia syndrome or a cardiomyopathy (genotype positive/phenotype negative (GP/PN)) [3,33]. The decision of sport eligibility in athletes with disease-causing or likely disease-causing DNA variants, but without evidence of disease, poses a challenge to the attending physician since there is still considerable debate over whether these patients should participate in competitive sport or not.

The European Society for Cardiology has traditionally held a restrictive position on this point, stating that GP/PN individuals should be barred from competitive sport and may participate only in recreational athletic activities [35]. This conservative attitude, which is now attenuated under certain conditions (see Section 7), is based mainly on two assumptions. First, participation in competitive sports might in and of itself trigger sudden death in patients with HCM [7], ARVC [52], or other inherited arrhythmia syndromes, such as CPVT [20–22], even when clinical signs are mild. Second, regular exercise training and competitive sports can indirectly trigger cellular mechanisms which may lead to the development of the cardiomyopathy phenotype (i.e. left ventricular hypertrophy or right ventricular dilation/dysfunction) or clinical evolution (i.e. tachyarrhythmia) in the presence of a predisposing gene abnormality [23]. Therefore, because the long-term consequences of an athletic lifestyle for gene carriers of cardiomyopathies or channelopathies (namely, phenotypic and clinical evolution in the presence of a susceptibility mutation) are still largely unresolved, the European recommendations have been more cautious and consistent with the practice endorsed by the sports medicine law in Italy. Recently, however, new research had been conducted regarding the natural history of inherited heart diseases which may help to expand tunderstanding of these rare entities [53], and some evidence regarding the safety of GP/PN athletes has been published.

In the field of inherited arrhythmias, a group of 70 GP/PN adolescent athletes with LQTS was followed for an average of 5.1 ± 2.9 years, and none experienced a sport-related event [54]. These results were replicated by Aziz et al. [55], who studied a cohort of 103 genotype-positive LQTS children who continued to practise their sport (both competitive and recreational) after the diagnosis. All patients were treated with beta blockers. Over an average of 7 years of follow-up (in 755 patient-years) no LQTS-related cardiac events/deaths were observed in treatment-compliant LQTS children while participating in sports.

With regard to cardiomyopathies, no adverse events were observed in two groups of GP/PN patients at risk for HCM with low rates of conversion to disease rates of 0% for 32 patients over an average 4 years of follow-up and 6% for 36 patients over 12 years of follow-up [31,56,57].

These data, together with the increasing cohort of individuals with genetically determined inherited heart diseases who are phenotypically normal, has led the American recommendations to conclude that there is insufficient evidence to preclude GP/PN individuals from physical activity.

According to the American experts, the possibility of participating in all competitive sports is considered 'reasonable' (class IIa) for asymptomatic GP/PN athletes who carry DNA variants associated with HCM and with all channelopathies, in the latter case advocating that appropriate precautionary measures are in place [49]. These measures include:

(1) electrolyte/hydration replenishment and avoidance of dehydration;
(2) acquisition of a personal **automatic external defibrillator** as part of the athlete's personal sports safety gear;
(3) establishment of an emergency action plan with the appropriate school or team officials.

In addition, some disease-specific indications are provided:

(1) avoidance of QT-prolonging drugs for athletes with LQTS (http://www.crediblemeds.org) and avoidance of drugs that exacerbate BrS in affected athletes (http://www.brugadadrugs.org), and
(2) avoidance or treatment of hyperthermia from febrile illnesses or training-related heat exhaustion or heat stroke for athletes with either LQTS or BrS.

Although no specific recommendations for GP/PN ARVC and DCM patients are provided in this documen [49], they can be extrapolated from the text. American Heart Association/American College of Cardiology (AHA/ACC) recommendations state that GP/PN ARVC athletes should receive continued follow-up 'because ARVC may progress phenotypically, and become more clinically apparent with time'. However, this permissive approach is contradicted within the very same document. The 'identification of a pathogenic mutation categorized as associated or probably associated with ARVC/D in the patient under evaluation' constitutes a major criterion for the diagnosis of ARVC [27], according to the most recent diagnostic criteria, and is even sufficient to establish a 'possible' diagnosis of ARVC. The American guidelines state that 'athletes with a possible diagnosis of ARVC should not participate in most competitive sports' [49], thereby contradicting de facto the practice of competitive sport in GP/PN ARVC subjects.

Finally, even though no clear indications exist in the American guidelines for GP/PN DCM patients, the document seems to limit any contraindications to competitive sport to only 'symptomatic athletes with DCM' [49].

Even though the American recommendations have made appreciable efforts to reduce the burden of sport disqualification for patients, some questions still remain.

First, with regard to the precautions suggested for GP/PN carriers of a variant related to channelopathies, we would like to point out that both the acquisition of a personal automatic external defibrillator and the establishment of an emergency action plan with the appropriate school or team officials pertain more to the environment and society overall than to the individual athlete. Along the same lines, the European Society of Cardiology has recently recommended that 'public access defibrillation is established at sites where cardiac arrest is relatively common and suitable storage is available (e.g. schools, sports stadiums, etc.)' [2]. Whether these measures of public awareness will impact the survival of cardiac arrest victims will be assessed by prospective studies.

Second, while the less stringent rules for HCM or BrS GP/PN subjects are understandable and have also been partially adopted by the European recommendations on sport eligibility (see Section 7), the indiscriminate deregulation of restrictions for all GP/PN channelopathies and the lack of clarity for GP/PN ARVC subjects appear less excusable.

In HCM, epidemiological data suggest that SCD in the absence of clinical risk factors is an extremely improbable event and the same concept is adopted by the '2014 ESC Guidelines on diagnosis and management of hypertrophic cardiomyopathy' [30], although with a lower strength for the recommendation (IIb in the European document and IIa in the 2015 AHA/ACC GL).

However, we believe that the 'one size fits all' outlook may not be acceptable for channelopathies and that it conflicts with the current recommendations of the ESC for the prevention of SCD [2].

In CPVT, it is known that the first manifestation of disease may be SCD, even in subjects with a previously negative exercise stress test [58]. Accordingly, the ESC guidelines for the prevention of SCD recommend that therapy with beta-blockers should be administered to 'genetically positive family members, even after a negative exercise test' [2].

Similarly, it is recognized that GP/PN LQTS subjects may suffer a cardiac arrest in a non-negligible proportion of cases and therefore should also receive beta-blockers, according to the current European guidelines [29]. In this group of patients the eligibility for competitive sport should be carefully evaluated by physicians experienced in managing LQTS patients (see Section 5).

With regard to ARVC mutation carriers, we believe that evidence from animal models [23] and human studies [6] sufficiently supports abstinence from strenuous/competitive sport in carriers of a pathogenic mutation, and therefore a more prudent approach is justified in these subjects and needs to be clearly stated.

Finally, it is essential to emphasize that the concept of 'phenotype negative' is extremely subjective. A CPVT patient is always 'phenotype negative' if he/she does not participate in an exercise stress test. Similarly, a patient with type 1 LQTS will be 'phenotype negative' if the ECG is recorded only at rest and the poor adaptation of QT interval during/after increase of the heart rate is not actively researched. An HCM or ARVC patient may be 'phenotype negative' if standard imaging is adopted, but more advanced clinical screening may be necessary to distinguish a truly phenotype-negative athlete from one with subtle evidence of disease. For example, cardiac magnetic resonance with contrast medium can detect abnormal morphology (e.g. myocardial crypts, elongated mitral valve leaflets, fibrosis, diastolic dysfunction) in genotype-positive HCM patients with no left ventricular hypertrophy [31].

Conclusions

The potential of genetic screening is evident in the field of sports medicine: it offers patients a way to identify inherited cardiovascular diseases early on in life before any other clinical signs and to implement protective measures if necessary, including discontinuation of competitive performance in a minority of cases. Two different approaches to genetic information are currently adopted on the two sides of the Atlantic Ocean. Up until now, the European Society of Cardiology has tended to consider all individuals who are carriers of a genetic defect associated with a primary arrhythmia syndrome (such as LQTS and CPVT) or with a cardiomyopathy (HCM or ARVC) to be potentially at risk, therefore restricting most of them from participation in competitive sport.

The American Heart Association/American College of Cardiology has instead embraced a more liberal approach with regard to these 'silent' mutation carriers, allowing them to participate in all competitive sport provided, by advising that some precautions are taken.

Both approaches are founded more on expert opinion than on clinical evidence. The more correct approach is probably a compromise beween the two, and the hope is that more data will be collected to quantify the risk of SCD in pre-symptomatic athletes and to allow a balanced and individualized approach towards sport eligibility.

Further reading

Ackerman MJ, Priori SG, Willems S, et al. HRS/EHRA expert consensus statement on the state of genetic testing for the channelopathies and cardiomyopathies. *Europace* 2011; 13: 1077–1109.

Elliott PM, Anastasakis A, Borger MA, et al. 2014 ESC Guidelines on diagnosis and management of hypertrophic cardiomyopathy: The Task Force for the Diagnosis and Management of Hypertrophic Cardiomyopathy of the European Society of Cardiology (ESC). *Eur Heart J* 2014; 35: 2733–79.

Maron BJ, Zipes DP, Kovacs RJ, et al. Eligibility and disqualification recommendations for competitive athletes with cardiovascular abnormalities: preamble, principles, and general considerations. A scientific statement from the American Heart Association and American College of Cardiology. *Circulation* 2015; 132: e256–61.

Pelliccia A, Fagard R, Bjornstad HH, et al. Recommendations for competitive sports participation in athletes with cardiovascular disease: a consensus document from the Study Group of Sports Cardiology of the Working Group of Cardiac Rehabilitation and Exercise Physiology and the Working Group of Myocardial and Pericardial Diseases of the European Society of Cardiology. *Eur Heart J* 2005; 26: 1422–45.

Priori SG, Blomstrom-Lundqvist C, Mazzanti A, et al. 2015 ESC guidelines for the management of patients with ventricular arrhythmias and the prevention of sudden cardiac death. *Eur Heart J* 2015; 36: 2793–867.

References

1. Collier R. Genetic tests for athletic ability: science or snake oil? *CMAJ* 2012; 184: E43–4.
2. Priori SG, Blomstrom-Lundqvist C, Mazzanti A, et al. 2015 ESC guidelines for the management of patients with ventricular arrhythmias and the prevention of sudden cardiac death. *Eur Heart J* 2015; 36: 2793–867.
3. Ackerman MJ, Priori SG, Willems S, et al. HRS/EHRA expert consensus statement on the state of genetic testing for the channelopathies and cardiomyopathies. *Europace* 2011; 13: 1077–1109.
4. Khan KM, Thompson AM, Blair SN, et al. Sport and exercise as contributors to the health of nations. *Lancet* 2012; 380: 59–64.
5. Eijsvogels TM, Fernandez AB, Thompson PD. Are there deleterious cardiac effects of acute and chronic endurance exercise? *Physiol Rev* 2016; 96: 99–125.
6. James CA, Bhonsale A, Tichnell C, et al. Exercise increases age-related penetrance and arrhythmic risk in arrhythmogenic right ventricular dysplasia/cardiomyopathy-associated desmosomal mutation carriers. *J Am Coll Cardiol* 2013; 62: 1290–7.
7. Maron BJ, Doerer JJ, Haas TS, et al. Sudden deaths in young competitive athletes: analysis of 1866 deaths in the United States, 1980–2006. *Circulation* 2009; 119: 1085–92.
8. Tester DJ, Ackerman MJ. The role of molecular autopsy in unexplained sudden cardiac death. *Curr Opin Cardiol* 2006; 21: 166–72.
9. Tester DJ, Ackerman MJ. Postmortem long QT syndrome genetic testing for sudden unexplained death in the young. *J Am Coll Cardiol* 2007; 49: 240–6.
10. Skinner JR, Crawford J, Smith W, et al. Prospective, population-based long QT molecular autopsy study of postmortem negative sudden death in 1 to 40 year olds. *Heart Rhythm* 2011; 8: 412–19.

11. Larsen MK, Nissen PH, Berge KE, et al. Molecular autopsy in young sudden cardiac death victims with suspected cardiomyopathy. *Forensic Sci Int* 2012; 219: 33–8.
12. Mazzanti A, Priori SG. Molecular autopsy for sudden unexplained death? Time to discuss pros and cons. *J Cardiovasc Electrophysiol* 2012; 23: 1099–1102.
13. Kim JH, Baggish AL. Differentiating exercise-induced cardiac adaptations from cardiac pathology: the 'grey zone' of clinical uncertainty. *Can J Cardiol* 2016; 32: 429–37.
14. Maron BJ, Pelliccia A. The heart of trained athletes: cardiac remodeling and the risks of sports, including sudden death. *Circulation* 2006; 114: 1633–44.
15. Pelliccia A, Culasso F, Di Paolo FM, Maron BJ. Physiologic left ventricular cavity dilatation in elite athletes. *Ann Intern Med* 1999; 130: 23–31.
16. Pelliccia A, Maron BJ, Culasso F, et al. Athlete's heart in women: echocardiographic characterization of highly trained elite female athletes. *JAMA* 1996; 276: 211–15.
17. Pelliccia A, Maron BJ, Culasso F, et al. Clinical significance of abnormal electrocardiographic patterns in trained athletes. *Circulation* 2000; 102: 278–84.
18. Basavarajaiah S, Wilson M, Whyte G, et al. Prevalence and significance of an isolated long QT interval in elite athletes. *Eur Heart J* 2007; 28: 2944–9.
19. Maron BJ. Distinguishing hypertrophic cardiomyopathy from athlete's heart physiological remodelling: clinical significance, diagnostic strategies and implications for preparticipation screening. *Br J Sports Med* 2009; 43: 649–56.
20. Coumel P. Catecholamine-induced severe ventricular arrhythmias with Adams–Stokes syndrome in children: a report of four cases. *Br Heart J* 1978; 40: 28–37.
21. Leenhardt A, Lucet V, Denjoy I, et al. Catecholaminergic polymorphic ventricular tachycardia in children: a 7-year follow-up of 21 patients. *Circulation* 1995; 91: 1512–19.
22. Priori SG, Napolitano C, Memmi M, et al. Clinical and molecular characterization of patients with catecholaminergic polymorphic ventricular tachycardia. *Circulation* 2002; 106: 69–74.
23. Kirchhof P, Fabritz L, Zwiener M, et al. Age- and training-dependent development of arrhythmogenic right ventricular cardiomyopathy in heterozygous plakoglobin-deficient mice. *Circulation* 2006; 114: 1799–1806.
24. Saberniak J, Hasselberg NE, Borgquist R, et al. Vigorous physical activity impairs myocardial function in patients with arrhythmogenic right ventricular cardiomyopathy and in mutation positive family members. *Eur J Heart Fail* 2014; 16: 1337–44.
25. Maron BJ, Pelliccia A, Spataro A, Granata M. Reduction in left ventricular wall thickness after deconditioning in highly trained Olympic athletes. *Br Heart J* 1993; 69: 125–8.
26. Bai R, Napolitano C, Bloise R, et al. Yield of genetic screening in inherited cardiac channelopathies: how to prioritize access to genetic testing. *Circ Arrhythm Electrophysiol* 2009; 2: 6–15.
27. Marcus FI, McKenna WJ, Sherrill D, et al. Diagnosis of arrhythmogenic right ventricular cardiomyopathy/dysplasia: proposed modification of the Task Force Criteria. *Eur Heart J* 2010; 31: 806–14.
28. Schwartz PJ, Priori SG, Spazzolini C, et al. Genotype–phenotype correlation in the long-QT syndrome: gene-specific triggers for life-threatening arrhythmias. *Circulation* 2001; 103: 89–95.
29. Priori SG, Schwartz PJ, Napolitano C, et al. Risk stratification in the long-QT syndrome. *N Engl J Med* 2003; 348: 1866–74.
30. Elliott PM, Anastasakis A, Borger MA, et al. 2014 ESC Guidelines on diagnosis and management of hypertrophic cardiomyopathy: The Task Force for the Diagnosis and Management of Hypertrophic Cardiomyopathy of the European Society of Cardiology (ESC). *Eur Heart J* 2014; **35**: 2733–79.
31. Thomas MJ, Battle RW. Something old, something new: using family history and genetic testing to diagnose and manage athletes with inherited cardiovascular disease. *Clin Sports Med* 2015; 34: 517–37.
32. Ackerman MJ, Priori SG, Willems S, et al. Heart Rhythm S, European Heart Rhythm A. HRS/EHRA expert consensus statement on the state of genetic testing for the channelopathies and cardiomyopathies. *Europace* 2011; 13: 1077–1109.
33. Priori SG, Wilde AA, Horie M, et al. Executive summary: HRS/EHRA/APHRS expert consensus statement on the diagnosis and management of patients with inherited primary arrhythmia syndromes. *Europace* 2013; 15: 1389–1406.
34. Hofman N, Tan HL, Alders M, et al. Active cascade screening in primary inherited arrhythmia syndromes: does it lead to prophylactic treatment? *J Am Coll Cardiol* 2010; 55: 2570–6.
35. Pelliccia A, Fagard R, Bjornstad HH, et al Recommendations for competitive sports participation in athletes with cardiovascular disease: a consensus document from the Study Group of Sports Cardiology of the Working Group of Cardiac Rehabilitation and Exercise Physiology and the Working Group of Myocardial and Pericardial Diseases of the European Society of Cardiology. *Eur Heart J* 2005; 26: 1422–45.
36. Sylvester J, Seidenberg P, Silvis M. The dilemma of genotype positive–phenotype negative hypertrophic cardiomyopathy. *Curr Sports Med Rep* 2014; 13: 94–9.
37. Suarez-Mier MP, Aguilera B, Mosquera RM, Sanchez-de-Leon MS. Pathology of sudden death during recreational sports in Spain. *Forensic Sci Int* 2013; 226: 188–96.
38. Anderson JH, Tester DJ, Will ML, Ackerman MJ. Whole exome molecular autopsy following exertion-related sudden unexplained death in the young. *Circ Cardiovasc Genet* 2016; 9: 259–65.
39. Charron P, Arad M, Arbustini E, et al. Genetic counselling and testing in cardiomyopathies: a position statement of the European Society of Cardiology Working Group on Myocardial and Pericardial Diseases. *Eur Heart J* 2010; 31: 2715–26.
40. Gimeno JR, Lacunza J, Garcia-Alberola A, et al. Penetrance and risk profile in inherited cardiac diseases studied in a dedicated screening clinic. *Am J Cardiol* 2009; 104: 406–10.
41. Prud'homme D, Bouchard C, Leblanc C, et al. Sensitivity of maximal aerobic power to training is genotype-dependent. *Med Sci Sports Exerc* 1984; 16: 489–93.
42. Bouchard C, An P, Rice T, et al. Familial aggregation of VO(2max) response to exercise training: results from the HERITAGE Family Study. *J Appl Physiol* (1985) 1999; 87: 1003–8.
43. Couture L, Chagnon M, Allard C, Bouchard C. More on red blood cell genetic variation in Olympic athletes. *Can J Appl Sport Sci* 1986; **11**: 16–18.
44. Webborn N, Williams A, McNamee M, et al. Direct-to-consumer genetic testing for predicting sports performance and talent identification: consensus statement. *Br J Sports Med* 2015; 49: 1486–91.

45. Bray MS, Hagberg JM, Perusse L, et al. The human gene map for performance and health-related fitness phenotypes: the 2006–2007 update. *Med Sci Sports Exerc* 2009; 41: 35–73.
46. Rankinen T, Fuku N, Wolfarth B, et al. No evidence of a common DNA variant profile specific to world class endurance athletes. *PLoS One* 2016; 11: e0147330.
47. Bouchard C, Sarzynski MA, Rice TK, et al. Genomic predictors of the maximal O(2) uptake response to standardized exercise training programs. *J Appl Physiol* (1985) 2011; 110: 1160–70.
48. Mattsson CM, Wheeler MT, Waggott D, et al. Sports genetics moving forward: lessons learned from medical research. *Physiol Genomics* 2016; 48: 175–82.
49. Maron BJ, Zipes DP, Kovacs RJ, et al. Eligibility and disqualification recommendations for competitive athletes with cardiovascular abnormalities: preamble, principles, and general considerations: a scientific statement from the American Heart Association and American College of Cardiology. *Circulation* 2015; **132**: e256–61.
50. Maron BJ, Zipes DP. Introduction: eligibility recommendations for competitive athletes with cardiovascular abnormalities-general considerations. *J Am Coll Cardiol* 2005; **45**: 1318–21.
51. Pelliccia A, Di Paolo FM, Quattrini FM, et al. Outcomes in athletes with marked ECG repolarization abnormalities. *N Engl J Med* 2008; 358: 152–61.
52. Corrado D, Basso C, Rizzoli G, et al. Does sports activity enhance the risk of sudden death in adolescents and young adults? *J Am Coll Cardiol* 2003; 42: 1959–63.
53. Mazzanti A, Kanthan A, Monteforte N, et al. Novel insight into the natural history of short QT syndrome. *J Am Coll Cardiol* 2014; 63: 1300–8.
54. Johnson JN, Ackerman MJ. Return to play? Athletes with congenital long QT syndrome. *Br J Sports Med* 2013; 47: 28–33.
55. Aziz PF, Sweeten T, Vogel RL, et al. Sports participation in genotype positive children with long QT syndrome. *JACC Clin Electrophysiol* 2015; 1: 62–70.
56. Gray B, Ingles J, Semsarian C. Natural history of genotype positive–phenotype negative patients with hypertrophic cardiomyopathy. *Int J Cardiol* 2011; 152: 258–9.
57. Jensen MK, Havndrup O, Christiansen M, et al. Penetrance of hypertrophic cardiomyopathy in children and adolescents: a 12-year follow-up study of clinical screening and predictive genetic testing. *Circulation* 2013; 127: 48–54.
58. van der Werf C, Nederend I, Hofman N, et al. Familial evaluation in catecholaminergic polymorphic ventricular tachycardia: disease penetrance and expression in cardiac ryanodine receptor mutation-carrying relatives. *Circ Arrhythm Electrophysiol* 2012; 5: 748–56.

SECTION 4

Cardiac diseases of interest in sports cardiology

4.1 **Myocardial and coronary diseases** *179*

4.1.1 Hypertrophic cardiomyopathy in athletes *179*
Aneil Malhotra and Sanjay Sharma

4.1.2 Arrhythmogenic cardiomyopathy and sudden death in young athletes: causes, pathophysiology, and clinical features *184*
Gaetano Thiene, Kalliopi Pilichou, Stefania Rizzo, and Cristina Basso

4.1.3 Myocarditis in athletes *201*
Martin Halle

4.1.4 Differentiating athlete's heart from left ventricular non-compaction cardiomyopathy *209*
Andrew D'Silva and Sanjay Sharma

4.1.5 Congenital coronary artery anomalies *217*
Cristina Basso, Carla Frescura, Stefania Rizzo, and Gaetano Thiene

4.2 **Valvular and aortic disease** *226*

4.2.1 Mitral valve prolapse in relation to sport *226*
Christian Schmied and Sanjay Sharma

4.2.2 Bicuspid aortic valve disease and competitive sports: key considerations and challenges *233*
Benjamin S. Wessler and Natesa G. Pandian

4.2.3 The athlete with congenital heart disease *238*
Guido E. Pieles and Graham Stuart

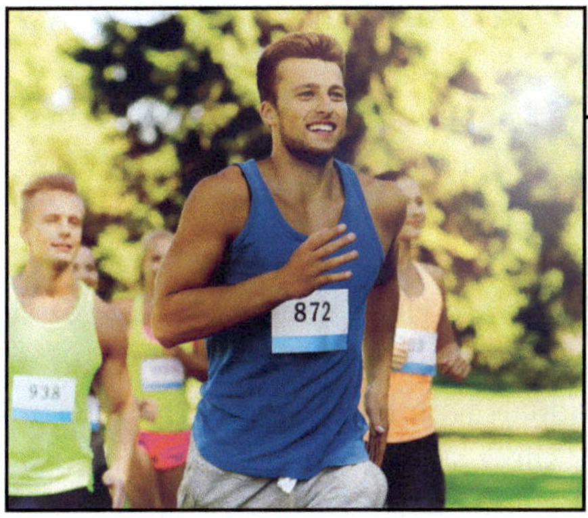

4.1

Myocardial and coronary diseases

Contents

4.1.1 **Hypertrophic cardiomyopathy in athletes** Aneil Malhotra and Sanjay Sharma *179*
4.1.2 **Arrhythmogenic cardiomyopathy and sudden death in young athletes: causes, pathophysiology, and clinical features** Gaetano Thiene, Kalliopi Pilichou, Stefania Rizzo, and Cristina Basso *184*
4.1.3 **Myocarditis in athletes** Martin Halle *201*
4.1.4 **Differentiating athlete's heart from left ventricular non-compaction cardiomyopathy** Andrew D'Silva and Sanjay Sharma *209*
4.1.5 **Congenital coronary artery anomalies** Cristina Basso, Carla Frescura, Stefania Rizzo, and Gaetano Thiene *217*

4.1.1 Hypertrophic cardiomyopathy in athletes

Aneil Malhotra and Sanjay Sharma

Introduction

Hypertrophic cardiomyopathy (HCM) is an inherited primary myocardial disorder that is characterized by left ventricular hypertrophy (LVH), impaired LV relaxation, and dynamic LV outflow tract obstruction (LVOTO) [1]. Just over 60% of cases can be explained by mutations within genes encoding sarcomeric contractile proteins [2]. A combination of myocyte disarray, fibrosis, small vessel disease, and altered calcium kinetics predisposes an affected individual to potentially fatal arrhythmias; sudden cardiac death (SCD) is the most feared complication, particularly in young individuals including athletes.

Prevalence of hypertrophic cardiomyopathy

Hypertrophic cardiomyopathy is one of the most common genetic diseases worldwide, with an autosomal dominant inheritance pattern and a prevalence of 1 in 500 [3]. The vast majority of affected individuals have a relatively benign disease course, and many cases are detected incidentally or during family screening. However, a minority die suddenly without warning, usually during the second and third decades of life. The risk of sudden death among exercising individuals is increased threefold, suggesting that the adrenergic surges from physical and metabolic stressors of exercise are a trigger for malignant tachyarrhythmias [4,5].

Hypertrophic cardiomyopathy in relation to sport

Hypertrophic cardiomyopathy is conventionally regarded as the commonest cause of SCD in young athletes (<35 years old) [6-8]. Based on the largest series of SCD in athletes (over 1800), HCM accounted for almost 40% of cases [8]. The vast majority of affected athletes are aged between 15 and 25 years. There is a strong male predisposition with a ratio of 9:1. Data from the UK and USA suggest that black athletes have a higher risk of exercise-related SCD caused by HCM than white athletes [9,10]. Most deaths occur in sports involving explosive bursts of sprinting, such as basketball and soccer. The majority of deaths occur during or immediately after sport and >80% of athletes are asymptomatic prior to the sentinel event.

Few studies have examined the prevalence HCM in highly trained athletes, and occasional case reports describe the presence of HCM in individuals with an active lifestyle who participate in sport. However, intuitively the combination of impaired myocardial relaxation and dynamic LVOTO is likely to select out the most affected individuals from highly competitive sport. In a study of over 3000 elite British athletes, only two were considered to have findings consistent with morphologically mild HCM, resulting in a prevalence of 1 in 1500 [7]. A similar prevalence based on history, examination, and 12-lead ECG was reported from the 25-year Italian screening programme of over 33,000 young athletes [11].

Diagnosis of hypertrophic cardiomyopathy in athletes

Hypertrophic cardiomyopathy is classically characterized by asymmetric septal hypertrophy with a maximum LV wall thickness ≥15mm in adults or a *Z* score >9 (Z score >2 in adolescents and children) [1]. Most affected individuals have a relatively small LV cavity size, a hyperdynamic systolic function, and impaired myocardial relaxation [12]. Approximately one-third of patients exhibit systolic anterior motion of the anterior mitral valve leaflet leading to dynamic LVOTO. The prevalence of LVOTO may be as high as 70% during exercise [13].

Differentiation of physiological LVH from HCM in athletes

Differentiation between physiological LVH as a response to regular intense bouts of exercise and morphologically mild HCM is crucial since an erroneous diagnosis has the potential for serious consequences [14]. For example, mislabelling an athlete with diagnosis of cardiomyopathy can lead to unnecessary disqualification from competitive sport, physical and psychological harm, and the potential loss of financial rewards. Conversely, false reassurance in an individual with HCM may jeopardize a young life.

It is well established that regular intensive exercise is associated with a 10–20% increase in LV wall thickness [12]. The vast majority of athletes have an LV wall thickness measurement within normal limits (7–12mm), but 2% of a large cohort of white male endurance athletes showed a wall thickness between 13 and 15mm, which is consistent with morphologically mild HCM [6,7]. The issue is more pertinent in black athletes who generally mount a greater hypertrophic response [15,16]. Previous studies of large cohorts of adult black male athletes have shown that 13–18% engaged in high dynamic sport revealed LV wall thickness measurements >12mm, although never exceeding 16mm [16]. The hypertrophic response is also observed in adolescent black males where 7% show an LV wall thickness of 13–15mm [16].

Conventional parameters used to distinguish physiological LVH from HCM are based on data from studies comparing athletes with physiological LVH with sedentary HCM patients [17,18]. In general, patients with HCM reveal asymmetric LVH, a smaller or not enlarged LV cavity, and abnormal indices of diastolic function. However, considering that athletes with HCM demonstrate a greater functional capacity than sedentary HCM patients [19], it is possible that individuals with HCM who have exercised since childhood may show structural and functional features that are conducive to augmentation of a large stroke volume during exercise. Recent studies have focused on direct comparisons between athletes with HCM and those with physiological LVH [19,20] to provide a clearer understanding of the morphological features of HCM in an exercising individual (➲ Fig. 4.1.1.1). Most data in athletes are derived from observational studies using echocardiography as the only imaging modality. In practice, however, diagnostic algorithms incorporating clinical symptoms and family history, ECG, cardiac imaging (echocardiography and CMR), and exercise stress testing are more useful for facilitating the differentiation (➲ Fig. 4.1.1.2).

Electrocardiogram

Although there are no specific electrocardiographic features to define HCM, abnormal T-wave inversion (TWI) is very common and was observed in over 80% of athletes with HCM in a recent study [21]. In another contemporary study of 106 athletes with HCM and 101 sedentary patients

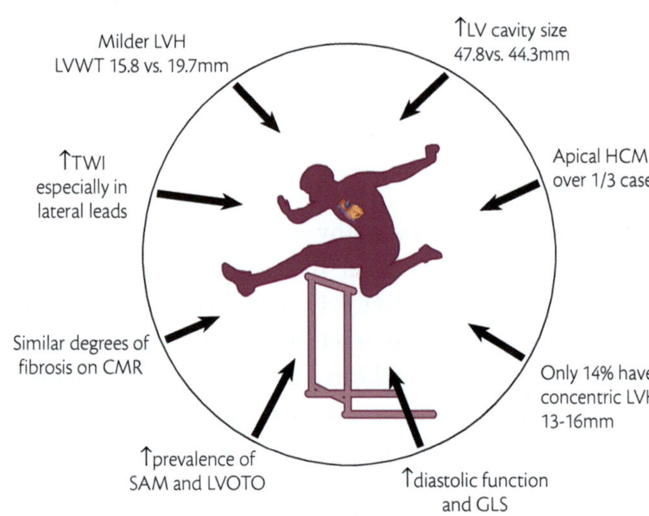

Fig. 4.1.1.1 Characteristics of athletes with hypertrophic cardiomyopathy: CMR, cardiac magnetic resonance imaging; ECG, electrocardiogram; GLS, global longitudinal strain; LV, left ventricular; LVH, left ventricular hypertrophy; LVOTO, left ventricular outflow tract obstruction; SAM, systolic anterior motion; TWI, T-wave inversion; VT, ventricular tachycardia.

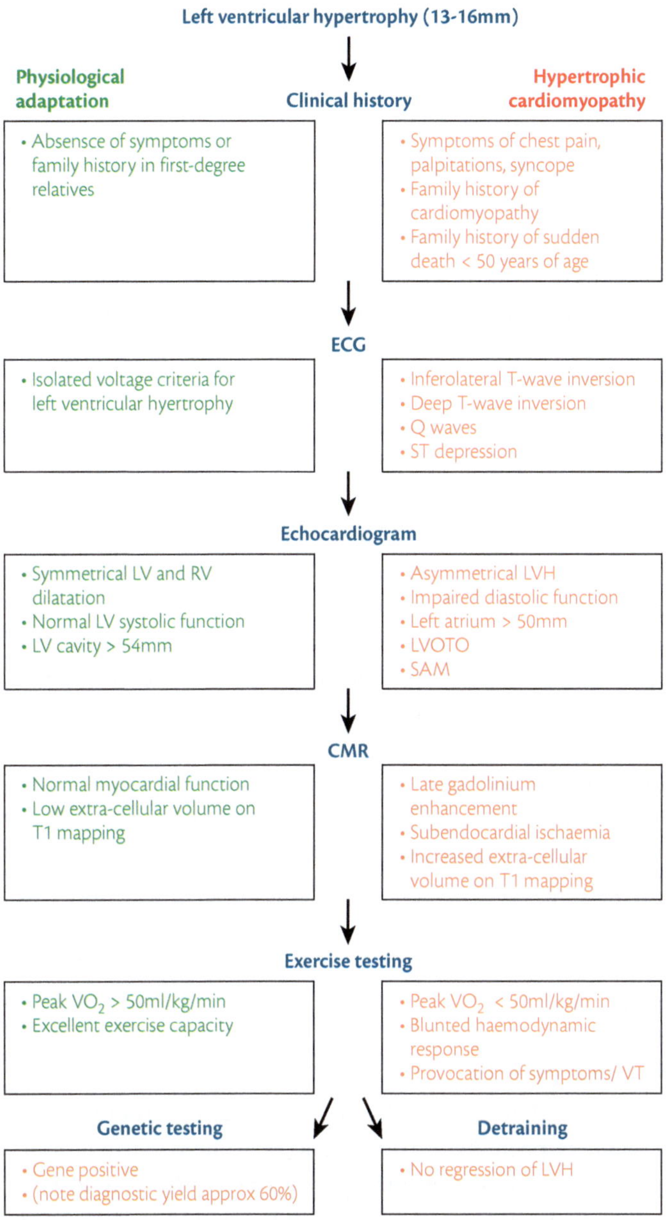

Fig. 4.1.1.2 Clinical tools to aid the differentiation of physiological left ventricular hypertrophy from morphologically mild hypertrophic cardiomyopathy: CMR, cardiac magnetic resonance imaging; ECG, electrocardiogram; LV, left ventricular; LVH, left ventricular hypertrophy; LVOTO, left ventricular outflow tract obstruction; RV, right ventricular hypertrophy; SAM, systolic anterior motion; VO_2, oxygen consumption; VT, ventricular tachycardia.

with HCM, TWI was more common in the affected athletes (96% vs 84%, $p = 0.003$) [19]. The majority of TWI in both groups was deep and affected the lateral leads. Over half of athletes with HCM also exhibited ST-segment depression, and a quarter revealed pathological Q waves. None of these changes were present in a smaller group of 55 healthy athletes with physiological LVH. A measure of caution is related to the presence in HCM patients of normal ECG patterns, or isolated increased R/S-wave voltages in a proportion of 5–10%.

Pattern and magnitude of left ventricular hypertrophy

Athletes with physiological LVH exhibited a homogenous and symmetrical increase in wall thickness. In contrast HCM is characterized relative to LV cavity size by bizarre patterns of hypertrophy that may be asymmetrical, septal, or apical. In addition, the sharp transition from a thickened LV segment to the contiguous ones is a common observation.

In a study comparing 106 athletes with HCM and 101 sedentary HCM patients, athletes with HCM exhibited a lesser degree of LVH (15.8mm vs 19.7mm, $p < 0.001$) and a third showed hypertrophy confined to the left ventricular apex [19]. Interestingly, only 14% of athletes with HCM had mild concentric LVH and would have fallen into the conventional grey zone between morphologically mild HCM and physiological LVH.

Left ventricular cavity size

The vast majority of athletes with physiological LVH demonstrate concomitant LV cavity enlargement ranging between 55 to 70mm [22]. In contrast, individuals with HCM generally have a small LV cavity size of <50mm. More recently, a study comparing 28 healthy athletes with 25 patients with HCM found that an LV cavity size <54mm distinguished pathology from physiology with a sensitivity and specificity of 100% [23]. However, in a study by Sheikh et al. [19], a few athletes with HCM showed an LV cavity even larger than 54mm. In athletes with HCM, with unimpaired physical performance, the enlarged LV cavity is probably a manifestation of adaptation to an increased cardiac workload associated with regular exercise, as opposed to sedentary patients with HCM where the LV dilatation is a marker of end-stage disease with decreased function and a marked reduction in functional capacity [24].

Indices of diastolic function and strain

Diastolic function is reduced in HCM patients because of impaired myocardial relaxation due to myofibre disarray, fibrosis, and impaired sarcoplasmic calcium kinetics. However, most athletes with HCM demonstrate normal diastolic function according to conventional parameters [20]. A study comparing 19 athletes with physiological LVH and 37 athletes with HCM showed that using $e' < 9$cm/s as a cut-off for pathology had a sensitivity of only 35%. The sensitivity fell further to 14% when using an E/e' ratio >12 as a marker of pathology. Moreover, using longitudinal function as a discriminating marker ($S' < 9$cm/s) had the highest sensitivity for identifying HCM in the athlete, albeit at 43%

with a specificity of 84%. Global longitudinal strain (GLS) of more than −10% resulted in a sensitivity of 87% and specificity of 95% for the diagnosis of HCM in a sedentary patient [25]. However, in an athlete a GLS of more than −15% is thought to suggest pathology.

Dynamic left ventricular outflow tract obstruction

Systolic anterior motion (SAM) of the mitral valve against the inter-ventricular septum, causing dynamic LVOTO, is present in approximately 25% of sedentary HCM individuals and up to 70% of cases during exercise [13]. Athletes with HCM do not usually reveal baseline or dynamic LVOTO.

CMR features

Cardiac magnetic resonance (CMR) is mandatory in all athletes with equivocal echocardiographic, ECG, or clinical findings. It has unrivalled value in excluding localized hypertrophy of the LV, which is not properly assessed by echocardiography, such as in the left ventricular apex or the anterolateral segment. Late enhancement after gadolinium infusion is suggestive of myocardial fibrosis, which would be more consistent with diagnosis of HCM.

Although myocardial fibrosis is thought to result in a non-compliant LV and impaired relaxation [26], a similar proportion of athletes with HCM and sedentary patients demonstrated late gadolinium enhancement (LGE) on CMR (33% vs 40.6%, $p = 0.258$) [19]. This highlights the role of CMR in those athletes in whom HCM is strongly suspected. It is plausible that despite similar magnitudes of scarring, athletes with HCM have a lower ischaemic burden in the absence of severe LVH and mechanical LVOTO.

CMR with T1 mapping and extracellular volume (ECV) content measurement has the potential of differentiating physiological LVH from mild HCM. Current data reveal that patients with HCM demonstrate high T1 signals and an increased ECV due to extracellular fibrosis and inflammation. In contrast, physiological LVH is due to an increase in cell size and a relative decrease in the ECV. A study of 30 endurance athletes and 15 sedentary patients revealed that the ECV component of LV mass was similar between athletes and controls, yet athletes showed a significantly higher indexed cellular mass than controls [27]. Furthermore, the highest performing athletes (peak oxygen consumption, VO_2max >60ml/min/kg) had the lowest ECV.

Another study by the same group investigated 16 patients with HCM and 10 athletes with physiological LVH. The HCM group had a higher ECV than the athletes and also demonstrated a strong correlation between ECV and wall thickness. In this study, an ECV of 22.5% differentiated physiological LVH from HCM with a sensitivity of 100% and specificity of 90% [27].

Response to exercise

Almost a quarter of HCM patients demonstrate an attenuated blood pressure response during exercise caused by abnormal vascular tone, small vessel ischaemia, or exertional LVOTO [28] segment depression. TWI or ventricular arrhythmias may also be observed. Athletes with physiological LVH, especially those competing in endurance sports, generally have an enlarged LV cavity and enhanced LV filling in diastole, enabling them to generate and maintain a large stroke volume and cardiac output throughout exercise, associated with a normal increase in systolic blood pressure during exercise (up to ≥200mmHg). A VO_2max of >50ml/kg/min or >120% of age-predicted value has traditionally been used to differentiate physiological LVH from disease [29]. This cut-off was based primarily on white male athletes. VO_2max variations for black athletes and those with HCM are yet to be validated.

The role of detraining

The complete cessation of exercise for 6–8 weeks reverses the structural and electrical changes of athlete's heart, with normalization of ECG repolarization changes and also regression of physiological LVH [30]. In contrast, an athlete with HCM is expected to show a persistent pathological phenotype [31[.

Molecular genetics

A variety of mutations in genes encoding structural and regulatory proteins of the cardiac sarcomere cause familial HCM. Genetic testing may play a role in the diagnosis of patients with morphologically mild LVH (13–16mm) and/or ECG repolarization changes. However, outside the context of family screening the diagnostic yield is low (about 25%). Furthermore, the increasing number of variants of uncertain clinical significance (VUSs) and the time lag before the results are available are important limitations on the indication of routine genetic analysis.

Exercise guidelines for athletes with hypertrophic cardiomyopathy

HCM is an extremely heterogeneous condition with a relatively good prognosis, but the link with SCD during sport means that any form of exercise prescription in such individuals is conservative. The main aim is to encompass as many preventable deaths as possible. Both the AHA/ACC and the ESC recommendations prohibit competitive sports involving medium to high dynamic/static components [32,33]. Indeed, competitive participation is limited to low dynamic and low static sports such as billiards, bowling, and golf.

Advances in molecular genetics mean that an increasing number of asymptomatic individuals are detected through cascade screening. In many circumstances such individuals do not reveal diagnostic phenotypic features of HCM. Exercise recommendations in such genotype positive/phenotype negative (GP/PN) individuals vary between the USA and Europe. The ESC recommendations adopt a conservative approach on the assumption that a genetic mutation might promote arrhythmogenesis, even in the absence of overt LVH. Echocardiographic and CMR studies have revealed subtle impairment of myocardial relaxation and a slight increase in the extracellular cardiac matrix in GP/PN patients [34,35]. Conversely, American studies in GGP/PN adolescents have revealed a low penetrance of disease over a 12-year follow-up with only two of 36 (6%) patients affected [36].

Based on these findings, it seems nowadays clinically sound to permit GP/PN individuals to participate in sports, including those with high dynamic and high static components, with the caveat of regular surveillance of the GP/PN athlete.

Conclusion

HCM has a broad spectrum of phenotypic expression, including a varied degree of LV hypertrophy and cavity remodelling, impaired diastolic function, dynamic left ventricular outflow tract obstruction, and microcirculatory coronary disease. HCM may be compatible even with unimpaired potential to augment stroke volume during exercise and achieve high peak oxygen consumption, and can be found in asymptomatic individuals regularly engaged in sport, although is conceivable that the combination of impaired myocardial relaxation and dynamic LVOTO probably selects out the most affected individuals from highly competitive sport. Differentiating physiological LVH from morphologically mild HCM in the athlete may be particularly challenging, and should be based on critical assessment of the different morphological, functional, and clinical criteria described here to aid the physician in making the correct diagnosis.

Further reading

Malhotra A, Sharma S. Distinguishing physiological left ventricular hypertrophy from hypertrophic cardiomyopathy in athletes. In Wilson MG, Drezner JA, Sharma S (eds), *IOC Manual of Sports Cardiology*. Chichester: Wiley Blackwell, 2017, pp.439–48.

Maron BJ, Doerer JJ, Haas TS, et al. Sudden deaths in young competitive athletes: analysis of 1866 deaths in the United States, 1980–2006. *Circulation* 2009; 119: 1085–92.

Pelliccia A, Maron BJ, Spataro A, et al. The upper limit of physiologic cardiac hypertrophy in highly trained elite athletes. *N Engl J Med* 1991; 324: 295–301.

Sheikh N, Papadakis M, Schnell F, et al. Clinical profile of athletes with hypertrophic cardiomyopathy. *Circ Cardiovasc Imaging* 2015; 8: e003454.

References

1. Elliott PM, Anastasakis A, Borger MA., et al. 2014 ESC Guidelines on diagnosis and management of hypertrophic cardiomyopathy: The Task Force for the Diagnosis and Management of Hypertrophic Cardiomyopathy of the European Society of Cardiology (ESC). *Eur Heart J* 2014: 1–55.
2. Watkins H, Ashrafian H, Redwood C, Inherited cardiomyopathies. *New Engl J Med.* 2011; 364: 1643–56.
3. Maron B, Gardin J, Flack J, et al. Prevalence of hypertrophic cardiomyopathy in a general population of young adults: echocardiographic analysis of 4111 subjects in the CARDIA Study. *Circulation* 1995; 92: 785–9.
4. Corrado D, Basso C, Rizzoli G, et al. Does sports activity enhance the risk of sudden death in adolescents and young adults? *J Am Coll Cardiol* 2003; 42: 1959–63.
5. Maron BJ. Contemporary insights and strategies for risk stratification and prevention of sudden death in hypertrophic cardiomyopathy. *Circulation* 2010; 121: 445–56.
6. Pelliccia A, Maron BJ, Spataro A, et al. The upper limit of physiologic cardiac hypertrophy in highly trained elite athletes. *N Engl J Med* 1991; 324: 295–301.
7. Basavarajaiah S, Wilson M, Whyte G, et al. Prevalence of hypertrophic cardiomyopathy in highly trained athletes: relevance to pre-participation screening. *J Am Coll Cardiol* 2008; 51: 1033–9.
8. Maron BJ, Doerer JJ, Haas TS, et al. Sudden deaths in young competitive athletes: analysis of 1866 deaths in the United States, 1980–2006. *Circulation* 2009; 199: 1085–92.
9. Maron BJ, Doerer JJ, Haas TS, et al. Sudden deaths in young competitive athletes: analysis of 1866 deaths in the United States, 1980–2006. *Circulation* 2009; 119:1085–92.
10. Harmon KG, Asif IM, Klossner D, Drezner JA. Incidence of sudden cardiac death in National Collegiate Athletic Association athletes. *Circulation* 2011; 123:1594–1600.
11. Corrado D, Basso C, Schiavon M, et al. Pre-participation screening of young competitive athletes for prevention of sudden cardiac death. *J Am Coll Cardiol* 2008; 52: 1981–9.
12. Pelliccia A, Maron BJ, Spataro A, et al. The upper limits of physiologic cardiac hypertrophy in highly trained elite athletes. *N Engl J Med* 1991; 324: 295–301.
13. Maron MS, Olivotto I, Zenovich AG, et al. Hypertrophic cardiomyopathy is predominantly a disease of left ventricular outflow tract obstruction. *Circulation* 2006; 114: 2232–9.
14. Bastiaenen R, Raju H, Sharma S, et al. Characterization of early repolarization during ajmaline provocation and exercise tolerance testing. *Heart Rhythm* 2013; 10: 247–54.
15. Basavarajaiah S, Boraita A, Whyte G, et al. Ethnic differences in left ventricular remodeling in highly-trained athletes relevance

to differentiating physiologic left ventricular hypertrophy from hypertrophic cardiomyopathy. *J Am Coll Cardiol* 2008; 51: 2256–62.
16. Sheikh N, Papadakis M, Carré F, et al. Cardiac adaptation to exercise in adolescent athletes of African ethnicity: an emergent elite athletic population. *Br J Sports Med* 2013; 47: 585–92.
17. Sharma S, Maron BJ, Whyte G, et al. Physiologic limits of left ventricular hypertrophy in elite junior athletes: relevance to differential diagnosis of athlete's heart and hypertrophic cardiomyopathy. *J Am Coll Cardiol* 2002; 40: 1431–6.
18. Vinereanu D, Florescu N, Sculthorpe N, et al. Differentiation between pathologic and physiologic left ventricular hypertrophy by tissue doppler assessment of long-axis function in patients with hypertrophic cardiomyopathy or systemic hypertension and in athletes. *Am J Cardiol* 2001; 88: 53–8.
19. Sheikh N, Papadakis M, Schnell F, et al. Clinical profile of athletes with hypertrophic cardiomyopathy. *Circ Cardiovasc Imaging* 2015; 8: e003454.
20. Malhotra A, Sheikh N, Dhutia H, et al. Differentiating physiological left ventricular hypertrophy from hypertrophic cardiomyopathy in athletes: proposed echocardiographic protocol. *Heart* 2014; 100(Suppl 3): A52.
21. Schnell F, Riding N, O'Hanlon R, et al. Recognition and significance of pathological T-wave inversions in athletes. *Circulation* 2015; 131: 165–73.
22. Spirito P, Pelliccia A, Proschan MA, et al. Morphology of the 'athlete's heart' assessed by echocardiography in 947 elite athletes representing 27 sports. *Am J Cardiol* 1994; 74: 802–6.
23. Caselli S, Maron MS, Urbano-Moral JA, et al. Differentiating left ventricular hypertrophy in athletes from that in patients with hypertrophic cardiomyopathy. *Am J Cardiol* 2014; 114: 1383–9.
24. Harris KM, Spirito P, Maron MS, et al. Prevalence, clinical profile, and significance of left ventricular remodeling in the end-stage phase of hypertrophic cardiomyopathy. *Circulation* 2006; 114: 216–25.
25. Butz T, van Buuren F, Mellwig KP, et al. Two-dimensional strain analysis of the global and regional myocardial function for the differentiation of pathologic and physiologic left ventricular hypertrophy: a study in athletes and in patients with hypertrophic cardiomyopathy. *Int J Cardiovasc Imaging* 2011; 27: 91–100.
26. Moreo A, Ambrosio G, De Chiara B, et al. Influence of myocardial fibrosis on left ventricular diastolic function: noninvasive assessment by cardiac magnetic resonance and echo. *Circ Cardiovasc Imaging* 2009; 2: 437–43.
27. Swoboda PP, McDiarmid AK, Erhayiem B, et al. Assessing myocardial extracellular volume by T1 mapping to distinguish hypertrophic cardiomyopathy from athlete's heart. *J Am Coll Cardiol* 2016; 67: 2189–90.
28. Kawasaki T, Azuma A, Kuribayashi T, et al. Vagal enhancement due to subendocardial ischemia as a cause of abnormal blood pressure response in hypertrophic cardiomyopathy. *Int J Cardiol* 2008; 129: 59–64.
29. Sharma S, Elliott PM, Whyte G, et al. utility of metabolic exercise testing in distinguishing hypertrophic cardiomyopathy from physiologic left ventricular hypertrophy in athletes. *J Am Coll Cardiol* 2000; 36: 864–70.
30. Basavarajaiah S, Wilson M, Junagde S, et al. Physiological left ventricular hypertrophy or hypertrophic cardiomyopathy in an elite adolescent athlete: role of detraining in resolving the clinical dilemma. *Br J Sports Med* 2006; 40: 727–9.
31. Pelliccia A. Remodeling of left ventricular hypertrophy in elite athletes after long-term deconditioning. *Circulation.* 2002; 105:944–9.
32. Maron BJ, Udelson JE, Bonow RO, et al. Eligibility and Disqualification Recommendations for Competitive Athletes with Cardiovascular Abnormalities: Task Force 3: Hypertrophic Cardiomyopathy, Arrhythmogenic Right Ventricular Cardiomyopathy and Other Cardiomyopathies, and Myocarditis: A Scientific Statement From the American Heart Association and American College of Cardiology. *Circulation* 2015; 132: e273–80.
33. Pelliccia A, Fagard R, Bjørnstad HH, et al. Recommendations for competitive sports participation in athletes with cardiovascular disease: a consensus document from the Study Group of Sports Cardiology of the Working Group of Cardiac Rehabilitation and Exercise Physiology and the Working Group of Myocardial and Pericardial Diseases of the European Society of Cardiology. *Eur Heart J* 2005; 26: 1422–45.
34. Ho CY, Lopez B, Coelho-Filo OR, et al. Myocardial fibrosis as an early manifestation of hypertrophic cardiomyopathy. *New Engl J Med* 2010, 362: 552–63.
35. Ho CY, Abbasi SA, Neilan TG, et al. T1 measurements identify extracellular volume expansion in hypertrophic cardiomyopathy sarcomere mutation carriers with and without left ventricular hypertrophy. *Circ Cardiovasc Imaging* 2013; 6: 415–22.
36. Jensen MK, Havndrup O, Christiansen M, et al. Penetrance of hypertrophic cardiomyopathy in children and adolescents: a 12-year follow-up study of clinical screening and predictive genetic testing. *Circulation* 2013; 127: 48–54.

4.1.2 Arrhythmogenic cardiomyopathy and sudden death in young athletes: causes, pathophysiology, and clinical features

Gaetano Thiene, Kalliopi Pilichou, Stefania Rizzo, and Cristina Basso

Introduction

Arrhythmogenic cardiomyopathy (AC) is a rare non ischaemic cardiomyopathy with a prevalence in the general population of 1:200 to 1:5000 [1,2]. Awareness that a disease affecting mainly the right ventricle could be a killer of young people and athletes first arose in the 1980s [3,4]. In the 1970s Fontaine and colleagues pioneered the concept of ventricular electrical instability originating in the right ventricle with premature ventricular beats/tachycardia with a left bundle branch block morphology [5]. Subsequently, Marcus et al. [6] described a disease with these ECG features in a seminal paper and named it right ventricular dysplasia; the disease was observed in adults and appeared not to have a malignant course. In 1988 Nava et al. [7] realized that this morbid entity was genetically transmissible with a Mendelian dominant pattern. However, it was not until 1988, in a paper by Thiene et al. [3] published in *The New England Journal of Medicine*, that it became clear that the disease is malignant and is a frequent cause of premature arrhythmic death, often precipitated by effort. The paper was accompanied by an editorial with the eloquent title 'Right ventricular cardiomyopathy: another cause of sudden death (SD) in the young' [8].

Corrado [9,10] focused on this disorder in athletes and demonstrated that, in Italy, it is a major cause of cardiac SD in athletes. The eligibility programme for sport activity had already been initiated in Italy. However, this cardiomyopathy was hidden and unknown, with apparently benign ECG signs (inverted T waves in precordial leads, premature ventricular beats), and some athletes were deemed eligible to participate in sport with catastrophic consequences.

Pathology

The morphological substrate of AC consists of fibrofatty tissue, which is the cause of electrical instability because of delayed impulse transmission within the ventricular myocardium and re-entry arrhythmias [3,11]. This affects mainly the free wall of the right ventricle, starting from the epicardium, and eventually becomes transmural, so it is easily accessible by bioptome in vivo.

The lack of myocardium accounts for ventricular dilatation and development of aneurysms at inflow, apex, and outflow tracts (the 'triangle of dysplasia') [6,11] (➔ Figs 4.1.2.1 and 4.1.2.2). The aneurysm of the inflow tract (diaphragmatic wall under the posterior leaflet of the tricuspid valve) is characteristic of the disease. The ventricular septum is usually spared. Histologically, the left ventricle is almost always involved (70% of cases), and when the disease is extensive it is biventricular (➔ Fig. 4.1.2.3) [11,12]. The involvement of the left ventricle is focal sub-epicardial, quite rarely transmural with aneurysms, and the term 'non-ischaemic left ventricular scar' has been proposed [13,14]. Rarely, only the left ventricle is affected (➔ Fig. 4.1.2.4). Accordingly, as identified by genotype–phenotype correlation studies, the disease may be right, left, or biventricular [15]. This is the reason why the term 'arrhythmogenic cardiomyopathy' has been introduced [16].

Pathobiology

The question is whether the absence of myocardium is congenital (dysplasia = maldevelopment), or the consequence of

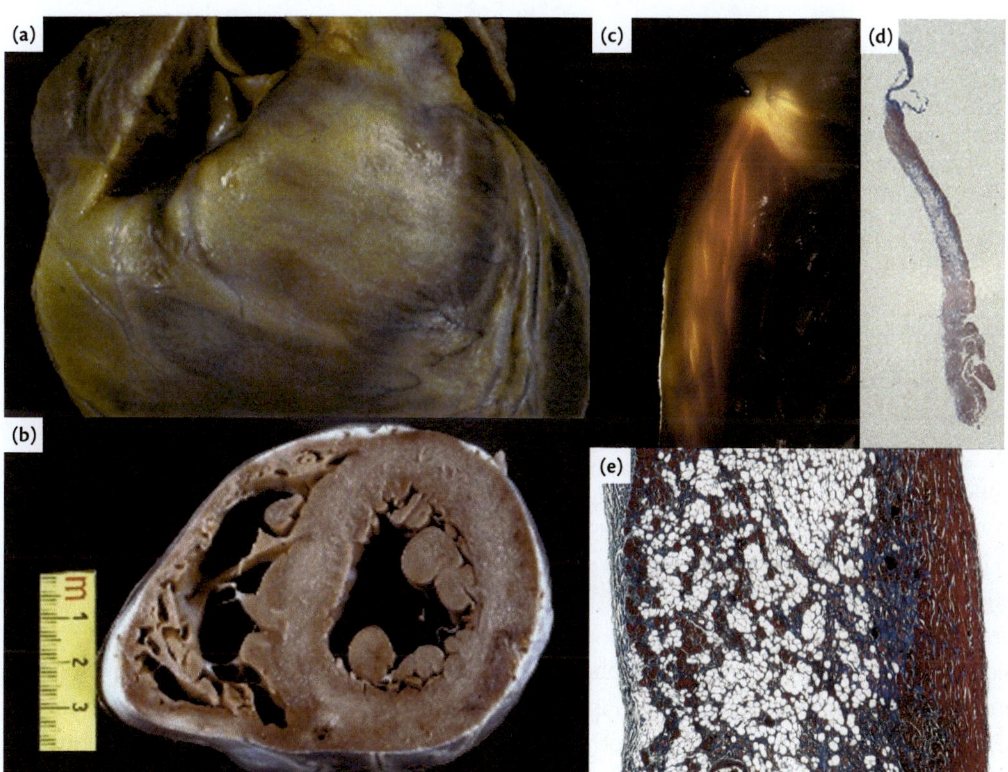

Fig. 4.1.2.1 Sudden cardiac death during exercise in a 26-year-old athlete with the regional form of AC. (a) Gross view of the heart specimen showing a yellow dilated pulmonary infundibulum. (b) Cross=section of the heart with normal left ventricle and ventricular septum and a focal involvement of the posterior right ventricular free wall in the absence of wall thinning. (c) Gross view of the pulmonary infundibulum showing a very thin, translucent free wall. (d) Panoramic histological view of the pulmonary infundibulum showing regional fibrofatty replacement (Heidenhain trichrome); (e) close-up of C (Heidenhain trichrome).

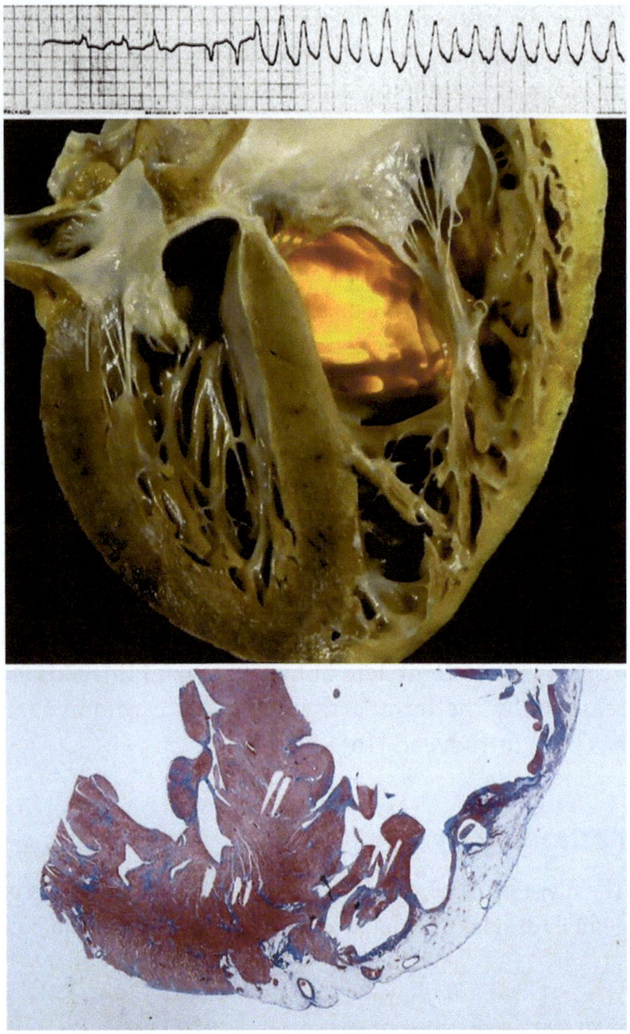

Fig. 4.1.2.2 Sudden cardiac death in a 25-year-old man with the diffuse form of AC. (a) ECG tracing of ventricular fibrillation. (b) Four-chamber section of the heart seen from behind. Note the translucent anterior infundibular wall. (c) Panoramic full-thickness histological sections of the apical segmentt. The transmural fibrofatty replacement of the right ventricle free wall is visible compared with a normal left ventricular and septal myocardium (Heidenhain trichrome).

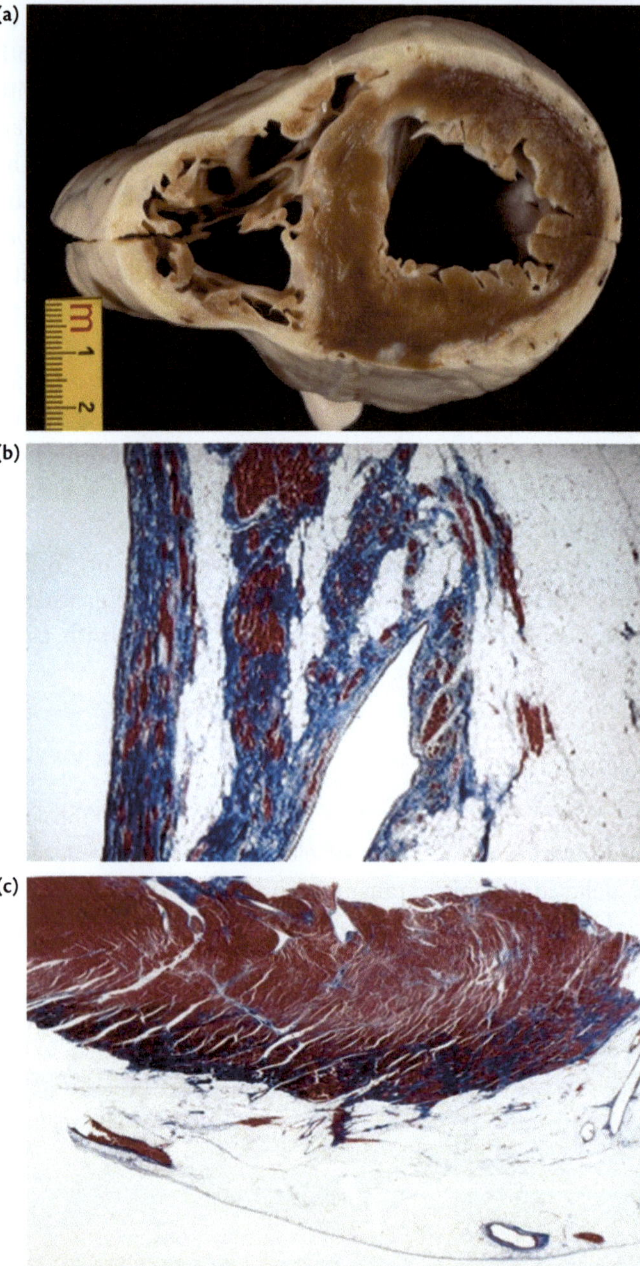

Fig. 4.1.2.3 Sudden cardiac death in a 39-year-old man with a family history of sudden death (two brothers) and complex arrhythmias. (a) Cross-section of the heart showing transmural fatty infiltration of the right ventricular free wall, sub-epicardial involvement of the left ventricle, and preserved ventricular septum. (b) Histological view of the right ventricular free wall showing transmural myocardial atrophy and massive fibrofatty replacement (Heidenhain trichrome). (c) Histological view of the left ventricular free wall showing fibrofatty replacement mostly confined to the sub-epicardial layer (Heidenhain trichrome).

genetically determined progressive cell death (dystrophy), or the sequel of inflammatory disease (myocarditis) with loss of the myocardium [11,16]. The phenotypic expression of the disease usually manifests in adolescence (➲ Fig. 4.1.2.5). Cell death due to apoptosis has been demonstrated both at post-mortem and in vivo, either in explanted hearts at the time of transplantation or in biopsy specimens [17]. Myocardial repair is characterized by both fibrous and fatty tissue taking the place of dying cardiomyocytes [18,19]. Occurrence of the fibrofatty tissue as a scarring sequel of myocarditis cannot be excluded in sporadic non-familial forms of AC. Otherwise, the frequent observation of lymphocytic infiltrates may be simply secondary to cell death (➲ Fig. 4.1.2.6) and the rarity of viral infection favours the hypothesis of inflammation as a reaction to spontaneous cell death [20]. Using histology, Basso et al. [11] demonstrated

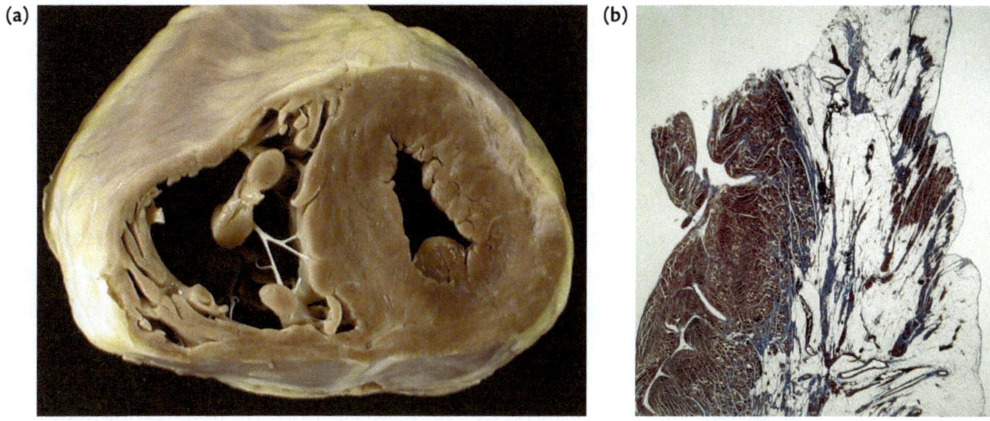

Fig. 4.1.2.4 Sudden cardiac death on effort in a 36-year-old man who was previously asymptomatic. (a) cross-section of the heart with normal appearance of the right ventricular and septal myocardium but whitish appearance of the lateral left ventricular free wall (outer layer) with preserved wall thickness. (b) Panoramic histological section of the lateral left ventricular free wall showing sub-epicardial fibrofatty replacement (Heidenhain trichrome).

that the phenomenon of progressive cell death is in keeping with a myocardial dystrophy, similar to that occurring in Duchenne's skeletal muscular dystrophy (11).

In view of the hereditary Mendelian transmission, the concept of 'genetically determined cardiomyopathy' has been put proposed, with a late phenotypic expression. However, since 1995 the disease has been universally considered to be a cardiomyopathy and is included as such in the WHO classification [21].

The genetics of AC: a desmosomal disease

It was nearly 20 years after the discovery of AC that the disease-causing genes were identified (➲ Fig. 4.1.2.7). A recessive variant was reported in 1986 in the island of Naxos by Nikos Protonotarios (cardiologist) and Adalena Tsatsopoulou (paediatrician) [22,23]. The Naxos disease is a cardio-cutaneous syndrome, with AC in the heart and palmo-plantar keratosis in the skin. What the skin and myocardium have in common is the cell junction

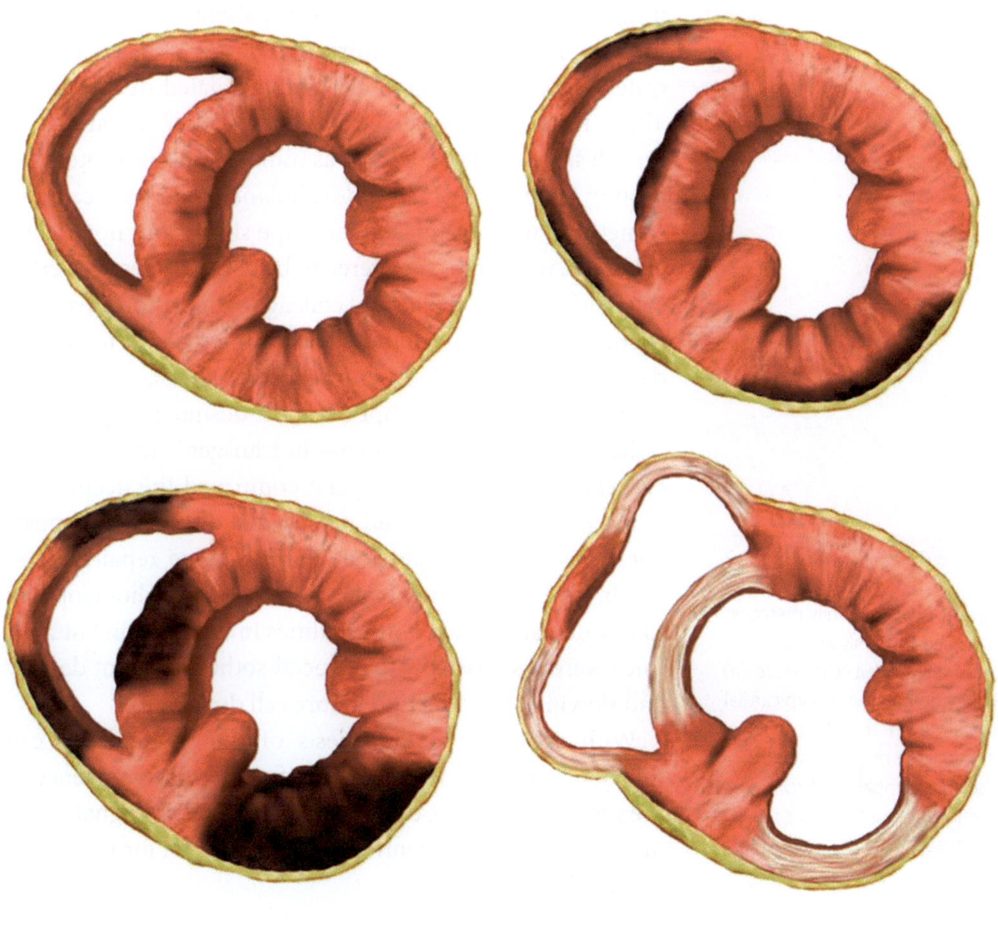

Fig. 4.1.2.5 AC is a progressive myocardial dystrophy (genetically determined cardiomyopathy) with onset after birth (usually during adolescence or young adulthood) with a wave front extending from the epicardium towards the endocardium.

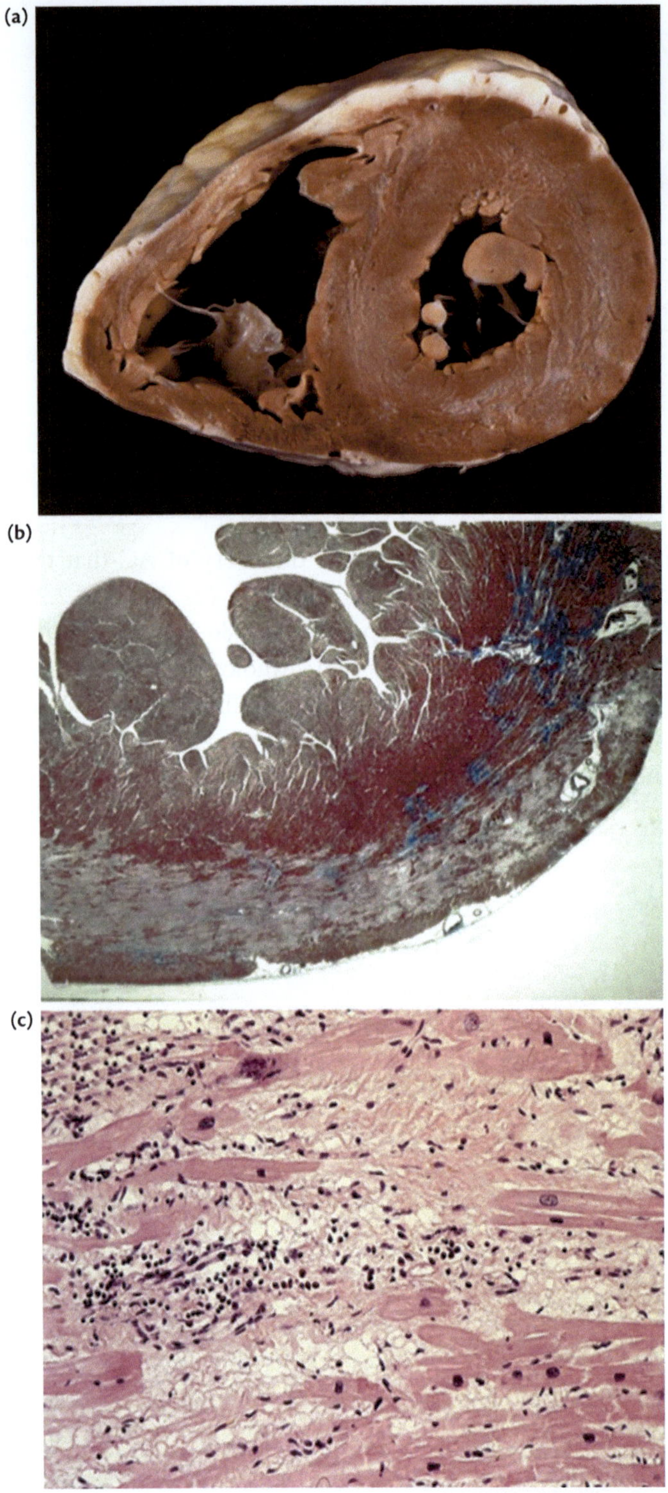

Fig. 4.1.2.6 Sudden cardiac death in a 15-year-old boy, a family member of a proband with demoplakin mutation, who died suddenly at rest despite negative cardiological pre-participation screening a year before. (a) Cross-section of the heart: only a grey band is evident in the sub-epicardial posterolateral region. (b) Panoramic histological view of the left ventricular wall showing a sub-epicardial band of acute–subacute myocyte necrosis with loose fibrous tissue and granulation tissue (Heidenhain trichrome). (c) Myocyte necrosis, myocytolysis, and polymorphous inflammatory infiltrates together with fibrous and fatty tissue repair are visible at higher magnification (haematoxylin–eosin).

apparatus, namely desmosomes. In 1996 a German group from Heidelberg observed that the absence of plakoglobin (PKG) in knockout mice significantly affects the formation of the desmosome, with fetal mice dying from cardiac rupture [24]. Moreover, the authors emphasized that 'in humans the PKG gene was located on chromosome 17q21, a region not yet identified in human cardiomyopathy patients ...'. This information did not escape the attention of the Greek group who in 1998, in association with McKenna and colleagues in London, demonstrated by linkage analysis in the Naxos families that the Naxos disease gene maps exactly to 17q21 [25]. In 2000 they found, by gene sequencing, a deletion of the PKG gene in that region, thus accounting for the Naxos cardio-cutaneous syndrome [26]. Meanwhile, another recessive cardio-cutaneous syndrome, with cardiac involvement equivalent to biventricular AC, known as Carvajal syndrome, was discovered in Ecuador and found to be associated with mutations of the desmoplakin gene [27–29]. This discovery prompted the Padua group to check on the dominant form of AC in families of the Veneto Region of Northeast Italy, and they also found mutations of the desmoplakin gene [30,31]. This confirmed that both the dominant and recessive forms of AC are a desmosome disease, as hypertrophic cardiomyopathy is a sarcomere disease [32]. Mutations of plakophilin-2, desmocollin-2, and desmoglein-2 were then identified in patients with dominant forms of AC, definitely confirming that AC is a genetic disorder of the cell junction at the intercalated disc [33–36]. There have been isolated reports of causal mutations in non-desmosomal genes, such as transmembrane protein 43, desmin, titin, lamin A/C, phospholamban and αT-catenin, sometimes with a clinical phenotype similar but not identical to AC, which are considered to be phenocopies or overlap syndromes [2,37]. Saffitz and colleagues in Boston have used immunohistochemical and electron microscopy to show a decrease of PKG and structural abnormalities, clearly indicating a mechanical disruption of the desmosome [29,38].

Recapitulation of the disease in transgenic mice by overexpression of the mutated gene confirmed the occurrence of a genetically determined myocardial disorder, with postnatal onset and progression, fibrous tissue repairing cell death, and development of biventricular cardiomyopathy [39]. Intercalated disc abnormalities in desmoglein2 mutant mice were associated with reduced sodium current density and slowing of conduction before cell death [40].

With regard to pathogenesis of the spontaneous cell injury, a transgenic mouse model first provided evidence of the suppression of the canonical Wnt/β-catenin signalling of nuclear PKG as representing a possible target for molecular therapy [41].

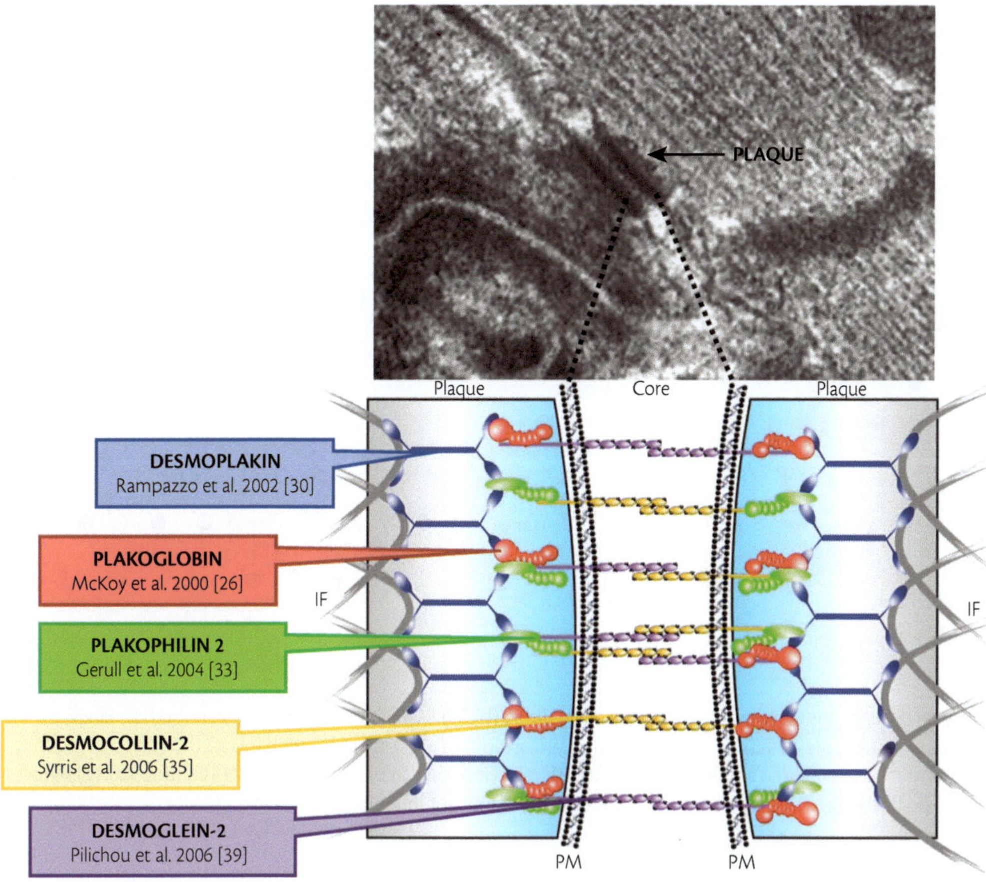

Fig. 4.1.2.7 AC is mainly a desmosomal disease, i.e. a disease of the intercellular junction.

Clinical diagnosis of AC

The challenge is the early detection of the disease phenotype as well as the identification of the gene mutation in the probands and carriers in the family by genetic screening (➔ Fig. 4.1.2.8) [1,2,37,42].

The phenotype consists of the following: (a) ECG depolarization–repolarization abnormalities with electrical instability of the ventricular myocardium; (b) dilatation and decreased ejection fraction of the right ventricle with segmental hypodyskinesia and aneurysm, sometimes leading to congestive heart failure in advanced stages; (c) fibrofatty myocardial replacement.

ECG abnormalities

Depolarization with delay in electrical impulse transmission within the myocardium and widening of the QRS complex, late potentials, and epsilon wave are the clue. Repolarization abnormalities are inverted T waves in the right precordial leads and non-ischaemic ST-segment elevation mimicking Brugada syndrome. Ventricular tachyarrhythmias (premature ventricular beats, sustained and non-sustained ventricular tachycardia) show typically a left bundle branch block morphology, meaning that their origin is from the right ventricle. Inverted T waves in inferior leads, with ventricular tachyarrhythmias of right bundle branch block morphology, are highly suspicious of the left ventricular variant of AC.

Electrical instability may evolve abruptly into ventricular fibrillation and cardiac arrest, which is the nightmare along with the natural history of the disease and the major target for SD prevention.

Morpho-functional abnormalities of the RV

In the past, RV angiography played a fundamental role in detecting RV dilatation, dyskinesia, and aneurysms. Two-dimensional echocardiography is able to visualize these abnormalities non-invasively and is easily repeatable in the follow-up of affected patients. However, tissue characterization is missing with 2D echocardiography.

Tissue characterization

This is only feasible using contrast-enhanced (CE) cardiac magnetic resonance (CMR) [43,44] and electro-anatomic mapping [45,46] and eventually by endomyocardial biopsy (EMB). Electro-anatomic voltage mapping is an invasive electrophysiological tool which is able to visualize

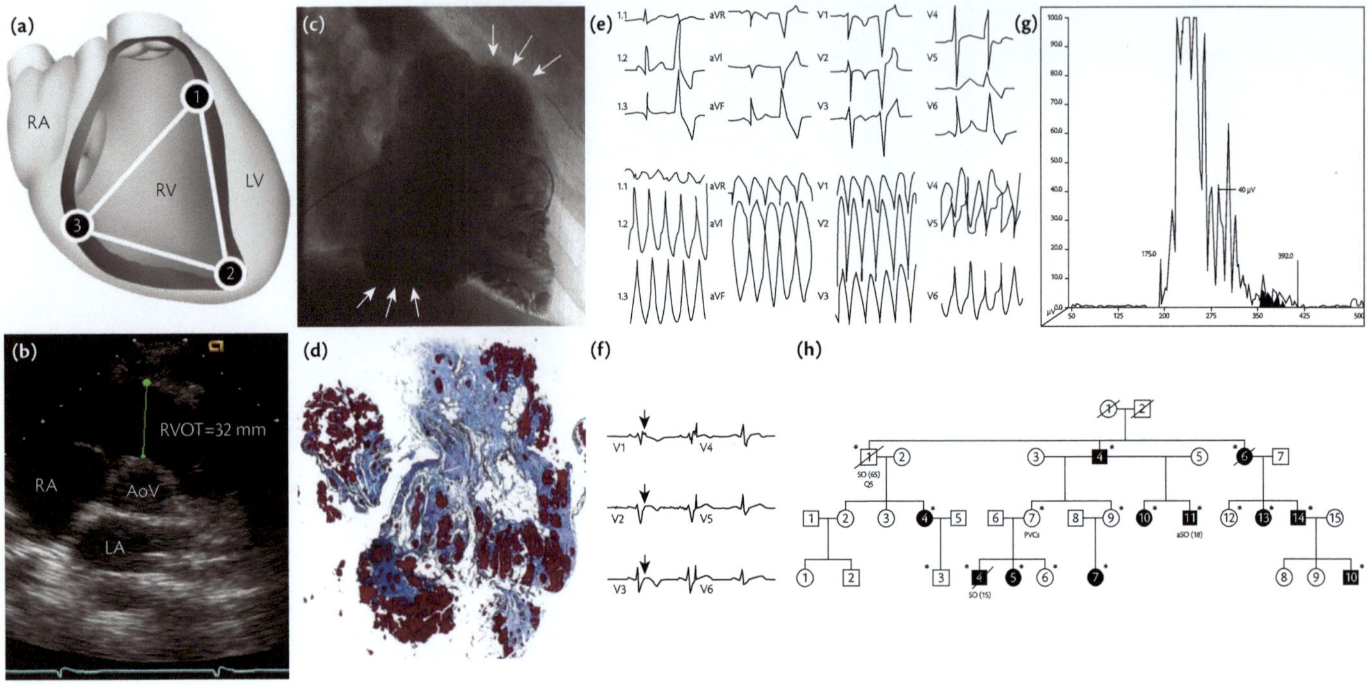

Fig. 4.1.2.8 Diagnostic tools for obtaining a clinical diagnosis of classical right ventricular AC. (a), (b), (c) RV dilatation and aneurysms in the triangle of dysplasia (echocardiography and angiography); (d) tissue characterization using endomyocardial biopsy; (e) 12-lead ECG with inverted T waves V1–V3, left bundle branch block morphology premature ventricular complexes, and VT; (f) post-excitation epsilon wave in precordial leads V1–V3 (arrows); (g) signal-averaged ECG with late potentials (40 Hz high-pass filtering); (h) family pedigree with autosomal dominant inheritance of the disease.

areas of the RV free wall with silent or decreased electrical activity due to myocardial loss/fibrofatty replacement (➲ Fig. 4.1.2.9). Since the RV free wall is thin and difficult to visualize because of the poor resolution power of the CMR, electro-anatomic mapping has been found to be superior in detecting scars in the RV [43,44]. The sensitivity is increased by the using unipolar or epicardial mapping [47]. However, as the LV is usually affected as well, and is the 'mirror' of the RV in CE-CMR, this imaging tool provides the best way of detecting left ventricular involvement, which is usually focal rather than transmural (➲ Fig. 4.1.2.10).

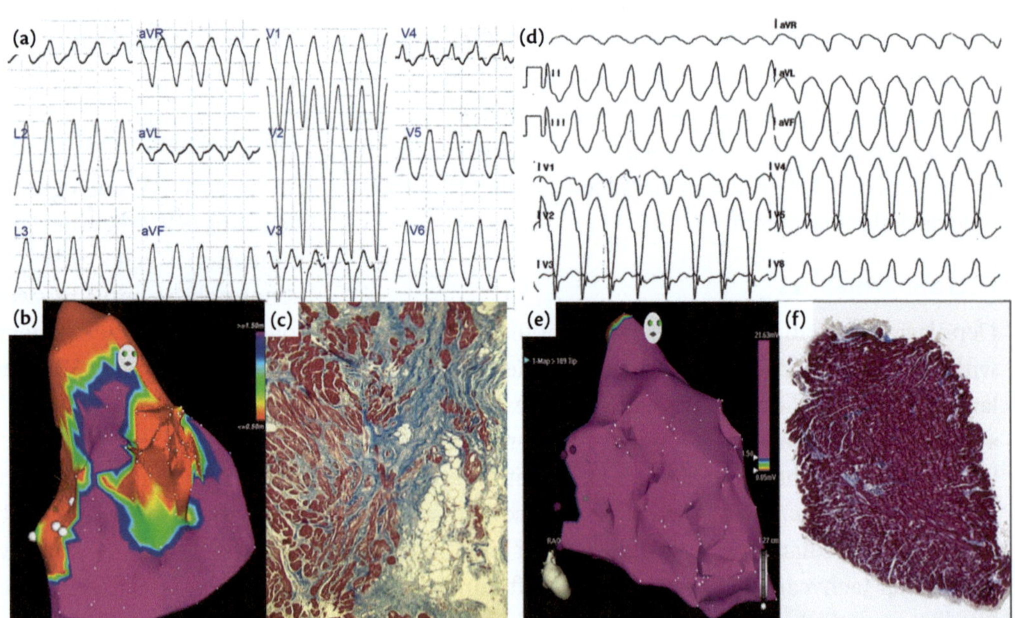

Fig. 4.1.2.9 Electro-anatomic mapping is a fundamental tool in differential diagnosis between AC (a), (b), (c) and phenocopies such as idiopathic right ventricular outflow tract (RVOT) tachycardia (d), (e), (f)).

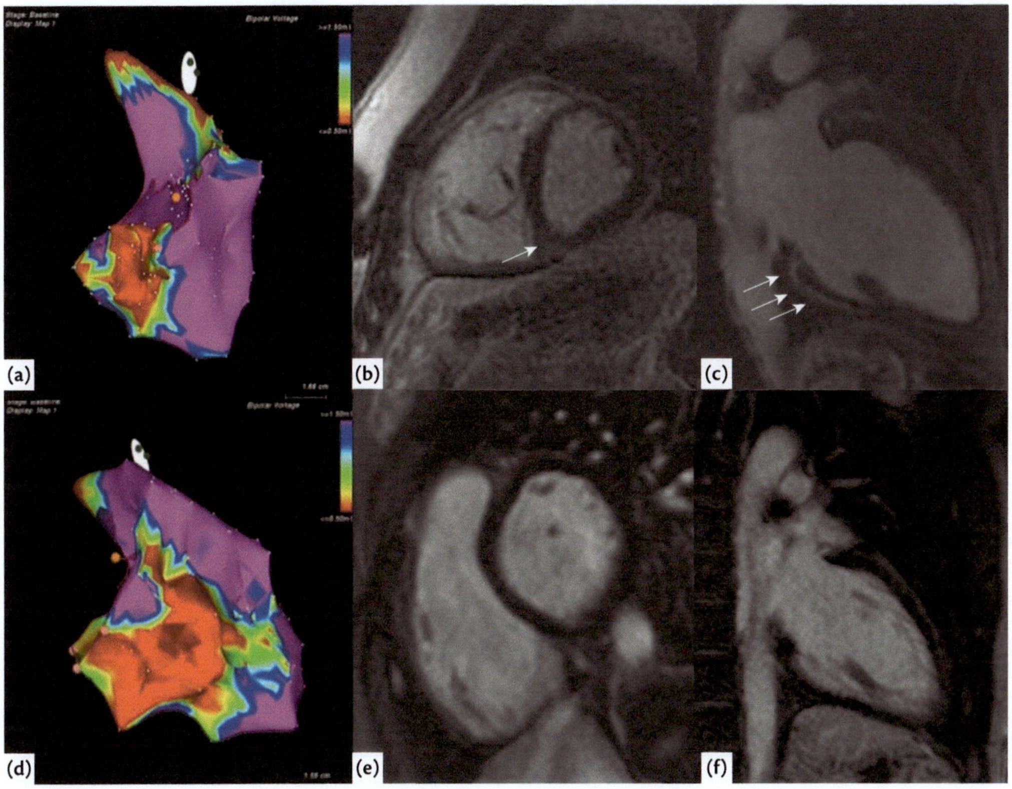

Fig. 4.1.2.10 Electro-anatomic mapping vs contrast-enhanced CMR in AC. The fibrofatty scar pathognomonic of AC is indirectly identifiable through either electro-anatomic voltage mapping as low-voltage areas (normal myocardium, purple), or CMR as late-enhancement areas. While the former is superior in detecting RV involvement ((a), (d)), the latter is often the only tool able to detect the frequent LV involvement (b), (c), (e), (f)).

EMB of the RV myocardium is the most specific method of diagnosing AC by establishing the presence of fibrofatty tissue or excluding 'phenocopies', although it has low sensitivity due to the segmental nature of the disease [48,49]. Residual myocardium less than 50% of the EMB sample has been demonstrated to be diagnostic [42,48] (➔ Figs 4.1.2.8 and 4.1.2.9).

Updated diagnostic criteria in which quantitative parameters were introduced with the aim of increasing sensitivity while maintaining specificity were proposed in 2010 [42]. They are organized in the following categories: (a) morphofunctional alterations by echocardiography and/or CMR and/or angiography;(b) tissue characterization by EMB; (c) repolarization abnormalities on ECG; (d) depolarization and conduction abnormalities on ECG; (e) ventricular arrhythmias; (f) family history including genetics. A definitive diagnosis is achieved in the presence of one major plus two minor criteria or four minor criteria from different categories (➔ Table 4.1.2.1).

Detection of AC in athletes

The Italian protocol for screening for sport eligibility, which includes both family history and ECG, may be sufficient to make the diagnosis when repolarization/depolarization abnormalities (➔ Figs 4.1.2.11 and 4.1.2.12) and arrhythmias are evident, and a family history exists [50]. The Italian protocol of pre-participation screening has successfully detected and disqualified athletes affected by the classical RV variant of AC. The rate of SD in athletes decreased from 4.0 to 0.4 deaths/100,000 athletes/year in the 22 years since the introduction of mandatory ECG at pre-participation screening, mostly because of the identification and disqualification of athletes found to be affected by cardiomyopathies, i.e. hypertrophic cardiomyopathy and AC [10]. However, the early stage of the classical RV AC variant, without dilatation and aneurysms, and the left ventricular variant may not be identificed at first-level pre-participation screening and require a high index of suspicion to proceed to second- and third-level investigations [14,51] (➔ Fig. 4.1.2.13).

The risk of SD from AC has been estimated to be 5.4 times greater during competitive sports than during sedentary activity (➔ Fig. 4.1.2.14) [9]. There are several possible reasons for such a propensity of AC to precipitate effort-dependent sudden cardiac arrest. Physical exercise acutely increases the RV afterload and cavity enlargement, which in turn may elicit ventricular arrhythmias by stretching the diseased RV myocardium. The advent of molecular genetics has provided new insights into the pathogenesis of AC, showing that it is a desmosomal disease. Therefore

Table 4.1.2.1. 2010 Task Force criteria for arrhythmogenic cardiomyopathy

I. Global or regional dysfunction and structural alterations			
Major			
	By 2D echo		
		Regional RV akinesia, dyskinesia, or aneurysm	
		and one of the following (end diastole):	
			◆ PLAX RVOT ≥32mm (corrected for body size [PLAX/BSA] ≥19 mm/m^2)
			◆ PSAX RVOT ≥36mm (corrected for body size [PSAX/BSA] ≥21mm/m^2)
			◆ or fractional area change ≤33%
	By CMR		
		Regional RV akinesia or dyskinesia or dyssynchronous RV contraction	
		and one of the following:	
			◆ Ratio of RV end-diastolic volume to BSA ≥110ml/m^2 (male) or ≥100ml/m^2 (female)
			◆ or RV ejection fraction ≤40%
	By RV angiography		
		Regional RV akinesia, dyskinesia, or aneurysm	
Minor			
	By 2D echo		
		Regional RV akinesia or dyskinesia	
		and one of the following (end diastole):	
			◆ PLAX RVOT ≥29 to <32mm (corrected for body size [PLAX/BSA] ≥16 to <19mm/m^2)
			◆ PSAX RVOT ≥32 to <36mm (corrected for body size [PSAX/BSA] ≥18 to <21mm/m^2)
			◆ or fractional area change >33% to ≤40%
	By CMR		
		Regional RV akinesia, dyskinesia, or dyssynchronous RV contraction	
		and one of the following:	
			◆ Ratio of RV end-diastolic volume to BSA ≥100 to <110ml/m^2 (male) or ≥90 to <100 ml/m^2 (female)
			◆ or RV ejection fraction >40% to ≤45%

II. Tissue characterization of wall		
Major		
	Fibrofatty replacement of myocardium on EMB	
		Residual myocytes <60% by morphometric analysis (or <50% if estimated), with fibrous replacement of the RV free wall myocardium in at least one sample, with or without fatty replacement of tissue on EMB
Minor		
		Residual myocytes <60% by morphometric analysis (or <50% if estimated), with fibrous replacement of the RV free wall myocardium in at least one sample, with or without fatty replacement of tissue on EMB

III. Repolarization abnormalities	
Major	
	◆ Inverted T waves in right precordial leads (V1, V2, and V3) or beyond in individuals >14 years of age (in the absence of complete right bundle branch block QRS ≥120ms)
Minor	
	◆ Inverted T waves in leads V1 and V2 in individuals >14 years of age (in the absence of complete right bundle branch block) or in V4, V5, or V6
	◆ Inverted T waves in leads V1, V2, V3, and V4 in individuals >14 years of age in the presence of complete right bundle branch block

Table 4.1.2.1. 2010 Task Force criteria for arrhythmogenic cardiomyopathy (*Continued*)

IV. Depolarization/conduction abnormalities	
Major	
	◆ Epsilon wave (reproducible low amplitude signals between end of QRS complex and onset of the T wave) in the right precordial leads (V1–V3)
Minor	
	◆ Late potentials by SAECG in at least one of three parameters in the absence of a QRS duration of ≥110ms on the standard ECG
	◆ Filtered QRS duration (fQRS) ≥114ms
	◆ Duration of terminal QRS <40 μV (low-amplitude signal duration) ≥38 ms
	◆ Root mean square voltage of terminal 40ms ≤20μV
	◆ Terminal activation duration of QRS ≥55ms measured from the nadir of the S wave to the end of the QRS, including R′, in V1, V2, or V3 in the absence of complete right bundle branch block

V. Arrhythmias	
Major	
	◆ Non-sustained or sustained ventricular tachycardia of left bundle branch morphology with superior axis (negative or indeterminate QRS in leads II, III, and aVF, and positive in lead aVL)
Minor	
	◆ Non-sustained or sustained ventricular tachycardia of RV outflow configuration, left bundle branch block morphology with inferior axis (positive QRS in leads II, III, and aVF and negative in lead aVL) or of unknown axis
	◆ >500 ventricular extrasystoles per 24 hours (Holter)

VI. Family history	
Major	
	◆ AC confirmed in a first-degree relative who meets current Task Force criteria
	◆ AC confirmed pathologically at autopsy or surgery in a first-degree relative
	◆ Identification of a pathogenic mutation† categorized as associated or probably associated with AC in the patient under evaluation
Minor	
	◆ History of AC in a first-degree relative in whom it is not possible or practical to determine whether he/she meets current Task Force criteria
	◆ Premature sudden death (35 years of age) due to suspected AC in a first-degree relative
	◆ AC confirmed pathologically or by current Task Force criteria in a second-degree relative

Two major, or one major and two minor, or four minor criteria: definite diagnosis of AC. One major and one minor, or three minor criteria: borderline diagnosis; One major, or two minor criteria from different categories: possible diagnosis.

impairment of myocyte cell–cell adhesion may lead to tissue and organ fragility, sufficient to promote myocyte death and subsequent fibrofatty repair, especially under conditions of mechanical stress like that occurring during competitive sports activity. Furthermore, a 'denervation supersensitivity' of the RV to catecholamines has been suggested to explain exercise-induced ventricular arrhythmias [52]. Sympathetic nerve trunks may be damaged and/or interrupted by the RV fibrofatty replacement, which progresses from the epicardium to the endocardium, resulting in a denervation supersensitivity to catecholamines. Arrhythmogenic mechanisms in the highly sensitive denervated myofibres include dispersion of refractoriness and re-entry, triggered activity, or both.

Risk stratification and prevention

The implantable cardioverter defibrillator (ICD) is the main tool for preventing SD. Clinical studies in patients affected by AC demonstrated that ICD delivered an appropriate shock for treatment of ventricular fibrillation or high rate ventricular tachycardia in 25% of people in a four-year

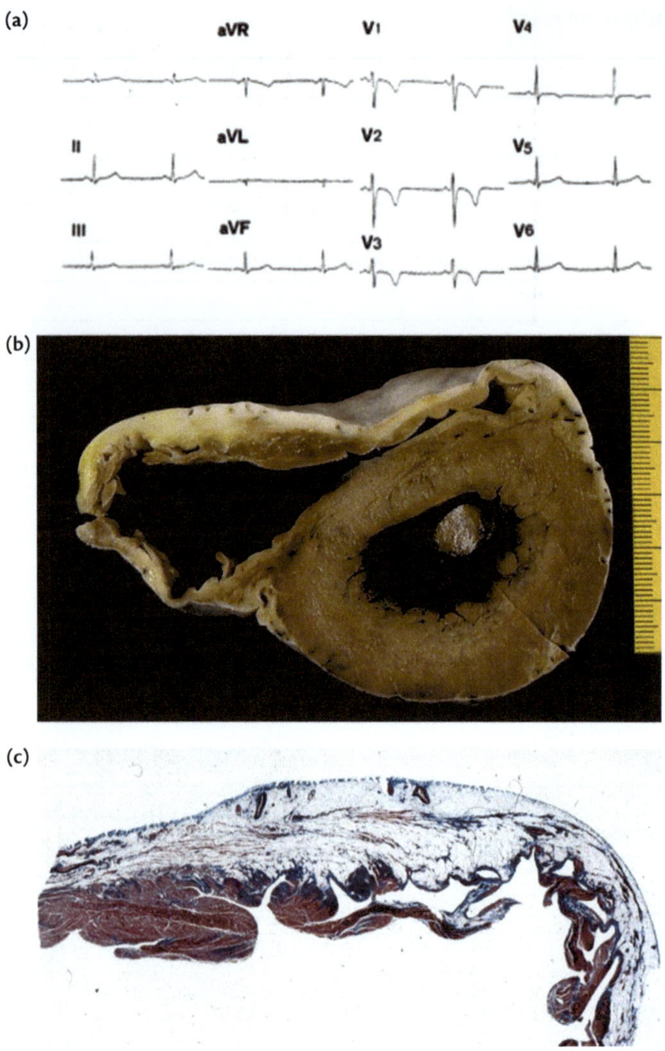

Fig. 4.1.2.11 Sudden cardiac death in a 17-year-old boy with diffuse form AC: (a) basal electrocardiogram showing inverted T wave in the right precordial lead up to V4; (b) gross view of the heart specimen, mid-ventricular cross-section showing aneurysms in the anterior and posterior right ventricular free walls and spotty involvement of the left ventricle; (c) histology of the anterior right ventricle with marked transmural fibrofatty replacement (Heidenhain trichrome).

follow-up, with successful restoration of sinus rhythm (➲ Fig. 4.1.2.15) [53,54]. ICD is truly life-saving; however, the indications for ICD depend on a precise risk stratification in which also the side effects are also considered. A consensus document, separating patients into those with a high annual SD risk (8–10%/year), an intermediate risk (1–2%/year), and a low risk (<1%/year), with ICD indication mandatory, individualized, and unjustified, respectively, has recently been published [55] (➲ Fig. 4.1.2.16). In particular, ICD is mandatory in AC patients with aborted SD, unstable sustained ventricular tachycardia, and cardiac syncope, but is unjustifiable in asymptomatic probands or relatives who are carriers of gene mutations. Compound and digenic heterozygosity was demonstrated to be a powerful risk factor for lifetime major arrhythmic events and SD, supporting the use of comprehensive genetic screening of desmosomal genes for arrhythmic risk stratification in AC [56].

Treatment

To date, only symptomatic therapy for arrhythmias is available because the precise pathogenic mechanisms of the onset and progression of theare still unknown (➲ Fig. 4.1.2.17) [57]. Effort and sport activity are triggers of ventricular tachyarrhythmias which can b fatal, so that life-style changes and disqualification from sport are life-saving per se. Drug therapy, particularly sotalol, and catheter ablation act on the arrhythmic mechanism [58]. Ablation interrupts the re-entry mechanisms of arrhythmias, but it is only temporarily effective and tachyarrhythmias may relapse [59]. ICD reverses ventricular fibrillation and high rate ventricular tachycardia to sinus rhythm. Provision of automated external defibrillators (AEDs) in sports ground is now legally mandatory in Italy,

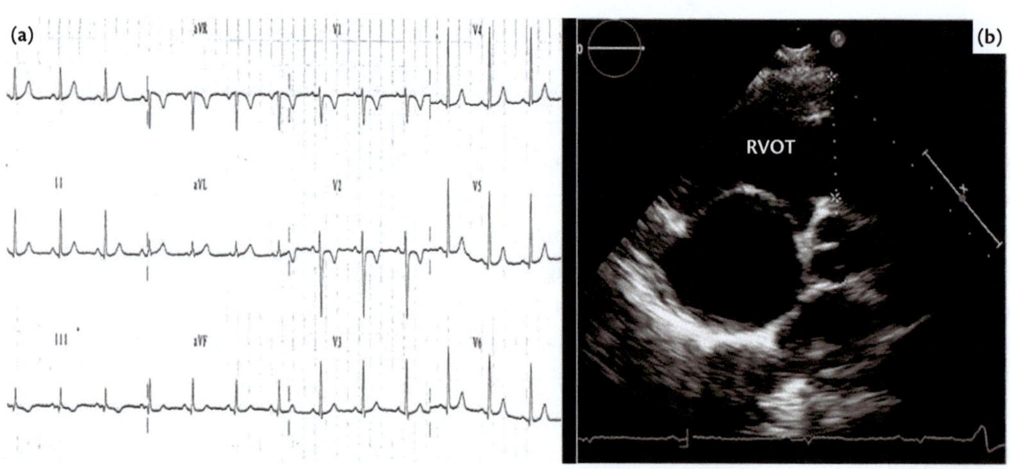

Fig. 4.1.2.12 ECG and echocardiographic findings in a 14-year-old male soccer player with AC who was disqualified from sport activity. (a) ECG shows T-wave inversion in right precordial leads (V_1–V_2); (b) echocardiographic examination reveals RV dilatation (RV outflow tract (RVOT) diameter of 39mm on end-diastolic parasternal short axis view), and RV dysfunction (akinesia of RVOT and posterobasal subtricuspid regions not shown).

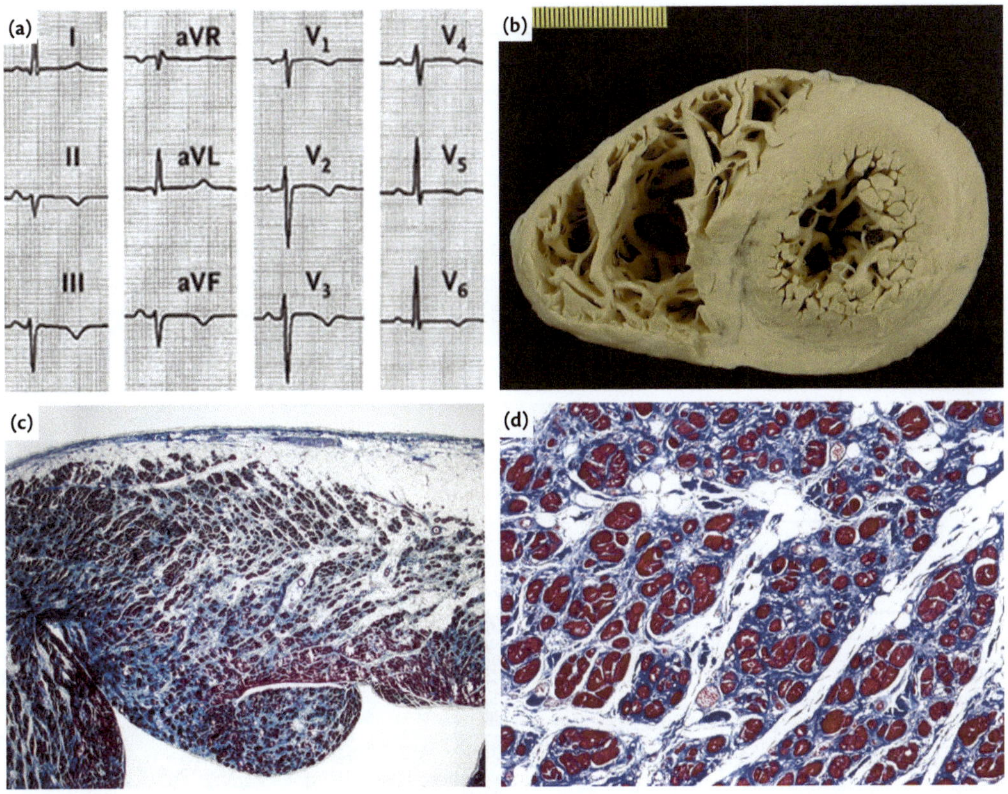

Fig. 4.1.2.13 A 24-year-old national-level canoeist who died suddenly during exercise 12 months after evaluation of undetected AC (normal 2D echocardiography): (a) 12-lead ECG shows diffuse T-wave inversion; (b) gross cardiac findings—cross-section of the heart with a dilated right ventricular chamber, hypertrophied subendocardial trabeculae, and a diffusely thinned (1.5mm in thickness) anterolateral wall (arrowheads) in the absence of aneurysm formation; (c) panoramic histological section of the right ventricular outflow tract showing diffuse fibrofatty replacement; (d) at higher magnification, surviving myocytes (red staining) are embedded within fibrous tissue (blue staining) and fat (white staining).

as is pre-participation screening including ECG. Coaches and players should be trained to use AEDs promptly [60,61].

In advanced AC with heart failure, anticoagulant therapy to prevent thrombus formation in the ventricular aneurysms/diskinetic areas and atrial appendage in the setting of atrial fibrillation is strongly indicated to prevent embolization and stroke [2,58]. In the setting of refractory heart failure or arrhythmic storms, cardiac transplant, to cut the Gordian knot, is the final option. Almost 4% of heart transplant cases are performed on AC patients with these characteristics [62]. Of course, the ideal therapy should be curative, addressing the aetiology and pathogenesis of the disease. Desmosomal gene transfer via injection of an adeno-vector, replacing the defective gene, is still a dream. It has been demonstrated as a promising therapy in catecholaminergic polymorphic ventricular tachycardia knock-in mice, both at birth in preventing onset of disease and in the adult by reverting the phenotype [63].

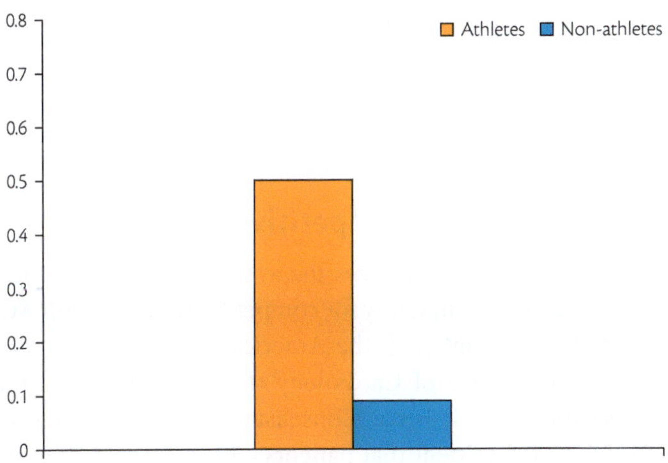

Fig. 4.1.2.14 Incidence and relative risk (RR) of sudden death from AC among young athletes and non-athletes.

Another ideal target is a drug able to stop onset and progression of the phenotype, namely to prevent cardiomyocyte death. Human-induced pluripotent stem cells (hiPSCs) are the new frontier [64–66]. Transforming dermal fibroblasts of AC patients with desmosome mutation, inducing stem cells and then mature cardiomyocytes, may serve to recapitulate the cellular AC phenotype of the patient himself and test an individualized drug therapy in vitro. The zebrafish is probably the ideal experimental model for bench investigation of AC because of its its rapid reproduction and the large number of animals available [67,68]. A drug able to modulate the intercalated disc by interfering with the suppression of canonical Wnt/β-catenin signalling and improving the ventricular ejection fraction has

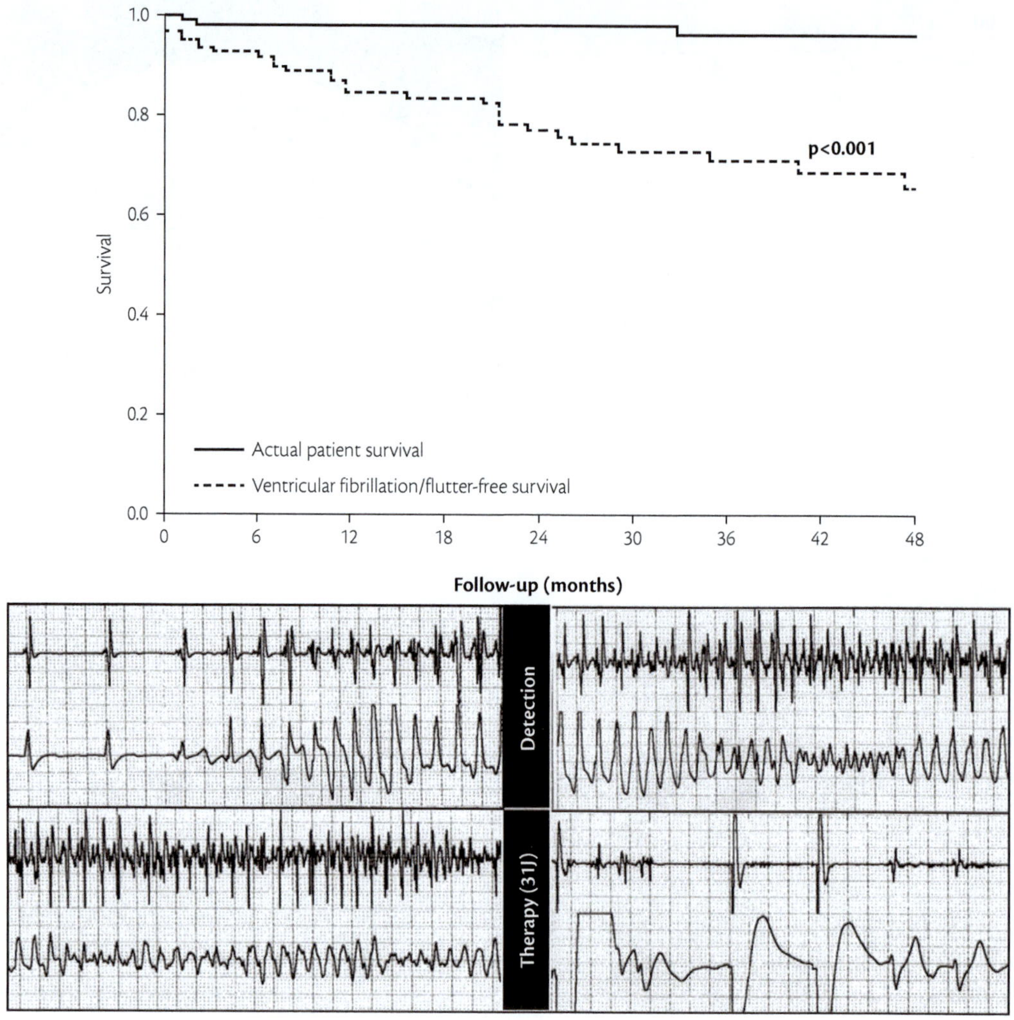

Fig. 4.1.2.15 Kaplan–Meier analysis of actual AC patient survival compared with survival free of ventricular fibrillation/flutter. The divergence of the lines reflects the estimated survival benefit of ICD therapy (25% life-saving effect). An ECG tracing of ventricular fibrillation with appropriate implantable cardioverter defibrillator discharge is also shown.

recently been discovered [67]. Molecular therapy is a new approach to curing and preventing SD replacing symptomatic treatment of arrhythmias.

Can AC be induced by exercise?

The question is whether chronic endurance sports can induce desmosomal stretch and accelerate the onset and progression of AC, as well as triggering electrical instability and SD. Tension is higher when the free wall is thinner (Laplace's law) and this may explain why the RV free wall is more vulnerable. The effect of exercise on individuals with AC is believed to be the promotion of breakdown of the desmosome, which eventually leads to fibrofatty replacement. Heterozygous PKG-deficient mice with demonstrated a clear propensity for developing AC phenotype following sustained exercise [69]. Endurance exercise accelerated cardiac remodelling in mice with over-expression of mutant desmoplakin associated with perturbed Wnt/β-catenin signalling [70]. Exercise has also been proved to increase penetrance and arrhythmic risk in human AC patients carrying desmosomal gene mutations [71–74]. However, the hypothesis of exercise-induced AC has recently been questioned [75,76]. Remodelling of the RV occurs in veteran elite endurance athletes, mimicking athlete's heart, in the absence of dysfunction or scarring [77,78].

Participation in competitive sport

➲ Table 4.1.2.2 summarizes the available consensus statements regarding eligibility for competitive athletes with AC: the ESC statement [79], the American Heart Association/ American College of Cardiology statement [80], and the International Task Force Consensus on the Treatment of AC [55]. It is evident that patients with definite AC (Class I) should avoid competitive sports. Possible exceptions are recreational low intensity sports such as billiards, bowls,

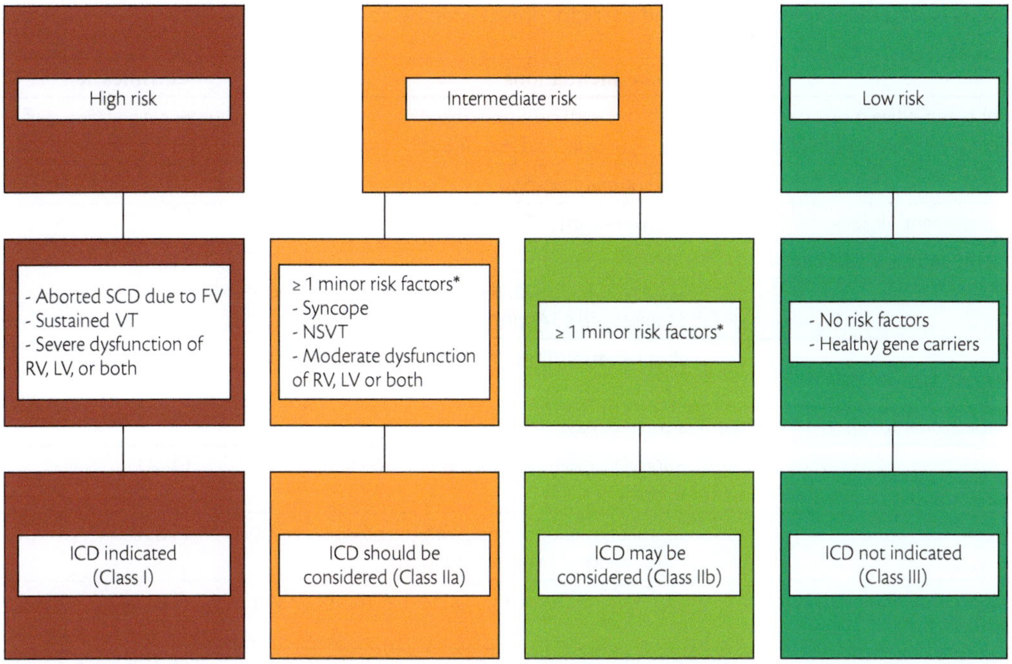

Fig. 4.1.2.16 Flowchart of risk stratification and indications for ICD in AC. The estimated risk of major arrhythmic events in the high risk category is >10%/year, in the intermediate risk category it ranges from 1% to 10%/year, and in the low risk category it is <1%/year. The high risk category includes patients who have experienced cardiac arrest due to VF or sustained VT and most benefit from ICD (estimated annual event rate >10%/year). The low risk category comprises probands and relatives without risk factors as well as healthy gene carriers (estimated annual event rate <1%/year) who do not require any treatment. The intermediate risk category includes AC patients with at least one risk factor, except those included in the high risk category (estimated annual event rate, 1–10%/year). The decision to implant an ICD in these patients should be made on an individual basis. SCD, sudden cardiac death; VF, ventricular fibrillation; VT, ventricular tachycardia; RV, right ventricle; LV, left ventricle.

and golf (class 1A sports). Participation in moderate to high intensity recreational sports is also discouraged. There is less evidence for the recommendations for restriction in asymptomatic gene carriers (genotype positive/phenotype negative) (Class IIa).

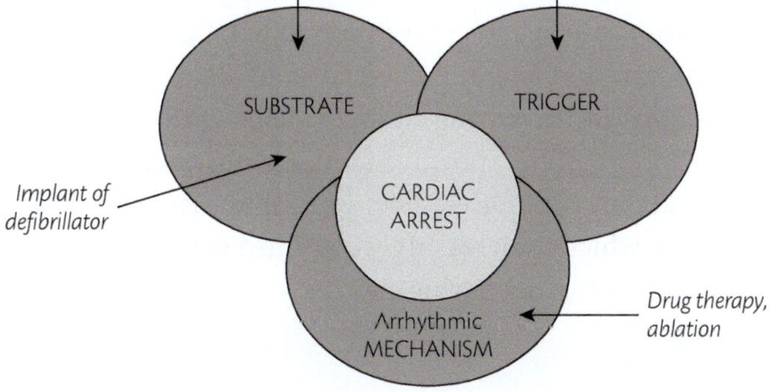

Fig. 4.1.2.17 Cardiac arrest is a combination of trigger, substrate, and arrhythmic mechanisms. Sport disqualification acts as a trigger, and drug therapy and ablation are palliative measures. A defibrillator clearly intervenes on the mode of cardiac arrest, namely ventricular fibrillation. The true method of disease prevention and cure should point to onset and progression of the substrate.

AC and sports cardiology: take home messages

1. AC is a major cause of SD in athletes since effort triggers life-threatening ventricular arrhythmias,because of the electrical instability milieu due to fibrofatty replacement. The risk of ventricular fibrillation is hangs over these athletes like the sword of Damocles.
2. Pre-participation screening, employing the use of ECG, is effective in detecting ECG abnormalities (large QRS, epsilon waves, inverted T waves on precordial leads, and left bundle branch block morphology ventricular arrhythmias) which should raise suspicion of the disease, and indicate additional second- and third-level investigations to obtain a definite diagnosis. The use of CMR, for with potential of detecting both morpho-functional and tissue composition abnormalities, including the overlooked left ventricular involvement, is probably becoming the diagnostic panacea. The mission of the sports cardiologist is not just to disqualify the athlete from sport or to confirm eligibility, but primarily to reach a diagnosis of the disease for appropriate therapy, as the disqualified athlete has now become a 'patient'.

Table 4.1.2.2 Consensus statements regarding AC and participation in exercise

Demographic	Recommendations	Classification
Recommendations for competitive sports participation in athletes with cardiovascular disease: a consensus document Study Group of Sports Cardiology of WG Cardiac Rehabilitation and Exercise Physiology and WG Myocardial and Pericardial Diseases ESC		
Definite AC	No competitive sports	
AHA/ACC Scientific Statement: Eligibility for Competitive Athletes with AC		
Athletes with possible, borderline, or definite AC	Participation in most competitive sports is not recommended, with the possible exception of low intensity class 1A sports	Class III
Athletes with AC	Prophylactic ICD placement to permit sports participation is not recommended	Class III
International Task Force Consensus Statement on the Treatment of AC		
Definite AC	Should not participate in competitive and/or endurance	Class I
Definite AC	Restrict athletic activities; with the possible exception of recreational low intensity sports	Class IIa
AC family members (gene carriers, negative phenotype)	Consider restriction on competitive sports activity	Class IIa
AC family members (negative genotype/phenotype)	Consider restriction on competitive sports activity	Class IIb

International Task Force Consensus Statement on the Treatment of AC (Class): Reproduced with permission from Corrado D, Wichter T, Link MS, et al. Treatment of Arrhythmogenic Right Ventricular Cardiomyopathy/Dysplasia: An International Task Force Consensus Statement. *Circulation*. Volume 36, Issue 46, pp. 441–53. Copyright © 2015 Oxford University Press and the European Society of Cardiology.

AHA/ACC Scientific Statement: Maron BJ, Udelson JE, Bonow RO, et al. Eligibility and disqualification recommendations for competitive athletes with cardiovascular abnormalities: Task Force 3: hypertrophic cardiomyopathy, arrhythmogenic right ventricular cardiomyopathy and other cardiomyopathies, and myocarditis: a scientific statement from the American Heart Association and American College of Cardiology. *J Am Coll Cardiol*, Volume 66, pp.2362–71. Copyright 2015 American Heart Association.

3. ICD is currently the main life-saving tool and should be employed according to risk stratification consensus criteria. An AED must be available in all sports grounds, and coaches and players themselves trained in its use. Prevention of SD by pre-participation screening and AED are not alternative procedures in sports practice, but should work together.
4. When AC is definitively diagnosed, since at least 60% of cases are heredo-familial and present desmosome gene or, more rarely, other gene mutations, genetic investigation should be carried out on the proband. If this is positive, cascade genetic screening should be performed on first-degree family members, associated with first- and second-level clinical study to discover asymptomatic carriers. This is a fundamental approach for primary prevention.
5. Basic research aimed at understanding the pathogenic mechanisms of AC should be encouraged, and sports cardiologists should be part of the interdisciplinary team for investigation and treatment.
6. There is clinical and experimental evidence, albeit controversial, that exercise with RV haemodynamic overload may favour onset and progression of AC, at least in genotype-positive patients. Reduction of sports activity will not only prevent abrupt onset of ventricular arrhythmias and risk of SD, but may also delay phenotype expression.
7. The rarer left ventricular variant (either isolated or dominant) with sub-epicardial focal fibrofatty scar ('non-ischaemic left ventricular scar') is not detected by ECG at first level pre-participation screening, which presents a major challenge for prevention of SD. Careful scrutiny of inferior and lateral ECG leads and widespread use of CE-CMR in the setting of low voltage QRS, repolarization abnormalities, positive family history, and syncopal episodes are all of great help in raising suspicion of this variant, which is increasingly identified in the clinical setting and risk of SD during exercise.

Further reading

Basso C, Bauce B, Corrado D, Thiene G. Pathophysiology of arrhythmogenic cardiomyopathy. *Nat Rev Cardiol* 2011; 9: 223–33.

Basso C, Corrado D, Marcus FI, et al. Arrhythmogenic right ventricular cardiomyopathy. *Lancet* 2009; 373:1289–1300.

Basso C, Thiene G, Valente M, et al. Arrhythmogenic right ventricular cardiomyopathy: dysplasia, dystrophy or myocarditis? *Circulation* 1996; 94: 983–91.

Corrado D, Basso C, Pavei A, et al. Trends in sudden cardiovascular death in young competitive athletes after implementation of a preparticipation screening program. *JAMA* 2006; 296: 1593–1601.

Corrado D, Wichter T, Link MS, et al. Treatment of arrhythmogenic right ventricular cardiomyopathy/dysplasia: an International Task Force Consensus Statement. *Circulation* 2015; 132: 441–53

James CA, Bhonsale A, Tichnell C, et al. Exercise increases age-related penetrance and arrhythmic risk in arrhythmogenic right ventricular dysplasia/cardiomyopathy-associated desmosomal mutation carriers. *J Am Coll Cardiol* 2013; 62: 1290–7.

Pilichou K, Thiene G, Bauce B, et al. Arrhythmogenic cardiomyopathy. *Orphanet J Rare Dis* 2016; 11: 33.

Thiene G, Nava A, Corrado D, et al. Right ventricular cardiomyopathy and sudden death in young people. *N Engl J Med* 1988; 318: 129–33.

Thiene G. The research venture in arrhythmogenic right ventricular cardiomyopathy: a paradigm of translational medicine. *Eur Heart J* 2015; 36: 837–46

Zorzi A, Perazzolo Marra M, Rigato I, et al. Nonischemic left ventricular scar as a substrate of life-threatening ventricular arrhythmias and sudden cardiac death in competitive athletes. *Circ Arrhythm Electrophysiol* 2016; 9: e004229.

References

1. Basso C, Corrado D, Marcus FI, et al. Arrhythmogenic right ventricular cardiomyopathy. *Lancet* 2009;373:1289–1300.
2. Pilichou K, Thiene G, Bauce B, et al. Arrhythmogenic cardiomyopathy. *Orphanet J Rare Dis* 2016; 11: 33.
3. Thiene G, Nava A, Corrado D, et al. Right ventricular cardiomyopathy and sudden death in young people. *N Engl J Med* 1988; 318: 129–33.
4. Thiene G. The research venture in arrhythmogenic right ventricular cardiomyopathy: a paradigm of translational medicine. *Eur Heart J* 2015; 36: 837–46.
5. Fontaine G, Frank R, Gallais-Hamonno F, et al. Electrocardiographic des potentials tardifs du syndrome de post-excitation. *Arch Mal Coeur* 1978; 8: 854–64.
6. Marcus FI, Fontaine G, Guiraudon G, et al. Right ventricular dysplasia. A report of 24 adult cases. *Circulation* 1982; 65: 384–98.
7. Nava A, Thiene G, Canciani B, et al. Familial occurrence of right ventricular dysplasia: a study involving nine families. *J Am Coll Cardiol* 1988; 12: 1222–8.
8. Maron BJ. Right ventricular cardiomyopathy: another cause of sudden death in the young. *N Engl J Med* 1988; 318: 178–9 (editorial).
9. Corrado D, Basso C, Rizzoli G, et al. Does sports activity enhance the risk of sudden death in adolescents and young adults? *J Am Coll Cardiol* 2003; 42: 1959–63.
10. Corrado D, Basso C, Pavei A, et al. Trends in sudden cardiovascular death in young competitive athletes after implementation of a preparticipation screening program. *JAMA* 2006; 296: 1593–1601.
11. Basso C, Thiene G, Valente M, et al. Arrhythmogenic right ventricular cardiomyopathy: dysplasia, dystrophy or myocarditis? *Circulation* 1996; 94: 983–91.
12. Corrado D, Basso C, Thiene G, et al. Spectrum of clinicopathologic manifestations of arrhythmogenic right ventricular cardiomyopathy/dysplasia: a multicenter study. *J Am Coll Cardiol* 1997; 30: 1512–20.
13. Pilichou K, Mancini M, Rigato I, et al. Nonischemic left ventricular scar: Sporadic or familial? Screen the genes, scan the mutation carriers. *Circulation* 2014; 130: e180–2.
14. Zorzi A, Perazzolo Marra M, Rigato I, et al. Nonischemic left ventricular scar as a substrate of life-threatening ventricular arrhythmias and sudden cardiac death in competitive athletes. *Circ Arrhythm Electrophysiol* 2016; 9: e004229.
15. Sen-Chowdhry S, Syrris P, Ward D, et al. Clinical and genetic characterization of families with arrhythmogenic right ventricular dysplasia/cardiomyopathy provides novel insights into patterns of disease expression. *Circulation* 2007; 115:1710–20.
16. Basso C, Corrado D, Thiene G. Arrhythmogenic right ventricular cardiomyopathy: what's in a name? From a congenital defect (dysplasia) to a genetically determined cardiomyopathy (dystrophy). *Am J Cardiol* 2010; 106: 275–7.
17. Valente M, Calabrese F, Angelini A, et al. In vivo evidence of apoptosis in arrhythmogenic right ventricular cardiomyopathy. *Am J Pathol* 1998; 152: 479–84.
18. d'Amati G, di Gioia CR, Giordano C, Gallo P. Myocyte transdifferentiation: a possible pathogenetic mechanism for arrhythmogenic right ventricular cardiomyopathy. *Arch Pathol Lab Med* 2000; 124: 287–90.
19. Sommariva E, Brambilla S, Carbucicchio C, et al. Cardiac mesenchymal stromal cells are a source of adipocytes in arrhythmogenic cardiomyopathy. *Eur Heart J* 2015; 37: 1835–46.
20. Calabrese F, Basso C, Carturan E, et al. Arrhythmogenic right ventricular cardiomyopathy/dysplasia: is there a role for viruses? *Cardiovasc Pathol* 2006; 15: 11–17.
21. Richardson P, McKenna WJ, Bristow M, ett al. Report of the 1995 WHO/ISFC Task Force on the definition and classification of cardiomyopathies. *Circulation* 1996; 93: 841–2.
22. Protonotarios N, Tsatsopoulou A, Patsourakos P, et al. Cardiac abnormalities in familial palmoplantar keratosis. *Br Heart J* 1986; 56: 321–6.
23. Protonotarios N, Tsatsopoulou A, Scampardonis G. Familial arrhythmogenic right ventricular dysplasia associated with palmoplantar keratosis. *N Engl J Med* 1988; 319: 174–6.
24. Ruiz P, Brinkmann V, Ledermann B, et al. Targeted mutation of plakoglobin in mice reveals essential functions of desmosomes in the embryonic heart. *J Cell Biol* 1996; 135: 215–25.
25. Coonar AS, Protonotarios N, Tsatsopoulou A, et al. Gene for arrhythmogenic right ventricular cardiomyopathy with diffuse nonepidermolytic palmoplantar keratoderma and woolly hair (Naxos disease) maps to 17q21. *Circulation* 1998; 97: 2049–58.
26. McKoy G, Protonotarios N, Crosby A, et al. Identification of a deletion in plakoglobin in arrhythmogenic right ventricular cardiomyopathy with palmoplantar keratoderma and wolly hair (Naxos disease). *Lancet* 2000; 355: 2119–24.
27. Carvajal-Huerta L. Epidermolytic palmoplantar keratoderma with woolly hair and dilated cardiomyopathy. *J Am Acad Dermatol* 1998; 39: 418–21.
28. Norgett EE, Hatsell SJ, Carvajal-Huerta L, et al. Recessive mutation in desmoplakin disrupts desmoplakin-intermediate filament interactions and causes dilated cardiomyopathy, woolly hair and keratoderma. *Hum Mol Genet* 2000; 9: 2761–6.

29. Kaplan SR, Gard JJ, Carvajal-Huerta L, et al. Structural and molecular pathology of the heart in Carvajal syndrome. *Cardiovasc Pathol* 2004; 13: 26–32.
30. Rampazzo A, Nava A, Malacrida S, et al. Mutation in human desmoplakin domain binding to plakoglobin causes a dominant form of arrhythmogenic right ventricular cardiomyopathy. *Am J Hum Genet* 2002; 71: 1200–6.
31. Bauce B, Basso C, Rampazzo A, et al. Clinical profile of four families with arrhythmogenic right ventricular cardiomyopathy caused by dominant desmoplakin mutations. *Eur Heart J* 2005; 26: 1666–75.
32. Maron BJ, Towbin JA, Thiene G, et al. Contemporary definitions and classification of the cardiomyopathies: an American Heart Association Scientific Statement from the Council on Clinical Cardiology, Heart Failure and Transplantation Committee; Quality of Care and Outcomes Research and Functional Genomics and Translational Biology Interdisciplinary Working Groups; and Council on Epidemiology and Prevention. *Circulation* 2006; 113: 1807–16.
33. Gerull B, Heuser A, Wichter T, et al. Mutations in the desmosomal protein plakophilin-2 are common in arrhythmogenic right ventricular cardiomyopathy. *Nat Genet* 2004; 36: 1162–4.
34. Pilichou K, Nava A, Basso C, et al. Mutations in desmoglein-2 gene are associated with arrhythmogenic right ventricular cardiomyopathy. *Circulation* 2006; 113: 1171–9.
35. Syrris P, Ward D, Evans A, et al. Arrhythmogenic right ventricular dysplasia/cardiomyopathy associated with mutations in the desmosomal gene desmocollin-2. *Am J Hum Genet* 2006; 79: 978–84.
36. Beffagna G, De Bortoli M, Nava A, et al. Missense mutations in desmocollin-2 N-terminus, associated with arrhythmogenic right ventricular cardiomyopathy, affect intracellular localization of desmocollin-2 in vitro. *BMC Med Genet* 2007; 8: 65.
37. Basso C, Bauce B, Corrado D, Thiene G. Pathophysiology of arrhythmogenic cardiomyopathy. *Nat Rev Cardiol* 2011; 9: 223–33.
38. Asimaki A, Tandri H, Huang H, et al. A new diagnostic test for arrhythmogenic right ventricular cardiomyopathy. *N Engl J Med* 2009; 360: 1075–84.
39. Pilichou K, Remme CA, Basso C, et al. Myocyte necrosis underlies progressive myocardial dystrophy in mouse dsg2-related arrhythmogenic right ventricular cardiomyopathy. *J Exp Med* 2009; 206: 1787–1802.
40. Rizzo S, Lodder EM, Verkerk AO, et al. Intercalated disc abnormalities reduced Na+ current density, and conduction slowing in desmoglein-2 mutant mice prior to cardiomyopathy changes. *Cardiovasc Res* 2012; 95: 409–18.
41. Garcia-Gras E, Lombardi R, Giocondo MJ, et al. Suppression of canonical Wnt/beta-catenin signaling by nuclear plakoglobin recapitulates phenotype of arrhythmogenic right ventricular cardiomyopathy. *J Clin Invest* 2006; 116: 2012–21.
42. Marcus FI, McKenna WJ, Sherrill D, et al. Diagnosis of arrhythmogenic right ventricular cardiomyopathy/dysplasia: proposed modification of the task force criteria. *Eur Heart J* 2010; 31: 806–14.
43. Perazzolo Marra M, Rizzo S, Bauce B, et al. Arrhythmogenic right ventricular cardiomyopathy: contribution of cardiac magnetic resonance imaging to the diagnosis. *Herz* 2015; 40: 600–6.
44. Perazzolo Marra M, Leoni L, Bauce B, et al. Imaging study of ventricular scar in arrhythmogenic right ventricular cardiomyopathy: comparison of 3D standard electroanatomical voltage mapping and contrast-enhanced cardiac magnetic resonance. *Circ Arrhythm Electrophysiol* 2012; 5: 91–100.
45. Corrado D, Basso C, Leoni L, et al. Three-dimensional electroanatomic voltage mapping increases accuracy of diagnosing arrhythmogenic right ventricular cardiomyopathy/dysplasia. *Circulation* 2005; 111: 3042–50.
46. Migliore F, Zorzi A, Silvano M, et al. Prognostic value of endocardial voltage mapping in patients with arrhythmogenic right ventricular cardiomyopathy/dysplasia. *Circ Arrhythm Electrophysiol* 2013; 6: 167–76.
47. Garcia FC, Bazan V, Zado ES, et al. Epicardial substrate and outcome with epicardial ablation of ventricular tachycardia in arrhythmogenic right ventricular cardiomyopathy/dysplasia. *Circulation* 2009; 120: 366–75.
48. Basso C, Ronco F, Marcus F, et al. Quantitative assessment of endomyocardial biopsy in arrhythmogenic right ventricular cardiomyopathy/dysplasia: an in vitro validation of diagnostic criteria. *Eur Heart J* 2008; 29: 2760–71.
49. Ladyjanskaia GA, Basso C, Hobbelink MG, et al. Sarcoid myocarditis with ventricular tachycardia mimicking ARVD/C. *J Cardiovasc Electrophysiol* 2010; 21: 94–8.
50. Migliore F, Zorzi A, Michieli P, et al. Prevalence of cardiomyopathy in Italian asymptomatic children with electrocardiographic T-wave inversion at preparticipation screening. *Circulation* 2012; 125: 529–38.
51. Pelliccia A, Di Paolo FM, Quattrini FM, et al. Outcomes in athletes with marked ECG repolarization abnormalities. *N Engl J Med* 2008; 358: 152–61.
52. Wichter T, Hindricks G, Lerch H, et al. Regional myocardial sympathetic dysinnervation in arrhythmogenic right ventricular cardiomyopathy. *Circulation* 1994; 89: 667–83.
53. Corrado D, Leoni L, Link MS, et al. Implantable cardioverter-defibrillator therapy for prevention of sudden death in patients with arrhythmogenic right ventricular cardiomyopathy/dysplasia. *Circulation* 2003; 108: 3084–91.
54. Corrado D, Calkins H, Link MS, et al. Prophylactic implantable defibrillator in patients with arrhythmogenic right ventricular cardiomyopathy/dysplasia and no prior ventricular fibrillation or sustained ventricular tachycardia. *Circulation* 2010; 122: 1144–52.
55. Corrado D, Wichter T, Link MS, et al. Treatment of arrhythmogenic right ventricular cardiomyopathy/dysplasia: an International Task Force Consensus Statement. *Circulation* 2015; 132: 441–53.
56. Rigato I, Bauce B, Rampazzo A, et al. Compound and digenic heterozygosity predicts life-time arrhythmic outcome and sudden cardiac death in desmosomal gene-related arrhythmogenic right ventricular cardiomyopathy. *Circ Cardiovasc Genet* 2013; 6: 533–42.
57. Thiene G, Rigato I, Pilichou K, et al. Arrhythmogenic right ventricular cardiomyopathy. What is needed for a cure? *Herz* 2012; 37: 657–62.
58. Rigato I, Corrado D, Basso C, et al. Pharmacotherapy and other therapeutic modalities for managing arrhythmogenic right ventricular cardiomyopathy. *Cardiovasc Drugs Ther* 2015; 29: 171–7.
59. Philips B, Madhavan S, James C, et al. Outcomes of catheter ablation of ventricular tachycardia in arrhythmogenic right ventricular dysplasia/cardiomyopathy. *Circ Arrhythm Electrophysiol* 2012; 5: 499–505.

60. Drezner JA, Rogers KJ. Sudden cardiac arrest in intercollegiate athletes: detailed analysis and outcomes of resuscitation in nine cases. *Heart Rhythm* 2006; 3: 755–9.
61. d'Amati G, De Caterina R, Basso C. Sudden cardiac death in an Italian competitive athlete: pre-participation screening and cardiovascular emergency care are both essential. *Int J Cardiol* 2016; 206: 84–6.
62. Thiene G, Angelini A, Basso C, et al. Novel heart diseases requiring transplantation. *Adv Clin Path* 1998, 2: 65–73.
63. Denegri S, Bongianino R, Lodola F, et al. Single delivery of an adeno-associated viral construct to transfer the CASQ2 gene to knock-in mice affected by cathecolaminergic polymorphic ventricular tachycardia is able to cure the disease from birth to advanced age. *Circulation* 2014; 129: 2673–81.
64. Takahashi K, Yamanaka S. Induction of pluripotent stem cells from mouse embryonic and adult fibroblast cultures by defined factors. *Cell* 2006; 126: 663–76.
65. Kim C, Wong J, Wen J, et al. Studying arrhythmogenic right ventricular dysplasia with patient-specific iPSCs. *Nature* 2013; 494: 105–10.
66. Murray CE, Pu WT. Reprogramming fibroblasts into cardiomyocytes. *N Engl J Med* 2011; 364: 177–8.
67. Asimaki A, Kapoor S, Plovie E, et al. Identification of a new modulator of the intercalated disc in a zebrafish model of arrhythmogenic cardiomyopathy. *Sci Transl Med* 2014; 6: 240–74.
68. Giuliodori A, Beffagna G, Marchetto G, et al. Loss of cardiac Wnt/β-catenin signalling in desmoplakin-deficient AC8 zebrafish models is rescuable by genetic and pharmacological intervention. *Cardiovasc Res* 2018; 114: 1082–97.
69. Kirchhof P, Fabritz L, Zwiener M, et al. Age- and training-dependent development of arrhythmogenic right ventricular cardiomyopathy in heterozygous plakoglobin-deficient mice. *Circulation* 2006; 114: 1799–1806.
70. Martherus R, Jain R, Takagi K, et al. Accelerated cardiac remodeling in desmoplakin transgenic mice in response to endurance exercise is associated with perturbed Wnt/β-catenin signaling. *Am J Physiol Heart Circ Physiol* 2016; 310: H174–87.
71. James CA, Bhonsale A, Tichnell C, et al. Exercise increases age-related penetrance and arrhythmic risk in arrhythmogenic right ventricular dysplasia/cardiomyopathy-associated desmosomal mutation carriers. *J Am Coll Cardiol* 2013; 62: 1290–7.
72. Ruwald AC, Marcus F, Estes NA, et al. Association of competitive and recreational sport participation with cardiac events in patients with arrhythmogenic right ventricular cardiomyopathy: results from the North American multidisciplinary study of arrhythmogenic right ventricular cardiomyopathy. *Eur Heart J* 2015; 36: 1735–43.
73. Perrin MJ, Angaran P, Laksman Z, et al. Exercise testing in asymptomatic gene carriers exposes a latent electrical substrate of arrhythmogenic right ventricular cardiomyopathy. *J Am Coll Cardiol* 2013; 62: 1772–9.
74. Sawant AC, Bhonsale A, te Riele AS, et al. Exercise has a disproportionate role in the pathogenesis of arrhythmogenic right ventricular dysplasia/cardiomyopathy in patients without desmosomal mutations. *J Am Heart Assoc* 2014; 3: e001471.
75. La Gerche A, Heidbuchel H, Burns AT, et al. Disproportionate exercise load and remodeling of the athlete's right ventricle. *Med Sci Sports Exerc* 2011; 43: 974–81.
76. La Gerche A, Claessen G, Dymarkowski S, et al. Exercise-induced right ventricular dysfunction is associated with ventricular arrhythmias in endurance athletes. *Eur Heart J* 2015; 36: 1998–2010.
77. Bohm P, Schneider G, Linneweber L, et al. Right and left ventricular function and mass in male elite master athletes: a controlled contrast-enhanced cardiovascular magnetic resonance study. *Circulation* 2016; 133: 1927–35.
78. Sanchis-Gomar F, López-Ramón M, Alis R, et al. No evidence of adverse cardiac remodeling in former elite endurance athletes. *Int J Cardiol* 2016; 222: 171–7.
79. Pelliccia A, Fagard R, Bjornstad HH, et al. Recommendations for competitive sports participation in athletes with cardiovascular disease: a consensus document from the Study Group of Sports Cardiology of the Working Group of Cardiac Rehabilitation and Exercise Physiology and the Working Group of Myocardial and Pericardial Diseases of the European Society of Cardiology. *Eur Heart J* 2005; 26: 1422–45.
80. Maron BJ, Udelson JE, Bonow RO, et al. Eligibility and disqualification recommendations for competitive athletes with cardiovascular abnormalities: Task Force 3: hypertrophic cardiomyopathy, arrhythmogenic right ventricular cardiomyopathy and other cardiomyopathies, and myocarditis: a scientific statement from the American Heart Association and American College of Cardiology. *J Am Coll Cardiol* 2015; 66: 2362–71.

4.1.3 Myocarditis in athletes

Martin Halle

Myocarditis: incidence and importance for sports cardiology

Acute and subacute myocarditis and perimyocarditis are the cause of sudden cardiac death in 5–25% of athletes [1–4]. The disease is not uncommon and accounts for up to 10% of autopsies in the general population [5,6].

Aetiology

In general, viral infections are responsible for the majority of cases of myocarditis, inducing inflammation of the myocardium with infiltration of inflammatory cells into muscle fibres and interstitium, causing oedema, muscle fibre membrane defects, and eventually apoptosis. All this creates an electrically unstable condition, which favours the development of atrial and ventricular tachyarrhythmias or conduction defects. When the extent of damage to the myocardial fibres is substantial, the process eventually evolves in dilatation and impairment of left ventricular function.

In contrast, pericarditis is primarily limited to the pericardium and pericardial sac; it does not affect the myocardial fibres, but rather induces pericardial inflammation with subsequent effusion. If both the myocardium and pericardium are affected, the disease state is termed perimyocarditis.

Clinically myocarditis and perimyocarditis may present in acute or chronic form, ranging from a pauci-symptomatic presentation to a clinical manifestation of severe heart failure. When dilated myopathy is detected, virus-induced cardiomyopathy is often a clinically derived diagnosis of exclusion, when other causes have been excluded.

Pathogens of myocarditis are mainly cardiotropic viruses, such as adenoviruses, enteroviruses (Coxsackie virus B3, hepatitis C or human immunodeficiency virus), parvovirus B19, or human herpes virus 6 [7]. Therefore, a myocardial manifestation of virus infection in athletes and active leisure-time sportsmen may be suspected particularly during or after an upper respiratory tract infection or gastroenteritis [7] or in those with lowered immune response. The proportion of individuals experiencing myocardial involvement during viral infection is estimated to be approximately 5%, but the majority of them will remain subclinical. As exercise may reduce immunological competence, particularly when performed with strenuous intensity and prolonged duration, it is possible that a locally confined and transient infection may spread, causing more severe disease states.

Other, less common, causes of myocarditis are [8]:

(1) bacterial (*Mycobacteria*, streptococcal species, *Mycoplasma pneumoniae*, *Treponema pallidum*);

(2) fungal (*Aspergillus*, *Candida*, *Coccidiodes*, *Cryptococcus*, *Histoplasma*);

(3) protozoal (*Trypanosoma cruzi*), parasitic (schistosomiasis, *Larva migrans*);

(4) toxic (anthracyclines, cocaine, interleukin-2);

(5) medication (sulfonamides, cephalosporins, diuretics, digoxin, tricyclic antidepressants, dobutamine);

(6) immunological (Churg–Strauss syndrome, inflammatory bowel disease, giant cell myocarditis, diabetes mellitus, sarcoidosis, systemic lupus erythematosus, thyrotoxicosis, Takayasu's arteritis, Wegener's granulomatosis).

Pathophysiology and phases of inflammation

Myocarditis follows a heterogeneous pattern of pathophysiology from viral infection to myocardial inflammation and apoptosis. The interplay between the myocardial microbial-induced agents and the different components of the patient's immune system determines the histological and clinical phenotype [7,9].

Viruses enter the body via the upper respiratory tract, bronchial tree, or gastrointestinal tract, where they may either penetrate the circulation and affect the heart directly or reside into the reticuloendothelial system (e.g. endothelial cells or bone marrow) as an extra-cardiac reservoir, maintaining the potential to infect myocardial fibres at any time later in life [6,8].

Viruses have a distinct pattern of infection. Enteroviruses such as Coxsackieviruses primarily infect myocytes inducing lytic processes, whereas erythroviruses such as parvovirus B19 only infect endothelial cells within the myocardium, thereby inducing apoptosis by endothelial dysfunction and secondary inflammation[7].

This acute phase of myocardial infection is followed by a phase of chronic inflammation with autoreactive immunopathogenesis. This may develop via a persistent viral infection, but is also found independently. This phase is of clinical importance as it determines mid- to long-term myocardial damage with clinical signs of impaired cardiac systolic function and arrhythmias [8].

Special aspects in athletes

Athletes are more exposed to microbes than the general population. There may be an increased risk of infection in certain sports such as orienteering (exposure to ticks and borreliosis) or contact sports with higher potential of droplet infection (e.g. boxing). Furthermore, elite athletes gather in large groups for training in extreme environments (e.g. skiers in Chile, cross-country skiers in Lapland), which further increases the likelihood of infection, and there is also the possibility of impaired immune competence, for example at higher altitudes during mountain training.

Additionally, elite athletes come from all over the world and sport events are organized globally, so that these athletes are all prone to potential infection by microbes during training and competition. These include bacterial infections such as tuberculosis, which is ubiquitous but is more common in third world countries, Chagas disease, which is primarily present in South America, and schistosomiasis (bilharziosis), which is present in Japan, China, Africa, Arabia, South America, and the Caribbean.

Athletes may also be taking medication, such as tricyclic antidepressants, or drugs, such as cocaine. Therefore it is crucial to take a thorough medical history, focusing particularly on travel schedules in the preceding months, in order to make a diagnosis. Thus physicians assessing athletes with cardiac problems should be familiar with characteristic signs and symptoms of diseases including those not commonly present in Europe.

A summary of viral myocarditis is given in ➲ Box 4.1.3.1.

Exercise and myocarditis

Clinical data linking strenuous prolonged exercise to manifestation of myocarditis and deterioration in health have not been assessed in humans, but clinical experience clearly

Box 4.1.3.1 Summary of viral myocarditis

- Pericarditis and myocarditis have to be differentiated, as pericarditis will not affect the myocardium and will have fewer complications.
- Myocardial involvement during viral infection is as large as 5% of the affected individuals.
- Viral myocarditis is primarily caused by parvovirus B19 or human herpes virus 6. Other major viruses are adenovirus and enterovirus such as Coxsackie virus B3.
- Susceptibility to pericarditis and myocarditis is increased after strenuous exercise/competition.
- Fifty per cent of cases of acute myocarditis resolve spontaneously.
- A detailed history, including travel to countries outside Europe, is important for reaching a diagnosis.

shows this relationship. Mild forms of myocarditis or perimyocarditis are more likely to be involved, because of their relatively high prevalence in athletes.

Animal studies indicate that a reduction of immune competence induced by exercise increases mortality in a murine model of Coxsackie virus B3 myocarditis [10,11]. In addition, it has been clearly shown that strenuous exercise may impair immunological competence, increasing the risk of upper respiratory tract infection [12] and possibly myocardial involvement. This is exaggerated in extreme environmental conditions.

Clinical presentation

Athletes are different from sedentary individuals with respect to their perception of clinical symptoms (see ➲ Box 4.1.3.2). As they have been exercising for decades and know their body extremely well at rest as well as its reaction during exercise and recovery, the perception of a mild general decline of exercise capacity or muscular strength, although expressed vaguely, can well be one of the early signs of myocardial involvement in myocarditis. These symptoms often represent a subacute state that will not be diagnosed immediately as myocarditis, as several clinical parameters, including ECG and echocardiography, may be unremarkable. In these cases athletes present with higher heart rates at rest and during comparable exercise intensities, experience muscle soreness, and reduced general 'drive'. In these conditions diagnosis of mild forms of perimyocarditis or myocarditis is difficult, particularly as symptoms include only reduced exercise performance and body discomfort, sometimes accompanied by mild depressive symptoms, which are also characteristic of an 'overtraining syndrome' whose cause is still unresolved but also includes viral pathogens. In all these cases myocarditis should be suspected and be at the top of a clinical work-up list for athletes.

Box 4.1.3.2 Symptoms of perimyocarditis in athletes

- New onset of angina in a young athlete without risk for ischaemic heart disease. Parvovirus B19 is prevalently inducing symptoms of angina because of endothelial involvement.
- Chest pain when lying on the left side in pericarditis.
- Increased resting and exercise heart rate.
- New onset of major conduction disturbances and arrhythmias.
- Impairment of overall exercise capacity.

Typical symptoms that are more straightforward for supporting the diagnosis of myocarditis are chest pain, particularly when lying on the left side in pericardial involvement, and palpitations caused by atrial as well as ventricular arrhythmias. Atrial fibrillation in young athletes is generally rare, but definitely requires a myocardial work-up, including CMR for excluding perimyocarditis (see Case 1 in ➲ Box 4.1.3.3 and Fig. 4.1.3.1). Episodes of atrial fibrillation are almost always self-limiting, lasting for only minutes, but remain indicative of perimyocarditis involving the area of the left atrium. Although the incidence of atrial fibrillation in older endurance athletes is greater and is not usually caused by acute viral myocarditis, the diagnosis of myocarditis has to be excluded. The diagnosis is clear when pericardial effusion is present in echocardiography.

New onset of ventricular arrhythmias at rest or during exercise in athletes should suggest a work-up for acute myocarditis. As athletes are very sensitive to their bodies, these ectopic beats are perceived as palpitations and will often lead to direct presentation to a physician for clinical work-up. Ventricular arrhythmias seem to be more or less independent of exercise. Interestingly, it is often observed that, in comparison with the resting state, the number of ventricular arrhythmias decreases rather than increases during exercise. This is usually different from coronary ischaemia where the number of arrhythmias increases during exercise. Because of a low resting heart rate, often <50bpm in endurance athletes, these ventricular ectopic beats may cause light-headedness, dizziness, or even presyncope.

On routine examination in pre-participation screening, athletes without major symptoms at rest or during exercise will be diagnosed by echocardiography, revealing a reduced left ventricular ejection fraction which is usually mild, but can sometimes be as low as 40%. Also, a pericardial effusion is easily diagnosed in a routine check-up by echocardiography.

Box 4.1.3.3 Case 1

A 20-year-old elite football player in the Russian national team was referred after T-wave alterations had been found in his resting ECG, a finding that had not been present the year before. Apart from general mild fatigue, the athlete had not experienced any specific symptoms such as palpitations, dizziness, or angina, and could not recall any recent acute infection or symptoms such as coughing, sore throat, or diarrhoea. Familial history of cardiac disease or sudden cardiac death was negative. ECG abnormalities included negative T waves in leads II, III, aVF, V4, V5, and V6 (➲ Fig. 4.1.3.1(a)). Echocardiography showed a borderline end-diastolic septal wall thickness (12mm), with normal systolic and diastolic function and no pericardial fluid. Further cardiological examinations, including a 24-hour Holter ECG and cardiac multi-slice computed tomography, which had been performed before in his home country, had not revealed any pathological findings (e.g. coronary sclerosis, aberrant coronary artery ostium, or coronary bridging). CMR was performed to exclude active myocarditis, and revealed signs of a subacute myocardial involvement (➲ Fig. 4.1.3.1b). Viral immune antibodies were negative for common cardiotropic viruses.

The athlete remained clinically stable during a period in hospital. He was advised to refrain from sports completely for six months and was judged not to be eligible for any competitive sport.

Re-evaluation after six months revealed constant abnormal ECG findings, but complete restitution of CMR abnormalities and no myocardial scarring. Because of the overall clinical picture the patient was considered to be eligible for competitive sports despite the remaining ECG changes with T inversions, but with the proviso that he had annual cardiological examination (including resting ECG, maximal ergometry, echocardiography and 24-hour Holter monitoring).

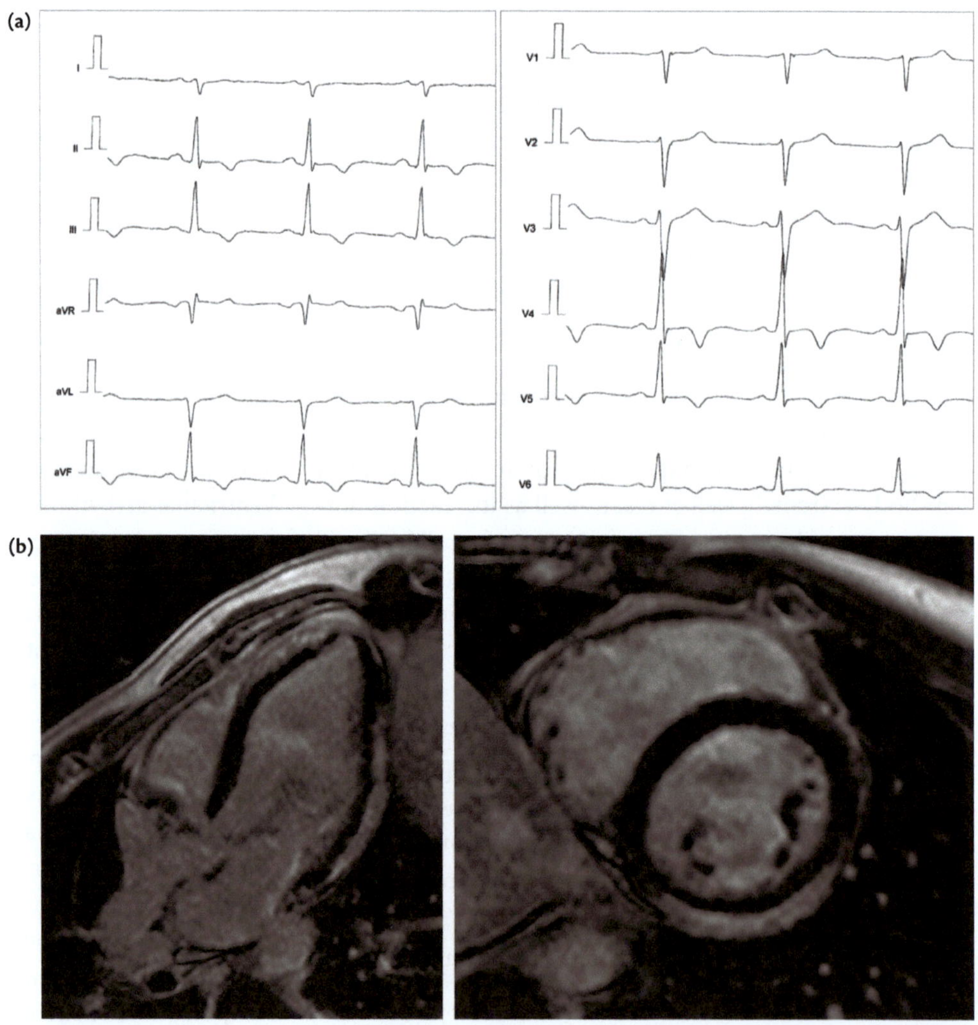

Fig. 4.1.3.1 (a) Typical signs for myocardial injury with inferolateral T waves. However, it is unclear whether this is cardiomyopathy or another form such as in myocarditis. (b) Typical CMR of lateral myocarditis with subendocardial late enhancement.

The effusion is usually small, but sometimes extends up to 1cm or more. In almost all cases a sound clinical work-up will not yield a specific viral antigen. Most of these athletes present in a subacute state of undetected myocarditis. Pericardial effusion will commonly resolve within a month, but can persist for several months in some cases.

Diagnostics

Clinical chemistry

Analyses for the diagnosis of myocarditis, including evidence for inflammation, cardiac biomarkers, and virus serology, are the same for both athletes and sedentary individuals, and include troponin I and CK-MB. However, cardiac markers such as CK, troponin I/T, and myoglobin may be physiologically elevated in athletes *after* an intensive training session or strenuous competition [13]. In addition, only approximately 25% of myocarditis cases reveal elevated troponin levels [14,15]. Virus serology is often inconclusive, and is not generally recommended as serology and endomyocardial biopsy (EMB) overlap in only 10% of the cases.

Resting ECG

Characteristic ECG abnormalities in myocarditis are tachycardia, atrial fibrillation, AV block, low voltage as in pericardial effusion, ST elevation in leads from different regions (lateral, inferior, posterior, anterior), T-wave inversions, and ventricular ectopy.

Atrial fibrillation or atrial ectopic beats, pericardial effusion, and ST elevation are more characteristic of pericarditis, whereas conduction abnormalities or ventricular ectopy are more often seen in myocarditis. ECG abnormalities may be present in combination and then often represent perimyocarditis (see Case 2 in ➲ Box 4.1.3.4 and Fig. 4.1.3.2).

Echocardiography

Echocardiography is mandatory and is a key diagnostic tool in the clinical work-up for myocarditis. Left ventricular ejection fraction and global or local impairment of LV function may be reduced in myocarditis. Regional as well as global impairment is observed. Sometimes a patchy pattern can be seen, mostly in the septal region, but a normal texture does not exclude acute or subacute myocarditis. A slight thickening of the myocardial wall associated with diastolic impairment may also be present. In an elite endurance athlete it is difficult to differentiate an LV dilatation as found in myocarditis from a physiological athlete's heart when previous examinations are not available for comparison.

In addition, a close evaluation of all four valves is mandatory to exclude bacterial endocarditis. A pericardial effusion will lead to the diagnosis of pericarditis. Stress-echocardiography will not yield additional information.

Exercise testing

Exercise testing is not a core diagnostic tool for assessing myocarditis. It rarely adds any diagnostic results beyond resting ECG. During the acute phase ergometry should not be performed, and in the subacute phase exertion should be limited to submaximal intensities. In subacute or healed myocarditis reduced frequency of ventricular ectopic beats is often observed during exercise.

Twenty-four hour Holter monitoring

Monitoring of arrhythmias is an important diagnostic tool in myocarditis and pericarditis during the acute phase

Box 4.1.3.4 Case 2

A 20-year-old national team alpine skier (20–25 hours training per week) presented to the emergency room with acute chest pain on the right side of the thorax after a strenuous exercise session, accompanied by a short period of approximately 10min of irregular and fast heart rate and palpitations. He had had a cold six days before admittance and had stopped training for four days, but then had started again with resistance training. On auscultation he had a regular pulse and pericardial rubbing, and clinical chemistry revealed an elevated C-reactive protein of 8mg/dl but negative cardiac biomarkers. ECG showed sinus rhythm but also ST elevation in almost all ECG leads (➲ Fig. 4.1.3.2(a)). Echocardiography was normal on first presentation, but a pericardial effusion developed during the subsequent two days. No ventricular arrhythmias were seen but a short period of self-limiting atrial fibrillation was detected during his first night in hospital. Anti-inflammatory medication relieved symptoms and a beta-blocker was tolerated initially, but the resting heart rate dropped to 45bpm after two weeks. All medication was then terminated.

Exercise was strictly avoided for six weeks. ECG and pericardial fluid normalized within this period and there was no recurrence of palpitations. Despite medical advice, the athlete started regular training at his own risk after six weeks and gradually increased the amount of aerobic exercise and resistance training because of the approaching competition season. On re-evaluation every six weeks, no pathology was diagnosed and the athlete completed the season without any problems (➲ Fig. 4.1.3.2(b)).

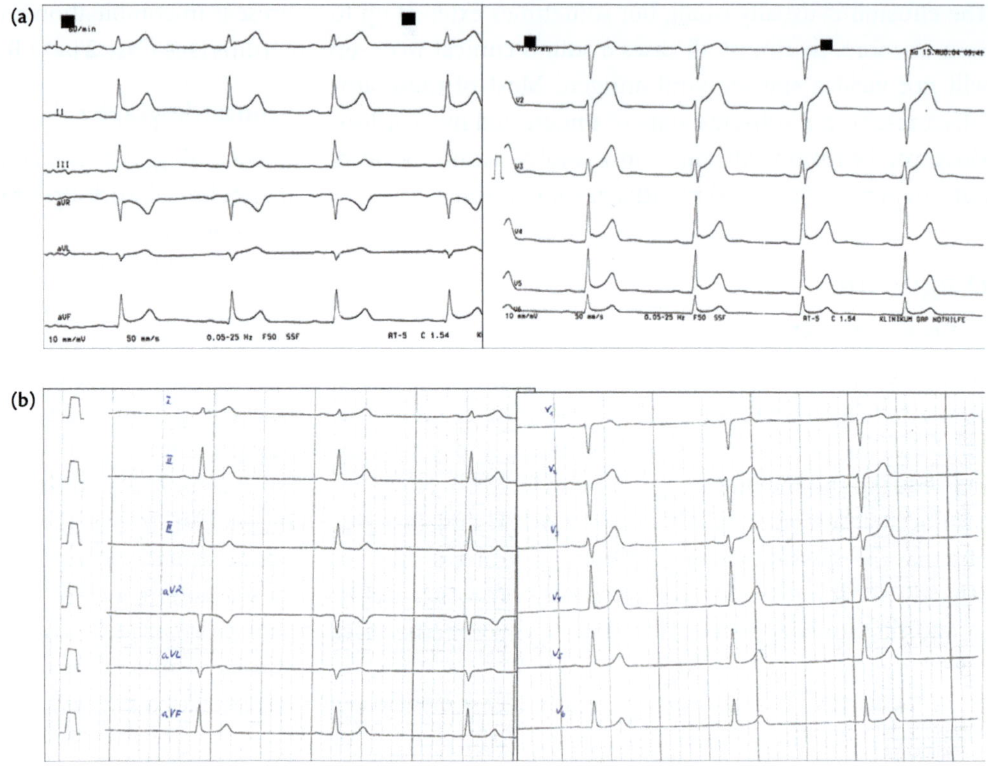

Fig. 4.1.3.2 (a) Typical ECG abnormalities in perimyocarditis with STelevation in most leads. (b) Resolution of ECG changes after two weeks.

and for follow-up. It should be included in the diagnostic work-up performed every six weeks during the first three months.

Cardiac magnetic resonance

CMR is the gold standard for assessing myocarditis because of its ability to assess myocardial oedema and scarring. Nevertheless it cannot replace myocardial biopsy for differentiating between different forms of myocarditis (e.g. giant cell myocarditis and others).

In myocarditis the most important CMR sequences are T2-weighted images for assessing myocardial oedema and late gadolinium enhancement (LGE) for assessing scarring (see Case 1 in ➲ Box 4.1.3.3). LGE reveals a typical sub-epicardial or patchy pattern distributed within the myocardium. LGE is usually localized within the lateral wall (see Case 1 in ➲ Box 4.1.3.3).

Ninety per cent of patients with acute myocarditis have a positive LGE [16]. Persistence of positive LGE is clinically valuable as it is the best predictor of death in patients with viral myocarditis [15] (see ➲ Box 4.1.3.5). It reveals a hazard ratio of 8.4 for all-cause mortality and 12.8 for cardiac mortality, findings which are independent of clinical symptoms. The sensitivity of LGE is approximately 50–60% [15,17]. When morphology and myocardial function are added to LGE, the sensitivity for myocarditis is 84% [15]. This is superior to functional parameters such as ejection fraction, enlargement of the left ventricle, or New York Heart Association (NYHA) class (HR 1.0–2.2. for cardiac mortality) [15]. The presence of LGE places a patient, irrespective of disease entity, at higher risk for sudden cardiac death (SCD). Occurrence of SCD in patients without LGE is very unlikely, even in the presence of impaired LV function [15].

Box 4.1.3.5 Clinical importance of late gadolinium enhancement[15]

- Sensitivity of CMR to detect myocarditis = 53% (100% EMB)
- Sensitivity of CMR + EF + morphology = 84%
- Presence of LGE → odds ratio of 24 for all-cause mortality
  → odds ratio of 37 for cardiac mortality
- LGE has a higher predictability of subsequent cardiac event than EF or NYHA
- Even in NYHA I/II 38% experienced cardiac death despite normal EF
- Positive LGE is NOT a predictor of incomplete recovery (NYHA>I)

Data from Grun S, Schumm J, Greulich S et al. Long-term follow-up of biopsy-proven viral myocarditis: predictors of mortality and incomplete recovery. *Journal of the American College of Cardiology*, Volume 59, pp. 1604–1615. Copyright © 2012 Elsevier.

Endomyocardial biopsy

EMB is the definitive test to confirm myocarditis. However, the indication remains limited and should be carried out in experienced centres, where it can be performed with a low rate of complications. In young individuals with significantly impaired myocardial function and new-onset heart failure it should be performed as soon as possible. CMR may help with guidance to the EMB site. EMB should not be performed in athletes with evidence of pericarditis in CMR without involvement of the myocardium (see ➲ Box 4.1.3.6).

Therapy

Therapy of myocarditis focuses on the treatment of heart failure following the 'unloading heart' principle when function is impaired [9]. Therefore exercise should be strictly avoided. In addition, medication is aimed at blocking neurohormonal activation. Anti-inflammatory treatment with non-steroidal anti-inflammatory drugs (NSAIDs) should be limited to patients with pericardial involvement and symptoms only. The lowest dose required to relieve symptoms should be followed. Colchicine has shown positive effects in both chronic and as acute forms. Immunosuppressive treatment by prednisolone or azathioprine, immunoglobulins, immuno-adsorption, or anti-viral treatment is still being evaluated in research settings. If there is evidence of giant cell myocarditis, this should be treated with prednisolone and azathioprine.

Box 4.1.3.6 Clinical and diagnostic work-up in athletes with suspion of myocarditis

- Myocarditis, pericarditis, and perimyocarditis should be clearly differentiated.
- Serology has a low sensitivity and is generally not recommended.
- Cardiac MR should be performed in *all* patients/athletes with suspected myocarditis.
- Ninety per cent of acute myocarditis reveal LGE in CMR (sub-epicardial, patchy pattern).
- Endomyocardial biopsy should be performed in those individuals with a clinically unstable condition and reduced ejection fraction. CMR is used to guide to the region of biopsy.
- Patients without LGE and EF>60% have a good prognosis.
- Patients with positive LGE should be followed closely. Repeated full cardiological work-up (ECG, echo, ergometry, clinical chemistry, 24-hour Holter and CMR) should be performed for re-evaluation after six months.
- Athletes with myocarditis can resume regular training after complete resolution of the process and at least after six months after clinical resolution of the disease, whereas athletes with pericarditis can return to competitive sports after three months.

Exercise recommendations

Prevention

As a myocardial manifestation of adenovirus and enterovirus infection may be suspected particularly during or after upper respiratory tract infection or gastroenteritis, athletes should be more cautious when they experience symptoms of coughing, sore throat, running nose, or diarrhoea. These viruses are not only cardiotropic, but may also cause peripheral muscle soreness and joint pain often accompanied by a general body tiredness. If this is present or even accompanied by sub-febrile temperatures, the athlete should completely refrain from any strenuous physical activity, as this may further impair immunological response and capacity by increasing the potential for systemic viral circulation and myocardial infection. In addition to this pathological mechanism of immunosuppression by exercise, other mechanisms include increased transition of viruses from the respiratory system to the circulation and impairment of the integrity of the gastro-intestinal tract.

Therefore athletes with a viral infection should be particularly cautious and refrain completely from exercise during the acute phase. The two key components that limit any intentional exercise are systemic tiredness and an increase in body temperature (which may only be slight). Exercise can be started again when these general symptoms of a cold have resolved. It is a generally accepted that a period of at least 3–5 days without symptoms should elapse before starting exercise of moderate intensity. In more severe cases this should be extended to 7–10 days. This strict regime can be modified when mild symptoms, such as those in a mild case of influenza, are present.

Exercise recommendation in myocarditis

In acute severe myocarditis, which has led to admission to hospital and even caused a reduction of left ventricular ejection fraction, exercise is strictly forbidden during the acute phase. The rest period depends on the severity and course of the disease. Therefore resumption of exercise strongly depends on clinical presentation, such as impairment of LV ejection fraction, arrhythmias, conduction ECG abnormalities, or pericardial effusion. In these cases exercise should not be started until six months after recovery [2,18].

Most athletes experience only mild forms of myocarditis, which do not require admission to hospital. However, intentional strenuous endurance exercise is strictly forbidden even in these mild forms. In addition, resistance exercise must not be performed until all symptoms have completely resolved.

Exercise can be increased slowly during the recovery phase. If all the pathologies have resolved, moderate exercise of short duration (e.g. 5–10min) can be performed more times daily. Recovery phases are also very important, and training days should be followed by resting or recovery days. Initial training intensity is strictly submaximal, with lactate levels below 2.0mmol/l or lower than VT1 in spiro-ergometry. Duration can be continuously increased. This should be the primary target before increasing the intensity of exercise.

Eligibility for competitive sports

The official guidelines of the European Association of Preventive Cardiology (EAPC), formerly EACPR, and the Scientific Statement of the American Heart Association [2] recommend that athletes with a diagnosis of myocarditis should be excluded from both competitive and amateur leisure-time sports activity for six months. This covers the whole spectrum of disease when the myocardium is involved, as best documented by CMR.

After this period all athletes should be re-evaluated prior to resuming competitive sports. During this phase clinically stable patients can perform daily activities such as cycling to work, walking, and similar activities. Intensity should clearly be limited to low-moderate physical activity. This intensity is best prescribed in the form of a maximal heart rate assessed in a sub-maximal exercise test (aerobic exercise capacity).

If the myocardium is unaffected and the disease is limited to the pericardium, as in pericarditis, athletes should also be excluded from competitive and amateur sports activities. The exclusion period is shorter than for myocarditis, and exclusion for competitive sports is recommended to be at least three months. If pericarditis leads to constrictive disease, then exercise is limited per se and treatment options should be evaluated.

If symptoms (overall reduced physical exercise capacity or more severe signs such as arrhythmias, impaired ejection fraction, or prolonged signs of myocardial involvement on CMR such as oedema) continue beyond these three or six months, then this period will have to be extended. A work-up for athletes is shown in ➲ Fig. 4.1.3.3.

It is of particular importance to specify activities regarding mode, duration, intensity, and frequency for elite athletes, as they have a different perception of 'low activity' than normal or sedentary patients. In some the advice of 'low activity' is perceived as 'cycling or running for an hour every day'. In addition, golf may be a form of exercise that is perceived by the physician from his or her experience as of low to moderate cardiopulmonary intensity. However, it must be realized that in elite sports even golf poses a cardiopulmonary strain, and training consists of additional types of exercise, such resistance exercise, on a daily basis. Therefore recommendations for elite athletes to return to participation in competitive sport should be prescribed cautiously (see ➲ Box 4.1.3.7).

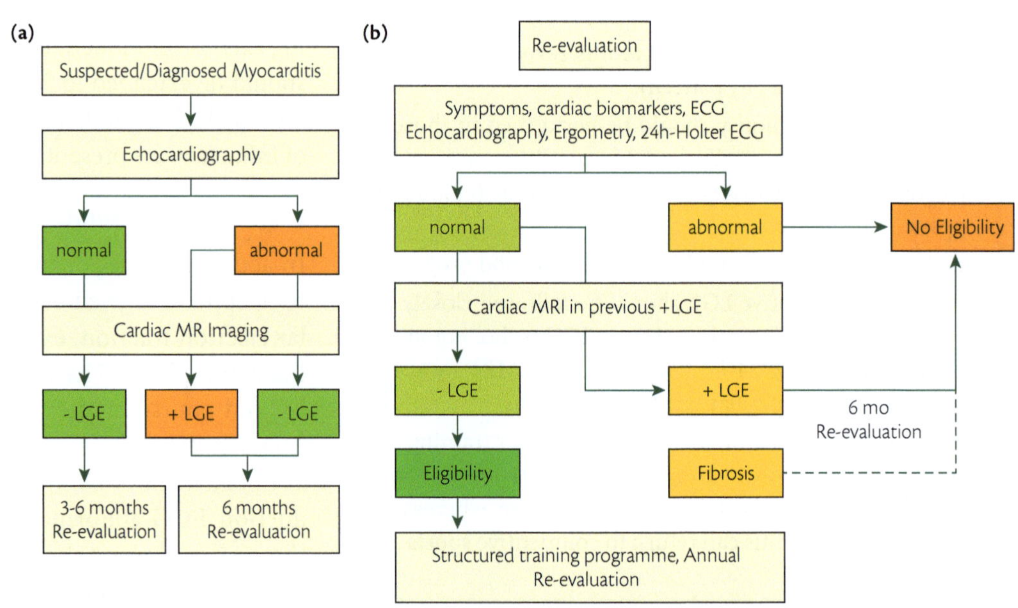

Fig. 4.1.3.3 (a) Assessment for myocarditis and sports eligibility. (b) Re-evaluation after six months for sports eligibility with diagnosis of myocarditis.

Box 4.1.3.7 Recommendations for return to sport

USA recommendations [2]

- No competitive sports for six months after probable or proven myocarditis
- Return to field decision guided by:
  - normal 12-lead ECG, but minor ECG alterations such as ST-T changes are not per se, the basis for restriction
  - normalization of serum markers of inflammatory or heart failure
  - exclusion of relevant arrhythmias by Holter ECG and exercise testing
  - normal echocardiography or radionuclide study at rest and with exercise

European Society of Preventive Cardiology [18]

- First follow-up six months after clinical onset of disease for myocarditis and three months for pericarditis
- Return-to-field decision guided by:
  - freedom from symptoms
  - normal 12-lead ECG
  - normal echocardiography
  - normal exercise testing
  - normal Holter ECG

Data from Maron BJ et al. Eligibility and Disqualification Recommendations for Competitive Athletes With Cardiovascular Abnormalities: Task Force 3: Hypertrophic Cardiomyopathy, Arrhythmogenic Right Ventricular Cardiomyopathy and Other Cardiomyopathies, and Myocarditis: A Scientific Statement From the American Heart Association and American College of Cardiology. *Circulation*, Volume 132, pp.273–80. Copyright © 2015 American Heart Association. Data from Pelliccia A, Corrado D, Bjornstad HH, Panhuyzen-Goedkoop N, Urhausen A, Carre F, Anastasakis A, Vanhees L, Arbustini E, Priori S. Recommendations for participation in competitive sport and leisure-time physical activity in individuals with cardiomyopathies, myocarditis and pericarditis. *Eur J Cardiovasc Prev Rehabil* 2006;13:876–85.

References

1. Maron BJ, Haas TS, Ahluwalia A, et al. Demographics and Epidemiology of Sudden Deaths in Young Competitive Athletes: From the United States National Registry. *Am J Med* 2016; 129: 1170–7.
2. Maron BJ, Udelson JE, Bonow RO, et al. Eligibility and Disqualification Recommendations for Competitive Athletes With Cardiovascular Abnormalities: Task Force 3: Hypertrophic Cardiomyopathy, Arrhythmogenic Right Ventricular Cardiomyopathy and Other Cardiomyopathies, and Myocarditis: A Scientific Statement From the American Heart Association and American College of Cardiology. *Circulation* 2015; 132: e273–80.
3. Maron BJ, Haas TS, Ahluwalia A, Rutten-Ramos SC. Incidence of cardiovascular sudden deaths in Minnesota high school athletes. *Heart Rhythm* 2013; 10: 374–7.
4. Maron BJ, Epstein SE, Roberts WC. Causes of sudden death in competitive athletes. *J Am Coll Cardiol* 1986; 7: 204–14.
5. Magnani JW, Dec GW. Myocarditis: current trends in diagnosis and treatment. *Circulation* 2006; 113: 876–90.
6. Cooper LT Jr. Myocarditis. *N Engl J Med* 2009; 360: 1526–38.
7. Caforio AL, Pankuweit S, Arbustini E, et al. Current state of knowledge on aetiology, diagnosis, management, and therapy of myocarditis: a position statement of the European Society of Cardiology Working Group on Myocardial and Pericardial Diseases. *Eur Heart J* 2013; 34: 2636–2648, 2648a–48d.
8. Schultheiss HP, Kuhl U, Cooper LT. The management of myocarditis. *Eur Heart J* 2011; 32: 2616–25.
9. Maisch B, Pankuweit S. Current treatment options in (peri)myocarditis and inflammatory cardiomyopathy. *Herz* 2012; 37: 644–56.
10. Friman G, Wesslen L, Karjalainen J, Rolf C. Infectious and lymphocytic myocarditis: epidemiology and factors relevant to sports medicine. *Scandinavian J Med Sci Sports* 1995; 5: 269–78.
11. Friman G, Wesslen L. Special feature for the Olympics. Effects of exercise on the immune system: infections and exercise in high-performance athletes. *Immunol Cell Biol* 2000;78: 510–22.
12. Scherr J, Nieman DC, Schuster T, et al. Nonalcoholic beer reduces inflammation and incidence of respiratory tract illness. *Med Sci Sports Exerc* 2012; 44: 18–26.
13. Scherr J, Braun S, Schuster T, et al. 72-h kinetics of high-sensitive troponin T and inflammatory markers after marathon. *Med Sci Sports Exerc* 2011; 43: 1819–27.
14. Pressler A, Schmid A, Freiberger V, et al. Myocarditis, myocardial fibrosis and eligibility for competitive sports. *Int J Cardiol* 2011; 152: 131–2.
15. Grun S, Schumm J, Greulich S, et al. Long-term follow-up of biopsy-proven viral myocarditis: predictors of mortality and incomplete recovery. *J Am Coll Cardiol* 2012; 59: 1604–15.
16. Mahrholdt H, Goedecke C, Wagner A, et al. Cardiovascular magnetic resonance assessment of human myocarditis: a comparison to histology and molecular pathology. *Circulation* 2004; 109: 1250–8.
17. Friedrich MG, Sechtem U, Schulz-Menger J, et al. Cardiovascular magnetic resonance in myocarditis: A JACC White Paper. *J Am Coll Cardiol* 2009; 53: 1475–87.
18. Pelliccia A, Corrado D, Bjornstad HH, et al. Recommendations for participation in competitive sport and leisure-time physical activity in individuals with cardiomyopathies, myocarditis and pericarditis. *Eur J Cardiovasc Prev Rehabil* 2006; 13: 876–85.

4.1.4 Differentiating athlete's heart from left ventricular non-compaction cardiomyopathy

Andrew D'Silva and Sanjay Sharma

Classification

Left ventricular non-compaction cardiomyopathy (LVNC) is the most recently described cardiomyopathy, but there remains academic disagreement regarding the aetiology of this disorder. The American Heart Association classified LVNC as a distinct genetic cardiomyopathy in 2006, whereas both the World Health Organization and the European Society of Cardiology acknowledge that, currently, there is insufficient evidence to recognize LVNC as a separate cardiomyopathy, stating that hypertrabeculation may merely be a congenital or acquired morphological trait shared by many phenotypically distinct cardiomyopathies [1]. As such, the position statements from these groups leave the entity of LVNC in the unclassified category.

Pathogenesis

The most popular theory concerning the genesis of LVNC is that the condition results from the arrest of myocardial compaction, which is the final stage of myocardial morphogenesis. The human embryo begins to develop myocardial trabeculations at the end of the fourth week of gestation. As these trabeculations mature, they develop deep recesses which communicate with the blood-filled cavity of the developing heart tube. It is speculated that this permits an increase in surface area to facilitate blood flow and subsequent myocardial cellular respiration during a period of increasing myocardial mass, whilst an epicardial coronary circulation is absent. Between the fifth and eight weeks of gestation, the trabecular myocardium undergoes compaction. This progresses from the epicardium to the endocardium, from the base to the apex, and from the septum to the lateral wall of the left ventricle, and coincides with the development of the epicardial coronary arteries, resulting in the supposition that the process may be hypoxia-driven [2].

This theory has attracted support as the appearance of the distinctive sinusoids and deep trabeculations on cardiac imaging in suspected LVNC cases are reminiscent of the embryonic architecture. In addition, as normal postnatal human cardiomyocytes are highly differentiated, they lose proliferative capacity, making the possibility of inducing such dramatic morphological appearances through the 'growth' of trabeculations unlikely. However, proof of an arrest in endomyocardial morphogenesis as the mechanism of LVNC is lacking, and cases have been described where non-compaction has only become evident after serial echocardiographic examinations with descriptions of an undulating and reversible phenotype. Such reports add weight to the possibility that left ventricular (LV) hypertrabeculation could be a morphological trait or epiphenomenon shared by distinct disease processes.

Insights have been gained with respect to the relationship between LV geometry and the appearance of increased trabeculation. Cardiac magnetic resonance (CMR) studies in LVNC and dilated cardiomyopathy patients have demonstrated that an increased LV sphericity is associated with increased global trabeculation [3]. A possible interpretation is that 'concealed' trabeculations may become manifest when the LV geometry is modified, particularly in heart failure where sphericity increases. This may explain the disappearance of LV trabeculation after successful heart failure treatment in some cases. Interestingly, global LV trabeculation appears to be influenced by LV sphericity but not by indexed LV end-diastolic volume, LV ejection fraction, or B-type natriuretic peptide levels [3].

Pronounced LV trabeculation and 'persistent intra-myocardial sinusoids' have been described in multiple congenital heart diseases, including atrial and ventricular septal defects, pulmonary stenosis, Ebstein's anomaly, and many others. When no other congenital heart lesion is present, LVNC is termed 'isolated', and this entity will be the focus of this chapter. Whilst the pathophysiological mechanisms underpinning 'isolated LVNC' and 'LVNC with congenital heart disease' are likely to be distinct, the presence of LV hypertrabeculation in combination with other cardiac diseases supports the possibility that LVNC is an overlap disorder [4]. Dysfunction of the sarcomere and sarcolemma are thought to activate a final common pathway resulting in the LVNC phenotype. This may explain how the phenotype can coexist with other cardiomyopathies involving the sarcomere and sarcolemma, such as hypertrophic cardiomyopathy, dilated cardiomyopathy, and restrictive cardiomyopathy.

Genetics

Genetic studies of patients with suspected or 'high probability' LVNC indicate significant genetic heterogeneity. The disorder has been linked to several different mutations in the sarcomeric, cytoskeletal, Z-line, and mitochondrial proteins. However, the molecular mechanisms and final common pathway that result in manifest LVNC remain undiscovered. The diagnostic yield of genetic testing is low, approximately 15–25% [5], although estimates between studies vary widely, mainly owing to differences in the populations studied. Most of the genes implicated in LVNC cases have been described in other cardiomyopathies, particularly dilated cardiomyopathy, hypertrophic cardiomyopathy, and restrictive cardiomyopathy. Moreover, investigations of first-degree relatives of LVNC patients often identify dilated cardiomyopathy or hypertrophic cardiomyopathy in other family members [6], supporting the view that LVNC has the potential to be a sarcolemmal or sarcomeric overlap disorder with shared molecular aetiology. Phenotypic expression can be extremely variable, despite a common genotype, and therefore may be influenced by background genetic modifiers, epigenetic factors, and haemodyamic and environmental factors. The most commonly reported mode of inheritance is autosomal dominant transmission with incomplete penetrance, although various other modes of inheritance have been reported at lower frequencies [6].

Given that myocardial and skeletal muscle cells share expression of many of the same genes, it is unsurprising that there is significant overlap between cardiomyopathy, muscular diseases, and neuromuscular diseases. In their case series Stollberger et al. [7] found that 82% of patients with LVNC had concomitant neuromuscular disorders, and they advocate careful neurological examination of all LVNC cases. However, this strength of association has not been replicated in other case series.

Prevalence

The true prevalence of LVNC is unknown. Current estimates are compiled from case series and observational cohort studies predominantly conducted in tertiary referral centres, resulting in significant case ascertainment, referral, recruitment, and publication biases. Published estimates suggest that the prevalence in the adult population could be between 0.014% [8] and 0.24% [9]. There are several reasons for variability across studies and some are worthy of mention.

First, earlier studies were significantly hampered in the detection of LVNC, a predominantly apically based disease, by technological weaknesses. The introduction of routine second-harmonic imaging to echocardiography in the late 1990s significantly improved endocardial boarder definition and the ability to visualize the cardiac apex. The result was a greater detection of cases and, with increased awareness of LVNC amongst cardiac sonographers, the reported prevalence increased further [9].

Second, despite technical developments, prevalence estimates will remain inaccurate whilst gold standard consensus criteria for the diagnosis do not exist. At present the diagnosis is based on the interpretation of imaging data alone. No weight is given to clinical information such as symptoms, family history, electrocardiographic information, or cardiac function. The imaging criteria that have been proposed are derived retrospectively from small cohorts without rigorous validation for their use in an unselected general population to which they are frequently applied. Kohli et al. [10] demonstrated this issue when echocardiographic criteria were applied to 199 patients with LV systolic impairment referred to a heart failure clinic at a London hospital. This group reported that 24% of this population satisfied one or more echocardiographic criteria for LVNC, and black patients fulfilled LVNC criteria at a frequency over double that of white patients. This raises serious questions as to whether current criteria are over-sensitive, and better understanding of the normal variation in LV trabeculation across ethnically diverse populations is needed. Progress in the elucidation of LVNC will remain hampered unless the diagnostic criteria can be substantially refined.

Clinical presentation

The clinical presentation of LVNC is highly variable. Owing to the same ascertainment bias that afflicts large case series and registries, caution must be exercised when interpreting reported frequencies of symptoms and complications.

Individuals with LVNC can be asymptomatic with normal LV systolic function. These individuals may be diagnosed incidentally when attending for echocardiography for other indications or on family screening of LVNC patients. Symptoms of LVNC may result from heart failure, arrhythmia, or systemic thromboembolism, which are the classically described triad. Heart failure with impaired systolic function comprises the majority of patients in the large registries, with mean LV ejection fractions reported as 31–46% (see Videos 4.1.4.1. and 4.1.4.2). Diastolic dysfunction is found in a high proportion and New York Heart Association (NYHA) class 3–4 symptoms in 30–48% [11].

A systematic overview of five large studies indicated that the resting ECG was found to be abnormal in 89% [12]. This finding is encouraging from the perspective of pre-participation screening of atletes, as it suggests that screening may identify athletes with LVNC and that a normal ECG may help to distinguish false-positive cases detected by over-sensitive imaging criteria. ECG abnormalities are variable and non-specific, including left bundle branch block, right bundle branch block, high-degree AV block, pathological Q waves, poor R wave progression, ST-segment changes, and T-wave inversion. Ventricular arrhythmias, particularly ventricular tachycardia have been reported at frequencies-ranging from 5% [12] to 9% [8], with non-sustained VT in as many as a third [12]. Atrial fibrillation has been documented in approximately 10% of registry patients, although even in sinus rhythm LVNC patients can experience systemic thromboembolism, which is reported in approximately 8% of them [12].

Mortality estimates for LVNC vary widely from 2% to 22% [11]; the most commonly reported mechanism of death is arrhythmic, with a significant proportion suffering a sudden cardiac death followed by pump failure. Although these early case series and registries suggest a poor prognosis, contemporary studies imply that the LVNC phenotype may not be so malignant. In a large multi-ethnic observational cohort, 26% of asymptomatic subjects satisfying a CMR-based definition of LVNC experienced a clinically benign course over a 10-year follow-up period, with no deterioration in LV function or adverse cardiac events [13]. Similarly, non-ischaemic dilated cardiomyopathy patients with marked LV hypertrabeculation have no difference in prognosis compared with those without [14].

Diagnosis: cardiovascular imaging criteria

The diagnosis of LVNC relies on cardiac imaging; however, current diagnostic criteria are highly controversial. Transthoracic echocardiography is the most common diagnostic modality owing to its widespread availability, low cost, and suitability for a wide range of patients and clinical environments. CMR studies of LVNC indicate that in the standard 17-segment LV model, the greatest extent of trabeculation is found at the cardiac apex [15,16]. Here, CMR has greater diagnostic strength and accuracy than echocardiography in imaging this portion of the heart. In addition to improving the detection of complications such as LV thrombi, CMR provides information on myocardial tissue characterization, such as the presence of focal fibrosis. Therefore these imaging modalities are complementary and both are valuable in improving the current understanding of this mysterious condition or shared morphological trait.

Echocardiographic criteria

The first criteria developed, which remain in clinical use, were proposed by Chin et al. [17] and based on a small cohort of eight, predominantly paediatric, patients. For consideration of LVNC the myocardium must have the appearance of a two-layered structure, comprising an epicardial compacted component and an endocardial non-compacted layer. This is a requirement for all the subsequent imaging criteria. This group formulated the ratio of the distance from the epicardial surface to the trough of the trabeculae (*X*) to the distance from the epicardial surface to the peak of the trabeculae (*Y*) (see ➲ Table 4.1.4.1). The measurement is made at end-diastole in either the apical four-chamber or subxiphoid view and a ratio of ≤0.5 discriminates between normal and LVNC cases in this cohort. The group acknowledged that discrimination of the epicardial surface was difficult at the apex and that this was associated with greater inter-observer variation [17].

The next echocardiographic criteria were proposed 11 years later and are arguably the most commonly used in clinical practice. Conscious that 'isolated' LVNC should be differentiated from congenital syndromes and other clinical entities, such as apical thrombi and hypertrophic cardiomyopathy, Jenni at al. [18] included additional stipulations in

Table 4.1.4.1 Echocardiographic and cardiac magnetic resonance diagnostic criteria for left ventricular non-compaction cardiomyopathy

	Chin et al. [17]	Jenni et al. [18]	Stollberger et al. [7]	Petersen et al. [15]	Jacquier et al. [16]
Patients (*n*)	8	34	62	7	16
Description of criteria	Bilayered myocardium *X*/*Y* ≤0.5	Bi-layered myocardium Perfusion of recesses Isolated finding *N*/*C* ≥2	More than three trabeculae seen in a single long-axis image	Bi-layered myocardium *N*/*C* >2.3	LV trabecular mass <20% of total myocardial mass
Cardiac phase	ED	ES	ED	ED	ED
Illustration	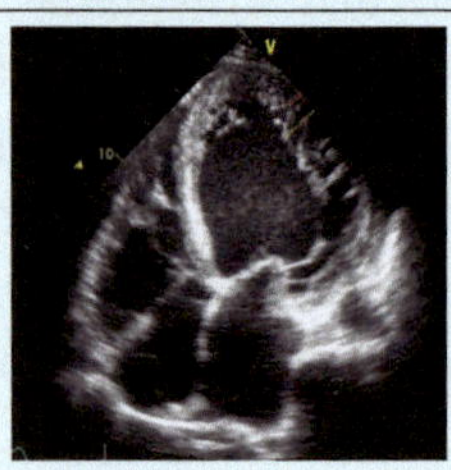	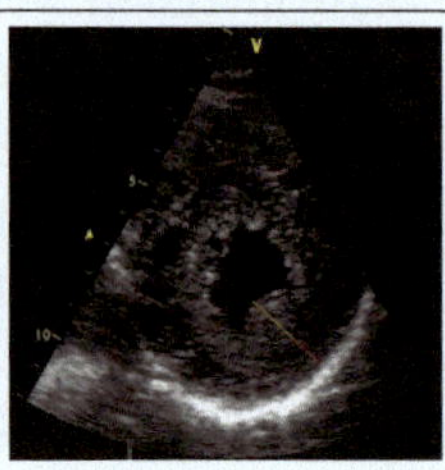	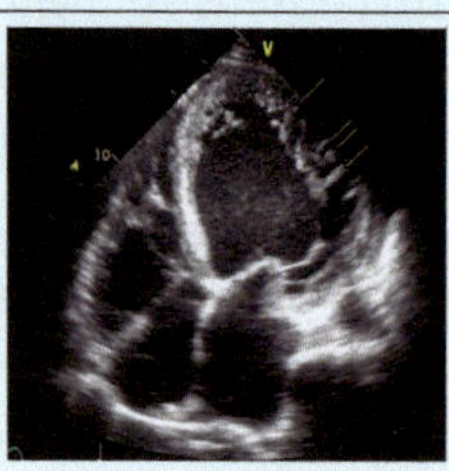	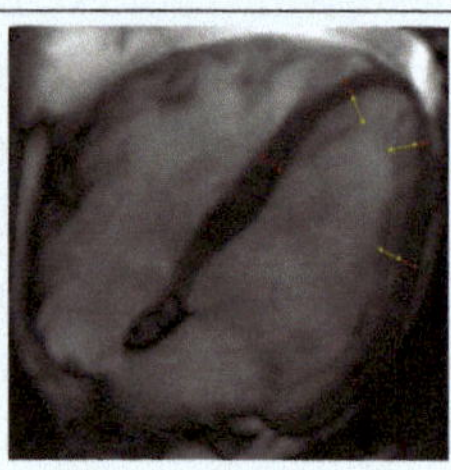	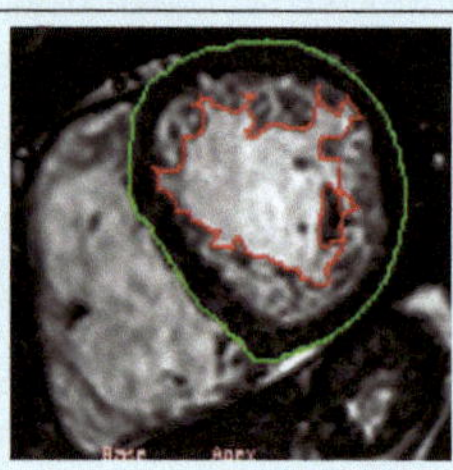

X, distance from epicardial layer to trabecular trough; *Y*, distance from epicardial layer to trabecular peak; *N*, thickness of non-compacted layer; *C*, thickness of compacted layer; ED, end-diastole; ES, end-systole.

Fig 4: Reprinted from *Journal of the American College of Cardiology*, Volume 64, Issue 19, Zemrak F, Ahlman MA, Captur G, Mohiddin SA, Kawel-Boehm N, Prince MR, et al. The relationship of left ventricular trabeculation to ventricular function and structure over a 9.5-year follow-up: the MESA study, pp. 1971-80. Copyright (2014), with permission from Elsevier.

Fig 5: Reproduced with permission from Jacquier, Alexis; Thuny, Franck. Measurement of trabeculated left ventricular mass using cardiac magnetic resonance imaging in the diagnosis of left ventricular non-compaction. *European Heart Journal*, Volume 31, Issue 9, Copyright © 2010 Oxford University Press and the European Society of Cardiology.

their criteria. The diagnosis of isolated LVNC requires the absence of other cardiac abnormalities and colour Doppler to demonstrate perfusion of the inter-trabecular recesses from the LV cavity. This group proposed measurement of the ratio of the thickest portion of the non-compacted (trabeculated) layer to the adjacent compacted myocardial layer. A ratio of ≥2 was used to distinguish LVNC from a small comparator group of patients with either dilated cardiomyopathy or hypertensive heart disease. This measurement is made in the parasternal short-axis view, but during end-systole rather than end-diastole. End-systole was chosen as it allowed the best visualization of the two myocardial layers but this is controversial and represents a significant departure from other criteria.

Stollberger et al. [7] took a different approach in developing their diagnostic criteria. This group began by viewing the problem from a histopathological perspective and appreciated the need to define normal trabeculation. Considering the findings of a large autopsy study including 474 normal human hearts, 97% had up to three prominent trabeculae, defined as discrete muscle bundles more than 2mm in diameter that stood out against the background left ventricular endocardium. This was the threshold above which abnormal hypertrabeculation could be defined. Noting that the distribution of LV trabeculation is highest from the papillary muscles to the apex, the criteria stipulated that more than three trabeculae should be visible in a single long-axis imaging plane. There was agreement that the inter-trabecular spaces should have demonstrable perfusion from the ventricular cavity, visualized on colour Doppler imaging. Later, the group added a non-compacted to compacted ratio of >2 to their criteria [19].

Cardiac magnetic resonance criteria

Petersen et al. [15] proposed the first CMR criteria. This group compared the findings from seven patients previously diagnosed with LVNC with a variety of cohorts that can be difficult to distinguish from LVNC when associated with prominent trabeculation. These included patients with dilated cardiomyopathy, hypertrophic cardiomyopathy, aortic stenosis, or hypertensive heart disease, normal healthy volunteers, and athletes. When LVNC patients were compared with subjects from these groups, the end-diastolic ratio of non-compacted to compacted layers was 60% greater. A cut-off point of >2.3 from any of the long-axis views during diastole, was chosen to generate the most favourable sensitivity and specificity for the detection of the LVNC patients in their cohort. Notably, the positive predictive value for this threshold was 75% in this study, suggesting that the potential for false-positive diagnoses in a quarter. These criteria were subsequently tested in a large multi-ethnic observational cohort, where 43% of subjects, without cardiac disease or hypertension, were found to have a two-layered myocardial appearance with a ratio >2.3 in at least one region and 5% in at least two regions [20].

A criticism of many of the proposed LVNC diagnostic imaging criteria is that they reduce the potential information that can be acquired from the three-dimensional beating heart into a one-dimensional length ratio with a binary cut-off between normality and disease. Jacquier et al. [16] proposed a more detailed method of measurement involving calculation of the global trabecular mass of the entire LV from the short-axis stack. This has the advantage of comprehensive assessment without confinement to a single LV view or segment and respects the continuous distribution of LV trabeculation in a population. Choosing a cut-off value with high sensitivity and specificity in their highly selected cohort, this group defined LVNC by a trabeculated LV mass above 20% of the total LV mass. However, other groups have reported that inter-observer variability is high when using this time-consuming method [21].

Another CMR approach to tackling the diagnostic problem of LVNC is to focus solely on the endocardium and disregard the length of the myocardial layers. Theoretically, increased LV trabeculation has the profound effect of increasing endocardial complexity through the presence of multiple deep recesses. These recesses can be regarded as complex repeating geometrical patterns that are self-similar across different scales, and this property can be utilized to calculate a fractal dimension. Captur et al. [22] used a box-counting method to calculate fractal dimensions in short-axis stack slices using a group of selected LVNC patients and a comparator healthy control group. An apical fractal dimension ≥1.3 was defined as the diagnostic cut off for discriminating LVNC from healthy controls.

Inter-observer disagreement contributes to diagnostic uncertainty, and a study with three operators having more than 20 years experience of using the echocardiographic criteria proposed by Stollberger et al. [19] found disagreement in 35% of cases. Even when the observers reviewed and discussed discordant cases together, 11% were still felt to be questionable [19]. In clinical practice, echocardiographers may advocate the employment of different diagnostic criteria for the identification of LVNC, and the correlation between criteria is poor [10]. This is not surprising as the criteria differ in what is measured, from which imaging plane, and in which phase of the cardiac cycle (see ➲ Table 4.1.4.2).

Table 4.1.4.2 Summary of a selection of the imaging diagnostic criteria for left ventricular non-compaction

Modality	Author	Year	No. of patients	Measurement	Imaging plane	Cardiac phase
Echo	Chin et al. [17]	1990	8	X/Y ≤0.5	LAx	ED
	Jenni et al. [18]	2001	34	N/C ≥2	SAx	ES
	Stollberger et al. [7]	2002	62	>3 trabeculations	LAx	ED
	Pignatelli et al. [26]	2003	36 children	N/C >1.4	LAx	ED
	Belanger et al. [27]	2008	60	N/C >2 plus area >5cm2	LAx + SAx	ES
	van Dalen et al. [28]	2008	10	LV twist–solid body rotation	SAx	ES and ED
CMR	Petersen et al. [15]	2005	7	N/C >2.3	LAx	ED
	Jacquier et al. [16]	2010	16	TM >20% total	SAx	ED
	Grothoff et al. [29]	2012	12	TM >25% and N/C ≥3	SAx + LAx	ED
	Captur et al. [22]	2013	30	Apical FD >1.3	SAx	ED
CT	Melendez-Ramirez et al. [30]	2012	10	N/C >2.2	SAx	ED

Echo, echocardiography; CMR, cardiac magnetic resonance; CT, computed tomography; X, distance from epicardial layer to trabecular trough; Y, distance from epicardial layer to trabecular peak; N, thickness of non-compacted layer; C, thickness of compacted layer; LAx, long-axis view; SAx, short-axis view/stack; ED, end-diastole; ES, end-systole.

Evaluation of the athlete: assessment and management

In a large observational cohort of 1146 athletes in the UK, echocardiographic criteria for LVNC were met in 8.1% of healthy athletes. Black athletes were more likely than white athletes to exhibit increased trabeculation [23]. The authors concluded that this finding most likely demonstrates a morphological epiphenomenon related to athletic cardiac remodelling in response to increased preload. In a more recent study of over 2500 Italian athletes (predominantly white) 1.4% showed trabeculations consistent with LVNC [24]. The epiphenomeon hypothesis is further supported by a study of 102 primagravida pregnant women. In this population, natural physiological changes result in a doubling of blood volume by the third trimester, where it was observed that 25% developed de novo trabeculation in the LV and 8% satisfied echocardiographic imaging criteria for LVNC despite having entirely normal LV morphology in the first trimester. This de novo hypertrabeculation also regressed post-partum, supporting the premise of a remodelling phenomenon, probably influenced by the changes in preload [25].

However, a diagnostic grey zone presents itself when athletes with LV hypertrabeculation show T-wave inversion on the ECG and/or mildly depressed LV systolic function (see Videos 4.1.4.3 and 4.1.4.4). This triad has been reported in 3.4% of black athletes and 0.5% of white athletes. T-wave inversion in black athletes is described elsewhere, but is more likely to be benign and training-related if confined to the anterior leads and preceded by convex ST-segment elevation. Mild depression of LV function at rest (EF 50–55%) can also be a feature of athlete's heart. This is more common in endurance athletes where a large LV cavity is capable of generating large stroke volume and cardiac output at rest without vigorous systolic excursion. Increased myocardial contractility and an increase in ejection fraction during exercise demonstrate that the apparently depressed LV systolic performance at rest is not representative of the true myocardial function in these athletes.

In order to distinguish between LVNC and the normal trabeculation of the athlete's heart, it is important to employ a multifaceted approach to be confident of the correct diagnosis. Symptoms including exercise intolerance, breathlessness, palpitation, or syncope warrant attention and will significantly raise the pre-test probability of underlying pathology in a suspected athlete. Similarly, a sinister family history of an inherited cardiomyopathy or sudden cardiac death influences the interpretation of abnormalities or variants detected on imaging, such as increased LV trabeculation. Any abnormality on the ECG that is not a normal variant may suggest underlying pathology and significantly impacts on the likelihood of disease.

For the athlete with prominent LV hypertrabeculation on echocardiography, additional echocardiographic parameters are essential for the assessment and distinction of the normal athletic heart from pathological LVNC. Common to many heart muscle diseases, LV systolic dysfunction, including longitudinal function, diastolic dysfunction, and abnormal myocardial deformation on strain imaging are commonly observed in LVNC patients. In contrast, by virtue of their training, athletes tend to have normal or supranormal values of the above indices, and those with an apparent mild reduction in LV systolic performance at rest demonstrate significant contractility reserve on exercise.

Demonstrable exercise-induced pathological arrhythmias, such as atrial fibrillation and ventricular tachycardia, suggest cardiomyopathy. Cardiopulmonary exercise testing can be valuable in the assessment of athletes with equivocal symptoms, ECG findings, or subtle imaging abnormalities. Depending on the degree of training and the discipline, athletes are expected to achieve peak oxygen consumption values well over 100% of that predicted for age and body size. As such, a peak oxygen consumption of <85% of the predicted value would be more suggestive of underlying cardiac pathology.

CMR also has an important role in differentiating the hypertrabeculated athlete's heart from LVNC. As well as imaging the extent of trabeculation in greater detail, CMR adds tissue characterization beyond the scope of echocardiography. The presence of late gadolinium enhancement suggests the presence of cardiomyopathy, as focal fibrosis is not a feature of the normal athlete's heart (see Fig. 4.1.4.1). Moreover, the distribution of delayed enhancement may assist in recognizing more subtle phenotypes of other cardiomyopathies, such as dilated cardiomyopathy and hypertrophic cardiomyopathy, which may overlap with LVNC. With evolving CMR technologies such as native T1 mapping, more methods may be available in the future to differentiate between the healthy athlete's heart, where T1 values are reduced, and cardiomyopathies, where disproportionate expansion of the extracellular matrix due to diffuse fibrosis can raise T1 values.

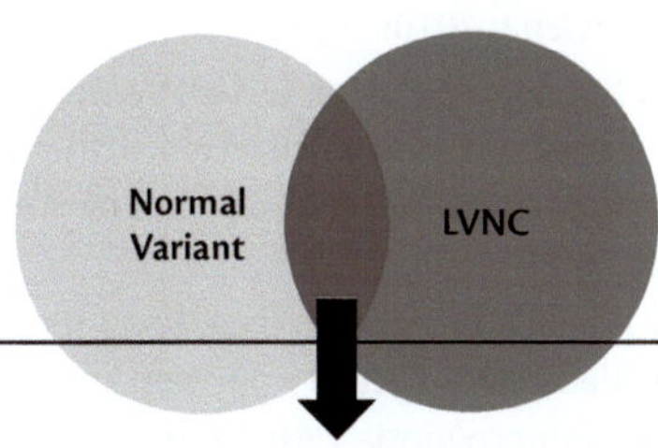

Normal Variant		LVNC
–	Symptoms	+
–	Family history	+
–	T wave inversion	+
–	LBBB	+
–	E' Lateral < 9 cm/sec	+
–	Peak VO_2 < 85%	+
–	↓ LVEF on exercise echo	+
–	Exercise induced VT/AF	+
–	Abnormal myocardial strain	+
–	Late Gadolinium Enhancement on CMR	+
–	Family member with similar features	+

Fig. 4.1.4.1 Proposed algorithm for the differentiation of pathological left ventricular non-compaction from physiological increases of LV trabeculation in the athlete. LVNC, left ventricular non-compaction cardiomyopathy; LBBB, left bundle branch block; VO_2, oxygen consumption; LVEF, left ventricular ejection fraction; VT, ventricular tachycardia; AF, atrial fibrillation; CMR, cardiac magnetic resonance.

A pragmatic approach to investigating the athlete with LV hypertrabeculation is through stratification based on the likelihood of underlying cardiomyopathy.

Asymptomatic athletes with normal LV systolic function, no family history of cardiomyopathy, and a normal ECG should be reassured that the imaging findings are likely to be a normal variant. Athletes with symptoms, a family history of cardiomyopathy, or ECG abnormality should undergo detailed evaluation with exercise testing (ideally cardiopulmonary exercise testing), CMR, and 24-hour Holter rhythm monitoring to look for further features of cardiomyopathy such as exercise limitation, myocardial fibrosis, or arrhythmias. Athletes with reduced LV systolic function which fails to improve on exercise should be evaluated comprehensively in the same way, with a high likelihood of LVNC (see Table 4.1.4.3). They should be followed up and managed in an inherited heart conditions clinic with tailored lifestyle advice and appropriate treatment based on their symptoms including evidence-based pharmacological therapies for LV systolic dysfunction.

LVNC patients are generally managed in the same way as dilated cardiomyopathy with indications for implantable cardioverter defibrillator and cardiac resynchronization therapy as for non-ischaemic cardiomyopathy. Cascade family screening should be offered, but at the present time genetic testing has no role in the identification of cases because of significant limitations in the current understanding of the genotype–phenotype correlation.

Exercise guidelines are similar to those for all primary cardiomyopathies (see Chapter 7.1). Athletes with definite diagnosis of LVNC should be advised against participation in competitive sports, with the exception of low dynamic and low static sporting disciplines (e.g. golf). Any individual presenting with a systemic thromboembolic event and satisfying imaging criteria for LVNC should be formally anticoagulated and presumed to have the disorder. Controversy remains as to whether all LVNC patients with reduced systolic function would benefit from anticoagulation.

Table 4.1.4.3 Proposed clinical risk stratification tool for the likelihood of left ventricular non-compaction cardiomyopathy when evaluating an athlete with increased left ventricular trabeculation

LVNC likehood	LV systolic impairment	Family history of LVNC	Systemic embolism	Abnormal ECG	Arrhythmia	CMR LGE
Low	–	–	–	–	–	–
Intermediate	Mild, improving on exercise	+/–	–	Any	Exercise-induced arrhythmia	+/–
High	Severe	+	+	LBBB, T-wave inversion	VT or AF	+

LVNC, left ventricular non-compaction cardiomyopathy; LV, left ventricular; ECG , electrocardiogram; LBBB, left bundle branch block; VT, ventricular tachycardia; AF, atrial fibrillation; CMR, cardiac magnetic resonance; LGE, late gadolinium enhancement.

Conclusion

The diagnosis of left ventricular non-compaction cardiomyopathy is challenging, and there is controversy as to whether the condition exists as a separate cardiomyopathy or as a shared morphological trait. Progress can only be made when the pathophysiological mechanisms underlying left ventricular non-compation are better understood, and this includes appreciation of the normal spectrum of left ventricular trabeculation and any factors that can influence changes in appearance. The field requires a refinement of diagnostic criteria in order to advance significantly, and at the present time clinicians must exercise their best judgement as to which individuals with left ventricular hypertrabeculation benefit from a diagnostic label and treatment, and for which such an approach would result in unnecessary harm. A multifaceted approach is required to provide the clinician with sufficient information on which to base decision-making and management.

Further reading

Gati S, Chandra N, Bennett RL, et al. Increased left ventricular trabeculation in highly trained athletes: do we need more stringent criteria for the diagnosis of left ventricular non-compaction in athletes? *Heart* 2013; 99: 401–8.

Kohli SK, Pantazis AA, Shah JS, et al. Diagnosis of left-ventricular non-compaction in patients with left-ventricular systolic dysfunction: time for a reappraisal of diagnostic criteria? *Eur Heart J* 2008; 29: 89–95.

Stollberger C, Gerecke B, Engberding R, et al. Interobserver agreement of the echocardiographic diagnosis of LV hypertrabeculation/noncompaction. *JACC Cardiovasc Imaging* 2015; 8: 1252–7.

Thavendiranathan P, Dahiya A, Phelan D, et al. Isolated left ventricular non-compaction controversies in diagnostic criteria, adverse outcomes and management. *Heart* 2013; 99: 681–9.

Towbin JA, Lorts A, Jefferies JL. Left ventricular non-compaction cardiomyopathy. *Lancet* 2015; 386: 813–25.

References

1. Elliott P, Andersson B, Arbustini E, et al. Classification of the cardiomyopathies: a position statement from the European Society Of Cardiology Working Group on Myocardial and Pericardial Diseases. *Eur Heart J* 2008; 29: 270–6.
2. Sedmera D, Pexieder T, Vuillemin M, et al. Developmental patterning of the myocardium. *Anat Rec* 2000; 258: 319–37.
3. Marchal P, Lairez O, Cognet T, et al. Relationship between left ventricular sphericity and trabeculation indexes in patients with dilated cardiomyopathy: a cardiac magnetic resonance study. *Eur Heart J Cardiovasc Imaging* 2013; 14: 914–20.
4. Towbin JA, Lorts A, Jefferies JL. Left ventricular non-compaction cardiomyopathy. *Lancet* 2015; 386: 813–25.
5. Olivotto I, d'Amati G, Basso C, et al. Defining phenotypes and disease progression in sarcomeric cardiomyopathies: contemporary role of clinical investigations. *Cardiovasc Res* 2015; 105: 409–23.
6. Hoedemaekers YM, Caliskan K, Michels M, et al. The importance of genetic counseling, DNA diagnostics, and cardiologic family screening in left ventricular noncompaction cardiomyopathy. *Circ Cardiovasc Genet* 2010; 3: 232–9.
7. Stollberger C, Finsterer J, Blazek G. Left ventricular hypertrabeculation/noncompaction and association with additional cardiac abnormalities and neuromuscular disorders. *Am J Cardiol* 2002; 90: 899–902.
8. Oechslin EN, Attenhofer Jost CH, et al. Long-term follow-up of 34 adults with isolated left ventricular noncompaction: a distinct cardiomyopathy with poor prognosis. *J Am Coll Cardiol* 2000; 36: 493–500.
9. Stollberger C, Finsterer J. Pitfalls in the diagnosis of left ventricular hypertrabeculation/non-compaction. *Postgrad Med J* 2006; 82: 679–83.
10. Kohli SK, Pantazis AA, Shah JS, et al. Diagnosis of left-ventricular non-compaction in patients with left-ventricular systolic dysfunction: time for a reappraisal of diagnostic criteria? *Eur Heart J* 2008; 29: 89–95.
11. Thavendiranathan P, Dahiya A, Phelan D, et al. Isolated left ventricular non-compaction controversies in diagnostic criteria, adverse outcomes and management. *Heart* 2013; 99: 681–9.
12. Bhatia NL, Tajik AJ, Wilansky S, et al. Isolated noncompaction of the left ventricular myocardium in adults: a systematic overview. *J Card Fail* 2011; 17: 771–8.
13. Zemrak F, Ahlman MA, Captur G, et al. The relationship of left ventricular trabeculation to ventricular function and structure over a 9.5-year follow-up: the MESA study. *J Am Coll Cardiol* 2014; 64: 1971–80.
14. Amzulescu MS, Rousseau MF, Ahn SA, et al. Prognostic impact of hypertrabeculation and noncompaction phenotype in dilated cardiomyopathy: a CMR study. *JACC Cardiovasc Imaging* 2015; 8: 934–46.
15. Petersen SE, Selvanayagam JB, Wiesmann F, et al. Left ventricular non-compaction: insights from cardiovascular magnetic resonance imaging. *J Am Coll Cardiol* 2005; 46: 101–5.

16. Jacquier A, Thuny F, Jop B, et al. Measurement of trabeculated left ventricular mass using cardiac magnetic resonance imaging in the diagnosis of left ventricular non-compaction. *Eur Heart J* 2010; 31: 1098–1104.
17. Chin TK, Perloff JK, Williams RG, et al. Isolated noncompaction of left ventricular myocardium: a study of eight cases. *Circulation* 1990; 82: 507–13.
18. Jenni R, Oechslin E, Schneider J, et al. Echocardiographic and pathoanatomical characteristics of isolated left ventricular non-compaction: a step towards classification as a distinct cardiomyopathy. *Heart* 2001; 86: 666–71.
19. Stollberger C, Gerecke B, Engberding R, et al. Interobserver agreement of the echocardiographic diagnosis of LV hypertrabeculation/ noncompaction. *JACC Cardiovasc Imaging* 2015; 8: 1252–7.
20. Kawel N, Nacif M, Arai AE, et al. Trabeculated (noncompacted) and compact myocardium in adults: the multi-ethnic study of atherosclerosis. *Circ Cardiovasc Imaging* 2012; 5: 357–66.
21. Fernández-Golfín C, Pachón M, Corros C, et al. Left ventricular trabeculae: quantification in different cardiac diseases and impact on left ventricular morphological and functional parameters assessed with cardiac magnetic resonance. *J Cardiovasc Med (Hagerstown)* 2009; 10: 827–33.
22. Captur G, Muthurangu V, Cook C, et al. Quantification of left ventricular trabeculae using fractal analysis. *J Cardiovasc Magn Reson* 2013; 15: 36.
23. Gati S, Chandra N, Bennett RL, et al. Increased left ventricular trabeculation in highly trained athletes: do we need more stringent criteria for the diagnosis of left ventricular non-compaction in athletes? *Heart* 2013; 99(6): 401–8.
24. Caselli S, Ferreira D, Kanawati E, et al. Prominent left ventricular trabeculations in competitive athletes: A proposal for risk stratification and management. *Int J Cardiol* 2016; 223: 590–5.
25. Gati S, Papadakis M, Papamichael ND, et al. Reversible de novo left ventricular trabeculations in pregnant women: implications for the diagnosis of left ventricular non-compaction in low risk populations. Circulation 2014; 130: 475–83.
26. Pignatelli RH, McMahon CJ, Dreyer WJ, et al. Clinical characterization of left ventricular noncompaction in children: a relatively common form of cardiomyopathy. *Circulation* 2003; 108: 2672–8.
27. Belanger AR, Miller MA, Donthireddi UR, et al. New classification scheme of left ventricular noncompaction and correlation with ventricular performance. *Am J Cardiol* 2008; 102: 92–6.
28. van Dalen BM, Caliskan K, Soliman OI, et al. Left ventricular solid body rotation in non-compaction cardiomyopathy: a potential new objective and quantitative functional diagnostic criterion? *Eur J Heart Fail* 2008; 10: 1088–93.
29. Grothoff M, Pachowsky M, Hoffmann J, et al. Value of cardiovascular MR in diagnosing left ventricular non-compaction cardiomyopathy and in discriminating between other cardiomyopathies. *Eur Radiol* 2012; 22:2699–709.
30. Melendez-Ramirez G, Castillo-Castellon F, Espinola-Zavaleta N, et al. Left ventricular noncompaction: a proposal of new diagnostic criteria by multidetector computed tomography. *J Cardiovasc Comput Tomogr* 2012; 6: 346–54.

➲ For additional multimedia materials please visit the online version of the book at http://www.oxfordmedicine.com/ escsportscardiology

4.1.5 Congenital coronary artery anomalies

Cristina Basso, Carla Frescura, Stefania Rizzo, and Gaetano Thiene

The estimated prevalence of congenital coronary artery anomalies (CAAs) in the general population is quite variable, depending on both the definition of a CAA and the source of data, and ranges from 0.21% to 5.79% [1–15]. Despite the low prevalence, CAAs are well recognized as a major cause of sudden cardiac death (SCD) in competitive athletes [16–29], accounting for about 17% of such deaths in the USA and 16% in Italy.

However, not all CAAs have the same prognostic impact, and each should be discussed individually, taking into account the symptoms and signs at clinical onset. Three main subgroups are recognized [30,31]:

(1) CAAs of origin and course
(2) CAAs of intrinsic anatomy
(3) CAAs of termination.

It is important to accept that different degrees of certainty (i.e. certain, highly probable, or uncertain) exist in defining the risk of SCD with various CAAs, and recommendations for management and sport eligibility need to be considered separately [32].

Coronary arteries of anomalous origin

Type 1A

The anomalous origin of a CA from the pulmonary artery, usually the left coronary (ALCAPA), also known as Bland–White–Garland syndrome, [33] is rarely observed in athletes [34] or reported as a cause of SCD in young adults [35]. The extent of the acquired collateral circulation between the coronary arteries is the major determinant of the clinical outcome, thus explaining why patients with well-formed collaterals have the 'adult type' of ALCAPA, and those without or with few collaterals have the 'infant type', with extensive myocardial infarction leading to congestive heart failure and/or SCD in early infancy or childhood [36–38]. However, the increased use of imaging modalities such as CT and CMR has led to more frequent identification of this CAA even in adults [39]. ALCAPA is listed among certain causes of SCD in the AECVP guidelines for autopsy investigation [32].

Type 1B

The anomalous origin of a CA from the wrong aortic sinus, either the left main CA from the right sinus or the right CA from the left sinus, is traditionally considered the CAA with highest risk of SCD. Despite a low prevalence in the general population (0.17%, 1.2%, and 0.17% in autopsy, angiography, and echocardiography studies, respectively) [15,40,41], these CAAs occur frequently in the athletic SCD population (12.2% vs 0.5% in non-athletic SCD), thus confirming that they are particularly likely to cause cardiac arrest during effort [27]. Ischaemia probably occurs in episodic bursts which may be cumulative with time. This is supported by observation of normal basal and effort ECG tracings together with signs of acute and/or chronic myocardial ischaemia at post-mortem examination in affected athletes [26].

Based on the course of the proximal tract of the anomalous CA, four anatomical subtypes of CAA with origin from the wrong aortic sinus are recognized: anterior to the pulmonary trunk (pre-pulmonic), posterior to the aorta (retro-aortic), septal (sub-pulmonic), and between the pulmonary artery and the aorta (inter-arterial) [30,31]. CAAs with an inter-arterial course carry the highest risk of ischaemia, particularly during exercise [16-18,26,42–46] (➔ Figs 4.1.5.1, 4.1.5.2, and 4.1.5.3). Several pathophysiological mechanisms have been postulated: compression of the anomalous CA between the aorta and the pulmonary artery occurring with increased cardiac output; the acute angle take-off of the anomalous CA; the intra-mural aortic course of the proximal tract of the anomalous CA; and a superimposed CA spasm or kinking [26,30]. Imaging features such as CA intussusception into the aortic wall, narrowing of the proximal anomalous CA, and asymmetrical compression of the anomalous CA with a slit-like lumen, particularly during systole and stress [30], are most probably due to the intra-mural aortic course [26].

The anomalous origin of the left CA from the right sinus and the anomalous origin of the right CA with an inter-arterial course are listed among the highly probable and uncertain causes of SCD, respectively [32]. The anomalous left CA is considered more malignant because of the larger amount of myocardium at risk of ischaemia, while anomalous right CA can often be an incidental finding [17].

Although SCD is frequently the first manifestation, it is not uncommon for alarming cardiac symptoms to occur in competitive athletes with wrong sinus CAA, suggesting that a history of exertional symptoms (i.e. syncope, palpitation, or chest pain) or signs always require exclusion of this CAA [26]. It is noteworthy that in our experience all available basal 12-lead and exercise ECGs are normal. Moreover, a review of the literature demonstrates that only 22% of young patients with CAA show ischaemic ECG changes on effort. Thus, if the index of suspicion is sufficiently high because of exertional syncope, palpitations, or chest pain, even in the setting of normal 12-lead and effort ECG, the origin and proximal course of the CA should be investigated initially by trans-thoracic or trans-oesophageal echocardiography [47–49]. Failure to demonstrate the CA ostia in a young person with syncope or angina should prompt further investigation

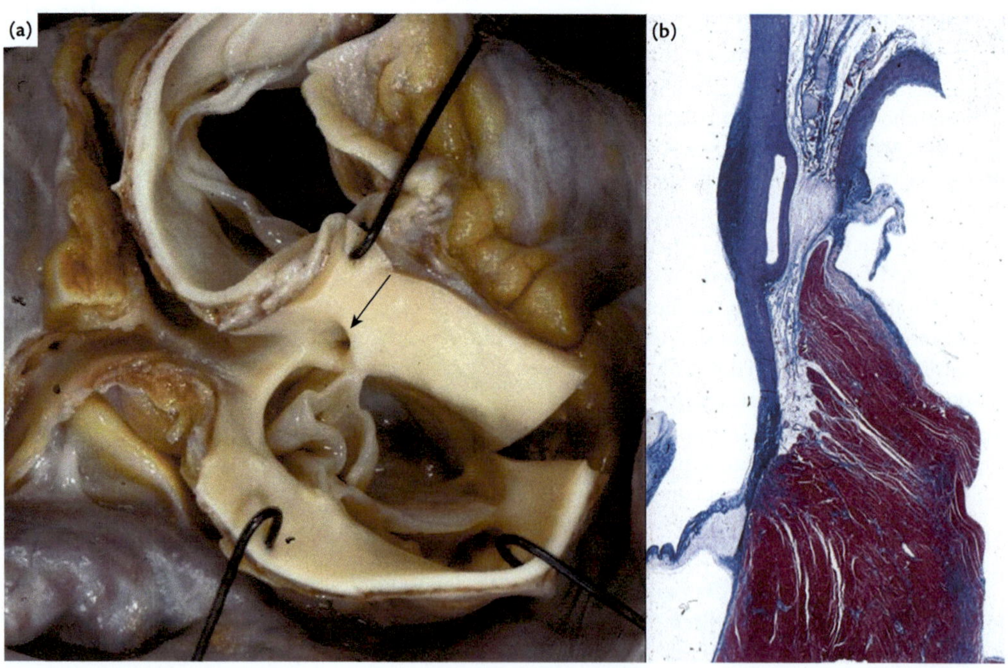

Fig. 4.1.5.1 A 22-year-old soccer player with wrong sinus CAA (right CA from the left sinus) who died suddenly during a game. (a) View of the aortic root (note the presence of two coronary ostia in the left sinus of Valsalva, with acute angle take-off of the anomalous right coronary artery (arrow)). (b) Longitudinal histological section of the aortic and pulmonary root showing the intra-mural course of an anomalous CA.

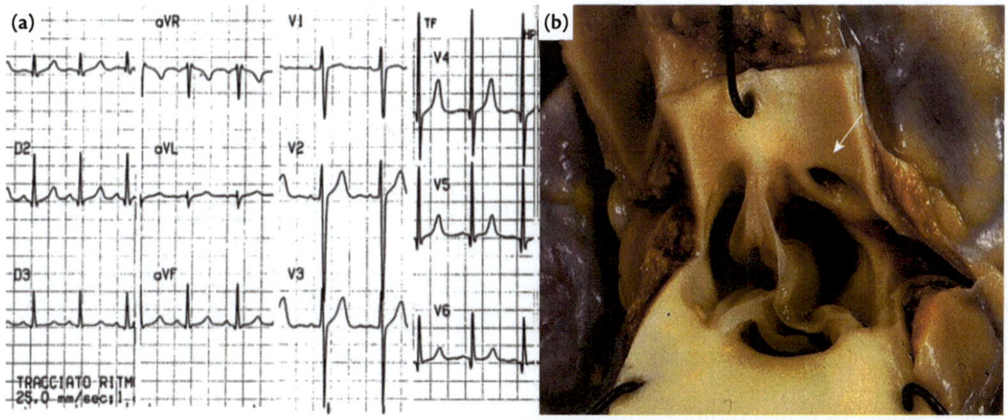

Fig. 4.1.5.2 A 15-year-old soccer player with wrong sinus CAA (left CA from the right sinus), a history of exertional syncope, and SCD during the second half of a game. (a) Normal 12-lead ECG performed 10 months before death as part of routine pre-participation screening.
(b) View of the aortic root. Note the right CA arising normally from the right aortic sinus (arrow), and the left main CA arising anomalously from the right sinus with an acute angle take-off producing a slit-like lumen.

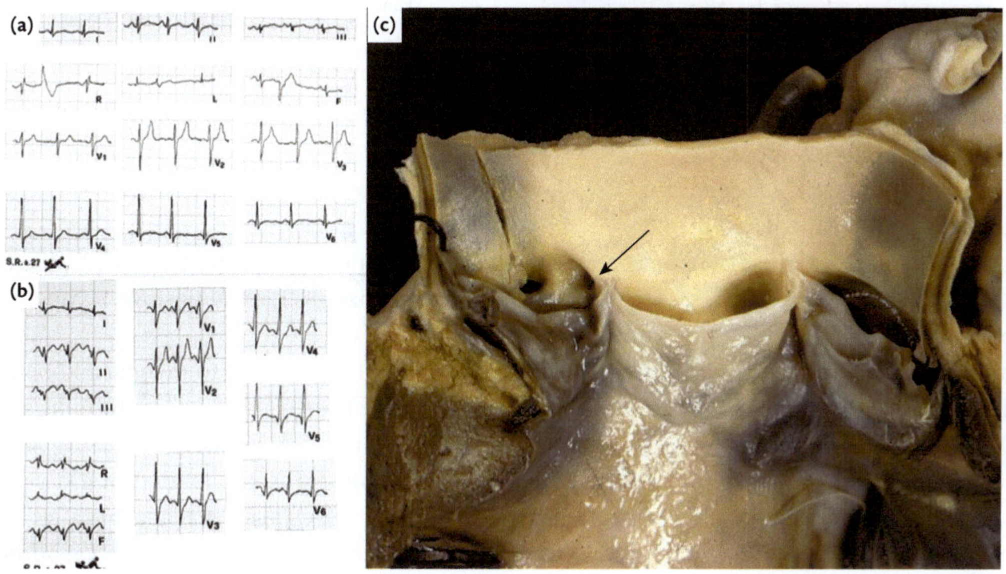

Fig. 4.1.5.3 A 27-year-old rugby player with wrong sinus CAA (right CA from the left sinus) who died suddenly during a game. (a) Basal 12-lead ECG with isolated premature ventricular beat. (b) Effort 12-lead ECG without any sign of myocardial ischaemia. (c) View of the aortic root. Note the presence of two coronary ostia in the left sinus of Valsalva, with an acute angle take-off of the anomalous right coronary artery (arrow).

by CMR and/or CT and eventually by angiography [50–52]. Evaluation of CAA can be performed by either CT or CMR with a class IIa/b recommendation according to the AHA Committee on Cardiovascular Imaging, although CMR is preferred because of radiation exposure concerns [53]. In Europe, CT the ESC Working Group on Nuclear Cardiology and Cardiac CT recommends angiography for all patients with a clinical suspicion of CAA [54].

Once diagnosed, wrong sinus CAAs require functional assessment, which is even more challenging. Nuclear exercise stress testing, coronary angiography, and intravascular ultrasound (IVUS) of the anomalous CA are used to achieve this [30]. Stress–rest ^{99m}Tc-sestamibi (^{99m}Tc-MIBI) myocardial perfusion SPECT, which is an established technique for the evaluation of the functional relevance of coronary stenosis, is currently used to investigate the functional relevance of known CAA, although the results are controversial [55,56]. A grading of CAA severity according to IVUS criteria, i.e. the amount of hypoplasia and the degree of lateral compression of the proximal vessel compared with the distal vessel, has also been proposed,. Combined fractional flow reserve (FFR) is also recommended for a more complete haemodynamic assessment of the CAA [57]. IVUS and FFR should be performed at both baseline and on dobutamine pharmacological stress.

A flowchart for diagnostic and functional assessment of suspected CAA is shown in ➲ Fig. 4.1.5.4.

Type 1C

All the remaining 'minor' anomalous coronary arteries originating from the aorta are considered to be uncertain causes of SCD [32].

The anomalous origin of the *left circumflex branch* from the right CA or the right sinus (estimated prevalence of 0.67%) is probably represents the most frequent CAA [18,58,59]. It is traditionally regarded as a benign condition, and is an incidental observation at autopsy or angiography. The anomalous CA branch shows a retro-aortic course to reach its normal distribution, and when arising from the right sinus with a separate ostium it can have an acute take-off. Since myocardial infarction or SCD cases in the absence of any other cause have been reported [16,17,60], each patient should be individually judged on the basis of symptoms and signs after exclusion of other causes.

The *anomalous left anterior descending artery* (LAD) from the right CA can have a pre-aortic (inter-arterial), pre-pulmonic (anterior), retro-aortic, or intra-septal course, with the anterior course being the most common. It is generally thought to be benign, but this may not not always be the case [61].

Single CA is the condition when only one CA originates from the aorta with a single ostium, and then takes the course of either the right or left CA and divides into two or three main coronary branches [62]. This is a very rare CAA seen in only 0.0024–0.044% of the population [63]. Patients are at risk when a coronary branch has an inter-arterial course or if they develop atherosclerotic disease when there are serious consequences because of the absence of collaterals.

High take-off is defined when a CA arise from the upper tubular portion of the aorta. It is a controversial cause of myocardial infarction and SCD [17]. The presence of a funnel-like ostium and a vertical intra-mural aortic course of the first tract of the anomalous CA have been anecdotically described as determinants of myocardial ischaemia.

In a postmortem analysis of athletes who died suddenly, *hypoplastic CAs* were reported in up to 5% [20]. The CA hypoplasia can manifest as a narrowed diameter (<1.5mm) or a shortened course, and typically targets one or two of the three major epicardial branches [64]. However, care should be taken not to confound extreme right or left dominant patterns with CA hypoplasia.

Anomalous course CAA (myocardial bridge)

Myocardial bridges, in the absence of any other structural anomaly, have been reported in approximately 5% of athletic field SCDs [20,21]. Effort-induced ischaemia has been attributed to tachycardia, which increases the myocardial oxygen requirement and reduces the diastolic coronary flow. Myocardial bridges consist of coronary segments, usually the LAD, which are surrounded by myocardium rather than running superficially in the epicardial fat (tunnelled CA or intra-mural course) [65,66] (➔ Fig. 4.1.5.5). Since many bridges have not haemodynamic consequences, the anatomic prevalence at post-mortem is higher than the angiographic one (15%-85% vs. 0.5%-2.5%) (65). These CAA are

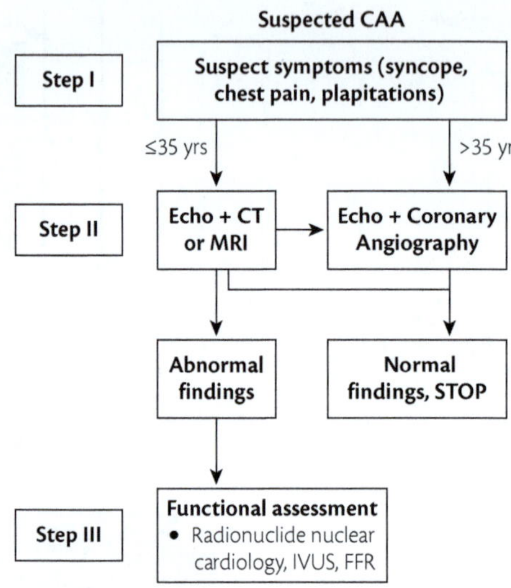

Fig. 4.1.5.4 Flowchart for diagnostic and functional assessment of suspected CAA.

increasingly detected even in asymptomatic patients due to the frequent use of coronary CT, thus posing therapeutic dilemmas.

Significant vessel constriction due to myocardial compression is present when there is a ≥70% systolic lumen reduction and persistent ≥35% reduction during mid to late diastole [67]. This transient angiographic sign, known as the 'milking effect', can be accentuated by intra-coronary nitroglycerin injection due to vasodilatation of the adjacent coronary segment. The clinical significance and pathophysiology of myocardial bridge is still a matter of debate. Myocardial ischaemia has been reported in patients with myocardial bridge in whom surgical debridging was effective in relieving both signs and symptoms [68–70]. Even SCD has been described, although the coexistence of hypertrophic cardiomyopathy should always be ruled out [20–22,71,72]. The length (2–3cm) and depth (2–3mm) of the myocardial bridge, together with histological features of disarray and fibrosis of the myocardium, can explain the compromised coronary flow [22,73]. Intravascular ultrasound studies have clearly shown that clinically significant myocardial bridges are characterized by phasic systolic compression, persistent reduction in diastolic lumen, increased blood flow velocities, retrograde systolic flow, and decreased coronary flow reserve [74–76].

As with other CAAs, the major challenge after diagnosis is functional assessment for management decisions [67,77], and there is no consensus on whether further diagnostic studies are needed in those with an 'incidental' finding of myocardial bridging.

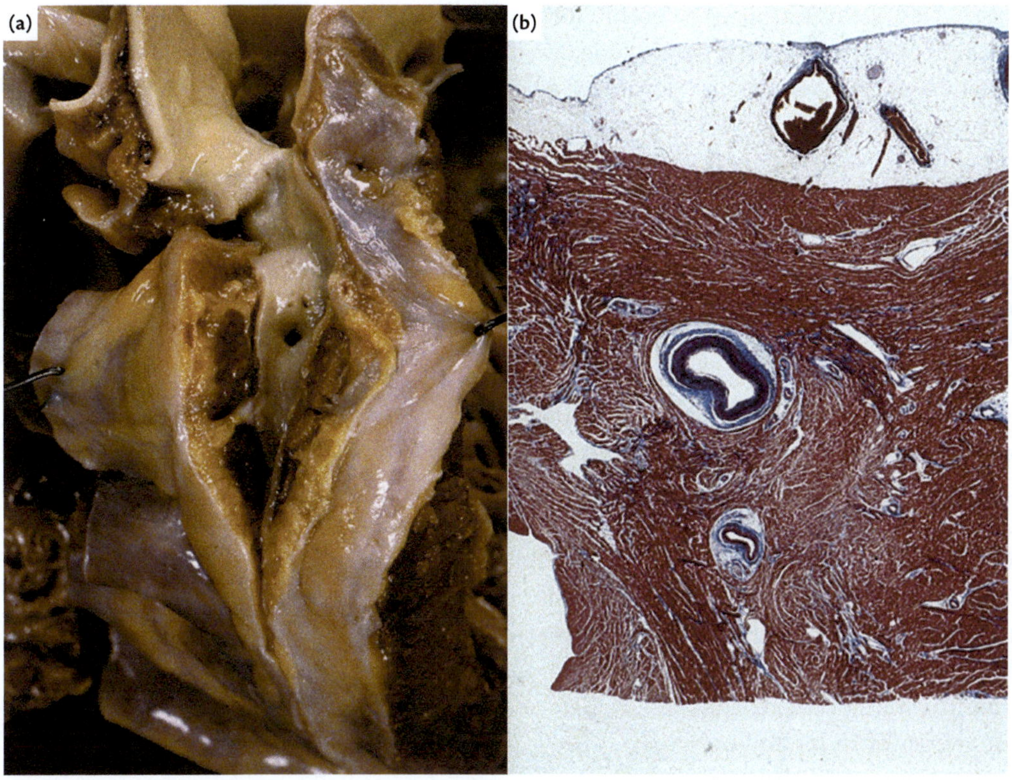

Fig. 4.1.5.5 A 35-year-old competitive athlete who died suddenly on effort. (a) Gross examination shows a deep intramyocardial course of the left anterior descending CA. (B) Histological section shows a thick myocardium encircling the coronary segments. Note the presence of disarray and interstitial fibrosis.

Coronary physiological measurements across a myocardial bridge during pharmacological infusion are useful, showing a distinctive flow velocity called the 'fingertip' phenomenon. To haemodynamically assess significant stenosis, FFR can be measured and a value <0.75 suggests the presence of ischaemia. Intravenous administration of dobutamine can lead to higher pressure gradients with angina symptoms in the setting of abnormal but non-ischaemic FFR (>0.80). An FFR of 0.75–0.80 represents a grey zone of ischaemia. Higher average peak velocity and greater pressure gradients with infusion of dobutamine compared with infusion of adenosine also suggest haemodynamically significant myocardial bridging. Finally, intra-coronary acetylcholine infusion (off-label use) could reveal endothelial dysfunctional or coronary vasospasm.

IVUS can detect the characteristic 'half-moon' sign, an echolucent area between the bridged coronary segment and epicardial tissue that persists throughout the cardiac cycle, and visualize proximal coronary segment atherosclerosis.

Finally, stress single-photon emission CT can assess reversible myocardial perfusion defects in patients with myocardial bridging, with a correlation between the amount of ischaemia and the degree of systolic luminal narrowing.

CA fistula

To the best of our knowledge, no athletic field SCD has been ascribed to CA fistula. It consists of a communication of one or two CAs with either a cardiac chamber or any of the great vessels and has been reported in up to 0.1–0.2% of selective coronary angiographies [1,78]. The haemodynamic consequences depend on the resistance (which is determined by fistula size, tortuosity, and length) and the site of drainage. The blood flow from the CA to a venous structure or right-sided cardiac chamber occurs throughout the cardiac cycle. With larger fistulas, a diastolic 'coronary steal' may exist, drawing blood away from the normal coronary tree, leading to symptoms and signs of myocardial ischaemia as well as chamber volume overload.

Small fistulas in asymptomatic children should be followed up for signs of increasing size and flow. It is recommended that early haemodynamically significant fistulas in both symptomatic and asymptomatic patients should be closed.

Clinical management of CAAs

Indications for the clinical management of CAA are derived from the 2008 AHA/ACC guidelines [79].

The definitive treatment for ALCAPA is surgical intervention with reconstruction of a dual coronary artery supply through direct reimplantation of the anomalous CA into the aorta or coronary bypass grafting (class IC recommendation). Furthermore, clinical evaluation with echocardiography and non-invasive stress testing every 3–5 years is indicated for adult survivors of ALCAPA repair,.

Patients with wrong sinus CAA can be managed medically, surgically, or even by percutaneous coronary intervention. Medical treatment consist of beta-blockers and avoidance of physical exercise. Surgical correction of wrong sinus CAA can be accomplished either by CA bypass grafting or newer techniques, such as reimplantation of the anomalous vessel in the proper coronary sinus or 'unroofing' the common wall between the aorta and the anomalous CA, resulting in a new orifice. According to the AHA/ACC 2008 guidelines [79], surgical coronary revascularization should be performed (Class I,B) in patients with any of the following indications: anomalous left main CA coursing between the aorta and the pulmonary artery; documented coronary ischaemia due to coronary compression (when coursing between the great arteries or in intra-mural fashion); anomalous origin of the right CA coursing between aorta and pulmonary artery with evidence of ischaemia.

Moreover, surgical coronary revascularization can be beneficial (Class IIa,C) in the setting of documented vascular wall hypoplasia, coronary compression, or obstruction to coronary flow, regardless of inability to document coronary ischaemia, and delineation of potential mechanisms of flow restriction via IVUS can be beneficial (Class IIa,C) in patients with documented wrong sinus CAA. Finally, surgical coronary revascularization may be appropriate (Class IIb,C) in patients with anomalous LAD coursing between the aorta and the pulmonary artery.

Treatment options for CA fistulas include surgical ligation, either isolated or in association with CA bypass grafting, and interventional closure with occlusion coils, umbrellas, vascular plugs, and covered stents [79]. The 2008 ACC/AHA guidelines (class I,C) indicate that if a continuous murmur is present, its origin should be defined by echocardiography, CMR, CT angiography, or cardiac catheterization. A large fistula, regardless of symptomatology, should be closed via either a transcatheter or a surgical route after delineation of its course and its potential to fully obliterate the fistula. A small to moderate fistula in the presence of documented myocardial ischaemia, arrhythmia, otherwise unexplained ventricular, systolic, or diastolic dysfunction or enlargement, or endarteritis should be closed via either a transcatheter or surgical approach after delineation of its course and its potential to fully obliterate the fistula. Clinical follow-up with echocardiography every 3–5 years can be useful for patients with small asymptomatic fistulas to exclude development of symptoms or progression of size or chamber enlargement that might alter management (Class IIa,C). Patients with small asymptomatic fistulas should not undergo closure (Class III,C).

Indications for therapy of myocardial bridges take into account the Schwarz classification [67,77]. Patients with an incidental finding of myocardial bridge on angiography and no objective signs of ischaemia (type A) need no treatment. Patients with ischaemia on stress test and objective signs of ischaemia (type B) and altered intra-coronary haemodynamics, quantitative coronary angiography, coronary flow reserve, or Doppler, with or without objective signs of ischaemia (type C), show significant symptomatic improvement with beta-blockers or calcium-channel blockers at five-year follow-up. Patients with type C myocardial bridge refractory to medical therapy can be considered for revascularization through myotomy, coronary artery bypass grafting, or percutaneous coronary intervention with stent implantation.

Guidelines for sport eligibility for athletes with CAA

To date, four official consensus documents/recommendations for sport eligibility in competitive athletes with CAA have been proposed. Obviously, these reflect different cultural, social, and legal backgrounds. They are as follows: the 36th Bethesda Conference, published in 2005 [80]; the Study Group of Sports Cardiology of the Working Group of Cardiac Rehabilitation and Exercise Physiology and the Working Group of Myocardial and Pericardial Diseases of the European Society of Cardiology (ESC), published in 2005 [81] and currently being revised; the fifth edition of the Italian Cardiological Guidelines for Sports Eligibility, published in 2017 [82], and the 2015 AHA/ACC scientific statement [83,84]. Eligibility recommendations for athletes with CAA are discussed and summarized in ➲ Chapter 7.1, Table 7.1.4.

Acknowledgement

This work was supported by the Registry of Cardio-cerebro-vascular Pathology, Veneto Region, Venice, Italy.

Further reading

Angelini P. Coronary artery anomalies: an entity in search of an identity. *Circulation* 2007; 115: 1296–1305.

Basso C, Maron BJ, Corrado D, Thiene G. Clinical profile of congenital coronary artery anomalies with origin from the wrong aortic sinus leading to sudden death in young competitive athletes. *J Am Coll Cardiol* 2000; 35: 1493–1501.

Basso C, Burke M, Fornes P, et al. Guidelines for autopsy investigation of sudden cardiac death. *Virchows Arch* 2008; 452: 11–18.

Corrado D, Basso C, Rizzoli G, et al. Does sports activity enhance the risk of sudden death in adolescents and young adults? *J Am Coll Cardiol* 2003; 42: 1959–63.

Maron B, Doerer J, Haas T, et al. Sudden deaths in young competitive athletes: analysis of 1866 deaths in the United States, 1980–2006. *Circulation* 2009; 119: 1085–92.

Pérez-Pomares JM, de la Pompa JL, Franco D, et al. Congenital coronary artery anomalies: a bridge from embryology to anatomy and pathophysiology: a position statement of the development, anatomy, and pathology ESC Working Group. *Cardiovasc Res* 2016; 109: 204–16.

Taylor AJ, Rogan KM, Virmani R. Sudden cardiac death associated with isolated congenital coronary artery anomalies. *J Am Coll Cardiol* 1992; 20: 640–7.

Thiene G, Corrado D, Basso C. *Sudden Cardiac Death in the Young and Athletes: Text Atlas of Pathology and Clinical Correlates*. Milan: Springer-Verlag, 2016.

Thiene G. Sudden cardiac death and cardiovascular pathology: from anatomic theater to double helix. *Am J Cardiol* 2014; 114: 1930–6.

Warnes C, Williams RG, Bashore TM, et al. ACC/AHA 2008 guidelines for the management of adults with congenital heart disease. *J Am Coll Cardiol* 2008; 52: e143–263.

References

1. Yamanaka O, Hobbs RE. Coronary artery anomalies in 126,595 patients undergoing coronary arteriography. *Cathet Cardiovasc Diagn* 1990; 21: 28–40.
2. Yildiz A, Okcun B, Peker T, et al. Prevalence of coronary artery anomalies in 12,457 adult patients who underwent coronary angiography. *Clin Cardiol* 2010; 33: E60–4.
3. Rigatelli G, Docali G, Rossi P, et al. Congenital coronary artery anomalies angiographic classification revisited. *Int J Cardiovasc Imaging* 2003; 19:3 61–6.
4. Harikrishnan S, Jacob SP, Tharakan J, et al. Congenital coronary anomalies of origin and distribution in adults: a coronary arteriographic study. *Indian Heart J* 2002; 54: 271–5
5. Garg N, Tewari S, Kapoor A, et al. Primary congenital anomalies of the coronary arteries: a coronary: arteriographic study. *Int J Cardiol* 2000; 74: 39–46.
6. Kardos A, Babai L, Rudas L, et al. Epidemiology of congenital coronary artery anomalies: a coronary arteriography study on a central European population. *Cathet Cardiovasc Diagn* 1997; 42: 270–5.
7. Wilkins CE, Betancourt B, Mathur VS, et al. Coronary artery anomalies: a review of more than 10,000 patients from the Clayton Cardiovascular Laboratories. *Tex Heart Inst J* 1988; 15: 166–73.
8. Zhang LJ, Yang GF, Huang W, et al. Incidence of anomalous origin of coronary artery in 1879 Chinese adults on dual-source CT angiography. *Neth Heart J*. 2010; 18: 466–70.
9. Cheng Z, Wang X, Duan Y, et al. Detection of coronary artery anomalies by dual-source CT coronary angiography. *Clin Radiol* 2010; 65: 815–22.
10. Erol C, Seker M. The prevalence of coronary artery variations on coronary computed tomography angiography. *Acta Radiol* 2012; 53: 278–84.
11. von Ziegler F, Pilla M, McMullan L, et al. Visualization of anomalous origin and course of coronary arteries in 748 consecutive symptomatic patients by 64-slice computed tomography angiography. *BMC Cardiovasc Disord* 2009; 9: 54.
12. Koşar P, Ergun E, Oztürk C, Koşar U. Anatomic variations and anomalies of the coronary arteries: 64-slice CT angiographic appearance. *Diagn Interv Radiol* 2009; 15: 275–83.
13. Duran C, Kantarci M, Durur Subasi I, et al. Remarkable anatomic anomalies of coronary arteries and their clinical importance: a multidetector computed tomography angiographic study. *J Comput Assist Tomogr* 2006; 30: 939–48.
14. Lipsett J, Cohle SD, Berry PJ, et al. Anomalous coronary arteries: a multicenter pediatric autopsy study. *Pediatr Pathol* 1994; 14: 287–300.
15. Alexander RW, Griffith GC. Anomalies of the coronary arteries and their clinical significance. *Circulation* 1956; 14: 800–5.
16. Roberts WC. Major anomalies of coronary arterial origin seen in adulthood. *Am Heart J* 1986; 111: 941–63.
17. Frescura C, Basso C, Thiene G, et al. Anomalous origin of coronary arteries and risk of sudden death: a study based on an autopsy population of congenital heart disease. *Hum Pathol* 1998; 29: 689–95
18. Roberts WC. Congenital coronary arterial anomalies unassociated with major anomalies of the heart and great vessels. In Roberts WC (ed), *Adult Congenital Heart Diseases*. Philadelphia, PA: FA Davis, 1987; 583–630.
19. Liberthson RR. Sudden death from cardiac causes in children and young adults. *N Engl J Med* 1996; 334:1039–44.
20. Maron BJ, Shirani J, Poliac LC, et al. Sudden death in young competitive athletes: clinical, demographic, and pathological profiles. *JAMA* 1996; 276: 199–204.
21. Maron B, Doerer J, Haas T, et al. Sudden deaths in young competitive athletes: analysis of 1866 deaths in the United States, 1980–2006. *Circulation* 2009; 119: 1085–92.
22. Corrado D, Thiene G, Cocco P, Frescura C. Non-atherosclerotic coronary artery disease and sudden death in the young. *Br Heart J* 1992; 68: 601–7.
23. Basso C, Frescura C, Corrado D, et al. Congenital heart disease and sudden death in the young. *Hum Pathol* 1995; 26: 1065–72.
24. Taylor AJ, Rogan KM, Virmani R. Sudden cardiac death associated with isolated congenital coronary artery anomalies. *J Am Coll Cardiol* 1992; 20: 640–7.
25. Burke AP, Farb A, Virmani R, et al. Sports-related and non-sports-related sudden cardiac death in young adults. *Am Heart J* 1991; 121: 568–75.
26. Basso C, Maron BJ, Corrado D, Thiene G. Clinical profile of congenital coronary artery anomalies with origin from the wrong aortic sinus leading to sudden death in young competitive athletes. *J Am Coll Cardiol* 2000; 35: 1493–1501.
27. Corrado D, Basso C, Rizzoli G, et al. Does sports activity enhance the risk of sudden death in adolescents and young adults? *J Am Coll Cardiol* 2003; 42: 1959–63.
28. Thiene G. Sudden cardiac death and cardiovascular pathology: from anatomic theater to double helix. *Am J Cardiol* 2014; 114: 1930–6.
29. Thiene G, Corrado D, Basso C. *Sudden Cardiac Death in the Young and Athletes: Text Atlas of Pathology and Clinical Correlates*. Milan: Springer-Verlag, 2016.

30. Angelini P. Coronary artery anomalies: an entity in search of an identity. *Circulation* 2007; 115: 1296–1305.
31. Pérez-Pomares JM, de la Pompa JL, Franco D, et al. Congenital coronary artery anomalies: a bridge from embryology to anatomy and pathophysiology. A position statement of the Development, Anatomy, and Pathology ESC Working Group. *Cardiovasc Res* 2016; 109: 204–16.
32. Basso C, Aguilera B, Banner J, et al. Association for European Cardiovascular Pathology. Guidelines for autopsy investigation of sudden cardiac death: 2017 update from the Association for European Cardiovascular Pathology. *Virchows Arch.* 2017; 471: 691–705.
33. Bland E, White P, Garland J. Congenital anomalies of the coronary arteries. *Am Heart J* 1933; 8: 797–801.
34. Facciorusso A, Lanna P, Vigna C, et al. Anomalous origin of the left coronary artery from the pulmonary artery in an elderly patient, football player in youth. *J Cardiovasc Med* 2008; 9: 1066–9.
35. Krexi L, Sheppard MN. Anomalous origin of the left coronary artery from the pulmonary artery (ALCAPA), a forgotten congenital cause of sudden death in the adult. *Cardiovasc Pathol* 2013; 22: 294–7.
36. Moodie DS, Fyfe D, Gill CC, et al. Anomalous origin of the left coronary artery from the pulmonary artery (Bland–White–Garland syndrome) in adult patients: long-term follow-up after surgery. *Am Heart J* 1983; 106: 381–8.
37. Dodge-Khatami A, Mavroudis C, Backer C. Anomalous origin of the left coronary artery from the pulmonary artery: collective review of surgical therapy. *Ann Thorac Surg* 2002; 74: 946–55.
38. Frommelt P, Frommelt M. Congenital coronary artery anomalies. *Pediatr Clin North Am* 2004; 51: 1273–88.
39. Yau JM, Singh R, Halpern EJ, Fischman D. Anomalous origin of the left coronary artery from the pulmonary artery in adults: a comprehensive review of 151 adult cases and a new diagnosis in a 53-year-old woman. *Clin Cardiol* 2011; 34: 204–10.
40. Engel HJ, Torres C, Page HL. Major variations in anatomical origin of the coronary arteries: angiographic observations in 4250 patients without associated congenital heart disease. *Cathet Cardiovasc Diagn* 1975; 1: 157–69.
41. Davis JA, Cecchin F, Jones TK, Portman MA. Major coronary artery anomalies in a pediatric population: incidence and clinical importance. *J Am Coll Cardiol* 2001; 37: 593–7.
42. Cheitlin MD, De Castro CM, McAllister HA. Sudden death as a complication of anomalous left coronary origin from the anterior sinus of Valsalva: a not-so-minor congenital anomaly. *Circulation* 1974; 50: 780–7.
43. Barth CW III, Roberts WC. Left main coronary artery originating from the right sinus of Valsalva and coursing between the aorta and pulmonary trunk. *J Am Coll Cardiol* 1986; 7: 366–73.
44. Liberthson RR, Dinsmore RE, Fallon JT. Aberrant coronary artery origin from the aorta: report of 18 patients, review of the literature and delineation of natural history and management. *Circulation* 1979; 59: 748–54.
45. Lim JC, Beale A, Ramcharitar S. Anomalous origination of a coronary artery from the opposite sinus. *Nat Rev Cardiol* 2011; 8: 706–19.
46. Cheitlin MD, MacGregor J. Congenital anomalies of coronary arteries: role in the pathogenesis of sudden cardiac death. *Herz* 2009; 34: 268–79.
47. Pelliccia A, Spataro A, Maron BJ. Prospective echocardiographic screening for coronary artery anomalies in 1,360 elite competitive athletes. *Am J Cardiol* 1993; 72: 978–9.
48. Maron BJ, Leon MB, Swain JA, et al. Prospective identification by two dimensional echocardiography of anomalous origin of the left main coronary artery from the right sinus of Valsalva. *Am J Cardiol* 1991; 68: 140–2.
49. Zeppilli P, Dello Russo A, Santini C, et al. In vivo detection of coronary artery anomalies in asymptomatic athletes by echocardiographic screening. *Chest* 1998; 114: 89–93.
50. Serota H, Barth CW III, Seuc CA, et al. Rapid identification of course of anomalous coronary arteries in adults: the 'dot and eye' method. *Am J Cardiol* 1990; 65: 891–8.
51. McConnell MV, Ganz P, Selwyn AP, et al. Identification of anomalous coronary arteries and their anatomic course by magnetic resonance coronary angiography. *Circulation* 1995; 92: 3158–62.
52. Mousseaux E, Hernigou A, Sapoval M, et al. Coronary arteries arising from the contralateral aortic sinus: electron beam computed tomographic demonstration of the initial course of the artery with respect to the aorta and right ventricular outflow tract. *J Thorac Cardiovasc Surg* 1996; 112: 836–40.
53. Bluemke DA, Achenbach S, Budoff M, et al. Noninvasive coronary artery imaging: magnetic resonance angiography and multidetector computed tomography angiography: a scientific statement from the American Heart Association Committee on Cardiovascular Imaging and Intervention, the Council On Cardiovascular Radiology and Intervention, and the Councils on Clinical Cardiology and Cardiovascular Disease in the Young. *Circulation* 2008; 118: 586–606.
54. Schroeder S, Achenbach S, Bengel F, et al. Cardiac computed tomography: indications, applications, limitations, and training requirements: report of a Writing Group deployed by the Working Group Nuclear Cardiology and Cardiac CT of the European Society of Cardiology and the European Council of Nuclear Cardiology. *Eur Heart J* 2008; 29: 531–56.
55. De Luca L, Bovenzi F, Rubini D, et al. Stress–rest myocardial perfusion SPECT for functional assessment of coronary arteries with anomalous origin or course. *J Nucl Med* 2004; 45: 532–6.
56. Uebleis C, Groebner M, von Ziegler F, et al. Combined anatomical and functional imaging using coronary CT angiography and myocardial perfusion SPECT in symptomatic adults with abnormal origin of a coronary artery. *Int J Cardiovasc Imaging* 2012; 28: 1763–74.
57. Sintek MA, Singh J, Billadello JJ. Dynamic evaluation of coronary anomalies originating from the opposite sinus of Valsalva (ACAOS). *Curr Treat Options Cardiovasc Med* 2015; 17: 47.
58. Page HL, Engel HJ, Campbell WB, Thomas CS. Anomalous origin of the left circumflex coronary artery: recognition, angiographic demonstration and clinical significance. *Circulation* 1974; 50: 768–73
59. Chaitman BR, Lespérence J, Saltiel J, Bourasse MG. Clinical, angiographic and hemodynamic findings in patients with anomalous origin of the coronary arteries. *Circulation* 1976; 53: 122–31.
60. Corrado D, Pennelli T, Piovesana P, Thiene G. Anomalous origin of the left circumflex coronary artery from the right aortic sinus of Valsalva and sudden death. *Cardiovasc Pathol* 1994; 3: 269–71.
61. Karabay KO, Bağirtan B, Erdim R, et al. A rare congenital coronary artery anomaly: anomalous of the left anterior descending

coronary artery arising from the right coronary artery and review of the literature. *Int J Cardiol* 2010; 140: e51–2.

62. Smith J. Review of single coronary artery with report of 2 cases. *Circulation* 1950; 1: 1168–75.
63. Desmet W, Vanhaecke J, Vrolix M, et al. Isolated single coronary artery: a review of 50,000 consecutive coronary angiographies. *Eur Heart J* 1992; 13: 1637–40.
64. Zugibe FT, Zugibe FT Jr, Costello JT, Breithaupt MK. Hypoplastic coronary artery disease within the spectrum of sudden unexpected death in young and middle age adults. *Am J Forensic Med Pathol* 1993; 14: 276–83.
65. Angelini P, Trivellato M, Donis J, Leachman RD. Myocardial bridges: a review. *Prog Cardiovasc* 1983; 26: 75–88.
66. Polacek P. Relation of myocardial bridges and loops on the coronary arteries to coronary occlusions. *Am Heart J* 1961; 61: 44–52.
67. Corban MT, Hung OY, Eshtehardi P, et al. Myocardial bridging: contemporary understanding of pathophysiology with implications for diagnostic and therapeutic strategies. *J Am Coll Cardiol* 2014; 63: 2346–55.
68. Feldman AM, Baughman KL. Myocardial infarction associated with a myocardial bridge. *Am Heart J* 1986; 111: 784–7.
69. Vasan RS, Bahl VK, Rajani M. Myocardial infarction associated with a myocardial bridge. *Int J Cardiol* 1989; 25: 240–1.
70. Faruqui AM, Maloy WC, Felner JM, et al. Symptomatic myocardial bridging of coronary artery. *Am J Cardiol* 1978; 41: 1305–9.
71. Basso C, Thiene G, Mackey-Bojack S, et al. Myocardial bridging, a frequent component of the hypertrophic cardiomyopathy phenotype, lacks systematic association with sudden cardiac death. *Eur Heart J* 2009; 30: 1627–34.
72. Morales AR, Romanelli R, Boucek RJ. The mural left anterior descending coronary artery, strenuous exercise and sudden death. *Circulation* 1980; 62: 230–7.
73. Ferreira AG, Trotter SE, Konig B, et al. Myocardial bridges: morphological and functional aspects. *Br Heart J* 1991; 66: 364–7.
74. Ge J, Erbel R, Rupprecht HJ, et al. Comparison of intravascular ultrasound and angiography in the assessment of myocardial bridging. *Circulation* 1994; 89: 1725–32.
75. Mohlenkamp S, Hort W, Ge J, Erbel R. Update on myocardial bridging. *Circulation* 2002; 106: 2616–22.
76. Bourassa MG, Butnaru A, Lespérance J, Tardif JC. Symptomatic myocardial bridges: overview of ischemic mechanisms and current diagnostic and treatment strategies. *J Am Coll Cardiol* 2003; 41: 351–9.
77. Schwarz ER, Gupta R, Haager PK, et al. Myocardial bridging in absence of coronary artery disease: proposal of a new classification based on clinical-angiographic data and long-term follow-up. *Cardiology* 2009; 112: 13–21.
78. Mangukia C. Coronary artery fistula. *Ann Thorac Surg* 2012; 93: 2084–92.
79. Warnes C, Williams RG, Bashore TM, et al. ACC/AHA 2008 guidelines for the management of adults with congenital heart disease. *J Am Coll Cardiol* 2008; 52: e143–263.
80. Maron BJ, Zipes DP. 36th Bethesda Conference: eligibility recommendations for competitive athletes with cardiovascular abnormalities. *J Am Coll Cardiol* 2005; 45: 2–64.
81. Pelliccia A, Fagard R, Bjørnstad HH, et al. Recommendations for competitive sports participation in athletes with cardiovascular disease: a consensus document from the Study Group of Sports Cardiology of the Working Group of Cardiac Rehabilitation and Exercise Physiology and the Working Group of Myocardial and Pericardial Diseases of the European Society of Cardiology. *Eur Heart J* 2005; 26: 1422–45.
82. Cardiovascular Guidelines for Eligibility in Competitive Sports (COCIS), 5th edn. Roma: CESI Ed., 2017.
83. Van Hare GF, Ackerman MJ, Evangelista JA, et al. Eligibility and disqualification recommendations for competitive athletes with cardiovascular abnormalities: Task Force 4: Congenital Heart Disease: A Scientific Statement From the American Heart Association and American College of Cardiology. *Circulation* 2015; 132: e281–91.
84. Thompson PD, Myerburg RJ, Levine BD, et al. Eligibility and disqualification recommendations for competitive athletes with cardiovascular abnormalities: Task Force 8: Coronary Artery Disease: A Scientific Statement From the American Heart Association and American College of Cardiology. *Circulation* 2015; 132: e310–14.

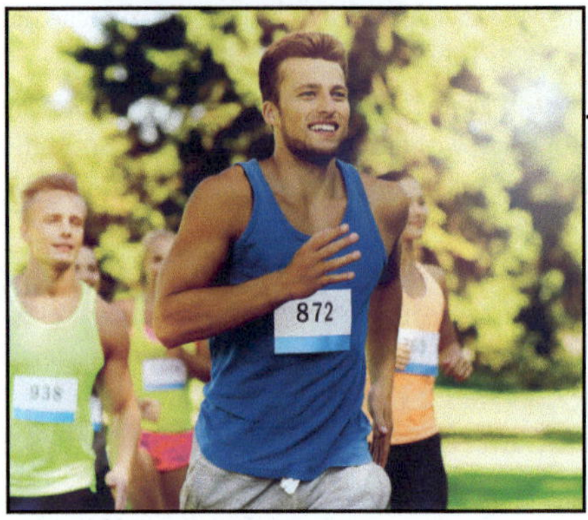

4.2

Valvular and aortic disease

Contents

4.2.1 **Mitral valve prolapse in relation to sport** Christian Schmied and Sanjay Sharma *226*
4.2.2 **Bicuspid aortic valve disease and competitive sports: key considerations and challenges** Benjamin S. Wessler and Natesa G. Pandian 233
4.2.3 **The athlete with congenital heart disease** Guido E. Pieles and Graham Stuart 238

4.2.1 Mitral valve prolapse in relation to sport

Christian Schmied and Sanjay Sharma

Introduction

Mitral valve prolapse (MVP) was first described by Barlow in 1960 and is one of the commonest structural abnormalities of the heart. The condition is characterized by myxoid degeneration of the mitral valve and appears to be more common in females. The vast majority of patients have a relatively benign natural history. However, a small proportion may develop severe mitral regurgitation (MR) due to degenerative disease or chordal rupture, infective endocarditis, embolic cerebrovascular accident, supraventricular and ventricular arrhythmias, and sudden cardiac death (SCD). Athletic training has the potential for expediting the degenerative process and a propensity for arrhythmias or even sudden death. This chapter will discuss the diagnosis, risk stratification, and eligibility criteria for participation in competitive sport.

Anatomy of the mitral valve

The mitral valve is a highly complex structure, and the evaluation of the valve as well as the severity of dysfunction and its underlying mechanisms can be challenging [1,2]. It consists of two anatomically different leaflets: a long narrow anterior leaflet and a shorter and wider posterior leaflet, which occupies a larger portion of the annular circumference. The leaflets are connected to the annulus, and their tips are attached to the chordae which join the papillary muscles. Mitral valve lesions are frequently associated with atrial and ventricular disease. Therefore the mitral valve is exposed to an interchange of different pathological structures and haemodynamic loading conditions. Because of the potential of the mitral valve apparatus to change its cellular matrix, it may undergo active structural changes [1–5]. Cardiac imaging has enabled detailed assessment of the mitral valve apparatus, particularly the complex interaction of the cardiopulmonary compartments [5]. In MVP, the leaflets are excessively long, and typically show myxomatous degeneration and increased leaflet compliance [6–8].

Nomenclature of mitral valve prolapse

The classification of MVP is based on echocardiographic findings. Morphologically, MVP can be divided into the classic (Barlow's disease) or the non-classic form. Classic MVP comprises excessively thickened leaflets (≥5mm) due to myxomatous degeneration from acidic mucopolysaccharidosis and >2mm systolic prolapse of the anterior and posterior leaflet into the left atrium. The non-classic form is characterized by thin, translucent, or minimally thickened leaflets (<5 mm) that are deficient in collagen, elastin, and proteoglycans. In this variant there is <2mm displacement of only one or two segments (most commonly the middle scallop of the posterior leaflet) and only moderate annular dilatation [9]. Billowing of the mitral leaflets describes a situation where the tips of leaflets remain in the left ventricle, while either one or both of the leaflets prolapse into the left atrium. Alternatively, cases of MVP which occur in the absence of concomitant cardiac disease or syndromes are considered as primary MVP. It is also recognised that MVP may be secondary to collagen diseases such as Marfan syndrome, Ehlers–Danlos syndrome, osteogenesis imperfecta, or pseudoxanthoma elasticum. MVP can also occur due to a primary genetic abnormality such as fibroelastin deficiency [10,11] or in the context of degenerative valvular disease such as the sequelae of rheumatic fever, infective endocarditis, and ischaemic heart disease.

Epidemiology

Reported prevalence of MVP depends on the definition of the disease and diagnostic criteria, and ranges from 2% to 15% [12–15]. Applying the currently accepted definition of MVP, the Framingham Heart Study reported an overall prevalence of 2.4% [12], of which 1.3% was classic MVP (leaflet thickness ≥5mm) and 1.1% was non-classic MVP (leaflet thickness <5mm). There is a trend towards a female preponderance [12] and the abnormality becomes more prevalent with age.

Mitral valve prolapse in relation to sport

The natural history of MVP is generally benign with MVP-related events of 0.2%/year [13,14]. However, MVP is the leading surgical indication for MR [15,16] and is the main structural abnormality complicated by infective endocarditis. Supraventricular tachycardia and ventricular arrhythmias are relatively common [17–20] and very occasionally the condition is implicated in SCD. The detection of young athletes with MVP is important, given the potential for avoiding some of these complications. One of the major challenges in all patients with MVP, including athletes, is to detect those who may be at risk of arrhythmogenic SCD.

Mitral valve prolapse and arrhythmias

One study showed that the prevalences of supraventricular arrhythmias and ventricular arrhythmias were 14% and 30%, respectively [19]. Premature ventricular contractions are the commonest rhythm disturbance and make up over two-thirds of all arrhythmic cases [20]. Individuals with moderate or severe mitral regurgitation are at the higher risk of ventricular arrhythmias, which usually arise from the left ventricle. In one study 34% of 35 patients judged to have idiopathic ventricular tachycardia exhibited MVP [21]. Early repolarization characterized by a notch at the end of the S wave or terminal slurring of the S wave has been reported to be more common in patients with MVP compared with healthy individuals with a structurally normal heart [22]. Inferior T-wave inversion is also more common in patients with MVP [17] and may be due to stretching of the posterior papillary muscle. These repolarization anomalies suggest that the mechanical effects of MVP create an arrhythmogenic milieu that may cause sustained and potentially life-threatening arrhythmias in some patients. An autopsy series has previously shown increased scarring in the inferobasal wall and papillary muscles in patients with MVP and SCD. The authors postulated that excessive stretch by the flail leaflets causing myocardial scarring promotes arrhythmogenesis [23]. In a more recent study the same group of researchers examined 36 living patients with arrhythmic MVP and confirmed the presence of inferobasal and papillary muscle fibrosis on cardiovascular magnetic resonance [24]. The authors also noted longer mitral valve annulus disjunction, presumably also due to stretch among patients with MVP and ventricular arrhythmias, compared with those without arrhythmia.

Sudden cardiac death in mitral valve prolapse

Although MVP is generally considered benign, numerous case reports have reported an association between this structural abnormality and SCD in relatively young individuals [25–28], and an overall annual mortality of 0.2–0.4%. In 1986, Jeratasey [27] reported 60 cases of MVP in association with SCD, but only four occurred in young individuals (<20 years old). One of these four individuals was a football player whose heart mass was 530g, suggesting that death may have been due to left ventricular hypertrophy rather than the valvular abnormality. Three of the 60 deaths occurred during exertion, two in athletes aged 39 and 31, and the third in the aforementioned football player aged 17 [27]. In a forensic autopsy series, MVP was reported in 5% of 2007 deaths. Among these, MVP was considered to be directly responsible for 17 (0.8%) deaths [29], indicating that it is the commonest congenital structural abnormality associated with sudden death.

The absence of a systematic registry for SCD in athletes in most countries means that the prevalence of MVP in athletes suffering a SCD is unknown. In the largest ever series of SCDs from the USA, which relied on a combination of autopsy reports and data from newspapers, insurance claims, and electronic search engines, MVP was involved in 4% of 842 SCDs in athletes [30]. In a recent study of 357 consecutive deaths among predominantly young athletes in the UK, where most deaths in Southeast England are referred for expert cardiac pathology, seven (2%) were due to MVP [31]. Between 1982 and 2004, in the Veneto region of Italy which has an established registry for SCD in athletes, it was reported that MVP caused five out of 41 (12%) deaths in athletes screened using history, examination, and ECG [32]. This proportion is probably higher because many other important cardiac diseases implicated in exercise-related SCD may have been excluded due to early detection during screening. However, MVP did not feature as a cause of death among 79 collegiate athletes in the USA [33]. Given its relatively high prevalence, it is difficult to be certain whether the detection of MVP in isolation can be considered to be the definite cause of sudden death. In one series of ambiguous autopsy where first-degree relatives of young victims of sudden cardiac death were screened for inherited arrhythmia syndromes, Brugada syndrome was diagnosed in one of three familes of victims of sudden death who revealed MVP [34]. Current consensus opinion states that in the event of a sudden cardiac arrest, death should only be attributed to MVP if there are redundant leaflets with thickening and regurgitation, or knowledge of previous ECGs showing ST and T-wave abnormalites or a prolonged QT interval [35]. However, this may overestimate the significance of MVP in athletic subjects since repolarization changes affecting the ST segment are common.

Risk factors for SCD in MVP

Several high risk factors have been reported for SCD in mitral valve prolapse. They include severe MR [15], impaired left ventricular function [15], bi-leaflet prolapse [23,36,37], ventricular premature complexes arising from the left ventricle (conducting with right bundle branch block or arising from the left fascicle), polymorphic ventricular extrasystoles [23], long mitral valve annulus disjunction, late gadolinium enhancement of the papillary muscles and inferobasal left ventricular wall [24], early repolarization changes, and a long QT interval.

Diagnosis of MVP

The diagnosis of MVP relies predominantly on echocardiography, although some affected individuals may express symptoms [1], rarely phenotypic features of Marfan syndrome and electrocardiographic abnormalities [22,27,35]. Patients with MVP may report sharp infra-mammary chest pain, breathlessness that is disproportionate to the level of exercise being performed, and palpitation even before the development of haemodynamically significant MR. Typical findings on auscultation include a mid-systolic click in the mitral area that may be accompanied by a mid-systolic murmur. The click is thought to be caused by snapping of the mitral chordae during systole when the valve prolapses into the atrium. The timing of the click is variable: In a sitting or standing position it classically occurs earlier in systole, while it can be heard later when the athlete is squatting [38]. However, once the valve becomes flail the murmur becomes pan-systolic and is usually indistinguishable from other causes of MR. These specific clinical situations suggest that diagnostic accuracy of auscultation in MVP is limited. Depending on the skills of the physician, the sensitivity and specificity vary from 52% to 100% and 66% to 73%, respectively [39]. Thus, while an integrative diagnostic approach is usual in daily practice the definite diagnosis is based on echocardiographic criteria.

Trans-thoracic echocardiography

Trans-thoracic echocardiography is the primary diagnostic tool for diagnosing MVP. Echocardiography provides information about the structure and function of the mitral valve, but also allows comprehensive evaluation of the sub-valvular complex, as well as the severity of MR and its haemodynamic consequences. Prolapse of the mitral valve is structurally and functionally defined by an abnormal systolic bulging of one or both leaflets towards the left atrium (≥2mm beyond a line connecting the annular hinge points in a parasternal long-axis view or apical three-chamber view) [39,40] (➔ Fig. 4.2.1.1).

The physiological 'saddle shape' of the mitral valve should not lead to an over-diagnosis without pathological displacement of the leaflets relative to the mitral annulus [11,40–42]. Findings from three dimensional echocardiography support this approach by demonstrating that MVP is defined most specifically by leaflet displacement relative to the anterior and posterior high points of the annular saddle when imaged in the long-axis views [43,44]. In addition to abnormal systolic bulging, further echocardiographic assessment of MVP also includes the evaluation of leaflet length and thickness and the diameter of the mitral annulus.

Assessment of mitral regurgitation and hemodynamic consequences

Mitral valve prolapse may progress to chordal rupture which most frequently affects the posterior leaflet and is generally associated with severe MR, adverse left ventricular

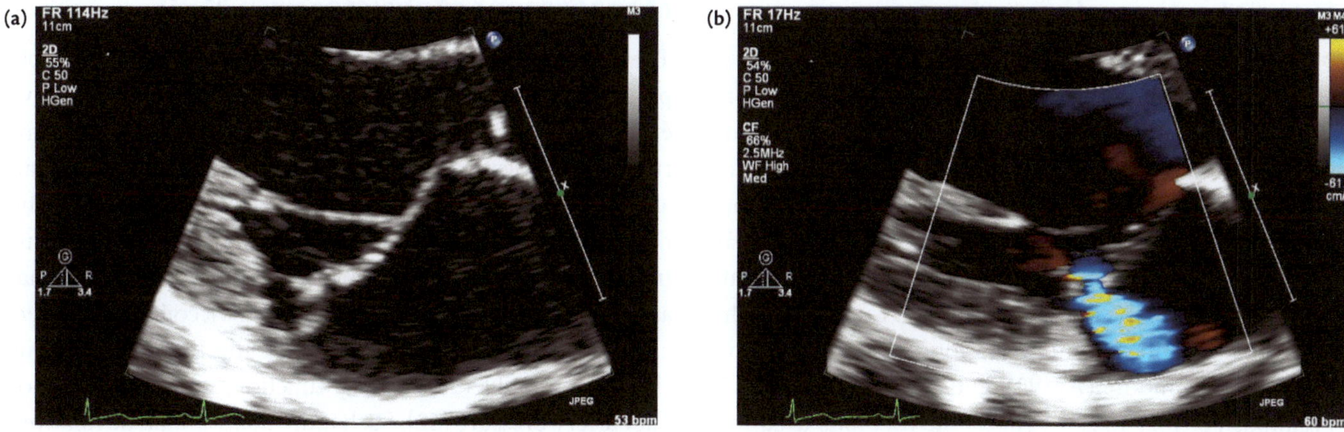

Fig. 4.2.1.1 (a) Parasternal long-axis view showing thickened and diffusely redundant myxomatous leaflets with prolapse of both mitral valve leaflets. (b) Parasternal long-axis colour Doppler in the same athlete exhibiting mild mitral regurgitation. Courtesy of the University Heart Center Zurich.

remodelling, and poor outcome without surgical intervention [45,46] (➲ Fig. 4.2.1.2).

The severity of MR due to failure of leaflet coaptation caused by chordal elongation or rupture and annular enlargement varies from mild to severe. Severe MR occurs in only 10% of patients, mostly due to flail leaflets [46]. Mitral regurgitation in patients with MVP is typically greatest in mid to late systole and therefore the regurgitant volume may be smaller than in pan-systolic regurgitation [47,48]. In athletes, the natural course of MR due to MVP may be affected by the type and intensity of exercise performed. Left ventricular remodelling due to athletic training itself may exacerbate malcoaptation through apical tethering.

The assessment of the severity of MR should integrate multiple echocardiographic parameters rather than one single measurement in order to minimize quantification errors. Individuals with chronic severe MR develop a compensatory increase in left ventricular size; however, it is important to recognize that a large proportion of athletic men with normal valves also reveal an enlarged left ventricular end-diastolic diameter. Furthermore, among athletes an enlarged left ventricle is accompanied by a normal and slightly depressed ejection fraction whereas individuals with MR show hyperdynamic left ventricular function until the later stages when left ventricular decompensation is associated with symptoms and reduced functional capacity. Quantification of MR using additional Doppler-based calculation of the regurgitant volume and the effective regurgitation orifice area can provide invaluable information about the severity of MR in athletes with MR and an enlarged left ventricle [49].

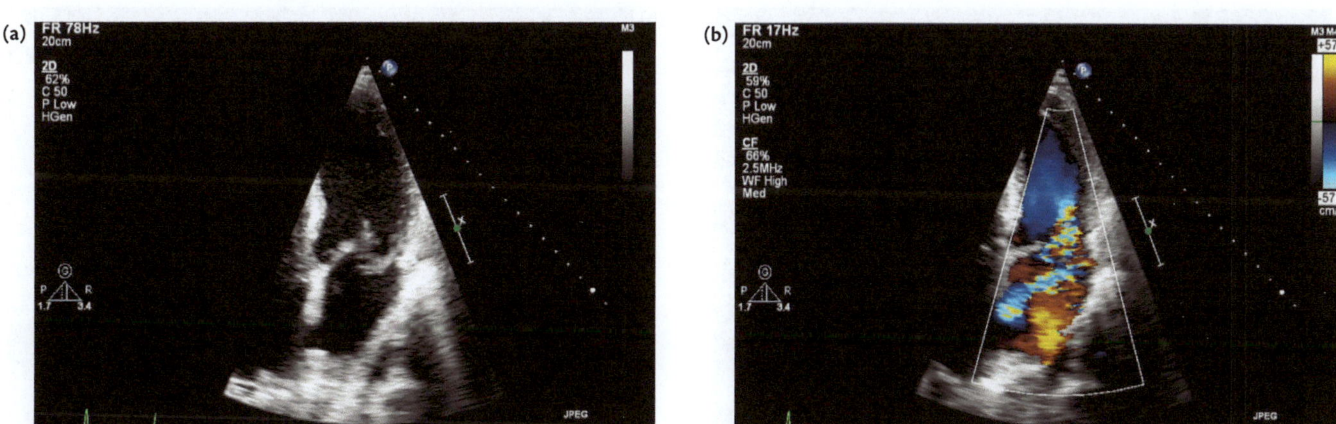

Figure 4.2.1.2 (a) Apical view demonstrating failure of coaptation due to chordal rupture with eversion of the free edge of the posterior leaflet into the left atrium. Chordal rupture affecting the posterior mitral leaflet is more common than with the anterior leaflet. (b) Apical view colour Doppler of the same athlete exhibiting severe pan-systolic mitral regurgitation.
Courtesy of the University Heart Center Zurich.

Advanced echocardiography

Trans-oesopageal echocardiography

In patients where trans-thoracic echocardiography is inconclusive or technically difficult, or when surgical intervention is being considered, knowledge of the particular individual mitral valve anatomy is necessary. Indeed, trans-oesophageal echocardiography (TOE) should be considered in all patients with moderate to severe MR. TOE allows accurate sub-classification of the lesion according to Carpentier, who first divided the anterior and posterior leaflets into antero-lateral (A1/P1), middle (A2/P2), and postero-medial (A3/P3) scallops (➲ Fig. 4.2.1.3). All classic methods used in a trans-thoracic approach can also be used in TOE to quantify MR. Because of its higher resolution, multiplane capabilities, and proximity to the mitral valve, TOE determines the severity of MR more accurately than trans-thoracic echocardiography [50] (➲ Fig. 4.2.1.4).

3D echocardiography

3D echocardiography, particularly real-time 3D-TOE, provides excellent assessment of the mitral valve complex. Real-time 3D-TOE has become routine in peri-operative and percutaneous mitral valve interventions and allows better assessment of dynamic mitral annulus function than conventional TOE (➲ Fig. 4.2.1.5).

Cardiovascular magnetic resonance

Although cardiovascular magnetic resonance imaging is an important tool in the assessment of cardiac disease and may enable quantification of mitral regurgitation, it is still not used routinely in the primary evaluation of MVP [51].

Management of athletes with MVP

The vast majority of patients with MVP have a favourable prognosis, although it is theoretically possible that intensive exercise may expedite the degenerative process, causing chord rupture and death from acute heart failure, or promote an arrhythmogenic substrate through mechanical stress of the flail leaflets on the papillary muscles and the adjacent ventricular myocardium. Current guidelines recommend that asymptomatic athletes with mild MR may continue to exercise without further investigation in the presence of sinus rhythm, normal left ventricular function, and resting pulmonary artery pressure [52]. Such individuals should be followed up annually with ECG and echocardiography as well as 24–48-hour Holter monitoring. It is our opinion that the detection of frequent ventricular premature complexes or complex ventricular arrhythmias during exercise in athletes with otherwise asymptomatic MVP with mild MR warrants assessment for myocardial scar with cardiac magnetic resonance, and that this condition is an indication to avoid intensive exercise.

Risk stratification

There is limited literature about risk stratification for identifying athletes with MVP who may be at risk of SCD. Based on the current information and the studies cited in this chapter, we consider symptomatic athletes, particularly those with intractable chest pain, palpitation, and syncope, and athletes with a family history of sudden death from MVP at high risk of an adverse event. Individuals with moderate or severe MR should abstain from moderate or high intensity exercise. Twelve-lead ECG evidence of T-wave inversion in the inferior and/or lateral leads, a prolonged QT interval or ventricular premature complexes with right bundle branch

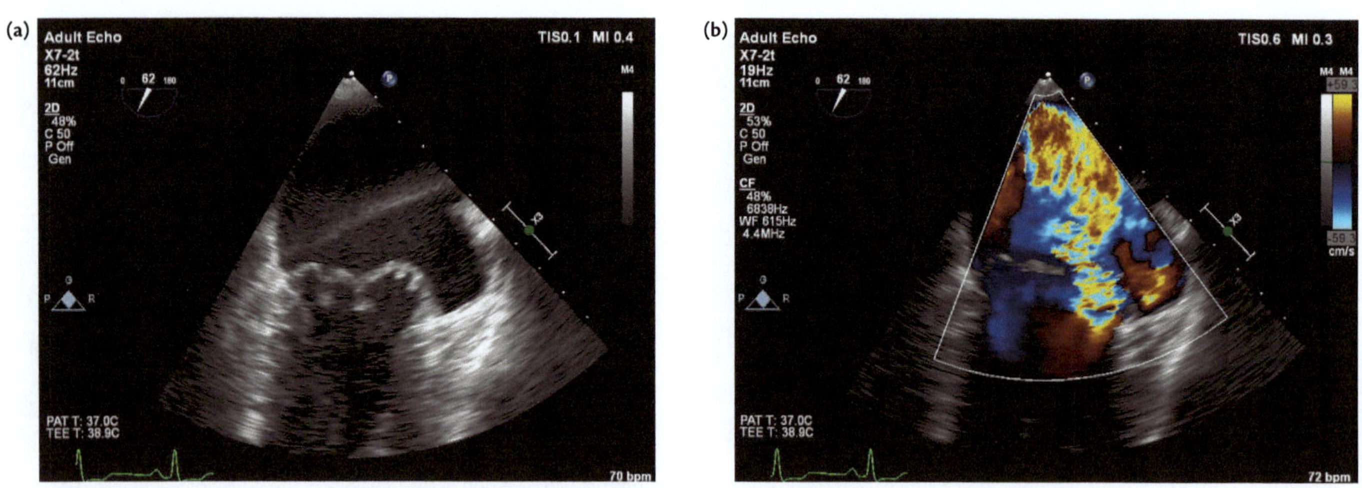

Fig. 4.2.1.3 (a)Trans-oesophageal echocardiography in an athlete with prolapse of the P1 and P3 posterior segments. (b) Trans-oesophageal echocardiography in the same athlete demonstrating severe mitral regurgitation.
Courtesy of the University Heart Center Zurich.

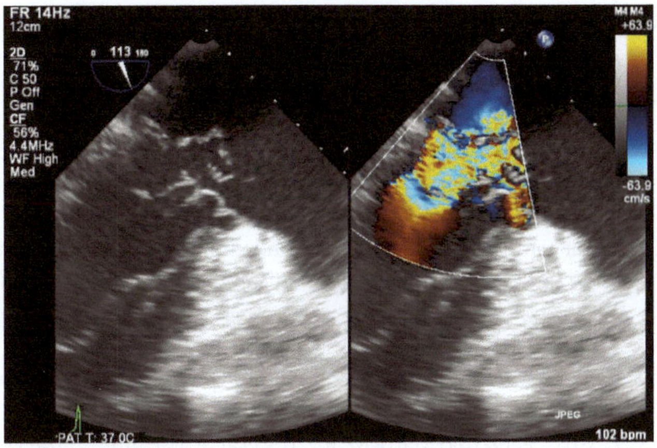

Fig. 4.2.1.4 Trans-oesophageal echocardiography in an athlete with prolapse of all three anterior segments (A1, A2, A3) and flail of the P3 segment of the posterior leaflet leading to severe pan-systolic mitral regurgitation ('colour compare' display)
Courtesy of the University Heart Center Zurich.

block or left ventricular fascicular morphology, and those with bi-leaflet MVP should be subject to Holter monitoring for 24–48 hours and cardiovascular magnetic resonance. The presence of frequent ventricular extra-systoles (>2000 per 24 hours), complex ventricular arrhythmias, or late gadolinium enhancement of the papillary muscles is an indication against competitive sports involving moderate or high intensity exercise (see also ➲ Chapter 7.1).

Surgery and return to sport

There is liitle evidence that pharmacological therapy influences the natural history of MVP. Surgical intervention is recommended for severe MR in all symptomatic patients and in asymptomatic patients with an LV ejection fraction between 30% and 50%, or with an LV end-systolic diameter ≥40mm. Mitral valve surgery is also reasonable with severe MR and normal left ventricular size and systolic function if the likelihood of a successful valve repair is >95% and estimated surgical mortality is <1% [53]. Athletes with a competent valve and preserved left ventricular function, normal resting pulmonary artery pressure, and a normal maximal exercise test can return to competition after 6 months once the sternotomy site has healed fully. Young athletes with mechanical valve prosthesis should be anticoagulated and should avoid all contact sports [52]. There is currently limited data to suggest that mitral valve repair or replacement alters arrhythmic risk in MVP.

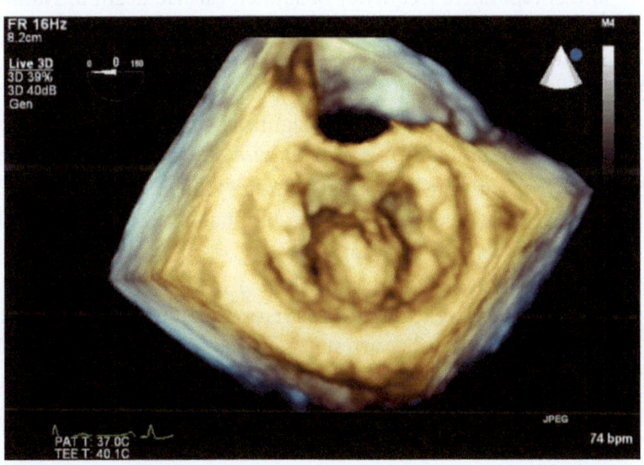

Fig. 4.2.1.5 3D trans-oesophageal echocardiography in an athlete demonstrating particular meso-systolic prolapse of the P2 segment.
Courtesy of the University Heart Center Zurich.

Other issues

Athletes with Marfan syndrome and MVP with mild mitral regurgitation should be assessed regarding the Marfan syndrome and managed according the current recommendations (see ➲ Chapter 7.1) [54]. Mitral valve prolapse is the commonest valvular abnormality potentially complicated by endocarditis, and this suspicion should arise in an athlete with protracted malaise, myalgia, and fever. Optimal dental hygiene is important for preventing endocarditis, although antibiotic prophylaxis may no longer be recommended.

Further reading

Addetia K, Mor-Avi V, Weinert L, et al. A new definition for an old entity: improved definition of mitral valve prolapse using three-dimensional echocardiography and color-coded parametric models. *J Am Soc Echocardiogr* 2014; 27: 8–16.

Avierinos JF, Gersh BJ, Melton LJ 3rd, et al. Natural history of asymptomatic mitral valve prolapse in the community. *Circulation* 2002; 106: 1355–61.

Basso C, Perazzolo Marra M, Rizzo S, et al. Arrhythmic mitral valve prolapse and sudden cardiac death. *Circulation* 2015; 132: 556–66.

Bonow RO, Nishimura RA, Thompson PD, Udelson JE. Eligibility and disqualification recommendations for competitive athletes with cardiovascular abnormalities. Task Force 5: Valvular Heart Disease. A Scientific Statement from the American Heart Association and American College of Cardiology. *J Am Coll Cardiol* 2015; 66: 2385–92

Dal-Bianco JP, Levine RA. Anatomy of the mitral valve apparatus: role of 2D and 3D echocardiography. *Cardiol Clin* 2013; 31: 151–64.

Finocchiaro G, Papadakis M, Robertus JL, et al. Etiology of sudden death in sports: insights from a United Kingdom regional registry. *J Am Coll Cardiol* 2016; 67: 2108–15.

Freed LA, Levy D, Levine RA, et al. Prevalence and clinical outcome of mitral-valve prolapse. *N Engl J Med* 1999; 341: 1–7.

Levine RA, Hagége AA, Judge DP, et al. f Mitral valve disease: morphology and mechanisms. *Nat Rev Cardiol* 2015; 12: 689–710.

Otani K, Takeuchi M, Kaku K, et al. Evidence of a vicious cycle in mitral regurgitation with prolapse: secondary tethering attributed to primary prolapse demonstrated by three-dimensional echocardiography exacerbates regurgitation. *Circulation* 2012; 126: S214–21.

Turker Y, Ozaydin M, Acar G, et al. Predictors of ventricular arrhythmias in patients with mitral valve prolapse. *Int J Cardiovasc Imaging* 2010; 26: 139–45.

References

1. Levine RA, Hagége AA, Judge DP, et al. Mitral valve disease: morphology and mechanisms. *Nat Rev Cardiol* 2015; 12:689–710.
2. Judge DP, Markwald RR, Hagége AA, Levine RA. Translational research on the mitral valve: from developmental mechanisms to new therapies. *J Cardiovasc Transl Res* 2011; 4: 699–701.
3. Roberts, R. Another chromosomal locus for mitral valve prolapse: close but no cigar. *Circulation* 2005; 112: 1924–6.
4. Ng CM, Cheng A, Myers LA, et al. TGF-beta-dependent pathogenesis of mitral valve prolapse in a mouse model of Marfan syndrome. *J Clin Invest* 2004; 114: 1586–92.
5. Dal-Bianco JP, Levine RA. Anatomy of the mitral valve apparatus: role of 2D and 3D echocardiography. *Cardiol Clin* 2013; 31: 151–64.
6. Barber JE, Kasper FK, Ratliff NB, et al. Mechanical properties of myxomatous mitral valves. *J Thorac Cardiovasc Surg* 2001; 122: 955–62.
7. Barber JE, Ratliff NB, Cosgrove DM 3rd, et al. Myxomatous mitral valve chordae. I: Mechanical properties. *J Heart Valve Dis* 2001; 10: 320–4.
8. Maslow AD, Regan MM, Haering JM, et al. Echocardiographic predictors of left ventricular outflow tract obstruction and systolic anterior motion of the mitral valve after mitral valve reconstruction for myxomatous valve disease. *J Am Coll Cardiol* 1999; 34: 2096–104.
9. Freed LA, Levy D, Levine RA, et al. Prevalence and clinical outcome of mitral-valve prolapse. *N Engl J Med* 1999; 341: 1–7.
10. Grau JB, Pirelli L, Yu PJ, et al. The genetics of mitral valve prolapse. *Clin Genet* 2007; 72: 288–95.
11. Glesby MJ, Pyeritz RE. Association of mitral valve prolapse and systemic abnormalities of connective tissue: a phenotypic continuum. *JAMA* 1989; 262: 523.
12. Procacci PM, Savran SV, Schreiter SL, Bryson AL. Prevalence of clinical mitral-valve prolapse in 1169 young women. *N Engl J Med* 1976; 294: 1086–8.
13. Freed LA, Benjamin EJ, Levy D, et al. Mitral valve prolapse in the general population: the benign nature of echocardiographic features in the Framingham Heart Study. *J Am Coll Cardiol* 2002; 40: 1298–1304.
14. Avierinos JF, Gersh BJ, Melton LJ 3rd, et al. Natural history of asymptomatic mitral valve prolapse in the community. *Circulation* 2002; 106: 1355–61.
15. Luxereau P, Dorent R, De Gevigney G, et al. Aetiology of surgically treated mitral regurgitation. *Eur Heart J* 1991;12(Suppl B): 2–4.
16. Waller BF, Morrow AG, Maron BJ, et al. Etiology of clinically isolated, severe, chronic, pure mitral regurgitation: analysis of 97 patients over 30 years of age having mitral valve replacement. *Am Heart J* 1982; 104: 276–88.
17. DeMaria AN, Amsterdam EA, Vismara LA, et al. Arrhythmias in mitral valve prolapse syndrome: prevalence, nature and frequency. *Ann Intern Med* 1976; 84: 656–60.
18. Winkle RA, Lopes MG, Fitzgerald JW, et al. Arrhythmias in patients with mitral valve prolapse. *Circulation* 1975; 52: 73–81.
19. Zuppiroli A, Mori F, Favilli S, et al. Arrhythmias in mitral valve prolapse: relation to anterior mitral leaflet thickening, clinical variables, and color Doppler echocardiographic parameters. *Am Heart J* 1994; 128: 919–27.
20. Turker Y, Ozaydin M, Acar G, et al. Predictors of ventricular arrhythmias in patients with mitral valve prolapse. *Int J Cardiovasc Imaging* 2010; 26: 139–45.
21. Ikeda T Mitral valve prolapse in idiopathic ventricular tachycardia: clinical and electrophysiological characteristics. *J Cardiol* 1991; 21: 717–26.
22. Peighambari MM, Alizadehasl A, Totonchi Z. Electrocardiographic changes in mitral valve prolapse syndrome. *J Cardiovasc Thorac Res* 2014; 6: 21–3.
23. Basso C, Perazzolo Marra M, Rizzo S, et al. Arrhythmic mitral valve prolapse and sudden cardiac death. *Circulation* 2015; 132: 556–66.
24. Perazzolo Marra M, Basso C, De Lazzari M, et al. Morphofunctional abnormalities of mitral annulus and arrhythmic mitral valve prolapse. *Circ Cardiovasc Imaging* 2016; 9: e005030
25. Chesler E, King RA, Edwards JE. The myxomatous mitral valve and sudden death. *Circulation* 1983; 67: 632–9.
26. Pocock WA, Bosman CK, Chesler E, et al. Sudden death in primary mitral valve prolapse. *Am Heart J* 1983; 107: 378–82.
27. Jeresaty RM. Mitral valve prolapse: definition and implications in athletes. *J Am Coll Cardiol* 1986; 7: 231–6.
28. Ahmed M, Roshdy A, Sharma R, Fletcher N. Sudden cardiac arrest and coexisting mitral valve prolapse: a case report and literature review. *Echo Res Pract* 2016; 3: D1–8.
29. Waller BF, Catellier MJ, Clark MA, et al. Cardiac pathology in 2007 consecutive forensic autopsies. *Clin Cardiol* 1992; 15: 760–5.
30. Maron BJ, Haas TS, Ahluwalia A, et al. Demographics and epidemiology of sudden deaths in young competitive athletes: from the United States National Registry. *Am J Med* 2016; 129: 1170–7.
31. Finocchiaro G, Papadakis M, Robertus JL, et al. Etiology of sudden death in sports: insights from a United Kingdom regional registry. *J Am Coll Cardiol* 2016; 67: 2108–15.
32. Corrado D, Basso C, Pavei A, et al. Trends in sudden cardiovascular death in young competitive athletes after implementation of a preparticipation screening program. *JAMA* 2006; 296: 1593–1601
33. Harmon KG, Asif IM, Maleszewski JJ, et al. Incidence, cause, and comparative frequency of sudden cardiac death in National Collegiate Athletic Association ATHLETES: A DECADE IN REView. *Circulation* 2015; 132: 10–19.
34. Papadakis M, Raju H, Behr ER, et al. Sudden cardiac death with autopsy findings of uncertain significance: potential for erroneous interpretation. *Circ Arrhythm Electrophysiol* 2013; 6: 588–96.
35. Survivors of out-of-hospital cardiac arrest with apparently normal heart: need for definition and standardized clinical evaluation. *Circulation* 1997; 95; 265–7.
36. Sriram CS, Syed FF, Ferguson ME, et al. Malignant bileaflet mitral-valve prolapse syndrome in patients with otherwise idiopathic out-of-hospital cardiac arrest. *J Am Coll Cardiol* 2013; 62: 222–30.
37. Vohra J, Sathe S, Warren R, et al. Malignant ventricular arrhythmias in patients with mitral valve prolapse and mild mitral regurgitation. *Pacing Clin Electrophysiol* 1993; 16: 387–93.
38. Barron JT, Manrose DL, Liebson PR. Comparison of auscultation with two-dimensional and Doppler echocardiography in patients with suspected mitral valve prolapse. *Clin Cardiol* 1988; 11: 401–6.

39. Levine, RA, Stathogiannis E, Newell JB, et al. Reconsideration of echocardiographic standards for mitral valve prolapse: lack of association between leaflet displacement isolated to the apical four chamber view and independent echocardiographic evidence of abnormality. *J Am Coll Cardiol* 1988; 11: 1010–19.
40. Addetia K, Mor-Avi V, Weinert L, et al. A new definition for an old entity: improved definition of mitral valve prolapse using three-dimensional echocardiography and color-coded parametric models. *J Am Soc Echocardiogr* 2014; 27: 8–16.
41. Devereux RB, Kramer-Fox R, Kligfield P. Mitral valve prolapse: causes, clinical manifestations, and management. *Ann Intern Med* 1989; 111: 305.
42. Levine RA, Triulzi MO, Harrigan P, Weyman AE. The relationship of mitral annular shape to the diagnosis of mitral valve prolapse. *Circulation* 1987; 75: 756–67.
43. Levine RA, Handschumacher MD, Sanfilippo AJ, et al. Three-dimensional echocardiographic reconstruction of the mitral valve, with implications for the diagnosis of mitral valve prolapse. *Circulation* 1989; 80: 589–98.
44. Otani K, Takeuchi M, Kaku K, et al. Evidence of a vicious cycle in mitral regurgitation with prolapse: secondary tethering attributed to primary prolapse demonstrated by three-dimensional echocardiography exacerbates regurgitation. *Circulation* 2012; 126: S214–21.
45. Ling LH, Enriquez-Sarano M, Seward JB, et al. Clinical outcome of mitral regurgitation due to flail leaflet. *N Engl J Med* 1996; 335: 1417–23.
46. Grigioni F, Tribouilloy C, Avierinos JF, et al. Outcomes in mitral regurgitation due to flail leaflets: a multicenter European study. *JACC Cardiovasc Imaging* 2008; 1: 133–41.
47. Schwammenthal E, Chen C, Benning F, et al. Dynamics of mitral regurgitant flow and orifice area: physiologic application of the proximal flow convergence method; clinical data and experimental testing. *Circulation* 1994; 90: 307–22.
48. Enriquez-Sarano M, Sinak LJ, Tajik AJ, et al. Changes in effective regurgitant orifice throughout systole in patients with mitral valve prolapse: a clinical study using the proximal isovelocity surface area method. *Circulation* 1995; 92: 2951–8.
49. Zoghbi WA, Enriquez-Sarano M, Foster E, et al. Recommendations for evaluation of the severity of native valvular regurgitation with two-dimensional and Doppler echocardiography. *J Am Soc Echocardiogr* 2003; 16: 777–802.
50. Pepi M, Tamborini G, Maltagliati A, et al. Head-to-head comparison of two- and three-dimensional transthoracic and transesophageal echocardiography in the localization of mitral valve prolapse. *J Am Coll Cardiol* 2006; 48: 2524.
51. Han Y, Peters DC, Salton CJ, et al. Cardiovascular magnetic resonance characterization of mitral valve prolapse. *JACC Cardiovasc Imaging* 2008; 1: 294.
52. Bonow RO, Nishimura RA, Thompson PD, Udelson JE. Eligibility and disqualification recommendations for competitive athletes with cardiovascular abnormalities. Task Force 5: Valvular Heart Disease. A Scientific Statement From the American Heart Association and American College of Cardiology. *J Am Coll Cardiol* 2015; 66: 2385–92.
53. Otto CM, Salerno C. Timing of surgery in asymptomatic mitral regurgitation. *N Engl J Med* 2005 352, 928–9.
54. Braverman AC, Harris KH, Kovacs RJ, Maron BJ. Eligibility and disqualification recommendations for competitive athletes with cardiovascular abnormalities: Task Force 7: Aortic Diseases, Including Marfan Syndrome. A Scientific Statement from the American Heart Association and American College of Cardiology. *J Am Coll Cardiol* 2015; 66: 2398–405.

4.2.2 Bicuspid aortic valve disease and competitive sports: key considerations and challenges

Benjamin S. Wessler and Natesa G. Pandian

Introduction

Sports activities have enriched human lives over millennia. However, if an athlete has a cardiac disorder, such as bicuspid aortic valve (BAV), it raises a number of questions. Let us start with a case study.

JW was 18 years old and had known about his heart murmur for four years. He was diagnosed with a BAV at age 14 when the murmur was detected, and his last echocardiogram, three years previously, demonstrated a peak velocity across his aortic valve (AoV) of 1.7m/s and median gradient of 16mmHg. His father had developed symptomatic aortic stenosis (AS) associated with BAV and underwent mechanical aortic valve replacement (AVR) at age 43. There was no family history of aortic dissection. JW was asymptomatic and played competitive basketball well. He was being recruited to play at a number of universities. JW (and his parents) sought opinions about the safety of competitive sports in light of this cardiovascular abnormality and want guidance on how he should proceed considering the risks (real and perceived) associated with his BAV, and the appropriateness and value (emotional and physical) of continued participation in high level competitive sports.

This chapter reviews the key concepts and important controversies that must be considered when taking care of patients with BAV who participate in competitive sports. It is not meant to be a comprehensive review, but instead highlights some of the major issues and controversies. With JW's case in mind, we review the salient clinical recommendations, pathophysiological issues, and important remaining controversies that inform decisions for patients with BAV who want to play competitive sports.

General approach

At first sight, recommendations for patients with BAV who play sports seem to be clear. Consistent with the current ACC/AHA consensus document on Eligibility and

Disqualification Recommendations for Competitive Athletes with Cardiovascular Abnormalities [1], our patient with asymptomatic mild AS (stage B), should proceed as follows.

1. An annual history and physical examination, and also Doppler echocardiography to identify progression of aortic stenosis.
2. Exercise testing to confirm that functional capacity is consistent with that required of the proposed competitive sport. During exercise testing note should be made of risk markers such as hypotension or electrocardiogram ischaemia and if no such markers are present it is reasonable to participate in all sports.
3. Serial follow-up to document increases in transvalvular gradient. As BAV disease is characterized by moderate stenosis, participation in competitive sports should be limited to low and moderate static exercise (e.g. equestrian, motorcycling, golf) or low and moderate dynamic exercise (e.g. table tennis, volleyball, fencing).
4. As stenosis progresses athletes who are asymptomatic with severe AS from BAV should not participate in competitive sports (except for very low intensity sports).

Unfortunately, each of these recommendations is supported by the lowest level of evidence (C, expert opinion), and without a clear evidence base, many questions remain. How do we tailor these recommendations to individuals [2]? Are there other important clinical concerns that should be considered? What recommendations can we make to our patient? Here, we review some of the background and challenges for clinicians and patients faced with this difficult clinical scenario.

Epidemiology of bicuspid aortic valve

BAV is the most common congenital abnormality, affecting 1–2% of the population (➲ Figs 4.2.2.1 and 4.2.2.2). Approximately 1 in 11 patients with bicuspid AoV have family members with the same disease, and males are more commonly affected (3:1 predominance). The clinical consequences of BAV disease most frequently occur in adulthood and relate to valve degeneration (resulting in stenosis) and complications related to the accompanying aortopathy (see next section). Early abnormalities are often progressive, as shown in a European cohort where the majority of patients with mild stenosis progressed to more severe disease over 30 years of follow-up [3]. Clinical consequences that occur at a younger age (and commonly arise during the years when patients play competitive sports) include the development of aortic insufficiency related to prolapsed leaflets and dilation of the aorta. Population studies show that non-valvular-associated lesions are common with this disease and affect approximately 50% of patients.

When evaluating patients with BAV, providers much always be aware that a BAV is seen with other syndromic diseases that should not be missed. These include concomitant cardiovascular pathology that involves other left-sided lesions, such as Turner syndrome (coarctation of the aorta), Shone syndrome (multiple obstructive left-sided lesions), and Williams syndrome (supravalular stenosis). Other lesions that may accompany bicuspid AoV include ventricular and atrial septal defects and patent ductus arteriosus, all of which can have important clinical consequences for the athlete with BAV.

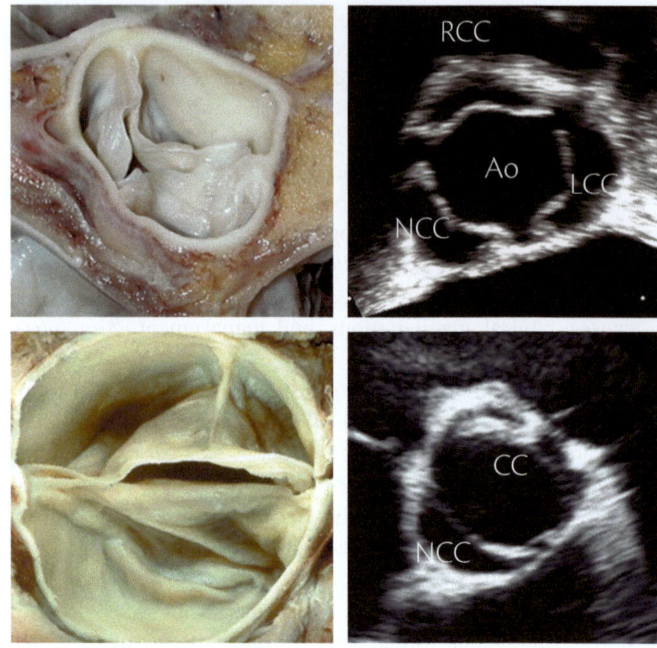

Fig. 4.2.2.1 Anatomical and 2D echocardiographic images of three-cuspid (top panel) and bicuspid (bottom panel) aortic valves: Ao, aorta; RCC, right coronary cusp; LCC, left coronary cusp; NCC, non-coronary cusp.

Pathophysiology of bicuspid aortic valve

There is a probable Mendelian pattern of inheritance for BAV, and therefore this phenotype clusters in families. While the actual events that lead to abnormal valve morphology are not known exactly, they probably occur early in fetal development since that is the time point when valve morphology is specified. The particular genetics involved are mechanistically complex [4], and some more recent studies suggest that BAV may result from a number of different potential mutations in various genes (only some of which have

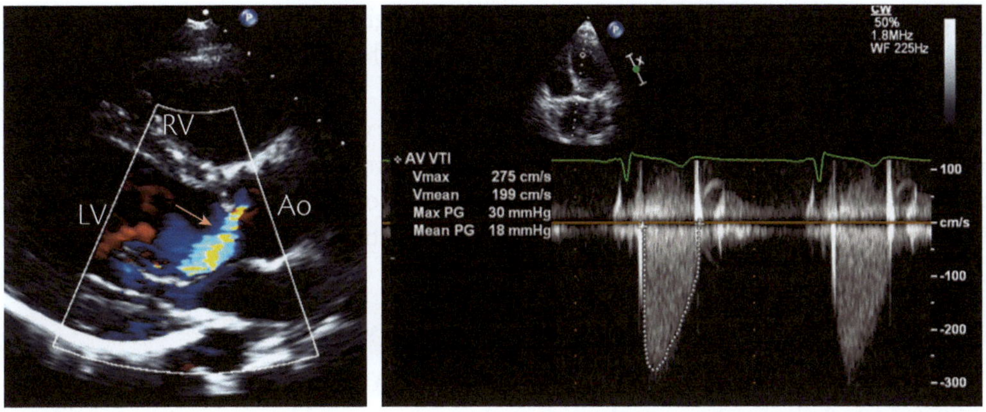

Fig. 4.2.2.2 Aortic regurgitation jet (arrow) in a subject with bicuspid aortic valve (left panel), and a Doppler echocardiographic recording depicting mild aortic stenosis in another subject (right panel); LV, left ventricle; RV, right ventricle; Ao, aorta.

been elucidated). One such example, *NOTCH1*, is a gene implicated in both abnormal aortic valve development and calcium regulation. Mutations at this site have been linked to the clinical changes that are commonly observed in these patients [5]. Indeed, other loci have been linked to the other cardiac abnormalities that are associated with BAV.

Degeneration of the AoV is probably due to abnormal haemodynamic shear stress that results from abnormal blood flow through a morphologically abnormal valve. Calcification is accelerated in this disease and affects patients at a younger age than does degenerative AoV disease; it is probably accelerated by endothelial dysfunction and active inflammation [6]. Aortic insufficiency can develop early due to prolapse of redundant leaflets and later due to dilation of the aortic root. The rate of intervention for isolated aortic insufficiency in the setting of BAV disease is generally quite low.

Beyond early aortic stenosis, bicuspid aortopathy represents perhaps the most important, feared, and most often overlooked lesion for these patients (generally) and for athletes with BAV (in particular). Dilation of the aorta (anywhere from the root to the aortic arch) is seen in approximately 50% of these patients [7]. Recent insights suggest that this dilation is distinct from the degenerative changes seen in patients without BAV, and the risk of dissection is probably different (and higher) at smaller diameters. Dilation often begins during childhood and relates to changes formerly called cystic medial necrosis. These pathological changes result from abnormal vascular smooth-muscle cell regulation within the media that leads to media disruption and ultimately decreased elasticity and integrity. Although the more proximal changes can be seen with trans-thoracic echocardiography, more distal ascending and arch lesions can be present and may be missed by this modality. To visualize these abnormalities additional imaging with CT or MRI should be considered.

Clinical course of patients with bicuspid aortic valve

Significant referral bias has influenced our understanding of this disease for years. Fortunately, we have gained recent insights into the natural history for asymptomatic patients with BAV (such as those participating in competitive sports). A large cohort of asymptomatic patients (n = 212) living in Olmsted County, Minnesota, USA were comprehensively studied at baseline and followed for development of symptoms and clinical events [8]. Some of the key findings from this study were that 15% of these patients had associated congenital abnormalities. Total follow-up for this cohort was 15 years (range 0.4–25 years) during which three deaths related to AoV pathology occurred (one each of endocarditis, aortic stenosis, and aortic regurgitation). Overall survival was 90% at 20 years after diagnosis, similar to the expected survival of the general population ($p = 0.72$). The rate of incident cardiovascular events was 33% at 20 years after diagnosis, and the most powerful predictor of cardiac events for this population was older age (HR 4.4; 95% confidence interval (CI) 2.4–7.9). Notably, hypertension and ascending aortic diameter were not significantly associated with cardiac events after controlling for other risk factors. Ascending aorta ≥40 mm at baseline did predict subsequent need for aortic surgery (HR 10.8; 95% CI 1.8–77.3). Notably, only eight patients in this cohort underwent ascending aortic surgery, and thus there is reasonable uncertainty associated with this effect size.

Given the prevalence of this disease and the generally benign course for asymptomatic patients, it is important to approach questions related to sports participation systematically and with attention to the potential risks specific to individual patients.

Sports for patients with cardiovascular disease

It is common for patients with cardiovascular disease (CVD), like the general population, to have a strong interest in participating in sports at all levels, and the physical and emotional benefits of such participation are well known [9]. A subset of this population become involved in highly competitive, highly dynamic sports. In clinical practice enquiries come from patients with underlying CVD that ranges from mild to severe and with interest in sports participation levels that range from recreational to competitive (and include possible injury). One important concern relating to competitive sports is whether or not participating athletes can gauge for themselves when exertion should stop. It is often the case with competitive sports that individuals are unable to exact stringent control over their level of exertion (and when to stop) [10]. Fortunately for patients and clinicians, significant work has been done to define these problems and offer guidance for eligibility and disqualification from competitive sports. The 16th, 26th, and 36th Bethesda Conferences have provided a framework for patients and clinicians to approach these issues as they enquire about various sporting activities in the setting of a variety of underlying CVDs. These important documents offer some guidance in the absence of clear evidence and rely largely on the opinions of thought leaders and evidence (when available). More recently the ACC/AHA Consensus Document on Eligibility and Disqualification Recommendations for Competitive Athletes With Cardiovascular Abnormalities offers an updated set of recommendations to help clinicians and patients as the epidemiology of cardiovascular diseases changes, interventions are more common (and have matured), and more and more (and younger) participants engage in competitive sports [10].

When considering the patient at the start of this chapter and his interest in competitive sports (with collision potential), it is important to characterize the type and risks of his chosen sport. In the current framework sports are grouped by their relative static vs dynamic muscle components [11]. Static muscle contractions stimulate skeletal muscle afferents that lead to significant and prolonged changes in blood pressure through the exercise pressor reflex, such as occurs typically in power disciplines. In contrast, dynamic exercise results in increased blood flow and thus demands an increase in cardiac output, such as occurs typically in endurance disciplines. While both these exercise types increase myocardial oxygen demand and left ventricle contractility, the mechanisms that lead to these changes vary. Since different sports have different relative contributions from these exercise components, their effects on the cardiovascular system vary. For instance, soccer is classified as a high dynamic component/low static component sport and thus has risks most closely aligned with the physiological changes that accompany dynamic exercises. Weightlifting is at the opposite end of the spectrum and American football lies somewhere in between. Ultimately, risk changes from minute to minute and position to position, depending on the actual activity/exertion being performed.

Screening athletes (with BAV)

There is broad recognition that pre-participation screening has the potential to mitigate sudden death risks in athletes across a broad range of sports. The exact form (and intensity) of such efforts is widely debated and remains highly variable and without consensus [9]. In the context of BAV this debate is important and unsettled. Detection of patients with BAV may occur through routine clinical encounters (where a murmur is appreciated), the history of known affected family members, or formal screening programmes that involve examinations plus or minus echocardiography. The risk for athletes is often not from the asymptomatic valve disease that might bring the patient to attention, but rather from haemodynamically significant valve disease with aortic stenosis and/or aortic regurgitation or associated lesions (specifically, common aortopathy) which might lead to dissection and sudden death. Rarer (but just as important) are the more distant lesions of cerebral aneurysms that are not routinely assessed and may pose significant risks to athletes playing contact sports.

For patients with BAV who are interested in participating in competitive contact sports it may be reasonable to pursue imaging tests to establish the presence or absence of all of these associated lesions so that risk assessments can be better individualized.

Aortopathy: when does risk increase?

Increasingly, it is being recognized that the aortic root dilation seen in patients with BAV behaves in a clinically similar way to patients with Marfan syndrome or other genetically mediated aortopathies. Specifically, a more aggressive threshold (aortic root diameter of 4.0–5.0cm) is considered as the threshold above which surgical intervention is recommended for these disease states [12]. This contrasts with the larger cut-off of >5.5cm for degenerative aortic dilation. More recent guidelines have addressed the same issue and recommended a different threshold (5.5cm or >5.0cm if there is a risk factor such as a family history of dissection or growth >0.5cm/year) [13]. These inconsistent recommendations left clinicians without clear guidance, and although this discrepancy was recently resolved [14] it shows that there is significant variability in risk and an unclear (and unlikely) threshold above which dissection risk clearly increases (and below which the risk is minimal).

Since it is unlikely that an individual's risk can be distilled to one threshold value (and that this value means the same thing for all patients), a more nuanced approach is appropriate. We agree with the most recent ACC/AHA guidelines which present aortic diameters corrected for age, sex, and body surface area (BSA) for patients with BAV [15]. Using a standardized Z-score allows aortic values to be interpreted in a patient-specific context. This exercise is made easy by a freely available downloadable calculator which is linked to these guidelines and allows the concept of a single threshold value that applies to all patients to be abandoned.

Legal concerns

It is the treating physician's goal to minimize the risks of sudden death for competitive athletes. To that end legal duty requires that physicians act in ways that are consistent with accepted practice standards and protect the best interests of the athlete [16]. Recommendations for patients with BAV should be consistent with valve and aorta guidelines, and ultimately tailored to individual sport demands and anatomical concerns. On an individual basis, when risks of injury or death in competitive sports are deemed too great (whatever this threshold value is for the treating clinician), recommendations against participating in competitive sports are reasonable despite the fact that they may be unpopular and be the cause of significant stress. Ultimately such decisions are designed to minimize inappropriate (i.e. overly conservative) disqualifications while keeping patients with known cardiovascular disease safe from the cardiovascular injury and sudden death risks associated with competitive sports.

For patients with BAV disease, this risk (and possible disqualification from participation) will relate most commonly to progressive valvular heart disease and ascending aorta dilation (and risk of dissection). Ultimately, legal debates with BAV will mirror other discussions where patient interests and autonomy and physician guidance and recommendations will come together within the local legal and participatory environments to inform decisions for or against participation.

Conclusion

The patient described at the start of this chapter was asymptomatic although he was interested in participating in a sport (basketball) with reasonable static and dynamic exercise components and also high collision potential. We would proceed with complete imaging to understand his ascending aorta anatomy and also the presence or absence of intra-cranial aneurysms. Once a baseline was obtained, we would repeat cardiovascular imaging (including aorta imaging) and exercise echocardiography annually while participation continued.

References

1. Bonow RO, Nishimura RA, Thompson PD, et al. Eligibility and disqualification recommendations for competitive athletes with cardiovascular abnormalities: Task Force 5: Valvular Heart Disease: A Scientific StatementfFrom the American Heart Association and American College of Cardiology. *Circulation* 2015; 132: e292–7.
2. Pelliccia A, Bjornstad HH, Anastassakis A, et al. Recommendations for competitive sports participation in athletes with cardiovascular disease. A Consensus Document from the Study Group of Sports Cardiology of the Working Group of Cardiac Rehabilitation and Exercise Physiology and the Working Group of Myocardial and Pericardial Diseases of the European Society of Cardiology. *Eur Heart J* 2005; 26: 1422–5.
3. Kitchiner D, Jackson M, Walsh K, et al. The progression of mild congenital aortic valve stenosis from childhood into adult life. *Int J Cardiol* 1993; 42: 217–23.
4. Cripe L, Andelfinger G, Martin LJ, et al. Bicuspid aortic valve is heritable. *J Am Coll Cardiol* 2004; 44: 138–43.
5. Garg V, Muth AN, Ransom JF, et al. Mutations in NOTCH1 cause aortic valve disease. *Nature* 2005; 437: 270–4.
6. Wallby L, Janerot-Sjöberg B, Steffensen T, Broqvist M. T lymphocyte infiltration in non-rheumatic aortic stenosis: a comparative descriptive study between tricuspid and bicuspid aortic valves. *Heart* 2002; 88: 348–51.
7. Verma S, Siu SC. Aortic dilatation in patients with bicuspid aortic valve. *N Engl J Med* 2014; 370: 1920–9.
8. Michelena HI, Desjardins VA, Avierinos J-F, et al. Natural history of asymptomatic patients with normally functioning or minimally dysfunctional bicuspid aortic valve in the community. *Circulation* 2008; 117: 2776–84.
9. Maron BJ, Levine BD, Washington RL, et al. Eligibility and disqualification recommendations for competitive athletes with cardiovascular abnormalities. Task Force 2: Preparticipation Screening for Cardiovascular Disease in Competitive Athletes: A Scientific Statement from the American Heart Association. *J Am Coll Cardiol* 2015; 66: 2356–61.
10. Maron BJ, Zipes DP, Kovacs RJ. Eligibility and disqualification recommendations for competitive athletes with cardiovascular abnormalities: preamble, principles, and general considerations. *Circulation* 2015; 132: e256–61.
11. Levine BD, Baggish AL, Kovacs RJ, et al. Eligibility and disqualification recommendations for competitive athletes with cardiovascular abnormalities. Task Force 1: Classification of Sports: Dynamic, Static, and Impact. *J Am Coll Cardiol* 2015; 66: 2350–5.
12. Hiratzka LF, Bakris GL, Beckman JA, et al. 2010 Guidelines for the diagnosis and management of patients with thoracic aortic disease. A Report of the American College of Cardiology

Foundation/American Heart Association Task Force on Practice Guidelines. *Circulation* 2010; 121: e266–369.
13. Nishimura RA., Otto CM, Bonow RO, et al. 2014 AHA/ACC guidelines for the management of patients with valvular heart disease: executive summary: a report of the ACC/AHA Task Force on Practice Guidelines. *J Am Coll Cardiol* 2014; 63: 2438–88.
14. Hiratzka LF, Creager MA, Isselbacher EM, Svensson LG. 2010 ACCF/AHA/AATS/ACR/ASA/SCA/SCAI/SIR/STS/SVM guidelines for the diagnosis and management of patients with thoracic aortic disease. Surgery for aortic dilatation in patients with bicuspid aortic valves: a statement of clarification from the ACC/AHA Task Force on Clinical Practice Guidelines. *Circulation* 2016; 133: 680–6.
15. Braverman AC, Harris KM, Kovacs RJ, et al. Eligibility and disqualification recommendations for competitive athletes with cardiovascular abnormalities. Task Force 7: Aortic Diseases, Including Marfan Syndrome: A Scientific Statement from the AHA and ACC. *Circulation* 2015; 132: e303–9.
16. Mitten MJ, Zipes DP, Maron BJ, Bryant WJ. Eligibility and disqualification recommendations for competitive athletes with cardiovascular abnormalities. Task Force 15: Legal Aspects of Medical Eligibility and Disqualification Recommendations: A Scientific Statement from the AHA. *Circulation* 2015; 132: e346–9.

4.2.3 The athlete with congenital heart disease

Guido E. Pieles and Graham Stuart

Introduction

With the success of cardiac surgical intervention, the number of teenagers and adults with congenital heart disease (CHD) is rising. Indeed, there are now many more adults than children with CHD—approximately 1 in 150 young adults have some form of CHD [1]. Regular physical exercise is an important lifestyle intervention that can improve quality of life in the CHD patient. Consequently, it is recommended that exercise advice and prescription should be an integral component of every patient encounter [2]. An increasing number of patients with CHD are participating in regular sport at levels ranging from gentle recreational activities to elite professional sport. The management of this complex group of athletes can pose significant challenges for the sports cardiologist.

Epidemiology of athletes with CHD

CHD can be defined as 'a structural abnormality of the heart or great vessels which is present at birth and is of current or future functional significance'. CHD is the most common birth defect and has a prevalence of 8–13 per 1000 live births [1]. Over 90% of CHD is diagnosed in the first year of life, with most palliative and corrective surgery performed in early childhood. Genes, environmental factors, and maternal infections contribute to a multifactorial aetiology [3]. A genetic origin has been established for many forms of CHD, and this is associated with a familial recurrence risk of 2–5%. Environmental factors include maternal diabetes, prescribed and recreational maternal drugs (e.g. diphenylhydantoin or alcohol/cocaine), and infective embryopathies (rubella, cytomegalovirus, Coxsackie, HIV). The adolescent and adult CHD population consists of mild unrepaired lesions, palliated and repaired CHD, and a small number of undiagnosed lesions with predominantly favourable physiology. In addition, there is a small population of patients with unrepaired CHD who have been judged too high risk for surgical intervention. This includes patients with pulmonary vascular disease (Eisenmenger syndrome) and others with complex cyanotic disease and reduced pulmonary blood flow.

Athletes with CHD encompass a wide variety of anatomical and pathophysiological subtypes. Moreover, there can be considerable variation between apparently similar diagnostic subgroups. For example, one athlete with tetralogy of Fallot and excellent haemodynamics may be able to compete at an elite level whereas another may have profound limitations due to heart failure symptoms or cardiac arrhythmias. Management of the athlete with CHD requires individually tailored lesion-specific treatment and follow-up.

Overall 90% of adults with CHD are in NYHA 1 or 2 [4] and can participate in some form of recreational sport and exercise. CHD athletes can be encountered at any level in sport ranging from disabled sporting disciplines (including Paralympic teams) to recreational, amateur, and even elite professional teams. They may present with a clear diagnosis and past medical history. Alternatively, they may present to sports cardiologists for the first time as apparently healthy athletes with new cardiovascular symptoms or with an abnormality on pre-participation screening. Under-diagnosis of CHD is common in some parts of the world. Thus, with the increasing number of African athletes competing in European countries, CHD is likely to be encountered with increasing frequency by the sports cardiologist. Every CHD athlete should have a good understanding of the underlying anatomical and pathophysiological diagnosis, and a personalized approach to exercise advice and prescription is essential. In many cases a joint assessment with a paediatric or congenital cardiologist will be required.

Approximately 25% of patients with CHD have an additional non-cardiac abnormality, and the sports cardiologist needs to consider this when assessing the athlete with CHD. This is also important in the disabled sport and Paralympic context. When assessing disabled athletes with a congenital anomaly, it is important for the sports medicine physician to be aware that they may have coexisting undiagnosed CHD.

Physical activity and sports in CHD

Most patients with CHD are sedentary and do not participate in regular exercise [2]. This may reflect over-protection by parents, clinicians, and other agencies such as schools and caregivers [5.6]. Moreover, there remains a lack of engagement in the need for exercise prescription in clinicians looking after CHD patients. In 2000, Swan and Hillis [7] reported that most adults with CHD received little or no exercise advice and most advice given was proscriptive. Little has changed since then, and even in the modern era many congenital heart units do not provide formal advice on exercise or sports participation [8]. Many children and young adults with CHD have reduced peak oxygen consumption, oxygen pulse, and ventilatory threshold compared with controls. Although this may be due to residual haemodynamic defects (including impaired pulmonary blood flow), Rosenblum et al. [9] demonstrated that reduced aerobic fitness in children and adults with CHD who have undergone complete surgical repair is usually due to physical deconditioning. In a comprehensive systematic review, Duppen et al. [10] demonstrated that exercise training programmes are safe and improve fitness in most adolescents and adults with CHD.

Regular exercise has multiple general health benefits for both the cardiovascular system and general health [11]. Muller et al. [12] demonstrated recently that the International Physical Activity Questionnaire (IPAQ) can be used successfully to record self-reported physical activity in adults with CHD. In this study of 786 adults with CHD, there was a clear correlation between achievement of recommended physical activity goals and improved physical and mental health related quality of life. Ideally, a specific exercise prescription should be given to every CHD patient by their cardiologist. However, this process is hampered by the lack of formal training in sports and exercise physiology received by most congenital cardiologists. Ideally, CHD patients should be provided with sports and exercise advice by an informed congenital cardiologist, but in the practice the input of a sports cardiologist and/or sport medicine specialist should be sought. It is likely that exercise participation will increase as knowledge of the multiple benefits of exercise in patients with CHD is disseminated [2].

Although regular physical activity and sport should be encouraged for most CHD patients, there is an important risk of long-term complications and problems such as heart failure, arrhythmias, and the need for re-operation (usually due to stenotic or regurgitant valves). The sports cardiologist must be alert to the presence of underlying CHD as intervention is usually required before the onset of major symptoms. For example, in athletes with tetralogy of Fallot, the main indication for pulmonary valve replacement is relatively subtle progressive change in right ventricular function, which can be identified by serial deterioration in cardiopulmonary exercise parameters. The presence of overt cardiovascular symptoms is a late feature which carries a poorer prognosis and may result in failure of right ventricular function to recover [13,14]. The wide diagnostic range and the need for individualized assessment require detailed knowledge of congenital heart disease, which can be a challenge to the sports physician and cardiologist. This highlights the need for close collaboration between the sports cardiologist and congenital heart specialist.

General exercise and sports participation guidance has been produced as part of the consensus management of adult CHD patients [14]. More specific eligibility and disqualification guidelines have been developed for competitive athletes with CHD [16]. These are largely consensus based and there is a need for evidence-based lesion-specific advice.

Exercise advice and the child with CHD

Exercise and training programmes can provide children with CHD with clear and sustained benefits, although these programmes are under-utilized [2,17]. Takken et al. [18] have developed lesion-specific recommendations for exercise participation and assessment for children with CHD, who should be encouraged to reach published activity guidelines (60min of moderate intensity exercise daily) to overcome the recognized risks of a sedentary lifestyle [6]. Exercise training programmes in children with CHD should be tailored to take account not only of the individual's disease subtype and current fitness level but also of deficiencies in other organ systems (pulmonary, musculoskeletal, neurological, and nutritional). Exercise advice should be an integral component of every clinic consultation [8]. Most children with fully repaired CHD can engage in sporting activities with minimal restriction. The main risk factors to consider are the potential for an exercise-induced arrhythmia, the use of medications such as warfarin where collision may be dangerous, the presence of a pacemaker or implantable device which might be damaged by collision, and the presence of an aortopathy. In general, aerobic exercise is preferable to isometric exercise because of the elevation of blood pressure and systemic vascular resistance which accompany isometric sports. Even in childhood, there is a considerable difference between the training requirements of recreational sport and those of elite age-group level competitive sport. This is discussed in detail in ➲ Chapter 1.2.3. There are no substantive studies which have investigated the effects of competitive training on cardiac physiology and cardiovascular risk in children with CHD.

Exercise advice and the adult with CHD

Exercise capacity is reduced in adults with CHD and this can lead to an impaired quality of life and long-term outcome. However, the degree of exercise limitation is extremely variable [19]. During routine follow-up review, the CHD patient should be asked about current sports and exercise participation. There is increasing scientific evidence for the sustained benefits of exercise in rehabilitation in adults with CHD [20], but few receive structured exercise training. A further problem is that exercise programmes in adults with CHD tend to consist of low intensity training protocols [18]. While these levels are safe, they have a low training effect. This has led to a scarcity of data on the cardiac adaptations which occur following high intensity training in athletes with CHD.

Using a pragmatic approach based on haemodynamic and electrophysiological parameters, Budts et al. [21] have recommended a stepwise approach to exercise prescription and advice for adults with CHD. This is summarized in ➲ Table 4.2.3.1. This approach prescribes exercise on the basis of the underlying physiology of the CHD patient rather than the anatomical defect or prior surgical intervention. This patient-centred approach should also consider patient preference (type of exercise/sport) as well as factors such as team or individual participation. It is important for the sports cardiologist to be familiar with the details of individual sports. For example, in the context of cycling, a CHD athlete may be advised to use smaller cog gearing with a higher cadence to increase the aerobic component and reduce the static component of the exercise stress while maintaining speed. Advice may need to be sought from sports professionals such as sport medicine specialists, strength and conditioning coaches, and physiotherapists. Budts et al. [21] stress that this stepwise approach may not be suitable for all CHD athletes and specifically does not apply to athletes with a congenital arrhythmia syndrome or congenital coronary anomaly.

Mortality risks of sudden cardiac death in CHD

Cardiovascular mortality accounts for 75% of all deaths in CHD, predominantly due to sudden cardiac death (SCD) (26%) and heart failure (21%) [22]. Despite this, the annual incidence of SCD in CHD is only 0.09% [23] and only 8% of deaths occur during exercise. Important risk factors for sudden death on exercise in CHD include increased age and complexity of disease, ventricular dysfunction, history of arrhythmias, pulmonary hypertension, degree of cyanosis, and presence of aortic disease [24]. The most common CHDs associated with sudden death in competitive athletes are abnormalities of coronary artery origin (which can be challenging to diagnose on screening), aortic

Table 4.2.3.1 Exercise prescription for congenital heart disease: stepwise assessment approach

Step	Description	Assessment technique/details
Step 1	History and physical examination	Include exercise/sports participation, medication, and detailed history of interventions
Step 2	Assessment of five baseline parameters	Ventricular function, pulmonary artery pressure, aortic size, arrhythmia risk and history, saturations at rest/exercise
Step 3	Decision on type of exercise	Type and intensity of sport; this should take into account static and dynamic components, risk of collision, risk of loss of consciousness, and patient preference
Step 4	Cardiopulmonary exercise testing	This should include assessment of exercise-induced arrhythmias, saturations on exercise, and blood pressure response to exercise
Step 5	Recommendation on relative intensity of exercise	This should take into account static and dynamic components of the sport and should be informed by knowledge from steps 1–4; details of exercise (e.g. team/solo, level of competition) should be taken into consideration.
Step 6	Follow-up	It is important to repeat each step in recognition that physiology changes with ageing and post-operative time.

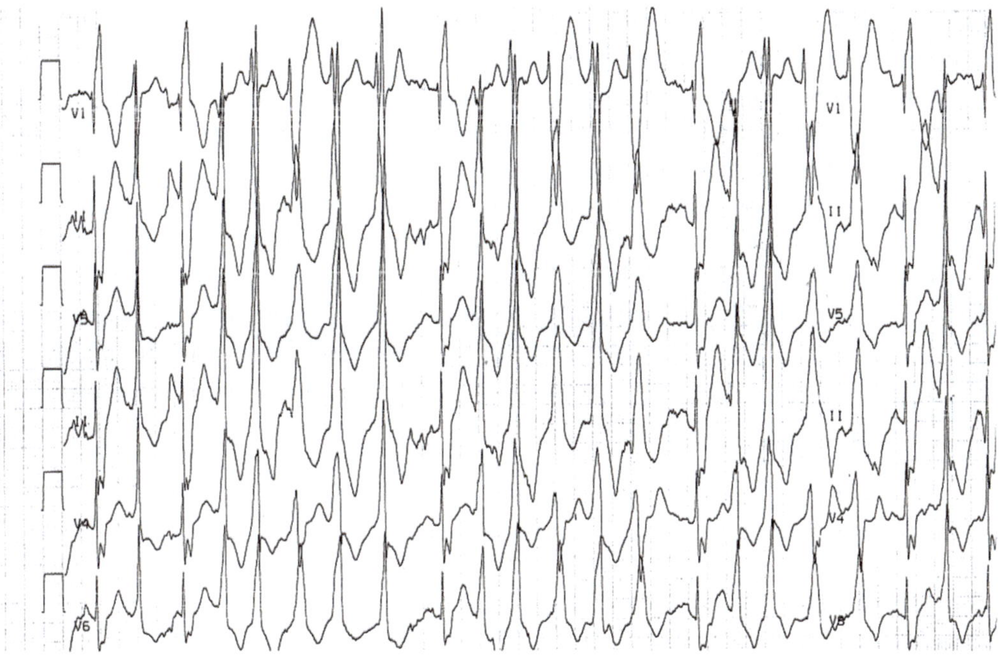

Fig. 4.2.3.1 Ventricular tachycardia in an 18-year-old asymptomatic girl with repaired tetralogy of Fallot and mild sub-aortic stenosis. Exercise stress testing can unmask latent exercise-induced arrhythmias.

stenosis, mitral valve prolapse, and aortic aneurysms [25]. In other congenital heart conditions, SCD is usually due to occurrence of a ventricular arrhythmia in a patient who has undergone surgical intervention. Extreme exercise can unmask an underlying arrhythmic tendency, and formal exercise stress testing can be useful in assessing this risk (➲ Fig. 4.2.3.1).

Sudden unexpected death is uncommon in children with CHD and rarely occurs during exercise. Jortveit et al. [26] reported an incidence of sudden unexpected death in only 0.2% of 11,272 children with CHD over a 15-year period. Only seven of these had a cardiac origin (0.07%) and none died during physical activity, although two were resuscitated following a cardiac arrest during sports. At present, most CHD follow-up data is confined to patients aged up to 40 years [27]. Although detailed follow-up data are slowly being gathered for this older ('geriatric') population with congenital heart disease, the precise risk factors for SCD in older CHD athletes are unclear [28].

Exercise pathophysiology in CHD

Quantitative exercise capacity is significantly reduced in most forms of adult CHD and this can lead to an impaired quality of life [19]. Even simple lesions such as an atrial septal defect or mild valve stenosis can influence performance in athletes with CHD. It is important for the sports cardiologist to understand the complex factors that can lead to reduced exercise capacity in athletes with CHD. While cardiac limitations are dominant, other organ system limitations (pulmonary, musculoskeletal) and cellular–metabolic dysfunction can contribute to exercise limitation.

Reduced VO_2max and peak oxygen pulse can indicate a reduced stroke volume response and are found in most forms of complex CHD but also in repaired tetralogy of Fallot, ventricular septal defect (VSD), aortic regurgitation, and post-operative coarctation of the aorta. The ventilatory anaerobic threshold in CHD is lower than in the normal population, and this can impair performance in many dynamic and steady rate exercise endurance sports. This is partly due to abnormalities in the metabolic and stress response pathways of the cardiac myocyte, but there is also a major skeletal muscle component. For example, recent work implicates a role for the myo-inhibitory cytokine myostatin in the regulation of both cardiac and skeletal muscle in CHD [29]. Similarly to heart failure syndrome, myostatin expression is reduced in CHD but can be increased by an exercise training programme [30] and may offer a potential therapeutic target in the future.

Reduction in ventilatory capacity and efficiency can also be the result of multiple sternotomies and thoracotomies. This may be exacerbated by phrenic palsy, which can occur as a long-term sequelae of surgery such as pulmonary artery banding or insertion of a systemic pulmonary artery shunt. In complex and cyanotic CHD, pulmonary gas exchange may be impaired due to ventilation–perfusion mismatch, which can persist despite correction of the cardiac defect [31].

Arrhythmias are common in adults with CHD and may be induced by exercise. While syncope and palpitations can occur, arrhythmias may be perceived as a reduced exercise tolerance, unexplained tiredness, or lethargy during exercise. Similarly, a blunted chronotropic response secondary to sinus node disease or conduction delay can lead to a reduction in performance. In the athlete with CHD, the sports cardiologist must have a high suspicion of arrhythmias when performance deteriorates.

Assessment of cardiac morphology and haemodynamics in the athlete with CHD

ECG

Because of congenital or post-operative changes, many athletes with CHD will fail standard pre-participation ECG screening [32]. Therefore ECG assessment in CHD should be interpreted in light of known lesion-specific ECG changes by a cardiologist experienced in the normal findings in CHD. Longitudinal ECG assessment is important as ECG changes may precede changes in structure. An echocardiogram should normally be carried out on the same occasion. The assessment of the athlete with CHD and symptoms of possible arrhythmic origin requires close collaboration between the congenital heart specialist and the sports cardiologist. Twenty-four hour ECG monitoring should be repeated annually in the athlete with significant CHD.

Trans-thoracic echocardiography

Trans-thoracic echocardiography is the first-line imaging modality in the assessment of the athlete with CHD. Guidelines for the performance of paediatric [33] and adult echocardiograms should be followed, but the assessment of the athlete with CHD requires considerable experience and an understanding of both sports cardiology and CHD. Trans-thoracic echocardiography can provide detailed information on cardiac anatomy, connection of extra-cardiac vessels to the heart, ventricular function, valves, and shunt lesions. Athletes with CHD should undergo echocardiographic examination annually, and more frequently if participating in high intensity training activities. Moreover, this assessment may need to be repeated more frequently in the context of complex CHD with reduced ventricular function, or if new symptoms occur.

Cardiac magnetic resonance (CMR) and computed tomography (CT)

The relevance and application of CMR in CHD is rapidly increasing [15]. CMR allows window-independent imaging, accurate delineation of detailed anatomy including 3D reconstruction, and tissue characterization and is the gold standard in ventricular and regurgitant volume quantification. The main use of CMR is in the quantitative assessment of RV and LV volumes, myocardial mass, myocardial scar (which may act as a trigger of arrhythmias), regurgitation fraction, and visualization of prosthetic materials (conduits) and underlying structural anomalies which cannot be clearly visualized using echocardiography (e.g. pulmonary veins, descending aorta size). Many criteria determining the timing of interventions in CHD are based on sequential CMR changes. The use of exercise imaging during CMR is in its infancy but promises to have considerable utility in the future assessment of the athlete with CHD. Newer techniques such as T1 weighting offer a huge potential to enable longitudinal assessment of diffuse fibrosis in the CHD population [34]. This could be of particular value for the CHD athlete.

Cardiac CT is the imaging modality of choice in the delineation of small anatomical structures such as coronary arteries and collateral arteries and for imaging parenchymal lung pathology. The main disadvantage of CT is radiation exposure; however, modern techniques have greatly reduced this. Crean [35] has reviewed the indications and respective benefits of CMR and CT in congenital heart disease in detail. CMR and CT imaging in the CHD patient should be performed in specialist CHD centres.

Cardiac catheterization

Diagnostic cardiac catheterization should be reserved for specific anatomical and physiological indications, such as coronary angiography, extra-cardiac collateral vessel angiography, shunt calculation, and measurement of pressure gradients and pulmonary vascular resistance. Most anatomical evaluation can be carried out using non-invasive techniques such as echocardiography or CMR. However, cardiac catheterization is still the investigation of choice in the assessment of pulmonary artery hypertension (PAH) and is essential prior to transcatheter interventions such as stent and valve implantation. Cardiac catheterization should only be performed in CHD centres with congenital surgical back-up facilities.

Functional and dynamic assessment of the athlete with CHD

Children above 10 years of age and adults with CHD who participate in regulated training and recreational and competitive sports should undergo a comprehensive annual assessment. This should include a detailed exercise history, including type, duration, and nature of exercise activity.

Clinical examination should include pulse oximetry, BP measurement, 12-lead ECG, and resting trans-thoracic echocardiography. The athlete should be asked about current medication and use of dietary supplements. A functional exercise assessment using treadmill or bicycle exercise ECG, cardiopulmonary exercise testing, and ideally exercise imaging is extremely helpful in evaluating the risks and benefits of exercise and in informing exercise prescription. In the athlete with deteriorating performance or exercise-related symptoms, an ECG should be obtained during exercise. Ideally this should be carried out during the athlete's chosen sport. This may involve use of a specific patient ECG monitor designed for ECG analysis during vigorous exercise.

Cardiopulmonary exercise testing (CPET)

Cardiopulmonary exercise testing has been used to risk stratify the adult with CHD and can predict outcome in many patient groups [31]. It is increasingly performed as a standard test for morbidity and mortality risk stratification in CHD, timing of intervention, and to correlate cardiac morphology and physiological function in CHD. Reference values for the adult CHD population are available [19] and recommendations exist for the paediatric CHD population [36]. While a single CPET can deliver important information on current functional capacity, repeated CPET assessment is invaluable and can monitor disease progression and inform success of interventions including an exercise training programme. Beyond an annual assessment, CPET should be performed in the athlete with CHD before and after an elective intervention and if significant changes in exercise performance, symptoms, or echocardiographic parameters are noted. CPET should always be combined with simultaneous exercise 12-lead ECG testing to allow assessment of underlying exercise-related arrhythmias. Indirect indices of cardiac performance can be deduced from CPET, but quantitative information on ventricular function remains limited.

Exercise (stress) echocardiography

In the athlete with CHD, exercise echocardiography can unmask subclinical ventricular dysfunction and valvar stenosis or regurgitation, which may not be apparent at rest. Traditionally, global and regional myocardial function was assessed qualitatively during exercise echocardiography, but this is strongly operator dependent. Tissue Doppler imaging and speckle-tracking echocardiography allow a quantitative evaluation of regional and global myocardial performance during exercise. In the athlete, exercise stress is superior to that of dobutamine stress, as it provokes physiological increases in preload and afterload in addition to increased cardiac contractility. This is important in patients with CHD where changes in loading characteristics are primary causes for ventricular dysfunction (as opposed to ischaemia). Although detailed normative data have not been established for all populations, load-independent parameters, such as isovolumic acceleration time or myocardial deformation, can provide information on the force–frequency relationship and contractility reserve during exercise stress. Novel assessment protocols combine myocardial performance assessment with simultaneous cardiopulmonary exercise testing, providing comprehensive data on cardiometabolic exercise response (➲ Fig. 4.2.3.2) [37].

General considerations in athletes with CHD

The age-specific assessment of the athlete with CHD

Athletes with CHD require an individualized assessment that takes into account the nature of the defect, the mode of corrective (or palliative) surgical and catheter interventions, residual lesions, haemodynamic state, and risk of arrhythmia. Importantly, resting assessment of these parameters is insufficient to comprehensively risk stratify athletes with CHD willing to participate in recreational and/or competitive sports. The recent EACPR recommendations on exercise prescription can help to risk stratify individuals [21] (➲ Table 4.2.3.1). The asymptomatic athlete with CHD may have residual intra-cardiac shunts (atrial septal defect, patent arterial duct, ventricular septal defect) or valve dysfunction but, in most cases, exercise participation can be recommended with minimal restriction. Undiagnosed structural lesions are rare in the childhood athlete, with the exception of anomalous coronary arteries which are the main risk for SCD. In young adult athletes with CHD, sequelae of previous surgery such as valvar incompetence and arrhythmias are the predominant problems. Ventricular dysfunction (systolic and diastolic) is encountered less often in the athlete population, but is prevalent in many non-athletes with CHD. Risk of arrhythmias and heart failure increases significantly in individuals with CHD aged over 35 years of life in CHD, and problems secondary to corrective or palliative procedures become a significant burden in the masters athlete with CHD. These include cardiac arrhythmias, left and particularly right systemic ventricular dysfunction, valvular incompetence, and obstruction of prosthetic conduits. Degenerative cardiac changes including coronary artery disease can develop in this group, although this is rare in cyanotic patients [38].

(a)
(b)

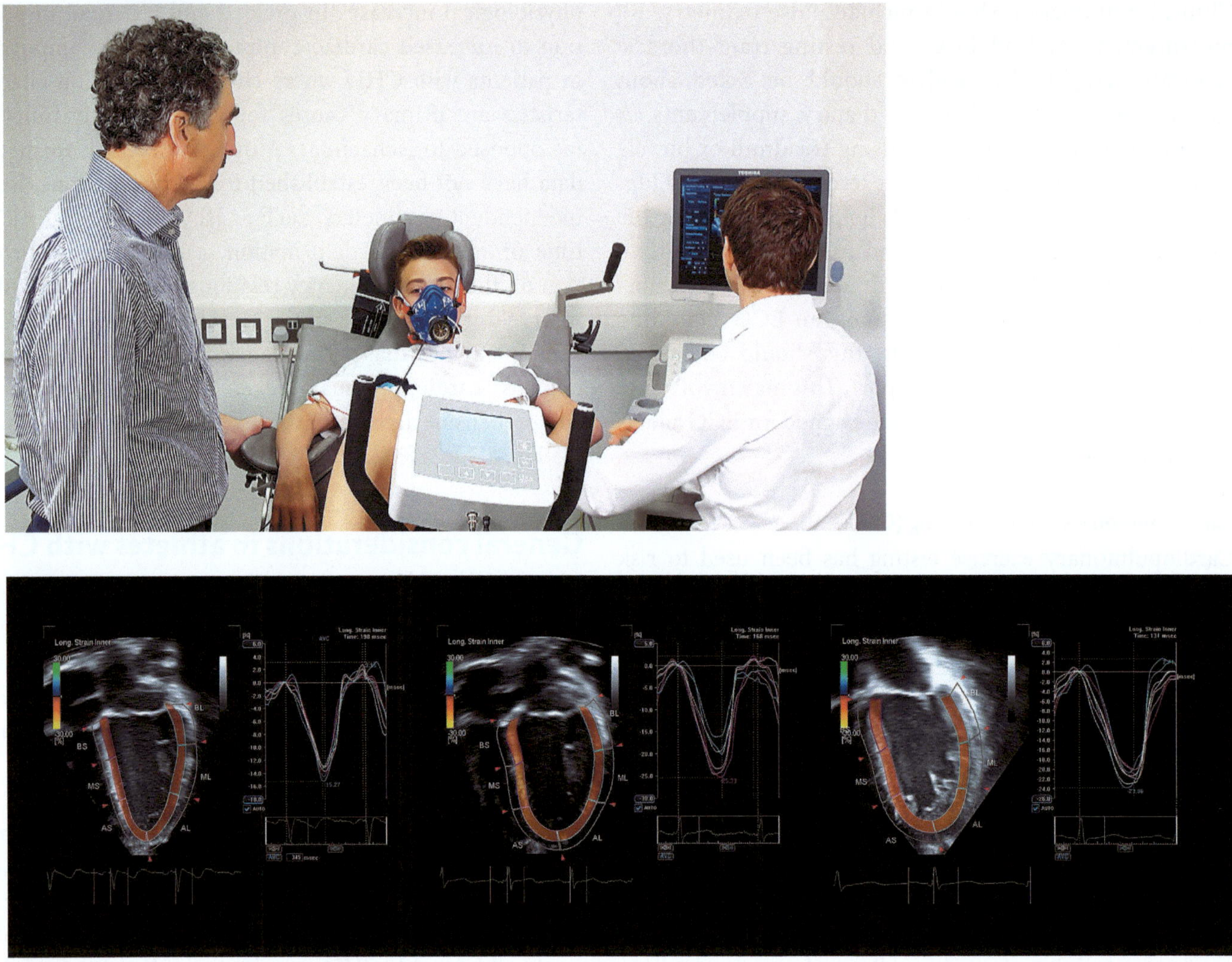

Fig. 4.2.3.2. Exercise stress echocardiography with simultaneous measurement of VO_2. (a) The simultaneous use of supine bicycle exercise echocardiography and measurement of oxygen consumption. (b) 2D wall motion tracking to serially assess myocardial strain reserve and directly correlate with metabolic exercise performance during exercise and recovery: LV peak longitudinal systolic strain at rest, HR 87/min (right panel), 50W, HR 90bpm (middle panel), at 100W, HR 117bpm (right panel).

Assessment of arrhythmias in CHD

Arrhythmias are the most common cause of emergency hospital admissions in adult patients with CHD [15]. They are most often the result of lesion-specific and surgical sequelae. Arrhythmias may be focal but are usually due to re-entry around surgical scars and natural anatomical barriers. Both atrial and ventricular arrhythmias can cause haemodynamic deterioration. Arrhythmias may also be caused by haemodynamic deterioration or subclinical heart failure. Guidelines for the assessment and treatment of arrhythmias in CHD have been published [39]. In the athlete with CHD, treatment may be hampered by the negative chronotropic effects of anti-arrhythmic drugs. Anti-arrhythmic agents like beta-blockers are unpopular as they may cause significant deterioration in athletic performance, and arrhythmia ablation may be a preferable option. Expert assessment and careful follow-up of the CHD athlete with an arrhythmia is essential. Assessment of arrhythmias in athletes with CHD should be performed at rest and during exercise (exercise 12-lead ECG, ECG Holter monitoring), and electrophysiology studies or loop recorder implantation should be considered in individual cases.

Heart failure in CHD

Careful longitudinal monitoring of LV and RV function and early diagnosis of dysfunction are important in the athlete with CHD. While heart failure therapy recommendations are similar to those for non-CHD patients, management of ventricular dysfunction in the athlete with CHD may differ significantly depending on individual aetiology and pathophysiology [15]. A wide range of pathological processes can lead to dysfunction, as virtually all forms of significant

CHD result in some degree of ventricular remodelling and adaptation that can become maladaptive and lead to cardiac failure. In non-corrected or non-palliated CHD, heart failure may occur due to pressure and volume overload of either ventricle. Post-operative long-term sequelae include myocardial scars, residual outflow tract and valvar stenosis, and regurgitation and intra-cardiac shunts. In addition, atrial and ventricular arrhythmias are major causes of subclinical or overt ventricular dysfunction. Exercise limitation is often the first symptom of ventricular dysfunction. In CHD athletes, ventricular dysfunction may affect both right and left ventricles, and this may lead to interventricular interaction with atypical heart failure symptoms [40]. Right ventricular (RV) assessment is important as several pathologies (e.g. tetralogy of Fallot, Fontan circulation, congenitally corrected transposition of the great arteries, Eisenmenger syndrome, and atrial septal defect) distort RV loading conditions and consequently RV function. Although acute RV failure is rare, chronic pre-load (volume) and after-load (pressure) increases are common. These can result in structural and functional maladaptation that lead to chronic and progressive RV failure. In turn this can affect LV performance because of the complex functional interaction that occurs between the two ventricles. This is particularly common when the RV supports the systemic circulation, for example after an atrial switch for transposition of the great arteries. The subpulmonary RV is more vulnerable than the systemic ventricle to acute load changes and changes in pulmonary vascular resistance, which occur during exercise. In the athlete with CHD, it is important to evaluate both ventricles by echocardiography annually and by cross-sectional imaging (CMR) every 2–3 years. Ideally, this should include regular dynamic functional (e.g. exercise) RV assessment.

Pulmonary arterial hypertension

Pulmonary arterial hypertension is an uncommon but severe complication of CHD. It usually occurs in the setting of a long-standing intra- or extra-cardiac communication (e.g. septal defects, patent arterial duct) which allows unrestricted volume and pressure overload. Over time this can result in fixed supra-systemic pulmonary artery pressures, elevated pulmonary vascular resistance, and reversal of shunting (Eisenmenger syndrome). The increase in RV afterload and RV pressure restricts the ability of the right ventricle to increase cardiac output through enhanced stroke volume. Moreover, the abnormal RV–LV interaction impairs LV filling and systemic cardiac output. This results in severely reduced exercise tolerance [19]. It is unlikely that patients with significant pulmonary vascular disease will be able to participate in recreational sport. Strenuous and competitive sports should be avoided in patients with PAH related to CHD, but there is emerging evidence to suggest that light dynamic and static exercise may be beneficial [41,16]. Gentle exercise should be selectively encouraged, although this will require careful monitoring.

Pulmonary artery pressures can elevate significantly in healthy athletes during exercise. Although this may lead to symptoms and reduced exercise performance, exercise-induced PAH is not considered to be a separate disease entity [41]. In the athlete with CHD, where even mild changes in PA pressures can unbalance haemodynamics, it is important to exclude PAH when performance decreases or there is a new onset of dyspnoea. Assessment should include evaluation of RV size, function and pressure, pulmonary and systemic venous flow dynamics, LV diastolic function, and diastolic ventricular interaction. A comprehensive assessment should include lung function tests, CPET, and catheter pulmonary vascular resistance study. Many athletes with CHD are at risk of developing late-onset PAH, even after surgical repair, and the sports cardiologist should be aware of this. The assessment of PAH should be part of every echocardiographic examination in athletes with CHD and also part of pre-competition screening.

The effects of high altitude on patients with CHD.

There are no guidelines addressing sports activities at moderate altitudes (1500–2500m above sea level) for patients with CHD. Hypobaric hypoxia leads to decreased oxygen consumption, decreased cardiac output, tachycardia, hypocapnia-mediated stroke volume decrease and a rise in pulmonary artery pressures in the acclimatization phase. Although patients with cyanotic CHD have an increased tolerance to normobaric hypoxia, an environment of hypobaric hypoxia can reduce oxygen tissue uptake significantly. This is a particular risk for patients with a univentricular circulation (Fontan palliation). The increase in pulmonary vascular resistance associated with moderate and extreme high altitude can lead to oxygenation impairment and reduced cardiac output. Patients with cyanotic or complex CHD should be advised not to engage in moderate or high intensity sporting activities at moderate altitude (1500–2500m), and should also be advised that they might become symptomatic even at rest. The benefits of high altitude training in athletes with complex CHD have not been assessed but, for many, this training modality should be avoided. Air travel is well tolerated, but travel to moderate altitude should be preceded by a full physiological assessment including lung function tests, CPET, and echocardiography. While travel above 2500m is generally not recommended in complex CHD, an informed decision should include individual assessment and patient-specific risk stratification.

Cardiac interventions in athletes with CHD—timing and risk stratification

The indications for and timing of surgical and transcatheter interventions in the athlete with CHD should follow consensus guidelines [15,42]. However, the congenital heart clinician, in collaboration with the sports cardiologist, must take into account the expectations and goals of the athlete which may differ significantly from those of the non-athlete. This is particularly important when considering surgical interventions. All interventions carry a small but significant risk, and the consequences may carry different significance for the athlete. Thus the ablation of a cardiac arrhythmia may carry a small risk of inducing heart block, which would require pacemaker implantation. The athlete with CHD may prefer to remain on medical therapy or opt for a lower-risk lower-efficacy procedure (e.g. cryoablation as opposed to radiofrequency ablation) if this reduces the need for a pacemaker which might curtail their sporting activities. On the other hand, the relative increase of physical fitness in the athlete with CHD may mask the significance of a haemodynamically important lesion, which left untreated might cause progressive irreversible damage. This reinforces the importance of serial assessment of exercise capacity and ventricular function. Finally, there is evidence that even simple lesions, which appear to have no haemodynamic significance at rest, can reduce exercise performance (e.g. a small intra-cardiac shunt or minor valve stenosis). While this does not present a significant morbidity risk to overall health, it might be a significant issue for the individual athlete. Therefore decisions on the timing of interventions in athletes with CHD should be made in collaboration with experts in sports and congenital cardiology and be based on longitudinal resting and exercise cardiac assessment.

Endocarditis prophylaxis

The risk of endocarditis is significantly higher in patients with CHD compared with the general population and varies between specific lesions. Risk may be lower in repaired CHD, but implantation of prosthetic conduits and valves poses an endocarditis risk in itself. Although antibiotic prophylaxis is contentious, primary prevention with good dental hygiene and appropriate treatment of skin infections is essential. In our view, high risk groups (prosthetic valves, residual shunts, previous endocarditis) should receive antibiotic prophylaxis before invasive dental procedures.

Athletic performance and complications/ risk stratification in common specific lesions

Simple shunt lesions with volume loading

Simple shunt lesions such as atrial septal defect (ASD), ventricular septal defect (VSD), and a patent arterial duct (PDA) are usually diagnosed and corrected in childhood. In the adult athlete haemodynamically significant unrepaired lesions will cause significant exercise intolerance, dyspnoea, recurrent respiratory infections, and palpitations (particularly in ASD). Atrial fibrillation, atrial flutter, paroxysmal intra-atrial re-entry tachycardia, and first-degree atrioventricular (AV) block are common in unrepaired ASD and also occur in repaired defects, although life-threatening ventricular arrhythmias are rare. Late-onset complete heart block can occasionally occur following VSD repair. A residual VSD or PDA will lead to left-sided volume load, and an ASD will cause right-sided volume overload.

Exercise capacity is reduced in unrepaired simple shunt lesions, including in patients without overt clinical exercise symptoms [4]. Symptoms should prompt urgent reassessment and closure of the defect unless there is a specific contraindication.

Atrioventricular septal defects (AVSD)

Exercise capacity in repaired AVSD can be moderately impaired as a result of ventricular dysfunction, elevated pulmonary vascular resistance, aortic valve regurgitation, or progressive sub-aortic stenosis. These residual lesions often warrant surgical re-intervention. Atrial arrhythmias and AV conduction defects can develop even years after repair. Life-threatening ventricular arrhythmias are rare but do occur.

Right ventricular outflow tract obstruction (Tetralogy of Fallot)

Most complications in tetralogy of Fallot are sequelae of primary or secondary surgical intervention. Arrhythmias cause significant morbidity, and atrial flutter, atrial fibrillation, and sustained ventricular tachycardia are observed in approximately 10% of patients 35 years after repair and the prevalence increases with age (➲ Fig. 4.2.3.1). Predictors for arrhythmias and associated SCD are moderate pulmonary or tricuspid incompetence, ventricular dysfunction, transannular patch repair, older age at repair, and QRS >180ms [43]. Exercise performance, which can be moderately reduced [19], is determined by RV dysfunction and resulting

RV–LV interaction [44]. Residual bioprosthetic conduit (valve) stenosis or regurgitation is common. Although it is often well tolerated, it causes progressive reduction in exercise capacity. In athletes, pulmonary valve replacement should be performed before symptoms occur. Rare but serious complications that are often clinically silent are aortic or pulmonary artery aneurysms. Aortic aneurysms can rupture and pulmonary artery aneurysms may cause symptoms of angina or dyspnoea during exercise secondary to coronary artery compression. Isolated pulmonary stenosis, even if mild, will reduce exercise performance.

Congenital aortic stenosis

Aortic stenosis (AS) is a cause of SCD in athletes [25]. Mild and moderate lesions have a low risk but disease can progress fast. Symptom assessment should be considered during both rest and exercise (ischemia, arrhythmias, reduced cardiac reserve). Athletes with severe or moderate AS with symptoms are not eligible for competitive sports, although they may not appear symptomatic. Treated congenital AS often shows residual stenosis or regurgitation, and a dilated aortic sinus or ascending aorta is seen in 45% after follow-up for a decade. Performance is mildly reduced in palliated lesions, as regurgitation and residual LV hypertrophy with subclinical diastolic function are the cause.

In the athlete, the choice of intervention should take into account the need to avoid a prosthetic valve and anticoagulation. Thus consideration should be given to interventions such as valvuloplasty or procedures such as the pulmonary autograft (Ross operation) where anticoagulation is not required.

Coarctation of the aorta and other aortic abnormalities

Coarctation is part of a generalized aortopathy and many problems persist following intervention. These include systemic hypertension, which may be very high during exercise. Aortic collaterals and premature coronary artery disease may also cause of impaired exercise performance. Aortic or cerebral aneurysms are a serious and progressive complication, and need to be actively sought (➔ Fig. 4.2.3.3). Arrhythmias are rare. Undiagnosed coarctation of the aorta may present with hypertension and it is important to exclude this diagnosis. There are often reduced femoral pulses with an intrascapular murmur, but both signs may be absent despite the presence of a significant coarctation. Aortic dilatation may occur, especially in the presence of a bicuspid aortic valve. Aortic dilatation is a feature of many congenital heart defects [45]. It is important to diagnose this in athletes as there is a small risk of aortic rupture.

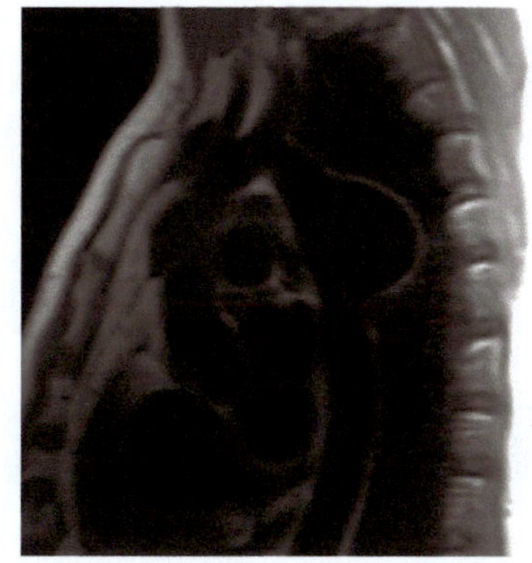

Fig. 4.2.3.3 Aneurysm of the descending aorta in a repaired coarctation of the aorta. This 3D CT reconstruction demonstrates a large aneurysm adjacent to a previously repaired coarctation of the aorta. This was asymptomatic but at high risk of rupture. It was successfully treated by transcatheter implantation of a covered stent.
Picture courtesy of Dr Nathan Manghat. Bristol Heart Institute.

Cyanotic lesions

Cyanosis in CHD is due to right-to-left shunting with deoxygenated blood entering the systemic circulation. Cyanotic patients require lifelong follow-up in specialized CHD centres. Exercise capacity is significantly reduced and 30% of adults with cyanotic heart disease will be in NYHA 3 [4]. This is due primarily to ventricular dysfunction and significantly reduced oxygen availability. Reduced exercise function is a strong predictor of outcome [31]. Cyanotic patients are usually only advised to participate in competitive sport of low static and dynamic intensity, but should eventually be encouraged to participate in light to moderate dynamic exercise after comprehensive assessment. Exercise advice should take into account the adaptive mechanisms to cyanosis, such as reduced cardiac exercise reserve (due to high resting cardiac output), erythrocytosis, and coagulopathy requiring optimal hydration at all times. This group includes patients with Eisenmenger syndrome and pulmonary vascular disease, and others with palliated conditions such as pulmonary atresia where corrective surgery has not been feasible. Some patients with complex cyanotic disease can reach old age and, although they have a significantly reduced exercise capacity, regular exercise can play an important social role as well as providing a potential health benefit, primarily by improving skeletal muscle efficiency (➔ Fig. 4.2.3.4).

Transposition of the great arteries (TGA)

In the current era, corrective surgery (arterial switch operation) is performed in the neonatal period. In an earlier surgical epoch, the atrial switch operation (Mustard or Senning operation) was used. The atrial switch operation

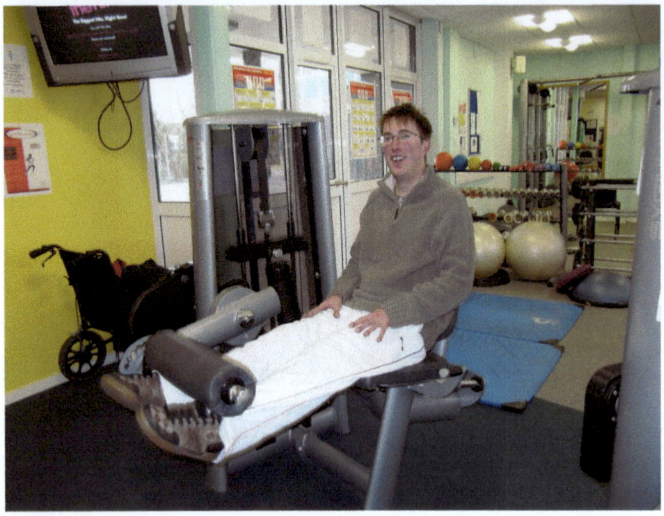

Fig. 4.2.3.4 Gentle weight training in complex congenital heart disease. Exercise participation has social as well as medical benefits. Note cyanosis and finger clubbing due to pulmonary atresia with ventricular septal defect. This had been palliated with a pulmonary to systemic artery shunt.

has significant complications which result in moderate to severe exercise intolerance. The most severe complication is progressive dysfunction of the systemic RV, aggravated by tricuspid regurgitation and residual shunts. Tachyarrhythmias including sustained atrial and ventricular arrhythmias occur, and the risk of SCD is significant. There is a small risk of coronary artery and branch pulmonary artery stenosis in TGA patients who have undergone an arterial switch. In addition, a small number develop an ascending aortopathy. Arrhythmias are less common. An exercise stress test should be carried out before participation in competitive exercise.

Congenitally corrected transposition of the great arteries (ccTGA)

Often surgery is not required in childhood and this diagnosis may be picked up as an incidental finding in adult life or during a pre-participation athletic screen. There may be coexistent lesions such as VSD or pulmonary or tricuspid valve abnormalities. Progressive (systemic) RV dysfunction, tricuspid regurgitation, and AV conduction defects may develop and are associated with a high morbidity in adulthood. RV failure and atrial and ventricular arrhythmias are the most serious complications during exercise. Exercise capacity may be moderately to severely limited but, in the absence of coexisting lesions or tricuspid regurgitation, exercise tolerance may be normal.

Fontan circulation.

A univentricular (Fontan) circulation is the result of a staged surgical approach to creating a direct connection of the systemic venous return to the pulmonary arteries; a single right or left ventricle supports the systemic circulation. This is the final surgical pathway for many complex forms of CHD characterized by an absent cardiac chamber or valve. The reduced ability to increase stroke volume, a blunted chronotropic response, residual shunting with cyanosis, and ventilatory and musculoskeletal impairment usually result in significantly reduced exercise capacity. However, some Fontan patients have managed to compete in certain endurance events, albeit at a low level of competition. Progressive sinus node dysfunction and intra-atrial re-entry tachycardias are common. The risk of exercise-induced life-threatening arrhythmias is low, but increases with the onset of progressive ventricular dysfunction. Jacobsen et al. [46] demonstrated that even this complex patient group may benefit from a structured exercise training programme, which results in improved quality of life and exercise ability. Furthermore, resistance training has been shown to augment the peripheral muscle pump with consequent improvements in cardiac output and exercise capacity [47].

Ebstein's Anomaly

Ebstein's anomaly is represented by displacement of the tricuspid valve (TV) leading to 'atrialisation' of the RV. Exercise performance in Ebstein's anomaly is determined by the severity of TV dysplasia, RV dysfunction, and inter-atrial shunting with cyanosis, and can vary from near normal to severe incapacity. Ebstein's anomaly is often associated with the presence of AV accessory pathways. This, in combination with atrial dilatation, may lead to a significant risk of arrhythmia.

Competition guidelines for patient guidelines with CHD

The first published guidelines for athletes with cardiovascular abnormalities did not include eligibility recommendations for patients with CHD. However, the unique challenge of sports participation in CHD was addressed subsequently [48,49]. These guidelines were based primarily on anatomical diagnosis and parameters such as the severity of the underlying lesion, the nature of the intervention, and known or identified complications. In general, these consensus guidelines state that many patients with CHD can participate in competitions and most should engage in recreational exercise activities, while acknowledging that little objective outcome data exist. These recommendations are based on insufficient evidence, and this was reiterated in the updated 2015 guidelines [16]. A detailed individual patient assessment is essential before specific sports participation can be recommended, and this is reiterated in the most recent guidelines.

Conclusion

Athletes with significant CHD are still relatively uncommon but are increasing in prevalence. They represent a wide spectrum of functional variation, with a variable risk of cardiac dysfunction and arrhythmias. The key message for the sports cardiologist is to be aware of the underlying diagnosis, the potential for change in functional impairment with time, the relatively high arrhythmia risk, and the need to ensure individualized assessment at rest and during exercise. Close collaboration with congenital heart specialists is recommended.

Further reading

Baumgartner H, Bonhoeffer P, de Groot NM, et al. ESC guidelines for the management of grown-up congenital heart disease (new version 2010). *Eur Heart J* 2010; 31: 2915–57.

Budts W, Borjesson M, Chessa M, et al. Physical activity in adolescents and adults with congenital heart defects: individualized exercise prescription. *Eur Heart J* 2013: 34: 3669–74.

Dimopoulos K, Okonko DO, Diller GP, et al. Abnormal ventilatory response to exercise in adults with congenital heart disease relates to cyanosis and predicts survival. *Circulation* 2006; 113: 2796–802.

Duppen N, Takken T, Hopman MT, et al. Systematic review of the effects of physical exercise training programmes in children and young adults with congenital heart disease. *Int J Cardiol* 2013; 168: 1779–87.

Khairy P, Van Hare GF, Balaji S, et al. PACES/HRS Expert Consensus Statement on the Recognition and Management of Arrhythmias in Adult Congenital Heart Disease. *Heart Rhythm* 2014; 11: e102–65.

Longmuir PE, Brothers JA, De Ferranti SD, et al. Promotion of physical activity for children and adults with congenital heart disease: a scientific statement from the American Heart Association. *Circulation* 2013; 127: 2147–59.

Pelliccia A, Zipes DP, Maron BJ. Bethesda Conference 36 and the European Society of Cardiology Consensus Recommendations revisited: a comparison of US and European criteria for eligibility and disqualification of competitive athletes with cardiovascular abnormalities. *J Am Coll Cardiol* 2008; 52: 1990–6.

Rhodes J, Ubeda Tikkanen A, Jenkins KJ. Exercise testing and training in children with congenital heart disease. *Circulation* 2010; 122: 1957–67.

Takken T, Giardini A, Reybrouck T, et al. Recommendations for physical activity, recreation sport, and exercise training in paediatric patients with congenital heart disease: a report from the Exercise, Basic & Translational Research Section of the European Association of Cardiovascular Prevention and Rehabilitation, the European Congenital Heart and Lung Exercise Group, and the Association for European Paediatric Cardiology. *Eur J Prev Cardiol* 2012; 19: 1034–65.

Warnes CA, Williams, RG, Bashore, TM, et al. ACC/AHA 2008 guidelines for the management of adults with congenital heart disease: executive summary. *Circulation* 2008; 118: 2395–451.

References

1. Marelli AJ, Ionescu-Ittu R, Mackie AS, et al. Lifetime prevalence of congenital heart disease in the general population from 2000 to 2010. *Circulation* 2014; 130: 749–56.
2. Longmuir PE, Brothers JA, De Ferranti SD, et al. Promotion of physical activity for children and adults with congenital heart disease: a scientific statement from the American Heart Association. *Circulation* 2013; 127: 2147–59.
3. Pierpont ME, Basson CT, Benson DW Jr, et al. Genetic basis for congenital heart defects: current knowledge: a scientific statement from the American Heart Association Congenital Cardiac Defects Committee, Council on Cardiovascular Disease in the Young. *Circulation* 2007; 115: 3015–38.
4. Inuzuka R, Diller GP, Borgia F, et al. Comprehensive use of cardiopulmonary exercise testing identifies adults with congenital heart disease at increased mortality risk in the medium term. *Circulation* 2012; 125: 250–9.
5. Moola F, Fusco C, Kirsh JA. The perceptions of caregivers toward physical activity and health in youth with congenital heart disease. *Qual Health Res* 2011; 21: 278–91.
6. Pieles GE, Horn R, Williams CA, Stuart AG. Paediatric exercise training in prevention and treatment. *Arch Dis Child* 2014; 99: 380–5.
7. Swan L, Hillis WS. Exercise prescription in adults with congenital heart disease: a long way to go. *Heart* 2000: 83: 685–7.
8. Williams CA, Gowing L, Horn R, Stuart AG. A survey of exercise advice and recommendations in United Kingdom paediatric cardiac clinics. *Cardiol Young* 2017; 27: 951–6.
9. Rosenblum O, Katz U, Reuveny R, et al. Exercise performance in children and young adults after complete and incomplete repair of congenital heart disease. *Pediatr Cardiol* 2015; 36: 1573–81.
10. Duppen N, Takken T, Hopman MT, et al. Systematic review of the effects of physical exercise training programmes in children and young adults with congenital heart disease. *Int J Cardiol* 2013; 168: 1779–87.
11. D'Silva A, Sharma S. Management of young competitive athletes with cardiovascular conditions. *Heart* 2017; 103: 463–73.
12. Müller JA, Berg T, Goeder A. et al. Physical activity in adults with congenital heart disease and associations with functional outcomes. *Heart* 2017; 103: 1117–28.
13. Therrien J, Siu SC, McLaughlin PR, et al. Pulmonary valve replacement in adults late after repair of tetralogy of Fallot. Are we operating too late? *J Am Coll Cardiol* 2000; 36: 1670–5.
14. Babu-Narayan SV, Diller GP, Gheta RR, et al. Clinical outcomes of surgical pulmonary valve replacement after repair of tetralogy of Fallot and potential prognostic value of preoperative cardiopulmonary exercise testing. *Circulation* 2014; 129: 18–27.
15. Baumgartner H, Bonhoeffer P, de Groot NM, et al. ESC guidelines for the management of grown-up congenital heart disease (new version 2010). *Eur Heart J* 2010; 31: 2915–57.
16. Van Hare GF, Ackerman MJ, Evangelista JA, et al. Eligibility and disqualification recommendations for competitive athletes with

cardiovascular abnormalities: Task Force 4: Congenital Heart Disease. *Circulation* 2015; 132: e281–91.

17. Tikkanen AU, Oyaga AR, Riano OA, et al. Paediatric cardiac rehabilitation in congenital heart disease: a systematic review. *Cardiol Young* 2012; 22: 241–50.
18. Takken T, Giardini A, Reybrouck T, et al. Recommendations for physical activity, recreation sport, and exercise training in paediatric patients with congenital heart disease: a report from the Exercise, Basic & Translational Research Section of the European Association of Cardiovascular Prevention and Rehabilitation, the European Congenital Heart and Lung Exercise Group, and the Association for European Paediatric Cardiology. *Eur J Prev Cardiol* 2012; 19: 1034–65.
19. Kempny A, Dimopoulos K, Uebing A, et al. Reference values for exercise limitations among adults with congenital heart disease. Relation to activities of daily life—single centre experience and review of published data. *Eur Heart J* 2012; 33: 1386–96.
20. Dua JS, Cooper AR, Fox KR, Stuart AG. Exercise training in adults with congenital heart disease: feasibility and benefits. *Int J Cardiol* 2010; 138: 196–205.
21. Budts W, Borjesson M, Chessa M, et al. Physical activity in adolescents and adults with congenital heart defects: individualized exercise prescription. *Eur Heart J* 2013; 34: 3669–74.
22. Oechslin EN, Harrison DA, Connelly MS, et al. 2000. Mode of death in adults with congenital heart disease. *Am J Cardiol* 2000; 86, 1111–6.
23. Koyak Z, Harris L, De Groot JR, et al. Sudden cardiac death in adult congenital heart disease. *Circulation* 2012; 126: 1944–54.
24. Diller GP, Baumgartner H. 2016. Sudden cardiac death during exercise in patients with congenital heart disease: the exercise paradox and the challenge of appropriate counselling. *Eur Heart J* 2016; 37: 627–9.
25. Maron BJ, Doerer JJ, Haas TS, et al. Sudden deaths in young competitive athletes: analysis of 1866 deaths in the United States, 1980–2006. Circulation 2009; 119; 1085–92.
26. Jortveit J, Eskedal L, Hirth A, et al. Sudden unexpected death in children with congenital heart defects. *Eur Heart J* 2016; 37: 621–6.
27. Verheugt CL, Uiterwaal CS, Grobbee DE, Mulder BJ. Long-term prognosis of congenital heart defects: a systematic review. *Int J Cardiol* 2008; 131; 25–32.
28. Afilalo J, Therrien J, Pilote L, et al. Geriatric congenital heart disease: burden of disease and predictors of mortality. *J Am Coll Cardiol* 2011; 58: 1509–15.
29. Bish LT, George I, Maybaum S, et al. Myostatin is elevated in congenital heart disease and after mechanical unloading. *PLoS One* 2011; 6: e23818.
30. Lenk K, Erbs S, Hollriegel R, et al. Exercise training leads to a reduction of elevated myostatin levels in patients with chronic heart failure. *Eur J Prev Cardiol* 2012; 19: 404–11.
31. Dimopoulos K, Okonko DO, Diller GP, et al. Abnormal ventilatory response to exercise in adults with congenital heart disease relates to cyanosis and predicts survival. *Circulation* 2006; 113: 2796–802.
32. Sharma S, Drezner JA, Baggish A, et al. International Recommendations for Electrocardiographic Interpretation in Athletes. *J Am Coll Cardiol* 2017; 69; 1057–75.
33. Lopez L, Colan SD, Frommelt PC, et al. Recommendations for quantification methods during the performance of a pediatric echocardiogram: a report from the Pediatric Measurements Writing Group of the American Society of Echocardiography Pediatric and Congenital Heart Disease Council. *J Am Soc Echocardiogr* 2010; 23; 465–95; quiz 576–7.
34. Riesenkampff E, Messroghli DR, Redington AN, Grosse-Wortmann L. Myocardial T1 mapping in pediatric and congenital heart disease. *Circ Cardiovasc Imaging* 2015; 8: e002504.
35. Crean A. Cardiovascular MR and CT in congenital heart disease. *Heart* 2007; 93: 1637–47.
36. Rhodes J, Ubeda Tikkanen A, Jenkins KJ. Exercise testing and training in children with congenital heart disease. *Circulation* 2010; 122: 1957–67.
37. Pieles GE, Gowing L, Forsey J, et al. The relationship between biventricular myocardial performance and metabolic parameters during incremental exercise and recovery in healthy adolescents. *Am J Physiol Heart Circ Physiol* 2015; 309: H2067–76.
38. Tarp JB, Jensen AS, Engstrom T, et al. Cyanotic congenital heart disease and atherosclerosis. *Heart* 2017; 103: 897–900.
39. Khairy P, Van Hare GF, Balaji S, et al. 2014. PACES/HRS expert consensus statement on the recognition and management of arrhythmias in adult congenital heart disease. *Heart Rhythm* 2014; 11: e102–65.
40. Friedberg MK, Redington AN. Right versus left ventricular failure: differences, similarities, and interactions. *Circulation* 2014; 129: 1033–44.
41. Galie N, Humbert M, Vachiery JL, et al. 2015 ESC/ERS guidelines for the diagnosis and treatment of pulmonary hypertension. *Eur Heart J* 2016; 37: 67–119.
42. Warnes CA, Williams RG, Bashore TM, et al. ACC/AHA 2008 guidelines for the management of adults with congenital heart disease: executive summary. *Circulation* 2008; 118: 2395–451.
43. Gatzoulis MA, Balaji S, Webber SA, et al. Risk factors for arrhythmia and sudden cardiac death late after repair of tetralogy of Fallot: a multicentre study. *Lancet* 2000; 356: 975–81.
44. Apitz C, Webb GD, Redington AN Tetralogy of Fallot. *Lancet* 2009; 374: 1462–71.
45. Kuijpers JM, Mulder BJ. Aortopathies in adult congenital heart disease and genetic aortopathy syndromes: management strategies and indications for surgery. *Heart* 2017; 103; 952–66.
46. Jacobsen RM, Ginde S, Mussatto K, et al. Can a home-based cardiac physical activity program improve the physical function quality of life in children with fontan circulation? *Congenit Heart Dis* 2016; 11: 175–82.
47. Cordina RL, O'Meagher S, Karmali A, et al. Resistance training improves cardiac output, exercise capacity and tolerance to positive airway pressure in Fontan physiology. *Int J Cardiol*; 2013; 168: 780–8.
48. Graham TP Jr, Driscoll DJ, Gersony WM, et al. Task Force 2: congenital heart disease. *J Am Coll Cardiol* 2005; 45: 1326–33.
49. Pelliccia A, Zipes DP, Maron BJ. Bethesda Conference 36 and the European Society of Cardiology Consensus Recommendations revisited a comparison of US and European criteria for eligibility and disqualification of competitive athletes with cardiovascular abnormalities. *J Am Coll Cardiol* 2008; 52: 1990–6.

SECTION 5

Rhythm disorders of interest in sports cardiology

5.1 **Channelopathy in athletes** *253*
Nicole M. Panhuyzen–Goedkoop and Arthur A.M. Wilde

5.2 **Ventricular tachyarrhythmias** *265*
Eduard Guasch and Lluís Mont

5.3 **Supraventricular tachyarrhythmias** *277*
Matthias Wilhelm

5.4 **Pre-excitation and conduction abnormalities** *288*
Pietro Delise

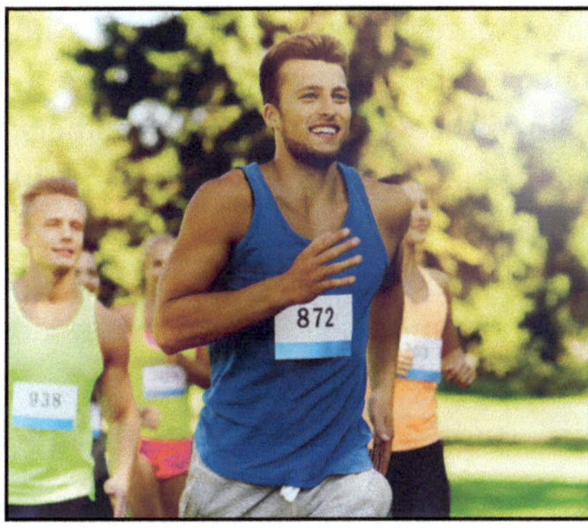

5.1

Channelopathy in athletes

Nicole M. Panhuyzen-Goedkoop and Arthur A.M. Wilde

Introduction

Channelopathies or ion-channel cardiac diseases are primary electrical disorders and belong to the inherited cardiac disorders. There are four major channelopathies: long QT syndrome (LQTS), short QT syndrome (SQTS), catecholaminergic polymorphic ventricular tachycardia (CPVT), and Brugada syndrome (BrS). Most channelopathies are transmitted as an autosomal dominant trait. Channelopathies are of special interest in sports cardiology because they predispose to life-threatening ventricular arrhythmia and are potentially lethal in relation to exercise. Idiopathic ventricular fibrillation is probably also an ion-channel cardiac disease, although only in some cases an underlying etiology is found. The prevalence of sudden cardiac death (SCD) due to channelopathy in young athletes is estimated to be 2–4% [1]. Most of these cases of SCD are caused by LQTS, with a reported incidence of 2% in the USA [1].

There are potential specific triggers in athletes that may provoke ventricular arrhythmia in ion-channel cardiac disease, inducing ventricular fibrillation (VF) and SCD. They include physical exercise in LQTS and CPVT, increased vagal tone at rest in BrS, immersion in (cold) water in LQTS, fever or hyperthermia in LQTS and BrS, and electrolyte and volume depletion in all channelopathies [2,3].

This chapter discusses the clinical presentation and management in athletes of the four major channelopathies: LQTS, SQTS, CPVT, and BrS.

Definitions

In accordance with the EHRA guidelines of 2013 and the ESC guidelines of 2015 we accept the following definitions for the four major channelopathies [4,5].

Long QT syndrome (LQTS)

LQTS is characterized by prolongation of the QT interval on repeated ECGs. The cut-off point of the QTc interval in athletes is discussed in the next section. The signature arrhythmia is torsades de pointes (TdP), which is a high rate polymorphic ventricular arrhythmia characterized by a shifting electrical axis. These arrhythmias can lead to loss of consciousness and in the most severe cases to SCD.

Short QT syndrome (SQTS)

SQTS is characterized by a short QTc-interval (≤330ms). It is also associated with a pro-arrhythmic substrate at both the atrial and the ventricular level.

Catecholaminergic polymorphic ventricular tachycardia (CPVT)

CPVT is an entity that only expresses itself in the setting of adrenergic stress. At rest the ECG is completely normal. The signature feature is an exercise/emotion-induced ventricular arrhythmia, initially starting with monomorphic ventricular ectopy and evolving into polymorphic couplets, triplets, and bidirectional (typical although rare) or polymorphic (more often) tachycardia with potential deterioration into VF. The disease manifests itself from age 5–6 years onwards.

Brugada syndrome (BrS)

BrS was originally described as an 'electrical disease' and is characterized by right precordial coved type or saddle-back type ST-segment elevation. Often there are also conduction abnormalities and there is a strong association with an increased risk of ventricular tachyarrhythmias, including VF. More recently it has become increasingly recognized that there are (discrete) structural abnormalities in the epicardial right ventricular outflow tract region.

Ion-channel cardiac disease

Long QT syndrome (LQTS)

Current internationally adopted guidelines in the general population define LQTS as the presence of a QTc interval ≥500ms on repeated ECGs without known cause (➔ Fig. 5.1.1) [4,5]. Patients with a pathogenic mutation are also diagnosed as LQTS patients, even in the presence of a normal QTc [4]. The Schwartz scoring system is still used, with 3.5 points as a cut-off value for the diagnosis of LQTS (modified Schwartz score) [5]. In this scoring system, among others, several electrocardiographic parameters are of importance in addition to clinical symptoms (and their characteristics) and details of the family history. If a QTc interval ≥500ms is already present on repeated ECGs the modified Schwartz score no longer contributes to the diagnosis of LQTS.

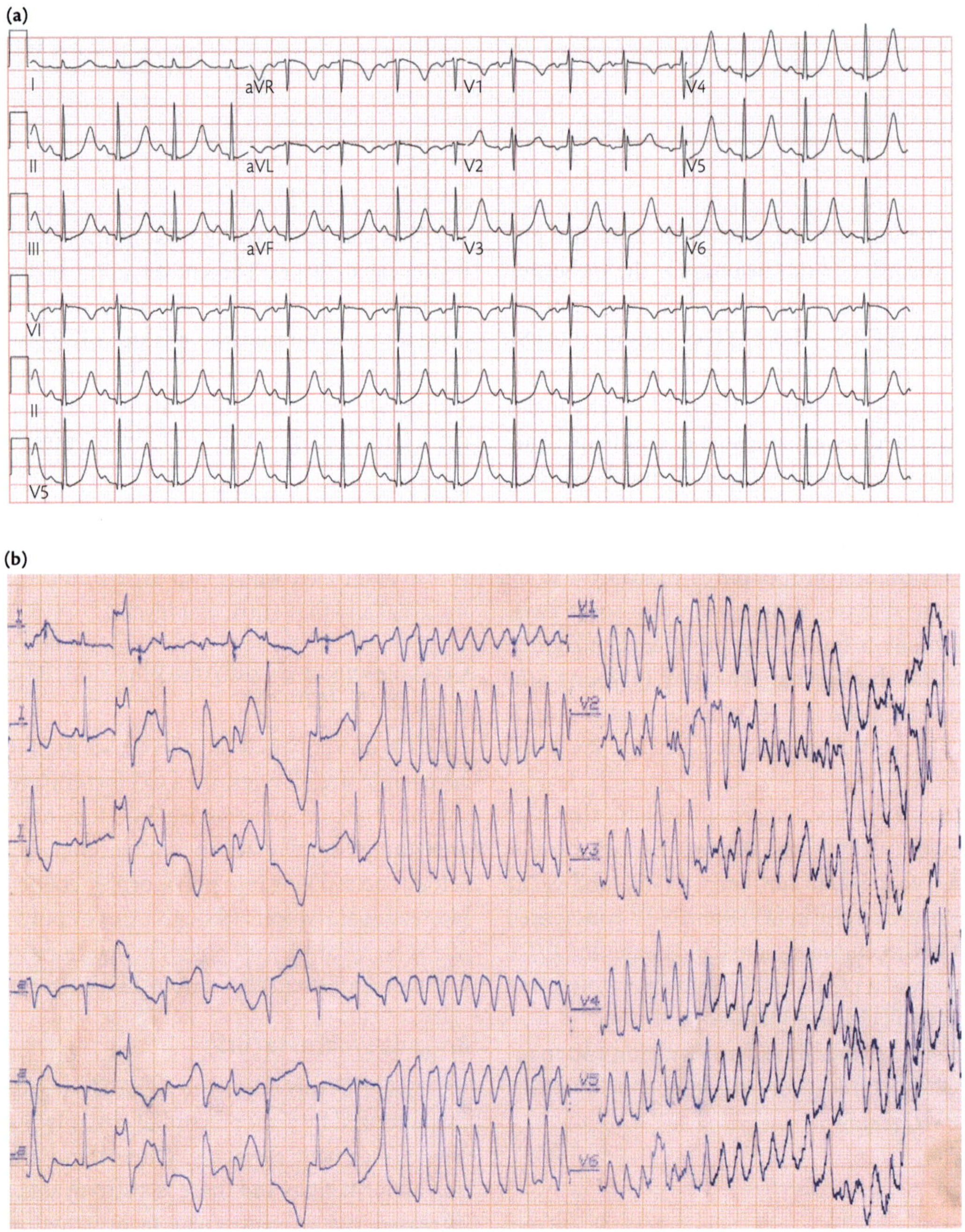

Fig. 5.1.1 (a) ECG of a 44-year-old woman with type 1 LQTS. The ECG shows sinus rhythm with a frequency around 100/bpm, normal conduction intervals, and abnormal repolarization. The T waves are wide and tall, which is typical for LQTS type 1, and the QTc is ±570ms. At a faster rate the QTc prolongation because more prominent. (b) The signature arrhythmia of LQTS, the torsades de pointes (TdP) arrhythmia, a high-rate polymorphic ventricular arrhythmia characterized by a shifting electrical axis.

Is the QTc interval cut-off point in the general population applicable to athletes?

Bazett's formula is commonly accepted as a tool to calculate the QT interval corrected for heart rate (QTc) [6]. The QT interval is assessed in a standard 12-lead ECG from lead II, or V5 or V6, using the longest value (➲ Fig 5.1.2). It is difficult to determine the end of the T wave because its morphology is not always a symmetrical deflection wave. The best option is to draw a tangent to the steepest last limb of the presumed T wave and the end is then defined as the intersection of this tangent with the baseline (➲ Fig. 5.1.2). Because the QT interval decreases with increasing heart rate, the measurement of the QT interval should be corrected for heart rate [6]. The RR′ interval is measured from the earliest onset of the preceding QRS to the earliest onset of the next QRS in milliseconds. The corrected QT is calculated using Bazett's formula:

$$QTc = QT / \sqrt{RR'}.$$

However, Bazett's formula may over-correct the QTc for heart rates >90bpm and under-correct for heart rates <60bpm. Holter monitoring can be used to calculate QTc at different heart rates. Although less accurate than a standardized 12-lead ECG for a single measurement, plotting the QT intervals against RR′ intervals over a longer period (i.e. the slope of the relation) may yield additional information, which needs to be elucidated by ongoing research. Exercise testing can be used to calculate QTc during exercise and recovery because standard 12-lead ECGs are available. However, the QT interval reacts slowly at higher heart rates (QT lag or QT hysteresis), resulting in possible misinterpretation of QTc [6].

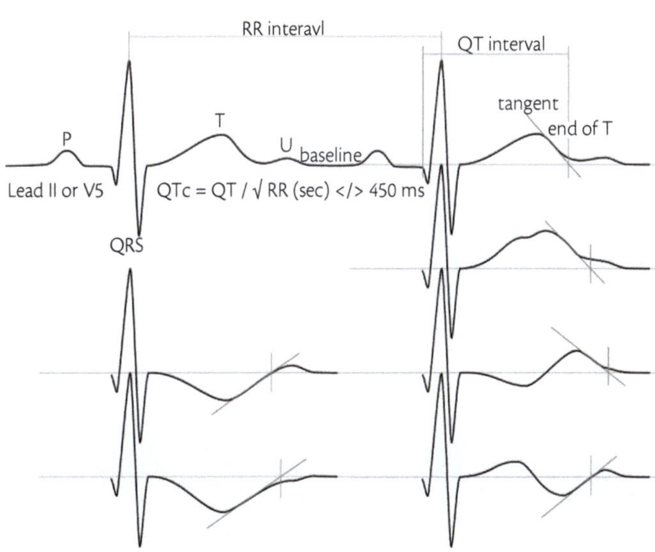

Fig. 5.1.2 Schematic illustration of the tangent method to define the end of the T wave in normal and abnormal TU morphologies, which then promotes the determination of the QTc interval.
Reproduced with permission from Arthur Wilde.

In addition to Bazett's formula there are other formulas for calculating QTc manually. None of the formulas calculates QTc accurately in bradycardia and tachycardia. Automated measurement of QTc requires visual confirmation of the T-wave morphology [6].

The main ion current responsible for the QT adaptation to heart rate is the catecholamine sensitive slow component of the delayed rectifier (i.e. I_{Ks}). In individuals with type 1 LQTS in whom this current is affected due to loss-of-function mutations in the gene encoding for this current, QT(c) shortening during exercise lags behind. This is associated with an increased risk of arrhythmias during exercise in LQTS1 individuals. In LQTS2, because of loss-of-function mutations in the gene encoding for the rapid component of the delayed rectifier (i.e. I_{Kr}), QT adaptation during exercise is in principle normal, although QTc intervals are generally longer. In LQTS3, because of gain-of-function mutations in the cardiac sodium channel, QT adaptation is completely normal and QT(c) intervals are mainly prolonged at slow heart rates. This translates into an increased likelihood for cardiac symptoms at a slow heart rate (i.e. during the night).

At the 36th Bethesda Conference cut-off points of QTc >470ms in males and QTc >480ms in females were estabished to distinguish between physiology and pathology in athletes [7]. In the Schwartz score, a QT interval >480ms is regarded as indicationg a high probability of LQTS [8]. Almost a decade ago the ESC Section on Sports Cardiology recommended a threshold for normal QTc of 440–470ms for men and 460–480ms for women [9]. The recent International Consensus Criteria [10] confirm suspicion of LQTS when QTc is longer than 470ms in men and 480ms in women, with a QTc interval ≥500ms indicating definite LQTS [11].

In a 10-year study of 2000 elite athletes, with a mean age of 20.2 years, a QTc interval of 460–570 ms was found in seven athletes [12]. In those with a QTc interval ≥500ms there were other confirmatory signs of LQTS (paradoxical prolongation of the QTc during exercise, gene mutation, and QTc prolongation in first-degree relatives). The authors concluded that if QTc is shorter than 500ms other LQTS features (e.g. symptoms or family history) are required to confirm the diagnosis of LQTS [12]. Hence, while a QTc interval ≥500ms in athletes should be regarded as diagnostic of LQTS, a QTc of 470–500ms in male athletes and 480–500ms in female athletes constitutes a 'grey zone' of high suspicion of LQTS and is an indication for further cardiac evaluation [4,7,12–16]. The Schwartz score system and details of the family history can be useful for estimating the exercise-related risk of cardiac events in this 'grey zone'.

Athletes with a QTc interval ≥500ms should be referred to a specialist for further evaluation and appropriate management, and should be withdrawn from sports participation during evaluation [5,16].

Symptoms

The symptoms of LQTS are periodic dizziness, syncopal attacks, and SCD. The signature arrhythmia of LQTS is torsades de pointes (TdP), which is a high rate polymorphic ventricular arrhythmia characterized by a shifting electrical axis. A short episode of TdP may even be asymptomatic or lead to a brief episode of dizziness. Longer episodes of TdP can lead to syncopal attacks, which may resemble an epileptic insult. A TdP arrhythmia can last for minutes and end spontaneously, but occasionally deteriorates into VF and the patient may eventually die in the absence of appropriate intervention.

Genetic counselling

In the mid-1990s the genetics underlying LQTS started to be unravelled. It soon became clear that mutations in various genes were involved (16 have been identified to date). Thus LQTS was subdivided into several subtypes with specific characteristics (LQTS1–LQTS16). The most frequent subtypes are LQTS1, LQTS2, and LQTS3, based on variants in the genes coding for the delayed rectifier (LQTS1, KCNQ1 coding for the ionic current I_{Ks}; LQTS2, KCNH2 coding for I_{Kr}) and the cardiac sodium channel SCN5a (LQTS3). The genetic subtype is highly relevant for the clinical presentation; for example, in LQTS1 an adrenergic trigger is responsible for over 90% of events, whereas these triggers are much less effective in the other main subtypes (≤60% in KCNH2 and ±30% in LQTS3). See Chapter 3.4.1 for the indications for genetic testing in LQTS.

Short QT syndrome (SQTS)

Short QT syndrome is a rare, albeit highly lethal, channelopathy. Only 100–200 cases have been described worldwide, subdivided into three genetic subtypes with mutations in KCNH2, KCNJ2, and KCNQ1. These mutations lead to enhanced repolarizing potassium currents, shortening the QT interval. SQTS has an autosomal dominant inheritance.

The QTc cut-off in SQTS in athletes

There is no definitive QTc cut-off which defines SQTS. In the most recent guideline document, QTc ≤330ms is considered diagnostic by itself, whereas QTc ≤360ms can be diagnostic in the presence of other clinical markers, i.e. familial sudden cardiac death or family members with an equally short QTc interval [4] (➲ Fig. 5.1.3).

In a 2–7-year follow-up study in a young population (ages 14–25 years) of 8,939 young athletes (72% male, 89% Caucasian), QTc was measured and compared with the current guidelines, the ESC recommendations, and the Seattle criteria [11,13,14,17]. The prevalence of SQTS was 8.6% using the ESC criteria (with a QTc interval cut-off of ≤380ms) and 17% using the Seattle criteria (with a QTc interval cut-off of ≤320ms) [11,14]. There was a slight male preponderance and ethnic differences in the QTc interval measured. African/Afro-Caribbean athletes were found to have a relatively shorter QTc than Caucasian athletes.

In a Finnish study of over 10,000 middle-aged individuals the prevalence of a QTc interval ≤320ms was 0.1%, and did not predict SCD [18]. In a Japanese study of over 10,000 people of all ages a QTc interval ≤300 ms was very rare (three cases), and was not associated with SCD or SQTS-related symptoms [19]. In a study of over 41,000 Swiss males the prevalence of a QTc interval ≤320ms was 0.02%, and no QTc intervals <300ms were measured [20]. In a computer-based ECG study in 1.7

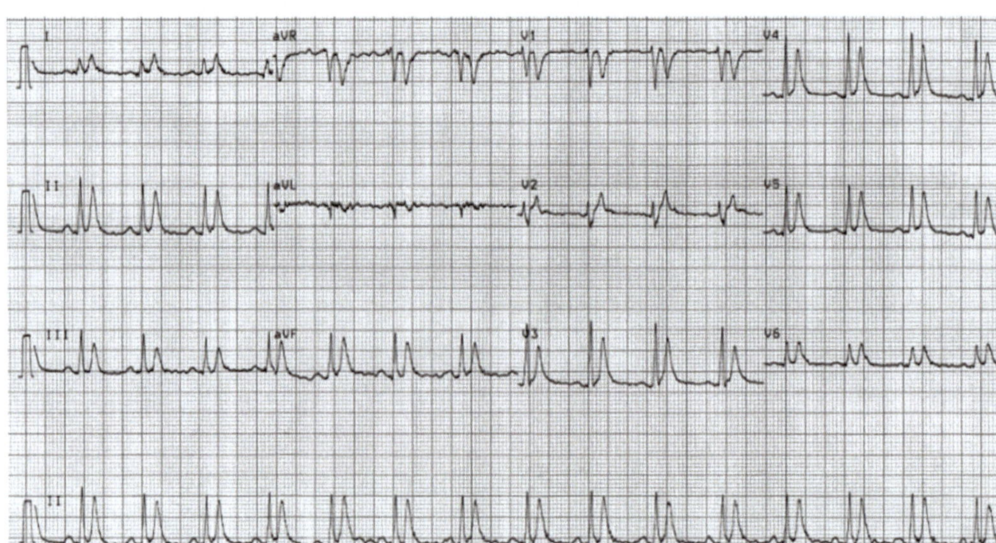

Fig. 5.1.3 Twelve-lead ECG recording with a short QT interval. The QT interval is 250ms and the QTc interval is 270ms. The tall peaked T waves in the precordial leads are characteristic of SQTS. Reproduced from *British Journal of Sports Medicine*, Electrocardiographic interpretation in athletes: the 'Seattle Criteria', Jonathan A Drezner et al., Volume 47, Issue 3, pp. 122–124. Copyright 2013, with permission from BMJ Publishing Group Ltd.

million people of all ages the prevalence of a QTc interval ≤300ms was very rare (0.7/100,000) [21]. A short QT interval was seen in people aged over 65 years with other ECG abnormalities and was associated with cardiac and non-cardiac disease [21]. No QTc intervals ≤300ms were recorded in the group aged below 17 years. In all these studies there was a male preponderance and the QTc interval in African/ Afro-Carribean people was relatively shorter than that in Caucasian [21], as was also seen in the study of athletes by Dhutia et al. [17]. A short QTc was not associated with an increased risk of SCD or SQTS-related symptoms in young athletes. However, if a short QT interval was found in the setting of a sudden cardiac arrest (SCA), there was an increased risk of (recurrent) SCD [21].

On the basis of these data it can be concluded that there is a high suspicion of SQTS in both African/Afro-Caribbean and Caucasian athletes with a QTc interval ≤320ms. They should be referred for additional cardiac evaluation, and restricted from participation in sports during evaluation [17–21].

In the overall population a cut-off point of ≤330 ms is defined as SQTS [5] Furthermore, when the ECG criterion of a short QT interval is observed in athletes with a good ventricular function and no arrhythmia at high heart rates (stress testing, Holter monitoring), the exercise-related risk for cardiac events is probably low. Follow-up is necessary at least every year in these athletes and in those athletes with a normal QTc interval but with a first-degree relative diagnosed with SQTS.

Symptoms

The symptoms of SQTS are palpitations, unexplained syncope, or SCD probably due to VF. The irregularity of the heart rhythm can occur during exercise, presenting as short episodes, but it may deteriorate into polymorphic VT (with syncope) and SCD when deterioration into VF has occurred.

Catecholaminergic polymorphic ventricular tachycardia (CPVT)

Catecholaminergic polymorphic ventricular tachycardia (CPVT) is an entity that only expresses itself in the setting of adrenergic stress. At rest the ECG is completely normal, although a relative bradycardia is common. CPVT is usually a disease with clinical manifestation at a young age (5–6 years onwards). The signature feature is an exercise/emotion-induced ventricular arrhythmia. Typically it starts with monomorphic ventricular ectopy at a specific heart rate that is quite consistent for a given patient. With ongoing exercise the ventricular ectopy becomes more complex, initially with polymorphic couplets and eventually polymorphic triplets and polymorphic tachycardias (➔ Fig 5.1.4). Deterioration into VF can occur. Most typically the clinical presentation is a bidirectional ventricular tachycardia.

CPVT is an autosomal dominant inherited trait with incomplete penetrance. The genetic basis is found in several genes that play a role in the calcium homeostasis of cardiac cells. The ryanodine receptor gene (RyR2) is involved in about two-thirds of successfully genotyped patients. An autosomal recessive form, more severe than the autosomal dominant variant, is associated with mutations in the CASQ2 gene.

CPVT is triggered by adrenergic stress. Therefore physical exercise should always be prohibited in these patients. Activities in which there is no physical effort (such as chess) can be allowed. However, it is difficult to predict the influence of psychological stress inducing adrenergic stimulation while participating in these games.

Anti-adrenergic interventions, including beta-blocker therapy and ablation of the left stellate ganglion, are very effective in reducing the arrhythmia burden.

(a)

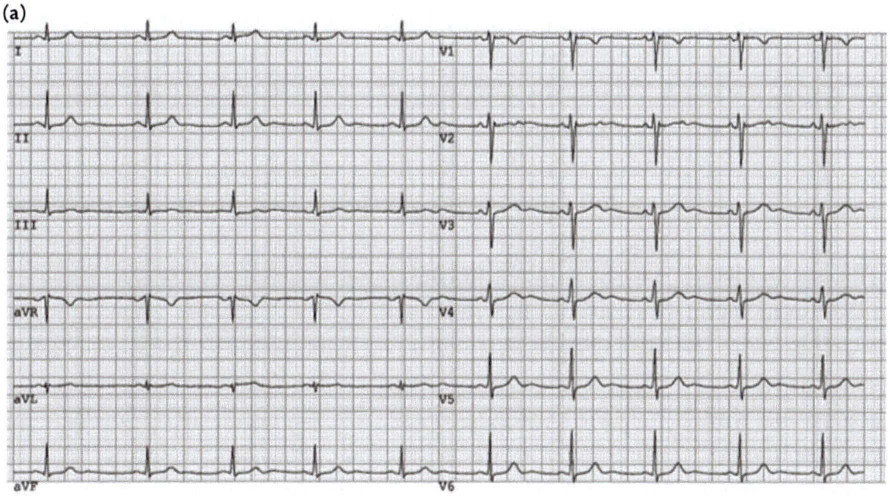

Fig. 5.1.4 Three 12-lead recordings obtained during an exercise test in a patient with CPVT. (a) A sinus arrhythmia with normal conduction intervals and normal repolarization.

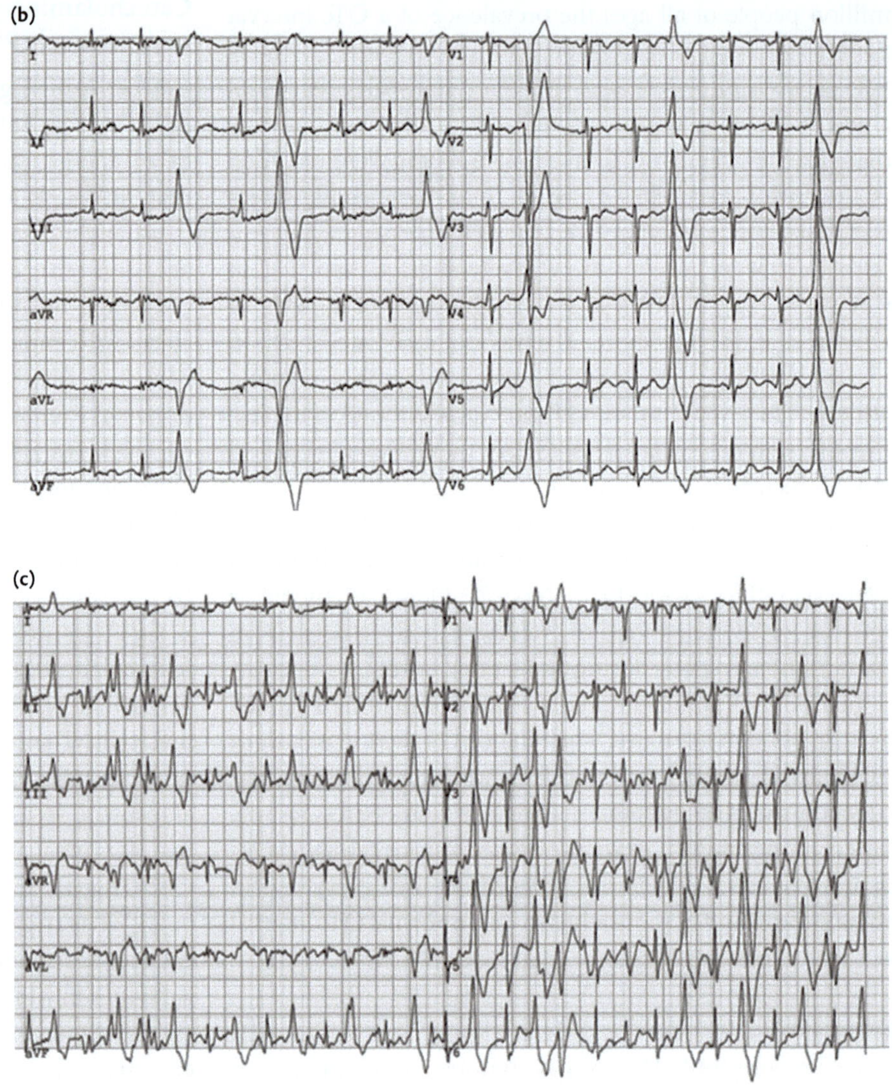

Fig. 5.1.4 *(Continued)*

(b) ECG taken during the initial few minutes of exercise. Single ectopics are seen with a polymorphic appearance. (c) ECG taken during ongoing exercise showing a bigeminy of ventricular extra-systoles and, in the initial part of the precordial leads, a polymorphic doublet. The patient was asymptomatic during this test.

Symptoms

The symptoms of CPVT are characterized by the ventricular arrhythmia occurring during the adrenergic state. At rest there are no symptoms. Episodic syncope can occur with the onset of ventricular arrhythmia during exercise or emotional stress with spontaneous recovery once the ventricular arrhythmia terminates. Longer-lasting ventricular arrhythmia can result in SCA when the ventricular arrhythmia deteriorates in VF.

Brugada syndrome (BrS)

Brugada syndrome (BrS) was originally described as an 'electrical disease' characterized by right precordial coved type or saddle-back type ST-segment elevation (➔ Fig. 5.1.5). Frequently, there are also conduction abnormalities at different cardiac levels and there is a strong association with an increased risk of ventricular tachyarrhythmias, including VF. BrS is associated with 4% of all SCDs in the general population [22]. More recently, it has become clear that there are discrete structural abnormalities, in particular located in the upper right ventricular anterior wall/outflow tract region [23]. These recent findings put BrS into a spectrum overlapping with arrhythmogenic right ventricular cardiomyopathy (ARVC) [24].

The arrhythmias in BrS are not particularly associated with adrenergic conditions such as exercise. On the contrary, most ventricular arrhythmic episodes and SCDs occur during the night at a time of increased vagal tone [25]. Increased vagal tone could be of relevance immediately after strenuous exercise, but clustering of immediate post-exercise arrhythmic events has not been reported to date. Hyperthermia (fever) in BrS may act as a trigger for the Brugada-associated ECG changes and/or ventricular arrhythmic episodes and for QTc prolongation [26,27]. The underlying mechanism potentially relates to the fact that sodium gating properties induced by an SNC5a mutation have been found to

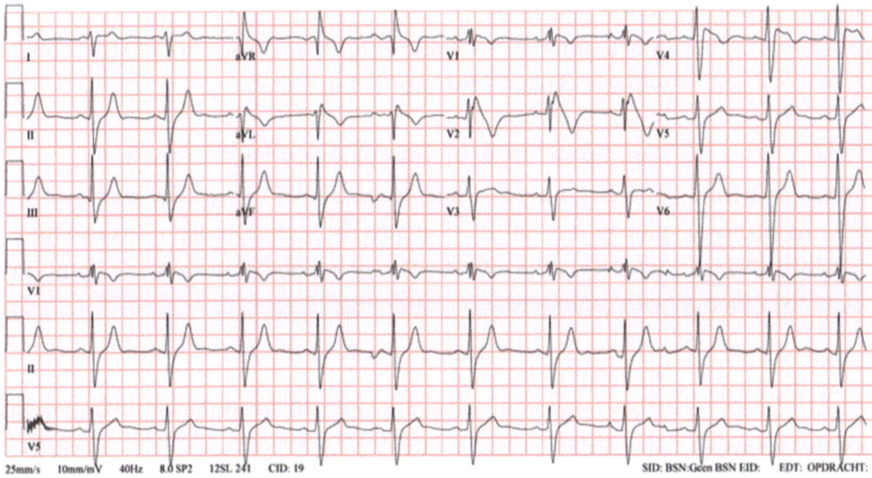

Fig. 5.1.5 ECG recording of Brugada syndrome (17-year-old boy, asymptomatic; positive family history for symptomatic Brugada syndrome).

be more prominent during fever [27]. Thus activities that may provoke increase in body temperature, which cannot be avoided during strenuous exercise, should be discouraged in BrS patients. In addition, there are also reports of potential pro-arrhythmic ECG changes during exercise in BrS patients [28]. However, at present there are no reports of exercise-induced arrhythmias in BrS patients.

The genetics of BrS is complex. A large number of genes have been implicated in its pathogenesis. However, the only gene with robust evidence for a potential pathogenic role is SCN5a (with mutations involving loss of sodium channel). The current hypothesis is that BrS is an oligogenetic disease, i.e. a disease based on a number of genetic variants with functional impact in several different genes [29].

Symptoms

The symptoms of BrS occur most frequently during rest or sleep. Most common are syncope and SCA, but 'nocturnal agonal respiration' can also occur during (self-terminating) ventricular arrhythmic episodes. Hyperthermia, such as that occurring during fever, can trigger ventricular arrhythmia and the patient can become symptomatic. Atrial fibrillation, which can be asymptomatic or present itself with irregular palpitations and/or reduced exercise tolerance in athletes, seems to be more frequent in patients with BrS.

In the absence of a type 1 ECG, which is required for the diagnosis of BrS, provocation with a sodium-channel blocker (ajmaline, flecainide) can be considered.

ECG changes in BrS

It is a challenge for the screening physician to recognize the Brugada ECG in athletes. In the right precordial leads there is a high take-off and downsloping ST-segment elevation of more than 2mm followed by a negative T wave in at least two contiguous leads [14] (➲ Fig. 5.1.5). Although there are several reports in the literature that a Brugada ECG can be identified with a higher placement of electrodes V1–V3 in the third and/or second intercostal space, this is not consistently observed in young athletes at eligibility screening. Therefore it is debatable whether higher placement of electrodes V1–V3 should be routinely performed in eligibility screening.

The Brugada ECG should be distinguished from a normal ECG in highly trained athletes. In athletes a J-point elevation with a convex ST-segment is regarded as a physiological cardiac adaptation [13]. This early repolarization pattern is present in almost all endurance athletes [30]. In a case–control study of 155 male Caucasian athletes and 50 sedentary controls, signs of Brugada-like ST-segment elevation without the definitive diagnosis of BrS was found in 8% of the male athletes [30]. No cardiac events had been reported in these athletes.

Athletes with spontaneous signs of a 'Brugada ECG' should be referred for further cardiac evaluation.

The risk of SCD in those with a Brugada ECG pattern only during class 1 provocation seems to be very low. Therefore, unless there are unexplained symptoms or a positive family history, ajmaline or flecainide testing should not be part of routine evaluation in athletes.

Loss-of-function sodium-channel mutations are also associated with the conduction delay (at all cardiac levels). These abnormalities usually worsen with increased heart rate. Such athletes should be discouraged from engaging in intensive exercise and sport activity as part of the disease management. In patients with overt SCN5a overlap syndromes, i.e. a combination with loss-of-function characteristics (sick sinus syndrome, conduction slowing throughout all cardiac compartments, BrS) and gain-of-function characteristics

(LQTS), management should probably also include restriction from intensive exercise and sport activity.

Eligibility screening in channelopathy

In many European countries there are recommendations for a uniform pre-participation and eligibility screening protocol in young athletes, including personal and family history, physical examination, and a 12-lead resting ECG [31] (see Chapter 7.1).

Personal and family history

Athletes with channelopathy can be completely asymptomatic before presentation with out-of-hospital cardiac arrest. They can have specific symptoms, such as palpitations, abnormal fatigue, (periodic) dizziness, syncopal attacks, and/or (near)syncope, and should be considered carefully during pre-participation evaluation.

If the family history reveals SCA or SCD at a young age the screening physician must be suspicious of an inherited electrical cardiovascular disease.

There are usually normal findings on physical examination in ion-channel cardiac disease.

Twelve-lead resting ECG

As noted in Chapter 2.1.1, it is important that the physician interpreting an athlete's ECG is familiar with the difference between sports-related or physiological electrical changes and pathological electrical changes, such as ion-channel cardiac disease [11,13,14] (➔ Figs 5.1.1, 5.1.3, 5.1.4, and 5.1.5) The ECG in eligibility screening is of utmost importance because ion-channel cardiac disease, such as LQTS and SQTS, can be detected with a 12-lead ECG at rest (➔ Figs 5.1.1 and 5.1.3). However, CPVT is typically provoked by adrenergic stimulation, such as exercise, and cannot be identified at rest (➔ Fig. 5.1.4). Likewise, BrS can be seen intermittently with a resting ECG (➔ Fig 5.1.5).

The ESC ECG criteria for athletes (2010) were updated by the Seattle criteria (2013), which have more recently been updated as the International Consensus Criteria [10].

Long QT syndrome

A QTc interval ≥500ms in athletes is definitive for diagnosis of LQTS, while a QTc interval ≥470ms in males and ≥480ms in females should raise suspicion of LQTS [12,14] (➔ Fig 5.1.1). Therefore athletes with a QTc interval ≥470ms in males and ≥480ms in females need further cardiac evaluation and risk assessment for cardiac events in relation to exercise. This is also supported by the recent AHA/ACC recommendations [16].

Short QT syndrome

A QTc interval ≤320ms is highly suspicious of SQTS in both white and black athletes (➔ Fig 5.1.3).

Catecholaminergic polymorphic ventricular tachycardia

There is a high suspicion of CPVT in athletes with a completely normal ECG at rest, but monomorphic ventricular ectopy at a specific heart rate which becomes more complex with ongoing exercise (➔ Fig 5.1.4).

Brugada syndrome

There is a high suspicion of BrS in athletes with a right precordial (leads V1-V2-V3) ST-segment elevation (➔ Fig. 5.1.5). The ST-segment elevation implies an early high take-off J wave (>2mm) with a downsloping ST-segment and a coved type negative T wave or saddle-back type positive T wave.

Athletes who suffer SCA without underlying structural disease are raises suspicion of ion-channel cardiac disease.

Additional cardiac evaluation in channelopathy

The ultimate goal of additional cardiac evaluation is to identify the disease and determine the risk of exercise-related cardiac events. Athletes with suspicion of ion-channel cardiac disease should be temporarily restricted from participation in sport and evaluated by a cardiologist, preferably with expertise in the field of sports medicine (sports cardiology) and/or channelopathy (electrophysiology).

Exercise stress testing and Holter monitoring

Additional cardiac evaluation consists of a sport-specific stress ECG until exertion and Holter monitoring to capture the rhythm or conduction problem. In type 1 LQTS the key feature at higher heart rates is a paradoxical increment of the QTc interval. If there is suspicion of CPVT, exercise stress testing and Holter monitoring at higher heart rates is necessary to establish the diagnosis.

Exercise stress testing also has the potential to reveal ventricular arrhythmia, particularly VT/VF at higher heart rates in LQTS, SQTS, and CPVT. The total number of ventricular ectopies (isolated, couplets, non-sustained or sustained VT) and the morphology of ventricular ectopy (monomorphic or polymorphic) can help to determine the diagnosis and also the risk of exercise-related cardiac events, such as SCA or SCD. If the total number of ventricular ectopies exceeds 1% (>2000 premature ventricular beats per 24 hours), particularly if seen at higher heart rates, the probability of having a disease increases.

Imaging with echocardiography and MRI

In channelopathy no structural morphological changes of the ventricles and atria, no valve incompetence, no congenital abnormalities, and especially no 'scar' or fibrosis (other than changes in myocardial wall thickness and cavity size as a part of physiological cardiac adaptation in athletes) are seen with the imaging techniques [32,33]. If a pathological structural morphological change in the heart is observed, the diagnosis of ion-channel cardiac disease is questionable. In BrS the diameters of the right ventricular outflow tract (RVOT), and sometimes even the diameters of the left ventricle, are at the upper limit of normal and, as already indicated, this disease entity might have an overlap with ARVC. Therefore, although more research is necessary, BrS is believed to be the only channelopathy with possible abnormal findings in imaging.

Electrophysiological study

Invasive electrophysiological (EP) studies with programmed electrical stimulation (PES) are not recommended for SCD risk stratification in channelopathy (class III indication, level of evidence C) [5]. An exception might be BrS, where the role of EP study for risk stratification is disputed, leading to a class IIb recommendation in the current guidelines [5].

Genetic counselling and family screening

Genetic testing is the final diagnostic tool for establishing the diagnosis. Details of the interpretation of genetic testing in athletes are given in Chapter 3.4.1. If diagnostic evaluation fails to detect a channelopathy in a highly suspicious athlete, an on-site automatic cardiac defibrillator (AED) can be a safe bystander on the field [34–37].

Athletes who have died suddenly should undergo an autopsy with extensive cardiac evaluation looking for the presence of an underlying cardiac disease. If there is no evidence for a structural heart disease, genetic testing of the deceased should be considered to identify inherited cardiac disease [38]. First-degree family members should also be screened [38]. The outcome of an autopsy and genetic testing and the results of family screening will have significant implications for the family members. This also applies when a first-degree relative dies suddenly in the absence of a structural heart disease, because the risk of SCD in the athletes with a positive family history is increased [39]. In Italy, autopsy is regulated by law [31,40]. However, autopsies are not performed routinely in all countries when an athlete dies suddenly. For example, in the Netherlands the family must give informed consent and cover the costs of autopsy. Thus a large number of autopsies are not performed and questions regarding the cause of death remain unanswered.

Management of athletes with channelopathy

Oral drug therapy and ICD implantation

In most patients with LQTS and CPVT pharmacological therapy (i.e. beta-blocker therapy) will suffice [5]. In particular, beta-blocker therapy is very effective in LQT1 patients, and should also be the first choice in LQT2 and LQT3. Surgical ablation of the left stellate ganglion is highly effective in cases of LQTS and CPVT where insufficient protection is provided by beta-blockers. An implantable cardioverter defibrillator (ICD) is sometimes needed, particularly for those who have been resuscitated (although exceptions can be made with respect to untreated LQT1 or CPVT patients) or those who remain symptomatic despite adequate beta-blocker therapy. In CPVT flecainide should be tried first in combination with beta-blocker therapy.

The efficacy of pharmacological therapy in SQTS has not been well studied. Sotalol and quinidine have been shown to prolong the QTc interval to some extent. Symptomatic patients will all end up with an ICD.

Symptomatic BrS patients should to be treated with an ICD. The acute management of arrhythmic storms requires intravenous isoprenaline and oral quinidine. Quinidine has also been shown to be effective in the long term.

Considerations on eligibility decision-making

Channelopathies are not (yet) curable. However, with current and new developments for diagnosis and treatment of channelopathy the risk of sports-related cardiac events can probably be better controlled. This means that sports restrictions need not be considered [9,16,31,41].

The original recommendations for sports participation in athletes with channelopathy were based on the ESC and Bethesda recommendations, and stated that roughly all athletes with a channelopathy with or without symptoms should be excluded from participation in sport [41,42]. These recommendations date from an era in which genetic testing was not widespread. Genetic testing leads to an increasing number of genotype positive/phenotype negative individuals with (concealed) channelopathy for whom the recommendations for sports participation are uncertain [41,42]. The recommendations are based on expert opinion, assuming an exercise-related pro-arrhythmic trigger for LQTS1 and CPVT [41,42] Furthermore, the ESC recommendations were mainly based on a large Italian pre-participation study in young athletes, excluding all athletes identified with electrical abnormalities from sports participation. In this screening study 0.6% of all disqualified athletes had LQTS [43]. During follow-up none of the disqualified LQTS athletes had a cardiac event or died suddenly.

In the meantime genetic testing is recommended in patients with channelopathy or suspicion of channelopathy, but there are few reports of exercise-related cardiac events in large cohorts [16,38] (see also, Chapter 3.4.1).

To date, there is only one observational study challenging the recommendations for sports participation in LQTS [44]. In a 10-year retrospective case record study of 157 LQTS gene-positive adolescent patients (mean age 17±11), athletic participation and LQTS-related events were reviewed. Athletes were informed in detail about the risk of sport participation and were not forced to continue participating in sports at any level of intensity if the athlete and both parents in the case of younger athletes agreed to this after reading the Bethesda conference guidelines. The athletes were treated with beta-blocker medications if possible and an ICD was implanted on an individual basis. They were advised to avoid QT-prolonging drugs, dehydration, exercise-related body heating, and electrolyte disturbances, and were instructed to carry an AED with them. Of 353 patients diagnosed with LQTS, 157 chose to continue sports participation, and 60 of them (31 females, mean age 12±7 years, with an average QTc of 501±46ms) participated in sport. During a mean follow-up of 5.5 years there was one cardiac event (0.33 events/year). The boy had already suffered from symptoms related to LQTS (unexplained fainting during physical and emotional stress) with a QTc of 490ms, and he suffered an aborted cardiac arrest when QTc increased to >550ms. During the study period he had two exercise-related appropriate VF-terminating ICD shocks, while being non-compliant using beta-blocker medication [44]. No events were registered in the genotype positive participants with QT intervals within the normal range. This study eventually showed that events are possible in patients with markedly prolonged QT interval and are unlikely to occur in genotype positive/phenotype negative individuals.

In a recent study among 63 adolescent patients with CPVT, 31 were athletes of a younger age [45]. At the time of the diagnosis 24 athletes were still active, and 21 of them continued competition after shared decision-making. Of these 21 athletes, 16 (76%) had experienced 32 CPVT-triggered events prior to diagnosis. During follow-up cardiac events occurred in three of the 21 athletes (14%), but none resulted in SCD [45]. The authors concluded that although undiagnosed and untreated CPVT is associated with a high risk of exercise-related cardiac events, the risk in well-treated and well-informed athletes with CPVT may be acceptable [45].

There are no similar reports describing continuation of sports participation challenging the current recommendations for sports participation in SQTS and BrS.

In an international ICD registry, athletes with an ICD (mean age 33 years (89 <20 years), 33% females) participating in organized (328) or high risk (44) sports were included [36] There were 60 competitive athletes. In the entire cohort there were 94 participants with an underlying cardiac diagnosis, 73 with LQTS, 10 with CPVT and seven with BrS. At an average follow-up of 31 months, no cardiac events were reported in relation to sports participation except VF terminating ICD shocks. These appropriate ICD shocks were observed in two patients with LQTS and one patient with CPVT. As a result of ICD shocks in 37 participants, 30% of them (3% of the total study population) decided to stop participating in sport [36]. The authors concluded that athletes with an ICD can participate in competitive sports without failure of lethal arrhythmia termination or physical injury [36]. However, this registry did not answer the question of whether an ICD in an athlete with a channelopathy provides sufficient protection to prevent SCD related to sports participation. The underlying cardiac disease ultimately determines the prognosis of the athlete/patient.

When an athlete with channelopathy suffers from symptoms such as syncope or aborted cardiac arrest, or ventricular arrhythmia detected during diagnostic work-up, he/she is at high risk for exercise-related cardiac events. These athletes, with phenotype positive but still unknown genotype, should temporarily be disqualified from sports participation. After genetic counselling and treatment with a beta-blocker and eventually an ICD, sports participation can be considered, but remains questionable because the protective effect of the treatment during exercise remains uncertain [44].

In conclusion, to date there is no evidence that athletes with channelopathy are always ineligible for sports participation. Eligibility decision-making for sports participation is based on the type of channelopathy, the presence of symptoms, genetic counselling, and family history, and cannot be solely based on the assumption that channelopathies induce exercise-related ventricular arrhythmia leading to SCA. It is clear that this field is still evolving, and in urgent need of more prospective data.

Return to play

Return to play is possible in athletes with suspected ion-channel disease if there is no evidence of its phenotypic expression. Follow-up with a 12-lead resting ECG, exercise stress testing, and Holter monitoring on a regular basis (at least annually) is recommended in these athletes.

Return to play in athletes identified with channelopathy can be considered if there is no ventricular arrhythmia with exercise stress testing or Holter monitoring, no complaints of periodic dizziness or syncope, and a normal physical performance in relation to athlete's type of sport, provided that the cardiac function is good. However, when there is SCD in a first degree relative, the physician should be cautious and eligibility should be assessed on an individual basis. Treatment options in channelopathy are oral drug medication, such as beta-blocker medication in LQTS and CPVT, and quinidine in SQTS. ICD implantation is indicated following aborted SCD. If there are no ventricular arrhythmia events during a period of three month after starting treatment, the athlete can eventually return to play [36].

Conclusion

Channelopathies or ion-channel cardiac diseases are primary electrical disorders and belong to the inherited cardiac disorders. The four major channelopathies (long QT syndrome, short QT syndrome, catecholaminergic polymorphic ventricular tachycardia, and Brugada syndrome) predispose to life-threatening ventricular arrhythmia, and are potentially lethal in relation to exercise. They have signature ECG changes and arrhythmias, which can be identified with a 12-lead resting ECG, Holter monitoring, and/or exercise stress testing.

Eligibility decision-making for sports participation is based on the type of channelopathy, the presence of symptoms, genetic counselling, and family history, and cannot be solely based on the assumption that channelopathies induce exercise-related ventricular arrhythmia leading to SCA. Eligibility decision-making should involve expert opinion from cardiologists with expertise in these rare syndromes. Athletes (and their parents in the case of a minor) are entitled to be given detailed information about the risk of sport participation and eligibility to continue sports participation at any level of intensity.

Further reading

Antonen O, Junttila MJ, Rissanen H, et al. Prevalence and prognostic significance of short QT interval in a middle aged Finnish population. *Circulation* 2007;116: 714–20.

Basavarajaiah S, Shah A, Sharma S. Sudden cardiac death in young athletes Heart 2007;93: 287–9

Drezner JA, Ackerman MJ, Cannon BC, et al. Abnormal electrocardiographic findings in athletes: recognising changes suggestive of primary electrical disease. *Br J Sports Med* 2013;47: 153–67.

Duhtia H, Malhotra A, Parpia S, et al. The prevalence and significance of a short QT interval in 18,825 low-risk individuals including athletes. *Br J Sports Med* 2016;50: 124–9.

Priori SG, Wilde AA, Horie M, et al. Executive summary: HRS/EHRA/APHRS Consensus Statement on the Diagnosis and Management of Patients with Inherited Primary Arrhythmia Syndromes. *Heart Rhythm* 2013;10: 1932–6.

References

1. Maron BJ, Doerer JJ, Haas TS, et al. Sudden deaths in young competitive athletes: analysis of 1866 deaths in the United States, 1980–2006. *Circulation* 2009;119: 1085–92.
2. Antzelevitch C, Brugada P, Borggrefe M. Brugada syndrome: report of the second consensus conference: endorsed by the Heart Rhythm Society and the European Heart Rhythm Association. *Circulation* 2005;111: 659–70.
3. Maron BJ. Sudden death in young athletes. *N Engl J Med* 2003;349: 1064–1075
4. Priori SG, Wilde AA, Horie M, et al. Executive summary: HRS/EHRA/APHRS Consensus Statement on the Diagnosis and Management of Patients with Inherited Primary Arrhythmia Syndromes. *Heart Rhythm* 2013;10: 1932–63.
5. Priori SG, Blömstrom-Lundqvist C, Mazzanti A, et al. 2015 ESC Guidelines for the management of patients with ventricular arrhythmias and the prevention of sudden cardiac death. *Eur Heart J* 2015;36: 2793–867.
6. Postema PG, Wilde AAM. The measurement of the QT interval. *Curr Cardiol Rev* 2014;10: 287–94.
7. Maron BJ, Zipes DP. Eligibility recommendations for competitive athletes with cardiovascular abnormalities. *J Am Coll Cardiol* 2005;45: 1312–75.
8. Schwartz PJ, Moss AJ, Vincent GM, Crampton RS. Diagnostic criteria for the long QT syndrome: an update. *Circulation* 1993;88: 782–4.
9. Heidbuchel H, Corrado D, Biffi A, et al. Recommendations for participation in recreational physical activity and competitive sports for patients with arrhythmias and potentially arrhythmogenic conditions. Part II: ventricular arrhythmias, channelopathies and implantable defibrillators. *Eur J Cardiovasc Prev Rehab* 2006;13: 676–86.
10. Sharma S, Drezner J, Baggish A, et al. International recommendations for electrocardiographic interpretation in athletes. *Eur Heart J* 2018;39: 1466–80.
11. Corrado D, Pelliccia A, Heidbuchel H, et al. Recommendations for interpretation of 12-lead electrocardiogram in the athlete. *Eur Heart J*2010:31: 243–59.
12. Basavarajaiah S, Shah A, Sharma S. Sudden cardiac death in young athletes. *Heart* 2007;93: 287–9.
13. Drezner JA, Ackerman MJ, Anderson J, et al. Electrocardiographic interpretation in athletes: the 'Seattle Criteria'. *Br J Sports Med* 2013;47: 122–4.
14. Drezner JA, Ackerman MJ, Cannon BC, et al. Abnormal electrocardiographic findings in athletes: recognising changes suggestive of primary electrical disease. *Br J Sports Med* 2013;47: 153–67.
15. Schwartz PJ, Priori SG, Spazzolini C. Genotype-phenotype correlation in the long-QT syndrome: gene-specific triggers for life-threatening arrhythmias. *Circulation* 2001;103: 89–95.

16. Ackerman MJ, Zipes DP, Kovacs RJ, Maron BJ. AHA/ACC Scientific Statement Eligibility and Disqualification Recommendations for Competitive Athletes With Cardiovascular Abnormalities: Task Force 10: The Cardiac Channelopathies *Circulation* 2015;132: e326–9.
17. Duhtia H, Malhotra A, Parpia S, et al. The prevalence and significance of a short QT interval in 18 825 low-risk individuals including athletes. *Br J Sports Med* 2016;50: 124–9.
18. Antonen O, Junttila MJ, Rissanen H, et al. Prevalence and prognostic significance of short QT interval in a middle aged Finnish population. *Circulation* 2007;116: 714–20.
19. Funada A, Hayashi K, Ino H, et al. Assessment of QT intervals and prevalence of short QT syndrome in Japan. *Clin Cardiol* 2008;31: 270–4.
20. Kobza R, Roos M, Niggli B, et al. Prevalence of long and short QT in a young population in 41,767 predominantly male Swiss conscripts. *Heart Rhythm* 2009;6: 652–7.
21. Iribarren C, Round AD, Peng JA, et al. Short QT in a cohort of 1.7 million persons: prevalence, correlates, and prognosis. *Ann Noninvasive Electrocardiol* 2014;19: 490–500.
22. Derval N, Simpson CS, Birnie DH, et al. Prevalence and characteristics of early repolarization in the CASPER registry: cardiac arrest survivors with preserved ejection fraction registry. *J Am Coll Cardiol* 2011;58: 722–8.
23. Nademanee K, Raju H, De Noronha S, et al. Fibrosis, connexin 43 and conduction abnormalities in the Brugada syndrome. *J Am Coll Cardiol* 2015;66: 1976–86.
24. Corrado D, Zorzi A, Cerrone M, et al. Relationship between arrhythmogenic right ventricular cardiomyopathy and Brugada syndrome: new insights from molecular biology and clinical implications. *Circ Arrhythm Electrophysiol* 2016;9: e003631.
25. Chung EH. Brugada ECG patterns in athletes. *J Electrocardiol* 2015;48: 539–43.
26. Amin AS, Meregalli PG, Bardai A, et al. Fever increases the risk of cardiac arrest in the Brugada syndrome. *Ann Int Med* 2008;149: 216–18.
27. Meregalli PG, Tan HL, Wilde AAM. Brugada syndrome: clinical and genetic aspects. InGussak I, Antzelevitch C (eds) *Electrical Diseases of the Heart* (2nd edn), Vol. 1. London: Springer-Verlag 2013, pp. 469–95.
28. Amin AS, de Groot EAA, Ruijter J, et al. Exercise-induced ECG changes in Brugada syndrome. *Circ Arrhythm Electrophysiol* 2009;2: 531–9.
29. Bezzina CR, Barc J, Mizusawa Y, et al. Common variants at SCN5A/SCN10A and HEY2 are associated with Brugada syndrome, a rare disease with high risk of sudden cardiac death. *Nat Genet* 2013;45: 1044–9
30. Bianco M, Bria S, Gianfelici A, et al. Does early repolarization in the athlete have analogies with the Brugada syndrome? *Eur Heart J*2001:22: 504–10.
31. Corrado D, Pelliccia A, Bjørnstad HH, et al. CV pre-participation screening of young competitive athletes for prevention of sudden death: proposal for a common European protocol. *Eur Heart J* 2005;26: 516–20.
32. Teske AJ, Prakken NH, De Boeck BW, et al. Effect of long term and intensive endurance training in athletes on the age related decline in left and right ventricular diastolic function as assessed by Doppler echocardiography. *Am J Cardiol* 2009;104: 1145–51.
33. Luijkx T. Cardiac MRI in athletes, PhD Thesis, Utrecht University, The Netherlands, 2012, ISBN: 978-90-5335-508-4.
34. Borjesson M, Serratosa L, Carré F, et al. Consensus document regarding cardiovascular safety at sports arenas. *Eur Heart J* 2011;32: 2119–24.
35. Drezner JA Preparing for sudden cardiac arrest—the essential role of automated external defibrillators in athletic medicine: a critical review. *Br J Sports Med* 2009;43: 702–7.
36. Lampert R, Olshansky B, Heidbuchel H, et al. Safety of sports for athletes with implantable cardioverter-defibrillators: results of a prospective, multinational registry. *Circulation* 2013;127: 2021–30.
37. Link MS, Myerburg RJ, Mark Estes III NA. Eligibility and disqualification recommendations for competitive athletes with cardiovascular abnormalities: Task Force 12: emergency action plans, resuscitation, cardiopulmonary resuscitation and automated external defibrillator. *J Am Coll Cardiol* 2015;21: 2434–8.
38. Ackerman MJ, Priori SG, Willems S, et al. HRS/EHRA expert consensus statement on the state of genetic testing for the channelopathies and cardiomyopathies. *Heart Rhythm* 2011;8: 1308–39.
39. Jouven X, Desnos M, Guerot C, Ducimetière P. Predicting sudden death in the population: the Paris Prospective Study I. *Circulation* 1999;99: 1978–83.
40. Corrado D, Basso C, Schiavon M, et al. Screening for hypertrophic cardiomyopathy in young athletes. *N Engl J Med* 1998;339: 364–9.
41. Pelliccia A, Fagard R, Bjornstad HH, et al. Recommendations for competitive sports participation in athletes with CV disease. *Eur Heart J* 2005;26: 1422–45.
42. Zipes DP, Ackerman MJ, Estes NAM 3rd, et al. Task Force 7: arrhythmias. *J Am Coll Cardiol* 2005;45: 1354–63.
43. Corrado D, Basso C, Pavei A, et al. Trends in sudden CV death in young competitive athletes after implementation of a pre-participation screening program. *JAMA* 2006;296: 1593–1601.
44. Johnson JN, Ackerman MJ. Return to play? Athletes with congenital long QT syndrome. *Br J Sports Med* 2013;47: 28–33.
45. Ostby SA, Bos JM, Owen HJ, et al. Competitive sports participation in patients with catecholaminergic polymorphic ventricular tachycardia: a single center's early experience. *J Am Coll Cardiol* 2016;2: 253–62.

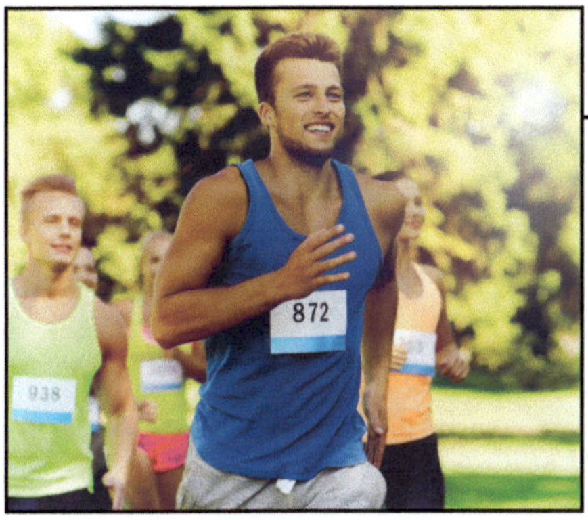

5.2

Ventricular tachyarrhythmias

Eduard Guasch and Lluís Mont

Introduction

Although the benefits of physical activity have been fully and extensively proved and are widely recognized, concerns about an increased risk of sudden cardiac death (SCD) in competitive athletes have been raised in the last two decades [1]. Extensive research has made apparent that most SCD events occur in individuals with an underlying previously undiagnosed cardiomyopathy. Physical activity is apparently increasing SCD risk in these individuals several-fold [2]. The cardiac conditions most frequently responsible for SCD in athletes are hypertrophic cardiomyopathy (HCM), arrhythmogenic right ventricle cardiomyopathy (ARVC), and coronary congenital abnormalities in young individuals (≤35 years old), and coronary artery disease (CAD) in master athletes (>35 years old) [3].

These concerns have led to the establishment of pre-participation screening programmes focusing on the identification of those cardiac conditions posing a risk for SCD [1]. Although concerns have been raised about costs and false-positive results [4], it has become clear that ECG produces a remarkable improvement in the diagnostic yield of screening programmes. ECG allows the identification of a variety of cardiomyopathies in their early subclinical stage [5]. Several expert consensus statements have developed classifications providing standardized ECG parameters which flag individuals at an increased risk of an underlying cardiomyopathy [6].

The prevalence of ventricular arrhythmia (VA) is increased in individuals with certain cardiac conditions [7] and might provide a means of early identification. In some cases, asymptomatic VA detected during a pre-participation screening programme is the first manifestation of an underlying heart disease which might put the athlete at an increased risk of SCD. Concern is greater for those athletes who develop symptomatic VA, as its impact on daily life and physical performance increases fears of SCD. Awareness of VA in athletes has been increased as recent data have suggested that strenuous physical activity might have a role in promoting a substrate for potentially lethal VA in otherwise healthy individuals, emphasizing the need for regular follow-up testing.

All these data emphasize the importance of appropriate screening for VA. However, prevalence of VA is also high in the healthy general population. Thus an increased risk of cardiomyopathy in athletes with VA needs to be weighted against the high prevalence of VA in the general population. Development of the most appropriate diagnostic and therapeutic approach for athletes with VA that identifies all athletes with cardiomyopathies but avoids unnecessary tests for healthy athletes has been a matter of concern for some time.

In this chapter, we will address the prognostic role of VAs and their diagnostic and therapeutic approach in athletes. The most prevalent causes of SCD in athletes are extensively addressed elsewhere in this book.

General insights into ventricular arrhythmias

Ventricular arrhythmias are an extensive concept encompassing dramatically different clinical presentations and prognostic impacts, ranging from single isolated ventricular premature beats (VPBs) (➲ Fig. 5.2.1(a) to non-sustained (<30s) ventricular tachycardia (➲ Fig. 5.2.1(b)) to sustained ventricular tachycardia (➲ Fig, 5.2.1(c)).

The morphology of ventricular beats identifies their origin in the ventricle. As a rule of thumb, ventricular arrhythmias arising from the LV will show a right bundle branch block (RBBB) morphology (➲ Fig. 5.2.1(a)), while those originating in the RV will show a left bundle branch block (LBBB)

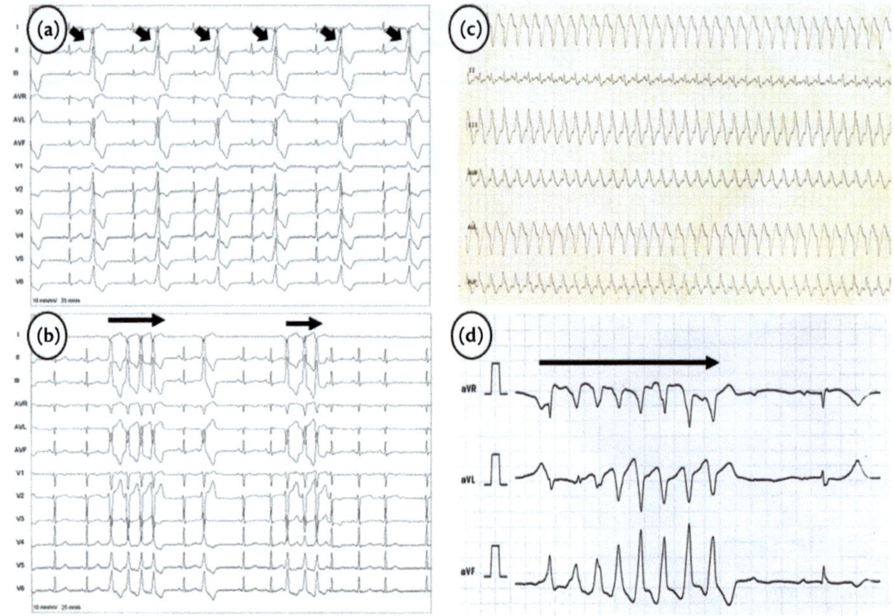

Fig. 5.2.1 ECG recordings of (a) a single isolated ventricular premature beat, (b) two short non-sustained monomorphic ventricular tachycardia events, (c) a sustained monomorphic ventricular tachycardia, and (d) a short polymorphic ventricular tachycardia.

morphology (➔ Fig. 5.2.1(b)). Ventricular arrhythmias originating in the LV outflow tract are a notable exception, as they frequently present with a LBBB-like morphology. Almost three-quarters of VPBs in apparently healthy athletes have a LBBB morphology [8–10], and in some studies the remainder have a fascicular origin [8] (see section on idiopathic ventricular arrhythmias).

Ventricular premature beats (VPBs) originating from a single focus show only one morphology (monomorphic); those with two or more morphologies are termed multifocal. Polymorphic ventricular tachycardia (VT) applies to those non-sustained or sustained events with beat-to-beat variations in ventricular beat morphologies (➔ Fig. 5.2.1(d)).

Prevalence of ventricular arrhythmias in the athlete

The prevalence of VAs largely depends on the duration of recording and individual factors such as age and comorbidities. Ventricular arrhythmias can be found in 1–6% of apparently healthy young and middle-aged individuals when screened with a 1–2-min 12-lead ECG recording [11,12], but in up to 70% when evaluated with a 24-hour Holter ECG. These arrhythmias are commonly monomorphic isolated ventricular premature beats (VPBs). It is unclear whether the VA burden in athletes is comparable to that in the general population. Some reports show that athletes are more frequently affected by ventricular arrhythmias [13], but most data suggest a similar prevalence of VA in athletes and non-athletes [14–16]. A small sample size in most studies and divergent methodologies limit our ability to draw accurate conclusions. Ventricular arrhythmia burden in athletes with frequent VAs tends to decrease over time after a deconditioning period [8,17]. This reduction appears to be more intense in those athletes with a more frequent VA at baseline [17,18]. Resumption of training is associated with a modest increase in VA burden [19]. Interestingly, it has been suggested that frequent VPBs tend to regress over time even in athletes who remain physically active [8,20]. Notably, the frequency of VA is not correlated with exercise-induced LV hypertrophy [21] or with cumulative lifetime hours of intense physical activity [22,23].

Diagnostic tests in athletes with ventricular arrhythmias

The identification of any VA in an athlete should always be carefully considered. Efforts should focus on SCD risk stratification, a process mainly determined by the identification of a possible cardiomyopathy. The minimum type of VA that merits further examination remains unknown. One or more PVBs in a standard 12-lead ECG predicted frequent VAs in a 24-hour Holter recording in elderly individuals in the general population [24]. The Seattle ECG criteria aim at providing a basis for a standardized unbiased approach to ECG interpretation in athletes. According to these criteria, two or more VPBs in a 10s recording justify further examination [6]. However, several factors will determine the depth of further examination based on a priori assessment of the risk of an underlying cardiomyopathy, as discussed in the section on clinical approach and management. In general, European scientific societies recommend that most athletes with VA should undergo 24-hour Holter monitoring, echocardiography, and an exercise test [25,26].

Resting 12-lead ECG should be carefully examined to identify any abnormalities while recognizing the physiological adaptation of athlete's heart [6]. Signs for the most common cardiomyopathies should be sought, including ischaemic heart disease, HCM, and ARVC, as well as primary arrhythmic syndromes such as Brugada syndrome and long or short QT syndrome (➲ Fig. 5.2.2). Prolonged ambulatory ECG recordings are strongly recommended in order to quantify VA burden and the presence of complex VAs. Twenty-four hour ECG Holter monitoring is usually sufficient for this purpose. However, a marked day-to-day variability in VA burden [27] is common, which should prompt considering regular follow-up of athletes with VA, particularly if there are clinic–ECG discrepancies.

Echocardiography is usually performed as a first-line technique to rule out structural heart disease, most commonly ischaemic cardiomyopathy, HCM, ARVC, or any valvular heart disease. The origin of both coronary arteries can be explored in a variable proportion of patients and an anomalous coronary origin confidently ruled out [28].

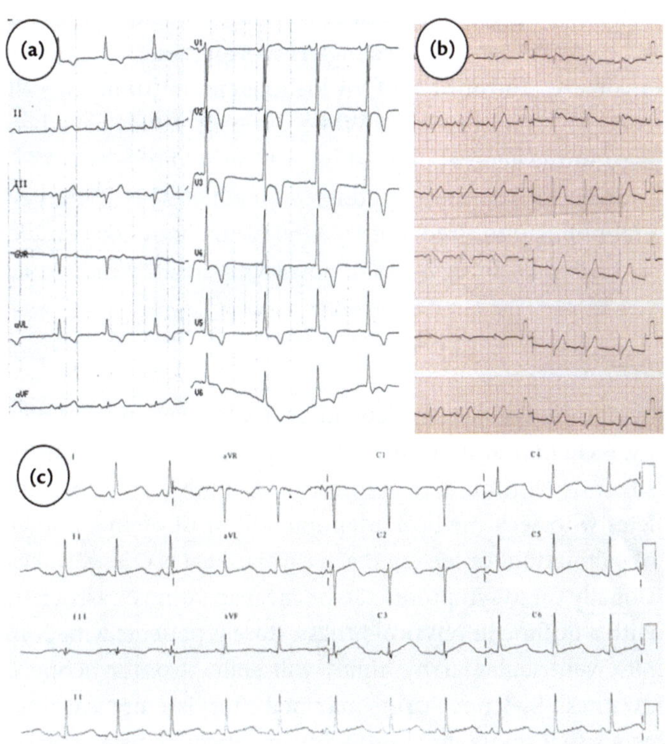

Fig. 5.2.2 Representative ECGs from patients with inherited cardiac conditions. (a) Hypertrophic cardiomyopathy. (b) Brugada syndrome and (c) long QT syndrome.

In certain cases with dubious results or very frequent or complex VAs, a deeper examination with cardiac magnetic resonance (CMR) provides a more accurate assessment of minor structural and functional abnormalities, and enables the evaluation of poor prognosis factors such as myocardial fibrosis [29].

Exercise testing assesses VA response to vigorous physical activity. In general, benign VAs tend to disappear during physical activity. Conversely, VPBs which increase in frequency or complexity during physical activity flag up those athletes with a greater likelihood of a cardiac condition. A thorough study is recommended in these individuals to rule out an underlying structural or molecular cardiac abnormality. Recent data have suggested that a stress echocardiogram test might be useful for identifying those athletes with an exercise-induced ARVC-like cardiomyopathy [30]. While healthy athletes will show improved RV function during effort [31], those with VA will fail to appropriately increase RV systolic function during exercise. Further studies are still required.

Clinical approach and management

The clinical, diagnostic, and therapeutic impact of VA in athletes is not homogenous. Depending on VA burden and morphology, athletes can be classified into one of the following diagnostic and prognostic categories that will be addressed in the following sections:

- athletes with infrequent VPBs
- athletes with frequent or complex VAs
- athletes with polymorphic VT.

A proposed schema for a diagnostic approach to athletes with ventricular arrhythmias is shown in ➲ Fig. 5.2.3.

Implications for and approach to athletes with infrequent ventricular premature beats

In general, those athletes with less than 2000 VPBs in 24 hours and no complex VAs (i.e. couplets or VT) are included in this group, which usually has a low SCD risk.

Symptoms

Infrequent VAs will remain clinically silent for long periods of time in most athletes. In this setting, ECG-based screening programmes might be able to identify these patients. Some patients might complain of palpitations, typically in quiet situations or when lying on the left side.

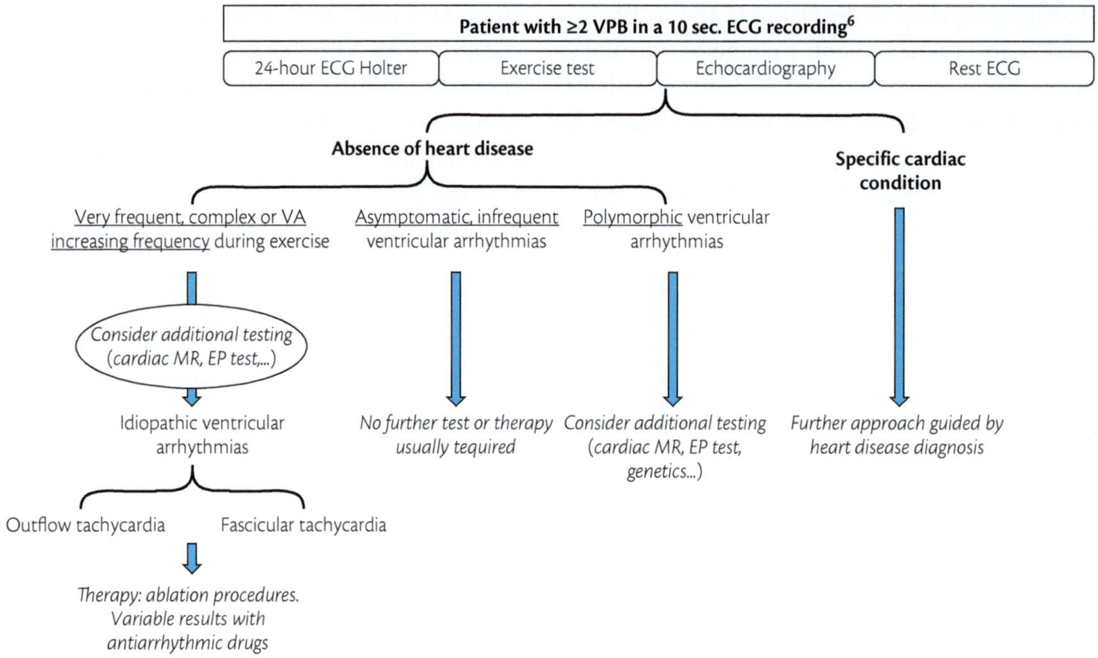

Fig. 5.2.3 Proposed diagnostic approach to patients with ventricular arrhythmias.

Prognosis

In the case of very infrequent ventricular arrhythmias (<100 VPBs in 24 hours) the risk of an underlying cardiomyopathy remains very low. In moderately frequent VPBs (100–2000 VPBs in 24 hours) a low, but significant, proportion of athletes will be diagnosed with a cardiac condition after a basic diagnostic work-up [9,10]. Multifocal VPBs have been associated with a worse outcome during follow-up than monomorphic VPBs, probably because of an increased prevalence of cardiomyopathies in these patients [32,33].

In the absence of an underlying cardiomyopathy, SCD risk is low and comparable with that of athletes without VA.

Management

In general, athletes without a heart disease who develop infrequent asymptomatic VPB should not receive antiarrhythmic therapy.

Eligibility for competitive sport

Athletes with infrequent VA are cleared for dynamic and/or intense competitive sport if VAs do not increase during exercise, the athlete remains asymptomatic, and a cardiomyopathy has been reasonably been ruled [25,26,34]. When a specific heart disease is diagnosed, it should guide further therapy and sport eligibility [25,34]. See also Chapter 7.1.

Implications for and approach to athletes with frequent or complex monomorphic ventricular arrhythmias

Patients with very frequent or complex (couplet, triplets, or VT) VAs are generally at a high risk of an underlying cardiomyopathy. The burden of VA included in the 'frequent VPB' concept is controversial. While different values have been used in the general population, a threshold of >2000 VPBs in 24 hours is commonly adopted for athletes [9]. In the general population, frequent (>30/60 VPBs/hour) or complex VAs are present in 2–9% of apparently healthy individuals [24,35].

Symptoms

Symptoms will largely depend on VA burden and complexity. As in non-athletic individuals, VAs may remain clinically silent or with mild symptoms in most athletes. Those athletes who seek medical attention will most often complain of palpitations or feeling that a cardiac beat is missing; occasionally these symptoms can be incapacitating or associated with a decline in physical fitness. Rarely, patients with complex ventricular arrhythmias will suffer from syncope or dizziness. Syncope during maximal effort is a medical emergency that should be thoroughly investigated, particularly if preceded by palpitations.

Approximately 15% of athletes [8] with persistent frequent VA will present progressive LV systolic dysfunction, known as VA-induced or VPB-induced cardiomyopathy. The total arrhythmic burden will determine the risk of VA-induced cardiomyopathy [36]; sustained or non-sustained VT should not be ignored. This emphasizes the need for regular ECG and echocardiographic follow-up in those athletes with frequent VA that persists over time [8].

The mechanisms of VA-induced cardiomyopathy remain largely unknown. A tachy/cardiomyopathy-like process has been suggested, but the 24-hour average heart rate is similar in affected and non-affected patients. Abnormal calcium handling has been suggested but has not been consistently demonstrated. Genetic factors are probably the most likely explanation for the large inter-individual variability in the development of VA cardiomyopathy.

A VA cardiomyopathy can develop in athletes even if the VA presents with a *benign* pattern, i.e. asymptomatic and disappearing during exercise [37]. In these individuals, abolishing VA usually improves and/or restores LV ejection fraction [37–40]. Elimination of VA and normalization of LV systolic function is better achieved with radiofrequency ablation procedures than with anti-arrhythmic drugs [41]. The VA burden threshold beyond which ablation might normalize cardiac function remains unclear. Initial investigations suggested that ablation should be performed in those individuals with >20% of premature ventricular contractions (PVCs) in 24-hour Holter ECG recordings [39], but recent data have shown that even those individuals with ≥13% of PVCs might improve their systolic function and haemodynamic status if ablated [38,42].

A critical issue in athletes presenting with a VA-induced cardiomyopathy is whether arrhythmias precede or are a consequence of LV dysfunction [37]. Mild degrees of LV dilation might be present in both circumstances. However, recent data show that most patients with a high burden of VA will clinically and haemodynamically benefit from VA ablation, regardless of whether structural heart disease is present [38]. This work supported radiofrequency ablation in all individuals with frequent ventricular arrhythmias (24-hour burden >13%) and LV systolic dysfunction, emphasizing the need for subsequent clinical and echocardiographic follow-up.

Prognosis

In general, the more frequent and complex VAs are, the higher the probability of being diagnosed with a cardiac condition. Up to 30% of athletes with very frequent VPBs (>2000/day) or non-sustained ventricular tachycardia have underlying potentially arrhythmogenic cardiomyopathies [9,10]. Sustained ventricular tachycardia is commonly associated with a structural heart disease. Frequent or complex ventricular arrhythmias that appear or increase during exercise should also raise suspicion of an underlying cardiac condition and prompt further and more detailed investigation [43]. A recent study used CMR in individuals with exercise-induced ventricular arrhythmias and an apparently normal heart to demonstrate a high burden of myocarditis sequelae [44].

In the absence of an underlying cardiomyopathy, SCD risk is low and comparable to that in athletes without VA. While some authors have reported a worse outcome for those apparently healthy individuals in the general population with frequent or complex VA [45], others have found a comparable prognosis in the two groups [35]. A high burden of undetected heart disease probably causes increased mortality in some cohorts [46] and emphasizes the need for comprehensive investigation in individuals with frequent or complex VA. In this regard, a well-characterized population of patients with frequent VPBs but no structural heart disease showed a low rate of serious cardiovascular complications [36]. In athletes, frequent VAs in the absence of a cardiomyopathy commonly regress after a variable deconditioning period (three to six months) and do not entail an adverse prognosis [17,47], even if sport is continued [8]. Nevertheless, regular follow-up is warranted in these athletes because of the risk of developing a VA-induced cardiomyopathy [8,37] or VA being an early manifestation of cardiomyopathies such as HCM or ARVC.

Concerns have been raised about VAs appearing or increasing their frequency during exercise in apparently healthy individuals. This is particularly noteworthy in athletes, in whom SCD is often triggered by bouts of physical activity. In the general population, frequent VPBs or non-sustained ventricular tachycardias occur in 1–4% of middle-aged individuals without apparent heart disease undergoing an exercise test [48–51]. The prognostic significance of exercise-induced VA in patients without detectable heart disease is controversial; data showing increased SCD risk [51,52] have not been consistently reproduced [48,50]. Once more, a high proportion of undetected cardiomyopathy has been claimed in those individuals with exercise-induced VA. Similar work in athletes in whom structural heart disease had been confidently excluded show that VA substantially increasing in frequency and/or complexity (>10 VPB, ventricular couplets or longer VA) during an exercise test are uncommon (<1%) but apparently benign [43,53]. Further studies involving larger cohorts are needed.

Management

Triggers for VA should be avoided; the role of caffeine avoidance remains controversial [54,55]. Beta-blockers or non-dihydropridinic calcium antagonists might be beneficial in some cases of symptomatic VPBs in otherwise healthy individuals. Class I antiarrhythmic drugs are a possible alternative in individuals with outflow tract ventricular tachycardia (OT-VT). Competitive athletes should be informed about the potential deleterious effects of beta-blockers on physical performance [56]. In addition, an updated version of the World Anti-Doping Agency (WADA) list of prohibited drugs should always be obtained and discussed.

Unfortunately, improvement after anti-arrhythmic drugs is limited. Ablation procedures are recommended in those athletes not willing to take chronic drug therapy or with incomplete symptom relief, and should be considered in those symptomatic individuals with very frequent monomorphic VA.

Eligibility for competitive sport

Complex VAs are cleared for competitive sport in the case of short idiopathic VA runs, if they do not increase during exercise, if they remain asymptomatic, and if a cardiomyopathy has reasonably been ruled out [25,26]. When a specific heart disease is diagnosed, it should guide further therapy and sport eligibility [25,34]. See also Chapter 7.1

Specific forms of interest in athletes with complex ventricular arrhythmias

Idiopathic ventricular arrhythmias

A large number of VAs in patients without a cardiomyopathy (idiopathic ventricular tachycardia) originate in the outflow tract of either ventricle (outflow tract-ventricular tachycardia (OT-VT)) or in the interventricular septum (fascicular ventricular tachycardia). Although their basic electrophysiological mechanisms are different, the two entities show common characteristics such as a benign prognosis, good response to verapamil, and a generally excellent outcome after radiofrequency ablation.

Right/left ventricular outflow-ventricular tachycardia

Ventricular tachycardia originating from either the right or the left ventricle outflow tract are the most common idiopathic VTs. Although exercise is the normal trigger for prolonged VT runs, other patients will experience a reduction or abolition during effort [57]. Outflow tract tachycardia characteristically present either as monomorphic (i.e. a single morphology) frequent isolated PVBs, non-sustained VT, or sustained VT. Acute termination by adenosine or verapamil is specific for OT-VT.

Both right and left ventricular OT-VT (RVOT-VT/LVOT-VT) typically present with a LBBB morphology and an inferior axis (predominant R wave in DII, DIII. and aVF leads). An early precordial transition during a VT episode (R larger than S in the V2 lead, i.e. R/S >1 in V2) suggests an LVOT origin (➲ Fig. 5.2.4(a)), while a late transition (R/S >1 in V4 or later) suggests an RVOT origin (➲ Fig. 5.2.4(b)). A variety of clinical parameters [58] and ECG parameters [59] have been proposed to aid in the non-invasive evaluation of its origin, particularly for patients with a transition (R/S>1) in V3 (Fig. 5.2.4 (c,d)). RVOT-VT and LVOT-VT share common electrophysiological mechanisms and properties [60]. However, in contrast with RVOT-VT, an LVOT origin is usually associated with elderly male patients with hypertension [58,60].

A common and clinically relevant concern is the differentiation between idiopathic RVOT, latent ARVC, and exercise-induced ARVC-like cardiomyopathy. Although all these conditions might present with similar ventricular tachycardia in the absence of overt right ventricle structural or functional abnormalities, long-term outcomes are dramatically distinguishable. Accordingly, the differentiation between idiopathic RVOT forms and early ARVC forms has attracted considerable attention [61–64]. Several strategies have been proposed to distinguish RVOT and latent ARVC. Right ventricle OT-VT generally presents with a single VT morphology, while two or more VT morphologies predict ARVC [65,66]. Ainsworth et al. [63] proposed an algorithm including QRS duration and axis to differentiate the two entities [63]. T-wave inversion in precordial leads has a high specificity for ARVC when used to discriminate patients with RVOT-VT [64,67], even in athletes [68]. Other ECG parameters such as S-wave upstroke duration in V1 might also aid in this purpose [64]. Although CMR might show minor structural abnormalities in patients with RVOT-VT [66], mild RV systolic dysfunction has recently been reported to be specific of early stages of ARVC [62]. In cases with uncertain diagnosis, an electrophysiological study might help: RF ablation effectively abolishes VAs in RVOT patients, whereas arrhythmia recurrences are common in ARVC patients. Even if the diagnosis of RVOT-VT seems certain, regular follow-up with a particular attention to the RV is recommended.

Prognosis for patients with RVOT-VT or LVOT-VT is generally excellent, with a low SCD risk. The acute success rate for RVOT-VT ablation is commonly >75% and the recurrence rate is 5–10%, with a low acute complication rate [69]. Conversely, beta-blockers, non-dihidropiridinic calcium antagonists and class I anti-arrhythmic drugs have a low success rate (≤50%).

Fascicular tachycardia

Fascicular tachycardias (FT-VT) are idiopathic VTs originating in the interventricular septum in which either the posterior (posterior fascicular tachycardia), in ~90% of cases, or the anterior (anterior fascicular tachycardia) fascicle of the conduction system participates in a re-entry

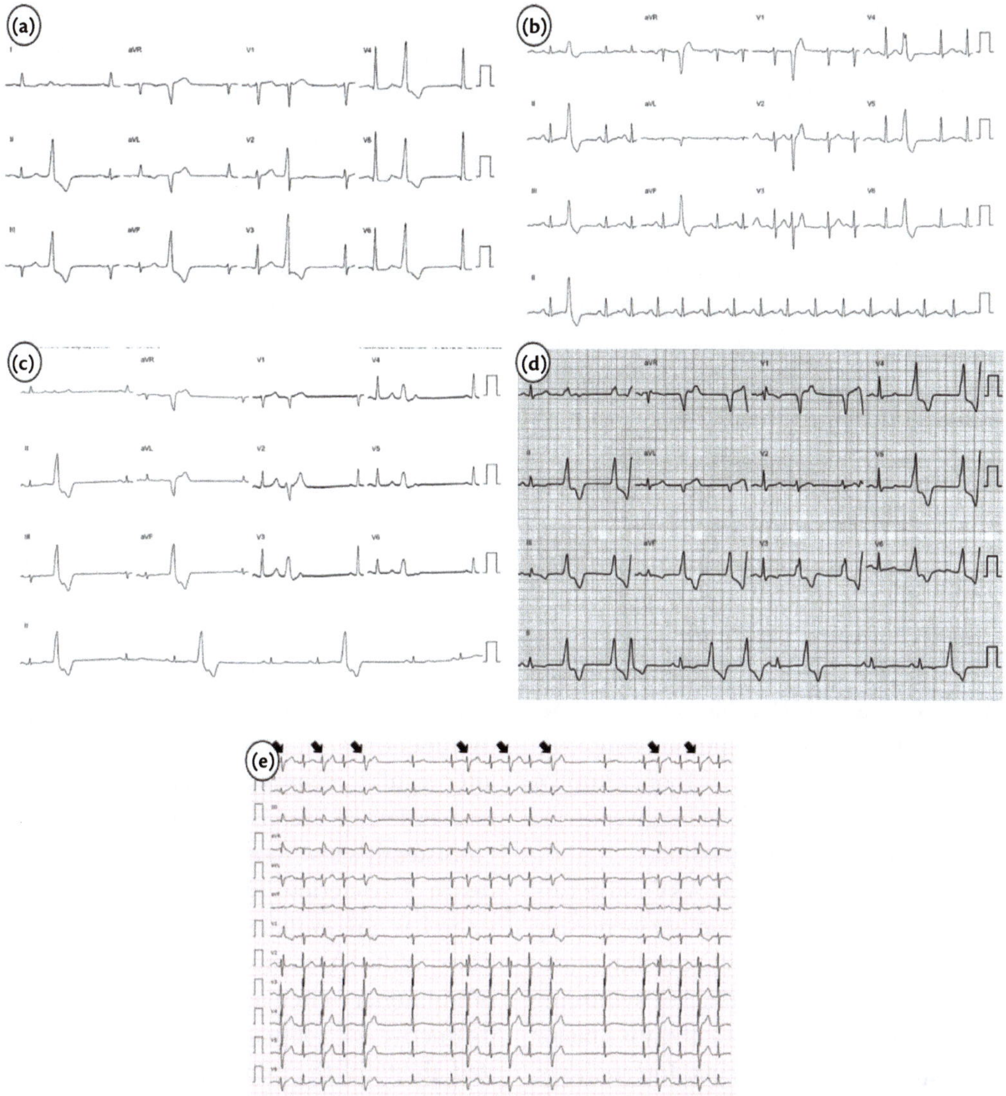

Fig. 5.2.4 Representative ECG showing characteristic idiopathic ventricular arrhythmias.

circuit. Taken together, the two FT-VT forms account for ~10% of idiopathic VT. Young and middle-aged men are characteristically affected. Although most FT-VT occurs at rest, physical activity can trigger some episodes.

Fascicular ventricular tachycardia features some characteristic ECG findings. Because FT-VT originates in the LV, FT-VT usually presents with an RBBB morphology with a left axis (posterior FT-VT) or right axis (anterior FT-VT) deviation. The QRS complex during VT is relatively narrow (usually <140ms) because of its proximity to the specific conduction system, allowing simultaneous RV and LV activation. Fast initial activation of the QRS is typical, with the interval between the beginning of the R wave and the nadir of the S wave uniformly being <80ms (➔ Fig. 5.2.4(e)). Verapamil characteristically terminates FT-VT. Taking all these characteristics together, it is not surprising that FT-VT is often misdiagnosed as a supraventricular tachycardia.

Anti-arrhythmic therapy usually involves calcium antagonists such as verapamil, although class I anti-arrhythmic drugs or beta-blockers are useful in a minority of cases. Radiofrequency ablation procedures are usually safe and effective in >85% of cases.

Ventricular arrhythmias in the presence of a cardiomyopathy

If frequent or complex VAs occur at rest [70,71] or during exercise [72,73] in patients with an underlying structural heart disease, they are at high risk of cardiovascular complications. The type of cardiomyopathy determines prognosis and eligibility for competitive sport.

Exercise as a cause of VA

Heidbüchel et al. [74] first identified a small subset of highly trained endurance athletes in whom VAs originate in a mildly dysfunctional RV and are associated with a poor prognosis involving an increased risk of haemodynamically unstable VT and SCD. Frequently, these athletes satisfy ARVC Task Force diagnostic criteria (~50–60% in selected populations [30,75,76]) and are diagnosed with ARVC ([77]. This was termed *exercise-induced ARVC-like cardiomyopathy*, since desmosomal mutations were only present in ≤13% of these athletes. Although some clinical and mechanistic data suggest that the *classic* and *gene-elusive ARVC* forms represent two extreme forms of the ARVC genetic, histological, and clinical continuum, this hypothesis has not yet been widely accepted and it is still not known whether the same diagnostic and therapeutic approach should be used in both cases.

Evidence for the exercise–ARVC spectrum

The contribution of physical activity to the creation or promotion of an arrhythmogenic ventricular substrate has been a matter of debate in recent years. The syndromic combination of VA, RV dysfunction, and an intense endurance training history has been named 'Heidbüchel syndrome'. Specifically, exercise might be the most important aetiological factor for unmasking ARVC in patients without a known predisposition or positive family history, or it might contribute to genetically determined ARVC progression.

The evidence for a pure exercise-induced ARVC-like cardiomyopathy is limited but has been continuously increasing in recent years [76]. A low burden of ARVC-causing mutations in a group of patients with Heidbüchel syndrome supports the proposal that intense physical activity is a major factor in ARVC pathology in some patients. Interestingly, mutations were absent in the best-trained individuals [75]. Consistent with this hypothesis, Sawant at al. [78] recently demonstrated a prominent history of endurance training in a cohort of patients with gene-elusive ARVC.

These results suggest a strong link between the genetic background and environmental factors in ARVC pathology. Experimental models provide an excellent opportunity for testing the complex genetic–environmental interactions in a controlled setting. Data from Benito et al. [79] supported a role for exercise as the single aetiological factor for an ARVC-like phenotype. A group of non-selected Wistar rats, without any genetic predisposition, underwent training on a treadmill for four months at very high-intensity. After the exercise period, researchers found that VA could be induced more readily in trained than in sedentary rats, and was accompanied by selective RV fibrosis and dysfunction.

Epidemiology

Exercise-induced ARVC-like cardiomyopathy is usually diagnosed in men in the fourth decade of life after a long history of high-intensity training, most commonly in endurance sports such as cycling, marathons, or triathlons [74,76,78]. The reasons for male predominance remain unexplored, but genetic factors and the low historical participation of women in highly demanding endurance sports have been proposed [80]. Several factors impede an accurate estimation of its prevalence, including the lack of well-defined diagnostic criteria, an extensive overlap with the classic form of ARVC, and subclinical effects [30]. Nevertheless, the small number of cases reported in the literature, mostly coming from a single centre, and the very low representation in SCD series suggest that exercise-induced ARVC-like cardiomyopathy is an uncommon disease with a relatively low impact on elite athletes.

Predominant role of RV in exercise-induced ARVC-like cardiomyopathy

The origin of VA in the RV of patients with potentially lethal VA was suspected on the basis of its LBBB morphology and a common association with a mild to moderate RV systolic dysfunction [74]. This results from selective RV damage after regular intense training. For a long time LV adaptation to a variety of exercise intensities was thoroughly studied, consistently showing a 'physiological' behaviour with no evidence of deleterious LV remodelling. However, the research focus has now switched from the LV to the atria and the RV. The specific RV shape, the thin wall, and the specific nature of pulmonary circulation physiology motivate a markedly distinctive RV adaptation to regular exercise [81]. The limited ability of the pulmonary circulation to accommodate large increases in stroke volume justifies an almost linear correlation between cardiac output and pulmonary pressure [30,82], a marked increase in RV pressure and wall stress [82], and an intensity-dependent impairment in RV systolic function after strenuous physical efforts [81,83,84].

It has been hypothesized that repetitive insults lead to selective RV ultrastructural damage which could result in an arrhythmogenic RV substrate [83], as shown in experimental models [79]. However, this has not yet been confirmed in humans. Increased fibrosis was found in an endocardial biopsy in five of ten athletes who suffered from right ventricle arrhythmias; inflammatory infiltrates were found in the remaining five patients [74].

Diagnosis

As exercise-induced ARVC-like cardiomyopathy is a relatively new entity, well-defined diagnostic criteria have not yet been established, although some patients will satisfy the ARCV Task Force criteria [77]. The evaluation of high intensity athletes with frequent or complex ventricular arrhythmias (particularly if asymptomatic), no overt structural heart disease, and no definite or probable ARVC diagnosis remains challenging. In this setting, RV systolic function assessment is critical, but requires complex echocardiography techniques. The RV systolic function remains near normal at rest in some patients with exercise-induced forms of ARVC [30], so mild degrees of dysfunction might easily be overlooked and considered part of the physiological athlete's heart. Recent work has suggested that the RV of athletes with exercise-induced ARVC-like cardiomyopathy will fail to improve the systolic function at mild to moderate exercise intensities [30], in contrast with healthy sedentary individuals or non-affected athletes [31]. However, its diagnostic accuracy needs to be tested prospectively and its role in daily clinical practice still needs to be established.

Therapeutic approach:

The therapeutic approach to patients with 'Heidbüchel syndrome' without a definitive ARVC diagnosis remains largely unknown. A therapeutic approach comparable to that of ARVC, including exercise cessation, is suggested for patients with a high degree of suspicion of exercise-induced ARVC or who are considered to be at high risk (i.e. presenting with syncope or other symptoms, with frequent or complex VAs, lack of RV increase in systolic function during exercise). Reduction of physical activity is associated with a lower incidence of VAs during follow-up [85], and results in an animal model suggest RV fibrosis regression with deconditioning [79].

Implications for and approach to athletes with polymorphic ventricular tachycardia

Polymorphic VT is frequently associated with an underlying cardiomyopathy, particularly if it is prolonged or occurs during physical activity. Structural heart disease underlies polymorphic VT in some patients. Transient acute ischaemic events should be explored. Primary arrhythmic syndromes, such as Brugada syndrome and long or short QT syndrome, should be thoroughly explored in rest ECG and/or provocation tests [86,87]. If there is a normal ECG and no structural heart disease is detected, catecholaminergic polymorphic ventricular tachycardia (CPVT) should be considered if polymorphic VT is observed during exercise. Bidirectional ventricular tachycardia is characteristic of CPVT [88]. Transitory causes of polymorphic VT merit special attention. Myocarditis and electrolytic disorders (e.g. those occurring after prolonged bouts of exercise) can potentially trigger severe polymorphic VA while active or ongoing, but might completely resolve after variable periods of time.

Symptoms

If prolonged, polymorphic VT usually entails haemodynamic instability and is associated with severe symptoms such as syncope or SCD.

Prognosis

Prognosis is determined by the underlying cardiomyopathy. A high risk of SCD is common in these patients.

Management

Athletes with polymorphic VT should be managed according to the specific approach of the specific cardiac condition.

Eligibility for competitive sport

Athletes diagnosed with most conditions associated with polymorphic VT (i.e. long QT syndrome, Brugada syndrome, CPVT, active myocarditis, high risk ischaemic heart disease) should refrain from dynamic competitive sport [25,26]. However, recent AHA/ACC guidelines are more permissive and consider allowing participation in competitive sports for some primary arrhythmic syndromes under certain circumstances, including some phenotype-negative channelopathies that have been diagnosed using a genetic test.

Competitive sports may also be considered (class IIb recommendation, level of evidence C) in previously symptomatic Brugada syndrome, early repolarization syndrome, or short or long QT syndrome, provided that precautionary measures have been adopted (such as AED available on site) and patients have been asymptomatic and receiving appropriate therapy for at least three months [32,89]. Competitive sports may be allowed after the resolution of a transitory aetiology of polymorphic VT, provided that VAs have regressed and are not provoked in an exercise test and any structural or functional abnormalities have normalized.

Further reading

Benito B, Gay-Jordi G, Serrano-Mollar A, et al. Cardiac arrhythmogenic remodeling in a rat model of long-term intensive exercise training. *Circulation* 2011; 123: 13–22.

Biffi A, Pelliccia A, Verdile L, et al. Long-term clinical significance of frequent and complex ventricular tachyarrhythmias in trained athletes. *J Am Coll Cardiol* 2002; 40: 446–52.

Guasch E, Mont L. Diagnosis, pathophysiology and management of exercise-induced arrhythmias. *Nat Rev Cardiol* 2016; 14: 88–101.

Heidbüchel H, Hoogsteen J, Fagard R, et al. High prevalence of right ventricular involvement in endurance athletes with ventricular arrhythmias: role of an electrophysiologic study in risk stratification. *Eur Heart J* 2003; 24: 1473–80.

La Gerche A, Burns AT, Mooney DJ, et al. Exercise-induced right ventricular dysfunction and structural remodelling in endurance athletes. *Eur Heart J* 2012; 33: 998–1006.

La Gerche A, Claessen G, Dymarkowski S, et al. Exercise-induced right ventricular dysfunction is associated with ventricular arrhythmias in endurance athletes. *Eur Heart J* 2015; 36: 1998–2010.

Sanz-de la Garza M, Rubies C, Batlle M, et al. Severity of structural and functional right ventricular remodeling depends on training load in an experimental model of endurance exercise. *Am J Physiol Heart Circ Physiol* 2017; 313: H459–68.

Guidelines and consensus statements

Mont L, Pelliccia A, Sharma S, et al. Pre-participation cardiovascular evaluation for athletic participants to prevent sudden death. *Europace* 2017; 19: 139–63.

Sharma S, Drezner JA, Baggish A, et al. International recommendations for electrocardiographic interpretation in athletes. *Eur Heart J* 2018; 39: 1466–80.

Zipes DP, Link MS, Ackerman MJ, et al. Eligibility and disqualification recommendations for competitive athletes with cardiovascular abnormalities: Task Force 9: Arrhythmias and Conduction Defects. *J Am Coll Cardiol* 2015; 66: 2412–23.

References

1. Corrado D, Basso C, Pavei A, et al. Trends in sudden cardiovascular death in young competitive athletes after implementation of a preparticipation screening program. *JAMA* 2006; 296: 1593–1601.
2. Corrado D, Basso C, Rizzoli G, et al. Does sports activity enhance the risk of sudden death in adolescents and young adults? *J Am Coll Cardiol* 2003; 42: 1959–63.
3. Harmon KG, Drezner JA, Wilson MG, Sharma S. Incidence of sudden cardiac death in athletes: a state-of-the-art review. *Heart* 2014; 100: 1227–34.
4. Steinvil A, Chundadze T, Zeltser D, et al. Mandatory electrocardiographic screening of athletes to reduce their risk for sudden death proven fact or wishful thinking? *J Am Coll Cardiol* 2011; 57: 1291–6.
5. Harmon KG, Zigman M, Drezner JA. The effectiveness of screening history, physical exam, and ECG to detect potentially lethal cardiac disorders in athletes: a systematic review/meta-analysis. *J Electrocardiol* 48: 329–38.
6. Drezner JA, Ackerman MJ, Anderson J, et al. Electrocardiographic interpretation in athletes: the 'Seattle criteria'. *Br J Sports Med* 2013; 47: 122–4.
7. Moss AJ, Davis HT, DeCamilla J, Bayer LW. Ventricular ectopic beats and their relation to sudden and nonsudden cardiac death after myocardial infarction. *Circulation* 1979; 60: 998–1003.
8. Delise P, Sitta N, Lanari E, et al. Long-term effect of continuing sports activity in competitive athletes with frequent ventricular premature complexes and apparently normal heart. *Am J Cardiol* 2013; 112: 1396–1402.
9. Biffi A, Pelliccia A, Verdile L, et al. Long-term clinical significance of frequent and complex ventricular tachyarrhythmias in trained athletes. *J Am Coll Cardiol* 2002; 40: 446–52.
10. Steriotis AK, Nava A, Rigato I, et al. Noninvasive cardiac screening in young athletes with ventricular arrhythmias. *Am J Cardiol* 2013; 111: 557–62.
11. Vitelli LL, Crow RS, Shahar E, et al. Electrocardiographic findings in a healthy biracial population. Atherosclerosis Risk in Communities (ARIC) Study Investigators. *Am J Cardiol* 1998; 81: 453–9.
12. Hiss RG, Lamb LE. Electrocardiographic findings in 122,043 individuals. *Circulation* 1962; 25: 947–61.
13. Palatini P, Maraglino G, Sperti G, et al. Prevalence and possible mechanisms of ventricular arrhythmias in athletes. *Am Heart J* 1985; 110: 560–7.
14. Bjørnstad H, Storstein L, Meen HD, Hals O. Ambulatory electrocardiographic findings in top athletes, athletic students and control subjects. *Cardiology* 1994; 84: 42–50.
15. Pigozzi F, Alabiso A, Parisi A, et al. Vigorous exercise training is not associated with prevalence of ventricular arrhythmias in elderly athletes. *J Sports Med Phys Fitness* 2004; 44: 92–7.
16. Talan DA, Bauernfeind RA, Ashley WW, et al. Twenty-four hour continuous ECG recordings in long-distance runners. *Chest* 1982; 82: 19–24.
17. Biffi A, Maron BJ, Verdile L, et al. Impact of physical deconditioning on ventricular tachyarrhythmias in trained athletes. *J Am Coll Cardiol* 2004; 44: 1053–8.
18. Delise P, Lanari E, Sitta N, et al. Influence of training on the number and complexity of frequent VPBs in healthy athletes. *J Cardiovasc Med (Hagerstown)* 2011; 12: 157–61.
19. Biffi A, Maron BJ, Culasso F, et al. Patterns of ventricular tachyarrhythmias associated with training, deconditioning and retraining in elite athletes without cardiovascular abnormalities. *Am J Cardiol* 2011; 107: 697–703.
20. Caselli L, Pieragnoli P, Ricciardi G, et al. Which factors predict the behavior of ventricular extrasystoles in athletes over time? *Scand J Med Sci Sports* 2014; 24: 395–9.
21. Biffi A, Maron BJ, Di Giacinto B, et al. Relation between training-induced left ventricular hypertrophy and risk for ventricular tachyarrhythmias in elite athletes. *Am J Cardiol* 2008; 101: 1792–5.
22. Rimensberger C, Carlen F, Brugger N, et al. Right ventricular adaptations and arrhythmias in amateur ultra-endurance athletes. *Br J Sports Med* 2014; 48: 1179–84.
23. Wilhelm M, Roten L, Tanner H, et al. Long-term cardiac remodeling and arrhythmias in nonelite marathon runners. *Am J Cardiol* 2012; 110: 129–35.
24. Sajadieh A, Nielsen OW, Rasmussen V, et al. Ventricular arrhythmias and risk of death and acute myocardial infarction in apparently healthy subjects of age >or=55 years. *Am J Cardiol* 2006; 97: 1351–7.
25. Pelliccia A, Fagard R, Bjørnstad HH, et al. Recommendations for competitive sports participation in athletes with cardiovascular disease. *Eur Heart J* 2005; 26: 1422–45.
26. Heidbüchel H, Corrado D, Biffi A, et al. Recommendations for participation in leisure-time physical activity and competitive sports of patients with arrhythmias and potentially arrhythmogenic conditions. Part II: Ventricular arrhythmias, channelopathies and implantable defibrillators. *Eur J Cardiovasc Prev Rehabil* 2006; 13: 676–86.
27. Michelson EL, Morganroth J. Spontaneous variability of complex ventricular arrhythmias detected by long-term electrocardiographic recording. *Circulation* 1980; 61: 690–5.
28. Wyman RA, Chiu RY, Rahko PS. The 5-minute screening echocardiogram for athletes. *J Am Soc Echocardiogr* 2008; 21: 786–8.

29. Schnell F, Claessen G, La Gerche A, et al. Subepicardial delayed gadolinium enhancement in asymptomatic athletes: let sleeping dogs lie? *BrJ Sports Med* 2016; 50: 111–17.
30. La Gerche A, Claessen G, Dymarkowski S, et al. Exercise-induced right ventricular dysfunction is associated with ventricular arrhythmias in endurance athletes. *Eur Heart J* 2015; 36: 1998–2010.
31. King G, Almuntaser I, Murphy RT, et al. Reduced right ventricular myocardial strain in the elite athlete may not be a consequence of myocardial damage. 'Cream masquerades as skimmed milk'. *Echocardiography* 2013; 30; 929–35.
32. Zipes DP, Link MS, Ackerman MJ, et al. Eligibility and disqualification recommendations for competitive athletes with cardiovascular abnormalities. Task Force 9: Arrhythmias and Conduction Defects. *J Am Coll Cardiol* 2015; 66: 2412–23.
33. Ephrem G, Levine M, Friedmann P, Schweitzer P. The prognostic significance of frequency and morphology of premature ventricular complexes during ambulatory Holter monitoring. *Ann Noninvasive Electrocardiol* 2013; 18: 118–25.
34. Maron BJ, Zipes DP, Kovacs RJ. Eligibility and disqualification recommendations for competitive athletes with cardiovascular abnormalities: preamble, principles, and general considerations. *J Am Coll Cardiol* 2015; 66: 2343–9.
35. Kennedy HL, Whitlock JA, Sprague MK, et al. Long-term follow-up of asymptomatic healthy subjects with frequent and complex ventricular ectopy. *N Engl J Med* 1985; 312: 193–7.
36. Niwano S, Wakisaka Y, Niwano H, et al. Prognostic significance of frequent premature ventricular contractions originating from the ventricular outflow tract in patients with normal left ventricular function. *Heart* 2009; 95: 1230–7.
37. Grazioli G, Fernández-Armenta J, Prat S, et al. Ablation of frequent premature ventricular complex in an athlete. *Scand J Med Sci Sports* 2015; 25: 876–9.
38. Penela D, Van Huls Van Taxis C, Aguinaga L, et al. Neurohormonal, structural, and functional recovery pattern after premature ventricular complex ablation is independent of structural heart disease status in patients with depressed left ventricular ejection fraction: a prospective multicenter study. *J Am Coll Cardiol* 2013; 62: 1195–1202.
39. Takemoto M, Yoshimura H, Ohba Y, et al. Radiofrequency catheter ablation of premature ventricular complexes from right ventricular outflow tract improves left ventricular dilation and clinical status in patients without structural heart disease. *J Am Coll Cardiol* 2005; 45: 1259–65.
40. Lubitz SA, Ozcan C, Magnani JW, et al. Genetics of atrial fibrillation: implications for future research directions and personalized medicine. *Circ Arrhythm Electrophysiol* 2010; 3: 291–9.
41. Bogun F, Crawford T, Reich S, et al. Radiofrequency ablation of frequent, idiopathic premature ventricular complexes: comparison with a control group without intervention. *Heart Ryythm* 2007; 4: 863–7.
42. Penela D, Acosta J, Aguinaga L, et al. Ablation of frequent PVC in patients meeting criteria for primary prevention ICD implant: safety of withholding the implant. *Heart Rhythm* 2015; 12: 2434–42.
43. Verdile L, Maron BJ, Pelliccia A, et al. Clinical significance of exercise-induced ventricular tachyarrhythmias in trained athletes without cardiovascular abnormalities. *Heart Rhythm* 2015; 12: 78–85.
44. Jeserich M, Merkely B, Olschewski M, et al. Patients with exercise-associated ventricular ectopy present evidence of myocarditis. *J Cardiovasc Magn Reson* 2015; 17: 100.
45. Bikkina M, Larson MG, Levy D. Prognostic implications of asymptomatic ventricular arrhythmias: the Framingham Heart Study. *Ann Intern Med* 1992; 117: 990–6.
46. Lee V, Hemingway H, Harb R, et al. The prognostic significance of premature ventricular complexes in adults without clinically apparent heart disease: a meta-analysis and systematic review. *Heart* 2012; 98: 1290–8.
47. Pelliccia A, Maron BJ, Di Paolo FM, et al. Prevalence and clinical significance of left atrial remodeling in competitive athletes. *J Am Coll Cardiol* 2005; 46: 690–6.
48. Marine JE, Shetty V, Chow G.V., et al. Prevalence and prognostic significance of exercise-induced nonsustained ventricular tachycardia in asymptomatic volunteers: BLSA (Baltimore Longitudinal Study of Aging). *J Am Coll Cardiol* 2013; 62: 595–600.
49. Yang JC, Wesley RC, Froelicher VF. Ventricular tachycardia during routine treadmill testing: risk and prognosis. *Arch Int Med* 1991; 151: 349–53.
50. Fleg JL, Lakatta EG. Prevalence and prognosis of exercise-induced nonsustained ventricular tachycardia in apparently healthy volunteers. *Am J Cardiol* 1984; 54: 762–4.
51. Jouven X, Zureik M, Desnos M, et al. Long-term outcome in asymptomatic men with exercise-induced premature ventricular depolarizations. *N Engl J Med* 2000; 343: 826–33.
52. Morshedi-Meibodi A, Evans JC, Levy D, et al. Clinical correlates and prognostic significance of exercise-induced ventricular premature beats in the community: the Framingham Heart Study. *Circulation* 2004; 109: 2417–22.
53. Fuchs T, Torjman A, Galitzkaya L, et al. The clinical significance of ventricular arrhythmias during an exercise test in non-competitive and competitive athletes. *Isr Med Assoc J* 2011; 13: 735–9.
54. Dixit S, Stein PK, Dewland TA, et al. Consumption of caffeinated products and cardiac ectopy. *J Am Heart Assoc* 2016; 5: e002503.
55. Newby DE, Neilson JM, Jarvie DR, Boon NA. Caffeine restriction has no role in the management of patients with symptomatic idiopathic ventricular premature beats. *Heart* 1996; 76: 355–7.
56. Atwood JE, Sullivan M, Forbes S, et al. Effect of beta-adrenergic blockade on exercise performance in patients with chronic atrial fibrillation. *J Am Coll Cardiol* 1987; 10: 314–20.
57. Mont L, Seixas T, Brugada P, et al. Clinical and electrophysiologic characteristics of exercise-related idiopathic ventricular tachycardia. *Am J Cardiol* 1991; 68: 897–900.
58. Penela D, De Riva M, Herczku C, et al. An easy-to-use, operator-independent, clinical model to predict the left vs right ventricular outflow tract origin of ventricular arrhythmias. *Europace* 2015; 17: 1122–8.
59. Betensky BP, Park RE, Marchlinski FE, et al. The V(2) transition ratio: a new electrocardiographic criterion for distinguishing left from right ventricular outflow tract tachycardia origin. *J Am Coll Cardiol* 2011; 57: 2255–62.
60. Iwai S, Cantillon DJ, Kim RJ, et al. Right and left ventricular outflow tract tachycardias: Evidence for a common electrophysiologic mechanism. *J Cardiovasc Electrophysiol* 2006; 17: 1052–8.

61. Finlay MC, Ahmed AK, Sugrue A, et al. Dynamic conduction and repolarisation changes in early arrhythmogenic right ventricular cardiomyopathy versus benign outflow tract ectopy demonstrated by high density mapping & paced surface ECG analysis. *PloS One* 2014; 9: 1–15.
62. Saberniak J, Leren IS, Haland TF, et al. Comparison of patients with early-phase arrhythmogenic right ventricular cardiomyopathy and right ventricular outflow tract ventricular tachycardia. *Eur Heart J Cardiovasc Imaging* 2017; 18: 62–9.
63. Ainsworth CD, Skanes AC, Klein GJ, et al. Differentiating arrhythmogenic right ventricular cardiomyopathy from right ventricular outflow tract ventricular tachycardia using multilead QRS duration and axis. *Heart Rhythm* 2006; 3: 416–23.
64. Nasir K, Bomma C, Tandri H, et al. Electrocardiographic features of arrhythmogenic right ventricular dysplasia/cardiomyopathy according to disease severity: a need to broaden diagnostic criteria. *Circulation* 2004; 110: 1527–34.
65. Niroomand F, Carbucicchio C, Tondo C, et al. Electrophysiological characteristics and outcome in patients with idiopathic right ventricular arrhythmia compared with arrhythmogenic right ventricular dysplasia. *Heart* 2002; 87: 41–7.
66. O'Donnell D, Cox D, Bourke J, et al. Clinical and electrophysiological differences between patients with arrhythmogenic right ventricular dysplasia and right ventricular outflow tract tachycardia. *Eur Heart J* 2003; 24: 801–10.
67. Morin DP, Mauer AC, Gear K, et al. Usefulness of precordial T-wave inversion to distinguish arrhythmogenic right ventricular cardiomyopathy from idiopathic ventricular tachycardia arising from the right ventricular outflow tract. *Am J Cardiol* 2010; 105: 1821–4.
68. Schnell F, Riding N, O'Hanlon R, et al. Recognition and significance of pathological T-wave inversions in athletes. *Circulation* 2015; 131: 165–73.
69. Calvo N, Jongbloed M, Zeppenfeld K. Radiofrequency catheter ablation of idiopathic right ventricular outflow tract arrhythmias. *Indian Pacing Electrophysiol* 2013; 13: 14–33.
70. Monserrat L, Elliott PM, Gimeno JR, et al. Non-sustained ventricular tachycardia in hypertrophic cardiomyopathy: an independent marker of sudden death risk in young patients. *J Am Coll Cardiol* 2003; 42: 873–9.
71. Doval HC, Nul DR, Grancelli HO, et al. Nonsustained ventricular tachycardia in severe heart failure. Independent marker of increased mortality due to sudden death. *Circulation* 1996; 94: 3198–203.
72. Gimeno JR, Tomé-Esteban M, Lofiego C, et al. Exercise-induced ventricular arrhythmias and risk of sudden cardiac death in patients with hypertrophic cardiomyopathy. *Eur Heart J* 2009; 30: 2599–605.
73. Perrin MJ, Angaran P, Laksman Z, et al. Exercise testing in asymptomatic gene carriers exposes a latent electrical substrate of arrhythmogenic right ventricular cardiomyopathy. *J Am Coll Cardiol* 2013; 62: 1772–9.
74. Heidbüchel H, Hoogsteen J, Fagard R, et al. High prevalence of right ventricular involvement in endurance athletes with ventricular arrhythmias: role of an electrophysiologic study in risk stratification. *Eur Heart J* 2003; 24: 1473–80.
75. La Gerche A, Robberecht C, Kuiperi C, et al. Lower than expected desmosomal gene mutation prevalence in endurance athletes with complex ventricular arrhythmias of right ventricular origin. *Heart* 2010; 96: 1268–74.
76. Ector J, Ganame J, van der Merwe N, et al. Reduced right ventricular ejection fraction in endurance athletes presenting with ventricular arrhythmias: a quantitative angiographic assessment. *Eur Heart J* 2007; 28: 345–53.
77. Marcus FI, McKenna WJ, Sherrill D, et al. Diagnosis of arrhythmogenic right ventricular cardiomyopathy/dysplasia: proposed modification of the task force criteria. *Circulation* 2010; 121: 1533–41.
78. Sawant AC, Bhonsale A, te Riele ASJM, et al. Exercise has a disproportionate role in the pathogenesis of arrhythmogenic right ventricular dysplasia/cardiomyopathy in patients without desmosomal mutations. *J Am Heart Assoc* 2014; 3: e001471.
79. Benito B, Gay-Jordi G, Serrano-Mollar A, et al. Cardiac arrhythmogenic remodeling in a rat model of long-term intensive exercise training. *Circulation* 2011; 123: 13–22.
80. Guasch E, Mont L. Exercise, sex and atrial fibrillation: arrhythmogenesis beyond Y-chromosome? *Heart* 2015; 101: 1607–9.
81. Elliott AD, La Gerche A. The right ventricle following prolonged endurance exercise: are we overlooking the more important side of the heart? A meta-analysis. *Br J Sports Med* 2015; 49: 724–9.
82. La Gerche A, Heidbüchel H, Burns AT, et al. Disproportionate exercise load and remodeling of the athlete's right ventricle. *Med Sci Sports Exerc* 2011; 43: 974–81.
83. La Gerche A, Burns AT, Mooney DJ, et al. Exercise-induced right ventricular dysfunction and structural remodelling in endurance athletes. *Eur Heart J* 2012; 33: 998–1006.
84. Sanz de la Garza M, Grazioli G, Bijnens BH, et al. Inter-individual variability in right ventricle adaptation after an endurance race. *Eur J Prev Cardiol* 2016; 23: 1114–24.
85. James CA, Bhonsale A, Tichnell C, et al. Exercise increases age-related penetrance and arrhythmic risk in arrhythmogenic right ventricular dysplasia/cardiomyopathy associated desmosomal mutation carriers. *J Am Coll Cardiol* 2013; 62: 1290–7.
86. Priori SG, Blomström-Lundqvist C, Mazzanti A, et al. 2015 ESC Guidelines for the management of patients with ventricular arrhythmias and the prevention of sudden cardiac death: The Task Force for the Management of Patients with Ventricular Arrhythmias and the Prevention of Sudden Cardiac Death of the Europe. *Eur Heart J* 2015; 36: 2793–867.
87. Priori SG, Wilde AA, Horie M, et al. HRS/EHRA/APHRS expert consensus statement on the diagnosis and management of patients with inherited primary arrhythmia syndromes. *Heart Rhythm* 2013; 10: 1932–63.
88. van der Werf C, Wilde AAM. Catecholaminergic polymorphic ventricular tachycardia: from bench to bedside. *Heart* 2013; 99: 497–504.
89. Ackerman MJ, Zipes DP, Kovacs RJ, Maron BJ. Eligibility and disqualification recommendations for competitive athletes with cardiovascular abnormalities. Task Force 10: The Cardiac Channelopathies. *J Am Coll Cardiol* 2015; 66: 2424–8.

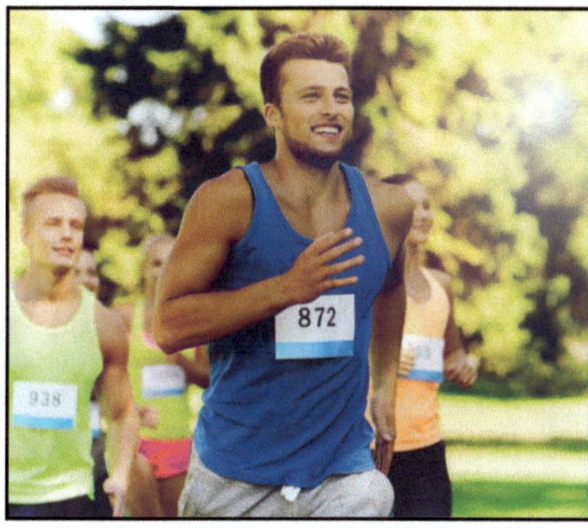

5.3

Supraventricular tachyarrhythmias

Matthias Wilhelm

Introduction

In an athletic population, the incidence of palpitations varies from 0.3% to as high as 70% depending on age and sport discipline [1]. A high proportion of athletes with palpitations have supraventricular tachyarrhythmias (SVTs) as the underlying electric disorder [1]. Among athletes referred to a specialized sports cardiology clinic, palpitations were the most common cardiac symptom (40%) and atrial fibrillation (AF) was the most prevalent diagnosis (7.5%) [2].

This chapter will discuss the different SVTs and the implications for treatment and sports participation in detail. It is based on the position paper of the European Study Group on Sports Cardiology 2006 [3], with appropriate modifications to accommodate newer evidence. The recent scientific statement from the American Heart Association and American College of Cardiology has also been considered [4]. European and American perspectives are similar in most parts and differ only in the risk stratification of *competitive* athletes with asymptomatic pre-excitation. This is elucidated in the section on asymptomatic ventricular pre-excitation, and in Chapter 5.4.

It should be noted that there is no clear division between recreational and competitive sports. Some individuals may engage in high intensity exercise during leisure-time activities. The physiological or pathophysiological implications of the two may be similar. Moreover, although the cardiovascular demand of different sports can be classified based on physiological characteristics (see Chapter 7.1), individual cardiac stress may vary and is influenced by changes in autonomic tone, hydration status, and electrolyte balance. Therefore, an individualized assessment of both the underlying condition and the type/intensity of the desired sports activity is required in every patient.

Diagnostic evaluation: general framework

If the personal history reveals *palpitations*, it is essential to ask the patient to define them as accurately as possible. Do they consist of (repetitive) premature beats or longer-lasting paroxysmal episodes, and is the heart rate during these episodes regular or not? Do they have a sudden onset and end (suggestive of atrioventricular nodal re-entrant tachycardia (AVNRT) or atrioventricular re-entrant tachycardia (AVRT)), or a *warm up* and *cool down* (suggestive of atrial tachycardia (AT)). In many cases, a patient will not complain about palpitations, but the history may reveal unspecific symptoms like lightheadedness, pre-syncope or syncope, unexplained weakness, fatigue, chest pain, or dyspnoea. These symptoms may be the only indicator of arrhythmia and therefore should be interpreted cautiously when noted in a physically active patient's history. Exercise-related syncope is rarely neurocardiogenic and should always lead to suspicion about an arrhythmic cause. Fast conduction of AF over an accessory pathway is an important differential diagnosis. The personal history should further enquire into the use of performance-enhancing or other drugs that may be pro-arrhythmic or could otherwise affect the heart (e.g. antibiotics, antidepressants, etc., but also smoking and alcohol consumption). Previous cardiovascular disease and cardiovascular risk factors should be investigated. Arterial hypertension is the most common risk factor in athletes and is a risk factor for AF [5].

Since symptoms do not distinguish between the different types of SVTs, a symptom–rhythm correlation should be obtained. Patients should be encouraged to have an ECG taken during palpitations or other non-specific symptoms, and physicians should then discuss the possibilities of documentation with them. An ambulatory 24-hour Holter recording can be used in patients with frequent (i.e. several episodes per week) but transient tachycardias. An

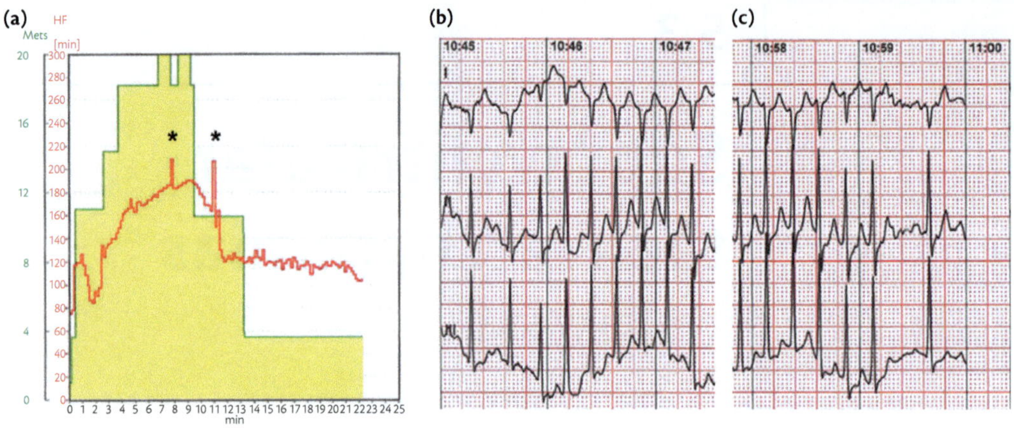

Fig. 5.3.1 Individualized treadmill protocol in a 22-year-old elite track and field athlete with palpitations on exertion. The athlete complained of repetitive episodes of self-limiting palpitations during high intensity running. Documented heart rate was 210bpm on his training monitor. Two exercise tests, one with a ramp protocol on a bicycle and one Bruce protocol on a treadmill, were uneventful. Two seven-day Holter monitorings showed normal sinus rhythm and revealed no arrhythmias. (a) An individualized treadmill protocol was chosen, based on the athlete's usual training, and two self-limiting supraventricular arrhythmias were induced (asterisks). (b) Sudden onset regular rhythm with 210bpm and (c) a sudden end were suggestive of an AV (nodal) re-entry tachycardia, which was confirmed during an electrophysiological study. The athlete was free from symptoms after ablation of the slow pathway.

event or wearable loop recorder is often more useful than a 24-hour recording in patients with less frequent arrhythmias. Implantable loop recorders may be helpful in selected cases with rare symptoms (i.e. fewer than two episodes per month) associated with severe symptoms [6].

Exercise testing may be indicated if symptom–rhythm correlation cannot be obtained from long-term ECG recordings. Regular ramp or step protocols (e.g. Bruce protocol) may not be sufficient to induce exercise-related arrhythmias, and individualized protocols based on the athlete's specific condition should be attempted (➔ Fig. 5.3.1).

Echocardiography can assess the presence or extent of structural heart disease. Rarely, persons with sustained forms of SVT, such as atrial flutter (AFL), AF, or permanent forms of atrial or junctional tachycardias (more common in young people) can present with a tachycardia-induced cardiomyopathy [6].

In some cases, it is advisable to perform laboratory analyses to rule out inflammation, anaemia with/without iron deficiency, hyperthyroidism, or electrolyte disorders as the underlying mechanism or trigger factor for selected SVTs (e.g. AFL, AF). Sinus tachycardia secondary to these laboratory abnormalities is an important differential diagnosis of SVTs.

An invasive electrophysiological (EP) study is indicated in some cases with persisting diagnostic uncertainty, despite non-invasive evaluation, or for prognostic reasons. Specific indications will be noted in the sections on the various arrhythmias. In selected arrhythmias the diagnostic evaluation can be followed by ablation of the arrhythmogenic substrate [6,7].

Apart from the initial evaluation, regular follow-up should be performed in patients/athletes with arrhythmias. They should also be advised to present for immediate re-evaluation if there is a recurrrence of symptoms, particularly if these are exercise-related. Patients need to be made aware of the importance of unspecific symptoms like sudden exertional fatigue or dyspnoea.

Atrial premature beats

Atrial premature beats (APBs) are a common finding in many athletes without any underlying cardiovascular abnormality, but only a few have more than 100 APBs in 24 hours [5]. An association between the APB burden and long-term endurance training has been found in some studies [9,10), but not in all [11]. APBs may be a trigger for other SVTs, especially AF [5]. However, APBs pass unnoticed in most patients, although they may lead to subjective palpitations without associated haemodynamic impairment.

Diagnostics

Usually, a careful history taking is indicative of the SVT's nature as isolated extrasystoles. Holter recording may be necessary to distinguish these from ventricular premature beats. Apart from a 12-lead ECG, physical examination, and thyroid function tests, no other cardiovascular assessments are indicated.

Treatment and exercise recommendations

In the absence of structural heart disease, no therapy is indicated. Participation in all sports, both *competitive* and *recreational*, is allowed.

Paroxysmal supraventricular tachycardias without ventricular pre-excitation

Paroxysmal supraventricular tachycardias (PSVT) *without* pre-excitation include (1) AVNRT, which is the most prevalent [12], (2) orthodromic AVRT with retrograde conduction over an accessory pathway (sometimes called *circus movement tachycardia*), or (3) an ectopic AT. When the accessory pathway is only capable of conduct from ventricles to atria, and hence shows no pre-excitation on the sinus rhythm ECG, it is denoted 'concealed' (meaning 'hidden'). When the accessory pathway also conducts antegradely, ventricular pre-excitation will be visible on the ECG during sinus rhythm. In this case the patient with PSVT has *Wolff–Parkinson–White syndrome*, which carries a risk of SCD and therefore is discussed in a separate section. Sports and exercise training are not associated with a higher risk for PSVT and its prevalence is comparable with that in the general population [8,10,11].

Diagnostics

Exclusion of pre-excitation and underlying structural heart disease is paramount during the diagnostic work-up of an athlete with PSVT. In some patients, however, pre-excitation may be minimal and apparently absent despite antegrade conduction over an accessory pathway (latent pre-excitation). It can be unmasked on a 12-lead ECG by manoeuvres that slow conduction through the AV node during sinus rhythm, such as carotid sinus massage or the intravenous administration of adenosine. Prolongation of the PR interval without a change in the QRS morphology, or transient AV block, rule out pre-excitation. In a patient with documented PSVTs, excluded pre-excitation, and excluded AFL, an invasive EP study is not necessary for differential diagnosis of the exact aetiology unless ablation is considered as the recommendations for sports participation do not depend on the type of underlying arrhythmia (AVNRT, AVRT over a concealed accessory pathway, or AT). In some patients with AT there may be more than one focus and/or this may be a hallmark of underlying cardiovascular disease. AT may also be associated with AF. Therefore diagnostic work-up in athletes in whom AT is diagnosed should evaluate these aspects.

Treatment and exercise recommendations

PSVTs without pre-excitation are generally considered to be benign arrhythmias, not associated with SCD if no structural heart disease is present. However, during physical activity and sympathetic stimulation the rates of both AVNRT and AVRT over a concealed accessory pathway increase. Exercise will also increase the ventricular rate during AT due to facilitation of an AV nodal conduction. This may lead to symptoms of haemodynamic compromise such as dizziness, acute fatigue, or syncope, even in the absence of structural heart disease.

If the patient wants to participate in *competitive* athletic activity, definitive treatment by ablation is recommended. Moreover, drug treatment may not be tolerated, may be illegal, or may even be dangerous during competitive sports (e.g. beta-blockers). If the ablation procedure is successful, the risk of recurrence is very low (<3%) and usually occurs within the first few months [6,15]. Therefore if no recurrences have developed after 1–3 months, competitive sports activity can be resumed for all types of sport and further follow-up is not required. Leisure-time and low to medium intensity training practice can generally be resumed after the puncture sites have healed, provided that there is no particular risk of arrhythmia recurring (e.g. history of exercise-related major (pre)syncope, findings at EP study, ease of ablation).

If the PSVTs are only sporadic and are not associated with haemodynamic consequences even when they develop during exercise, or if ablation is not successful, sports activity is allowed when there is no increased risk due to loss of consciousness (unlike in pilots, motorsports drivers, parachute jumpers, divers, and mountain climbers). Exercise should be stopped as soon as palpitations arise, but can be resumed after they cease. An annual follow-up is necessary.

If the patient only wants to perform *leisure-time activities* and lower-level sports and there are no associated symptoms during tachycardia, participation is allowed and he/she only needs to be instructed to stop physical activity as soon as palpitations occur. Prophylactic drug treatment with beta-blockers or non-dihydropyridine calcium-channel antagonists can be considered, although it has limited efficacy, will not be well tolerated, and may need to be continued lifelong. Class I drugs generally play no role in the management of regular PSVTs. Therefore in a recreational athlete with recurrence of PSVTs despite maintenance treatment with beta-blockers or non-dihydropyridine calcium-channel antagonists, ablation should be considered as the definitive treatment. Ablation can also be the patient's preference as first-choice therapy after discussion with the physician because of the likelihood of a long-term cure, its high efficacy (>98% for AVNRT and AVRT, >85% for AT), and the relatively rare incidence of complications in experienced centres [6,15]. Complications mainly consist of AV block (requiring pacemaker implantation, <1%) or perforation with cardiac tamponade. In selected cases with an increased risk of complete AV block (e.g. para-Hisian accessory pathways or certain forms of atypical AVNRT) cryo-ablation could be an alternative to radiofrequency (RF) ablation, although its superiority over RF energy with respect to the risk of AV block has not been demonstrated and the long-term recurrence rate may be higher [16].

Paroxysmal supraventricular tachycardias with ventricular pre-excitation (Wolff–Parkinson–White syndrome)

Wolff–Parkinson–White (WPW) syndrome is defined as the presence of PSVTs in a patient with ventricular pre-excitation, which are due to an accessory pathway with antegrade conduction. The prevalence of pre-excitation in the general population varies from 0.1% to 0.3% [17,18], and it seems to be the same in athletic populations [19]. The risk of sudden death in patients with pre-excitation varies from 0.15% to 0.20% in population-based studies, but has been reported to be around 2% in symptomatic patients [20].

Accessory-pathway-dependent arrhythmias include AVRTs that are either orthodromic or antidromic. However, WPW patients may also develop other arrhythmias, such as AF, which can lead to fast ventricular rhythms and syncope (➲ Fig. 5.3.2). Rapid antegrade conduction over the accessory pathway may degenerate into ventricular fibrillation and lead to sudden cardiac death (SCD) [20]. It has been estimated that a third of patients with WPW syndrome may develop AF. There is still discussion as to how far patients with WPW syndrome have an increased risk for AF per se (e.g. due to secondary degeneration of AVRT); nevertheless, exercise has been reported to be associated with an increased risk of ventricular arrhythmias and SCD in this context. The majority of sudden deaths occur during exercise or under emotional stress [20]. Moreover, athletes may have an increased risk of AF (see section on atrial fibrillation and atrial flutter) even after retiring from high level competitive sports. Therefore sports activity in the presence of overt pre-excitation may expose the athlete to an increased risk of SCD if the accessory pathway has the potential for fast antegrade conduction.

Diagnostics

Evaluation of the athlete with ventricular pre-excitation should exclude an associated structural cardiac disease, such as hypertrophic cardiomyopathy or Ebstein anomaly, by physical examination, 12-lead ECG, and echocardiogram.

The risk of development of ventricular fibrillation secondary to AF depends on the antegrade refractory period of the accessory pathway. The refractory period is modulated by autonomic tone. Although non-invasive measurements may indicate a long refractory period (e.g. when there is intermittent pre-excitation during sinus rhythm on ECG or

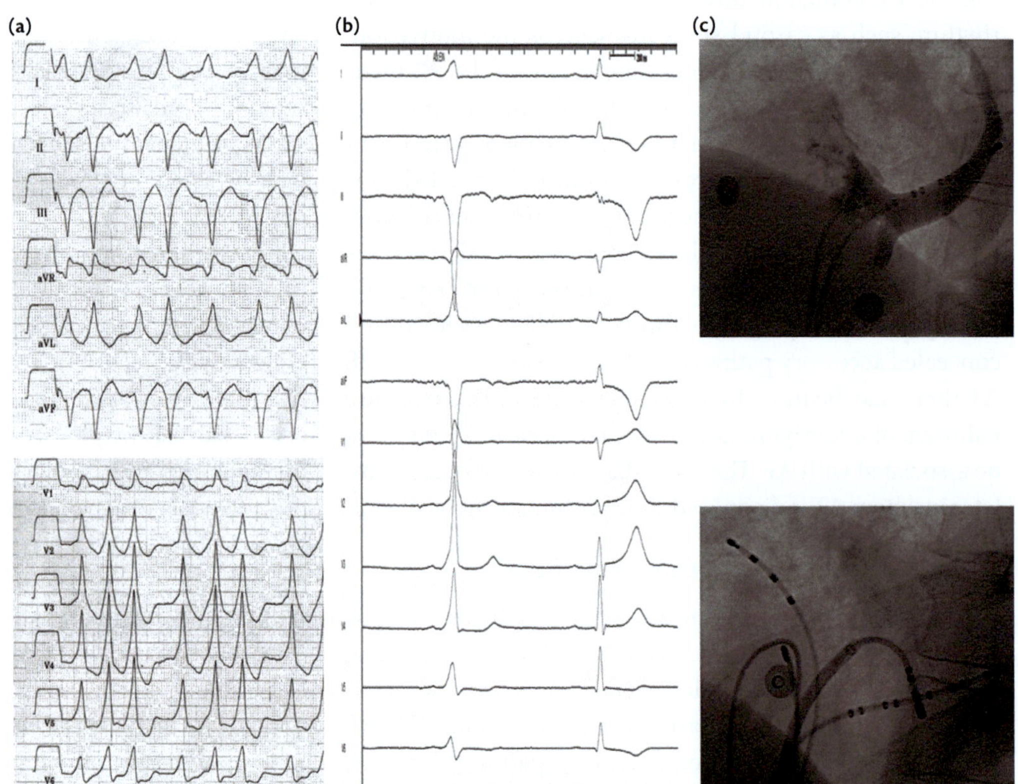

Fig. 5.3.2 Amateur athlete with pre-syncope during a marathon. (a) The ECG in the emergency department showed a fast broad-complex tachycardia with irregular rhythm (FBI), which turned out to be atrial fibrillation in the presence of an accessory pathway. Cardioversion was performed. (b) ECG during the electrophysiological study. The left beat shows pre-excitation with a similar pattern to the initial tachyarrhythmia. The right beat shows the successful ablated accessory pathway. (c) left anterior oblique projection of the heart with the ablation catheter in an inferior position in the left atrium.

Holter, or when pre-excitation suddenly disappears during sinus tachycardia on an exercise test), the conditions existing during competitive events cannot be fully reproduced under laboratory conditions.

Treatment and exercise recommendations

Ablation of the accessory pathway is mandatory in *competitive* and *recreational* athletes with pre-excitation and documented arrhythmias. In the case of only sporadic episodes of palpitations, good haemodynamic tolerance (even during exercise), and/or anticipation of an ablation procedure with increased risk (e.g. anteroseptal accessory pathway), management can be guided by assessment of the antegrade conduction characteristics of the accessory pathway by non-invasive testing or an invasive EP study. When these assessments reveal a long refractory period, and hence a low risk of sudden death, continuation of sports activity is allowed without ablation (with instructions to stop sports on recurrence of palpitations and to have an anual re-evaluation). However, when arguments are present for an increased risk of sudden death, ablation is mandatory.

Resumption of *leisure-time activities* and low to medium intensity training practice can generally be resumed after the puncture sites have healed, provided that there is no particular risk of recurrence of arrhythmia (e.g. a history of exercise-related major (pre)syncope, findings from EP study, ease of ablation) when an individualized approach is warranted. Resumption of competitive sports (see also Chapter 7.1) is possible after one to three months, but with further ECG control at six months and a year (given the very small risk of late recurrence of pre-excitation).

Asymptomatic ventricular pre-excitation

Ventricular pre-excitation may be diagnosed in an asymptomatic athlete during pre-participation screening (➔ Fig. 5.3.3). In the absence of structural heart disease it carries a small but definite risk of SCD, and consequently needs careful evaluation and risk stratification. Sudden death may be the first manifestation of the WPW syndrome in about half of WPW patients, and it usually presents during exercise or emotional stress [20].

Diagnostics

European and American recommendations differ with regard to risk stratification in *competitive* athletes. While the European perspective is that an EP study is warranted in all *competitive* athletes, the American approach is to perform an exercise test and determine whether the pre-excitation abruptly terminates at low heart rates. Invasive EP study is only recommended for those athletes where risk is unclear [3,4].

Inducibility of AVRT or atrial fibrillation [21], a pre-excited R–R <240ms at baseline or <220ms during isoproterenol infusion, an antegrade refractory period <250ms at baseline [22], the presence of multiple accessory pathways, or a septal location (mainly posteroseptal and midseptal) [20] are the electrophysiological parameters considered to be associated with an increased risk of sudden death [23].

In *recreational* athletes, risk assessment can first be pursued via non-invasive testing, looking for intermittent pre-excitation on ECG or Holter, the disappearance of pre-excitation after administration of a low dose of class I drugs,

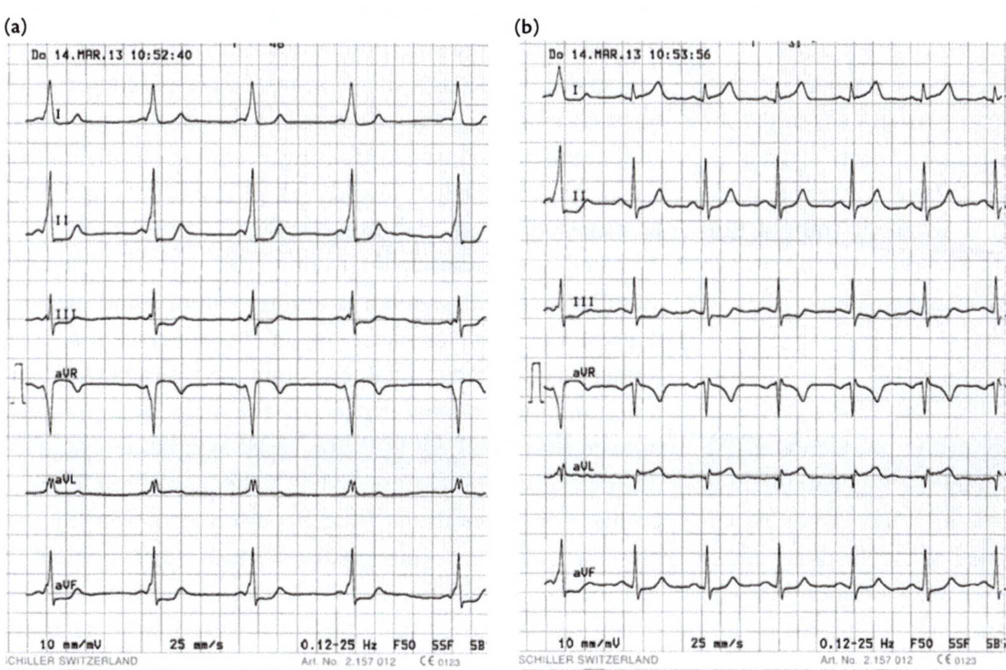

Fig. 5.3.3 A 25-year-old track and field athlete with intermittent asymptomatic pre-excitation. (a) Resting ECG performed during pre-participation screening: heart rate 58bpm, short PR interval and clearly visible delta wave in all leads, associated with ST depressions in the inferior leads. (b) After body movement: heart rate 80bpm, PR interval 146ms, no delta wave. No ablation was performed.
Courtesy of Boris Gojanovic.

or its abrupt disappearance during exercise testing [23]. The sensitivity of non-invasive screening for fast antegrade conduction is good but its specificity is low [22], so that about half the patients will need a subsequent EP study to rule out an increased risk of sudden death.

Treatment and exercise recommendations

In *competitive* athletes with an increased risk of sudden death, ablation of the accessory pathway is mandatory given its high success rate and low incidence of complications. Moreover, the efficacy and safety of anti-arrhythmic drug (AAD) treatment has never been proved in WPW patients in general or athletes in particular. Ablation can also be considered in others because about 3.5% of non-inducible patients may become symptomatic during follow-up. However, the risks of ablation should be weighed against the benefits, after extensive discussion with the athlete, and the decision should be made on an individual basis. For athletes who refuse ablation, or if the procedure is associated with a high risk (e.g. anteroseptal accessory pathways), competitive sport activities are allowed when the EP study demonstrates the absence of parameters for risk and when the sports discipline does not put the athlete at risk when there is a loss of consciousness (e.g. pilots etc.).

In *recreational* athletes, when AVRTs are inducible or when they have an accessory pathway with a short antegrade refractory period, ablation is mandatory. When AVRTs are not inducible, the decision to ablate or not ablate should depend on individual assessment.

In patients performing sports activities in which there is an increased risk of accidents when they lose consciousness (e.g. pilots), ablation is mandatory even when it is not inducible.

It should be noted that, in children younger than 12 years, the risk of AF-induced ventricular arrhythmias and sudden death is very low. A conservative approach is generally recommended in this age group, although a recent study [24] suggested that prophylactic assessment and ablation reduces the risk of sudden death. The risk–benefit ratio of this approach on a large scale needs further study.

Atrial fibrillation and atrial flutter

Young, competitive athletes have a low prevalence of AF (0.3%), comparable with the general population [14]. Moreover, light to moderate physical activities are associated with a significantly lower risk of AF in older adults [25]. However, there is evidence for an association between vigorous physical activities, particularly long-term endurance sport practice, and a higher risk of AF and AFL in the ageing athlete [11,13,26–34]. For a review of these studies, see [5,35,36]. Karjalainen et al. [26] were the first to report a 5.5-fold increased risk of AF in veteran orienteers (mean age 52±10 years) compared with age-matched controls, despite fewer risk factors for AF. AFL was also documented in three athletes [26]. The prevalence of AF was 5.3% in orienteers compared with 0.9% in controls, reflecting the rate usually expected in this age group [37]. Age, volume, intensity, type, and level of sport may contribute to AF risk. Compared with controls, the risk of AF was increased 1.7-fold (95% CI, 1.2–2.3) in vigorous joggers (<50 years) [33] and 8.8-fold (95% CI, 1.3–61.3) in marathon runners (mean age 39±9 years) [31]. In long-term cross-country skiers (mean age 69.5±10.2 years) the prevalence of AF was as high as 16.7% during a follow-up of 28–30 years [34]. In a systematic review and meta-analysis including 655 athletes and 895 controls (mean age 51±9 years), the overall risk for AF was significantly higher in the athletes than in the controls (odds ratio 5.3, 95% CI 3.6–7.9), with a striking male predominance (93%) [38]. In former professional cyclists (mean age 66±7 years) the prevalence of AFL was higher than that of AF (6.5% vs 3.2%) [11].

AFL is usually the manifestation of a counterclockwise (rarely, clockwise) macro re-entrant circuit around the tricuspid valve. AF can be induced and sustained by rapid focal firing (predominantly from the pulmonary veins) or by multiple micro re-entrant circuits in the left atrium [39,40]. AFL may be present together with AF or develop after the administration of class I AADs for AF [41,42]. The arrhythmia may be life-threatening during exertion due to 1:1 conduction to the ventricles under high sympathetic tone.

The reasons for an association of AF and AFL with vigorous exercise are probably complex: An animal model suggested that chronic endurance exercise increases AF susceptibility through atrial remodelling (dilatation and fibrosis) and vagal enhancement [43]. Cardiac structural adaptation to endurance training apears to contribute to the atrial substrate for AF and AFL [9,31,34] (➲ Fig. 5.3.4). In one study, male endurance athletes showed more pronounced atrial remodelling, compared with their female counterparts with similar training volume and performance. Male athletes had a higher blood pressure at rest, higher markers of sympathetic tone, and an altered diastolic function, possibly explaining the male predominance in exercise-related AF [44]. Increased sympathetic activity during exercise may trigger AF in patients with underlying predisposing conditions (like hypertension), whereas an increased vagal tone may predispose to AF development at rest. In some patients AF may develop secondary to atrial ectopy, atrial tachycardia, or PSVTs, with or without overt pre-excitation, because of an underlying cardiomyopathy,

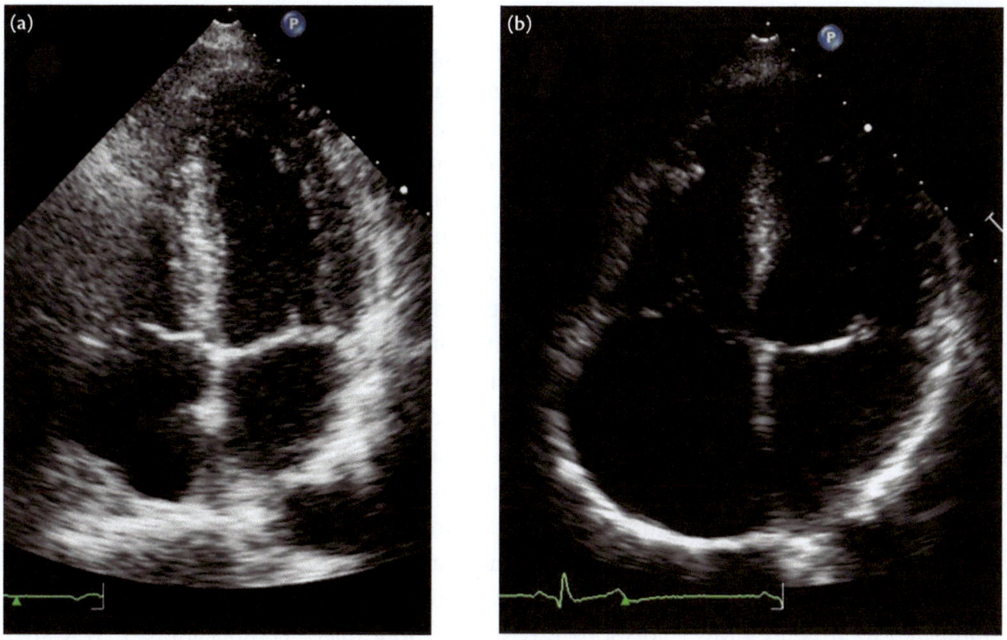

Fig. 5.3.4 Atrial remodelling in two participants in a 10-mile race. (a) A 45-year-old leisure-time runner: finishing time 92min; 1040 hours cumulative lifetime training; no marathon participation; no atrial dilatation (right atrium 21ml/m^2, left atrium 20ml/m^2). (b) A 43-year-old semi-competitive athlete: finishing time 54 min; 11,960 hours cumulative lifetime training; 30 marathon participations; biatrial dilatation (right atrium, 51ml/m^2, left atrium 35ml/m^2); history of paroxysmal atrial flutter and atrial fibrillation.

silent myocarditis, or other structural heart disease [45]. Sports participation may accelerate the development and progression of AF due to other underlying causes. The role of performance-enhancing drugs, such as anabolic steroids, in the development of the AF substrate or in triggering the arrhythmia is largely unknown [46].

Diagnostics

Based on the athletes' history, AF and AFL can be categorized as *first onset*, *paroxysmal*, or *persistent* (i.e. requiring chemical or electrical cardioversion). *Permanent* AF is defined as accepted chronic AF, where catheter ablation was not intended or not successful. *Permanent* AFL is rare due to the high success rate of catheter ablation (see the next section on treatment and exercise recommendations) [40]. AF-related symptoms can be classified according to the European Heart Rhythm Association (EHRA) score, ranging from EHRA I—no symptoms, to EHRA IV—disabling symptoms with discontinuation of daily activities [40].

Usually, progression in frequency and duration of AF episodes over time can be expected unless a specific aetiological cause can be identified and cured (e.g. hyperthyroidism, illegal drug use, myocarditis). Diagnostic assessment should focus on the exclusion of risk factors for AF and AFL (e.g. hypertension) and structural heart disease (e.g. myocarditis or cardiomyopathy). Rapid atrioventricular (AV) conduction through the AV node during physical activity may lead to symptoms of haemodynamic impairment such as dizziness, syncope, or sudden extreme fatigue. A careful history and, if possible, ECG recording during such circumstances (exercise test, Holter monitoring, long-term event recorder) will help to guide treatment.

Treatment and exercise recommendations

Patients with a history of AF and/or AFL should be instructed to stop physical activity on the emergence of palpitations or other major symptoms. If a primary cause for AF is present, competitive or leisure-time sports participation should be temporarily suspended but can be resumed after the cause has been corrected and stable sinus rhythm has been present formore than two months. Hence sports participation will also be guided by these underlying conditions. In the absence of primary disorders or major cardiac disease, recommendations for *competitive sports* or *leisure-time activities* will largely depend on the type of AF (first onset, paroxysmal, persistent, permanent) and on the ventricular rate during AF episodes, especially during high intensity exercise. In patients with a single episode of AF or with only very sporadic paroxysms, resumption of all sports activities without treatment can be considered when stable rhythm has been present for more than three months and the AF episodes have not led to major haemodynamic impairment. If the athlete has recurrences, and in particular if he/she is symptomatic during episodes of AF due to a fast ventricular response with haemodynamic impairment (EHRA score >1), treatment is mandatory for sports continuation.

Two treatment strategies, *rate control* and *rhythm control*, have to be discussed with the athlete [7,40]. Moreover, given the causal relationship between endurance sport practice and AF and AFL, reduction of training volume and intensity should also be discussed and the possibility of alternative exercise forms with lower cardiovascular demands should be addressed. However, in clinical practice most athletes will prefer to continue with their sports activities on the same level.

The therapeutic goal of *rate control* is difficult to reach in athletes since beta-blockers will not be well tolerated (or are even prohibited in the special case of competitive athletes), and digoxin or non-dihydropyridine calcium-channel antagonists alone may not be potent enough to slow heart rate during exertional AF. Often a combination of bradycardic agents is needed, with individually titrated therapy avoiding sinus bradycardia at rest or chronotropic incompetence during exercise [40]. When the heart rate during recurrent paroxysms of AF (or during permanent AF) is acceptable at maximal physical performance in any given athlete and there are no signs of haemodynamic impairment, sports activity can be resumed at any level.

The *rhythm control* strategy is indicated in athletes with symptomatic AF (EHRA score ≥2) despite adequate or non-tolerated rate control. It includes class I AADs (e.g. disopyramide, flecainide, or propafenone), class 3 AADs (e.g. sotalol or amiodarone), and/or catheter ablation. Sotalol may be preferred for adrenergically mediated AF, disopyramide for vagally mediated AF, flecainide or propafenone for undetermined AF, and amiodarone as a second choice [40]. Amiodarone-related phototoxicity and photoallergic reactions may limit its applicability in athletes involved in outdoor sports such as cross-country skiing or triathlon [47]. In general, at least one course of AAD therapy should be attempted prior to catheter ablation. However, in selected athletes with severely impaired physical performance and intention to continue competitive sports, catheter ablation may be used as a first-line strategy [7].

In some athletes with paroxysmal AF, class I AADs can only be used for acute reconversion therapy as a 'pill in the pocket' strategy [48]. It is prudent to instruct these patients to refrain from sports as long as the arrhythmia persists, and until one to two half-lives of the AAD have elapsed.

Caution in the use of class I AADs as monotherapy in patients with AF should specifically be mentioned. These drugs may prevent AF recurrences. However, they can convert AF into slow AFL, which may conduct 1:1 to the ventricles during situations with high sympathetic tone [41,42]. Impregnation of the ventricles with the class I drug will result in broad QRS complexes (resembling ventricular tachycardia) and profound negative inotropic effects leading to cardiogenic shock and even sudden death. Therefore class I AADs should be combined with drugs slowing AV conduction (e.g. beta-blockers or non-dihydropyridine calcium-channel antagonists). Prophylactic ablation of the flutter circuit may be considered in athletes in whom therapy with class I drugs is indicated. The 'hybrid' therapy of class I drugs and ablation of flutter may obviate the need for maintenance therapy with bradycardic agents [49,50].

Regular ECG monitoring is recommended in athletes undergoing AAD therapy. An increase in QRS duration of >25% on therapy compared with baseline is a sign of potential risk of pro-arrhythmia and the drug should be stopped or its dose reduced [40].

Given the difficulties of treating athletes with AF with AADs, non-pharmacological options such as pulmonary vein isolation [51] or other extensive left atrial catheter ablation approaches [52] should be considered, especially in athletes with severe symptoms and in whom AF is induced by focal atrial tachycardia. Furlanello et al. [53] reported studies of radiofrequency catheter ablation for AF in 20 competitive athletes with disabling symptoms. The success rate after a mean of two ablations was 90% without major complications [53]. Calvo et al. [54] analysed a series of AF ablations in 182 consecutive patients, 59% with *lone AF*, and 39% of those classified as endurance athletes (endurance sport activity >3 hours per week for at least 10 years). A second ablation was necessary in 37% of patients to achieve a 72% overall probability of freedom from AF at 1 year. Circumferential pulmonary vein ablation was as effective in AF secondary to endurance sport practice as in other aetiologies of AF. Koopman et al. [55] compared the procedural outcome of 94 athletes (>3 hours training per week for >10 years or more than 1500 lifetime training hours, 63% endurance athletes) with 41 controls. The final outcome after a mean of 1.2±0.5 ablations was similar for endurance athletes, non-endurance athletes, and controls (87%, 84%, and 85%, respectively, after 3 years of follow-up). Despite these encouraging results it must be remembered that these ablation studies did not include high level endurance athletes who may exhibit more pronounced atrial remodelling (➲ Fig. 5.3.4), predisposing to a lower procedural success [56]. Moreover, possible complications, such as pulmonary vein stenosis, cardiac tamponade, stroke, and LA–oesophageal fistula have to be discussed with the patient before an ablation strategy is chosen [37]. After a successful ablation procedure and absence of symptomatic recurrences for at least three months, resumption of all sports activity seems to be warranted, but the athletes should be followed up closely (i.e. every six months in the first year and than every year) (see also Chapter 7.1).

In contrast with AF ablation, catheter ablation of the isthmus is a highly effective and safe therapy for AFL and therefore is recommended as first-line therapy in both *competitive* and *leisure-time* athletes. In non-athletes, recurrence rates are low (3–11%) and are rare beyond three months [57,58]. However, high-level endurance athletes may have a massively enlarged right atrium (➲ Fig. 5.3.4), which possibly adversely affects procedural success and long-term results. Non-competitive sports participation can be allowed early after ablation unless symptoms of major haemodynamic impairment were present during exercise before ablation, and resumption of competitive sports activity is possible after three months free from AFL [3] (see also Chapter 7.1).

Some athletes with successful AFL ablation will develop paroxysmal or persistent AF during follow-up [59]. A history of endurance sports has been identified in multivariate analysis as an independent risk factor for AF development after AFL ablation, indicating common functional (autonomic nervous) and/or structural mechanisms in their pathogenesis [30]. Therefore recommendations for AF are also valid for athletes with AFL. In the presence of combined AFL and AF, a 'hybrid therapy', including isthmus ablation and continuation of drug therapy or catheter ablation for AF, is recommended [49,50].

Stroke risk has to be assessed in all athletes with AF and AFL, independent of whether the rate or rhythm control strategy is used. In athletes aged <65 years with *lone* AF (i.e. non-valvular AF and no structural heart disease) no anti-thrombotic therapy is indicated. In athletes aged ≥65 years and with a CHA_2DS_2-VASc score ≥1 oral anticoagulant therapy, preferably with a novel oral anticoagulant (NOAC) should be initiated [7]. Anticoagulant therapy excludes these athletes from competitive sports with a risk of bodily collision or trauma (e.g. ice hockey). However, veteran athletes (>65 years) rarely perform these sports.

Further reading

Blomstrom-Lundqvist C, Scheinman MM, Aliot EM, et al. ACC/AHA/ESC guidelines for the management of patients with supraventricular arrhythmias: executive summary. *J Am Coll Cardiol* 2003; 42: 1493–1531.

Calvo N, Brugada J, Sitges M, Mont L. Atrial fibrillation and atrial flutter in athletes. *Br J Sports Med* 2012; 46 (Suppl 1): i37–43.

Camm AJ, Kirchhof P, Lip GY, et al. Guidelines for the management of atrial fibrillation: Task Force for the Management of Atrial Fibrillation of the European Society of Cardiology (ESC). *Eur Heart J* 2010; 31: 2369–429.

Camm AJ, Lip GY, De Caterina R, et al. 2012 focused update of the ESC Guidelines for the management of atrial fibrillation: an update of the 2010 ESC Guidelines for the management of atrial fibrillation. *Eur Heart J* 2012; 33: 2719 47.

Mont L, Elosua R, Brugada J. Endurance sport practice as a risk factor for atrial fibrillation and atrial flutter. *Europace* 2009; 11: 11–17.

Page RL, Joglar JA, Caldwell MA, et al. 2015 ACC/AHA/HRS guideline for the management of adult patients with supraventricular tachycardia. *J Am Coll Cardiol* 2016; 67: e27–115.

Wilhelm M. Atrial fibrillation in endurance athletes. *Eur J Prev Cardiol* 2013; 21: 1040–8.

References

1. Lawless CE, Briner W. Palpitations in athletes. *Sports Med* 2008; 38: 687–702.
2. Kaiser-Nielsen LV, Tischer SG, Prescott EB, Rasmusen HK. Symptoms, diagnoses, and sporting consequences among athletes referred to a Danish sports cardiology clinic. *Scand J Med Sci Sports* 2017; 27, 115–23.
3. Heidbüchel H, Panhuyzen-Goedkoop N, Corrado D, et al. Recommendations for participation in leisure-time physical activity and competitive sports in patients with arrhythmias and potentially arrhythmogenic conditions> Part I: Supraventricular arrhythmias and pacemakers. *Eur J Cardiovasc Prev Rehabil* 2006; 13: 475–84.
4. Zipes DP, Link MS, Ackerman MJ, et al. Eligibility and disqualification recommendations for competitive athletes with cardiovascular abnormalities: Task Force 9: Arrhythmias and Conduction Defects. *J Am Coll Cardiol* 2015; 66: 2412–23.
5. Wilhelm M. Atrial fibrillation in endurance athletes. *Eur J Prev Cardiol* 2013; 21: 1040–8.
6. Blomstrom-Lundqvist C, Scheinman MM, Aliot EM, et al. ACC/AHA/ESC guidelines for the management of patients with supraventricular arrhythmias: executive summary. *J Am Coll Cardiol* 2003; 42: 1493–1531.
7. Camm AJ, Lip GY, De Caterina R, et al. 2012 focused update of the ESC Guidelines for the management of atrial fibrillation: an update of the 2010 ESC Guidelines for the management of atrial fibrillation. *Eur Heart J* 2012; 33: 2719–47.
8. Talan DA, Bauernfeind RA, Ashley WW, et al. Twenty-four hour continuous ECG recordings in long-distance runners. *Chest* 1982; 82: 19–24.
9. Wilhelm M, Roten L, Tanner H, et al. Atrial remodeling, autonomic tone, and lifetime training hours in nonelite athletes. *Am J Cardiol* 2011; 108: 580–5.
10. Bjornstad H, Storstein L, Meen HD, Hals O. Ambulatory electrocardiographic findings in top athletes, athletic students and control subjects. *Cardiology* 1994; 84: 42–50.
11. Baldesberger S, Bauersfeld U, Candinas R, et al. Sinus node disease and arrhythmias in the long-term follow-up of former professional cyclists. *Eur Heart J* 2008; 29: 71–8.
12. Wu D, Denes P, Amat-y-Leon F, et al. Clinical, electrocardiographic and electrophysiologic observations in patients with paroxysmal supraventricular tachycardia. *Am J Cardiol* 1978; 41: 1045–51.
13. Andersen K, Farahmand B, Ahlbom A, et al. Risk of arrhythmias in 52,755 long-distance cross-country skiers: a cohort study. *Eur Heart J* 2013; 34: 3624–31.
14. Pelliccia A, Maron BJ, Di Paolo FM, et al. Prevalence and clinical significance of left atrial remodeling in competitive athletes. *J Am Coll Cardiol* 2005; 46: 690–6.
15. Page RL, Joglar JA, Caldwell MA, et al. 2015 ACC/AHA/HRS guideline for the management of adult patients with supraventricular tachycardia. *J Am Coll Cardiol* 2016; 67: e27–115
16. Deisenhofer I, Zrenner B, Yin YH, et al. Cryoablation versus radiofrequency energy for the ablation of atrioventricular nodal reentrant tachycardia (the CYRANO Study): results from a large multicenter prospective randomized trial. *Circulation* 2010; 122: 2239–45.

17. Sorbo MD, Buja GF, Miorelli M, et al. [The prevalence of the Wolff-Parkinson-White syndrome in a population of 116,542 young males]. *G Ital Cardiol* 1995; 25: 681–7.
18. Sano S, Komori S, Amano T, et al. Prevalence of ventricular pre-excitation in Japanese schoolchildren. *Heart* 1998; 79: 374–8.
19. Corrado D, Basso C, Pavei A, et al. Trends in sudden cardiovascular death in young competitive athletes after implementation of a preparticipation screening program. *JAMA* 2006; 296: 1593–1601.
20. Timmermans C, Smeets JL, Rodriguez LM, et al. Aborted sudden death in the Wolff-Parkinson-White syndrome. *Am J Cardiol* 1995; 76: 492–4.
21. Pappone C, Santinelli V, Rosanio S, et al. Usefulness of invasive electrophysiologic testing to stratify the risk of arrhythmic events in asymptomatic patients with Wolff-Parkinson-White pattern: results from a large prospective long-term follow-up study. *J Am Coll Cardiol* 2003; 41: 239–44.
22. Gaita F, Giustetto C, Riccardi R, et al. Stress and pharmacologic tests as methods to identify patients with Wolff-Parkinson-White syndrome at risk of sudden death. *Am J Cardiol* 1989; 64: 487–90.
23. Wellens HJ, Rodriguez LM, Timmermans C, Smeets JP. The asymptomatic patient with the Wolff-Parkinson-White electrocardiogram. *Pacing Clin Electrophysiol* 1997; 20: 2082–6.
24. Pappone C, Manguso F, Santinelli R, et al. Radiofrequency ablation in children with asymptomatic Wolff-Parkinson-White syndrome. *N Engl J Med* 2004; 351: 1197–1205.
25. Mozaffarian D, Furberg CD, Psaty BM, Siscovick D. Physical activity and incidence of atrial fibrillation in older adults: the cardiovascular health study. *Circulation* 2008; 118: 800–7.
26. Karjalainen J, Kujala UM, Kaprio J, et al. Lone atrial fibrillation in vigorously exercising middle aged men: case-control study. *BMJ* 1998; 316: 1784–5.
27. Mont L, Sambola A, Brugada J, et al. Long-lasting sport practice and lone atrial fibrillation. *Eur Heart J* 2002; 23: 477–82.
28. Hoogsteen J, Schep G, Van Hemel NM, Van Der Wall EE. Paroxysmal atrial fibrillation in male endurance athletes: a 9-year follow up. *Europace* 2004; 6: 222–8.
29. Elosua R, Arquer A, Mont L, et al. Sport practice and the risk of lone atrial fibrillation: a case-control study. *Int J Cardiol* 2006; 108: 332–7.
30. Heidbüchel H, Anné W, Willems R, et al. Endurance sports is a risk factor for atrial fibrillation after ablation for atrial flutter. *Int J Cardiol* 2006; 107: 67–72.
31. Molina L, Mont L, Marrugat J, et al. Long-term endurance sport practice increases the incidence of lone atrial fibrillation in men: a follow-up study. *Europace* 2008; 10: 618–23.
32. Mont L, Tamborero D, Elosua R, et al. Physical activity, height, and left atrial size are independent risk factors for lone atrial fibrillation in middle-aged healthy individuals. *Europace* 2008; 10: 15–20.
33. Aizer A, Gaziano JM, Cook NR, et al. Relation of vigorous exercise to risk of atrial fibrillation. *Am J Cardiol* 2009; 103: 1572–7.
34. Grimsmo J, Grundvold I, Maehlum S, Arnesen H. High prevalence of atrial fibrillation in long-term endurance cross-country skiers: echocardiographic findings and possible predictors: a 28–30 years follow-up study. *Eur J Cardiovasc Prev Rehabil* 2010; 17: 100–5.
35. Mont L, Elosua R, Brugada J. Endurance sport practice as a risk factor for atrial fibrillation and atrial flutter. *Europace* 2009; 11: 11–17.
36. Calvo N, Brugada J, Sitges M, Mont L. Atrial fibrillation and atrial flutter in athletes. *Br J Sports Med* 2012; 46 (Suppl 1): i37–43.
37. Feinberg WM, Blackshear JL, Laupacis A, et al. Prevalence, age distribution, and gender of patients with atrial fibrillation. Analysis and implications. *Arch Intern Med* 1995; 155: 469–73.
38. Abdulla J, Nielsen JR. Is the risk of atrial fibrillation higher in athletes than in the general population? A systematic review and meta-analysis. *Europace* 2009; 11: 1156–9.
39. Nattel S, Burstein B, Dobrev D. Atrial remodeling and atrial fibrillation: mechanisms and implications. *Circ Arrhythm Electrophysiol* 2008; 1: 62–73.
40. Camm AJ, Kirchhof P, Lip GY, et al. Guidelines for the management of atrial fibrillation: the Task Force for the Management of Atrial Fibrillation of the European Society of Cardiology (ESC). *Eur Heart J* 2010; 31: 2369–429.
41. Kawabata M, Hirao K, Horikawa T, et al. Syncope in patients with atrial flutter during treatment with class Ic antiarrhythmic drugs. *J Electrocardiol* 2001; 34: 65–72.
42. Brembilla-Perrot B, Houriez P, Beurrier D, et al. Predictors of atrial flutter with 1:1 conduction in patients treated with class I antiarrhythmic drugs for atrial tachyarrhythmias. *Int J Cardiol* 2001; 80: 7–15.
43. Guasch E, Benito B, Qi X, et al. Atrial fibrillation promotion by endurance exercise: demonstration and mechanistic exploration in an animal model. *J Am Coll Cardiol* 2013; 62: 68–77.
44. Wilhelm M, Roten L, Tanner H, et al. Gender differences of atrial and ventricular remodeling and autonomic tone in nonelite athletes. *Am J Cardiol*2011: 108; 1489–95.
45. Furlanello F, Bertoldi A, Dallago M, et al. Atrial fibrillation in elite athletes. *J Cardiovasc Electrophysiol* 1998; 9 (8 Suppl): S63–8.
46. Sullivan M, Martinez CM, Gallagher EJ. Atrial fibrillation and anabolic steroids. *J Emerg Med* 1999; 17: 851–7.
47. Jaworski K, Walecka I, Rudnicka L, et al. Cutaneous adverse reactions of amiodarone. *Med Sci Monit* 2014; 20: 2369–72.
48. Alboni P, Botto GL, Baldi N, et al. Outpatient treatment of recent-onset atrial fibrillation with the 'pill-in-the-pocket' approach. *N Engl J Med* 2004; 351: 2384–91.
49. Nabar A, Rodriguez LM, Timmermans C, et al. Effect of right atrial isthmus ablation on the occurrence of atrial fibrillation: observations in four patient groups having type I atrial flutter with or without associated atrial fibrillation. *Circulation* 1999; 99: 1441–5.
50. Reithmann C, Dorwarth U, Dugas M, et al. Risk factors for recurrence of atrial fibrillation in patients undergoing hybrid therapy for antiarrhythmic drug-induced atrial flutter. *Eur Heart J* 2003; 24: 1264–72.
51. Haissaguerre M, Jais P, Shah DC, et al. Spontaneous initiation of atrial fibrillation by ectopic beats originating in the pulmonary veins. *N Engl J Med* 1998; 339: 659–66.
52. Pappone C, Oreto G, Rosanio S, et al. Atrial electroanatomic remodeling after circumferential radiofrequency pulmonary vein ablation: efficacy of an anatomic approach in a large cohort of patients with atrial fibrillation. *Circulation* 2001; 104: 2539–44.

53. Furlanello F, Lupo P, Pittalis M, et al. Radiofrequency catheter ablation of atrial fibrillation in athletes referred for disabling symptoms preventing usual training schedule and sport competition. *J Cardiovasc Electrophysiol* 2008; 19: 457–62.

54. Calvo N, Mont L, Tamborero D, et al. Efficacy of circumferential pulmonary vein ablation of atrial fibrillation in endurance athletes. *Europace* 2010; 12: 30–6.

55. Koopman P, Nuyens D, Garweg C, et al. Efficacy of radiofrequency catheter ablation in athletes with atrial fibrillation. *Europace* 2011; 13: 1386–93.

56. Boersma LV. Atrial fibrillation ablation in athletes: an Olympic challenge? *Europace* 2010; 12: 3–4.

57. Schmieder S, Ndrepepa G, Dong J, et al. Acute and long-term results of radiofrequency ablation of common atrial flutter and the influence of the right atrial isthmus ablation on the occurrence of atrial fibrillation. *Eur Heart J* 2003; 24: 956–62.

58. Hsieh MH, Tai CT, Chiang CE, et al. Recurrent atrial flutter and atrial fibrillation after catheter ablation of the cavotricuspid isthmus: a very long-term follow-up of 333 patients. *J Interv Card Electrophysiol* 2002; 7: 225–31.

59. Anné W, Willems R, van der Merwe N, et al. Atrial fibrillation after radiofrequency ablation of atrial flutter: preventive effect of angiotensin converting enzyme inhibitors, angiotensin II receptor blockers, and diuretics. *Heart* 2004; 90: 1025–30.

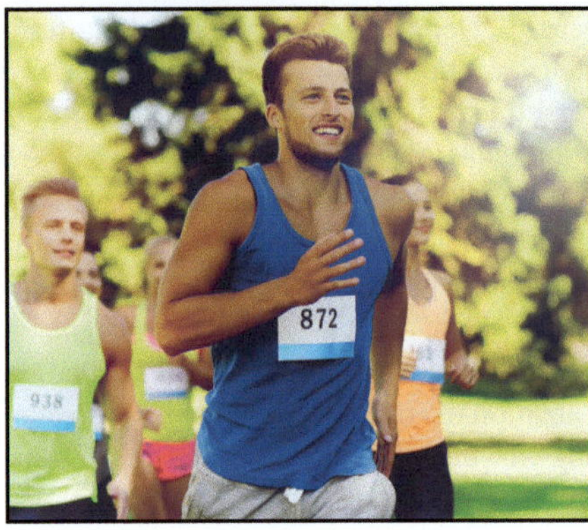

5.4

Pre-excitation and conduction abnormalities

Pietro Delise

Introduction

Ventricular pre-excitation (Wolff–Parkinson–White (WPW) ECG pattern) and conduction abnormalities may be discovered during cardiovascular pre-participation screening in athletes.

The WPW pattern has a prevalence of about 1 in 1000, while the prevalence of conduction abnormalities depends on the type of defect. For example, left bundle branch block (LBBB) has a prevalence of 1 in 1000, while right bundle branch (RBBB) has a prevalence of 1 in 100 [1] (➲ Table 5.4.1). Therefore, in large populations of subjects undergoing cardiovascular screening, it is not unusual to identify subjects with such abnormalities who require a prognostic evaluation and appropriate advice about their eligibility to participate in sport.

Pre-excitation

The pre-excitation ECG pattern (WPW) is due to the congenital presence of accessory pathways (Kent bundle) which connect one atrium to a ventricle, producing an electric bypass over the normal conduction system. Accessory pathways are located around the mitral annulus (60%), in the atrial septum (30%), or around the tricuspid annulus (10%) [2] (➲ Fig. 5.4.1).

In a third of cases a WPW pattern identfied at birth spontaneously disappears before the age of 6 years [3–5]. The WPW pattern continues to decline with age. and it is very rare in the elderly (its prevalence in males is 2.8 in 1000 at 20–29 years and 0.5 in 1000 at 60 years; in female its prevalence is 1.1 in 1000 and 0.5 in 1000, respectively) [6].

Patients with the WPW pattern can also present with symptoms due to arrhythmias [2,7–10]. The most common arrhythmia is orthodromic atrioventricular re-entrant tachycardia (O-AVRT) which is benign [7]. It is due to a macro re-entry in which anterograde conduction occurs via the AV node (AVN) and retrograde conduction occurs via the accessory pathway (➲ Fig. 5.4.2). Antidromic AVRT is very rare and is also due a macro re-entry in the reverse sense with respect to O-AVRT. In the former case QRS is narrow during tachycardia, whereas in the latter it is pre-excited.

Patients with the WPW pattern may present with high frequency atrial fibrillation [8–12]. Generally atrial fibrillation is triggered by an O-AVRT [13,14] (➲ Figs 5.4.2 and 5.4.3). Furthermore, in subjects with short anterograde refractory period of the Kent bundle, atrial fibrillation may degenerate into ventricular fibrillation, possibly leading to sudden death [15–17].

Not all subjects with the WPW pattern on 12-lead ECG are symptomatic. On the contrary, over 90% of children, about 65% of adolescents and teenagers, and about 40% of the over-thirties are asymptomatic [4,5,18]. These data reveal that the asymptomatic condition is far from rare. However, it can also be deduced from these data that there is no guarantee that asymptomatic subjects will remain so, particularly if they are young. Indeed, symptoms may appear at any stage of life. In a long-term prospective study, Munger et al. [19] found that the mean age of onset of symptoms is 28 years, but the majority of subjects aged over 40 years remain asymptomatic.

While the absence of symptoms may be only a temporary condition in some asymptomatic subjects, in others it persists over time because the accessory pathway does not have retrograde conduction. In a pooled analysis [20] of five studies [14,21–24], we found this condition in 46% of asymptomatic adults. Under this condition O-AVRT cannot occur and atrial fibrillation is less likely. However, if it does occurs it can still be malignant if rapid anterograde conduction over the accessory pathway is present.

Table 5.4.1 Prevalence of ECG abnormalities in an unselected population of 32,652 young subjects during pre-participation cardiovascular screening

	Number	Prevalence
Total	32,652	
Negative T waves in precordial/standard leads	751	2.3%
Right bundle branch block	351	1%
Left anterior hemiblock	162	0.5%
Left bundle branch block	19	0.1%
Wolff–Parkinson–White	42	0.1%
Others (incomplete RBBB, prolonged PR interval, early repolarization pattern)	2280	7%

Reproduced with permission frozm Pelliccia, Antonio; Culasso, Franco. Prevalence of abnormal electrocardiograms in a large, unselected population undergoing pre-participation cardiovascular screening. *European Heart Journal*, Volume 28, Issue 16. Copyright © 2007 Oxford University Press and the European Society of Cardiology.

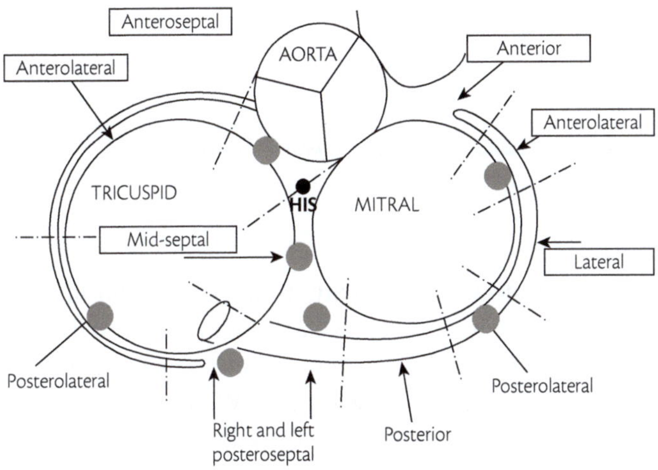

Fig. 5.4.1 Possible locations of accessory pathways around the mitral valve, the tricuspid valve, and the inter-atrial septum.

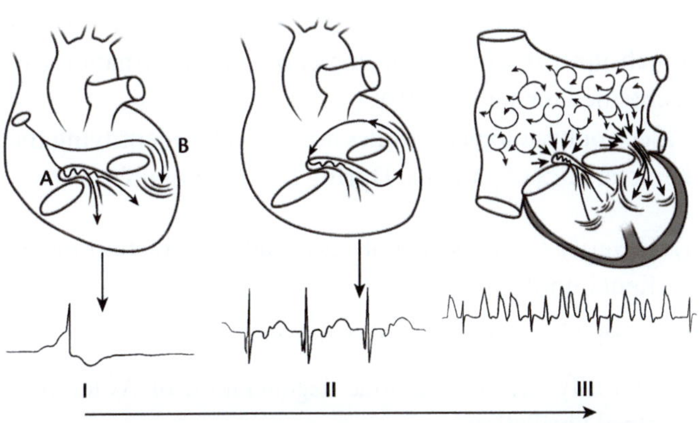

Fig. 5.4.2 The WPW ECG pattern is due to the presence of an anomalous pathway which connects an atrium to a ventricle (I). O-AVRT is due to a macro re-entry involving the normal conduction system in the anterograde direction and the anomalous pathway in the retrograde direction (II). In WPW syndrome atrial fibrillation (III) is generally triggered by O-AVRT. Note that during O-AVRT the QRS is narrow while during atrial fibrillation it is wide and the rhythm is irregular.

Clinical characteristics of WPW patients with cardiac arrest

Analysis [20] of data pooled from three large studies of case records [16,17,25], including 63 adult WPW subjects resuscitated after cardiac arrest, revealed the following main findings.

1. Cardiac arrest can occur at any age, but generally happens around the age of 20–30 years.
2. In 73% of cases, it occurs in symptomatic subjects.
3. It particularly strikes those who have already suffered episodes of atrial fibrillation (up to 70%).
4. Cardiac arrest may be the first clinical manifestation in subjects who are asymptomatic or unaware of their anomaly in a mean 27% of cases (12% [16], 26% [17], and 53% [25]).

The last observation raised diffuse alarm because many concluded that one in four of WPW patients who die have no prodromal symptoms.

However, it should be emphasized that this conclusion is the result of an arbitrary extrapolation of what was reported in the studies cited above. For example, Timmermans et al. [25], stated that 'In over 50% of cases, cardiac arrest occurs in subjects who are unaware of their condition'. But this does not mean that these subjects were totally asymptomatic. Indeed, a subject with WPW may well be unaware of his own anomaly, but be symptomatic without knowing why.

Incidence of sudden cardiac death in asymptomatic patients with the WPW pattern

The data on adults are fairly abundant and suggest a very low risk of sudden cardiac death (SCD) in asymptomatic subjects. In a cumulative analysis [20] of 13 studies published

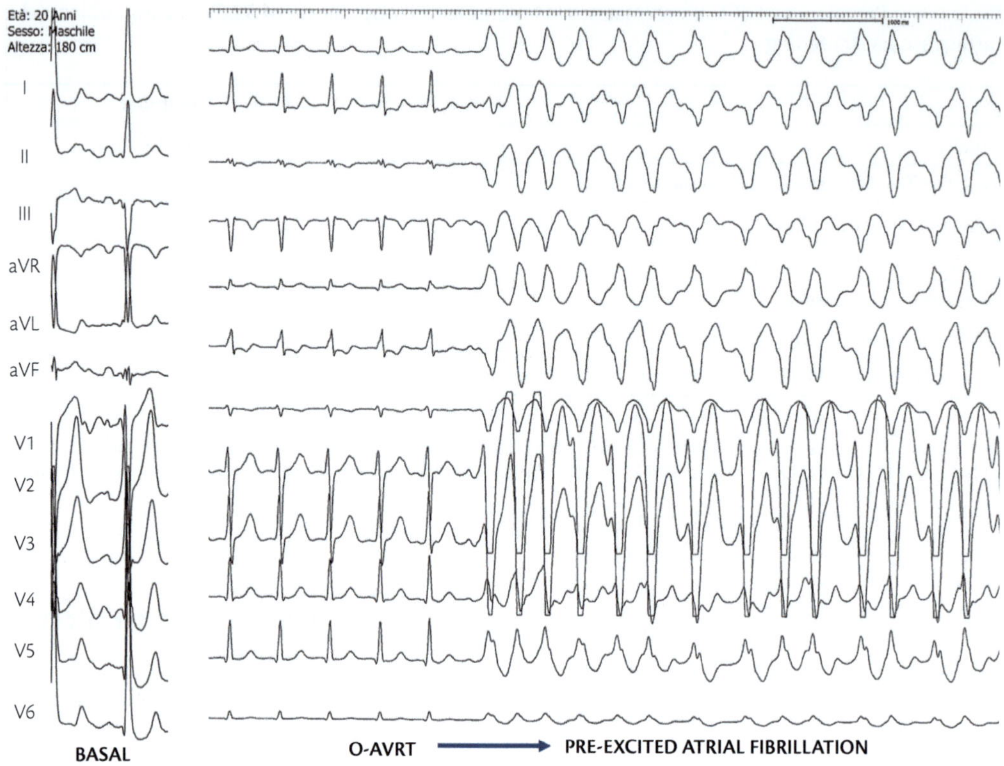

Fig. 5.4.3 Patients with the WPW ECG pattern and frequent episodes of palpitations. During the electrophysiological study an ortodromic O-AVRT is induced by extra-atrial stimuli. Note the narrow QRS during O-AVRT. After few seconds O-AVRT triggers atrial fibrillation conducted to the ventricles through the anomalous pathway. Note the wide QRS which resembles the QRS during sinus rhythm.

between 1964 and 2001 [13,16,19,21–24,26–31], which included 749 patients prospectively followed up for a total of 6724 years, we found a 0% incidence of sudden death.

In a recent meta-analysis conducted in 20 studies reporting 8822 person-years of follow-up Obeyeseker et al. [32] found an incidence of SCD of 0.86 in 1000 patients per year. However, in the same study a discrepancy was found between non-Italian and Italian studies [33,34], which showed incidences of SCD of 0.26 and 2.55, respectively, in 1000 patients per year. The over-estimation of incidence of SCD in Italian studies [33,34] may be due to the fact that three of the four patients who suffered a cardiac arrest, although asymptomatic on enrolment, had had at least one episode of atrial fibrillation before the fatal, or potentially fatal, event. As a consequence,these patients, although asymptomatic at enrolment, could no longer be regarded as asymptomatic from the first episode of atrial fibrillation.

Fewer data on children are available. In a meta-analysis reporting 2900 person-years of follow-up, Obeyeseker et al. [32] found an incidence of SCD in children of 1.93 in 1000 patients per year.

Is it possible to predict the risk of arrhythmias in asymptomatic subjects with the WPW pattern?

Cardiac arrest in WPW is generally linked to a cascade of events. The prime mover is AVRT which, in the presence of elevated atrial vulnerability, triggers atrial fibrillation [13,16,35] (➲ Figs 5.4.2 and 5.4.3). This may in turn degenerate into ventricular fibrillation if the anomalous pathway has brief anterograde refractoriness. While all the factors discussed so far are important, there is no doubt that, for cardiac arrest to occur, brief refractoriness of the anomalous pathway is absolutely essential [16].

A low risk of high frequency atrial fibrillation (i.e. a short refractory period of Kent bundle) can be predicted from the basal ECG in intermittent WPW and/or when pre-excitation abruptly disappears during effort. No information can be obtained for stable WPW.

Electrophysiological studies are useful for identifying the characteristics of patients. During EPS it is possible:

(1) to verify the presence of retrograde conduction of the Kent bundle
(2) to establish the inducibility of AVRT
(3) to verify the spontaneous degeneration of AVRT into atrial fibrillation
(4) to state atrial vulnerability (i.e. easy inducibility of atrial fibrillation and its duration and/or spontaneous resolution)
(5) to calculate the anterograde effective refractory period of the Kent bundle.

The simplest way to evaluate the last of these parameters is to calculate the shortest RR interval between the pre-excited complexes during induced atrial fibrillation or high rate atrial pacing.

All these evaluations can be usefully repeated during catecholamine infusion or during effort (in the case of trans-oesophageal EPS). In fact physical activity (by increasing catecholamine) not only facilitates the inducibility of AVRT, but can also significantly reduce the anterograde effective refractory period of the accessory pathway, increasing heart rate during atrial fibrillation.

The anterograde refractory period of the Kent bundle is considered the most important parameter for predicting the risk of SCD. In fact, in patients resuscitated after cardiac arrest (almost always during induced atrial fibrillation) the shortest RR intervals are <250ms, and even <200ms in the majority of cases [16,21,36]. In children, the cut-off is lower (200ms and 170 ms, respectively) [37]. Moreover, sustained atrial fibrillation is easily inducible in patients resuscitated after cardiac arrest, and frequently spontaneously degenerates into atrial fibrillation during EPS-induced AVRT [33–35].

Unfortunately, the most important parameter assumed as a predictor of risk of SCD, despite its high sensitivity, has a very low specificity. Indeed, short RR intervals (<250ms) during atrial fibrillation are very frequently observed in asymptomatic patients without cardiac arrest (~50%) [13], which conflicts with the very low incidence of cardiac arrest in this population [20,32].

Recommendations for competitive sport in asymptomatic athletes with the WPW pattern

Italian [38,40], European [41,42], and US guidelines [43] all state that symptomatic subjects are not eligible to participate in competitive sport. All the guidelines recomment the use of EPS to stratify the risk in asymptomatic subjects (see also Chapter 7.1). The Italian and European guidelines recommend EPS after the age of 12 years. Both endocavitary (E-EPS) and trans- oesophageal (T-EPS) electrophysiological study can be performed.

T-EPS [44] is able to provide the main parameters for risk stratification: the inducibility of AVRT, atrial vulnerability, and the shortest RR intervals during induced atrial fibrillation. The examination can be carried out both in basal conditions and during exercise testing or catecholamine infusion. T-EPS is a low-cost procedure that can easily be performed even in small facilities, does not require exposure to radiation, and is well accepted by patients. As a consequence, it was widely adopted in Italy in the 1980s and 1990s [38,40].

In Italian and European guidelines [38–42] the following asymptomatic athletes are considered to be fully eligible for participation in sport:

- AVRT non-inducible
- no high atrial vulnerability
- shortest RR interval during induced AF (or effective refractory period of anomalous pathway) ≥250ms in the basal state and ≥210 msec during effort or catecholamine infusion

In Italian and European guidelines the following asymptomatic athletes may be restricted from participation in competitive sport:

- AVRT inducible
- high atrial vulnerability
- shortest RR interval during induced AF (or effective refractory period of anomalous pathway) <250ms in the basal state and <210ms during effort or catecholamine infusion.

In the US guidelines catheter ablation is suggested in the presence of shortest RR intervals <250ms during induced atrial fibrillation.

Conduction abnormalities

Conduction abnormalities (first or second degree AV block, left fascicular blocks, right and left bundle branch blocks) may be found by chance during pre-participation screening in asymptomatic athletes [1]. Their incidence varies according to the type of conduction abnormality (Table 5.4.1).

First-degree AV block is frequent in aerobic athletes, who can also have periods of second-degree AV block (Mobitz 1) or advanced AV block. The more advanced degrees of AV block are generally observed during night. As a rule, in the absence of heart disease AV node conduction normalizes during effort. Incomplete RBBB is also frequent in athletes. However, other blocks are rare: RBBB (1%) (➔ Fig. 5.4.4); fascicular blocks (i.e. left anterior fascicular block (LAFB), left posterior fascicular block (LPFB), or RBBB plus fascicular blocks) (0.5%) (➔ Fig. 5.4.5); LBBB (0.1%) (➔ Fig. 5.4.6).

All these conduction abnormalities can be due to heart disease, which should be excluded by appropriate instrumental investigations. In particular LBBB, RBBB + LAFB, and RBBB + LPFB require instrumental investigation (i.e. cardiac magnetic resonance and/or coronary CT angiography) in addition to echocardiography and Holter monitoring (➔ Fig. 5.4.6).

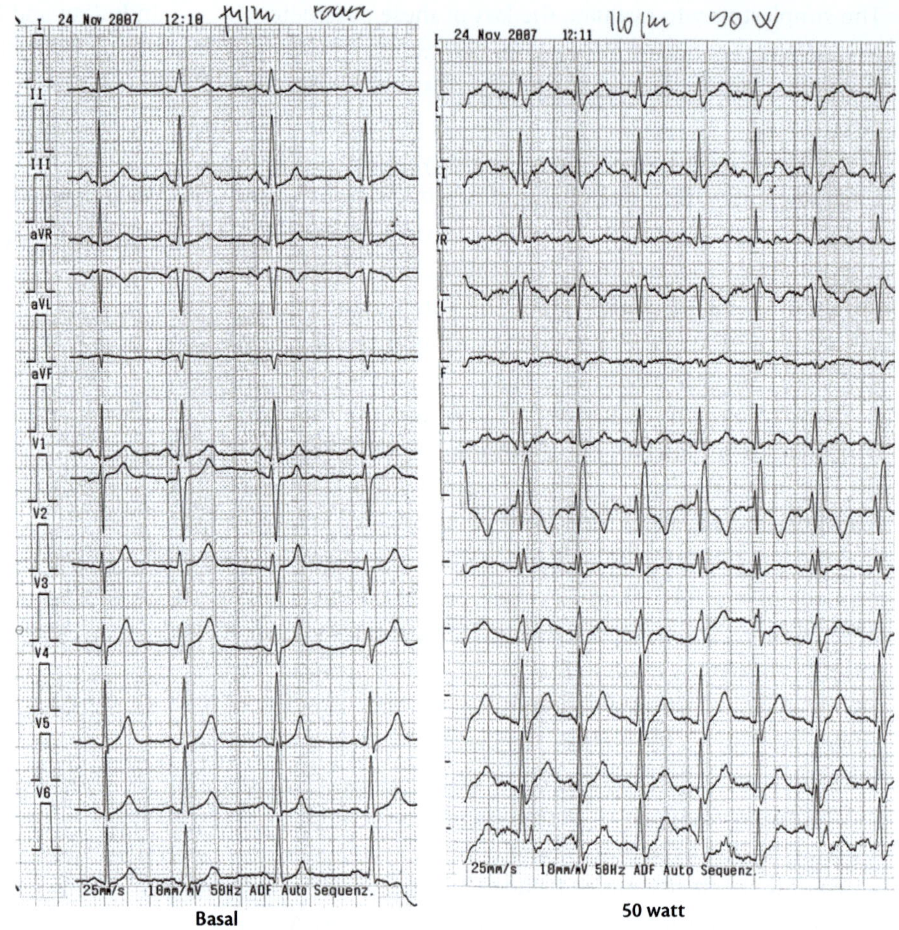

Fig. 5.4.4 Male, 30 years: soccer player; no heart disease; asymptomatic; during effort presents a tachycardia-dependent RBBB. After six months developed a stable RBBB

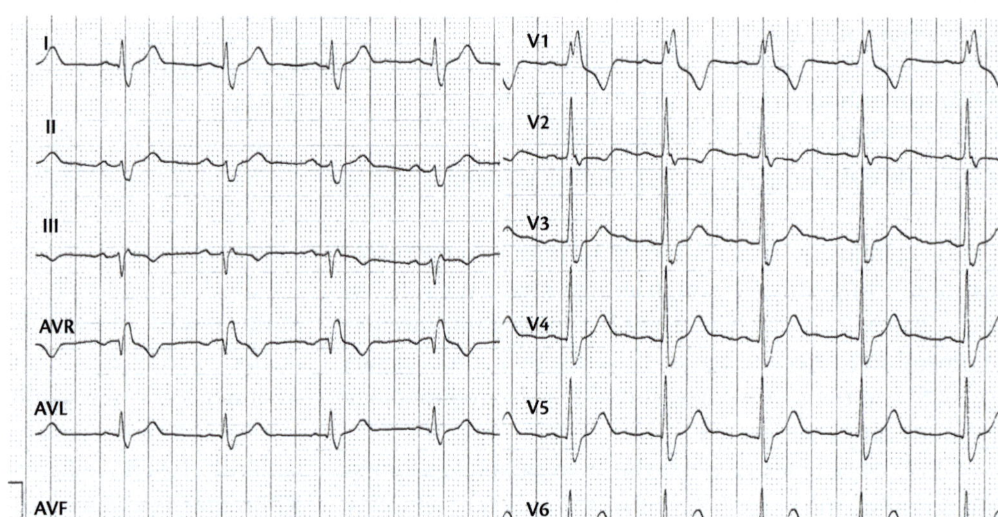

Fig. 5.4.5 Male, 40 years: skindiver; asymptomatic; no heart disease. RBBB + LAH discovered during cardiovascular screening.

In the absence of organic heart disease, conduction abnormalities may be related to familial genetic diseases involving ion channels (Lenègre disease) (➲ Fig. 5.4.7). A number of studies have demonstrated that Lenègre disease may be due to mutations of genes encoding SCN5A or modulating (SCN10A, SCN1B-SCN4B) Na^+ channels [45–48]. A defect in these genes can also be found in Brugada syndrome and LQTS [47,49].

It has been demonstrated that in families with a defective SCN5A gene some members are affected by Brugada

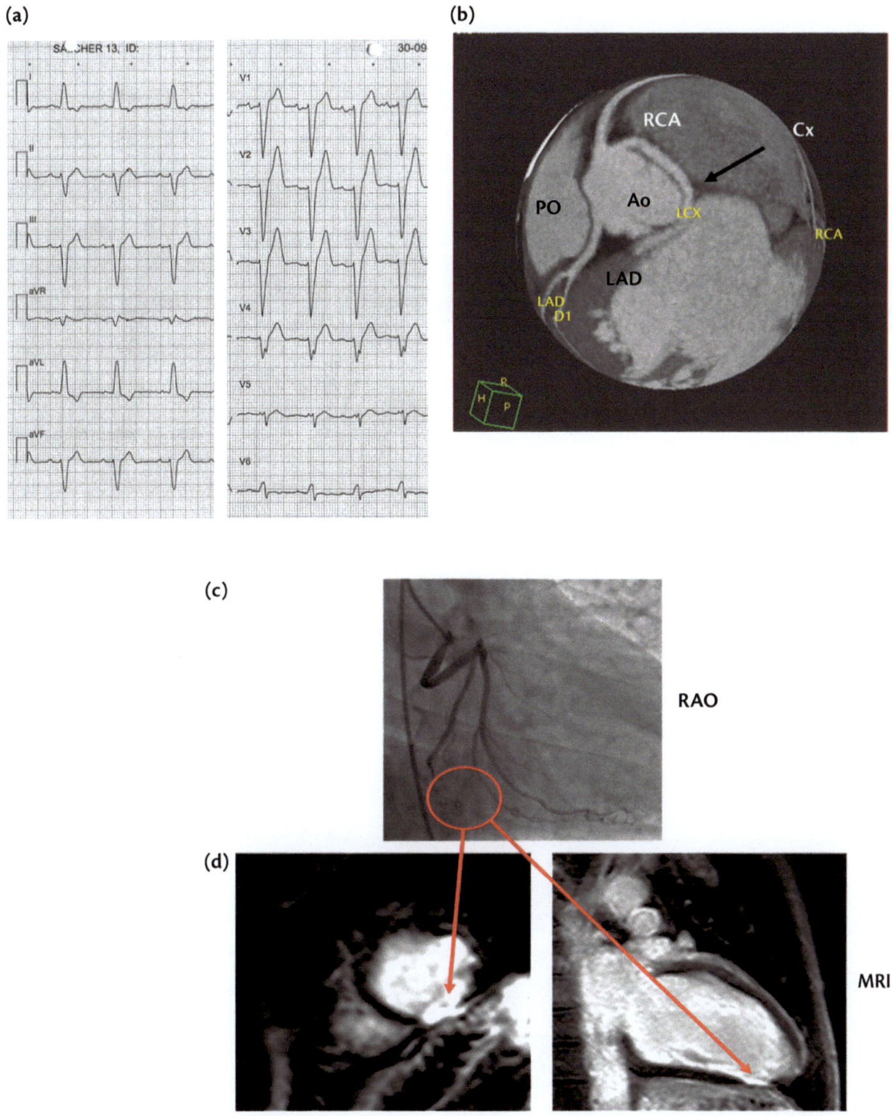

Fig. 5.4.6 (a) Male, 22 years; professional soccer player; asymptomatic. LBBB discovered by chance. Coronary CT angiography showed an anomalous origin of left circumflex from right coronary sinus. (b) Same case as in (a). Coronary angiography (RAO) (c) confirms that the left circumflex artery arises from the right coronary sinus and has a narrow angle in the first part. MRI after gadolinium shows a late enhancement in the posterolateral left ventricle (d).

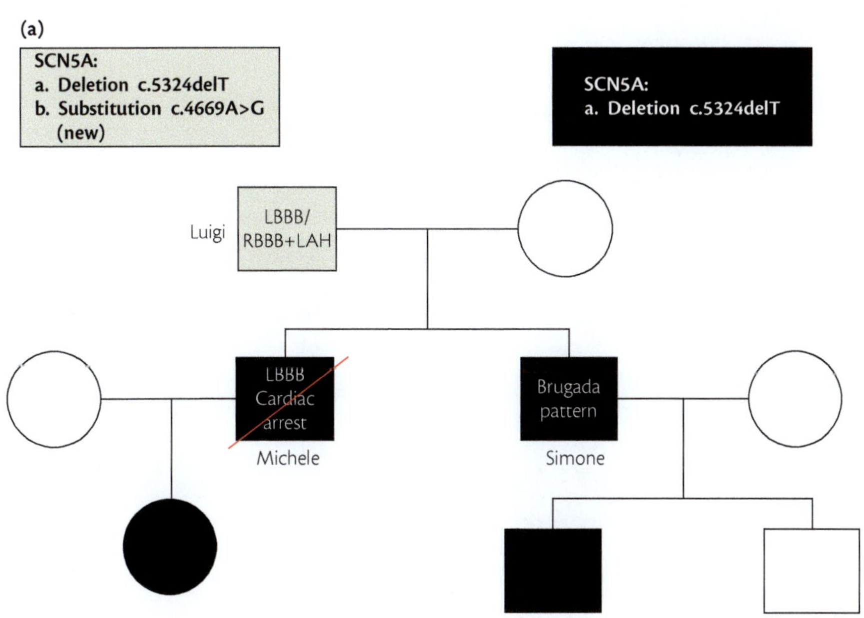

Fig. 5.4.7 (a) Pedigree of family S. Black shading, males and females with a single mutation of the SCN5A gene; grey shading subject with two mutations. Simone (aged 37) has a typical Brugda type 1 ECG pattern induced by flecainide. Michele has an LBBB and suffered resuscitated cardiac arrest at age 34 years. Their father, Luigi, has had an LBBB since the age of 30. At age 65 he developed bilateral BBB and had a pacemaker implantation.

(b)

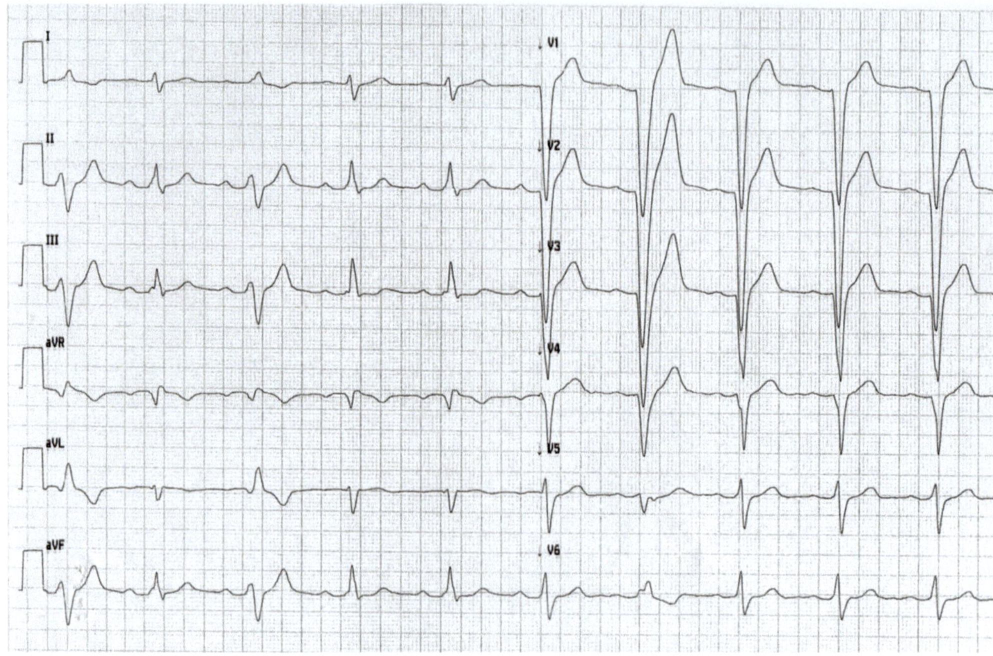

(c)

A

B

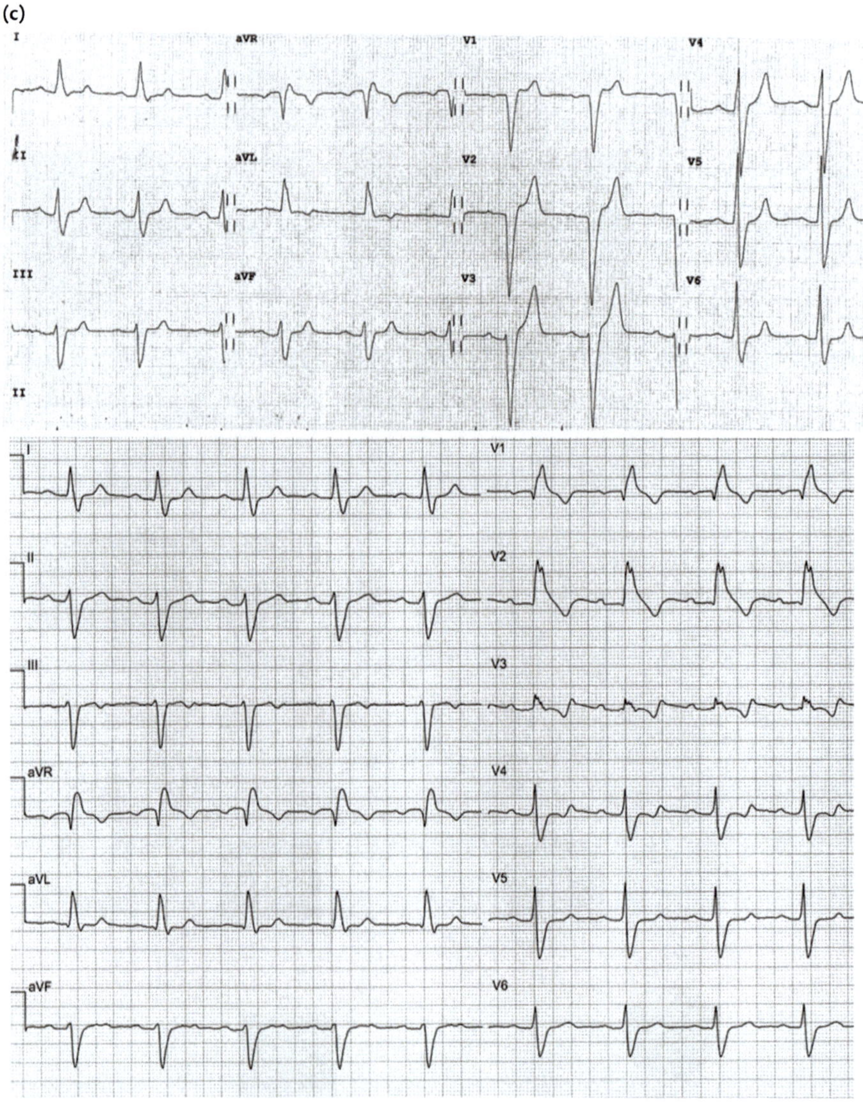

Fig. 5.4.7 ***(Continued)***

(b) ECG for Michele showing the LBBB with alternating left axis deviation. (c) ECGs for Luigi at (A) age 30 showing an LBBB, and (B) age 65 showing RBBB + LAH. Because of the bilateral branch conduction defects a pacemaker was implanted.

syndrome and others by Lenègre disease [50]. In addition, patients with a defect of SCN5A may have Brugada syndrome alone or associated with conduction defects [51]. Therefore when a subject with rare conduction abnormalities is discovered, familial screening should be performed.

The prognostic significance of fascicular conduction defects in the young in the absence of heart disease is not clearly established. In Lenègre disease the conduction defect may worsen, degenerating to an advanced AV block in the elderly [45].

Recommendations for competitive sport in asymptomatic athletes with conduction abnormalities

In Italian [38–40], European [41,42], and US [43] guidelines, asymptomatic subjects, in the absence of heart disease, are eligible to participate in any sport under the following conditions: first- or second-degree AV block when AV conduction normalizes during effort and when pauses during Holter monitoring are <3s.

In more recent Italian guidelines [39], asymptomatic subjects with RBBB, LAH, LPH, and LBBB can participate in all sports in the absence of heart diseases, including genetic disease, such as Lenègre disease, and without episodes of AV block.

In US guidelines [43] asymptomatic subjects with LBBB can participate in all sports in the absence of episodes of AV block in Holter monitoring. (See also Chapter 7.1.)

Further reading

Biffi A, Delise P, Zeppilli P., et al. Italian cardiological guidelines for sports eligibility in athletes with heart disease. Part 2. *J Cardiovasc Med* 2013; 14: 500–15.

Delise P, Sciarra L. Asymptomatic Wolff-Parkinson-White: what to do? Extensive ablation or not. *J Cardiovasc Med* 2007; 8: 668–74.

Goudevenos JA, Katsouras CS, Graekas G, et al. Ventricular pre-excitation in the general population: a study on the mode of presentation and clinical course. *Heart* 2000; 83: 29–34.

Pelliccia A, Culasso F, Di Paolo FM, et al. Prevalence of abnormal electrograms in a large, uselected population undergoing pre-participation cardiovascular screening. *Eur Heart J* 2007; 28: 2006–10.

Zipes D, Link MS, Ackermn MJ, et al. Elegibility and disqualification recommendations for competitive athletes with cardiovascular abnormalities:Task Force 9: Arrhythmias and Conduction Defects. *Circulation* 2015; 132: e315–25.

References

1. Pelliccia A, Culasso F, Di Paolo FM., et al. Prevalence of abnormal electrograms in a large, unselected population undergoing pre-participation cardiovascular screening. *Eur Heart J* 2007; 28: 2006–10
2. Delise P. *Sport e Aritmie*.Rome: CESI, 2011.
3. Giardina AC, Ehlers KH, Engle MA. Wolff-Parkinson-White syndrome in infants and children. *Br Heart J* 1972; 34: 839–46.
4. Deal B, Keane J, Gillette P, Garson A. Wolff-Parkinson-White syndrome and supraventricular tachycardia during infancy: management and follow up. *J Am Coll Cardiol* 1985; 5: 130–5.
5. Becquart J, Vaksmann G, Becquart U, Dupuis C. Long term follow up of Wolff-Parkinson-White syndrome discovered in infancy. *Arch Mal Coeur Vaiss* 1988; 81: 695–700.
6. Guize L, Soria R, Chaouat JC, et al. Prevalence and course of Wolff-Parkinson-White syndrome in a population of 138048 subjects. *Ann Med Intern (Paris)* 1985; 136: 474–8.
7. Durrer D, Schoo L, Schuilenburg RM, Wellens HJ. The role of premature beats in the initiation and the termination of supraventricular tachycardia in the Wolff-Parkinson-White syndrome. *Circulation* 1967; 34: 644–56.
8. Wellens HJ, Durrer D. Wolff-Parkinson-White syndrome and atrial fibrillation. *Am J Cardiol* 1974; 34: 777–83.
9. Campbell RW, Smith RA, Gallagher JJ, et al. Atrial fibrillation in the preexcitation syndrome. *Am J Cardiol* 1977; 40: 514–20.
10. Bauernfeind RA, Wyndham CR, Swiryn SP, et al. Paroxysmal atrial fibrillation in the Wolff-Parkinson-White syndrome. *Am J Cardiol* 1981; 47: 562–9.
11. Morady F, Sledge C, Shen E, et al. Electrophysiologic testing in the management of patients with the Wolff-Parkinson-White syndrome and atrial fibrillation. *Am J Cardiol* 1983; 51: 1623–9.
12. Waspe L, Brodman R, Kim S, Fisher J. Susceptibility to atrial fibrillation and ventricular tachyarrhythmias in the Wolff-Parkinson-White syndrome: role of the accessory pathway. *Am Heart J* 1986; 112: 1141–52.
13. Delise P, D'Este D, Bonso A, et al. Different degrees of risk of high-frequency atrial fibrillation in symptomatic and asymptomatic WPW syndrome: electrophysiologic evaluation. *G Ital Cardiol* 1987; 17: 127–33.
14. Delise P, Bonso A, D'Este D, et al. Prognostic value of the electrophysiologic evaluation of atrial vulnerability in the WPW syndrome. *Eur Heart J* 1989; 10: 397.
15. Dreifus LS, Haiat R, Watanabe Y, et al. Ventricular fibrillation: a possible mechanism of sudden death in patients with Wolff-Parkinson-White syndrome. *Circulation* 1971; 43: 520–7.
16. Klein GJ, Bashore TM, Sellers TD, et al. Ventricular fibrillation in the Wolff-Parkinson-White syndrome. *N Engl J Med* 1979; 301: 1080–5.
17. Montoya PT, Brugada P, Smeets JC et al. Ventricular fibrillation in the Wolff-Parkinson-White syndrome. *Eur Heart J* 1991; 12: 144–50.
18. Soria R, Guize L, Chretien JM, et al. The natural history of 270 cases of Wolff-Parkinson-White syndrome in a survey of the general population. *Arch Mal Coeur Vaiss* 1989; 82: 331–6.
19. Munger TM, Packer DL, Hammill SC, et al. A population study of the natural history of Wolff-Parkinson-White syndrome in Olmsted County, Minnesota, 1953–1989. *Circulation* 1993; 87: 866–73.
20. Delise P, Sciarra L. Asymptomatic Wolff-Parkinson-White: what to do? Extensive ablation or not. *J Cardiovasc Med* 2007; 8: 668–74
21. Milstein S, Sharma AD, Klein GJ. Electrophysiologic profile of asymptomatic Wolff-Parkinson-White pattern. *Am J Cardiol* 1986; 57: 1097–1103.

22. Satoh M, Aizawa Y, Funazaki T, et al. Electrophysiologic evaluation of asymptomatic patients with the Wolff-Parkinson-White pattern. *Pacing Clin Electrophysiol* 1989; 12: 413–20.
23. Leitch JW, Klein GJ, Yee R, Murdock C. Prognostic value of electrophysiology testing in asymptomatic patients with Wolff-Parkinson-White pattern. *Circulation* 1990; 82: 1718–23.
24. Bertaglia E, Delise P, Coro L, et al. Valore prognostico della valutazione elettrofisiologica poliparametrica in giovani sportivi asintomatici con sindrome di Wolff-Parkinson-White. *Int J Sports Cardiol* 1998; 7: 29–34.
25. Timmermans C, Smeets JL, Rodriguez LM, et al. Aborted sudden death in the Wolff-Parkinson-White syndrome. *Am J Cardiol* 1995; 76: 492–4.
26. Smith RF. The Wolff-Parkinson-White syndrome as an aviation risk. *Circulation* 1964; 29: 672–9.
27. Fukatani M, Tanigawa M, Mori M, et al. Prediction of a fatal atrial fibrillation in patients with asymptomatic Wolff-Parkinson-White pattern. *Jpn Circ J* 1990; 54: 1331–9.
28. Beckman KJ, Gallastegui JL, Bauman JL, Hariman RJ. The predictive value of electrophysiologic studies in untreated patients with Wolff-Parkinson-White syndrome. *J Am Coll Cardiol* 1990; 15: 640–7.
29. Brembilla-Perrot B, Ghawi R. Electrophysiological characteristics of asymptomatic Wolff-Parkinson-White syndrome. *Eur Heart J* 1993; 14: 511–15.
30. Goudevenos JA, Katsouras CS, Graekas G, et al. Ventricular pre-excitation in the general population: a study on the mode of presentation and clinical course. *Heart* 2000; 83: 29–34.
31. Fitzsimmons PJ, McWhirter PD, Peterson DW, Kruyer WB. The natural history of Wolff-Parkinson-White syndrome in 228 military aviators: a long-term follow-up of 22 years. *Am Heart J* 2001; 142: 530–6.
32. Obeyesekere MN, Leong-Sit P, Massel D, et al. Risk of arrhythmias and sudden death in patients with asymptomatic preexcitation: a meta-analysis. *Circulation* 2012; 2308–15.
33. Pappone C, Santinelli V, Rosanio S, et al. Usefulness of invasive electrophysiologic testing to stratify the risk of arrhythmic events in asymptomatic patients with Wolff-Parkinson-White pattern: results from a large prospective long-term follow-up study. *J Am Coll Cardiol* 2003; 41: 239–44.
34. Pappone C, Santinelli V, Manguso F, et al. A randomized study of prophylactic catheter ablation in asymptomatic patients with the Wolff-Parkinson-White syndrome. *N Engl J Med* 2003; 349: 1803–11.
35. Vergara G, Delise P. Wolff-Parkinson-White syndrome. *G Ital Cardiol* 1989; 19: 234–44.
36. Sharma AD, Yee R, Guiraudon G, Klein GJ. Sensitivity and specificity of invasive and noninvasive testing for risk of sudden death in Wolff-Parkinson-White syndrome. *J Am Coll Cardiol* 1987; 10: 373–81.
37. Bromberg BI, Lindsay BD, Cain ME, Cox JL. Impact of clinical history and electrophysiologic characterization of accessory pathways on management strategies to reduce sudden death among children with Wolff-Parkinson-White syndrome. *J Am Coll Cardiol* 1996; 27: 690–5.
38. Delise P, Guiducci U, Zeppilli P, et al. Cardiological guidelines for competitive sports elegibility. *Ital Heart J* 2005; 6: 661–702.
39. Biffi A, Delise P, Zeppilli P, et al. Italian cardiological guidelines for sports eligibility in athletes with heart disease. Part 1. *J Cardiovasc Med* 2013; 14: 477–99.
40. Biffi A, Delise P, Zeppilli P, et al. Italian cardiological guidelines for sports eligibility in athletes with heart disease. Part 2. *J Cardiovasc Med* 2013; 14: 500–15
41. Pelliccia A, Fagard R, Bjornstad, et al. Recommendations for competitive sports participation in athletes with cardiovascular disease. *Eur Heart J* 2005; 26: 1422–45.
42. Heidbüchel H, Panhuyzen-Goedkop N, Corrado D, et al. Recommendations for participation in leasure-time physical activity and competitive sports in patients with arrhythmias and potentially arrhythmogenic conditions. Part I: Supraventricular arrhythmias and pacemaker. *Eur J Cardiovasc Prev Rehabil* 2006; 13: 475–84.
43. Zipes D, Link MS, Ackerman MJ, et al. Eligibility nd disqualification recommendations for competitive athletes with cardiovascular abnormalities:Task Force 9: Arrhythmias and conduction defects. *Circulation* 2105; 132: e315–25.
44. Vergara G, Furlanello F, Disertori M, et al. Induction of supraventricular tachyarrhythmias at rest and during exercise with transesophageal atrial pacing in the electrophysiological evaluation of asymptomatic athletes with Wolff-Parkinson-White syndrome. *Eur Heart J* 1988; 9: 1119–25.
45. Probst V, Kyndt F, Potet F, et al. Haploinsufficiency in combination with aging causes SCN5A-linked hereditary Lenègre disease. *J Am Coll Cardiol* 2003; 41: 643–52.
46. Wilde A, Brugada R. Phenotypical manifestations of mutations in the genes encoding subunits of the cardiac sodium channel. *Circ Res* 2011; 108: 884–7.
47. Zumhagen S, Veldkamp MV, Stallmeyer B, et al. A Heterozygous deletion mutation in the cardiac channel gene SCN5A with loss-and gain-of-function characteristics manifests as isolated conduction disease, without signs of Brugada or long QT syndrome. *PLoS One* 2013; 8: e67963
48. Probst V, Alloui M, Sacher F, et al. Progressive cardiac conduction defect is the prevailing phenotype in carriers of a Brugada syndrome SCN5A mutation. *J Cardiovasc Electrophysiol* 2006; 17: 270–5.
49. Saber S, Amarouch MY, Fazelifar AF, et al. Complex genetic background in a large family with Brugada syndrome. *Physiol Rep* 2015: 3; e12256.
50. Kyndt F, Probst V, Potet F, et al. Novel SCN5A mutation leading either to isolated cardiac conduction defect or Brugada syndrome in a large French family. *Circulation* 2001; 104: 30181–6.
51. Maury P, Rollin A, Sacher F, et al. Prevalence and prognostic role of various conduction disturbances in patients with the Brugada syndrome. *Am J Cardiol* 2013; 112: 1384–9.

SECTION 6

Sudden cardiac death in athletes

6.1 Incidence of sudden cardiac death in athletes *299*
Jonathan A. Drezner and Kimberly G. Harmon

6.2 Cardiovascular causes of sudden death in athletes *309*
Cristina Basso, Stefania Rizzo, and Gaetano Thiene

6.3 The risk, aetiology, clinical features, management, and prevention of exercise-related sudden cardiac death and acute cardiac events in adult athletes *321*
Paul D. Thompson

6.4 Less frequent causes of sudden cardiac death *328*

6.4.1 Less frequent causes of SCD (commotio cordis): non-cardiac causes (drug abuse, hyperpyrexia, rhabdomyolysis, sickle cell anaemia)— Part 1 *328*
Erik Ekker Solberg and Paolo Emilio Adami

6.4.2 Less frequent causes of SCD (aortic rupture): non-cardiac causes (asthma, extreme environmental conditions (heat, cold, altitude))—Part 2 *332*
Erik Ekker Solberg and Paolo Emilio Adami

6.5 Pre-participation screening of young competitive athletes *339*
Domenico Corrado and Alessandro Zorzi

6.6 Cardiovascular screening of adult/senior competitive athletes *352*
Luc Vanhees and Mats Börjesson

6.7 Cardiovascular screening of children and adolescent athletes (<14 years) *359*
Massimo Chessa, Werner Budts, and Javier Fernandez Sarabia

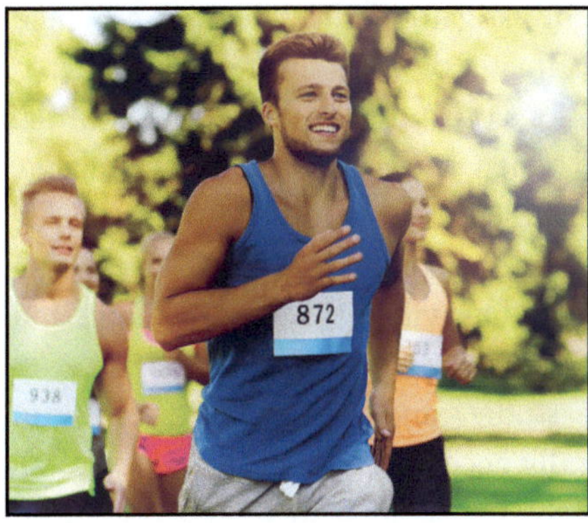

6.1

Incidence of sudden cardiac death in athletes

Jonathan A. Drezner and Kimberly G. Harmon

Introduction

Sudden cardiac arrest (SCA) is the leading cause of sudden death in young athletes (<35 years) during sports and exercise [1–3]. Current estimates of the incidence of sudden cardiac death (SCD) in athletes range from almost 1 in a million [4] to 1 in 23,000 [5] athletes per year, while some specific athlete populations are reported at even higher risk (1 in 3000) [1]. Differences in current estimates are largely due to inconsistent methodology and heterogeneous population comparisons.

Sudden cardiac arrest and death (SCA/D) is often caused by a genetic, structural, or electrical cardiac disorder [2,3,6–9], although autopsy-negative sudden unexplained death is reported on post-mortem examination in up to 44% of presumed SCA/D cases [2,7–11). The prevalence of cardiac conditions associated with SCA/D in young athletes is approximately 0.3%, which is supported by studies using non-invasive evaluation tools to identify cardiac disorders at elevated risk in young athletes [12–20]. In athletes with predisposing conditions, exercise can unmask occult cardiac disease to precipitate SCA [21]. Importantly, not all athletes with a condition associated with SCA will go on to have a cardiovascular event, but the tragic impact of SCD in young athletes has led to intense debate regarding the most effective screening programmes.

A precise understanding of the frequency of these catastrophic events is needed to fully assess the need for and required rigour of potential prevention strategies. This chapter reviews the incidence of SCD in athletes and examines the impact of study methodology and differences based on gender, race, sport, and geographic region.

Impact of study methodology

Estimates of the rate of SCA/D in athletes vary widely and are greatly affected by study methodology. To correctly calculate the incidence of SCA/D requires an accurate means of case identification (numerator) and an exact estimate of the athlete population being studied (denominator). Because reporting of SCA/D in athletes is not obligatory in most countries, many incidence studies risk under-estimating the true incidence because of incomplete case ascertainment. For instance, studies using media reports as their main source of case capture identify only 5–56% of SCD cases, even in high profile competitive athletes [1,8,22,23]. Use of catastrophic insurance claims performs even more poorly. In one study, use of catastrophic insurance claims as the only method for case identification missed 83% of SCD cases and 92% of all SCA/D cases in Minnesota high school athletes [24,25] Thus, when evaluating incidence estimates, one must assess the thoroughness of the methods used for case identification.

The denominator used in incidence calculations has an equally important role in producing accurate estimates. The athlete population being studied needs to be precisely defined, ideally with tabulated individual athlete data and demographics that is updated each year of the study. Investigations using census population statistics, cross-sectional surveys, or self-reported athlete participation data, or that extrapolate athlete population statistics from a single year across a wide study period, all contribute to inaccuracies and less reliable calculations.

Other athlete population parameters also need to be well defined to best interpret study results. Does the study include all cases of SCA/D (survivors plus deaths) or only cases that result in death? Does the study include all cases of SCA/D at any time (i.e. during exercise, rest, and sleep) or only those that occur during exercise and sport? As an example, one study with methodological limitations included only cases that occurred on a school campus during formal sports participation and were reported in a school insurance claim [24] These limitations led to a substantial under-estimate of the true incidence of SCA/D in the study population [25]. Studies indicate that 56–80% of SCA/D in young athletes occurs during exercise, with the remainder considered non-exertional [2,3,26].

Age is also a significant variable influencing SCA/D incidence calculations. Young pre-adolescent athletes may not manifest genetic cardiac disorders until physical maturation or young adulthood. Thus, both the risk and incidence of SCA/D may be different in young athletes aged 12–18 years than in those aged 18–24 years. In addition, it is well established that the risk of atherosclerotic coronary artery disease (CAD) increases considerably above the age of 30–35 years [23,27] Thus, studies that span a wide age range and include older athletes may mis-estimate the risk in younger athlete groups. For example, one study from Israel used a retrospective search of two newspapers over a 24-year time frame to evaluate the impact of a national screening programme [28]. The study methodology was fatally flawed in both the accuracy of case ascertainment and the inclusion of a wide age range from 12 to 44 years [29]. Even though the study did not provide reliable conclusions, it still reported a relatively high incidence of SCD because the older age range was included. Therefore a narrow age range will provide the most accurate incidence estimates for specific athlete populations. However, most studies have a broad age range and variable methodology, making interpretation and comparisons difficult.

Incidence of SCD in athletes

The first estimates of SCD incidence emerged in the 1990s (see ➲ Table 6.1.1). Initial studies using newspaper clippings and search of media reports approximated the risk of SCD in athletes at 1 in 200,000 athletes per year [30,31]. More recent studies and a closer examination of methodologies have challenged this estimate as too low [1,2,26,32,33] In a 10-year examination of SCD in US college athletes using multiple data sources for case identification and precise student-athlete population statistics, investigators reported an overall risk of SCD of 1 in 54,000 [2]. Males were at higher risk than females (1 in 38,000 versus 1 in 122,000), and black athletes were at higher risk than Caucasian athletes (1 in 21,000 versus 1 in 68,000) [2]. In this study, male basketball players had the highest annual risk of SCD (1 in 9,000), and the risk in male black basketball players was 1 in 5,300 [2]. The higher risk of SCD in male, black, and basketball athletes has been corroborated in a second independent study examining SCD in US college athletes [26].

Unfortunately, the low event rate (1 in 200,000) first reported has been perpetuated in the sports cardiology community by some investigators who have not accepted more contemporary estimates or not thoroughly considered the impact and limitations of study methodology on initial estimates [34]. Indeed, when one considers that the relative risk of SCD in specific athlete populations is up to 19 times higher than the risk in other athlete groups, it seems that this differential risk should heavily influence the choice and intensity of the prevention strategies employed [35].

Based on available studies and a systematic review of the literature, a generally accepted annual incidence of all SCA/D is approximately 1 in 80,000 in high-school-aged athletes and 1 in 50,000 in college-aged athletes [36]. Limited estimates are available for youth and professional athletes.

Impact of gender, race, and sport

Evidence clearly supports the contention that athletes display a differential risk for SCA/D based on gender, race, sport, and level of play [1,2,24–26,30,31,37–39] (see ➲ Table 6.1.1). Incidence rates are consistently higher in males than in females, with a relative risk ranging from 3:1 to 9:1 (male:female) [2,14,21,25,30,31,38]. Black college athletes from all sports have a reported SCD risk 3.2 times that of their Caucasian peers [2]. Robust data from independent datasets further supports the observation that some athlete groups have a substantially higher risk than others [2,26]. In the USA, male black college basketball players have the highest reported risk of SCD at 1 in 5,300 per year, and male college basketball players of any race or division have the highest risk compared with all other sports (1 in 9,000 per year) [2]. Studies in the USA consistently report that two sports alone, male basketball and American football, account for 50–61% of all identified cases of SCA/D [2,3,26] The reasons for these differences based on gender, race, and sport are not well understood and require additional study.

Geographic differences

Limited data are available to suggest that there are major geographical differences in the incidence of SCA/D in athletes that are not accounted for by differences in race or study methodology. A 25-year prospective study from the Veneto region of Italy, utilizing a mandatory reporting system of SCD, found an overall incidence of 1 in 25,000 athletes per year (ages 12–35) before implementation of a national screening programme [14]. In Israel, an overall incidence of 1 in 38,000 was reported, although this study had limited means of case identification and a wide age range (12–44 years) [28]. In Denmark, a retrospective review of death certificates reported a lower rate of sports-related SCD of

Table 6.1.1 Incidence of sudden cardiac arrest and death in athletes

Study	Study design and population	Case identification	Denominator	Exertional SCD or all SCD?	SCD or all SCA/D?	Study years	Age range (years) No. of cases	Annual incidence
Van Camp et al. 1996 [30]	Retrospective cohort: high school and college athletes	National Center for Catastrophic Sports Injury Research and media reports	Data from NCAA, NFHS, NAIA, and NJCAA, added together with conversion factor (1.9 for high school and 1.2 for college) used to account for multisport athletes 'based on discussions with representatives from the national organizations'	Exertional	SCD	1983–93	13–24; N = 160	**College + high school** Overall 1:188,000 Male 1:134,000 Female 1:752,000 **High school** Overall 1:213,000 Male 1:152,000 Female 1:861,000 **College** Overall 1:94,000 Male 1:69,000 Female 1:356,000
Maron et al. 1998 [31]	Retrospective cohort: Minnesota high school athletes	Catastrophic insurance claims	Minnesota State High School League (estimated using conversion factor of 2.3 to account for multisport athletes)	Exertional only during school-sponsored sport	SCD	1985–97	16–17; N = 3	**High school** Overall 1:217,000 Male 1:129,000 Female: 0
Corrado et al. 2003 [6]	Prospective cohort: athletes and non-athletes in the Veneto Region of Italy	Mandatory reporting of sudden death	Registered athletes in the Sports Medicine Database of the Veneto Region of Italy and the Italian Census Bureau	All	SCD	1979–99	12–35; N = 51 12–35; N = 208	**Athletes** Overall 1:47,000 Male 1:41,000 Female 1:93,000 **Non-athletes** Overall 1:143,000
Drezner 2005 [50]	Retrospective survey: college athletes	Survey of NCAA Division I institutions (244/326 responded)	Reported number of athletes	All	SCD	—	N=5	**College** Overall 1:67,000
Corrado et al. 2006 [14]	Prospective cohort: athletes and non-athletes in the Veneto Region of Italy	Mandatory reporting to the Registry of Juvenile Sudden Death	Registered athletes in the Sports Medicine Database of the Veneto Region of Italy and the Italian Census Bureau	All	SCD	1979–2004	12–35; N = 55 12–35; N=265	**Athletes** 1:24,000 (pre-screen) 1:233,000 (post-screen) **Non-athletes** 1:127,000 (unscreened)
Maron et al. 2009 [3]	Retrospective cohort; amateur and competitive athletes	US Registry for Sudden Death in Athletes	An estimated 10.7 million participants per year ≤39 years of age in all organized amateur and competitive sports	All	SCA + SCD	1980–2006	8–39; N = 1046	**Athletes** 1:164,000

Table 6.1.1 Incidence of sudden cardiac arrest and death in athletes *(Continued)*

Drezner et al. 2009 [5]	Cross-sectional survey: high school athletes	Survey of 1710 high schools with AEDs	Reported number of student athletes	All cases occurring on campus	SCA + SCD	2006–7	14–17; N = 14	**High school** 1:23,000 (SCA + SCD) 1:64,000 (SCD)
Holst et al. 2010 [8]	Retrospective cohort: athletes and general population in Denmark	Review of death certificates, Cause of Death Registry, and National Patient Registry in Denmark	Interview data of people age 16–35 years from the National Danish Health and Morbidity Study	Sports-related SCD in athletes versus all SCD in the general population	SCD	2000–6	12–35; N = 15 12–35; N = 428	**Athletes** 1:83,000 **General population** 1:27,000
Marijon et al. 2011 [48]	Prospective cohort: general population in France	Data from emergency medical system	General population statistics, data from the Ministry of Health and Sport to estimate young competitive athlete population	Sports-related SCA or SCD with moderate or vigorous exercise	SCA + SCD	2005–10	10–75; N = 820 10–35; N = 50	**General population** 1:217,000 **Young competitive athlete** 1:102,000 **Young non-competitive athlete** 1:455,000
Steinvil et al. 2011 [28]	Retrospective cohort: athletes in Israel	Retrospective review of two Israeli newspapers	Competitive athletes registered in the Israel Sport Authority in 2009; extrapolated these data for previous 24 years based on the growth of the Israeli population (age 10–40) from the Central Bureau of Statistics; allowed for a presumed doubling of the sporting population aged over 24 years	All	SCD	1985–2009	12–44; N = 24	**Athletes** 1:38,000
Harmon et al. 2011 [1]	Retrospective cohort: college athletes	Parent Heart Watch database, NCAA resolutions list, catastrophic insurance claims	Participation data from the NCAA	All	SCD	2004–8	18–26; N = 37	**College** Overall 1:43,000 Male 1:33,000 Female 1:76,000 Black 1:17,000 White 1:58,000 Male, black 1:13,000 Male, basketball 1:7000 Male, Div. I basketball 1:3,000

Table 6.1.1 Incidence of sudden cardiac arrest and death in athletes *(Continued)*

Maron et al. (2013) [37]	Retrospective cohort: Minnesota high school athletes	US Registry for Sudden Death in Athletes	Minnesota State High School League statistics (estimated using conversion factor of 2.3 to account for multisport athletes)	All	SCD	1986–2011	12–18; N = 13	**High school** Overall 1:150,000 Male 1:83,000 Female 0
Roberts and Stovitz 2013 [24]	Retrospective cohort: Minnesota high school athletes	Catastrophic insurance claims	Minnesota State High School League statistics (sum of unduplicated athletes 1993–4 to 2011–12 school years)	Exertional only during school-sponsored sport	SCD	1993–2012	12–19; N = 4	**High school** 1:417,000 (1993–2012) 1:909,000 (2003–12) Female 0
Maron et al. 2014 [26]	Retrospective cohort: college athletes	US Registry for Sudden Death in Athletes and NCAA resolutions list	Participation data from the NCAA	All	SCD	2002–11	17–26; N = 64	**College** Overall 1:63,000 Male 1:56,000 Female 1:333,000 Black 1:26,000 White 1:143,000
Toresdahl et al. 2014 [38]	Prospective observational: high school students and student athletes	2149 high schools monitored for SCA events on school campus	Reported number of students and student athletes	All cases occurring on school campus	SCA + SCD	2009–11	14–18; N = 44	**Student-athlete** Overall 1:88,000 Male 1:58,000 Female 1:323,000 **Student non-athlete** Overall 1:326,000 Male 1:286,000 Female 1:357,000
Drezner et al. 2014 [25]	Retrospective cohort: Minnesota high school athletes	Public media reports	Minnesota State High School League statistics (sum of unduplicated athletes 2003–4 to 2011–12 school years)	All	SCA + SCD	2003–12	14–18; N = 13	**High School** Overall 1:71,000 Female 0 Male, basketball 1:21,000
Harmon et al. 2014 [39]	USA	Public media reports	Participation data from the NFHS	All	SCA + SCD	2007–13	14–18; N = 109	**High school** Overall 1:67,000 Male 1:45,000 Female 1:238,000 Male, basketball 1:37,000
Risgaard et al. 2014 [23]	Retrospective cohort: competitive and non-competitive athletes in Denmark	Review of death certificates and the Danish National Patient Registry	Competitive and non-competitive athlete populations in Denmark estimated based on survey data from the Danish National Institute of Public Health	Sports-related SCD in competitive versus non-competitive athletes	SCD	2007–9	12–35; N = 44	**Competitive athlete** 1:213,000 **Non-competitive athlete** 1:233,000

Table 6.1.1 Incidence of sudden cardiac arrest and death in athletes *(Continued)*

Harmon et al. 2015 [2]	Retrospective cohort: athletes	Parent Heart Watch database, NCAA resolutions list, catastrophic insurance claims	Participation data from the NCAA	All	SCD	2003–13	17–26; N = 79	**College** Overall 1:53,000 Male 1:38,000 Female 1:122,000 Black 1:21,000 White 1:68,000 Football 1:36,000 Male, soccer 1:24,000 Male, black 1:16,000 Male, basketball 1:9,000 Male, black, basketball 1:5,300 Male, Div. I basketball 1:5,200
Bohm et al. 2016 [41]	Prospective cohort: sports-related SCD in all persons in Germany	Voluntary reporting to German National Registry, web-based media search, regional institutes	Physical activity estimated from the German Health Update study and extrapolated to population data from the German Federal Statistical Office	Sports-related SCD	SCD	2012–14	10–79; N = 144	**Sports participants** 1:1,200,000
Maron et al. 2016 [47]	Retrospective cohort	Records of the Medical Examiner	Data from the Minnesota Department of Education, National Center for Education Statistics, and the Minnesota State High School League for Hennepin County, Minnesota	All	SCD	2000–14	14–23; N = 27	**Non-athlete** 1:39,000 **Athlete** 1:121,000

1 in 83,000 in persons aged 12–35 years [8]. This study and other reports from Minnesota, which has a large population of Scandinavian descent, have suggested that the risk of SCD may be lower within this geographic region [37,40] In Germany, a population-based prospective nationwide registry of sports-related SCD, with voluntary reporting of cases in both recreational and competitive athletes, found the overall incidence of SCD in sports participants aged 18–79 years (average age 47) to be 1 in 1.2 per million per year [41].

Athletes versus other populations

Current epidemiological studies provide a mixed understanding of the comparative risk of SCA/D in athletes versus non-athletes (see Tables 6.1.1 and 6.1.2, and Fig. 6.1.1). In general, the estimated incidence range of SCA/D in the general population of adolescents and young adults overlaps with the estimated incidence range of SCA/D in adolescent and young adult athletes [38,42–46]. One comprehensive prospective study spanned 30 years and reported a SCA/D rate of 1 in 69,000 in 14–24 year olds and 1 in 22,000 in 25-35-year olds in King County, Washington, but did not report the rate of sports-related SCA/D.[45].

Few studies have directly compared the incidence of SCA in a general population of young people versus young athletes. A prospective study monitoring SCA in US high schools found that student athletes were 3.7 times more likely to suffer SCA on school campus than non-athlete peers

Table 6.1.2 Incidence of sudden cardiac arrest and death in the general and active adult populations

Study	Study design and population	Case identification	Denominator	Exertional SCD orall SCD?	SCD or all SCA/D?	Study years	Age range (years) No. of cases	Annual incidence
General population								
Papdakis 2009 [51]	Retrospective cohort, UK	Review of death certificates	Population statistics	All	SCD	2002–5	1–34; *N* = 3409	1:55,000
Atkins et al. 2009 [42]	Prospective population cohort study, USA	EMS database of out-of-hospital cardiac arrest	Population statistics	All	SCA + SCD	2005–7	12–19; *N* = 114	1:27,000
Chugh et al. 2009 [43]	Prospective population based, Oregon, USA	Data from EMS, Medical Examiner, and area hospitals	Population statistics from Multnomah County, Oregon	All	SCA + SCD	2002–5	10–14; *N* = 2	1:59,000
Solberg 2010 [52]	Retrospective cohort, Norway	Norwegian Cause of Death Registry validated with autopsy and medical records	Population statistics	Exertional	SCD	1979–98	15–34; *N* = 23	1:111,000
Margey 2011 [53]	Retrospective cohort, Ireland	Review of death certificates with autopsy confirmation	Population statistics	All	SCD	2005–7	15–35; *N* = 116	Overall 1:35,000 Male 1:20,000 Female 1:77,000
Cooper et al. 2011 [44]	Retrospective cohort, USA	Automated data from four health plans	Computerized healthrecords	All	SCA + SCD	1986–2005	2–24; *N* = 33	1:78,000
Meyer et al. 2012 [45]	Prospective population based; Washington State, USA	EMS cardiac arrest database over 30 years	Population statistics from King County, Washington	All	SCA + SCD	1980-2009	14–35; *N* = 305	Age 14–24 1:69,000 Age 25–35 1:23,000
Pilmer 2013 [54]	Retrospective cohort, Ontario, Canada	Coroner's database	Population statistics	All	SCD	2008	2–40; *N* = 174	1:34,000
Pilmer 2014 [55]	Retrospective cohort, Ontario, Canada	Coroner's database	Population statistics	All	SCD	2005–9	1–19; *N* = 116	1:128,000
Winkle 2014 [56]	Retrospective cohort, Denmark	Review of death certificates, autopsy reports, and health records	Population statistics	All	SCD	2000–6	1–18; *N* = 62	1:90,909
Active adult population: US military and firefighters								
Eckart et al. 2004 [49]	Retrospective cohort, US military recruits	Mandatory reporting of all deaths to Department of Defense Registry with autopsy data	Department of Defense	All	SCD	1977–2001	18–35; *N* = 108	**Military recruits** 1:15,000 (cardiac)1:9000 (cardiac + idiopathic)
Eckart et al. 2011 [27]	Retrospective cohort, US active military personnel	Mandatory reporting of all deaths to Department of Defense Registry with autopsy data	Department of Defense statistics	All	SCD	1998–2008	18–35; *N* = 298	**Military Personnel** **Male** Age <20, 1:30,000 Age 20–24, 1:41,000 Age 25–29, 1:30,000 Age 30–35, 1:25,000 **Female** Age <20, 1:20,000 Age 20–24, 1:92,000 Age 25–29, 1:161,000 Age 30–35, 1:147,000
Farioli et al. 2015 [46]	Retrospective cohort; USA	USA Fire Administration and the National Institute for Occupational Safety and Health Fire Fighter Fatality Investigation and Prevention Program	Current population survey of the number of US career firefighters	All	SCD	1998–2012	18–34; *N* = 14	**Firefighters** Age 18–24, 1:19,000 Age 25–34, 1:26,000

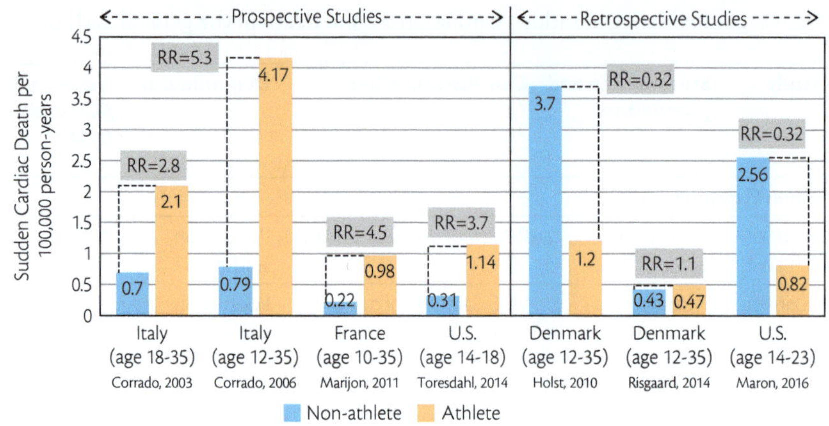

Fig. 6.1.1 Relative risk of sudden cardiac arrest and death in athletes versus non-athletes.

[38]. However, this study did not account for activities off campus, and thus did not allow an absolute risk comparison between groups. In contrast, a retrospective study comparing the risk of SCD in adolescent and young adult athletes versus non-athletes in Hennepin County, Minnesota, found a higher incidence of SCD in non-athletes [47]. This study was limited by population estimates of the athletes and non-athletes at risk and by unclear methodology to confirm if cases participated in an organized sport.

In a prospective cohort study from the Veneto region of Italy, a higher risk of SCD (relative risk 2.8) was found in competitive athletes than in age-matched sedentary controls (age 12–35 years) [6]. In France, a 5-year prospective observational study reported that the relative risk of sudden death was 4.5 times higher in young competitive athletes (age 10–35 years) than in recreational sports participants of the same age [48]. In contrast, investigators from Denmark who performed a retrospective review of death certificates reported a rate of SCD in athletes aged 12–35 years that was 3.3 times lower than that in the general population [8]. A follow-up study from Denmark reported no difference in the rate of sports-related SCD in competitive versus non-competitive athletes aged 12–35 years [23]. However, this study involved a retrospective review of death certificates to establish the numerator and self-reported survey data on athletic participation extrapolated to population census data to establish the denominator; thus the methodology used raises uncertainty in the results. Notably, in this study only 2 of 44 (<5%) cases of sports-related SCD were identified via an extensive media search [23].

It is noteworthy that all prospective studies using similar methodology to monitor cases of SCA/D in both athletes and non-athletes have found the relative risk of SCA/D to be higher in athletes than in non-athletes [6,14,38,48] (➔ Fig. 6.1.1) In contrast, all retrospective studies using a review of death certificates to identify and categorize cases and less reliable methodology to estimate and extrapolate the athlete and non-athlete populations have found athletes to be at lower risk [8,23,47] (➔ Fig. 6.1.1).

Studies in other active young adult populations, such as the US military and firefighters, have demonstrated higher rates of SCD, comparable to rates in college male athletes [27,46,49] (➔ Table 6.1.2) The higher rates in these active young adult populations may be due to the older age range (18–35 years) as well as use of mandatory reporting systems allowing for more precise case capture. The US military employs mandatory reporting of deaths with standard autopsy protocols and has clearly defined denominators. Military personnel undergo regular intense physical training, especially for recruits during basic training (median age 19 years). In a retrospective cohort study of 6.3 million recruit years over 25 years, the rate of SCD in military recruits was 1 in 10,000 [49]. In a follow-up study examining the rate of SCD in active duty military personnel who undergo regular physical activity but not necessarily the intense activity experienced during basic training, the rate of SCD was approximately 1 in 30,000 in persons aged 18–30 [27]. As expected, the incidence of SCD increased in older military personnel (>30 years) due to death secondary to atherosclerotic heart disease [27].

Conclusions

Estimates of the rate of SCA/D in athletes vary widely and are affected by study methodology, the reliability and means of case identification, age range, the accuracy of population denominators, the inclusion or exclusion of cardiac arrest with survival, and cases occurring at rest or outside exercise. To fully understand the cardiovascular risks in athletes and the potential to prevent major cardiovascular events through screening, incidence estimates should include both SCA survivors and SCD cases occurring at any time (i.e. exercise, rest, or sleep). A currently acceptable annual incidence of all SCA/D is approximately 1 in 80,000 in high-school-aged athletes and 1 in 50,000 in college-aged athletes [36]. Males, black athletes, and male basketball players are at higher risk of SCA/D. Although many questions and challenges to more intensive cardiovascular prevention in athletes exist, both scientific limitations and misinterpretations have perpetuated an under-estimate of SCA/D in athletes, and perhaps impeded progress toward the evaluation and implementation of more effective preventive programmes. Additional research is needed to better understand the incidence of SCA/D in different athlete populations.

Further reading

Drezner JA, Harmon KG, Borjesson M. Incidence of sudden cardiac death in athletes: where did the science go? *Br J Sports Med* 2011; 45: 947–8.

Drezner JA, Harmon KG, Marek JC. Incidence of sudden cardiac arrest in Minnesota high school student athletes: the limitations of catastrophic insurance claims. *J Am Coll Cardiol* 2014; 63: 1455–6.

Drezner JA, Harmon KG, Asif IM, Marek JC. Why cardiovascular screening in young athletes can save lives: a critical review. *Br J Sports Med* 2016; 50: 1376–8.

Drezner JA, O'Connor FG, Harmon KG, et al AMSSM Position Statement on Cardiovascular Preparticipation Screening in Athletes: current evidence, knowledge gaps, recommendations and future directions. *Clin J Sport Med* 2016; 26: 347–61.

Harmon K, Asif I, Klossner D, Drezner J. Incidence of sudden cardiac death in NCAA athletes. *Circulation* 2011; 123: 1594–1600.

Harmon KG, Drezner JA, Wilson MG, Sharma S. Incidence of sudden cardiac death in athletes: a state-of-the-art review. *Br J Sports Med* 2014; 48: 1185–92.

Harmon KG, Asif IM, Maleszewski JJ, et al. Incidence, etiology, and comparative frequency of sudden cardiac death in NCAA athletes: a decade in review. *Circulation* 2015; 132: 10–19.

Harmon KG, Asif IM, Maleszewski JJ, et al. Incidence and etiology of sudden cardiac arrest and death in high school athletes in the United States. *Mayo Clin Proc* 2016; 91: 1493–1502.

Toresdahl BG, Rao AL, Harmon KG, Drezner JA. Incidence of sudden cardiac arrest in high school student athletes. *Heart Rhythm* 2014; 11: 1190–4.

References

1. Harmon KG, Asif IM, Klossner D, Drezner JA. Incidence of sudden cardiac death in National Collegiate Athletic Association athletes. *Circulation* 2011; 123: 1594–1600.
2. Harmon KG, Asif IM, Maleszewski JJ, et al. Incidence, cause, and comparative frequency of sudden cardiac death in National Collegiate Athletic Association athletes: a decade in review. *Circulation* 2015; 132: 10–19.
3. Maron BJ, Doerer JJ, Haas TS, et al. Sudden deaths in young competitive athletes: analysis of 1866 deaths in the United States, 1980–2006. *Circulation* 2009; 119: 1085–92.
4. Roberts WO, Stovitz SD. Incidence of sudden cardiac death in Minnesota high school athletes 1993–2012 screened with a standardized pre-participation evaluation. *J Am Coll Cardiol* 2013; 62: 1298–1301.
5. Drezner JA, Rao AL, Heistand J, et al. Effectiveness of emergency response planning for sudden cardiac arrest in United State s high schools with automated external defibrillators. *Circulation* 2009; 120: 518–25.
6. Corrado D, Basso C, Rizzoli G, et al. Does sports activity enhance the risk of sudden death in adolescents and young adults? *J Am Coll Cardiol* 2003; 42: 1959–63.
7. de Noronha SV, Sharma S, Papadakis M, et al. Aetiology of sudden cardiac death in athletes in the United Kingdom: a pathological study. *Heart* 2009; 95: 1409–14.
8. Holst AG, Winkel BG, Theilade J, et al. Incidence and etiology of sports-related sudden cardiac death in Denmark: implications for preparticipation screening. *Heart Rhythm* 2010; 7: 1365–71.
9. Suarez-Mier MP, Aguilera B, Mosquera RM, Sanchez-de-Leon MS. Pathology of sudden death during recreational sports in Spain. *Forensic Sci Int* 2013; 226: 188–96.
10. Ullal AJ, Abdelfattah RS, Ashley EA, Froelicher VF. Hypertrophic cardiomyopathy as a cause of sudden cardiac death in the young: a meta-analysis. *Am J Med* 2016; 129: 486–96.
11. Finocchiaro G, Papadakis M, Robertus JL, et al. Etiology of sudden death in sports: insights from a United Kingdom Regional Registry. *J Am Coll Cardiol* 2016; 67: 2108–15.
12. Maron BJ, Friedman RA, Kligfield P, et al. Assessment of the 12-lead electrocardiogram as a screening test for detection of cardiovascular disease in healthy general populations of young people (12–25 years of age): a scientific statement from the American Heart Association and the American College of Cardiology. *J Am Coll Cardiol* 2014; 64: 1479–1514.
13. Fuller CM, McNulty CM, Spring DA, et al. Prospective screening of 5,615 high school athletes for risk of sudden cardiac death. *Med Sci Sports Exerc* 1997; 29: 1131–8.
14. Corrado D, Basso C, Pavei A, et al. Trends in sudden cardiovascular death in young competitive athletes after implementation of a preparticipation screening program. *JAMA* 2006; 296: 1593–1601.
15. Wilson MG, Basavarajaiah S, Whyte GP, et al. Efficacy of personal symptom and family history questionnaires when screening for inherited cardiac pathologies: the role of electrocardiography. *Br J Sports Med* 2008; 42: 207–11.
16. Bessem B, Groot FP, Nieuwland W. The Lausanne recommendations: a Dutch experience. *Br J Sports Med* 2009; 43: 708–15.
17. Hevia AC, Fernandez MM, Palacio JM, et al. ECG as a part of the preparticipation screening programme: an old and still present international dilemma. *Br J Sports Med* 2011; 45: 776–9.
18. Baggish AL, Hutter AM Jr, Wang F, et al. Cardiovascular screening in college athletes with and without electrocardiography: a cross-sectional study. *Ann Intern Med* 2010; 152: 269–75.
19. Fudge J, Harmon KG, Owens DS, et al. Cardiovascular screening in adolescents and young adults: a prospective study comparing the Pre-participation Physical Evaluation Monograph 4th Edition and ECG. *Br J Sports Med* 2014; 48: 1172–8.
20. Drezner JA, Prutkin JM, Harmon KG, et al. Cardiovascular screening in college athletes. *J Am Coll Cardiol* 2015; 65: 2353–5.
21. Maron BJ. Sudden death in young athletes. *N Engl J Med* 2003; 349: 1064–75.
22. Risgaard B, Tfelt-Hansen J, Winkel BG. Sports-related sudden cardiac death. How to prove an effect of preparticipation screening? *Heart Rhythm* 2016; 13: 1560–2.

23. Risgaard B, Winkel BG, Jabbari R, et al. Sports-related sudden cardiac death in a competitive and a noncompetitive athlete population aged 12 to 49 years: data from an unselected nationwide study in Denmark. *Heart Rhythm* 2014; 11: 1673–81.
24. Roberts WO, Stovitz SD. Incidence of sudden cardiac death in Minnesota high school athletes 1993–2012 screened with a standardized pre-participation evaluation. *J Am Coll Cardiol* 2013; 62: 1298–1301.
25. Drezner JA, Harmon KG, Marek JC. Incidence of sudden cardiac arrest in Minnesota high school student athletes: the limitations of catastrophic insurance claims. *J Am Coll Cardiol* 2014; 63: 1455–6.
26. Maron BJ, Haas TS, Murphy CJ, et al. Incidence and causes of sudden death in U.S. college athletes. *J Am Coll Cardiol* 2014; 63: 1636–43.
27. Eckart RE, Shry EA, Burke AP, et al. Sudden death in young adults an autopsy-based series of a population undergoing active surveillance. *J Am Coll Cardiol* 2011; 58: 1254–61.
28. Steinvil A, Chundadze T, Zeltser D, et al. Mandatory electrocardiographic screening of athletes to reduce their risk for sudden death proven fact or wishful thinking? *J Am Coll Cardiol* 2011; 57: 1291–6.
29. Drezner JA, Harmon KG, Borjesson M. Incidence of sudden cardiac death in athletes: where did the science go? *Br J Sports Med* 2011; 45: 947–8.
30. Van Camp SP, Bloor CM, Mueller FO, et al. Nontraumatic sports death in high school and college athletes. *Med Sci Sports Exerc* 1995; 27: 641–7.
31. Maron BJ, Gohman TE, Aeppli D. Prevalence of sudden cardiac death during competitive sports activities in Minnesota high school athletes. *J Am Coll Cardiol* 1998; 32: 1881–4.
32. Drezner JA, Harmon KG, Borjesson M. Incidence of sudden cardiac death in athletes: where did the science go? *Br J Sports Med* 2011; 45: 947–8.
33. Drezner JA, Harmon KG, Marek JC. Incidence of sudden cardiac arrest in Minnesota high school student athletes: the limitations of catastrophic insurance claims. *J Am Coll Cardiol* 2014; 63: 1455–6.
34. van Brabandt H, Desomer A, Gerkens S, Neyt M. Harms and benefits of screening young people to prevent sudden cardiac death. *BMJ* 2016; 353: i 1156.
35. Drezner JA, Harmon KG, Asif IM, Marek JC. Why cardiovascular screening in young athletes can save lives: a critical review. *Br J Sports Med* 2016; 50: 1376–8.
36. Harmon KG, Drezner JA, Wilson MG, Sharma S. Incidence of sudden cardiac death in athletes: a state-of-the-art review. *Br J Sports Med* 2014; 48: 1185–92.
37. Maron BJ, Haas TS, Ahluwalia A, Rutten-Ramos SC. Incidence of cardiovascular sudden deaths in Minnesota high school athletes. *Heart Rhythm* 2013; 10: 374–7.
38. Toresdahl BG, Rao AL, Harmon KG, Drezner JA. Incidence of sudden cardiac arrest in high school student athletes on school campus. *Heart Rhythm* 2014; 11: 1190–4.
39. Harmon KG, Asif IM, Ellenbogen R, Drezner JA. The incidence of sudden cardiac arrest in United States high school athletes. *Br J Sports Med* 2014; 48: 605.
40. Maron BJ, Haas TS, Doerer JJ, et al. Comparison of U.S. and Italian experiences with sudden cardiac deaths in young competitive athletes and implications for preparticipation screening strategies. *Am J Cardiol* 2009; 104: 276–80.
41. Bohm P, Scharhag J, Meyer T. Data from a nationwide registry on sports-related sudden cardiac deaths in Germany. *Eur J Prev Cardiol* 2016; 23: 649–56.
42. Atkins DL, Everson-Stewart S, Sears GK, et al. Epidemiology and outcomes from out-of-hospital cardiac arrest in children: the Resuscitation Outcomes Consortium Epistry-Cardiac Arrest. *Circulation* 2009; 119: 1484–91.
43. Chugh SS, Reinier K, Balaji S, et al. Population-based analysis of sudden death in children: the Oregon Sudden Unexpected Death Study. *Heart Rhythm* 2009; 6: 1618–22.
44. Cooper WO, Habel LA, Sox CM, et al. ADHD drugs and serious cardiovascular events in children and young adults. *N Engl J Med* 2011; 365: 1896–1904.
45. Meyer L, Stubbs B, Fahrenbruch C, et al. Incidence, causes, and survival trends from cardiovascular-related sudden cardiac arrest in children and young adults 0 to 35 years of age: a 30-year review. *Circulation* 2012; 126: 1363–72.
46. Farioli A, Christophi CA, Quarta CC, Kales SN. Incidence of sudden cardiac death in a young active population. *J Am Heart Assoc* 2015; 4(6): e 001818.
47. Maron BJ, Haas TS, Duncanson ER, et al. Comparison of the frequency of sudden cardiovascular deaths in young competitive athletes versus nonathletes: should we really screen only athletes? *Am J Cardiol* 2016; 117: 1339–41.
48. Marijon E, Tafflet M, Celermajer DS, et al. Sports-related sudden death in the general population. *Circulation* 2011; 124: 672–81.
49. Eckart RE, Scoville SL, Campbell CL, et al. Sudden death in young adults: a 25-year review of autopsies in military recruits. *Ann Intern Med* 2004; 141: 829–34.
50. Drezner JA, Rogers KJ, Zimmer RR, Sennett BJ. Use of automated external defibrillators at NCAA Division I universities. *Med Sci Sports Exerc* 2005; 37: 1487–92.
51. Papadakis M, Sharma S, Cox S, et al. The magnitude of sudden cardiac death in the young: a death certificate-based review in England and Wales. *Europace* 2009; 11: 1353–8.
52. Solberg EE, Gjertsen F, Haugstad E, Kolsrud L. Sudden death in sports among young adults in Norway. *Eur J Cardiovasc Prev Rehabil* 2010; 17: 337–41.
53. Margey R, Roy A, Tobin S, et al. Sudden cardiac death in 14- to 35-year olds in Ireland from 2005 to 2007: a retrospective registry. *Europace*. 2011; 13: 1411–18.
54. Pilmer CM, Porter B, Kirsh JA, et al. Scope and nature of sudden cardiac death before age 40 in Ontario: a report from the Cardiac Death Advisory Committee of the Office of the Chief Coroner. *Heart Rhythm* 2013; 10: 517–23.
55. Pilmer CM, Kirsh JA, Hildebrandt D, et al. Sudden cardiac death in children and adolescents between 1 and 19 years of age. *Heart Rhythm* 2014; 11: 239–45.
56. Winkel BG, Risgaard B, Sadjadieh G, et al. Sudden cardiac death in children (1–18 years): symptoms and causes of death in a nationwide setting. *Eur Heart J* 2014; 35: 868–75.

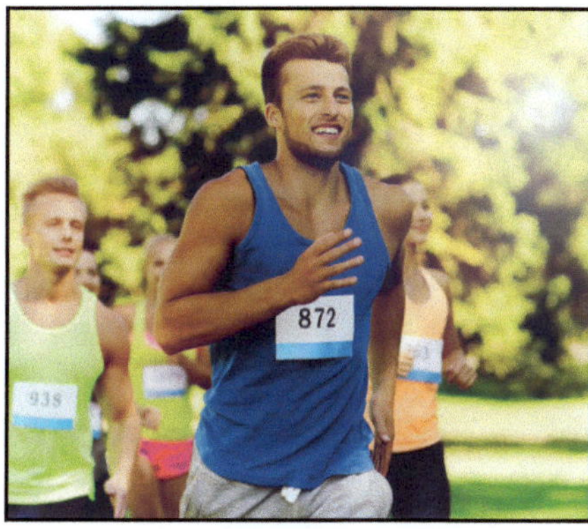

6.2

Cardiovascular causes of sudden death in athletes

Cristina Basso, Stefania Rizzo, and Gaetano Thiene

Introduction

Sudden cardiac death (SCD) is usually the result of an interaction between transient acute events ('trigger') and either structural or non-structural cardiovascular abnormalities ('substrate'). The structural culprit is located in any of the cardiovascular components, i.e. aorta, coronary arteries, myocardium, valves, conduction system, ion channels [1–4]. Epidemiological studies demonstrated that the occurrence of SCD in athletes is nearly three times greater than that in non-athletes [5]. In other words, sport activity, whether competitive or not, adds a significant risk if the athletes are affected by concealed cardiac diseases. Triggers of SCD in young competitive athletes include exercise-related sympathetic stimulation, abrupt haemodynamic changes, and myocardial ischaemia [6,7]. Dehydration, hyperpyrexia, electrolyte imbalances, and increased platelet aggregation with exercise may play also a role.

In this chapter, we will review the various structural diseases associated with a risk of SCD in athletes and discuss the reasons for disparity among available published studies, thus raising the need for uniform reporting. Identifying causes of SCD in the athletic population is important for guiding preventive measures.

Atherosclerotic coronary artery disease

Atherosclerotic coronary artery disease is the most common cause of sports-related SCD in older people. It is identified in more than 80% of cases, for whom arrhythmic SCD may be the earliest manifestation of an ongoing acute myocardial infarction. Coronary artery pathology consists of single or multivessel atherosclerotic disease with thrombotic occlusion of a coronary segment, which produces a sharp interruption of regional myocardial blood flow [8–10] (➲ Fig. 6.2.1). Thrombus may precipitate onto a ruptured atherosclerotic plaque or an endothelial erosion. Rupture affects plaque with lipid-rich cores and thin fibrous caps. Erosion is usually the consequence of inflammation and may involve a fibrocellular plaque devoid of lipids [11,12]. In a comparative autopsy study of atherosclerotic plaques in men who suffered coronary SCD on effort vs. at rest, acute plaque rupture was significantly more prevalent in the former (68% vs 23%, respectively) [9]. Moreover, plaque rupture on effort occurred in the central thin-cap at difference from plaque rupture at rest, typically occurring in the so-called shoulder region. On the basis of these findings, the authors suggested that haemodynamic factors contribute to stress-related plaque rupture in sports-related SCD.

Coronary SCD in the young is usually due to accelerated coronary atherosclerosis; occlusive thrombosis or healed myocardial infarction are rarely observed [13]. Indeed, unlike SCD in adult and elderly patients, which is mostly associated with multivessel disease and an occlusive or mural thrombus [8–12], coronary SCD in young patients is rarely precipitated by coronary thrombosis [13]. Rather, the pathology usually consists of a single obstructive plaque (>70% luminal stenosis) located at the first tract of the left anterior descending coronary artery (➲ Fig. 6.2.2). The plaque is mainly fibrocellular and devoid of atheroma, fissuring, or thrombosis [13,14]. Preservation of the tunica media, absence of thrombosis, and frequent episodes of variant angina are all features in keeping with a transient ischaemic episode, most probably attributable to coronary vasospasm [1–3, 15]. Temporary myocardial ischaemia, occurring in the setting of either stable (on effort) or unstable (at rest) angina pectoris, may trigger fatal arrhythmias in the absence of overt myocardial damage, or, more probably, in the presence of patchy contraction band necrosis

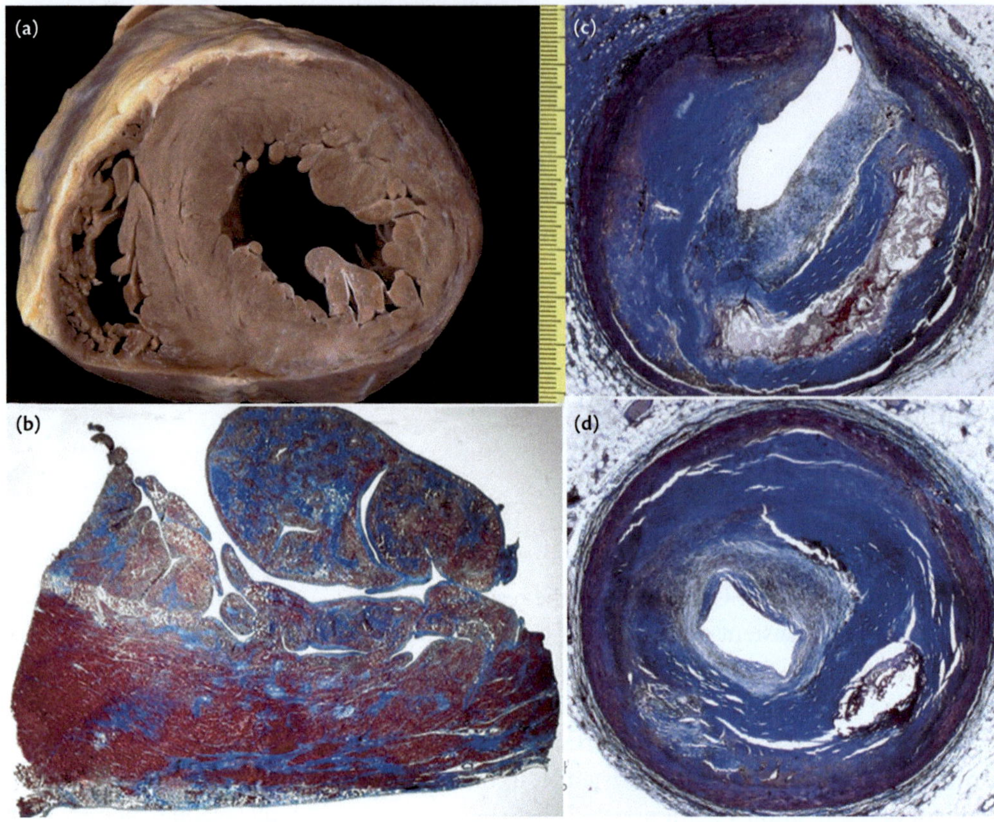

Fig. 6.2.1 Sudden cardiac death on effort in a 58-year-old man with concealed previous myocardial infarction due to multi-vessel atherosclerotic coronary artery disease. (a) Transverse section of the heart specimen showing thinning of the posterolateral left ventricular free wall with scarring. (b) Sub-endocardial and patchy transmural replacement type fibrosis is visible on the panoramic histological section of the posterolateral left ventricular free wall (Heidenhain trichrome). (c), (d) Transverse sections of the anterior descending and circumflex branches of the left coronary artery showing critical stenosis due to eccentric and concentric fibro-atheromatous plaques (Heidenhain trichrome).

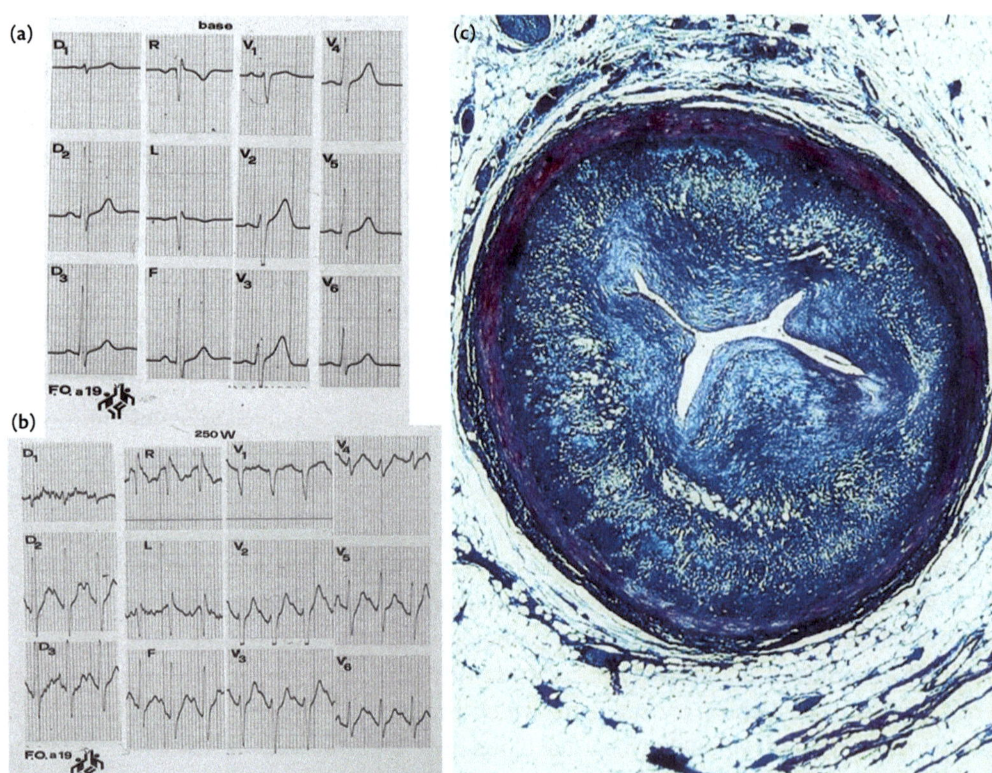

Fig. 6.2.2 Sudden cardiac death of a 19-year-old basketball player during a game due to accelerated atherosclerotic coronary artery disease. (a) Normal basal 12-lead ECG. (b) Effort 12-lead ECG without any sign of myocardial ischaemia. (c) Histological section of the proximal left anterior descending coronary artery; note the critical luminal stenosis due to a concentric, mostly fibrocellular, atherosclerotic plaque (Heindenhain trichrome).

sufficient to account for slow conduction unidirectional block and re-entry phenomena.

Risk factors for accelerated atherosclerotic coronary artery disease are not easily recognizable in young SCD victims because of the absence of clinical information and laboratory tests, even in athletes. Among the risk factors, cocaine and other illicit drugs such as anabolic steroids should be always considered in young adults and athletes [16,17].

Acute ischaemic damage of the myocardium accounts for automaticity or slow conduction, leading to unidirectional blocks, re-entry circuits, and ventricular tachyarrhythmias. Asystole, due to impairment of sinus and AV node perfusion, can be the presentation of the coronary thrombosis that affects the right coronary artery in a right dominant circulation or the left circumflex artery in a left dominant pattern [18].

Life-threatening ventricular tachyarrhythmias arise in patients with myocardial scars from previous infarction, and result from a slowing of conduction and the onset of re-entry circuits at the border between normal myocardium and scar, as well as a zigzag propagation of the impulse within the fibrotic area.

Non-atherosclerotic coronary artery disease

A more detailed description is given in ➲ Chapter 4.1.5. People with an anomalous coronary artery origin from the wrong aortic sinus, either the right coronary artery from the left sinus or the left coronary artery from the right sinus, with an inter-atrial course, have a greater risk of arrhythmic cardiac arrest (➲ Fig. 6.2.3). SCD results from myocardial ischaemia precipitated during exercise, due to an abnormal coronary ostium with an acute angle take-off, an intra-mural aortic course with a slit-like lumen, compression of the anomalous vessel between the aorta and pulmonary artery, and/or coronary spasm [19–22]. This cardiovascular substrate is reported as a major cause of SCD in both the Italian and US series [5,23].

A condition of purely anomalous course is the myocardial bridge. An epicardial coronary stem, usually the left anterior descending coronary artery, may run deep into the myocardium, demonstrating an intra-mural course. It was originally regarded as an important cause of SCD on effort [24), but this is now questioned, even when it is associated with hypertrophic cardiomyopathy, in the absence of clear-cut signs and symptoms of myocardial ischaemia [25,26].

Finally, acquired coronary artery diseases other than atherosclerosis, even though they are exceptional, may account for life-threatening arrhythmias due to ischaemic injury. They include coronary embolism, spontaneous dissection, and arteritis.

Cardiomyopathies

A 'primarily' arrhythmic myocardium can account for cardiac arrest in the athlete. While dilated cardiomyopathy and restrictive cardiomyopathy are typically characterized by congestive heart failure and SCD is exceedingly rare, the natural history of hypertrophic cardiomyopathy (HCM) and arrhythmogenic cardiomyopathy (AC) is usually marked by ventricular arrhythmias with SCD even as a first clinical manifestation [27,28]. These cardiomyopathies have been consistently implicated as the leading cause of sports-related cardiac arrest in the young, with HCM accounting for more than a third of fatal cases in the USA [23] and AC for approximately a quarter in the Veneto region of Italy [5].

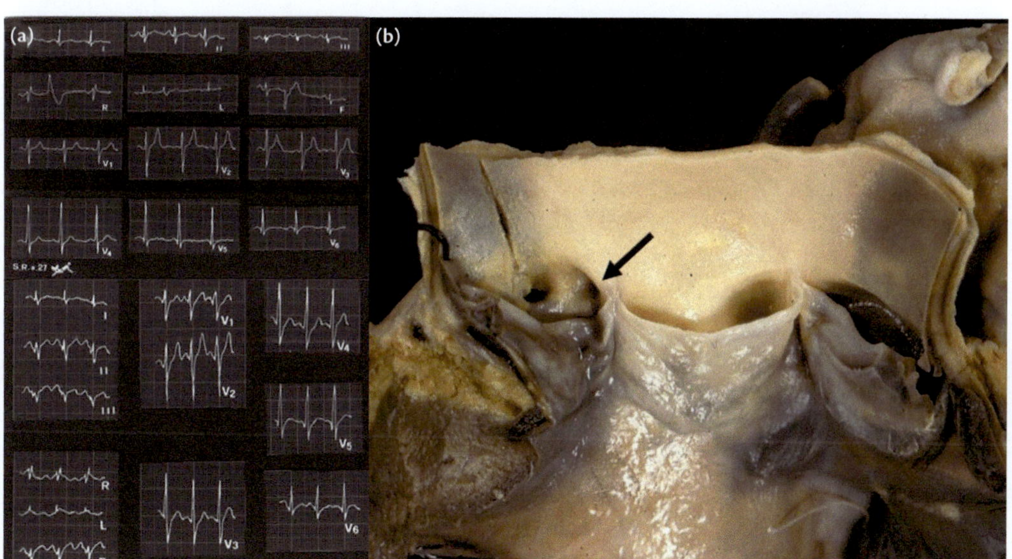

Fig. 6.2.3 Sudden cardiac death of a 27-year-old rugby player during a game due to anomalous coronary artery origin. (a) Basal 12-lead ECG with isolated premature ventricular beat, and effort 12-lead ECG with no sign of myocardial ischaemia. (b) View of the aortic root; note the presence of two coronary ostia in the left sinus of Valsalva, with an acute angle take-off of the anomalous right coronary artery (arrow).

HCM in young SCD victims is characterized by either symmetric or asymmetric left ventricular hypertrophy, with a wide regional distribution, usually in the basal portion of the ventricular septum but also in the anterior free wall and apex [29,30] (➲ Fig. 6.2.4). The septal bulging, with or without fibrous thickening of the septal endocardium and anterior mitral valve leaflet, may create sub-aortic obstruction with left ventricular outflow tract gradient. Histology typically shows myocardial disarray (i.e. myocytes spatially arranged in a chaotic manner) and interstitial fibrosis [31,32]. Myocyte necrosis and replacement-type (i.e. scarring) fibrosis are frequent findings in SCD victims in the absence of atherosclerotic coronary disease [30,33,34]. Small-vessel disease, myocardial bridging, and elevated intra-myocardial diastolic pressure have been advocated to account for impaired myocardial perfusion [25,30,34]. The combination of myocardial disarray and replacement fibrosis provides an ideal substrate for inhomogeneous intraventricular conduction and re-entry phenomena.

A precise diagnosis of HCM is of utmost value since it is a heredo-familial genetically determined cardiomyopathy. Therefore HCM should be distinguished from idiopathic left ventricular hypertrophy, which has been reported in young people and athletes who died suddenly [23]. Whether individuals with this condition are at risk of SCD is still a matter of debate, and differential diagnosis from 'athlete hearts' is also a challenge at post-mortem [35,36]. It is characterized by concentric symmetric left ventricular hypertrophy, with a degree of hypertrophy beyond that seen in trained athletes (i.e. left ventricular thickness >15 mm), in the absence of predisposing conditions (aortic valve stenosis, isthmal coarctation, systemic hypertension). Furthermore, different from HCM, there is no evidence macroscopically of sub-aortic plaque and mitral valve disease, or histologically of myocardial disarray, fibrosis, and small vessel disease.

AC, which is a leading cause of SCD in young people and athletes in the Italian series, is also a genetically determined cardiomyopathy, characterized by myocardial atrophy and fibro-fatty replacement, more often of the right ventricular free wall [37,38]. At gross examination, heart weight is usually within normal limits and the right ventricle appears yellow or whitish with a thinned wall. Right ventricular aneurysms have been reported in nearly 50% of cases, typically located at the postero-inferior wall, the apex, and the infundibulum ('triangle of dysplasia') [39,40] (➲ Fig. 6.2.5). At histology, the fibro-fatty tissue replacement has a typical location in the sub-epicardial–mid-mural myocardial layers with a wavefront extension towards the endocardium; focal myocarditis with myocyte death is often observed. Although the right ventricular free wall is the classic location, the left

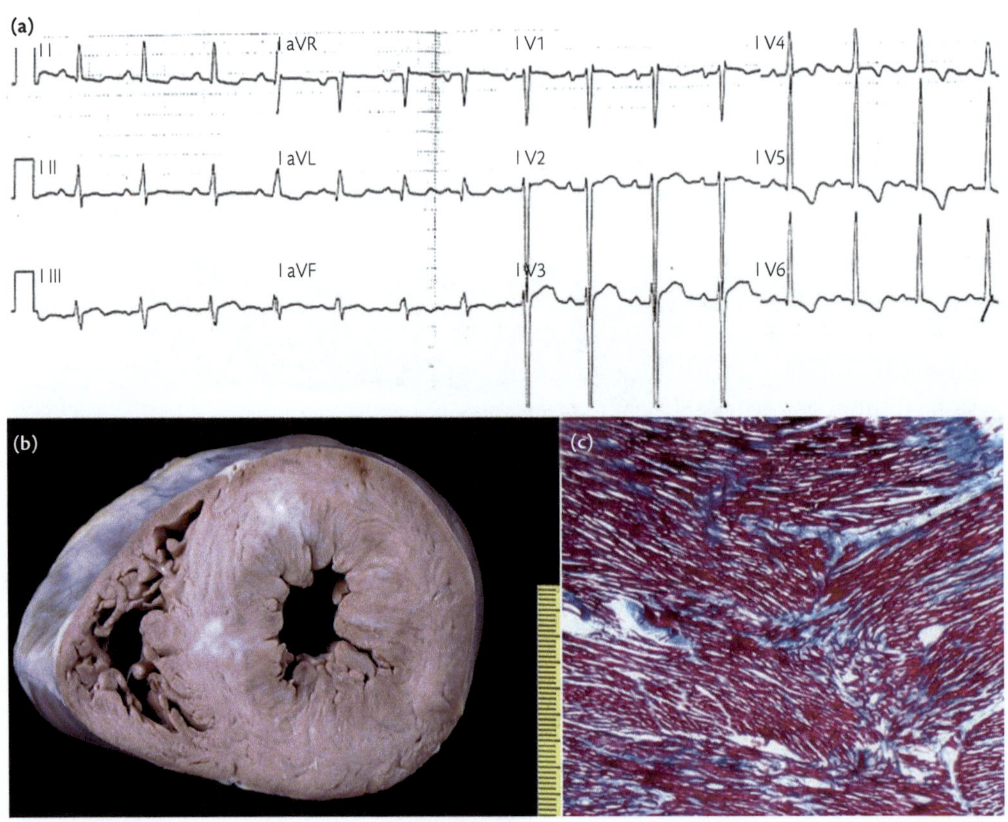

Fig. 6.2.4 Sudden cardiac death of a 15-year-old athlete during cycling due to hypertrophic cardiomyopathy. (a) Twelve-lead ECG shows deep inverted T waves on V4–V6. (b) Cross-section of the heart demonstrates asymmetric septal hypertrophy with grossly visible myocardial scars. (c) Histology shows extensive myocardial disarray.

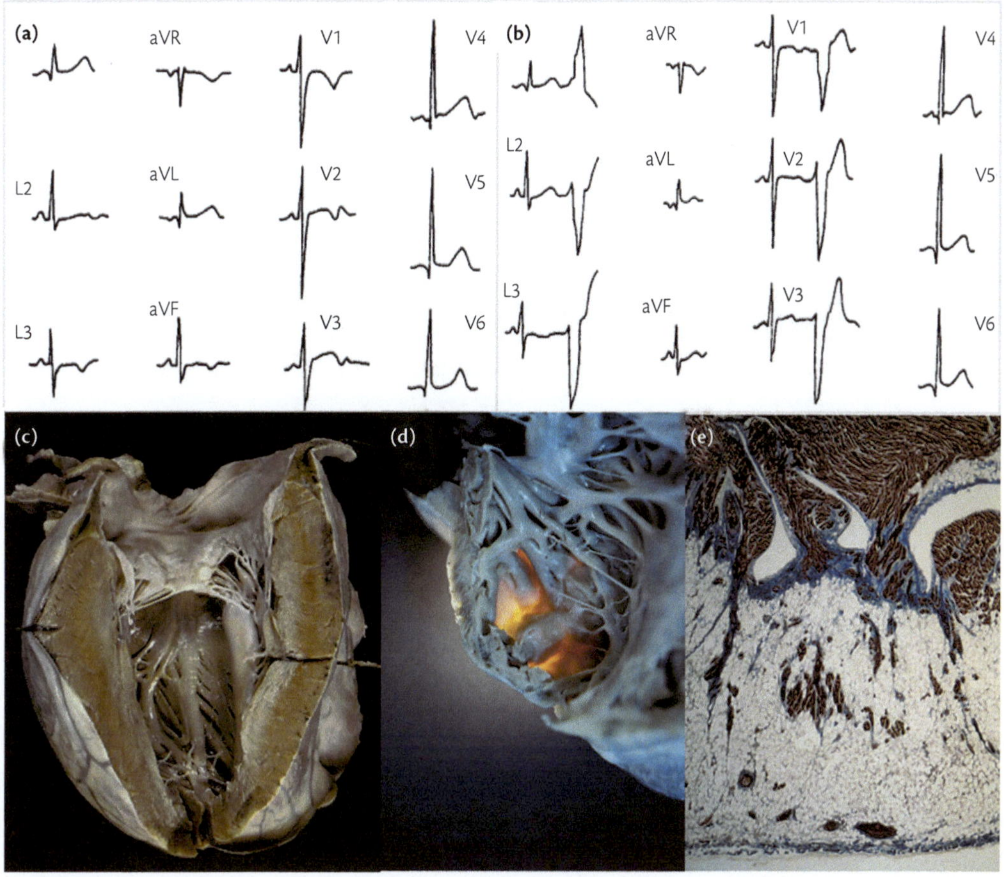

Fig. 6.2.5 Sudden cardiac death in a 30-year-old competitive athlete who died suddenly during a soccer game due to arrhythmogenic cardiomyopathy (late eighties, early screening). (a) Note the inverted T waves in the right precordial leads. (b) Stress test ECG: a single premature ventricular beat with left bundle branch block morphology. (c) At post-mortem, the left ventricle was normal. (d) The right ventricle shows a typical inferior aneurysm. (e) At histology, transmural fibro-fatty replacement of the right ventricular free wall (Heidenhain trichrome).

ventricle may also be affected and even be dominant, with an unusual distribution of the fibro-fatty tissue in the subepicardium of the posterolateral wall [37,38,41,42]. In the last 10 years, a marked reduction in the number of athletes who died suddenly with the classical AC variant has been observed in the Italian SCD Registry owing to the increased detection of affected people at pre-participation screening; in contrast, the left ventricular AC variant still kills athletes since it is not usually identified by current diagnostic criteria [43,44,unpublished data].

Myocarditis is usually accompanied by clinical signs of systolic dysfunction and ventricular dilatation. Prodromes may consist of a flu-like illness a few days before death, syncopal episodes, and premature ventricular beats. However, clinical presentation may even be arrhythmic, without heart failure. SCD may occur in either the active or healed phases as a consequence of life-threatening ventricular arrhythmias which develop in the setting of inflammatory infiltrates, interstitial oedema, and myocardial necrosis, with or without fibrosis (acute and chronic myocarditis) (45–47) (see ➲ Fig.6.2.6). The strongest evidence that subclinical myocarditis can cause ventricular fibrillation comes from a US autopsy series on army recruits in which 40% of those who died suddenly had histological evidence of myocarditis [48]. However, the wide variability in the prevalence of myocarditis as the cause of SCD in published series raises questions about the homogeneity of histological diagnostic criteria [26]. Rare interstitial lymphocytes ($<7/mm^2$) are a normal finding, and should not be interpreted as a sign of myocarditis. The gross appearance of the heart is not distinctive and its weight may be within normal values. Histology typically discloses patchy inflammatory infiltrates, either polymorphous or lymphocytic. SCD as a consequence of patchy giant cell myocarditis as well as eosinophilic myocarditis, in the setting of allergic conditions, has also been reported. Evidence of viral myocardial infection is often found by employing molecular biology techniques [47]. The report of an increased SCD rate among young Swedish elite orienteers with histopathological evidence of myocarditis and serological demonstration of antibodies to Chlamydia pneumoniae should be noted [49,50].

In addition to molecular studies, toxicological investigation is mandatory to rule out unnatural causes, particularly in young competitive athletes. For instance, myocarditis is a well-known cocaine-related cardiovascular complication [51,52]. Excess catecholamines leading to myocyte damage

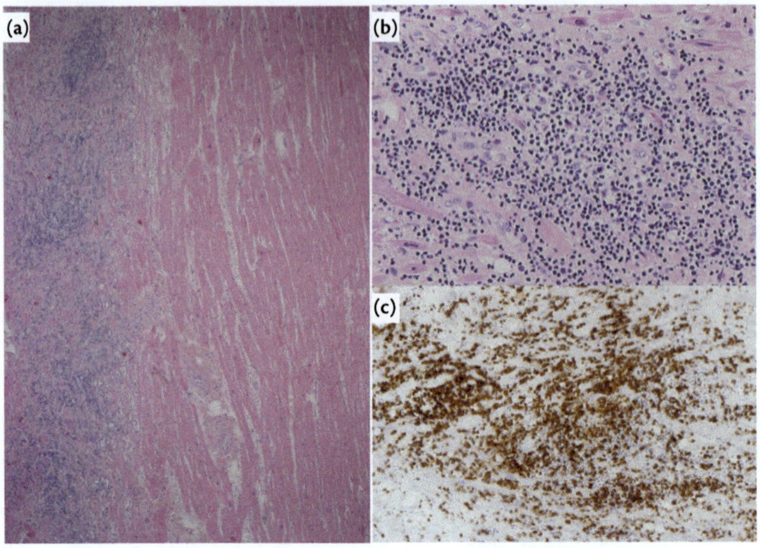

Fig. 6.2.6 Sudden cardiac death on effort in a 22-year-old basketball player due to myocarditis. (a) Histology of the left ventricle: note the interstitial oedema and massive inflammatory infiltrates in the outer layer of the left ventricular free wall (haematoxylin–eosin). (b) At higher magnification, diffuse polymorphous cell inflammatory infiltrates associated with myocyte necrosis (haematoxylin–eosin). (c) Abundant T-lymphocytes are revealed by CD3 immunostaining.

due to calcium overload or transient coronary vasoconstriction are possible pathophysiological mechanisms. It is still a matter of debate whether inflammatory infiltrates are a secondary reaction to myocyte death or a primary hypersensitivity reaction to cocaine. Anabolic androgenic steroids have also been associated with lymphocytic myocarditis [53]. Finally, eosinophilic infiltrates usually suggest allergic diathesis or reaction to drug therapy.

Valve diseases

Aortic stenosis, mitral valve prolapse, and Ebstein malformation of the tricuspid valve have been all associated with SCD in the young and athletes.

In aortic stenosis, elevated ventricular systolic pressure as well as increased myocardial mass and stiffness may account for both raised oxygen consumption and reduced coronary reserve and provide a substrate for myocardial ischaemia, particularly in the sub-endocardium, even in the absence of coronary artery disease. While aortic stenosis in the elderly is usually due to dystrophic calcification of a tricuspid or bicuspid aortic valve, in the young it is mostly related to congenital unicuspid or bicuspid conditions [54]. However, nowadays aortic stenosis is an uncommon cause of SCD because of improved identification of patients at risk, sports restriction, and timely surgical intervention [1–3]. Pre-participation screening, including physical examination with heart murmur, can identify this condition early, thus explaining why it is rarely found as a cause of SCD in athletes.

Mitral valve prolapse is the most common valve disease with an estimated prevalence of 2–3% in the general population. SCD is rarely reported in the young and athletes and may be a mechanical complication (i.e. chordal rupture) or, more frequently, the consequence of life-threatening ventricular arrhythmias. Autonomic nervous system dysfunction, conduction system and myocardial diseases have been advanced as possible aetiopathogenetic mechanisms. In particular, we have demonstrated the presence of replacement-type fibrosis at the level of papillary muscles and the infero-basal left ventricular wall as the ideal substrate for electrical instability in SCD victims with mitral valve prolapse [55].

Aortic dissection

Aortic rupture in the young is usually the consequence of dissection complicating either genetic or congenital anomalies, such as familial dissecting aneurysms, Marfan, Loeys–Dietz, and Ehlers–Danlos syndromes, isthmal coarctation, and bicuspid aortic valve [54]. The dissection may involve the entire aorta (type I), the ascending intra-pericardial segment (type II), or the descending thoracic aorta (type III). The location of the dissection in the outer media, close to the adventitia, makes the intra-mural haematoma prone to external rupture, with haemopericardium and cardiac tamponade or haemothorax, particularly of the left pleural cavity, leading to fatal haemorrhagic shock. Retrograde dissection towards the aortic root may give rise to other mechanisms of SCD, such as myocardial ischaemia due to coronary ostia involvement, acute aortic incompetence due to valve cusp detachment, or AV block and cardiac asystole due to haemorrhagic infiltration of the atrial septum.

Wolff–Parkinson–White syndrome

Wolff–Parkinson–White syndrome is a cardiac conduction system disorder characterized by abnormal accessory pathways (Kent fascicles) between the atria and the ventricles [56]. Patients usually present with palpitations, pre-syncope, or syncope due to supraventricular tachycardia. Although rare, SCD may be the first manifestation of this conduction system disease, also on effort. The diagnosis is based upon detection of characteristic ECG changes, which include a delta wave, a short PR interval, and a widened QRS complex. This explains why this disease is not listed among cardiovascular causes of SCD in countries where the ECG is a fundamental part of the pre-participation screening for competitive athletes.

SCD with a structurally normal heart

In a widely variable proportion of SCD cases, underlying the shortcomings of different methodology and source of data, the cause is not identified. In other words, no apparent organic substrate is detected by traditional investigations (normal heart or unexplained SCD or mors sine materia), and SCD is ascribable merely to an abrupt functional disorder [57]. Post-mortem genetic analysis is recommended in such cases ('molecular autopsy'), as well as careful collection and reading of the available ECG tracings and cardiological screening of first-degree family members to look for ion-channel diseases (long QT, short QT, Brugada syndromes, and catecholaminergic polymorphic ventricular tachycardia) [58–62]. The circumstances of death are of utmost importance for addressing the investigation [26]. However, after the initial emphasis on post-mortem genetic investigation, caution is needed because of the difficulties in interpreting the pathogenic significance of gene mutations in the absence of a clear-cut phenotype, positive family history, and family members available for cascade genetic and cardiological screening for co-segregation analysis.

Finally, SCD during sport can also be the result of a non-penetrating blow to the chest wall (commotio cordis), which can trigger abrupt ventricular fibrillation in the absence of any cardiac structural lesions [63].

The need for uniform registration of causes of SCD in athletes

This discrepancy among SCD series in different countries may be explained by several factors (➔ Table 6.2.1) [3,5,26,64–77].

First, a review of the publications on the topic of SCD in the athlete clearly shows that there is a wide variability in the definition of the athletic population, with some including recreational sport activity and others including only competitive sport [78].

The population age range is also quite different when comparing series of SCD in athletes. Master athletes (>35 years) have a 4-5 times higher rate of SCD than younger age athletes (<35 years), and this mostly reflects a higher burden of ischaemic heart disease which increases exponentially with age [79]. Thus, when considering the aetiology of SCD in the young, the upper age limit should be examined carefully to avoid any bias.

In terms of ethnicity, the Northeast Italy experience prospectively investigated a consecutive series of SCD occurring in young people in a well-defined geographical area with a homogeneous ethnic group. In contrast, US and UK series are more heterogenous, and athletes of black ethnicity appear to have a higher incidence of SCD than Caucasian athletes. Black US college athletes have about a 3–5 times higher risk of SCD than white athletes.

Large differences in the source of data for case identification exist among published series/registries of SCD in the young, including athletes. Most of studies rely on death certificates, and there is a lack of standardization in death certificate coding. Furthermore, very few studies have reported estimates from primary data [78].

Even when SCD series are based upon autopsy examination, a wide variability of the procedures in post-mortem assessments can be observed. Any study based on a retrospective review of autopsy reports has an intrinsic limitation. The quality of assessment by the forensic pathologist who performs the initial examination in most cases of SCD is also questionable, since he/she may have limited experience with the diagnoses of conditions predisposing to SCD in athletes [3,26,80,81]. Moreover, the autopsies are usually performed by different examiners, including local pathologists and medical examiners with variable training and expertise, and there may also be differences in the investigation protocol. The information provided in the autopsy report also varies considerably. In the Italian study, morphological examination of all hearts was performed according to a standard protocol by the same group of experienced cardiovascular pathologists in order to obtain a higher level of confidence in the results. The general level of expertise for cardiovascular pathology among UK and US medical examiners has been questioned [81]. As demonstrated, there is a large disparity (up to 40%) with respect to the potential cause of SCD when comparing reports from specialized cardiac pathologists versus

Table 6.2.1 Sudden cardiac death related to sports activity: published series

Study	Time interval	Population	Source of data	Number	Age range	CAD	CCA	HCM	AC	ILVH	DCM	MYO	UNEX
Burke et al. 1991 [64]	1981–8	Maryland USA: forensic, exercise-related SD	Retrospective, autopsy-based AFIP review	34	14–40	26	12	24	3	9		6	18
Van Camp, et al. 1995 [65]	1983–93	USA, high school and college athletes sports SD	Retrospective, NCAA, nfshsa, naia, njcaa	1071	13–24	2.8	14.9	47.6	0.9	4.7	4.7	6.5	6.5
Corrado et al. 2003 [5]	1979–99	Northeast Italy, PPS athletes SD	Prospective, single centre, autopsy-based	56	12–35	18	16	1.8	21.4	–	1.8	8.9	3.6# (1 LQT)
Maron et al. 2009 [66]	1980–2006	US competitive athletes SD (including aborted SD)	Retrospective, National Registry, variety of sources/ databases	6902	8–39	3.3	20.5	36	4.3	8.2	2	5.9	4
De Noronha et al. 2009 [67]	1996–2008	UK, amateur athletes SD	Retrospective, CRY, referral	89	7–35	–	6.7	12.3	10.1	24.7	–	3.3	29.2
Solberg et al. 2010 [68]	1990–7	Norway, SD during sport	Retrospective, Cause of Death Registry (death certificates)	23	15–34	52	4.3	4.3	–	–		21.7	–
Holst et al. 2010 [69]	2000–6	Denmark, athletes, SD during sport	Retrospective, death certificates	15	12–35	13.3	6.6	6.6	26.6	6.6	–	6.6	26.6
Marijon et al. 2011 [70]	2005–10	France, sports-related SD (including aborted SD)	Prospective, National Ambulance Service reporting, web based screening of media releases	50	10–35	6	–4	145	4	–	4	4	487 (including ion-channel, primary VF, early rep)
Suarez-Mier et al. 2013 [71]	1995–2010	Madrid, Spain SD during sport	Retrospective, single centre, autopsy-based	81	9–35	13.5	6.1	9.8	14.8	8.6	2.4	4.9	23.4
Maron et al. 2014 [72]	2002–2011	US College athletes SD	Prospective and retrospective, US National Registry SD athlete, NCAA	643	17–26	10.5	17	44.6	6.3	–	4.2	4.2	2.17 (LQT)
Risgaard et al. 2014 [73]	2007–2009	Sport-related SD, Denmark, nationwide,	Retrospective, death certificates, autopsy reports (80%)	44	12–49	34	2.3	2.3	11	96	–	4.5	9
Harmon et al. 2014 [74]	2004–8	US, college athletes SD	Retrospective, NCAA, PHW	45	17–24	5	14	3	3	8	8	8	347

Table 6.2.1 Sudden cardiac death related to sports activity: published series *(Continued)*

Harmon et al. 2015 [75]	2003–13	US, college athletes SD	Retrospective, NCAA, PHW	79	17–24	9	11	8	5	8		9	267#
Chappex et al. 2015 [76]	1995–2010	Lausanne, Switzerland, SD during sport activity	Retrospective, single centre, autopsy based	22	10–50	27	4.5	18 (hypertrophic heart)	13.6	–	–	9	22.7
Finocchiaro et al. 2016 [77]	1994–2014	London, CRY SD during sport activity	Retrospective, coroner autopsy based, referral to CRY	79 179	7–17 18–35	−2	114	68	6 14	10 14	– 0.5	22	44 56

[1]24 excluded because autopsy not performed or report not available.[2]Additional 359 are considered cardiovascular event but there is no precise diagnosis due to autopsy not performed, or no access to post-mortem, or ambiguous or insufficient description.[3]47 confirmed cardiovascular, 17 presumed cardiovascular.[4]Sixcongenital heart disease, not otherwise specified.[5]Including possible HCM.[6]Left ventricular hypertrophy not otherwise specified, 9%.[7]Including in vivo diagnosis of ion-channel disease.

AC, arrhythmogenic cardiomyopathy; CAD, coronary artery disease; CCA, congenital coronary anomalies; CRY, cardiac risk in the young; DCM, dilated cardiomyopathy; HCM, hypertrophic cardiomyopathy; ILVH, idiopathic left ventricular hypertrophy; LQT, long QT syndrome; MYO, myocarditis; njcaa, National Junior College Athletic Association; nfshsa, National Federation of State High School Associations; naia, National Association of Intercollegiate Athletes; NCAA, National Collegiate Athletic Association (media report, NCAA database, insurance claims, autopsy reports); PHW, Parent Heart Watch (national non-profit organization); PPS, pre-participation screening with ECG; SD, sudden death; Unex, unexplained; VF, ventricular fibrillation.

reports from general pathologists [35]. General pathologists are more likely to ascribe death to structural causes rather than designate the heart as normal, by attributing, for instance, isolated fatty infiltration of the right ventricle to AC and left ventricular hypertrophy to HCM. On the other hand, it is possible that a more specific cause of SCD could have been found in many unexplained SCD cases if a more detailed and comprehensive autopsy had been performed [35]. In our experience, more than two-thirds of SCD cases initially categorized as 'normal heart' were eventually found to have structural heart diseases after a careful specialized cardiac examination [46]. If a referral system in which local pathologists perform the autopsy, including cardiac examination, before referring the heart is used, the risk of referral bias is high. In fact, local pathologists are more likely to refer challenging cases, such as athletes with ambiguous autopsy findings or normal heart, while coronary atherosclerosis and HCM may be under-represented [77].

The almost total absence of atherosclerotic coronary artery disease in the UK [67,77], French [70], and US series [66], despite a study population age upper limit of 35–39 years is noteworthy. These data support the issues of the poor quality of autopsy and/or the unreliability of certificates of death, as well as selection bias.

Finally, pre-participation screening obviously modifies the distribution of the aetiology of SCD. Once identified, athletes affected by cardiovascular diseases that may convey a greater risk of SCD may be disqualified from sport activity. Thus the aetiology and incidence figures of SCD in countries in which pre-participation screening is mandatory are altered by the exclusion of cardiovascular causes which are easily identifiable. This is the case of Italy, where a systematic pre-participation screening, based on 12-lead ECG in addition to history and physical examination, has been the practice since 1982 [4–7]. This screening strategy has proved to be effective in the identification of athletes with previously undiagnosed HCM, thanks to the high sensitivity of 12-lead ECG. A time-trend analysis of the incidence of SCD in young competitive athletes age 12–35 years in the Veneto region of Italy between 1979 and 2004 demonstrated a sharp decline of SCD in athletes after the introduction of the nationwide screening programme in 1982. Most of the mortality reduction was attributable to fewer deaths from HCM and AC [4,82]. A parallel analysis of the causes of disqualifications from competitive sports at the Center for Sports Medicine in the Padua country area showed that the proportion of athletes identified and disqualified for cardiomyopathies doubled from the early- to the late-screening period. This indicates that mortality reduction was a reflection of a lower incidence of SCD from cardiomyopathies, as a result of increasing identification over time of affected athletes at preparticipation screening.

In conclusion, proper understanding of the incidence and pathogenesis of SCD in the athlete is essential for screening and prevention strategies. Standardized autopsy protocols, including post-mortem genetic testing, should be followed in any SCD case [78]. Autopsies should be performed either locally, when available, or at specialized centres with cardiovascular pathology expertise [26]. Centralized data collection with mandatory reporting of deaths and standardized protocols at national level would significantly improve the quality of information and our understanding of the causes of SCD in young athletes.

Further reading

Basso C, Aguilera B, Banner J, et al.; Association for European Cardiovascular Pathology. Guidelines for autopsy investigation of sudden cardiac death: 2017 update from the Association for European Cardiovascular Pathology. *Virchows Arch* 2017; 471: 691–705.

Basso C, Carturan E, Pilichou K, et al. Sudden cardiac death with normal heart: molecular autopsy. *Cardiovasc Pathol* 2010; 19: 321–5.

Basso C, Corrado D, Rossi L, Thiene G Ventricular preexcitation in children and young adults: atrial myocarditis as a possible trigger of sudden death. *Circulation* 2001; 103: 269–75.

Basso C, Maron BJ, Corrado D, Thiene G Clinical profile of congenital coronary artery anomalies with origin from the wrong aortic sinus leading to sudden death in young competitive athletes. *J Am Coll Cardiol* 2000; 35: 1493–1501.

Basso C, Perazzolo Marra M, et al. Arrhythmic mitral valve prolapse and sudden cardiac death. *Circulation* 2015; 132: 556–66.

Basso C, Thiene G, Corrado D, et al. Hypertrophic cardiomyopathy and sudden death in the young: pathologic evidence of myocardial ischemia. *Hum Pathol* 2000; 31: 988–98.

Corrado D, Basso C, Pavei A, et al. Trends in sudden cardiovascular death in young competitive athletes after implementation of a preparticipation screening program. *JAMA* 2006; 296: 1593–1601.

Corrado D, Basso C, Rizzoli G, et al. Does sports activity enhance the risk of sudden death in adolescents and young adults ? *J Am Coll Cardiol* 2003; 42: 1959–63.

Thiene G, Corrado D, Basso C *Sudden Cardiac Death in the Young and Athletes*. Milan: Springer, 2016.

Thiene G Sudden cardiac death and cardiovascular pathology: from anatomic theater to double helix. Am J Cardiol 2014; 114: 1930–6.

References

1. Thiene G, Carturan E, Corrado D, Basso C. Prevention of sudden cardiac death in the young and in athletes: dream or reality? *Cardiovasc Pathol* 2010; 19: 207–17.
2. Thiene G. Sudden cardiac death and cardiovascular pathology: from anatomic theater to double helix. *Am J Cardiol* 2014; 114: 1930–6.
3. Thiene G, Corrado D, Basso C. Sudden Cardiac Death in the Young and Athletes. *Milan: Springer*, 2016.
4. Corrado D, Basso C, Pavei A, et al. Trends in sudden cardiovascular death in young competitive athletes after implementation of a preparticipation screening program. *JAMA* 2006; 296: 1593–1601.
5. Corrado D, Basso C, Rizzoli G, et al. Does sports activity enhance the risk of sudden death in adolescents and young adults? *J Am Coll Cardiol* 2003; 42: 1959–1963.
6. Corrado D, Basso C, Thiene G. Sudden death in young athletes. *Lancet* 2005; 366(Suppl 1): S47–8.
7. Corrado D, Basso C, Schiavon M, et al. Pre-participation screening of young competitive athletes for prevention of sudden cardiac death. *J Am Coll Cardiol* 2008; 52: 1981–9.
8. Thompson PD, Funk EJ, Carleton RA, et al. Incidence of death during jogging in Rhode Island from 1975 through 1980. *JAMA* 1982; 247: 2535–8.
9. Burke AP, Farb A, Malcom GT, et al. Plaque rupture and sudden death related to exertion in men with coronary artery disease. *JAMA* 1999; 281: 921–6.
10. Davies MJ, Thomas A. Thrombosis and acute coronary-artery lesions in sudden cardiac ischemic death. *N Engl J Med* 1984; 310: 1137–40.
11. van der Wal AC, Becker AE, van der Loos CM, Das PK. Site of intimal rupture or erosion of thrombosed coronary atherosclerotic plaques is characterized by an inflammatory process irrespective of the dominant plaque morphology. *Circulation* 1994; 89: 36–44.
12. Farb A, Burke AP, Tang AL, et al. Coronary plaque erosion without rupture into a lipid core. A frequent cause of coronary thrombosis in sudden coronary death. *Circulation* 1996; 93: 1354–63.
13. Corrado D, Basso C, Poletti A, et al. Sudden death in the young: is coronary thrombosis the major precipitating factor? *Circulation* 1994; 90: 2315–23.
14. Corrado D, Thiene G, Buja GF, et al. The relationship between growth of atherosclerotic plaques, variant angina and sudden death. *Int J Cardiol* 1990; 26: 361–7.
15. Tavora F, Cresswell N, Li L, et al. Sudden coronary death caused by pathologic intimal thickening without atheromatous plaque formation. *Cardiovasc Pathol* 2011; 20: 51–7.
16. Lucena J, Blanco M, Jurado C, et al. Cocaine-related sudden death: a prospective investigation in south-west Spain. *Eur Heart J* 2010; 31: 318–29.
17. Montisci M, Thiene G, Ferrara SD, Basso C. Cannabis and cocaine: a lethal cocktail triggering coronary sudden death. *Cardiovasc Pathol* 2008; 17: 344–6.
18. Thiene G, Rizzo S, Basso C. Pathology of sudden death, cardiac arrhythmias and conduction systems. In Buja M, Butany J (eds), *Cardiovascular Pathology*. Amsterdam: Elsevier, 2016, pp. 361–433.
19. Thiene G, Basso C. Sudden coronary death—not always atherosclerotic. *Heart* 2010; 96: 1084–5.
20. Basso C, Maron BJ, Corrado D, Thiene G. Clinical profile of congenital coronary artery anomalies with origin from the wrong aortic sinus leading to sudden death in young competitive athletes. *J Am Coll Cardiol* 2000; 35: 1493–1501.
21. Hill SF, Sheppard MN. A silent cause of sudden cardiac death especially in sport: congenital coronary artery anomalies. *Br J Sports Med* 2014; 48: 1151–6.
22. Taylor AJ, Rogan KM, Virmani R. Sudden cardiac death associated with isolated congenital coronary artery anomalies. *J Am Coll Cardiol* 1992; 20: 640–7.
23. Maron BJ. Sudden death in young athletes. *N Engl J Med* 2003; 349: 1064–75.
24. Morales AR, Romanelli R, Boucek RJ. The mural left anterior descending coronary artery, strenuous exercise and sudden death. *Circulation* 1980; 62: 230–7.
25. Basso C, Thiene G, Mackey-Bojack S, et al. Myocardial bridging, a frequent component of the hypertrophic cardiomyopathy phenotype, lacks systematic association with sudden cardiac death. *Eur Heart J* 2009; 30: 1627–34.

26. Basso C, Aguilera B, Banner J, et al.; Association for European Cardiovascular Pathology. Guidelines for autopsy investigation of sudden cardiac death: 2017 update from the Association for European Cardiovascular Pathology. *Virchows Arch* 2017; 471: 691–705.
27. Elliott PM, Anastasakis A, Borger MA, et al. 2014 ESC Guidelines on diagnosis and management of hypertrophic cardiomyopathy: the Task Force for the Diagnosis and Management of Hypertrophic Cardiomyopathy. *Eur Heart J* 2014; 35: 2733–9
28. Basso C, Corrado D, Bauce B, Thiene G. Arrhythmogenic right ventricular cardiomyopathy. *Circ Arrhythm Electrophysiol* 2012; 5: 1233–46.
29. Teare D. Asymmetrical hypertrophy of the heart in young adults. *Br Heart J* 1958; 20: 1–8.
30. Basso C, Thiene G, Corrado D, et al. Hypertrophic cardiomyopathy and sudden death in the young: pathologic evidence of myocardial ischemia. *Hum Pathol* 2000; 31: 988–98.
31. Maron BJ, Roberts WC. Quantitative analysis of cardiac muscle cell disorganization in the ventricular septum of patients with hypertrophic cardiomyopathy. *Circulation* 1979; 59: 689–706.
32. Maron BJ, Anan TJ, Roberts WC. Quantitative analysis of the distribution of cardiac muscle cell disorganization in the left ventricular wall of patients with hypertrophic cardiomyopathy. *Circulation* 1981; 63: 882–94.
33. Maron BJ, Epstein SE, Roberts WC. Hypertrophic cardiomyopathy and transmural myocardial infarction without significant atherosclerosis of the extramural coronary arteries. *Am J Cardiol* 1979; 43: 1086–1102.
34. Maron BJ, Wolfson JK, Epstein SE, Roberts WC. Intramural ('small vessel') coronary artery disease in hypertrophic cardiomyopathy. *J Am Coll Cardiol* 1986; 8: 545–57.
35. de Noronha SV, Behr ER, Papadakis M, et al. The importance of specialist cardiac histopathological examination in the investigation of young sudden cardiac deaths. *Europace* 2014; 16: 899–907.
36. Papadakis M, Raju H, Behr ER, et al. Sudden cardiac death with autopsy findings of uncertain significance: potential for erroneous interpretation. *Circ Arrhythm Electrophysiol* 2013; 6: 588–96.
37. Basso C, Corrado D, Marcus FI, et al. Arrhythmogenic right ventricular cardiomyopathy. *Lancet* 2009; 373: 1289–1300.
38. Pilichou K, Thiene G, Bauce B, et al. Arrhythmogenic cardiomyopathy. *Orphanet J Rare Dis* 2016; 11: 33.
39. Thiene G, Nava A, Corrado D, et al. Right ventricular cardiomyopathy and sudden death in young people. *N Engl J Med* 1988; 318: 129–33.
40. Basso C, Thiene G, Corrado D, et al. Arrhythmogenic right ventricular cardiomyopathy: Dysplasia, dystrophy, or myocarditis? *Circulation* 1996; 94: 983–91.
41. Lobo F, Silver MD, Butany J, Heggtviet HA. Left ventricular involvement in right ventricular dysplasia/cardiomyopathy. *Can J Cardiol* 1999; 15: 1239–47.
42. Tavora F, Zhang M, Franco M, et al. Distribution of biventricular disease in arrhythmogenic cardiomyopathy: an autopsy study. *Hum Pathol* 2012; 43: 592–6.
43. Marcus FI, McKenna WJ, Sherrill D, et al. Diagnosis of arrhythmogenic right ventricular cardiomyopathy/dysplasia: proposed modification of the Task Force Criteria. *Circulation* 2010; 121: 1533–41.
44. d'Amati G, De Caterina R, Basso C. Sudden cardiac death in an Italian competitive athlete: pre-participation screening and cardiovascular emergency care are both essential. *Int J Cardiol* 2016; 206: 84–6.
45. Basso C, Calabrese F, Corrado D, Thiene G. Postmortem diagnosis in sudden cardiac death victims: macroscopic, microscopic and molecular findings. *Cardiovasc Res* 2001; 50: 290–330.
46. Corrado D, Basso C, Thiene G. Sudden cardiac death in young people with apparently normal heart. *Cardiovasc Res* 2001; 50: 399–408.
47. Basso C, Calabrese F, Angelini A, et al. Classification and histological, immunohistochemical, and molecular diagnosis of inflammatory myocardial disease. *Heart Fail Rev* 2013; 18: 673–81.
48. Phillips M, Robinowitz M, Higgins JR, et al. Sudden cardiac death in Air Force recruits. *JAMA* 1986; 256: 2696–9.
49. Wesslén L, Påhlson C, Friman G, et al. Myocarditis caused by Chlamydia pneumoniae (TWAR) and sudden unexpected death in a Swedish elite orienteer. *Lancet* 1992; 340: 427–8
50. Wesslén L, Påhlson C, Lindquist O, et al. An increase in sudden unexpected cardiac deaths among young Swedish orienteers during 1979–1992. *Eur Heart J* 1996; 17: 902–10.
51. Karch SB, Billingham ME. The pathology and etiology of cocaine-induced heart disease. *Arch Pathol Lab Med* 1988; 112: 225–30.
52. Pilgrim JL, Woodford N, Drummer OH. Cocaine in sudden and unexpected death: a review of 49 post-mortem cases. *Forensic Sci Int* 2013; 227: 52–9.
53. Montisci M, El Mazloum R, Cecchetto G, et al. Anabolic androgenic steroids abuse and cardiac death in athletes: morphological and toxicological findings in four fatal cases. *Forensic Sci Int* 2012; 217: e13–18.
54. Basso C, Frescura C, Corrado D, et al. Congenital heart disease and sudden death in the young. *Hum Pathol* 1995; 26: 1065–72.
55. Basso C, Perazzolo Marra M, Rizzo S, et al. Arrhythmic mitral valve prolapse and sudden cardiac death. *Circulation* 2015; 132: 556–66.
56. Basso C, Corrado D, Rossi L, Thiene G. Ventricular preexcitation in children and young adults: atrial myocarditis as a possible trigger of sudden death. *Circulation* 2001; 103: 269–75.
57. Basso C, Carturan E, Pilichou K, et al. Sudden cardiac death with normal heart: molecular autopsy. *Cardiovasc Pathol* 2010; 19: 321–5.
58. Priori SG, Wilde AA, Horie M, et al. Executive summary: HRS/EHRA/APHRS expert consensus statement on the diagnosis and management of patients with inherited primary arrhythmia syndromes. *Heart Rhythm* 2013; 10: e85–108.
59. Tester DJ, Medeiros-Domingo A, Will ML, et al. Cardiac channel molecular autopsy: insights from 173 consecutive cases of autopsy-negative sudden unexplained death referred for post-mortem genetic testing. *Mayo Clin Proc* 2012; 87: 524–39.
60. Semsarian C, Ingles J, Wilde AA. Sudden cardiac death in the young: the molecular autopsy and a practical approach to surviving relatives. *Eur Heart J* 2015; 36: 1290–6.
61. Hofman N, Tan HL, Alders M, et al. Yield of molecular and clinical testing for arrhythmia syndromes: report of 15 years' experience. *Circulation* 2013; 128: 1513–21.

62. Behr E, Wood DA, Wright M, et al. Cardiological assessment of first-degree relatives in sudden arrhythmic death syndrome. *Lancet* 2003; 362: 1457–9.
63. Maron BJ, Estes NA 3rd. Commotio cordis. *N Engl J Med* 2010; 362: 917–27.
64. Burke AP, Farb A, Virmani R, et al. Sports-related and non-sports-related sudden cardiac death in young adults. *Am Heart J* 1991; 121: 568–75.
65. Van Camp SP, Bloor CM, Mueller FO, et al. Non-traumatic sports death in high school and college athletes. *Med Sci Sports Exerc* 1995; 27: 641–7.
66. Maron BJ, Doerer JJ, Haas TS, et al. Sudden deaths in young competitive athletes: analysis of 1866 deaths in the United States, 1980-2006. *Circulation* 2009; 119: 1085–92.
67. de Noronha SV, Sharma S, Papadakis M, et al. Aetiology of sudden cardiac death in athletes in the United Kingdom: a pathological study. *Heart* 2009; 95: 1409–14.
68. Solberg EE, Gjertsen F, Haugstad E, Kolsrud L. Sudden death in sports among young adults in Norway. *Eur J Cardiovasc Prev Rehabil* 2010; 17: 337–41.
69. Holst AG, Winkel BG, Theilade J, et al. Incidence and etiology of sports-related sudden cardiac death in Denmark—implications for preparticipation screening. *Heart Rhythm* 2010; 7: 1365–71.
70. Marijon E, Tafflet M, Celermajer DS, et al. Sports-related sudden death in the general population. *Circulation* 2011; 124: 672–81.
71. Suárez-Mier MP, Aguilera B, Mosquera RM, Sánchez-de-León MS. Pathology of sudden death during recreational sports in Spain. *Forensic Sci Int* 2013; 226: 188–96.
72. Maron BJ, Haas TS, Murphy CJ, et al. Incidence and causes of sudden death in U. S. college athletes. *J Am Coll Cardiol* 2014; 63: 1636–43.
73. Risgaard B, Winkel BG, Jabbari R, et al. Sports-related sudden cardiac death in a competitive and a noncompetitive athlete population aged 12 to 49 years: data from an unselected nationwide study in Denmark. *Heart Rhythm* 2014; 11: 1673–81.
74. Harmon KG, Drezner JA, Maleszewski JJ, et al. Pathogeneses of sudden cardiac death in national collegiate athletic association athletes. *Circ Arrhythm Electrophysiol* 2014; 7: 198–204.
75. Harmon KG, Asif IM, Maleszewski JJ, et al. Incidence, cause, and comparative frequency of sudden cardiac death in National Collegiate Athletic Association athletes: a decade in review. *Circulation* 2015; 132: 10–19.
76. Chappex N, Schlaepfer J, Fellmann F, Bhuiyan ZA, Wilhelm M, Michaud K. Sudden cardiac death among general population and sport related population in forensic experience. *J Forensic Leg Med* 2015; 35: 62–85.
77. Finocchiaro G, Papadakis M, Robertus JL, et al. Etiology of sudden death in sports: insights from a United Kingdom regional registry. *J Am Coll Cardiol.* 2016; 67: 2108–15.
78. Solberg EE, Borjesson M, Sharma S, et al. Sudden cardiac arrest in sports- need for uniform registration: a position paper from the Sport Cardiology Section of the European Association for Cardiovascular Prevention and Rehabilitation. *Eur J Prev Cardiol* 2016; 23: 657–67.
79. Chugh SS, Weiss JB. Sudden cardiac death in the older athlete. *J Am CollCardiol* 2015; 65: 493–502.
80. Sheppard MN. Aetiology of sudden cardiac death in sport: a histopathologist's perspective. *Br J Sports Med* 2012; 46(Suppl 1): i15–21.
81. Friedewald VE, Maron BJ, Roberts WC. The editor's roundtable: sudden cardiac death in athletes. *Am J Cardiol* 2007; 100: 1451–9.
82. Corrado D, Basso C, Schiavon M, Thiene G. Screening for hypertrophic cardiomyopathy in young athletes. *N Engl J Med* 1998; 339: 364–9.

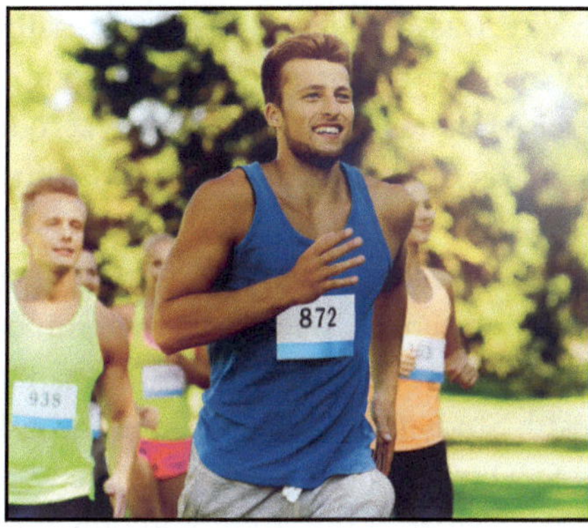

6.3

The risk, aetiology, clinical features, management, and prevention of exercise-related sudden cardiac death and acute cardiac events in adult athletes

Paul D. Thompson

Introduction and definitions

Many studies have demonstrated that exercise acutely increases the risk of acute myocardial infarction (AMI) [1–3] and sudden cardiac death (SCD) [4–7] in adults. 'Adult' is variously defined as age over 30, 35, or 40 years [8], and a cardiac event is generally considered to be exercise related if the event or its symptoms start during, or within an hour after, exercise [9]. Most studies have also examined the risk of vigorous exercise, usually defined as activities requiring ≥6 METs, where a MET (metabolic equivalent)is the energy cost of an average person sitting at rest or 3.5ml O_2/kg/min. This definition of activity is required because exercise-related cardiac events are so rare that large epidemiological studies are needed and measurements of individual capacity are not feasible. Nevertheless, the cardiac risks of exercise are probably determined less by the absolute work rate and more by the work rate relative to the individual's maximum capacity, since increases in heart rate, systolic blood pressure, and catecholamine concentrations are all more closely related to the relative work rate of the individual than to the absolute work rate of exercise.

The risk of exertion-related acute myocardial infarction

The Determinants of Myocardial Infarction Onset Study (ONSET) [2] asked 1228 patients with AMI about their habitual physical activity level as well as their activity in the 26 hours before their AMI. ONSET compared the frequency of heavy physical exertion in the hour before the AMI using a case cross-over design, in which the patient served as their own control. Heavy physical exertion was defined as any activity requiring ≥6 METs. Patients reported heavy physical exertion before their AMI in 4.4% of cases. The relative risk of an exercise-related AMI was 3.9 times higher than at other times (95% confidence limits (CI), 4.6–7.7). This risk decreased progressively from 107 to 19.4 to 8.6 to 2.4 as the frequency of exertion increased from zero to 1–2, to 3–4, to >5 times weekly, demonstrating that higher frequencies of heavy physical exertion are associated with a lower risk of an exercise-related event (➲ Fig. 6.3.1).

Similarly, the Triggers and Mechanisms of Myocardial Infarction Study (TRIMM) [3] interviewed 1194 patients with AMI and used both a standard case–control and a case cross-over design to evaluate the frequency of physical exertion before the AMI. More patients (7.1%) than controls (3.9%) reported physical exertion ≥6 METS at the onset of their AMI, indicating that vigorous exertion increased the risk 2.1-fold (CI, 1.1–3.6). The increased risk was also 2.1-fold greater with case cross-over analysis (CI, 1.6–3.1). The risk of an exercise-related AMI was 6.9-fold greater than during less vigorous activity in those exercising less than four times weekly, but only 1.3-fold higher in those

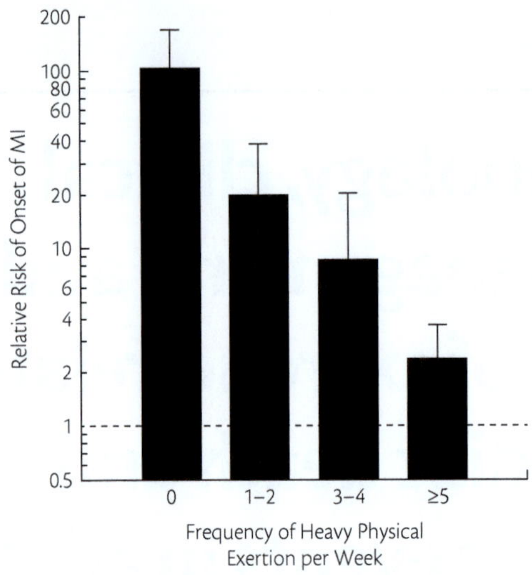

Fig. 6.3.1 The vertical bars represent the risk of an acute myocardial infarction (AMI) during heavy physical exertion relative to an AMI at other times (dotted horizontal line) according to the frequency of usual heavy physical exertion from none to more than five times weekly. The T bars represent 95% confidence limits. The vertical scale is logarithmic.
Reproduced with permission from Mittleman MA, Maclure M, Tofler GH, Sherwood JB, Goldberg RJ, Muller JE. Triggering of acute myocardial infarction by heavy physical exertion. Protection against triggering by regular exertion. Determinants of Myocardial Infarction Onset Study Investigators. *N Engl J Med* 1993 Dec 2; 329(23): 1677–83.

exercising more frequently. This again shows that exercise acutely increases the risk, but that habitual exertion reduces the risk of an exercise-related event.

The risk of exertion-related sudden cardiac death

The Physicians' Health Study used physicians as their own control in a nested case–control design to determine the risk of exercise-related SCD [4]. At the start of the study-physicians were asked how often they exercised enough to work up a sweat. Working up a sweat was considered vigorous exercise. The duration of each exercise session was estimated as 1 hour, comprising 30 minutes of exercise and 30 minutes of a post-exertion risk period. The frequency of exercise-related SCDs was compared between the hour of exercise and the hours before and after exercise. There were only 23 exercise-related, and 99 non-exercise-related, SCDs among the 21,481 male physicians over the 12 years of the study. Seventeen exercise-related SCDs occurred during the exercise and six occurred immediately after exercise. The risk of SCD was 16.9% higher during exercise than during the comparison hours (CI, 10.5–27%). The absolute risk was low, with only one death per 1.4 million hours of vigorous exertion, but the risk of a non-exercise-related SCD was even less, at one death per 19 million hours. Increasing baseline physical activity was associated with decreasing risk of exercise-related SCD, with the risk dropping from 74 to 19 to 11 as the exercise frequency increased from zero to 1–4, to >5 sessions per week, again showing that habitual exercise reduced the risk of an exercise-related SCD.

Vigorous exercise also increases the risk of SCD in women, but both the absolute number of SCDs and the magnitude of the exercise-induced increase are markedly lower than in men. The Nurses' Health Study (NHS) determined the risk of an exercise-related SCD in 84,888 nurses [7]. There were only 288 SCDs over the 24 years of the study, and only nine occurred during exertion requiring ≥6 METs. The NHS also used a nested case–control design and demonstrated that the risk of SCD was 2.38 times higher (CI, 1.23–4.6) during exercise than during the comparison periods. As with men, the risk of an exercise-related event decreased with increasing activity. Women exercising for more than 2 hours weekly had no increase in SCD with exertion.

The absolute risk of exercise-related SCD and AMI

The absolute risk of SCD during exercise is low and has been estimated as one death per year for every 15,000 [6] to 18,000 [5] ostensibly healthy individuals. There are problems with these estimates. Both studies are small, based on only ten [6] and nine [5] cases, so they have wide confidence limits. These are also old studies and may not reflect the present where better atherosclerosis prevention strategies have reduced the prevalence of CAD. However, we are unaware of more recent estimates of the absolute risk of exercise-related SCDs in unselected populations of exercising individuals. The absolute risk of exercise-related AMI has also not, to our knowledge, been clearly defined in the general population. However, the risk may be substantial, and has been estimated at 1 AMI in 593–3852 active individuals per year [10].

Aetiologey of exercise-related cardiac events in adults

Atherosclerotic coronary artery disease (CAD) is the predominant cause of exercise-related sudden cardiac events in adult and senior athletes, and is responsible for 84% of such deaths [11]. This seems paradoxical because increasing amounts of physical activity are associated overall with a reduced incidence of CAD [12]. Exercise training also produces beneficial changes in several CAD risk factors, including reductions in serum glucose and triglycerides, and blood pressure, and increases in high density lipoprotein cholesterol (HDL-C) [13], and participation in exercise-based cardiac rehabilitation after a CAD event decreases the number of subsequent events [14]. Nevertheless, and despite these long-term benefits, vigorous physical activity increases the risk of AMI and SCD as discussed above.

The immediate cause of SCD in adults depends on the individual's clinical history. The majority of adults who develop an exercise-related SCD have occult undiagnosed CAD, but up to 30% may have no diagnosed cause, and the remainder have dilated or hypertrophic cardiomyopathy, congenital heart disease, or other cardiac disease (➔ Fig. 6.3.2) [11].

Most AMIs and SCDs unrelated to exercise in the asymptomatic general population are due to acute coronary plaque rupture or erosion with acute thrombosis. In contrast, SCD among the general population with diagnosed CAD often occurs without evidence of an acute coronary lesion, suggesting that ventricular fibrillation from scar or ischaemia was responsible.

Exercise-related AMIs in previously asymptomatic individuals [1], including rare reports in athletes [1,15], are most commonly associated with plaque rupture and acute coronary thrombosis. Such individuals have less extensive CAD than those whose AMI was not exercise related, suggesting that exercise incited the acute event [1]. In contrast, an acute coronary lesion is found in only approximately 15% of all sport-related sudden cardiac arrests (SCAs) [11]. An additional 45% of all sport-related deaths have evidence of chronic CAD [11], suggesting that a cardiac arrhythmia from exercise-induced ischaemia or a myocardial scar caused the arrest. Thus it appears that exercise-related AMI in asymptomatic subjects is often due to acute plaque rupture and thrombosis, whereas exercise-related SCD and SCA are most frequently associated with chronic, and not acute, CAD.

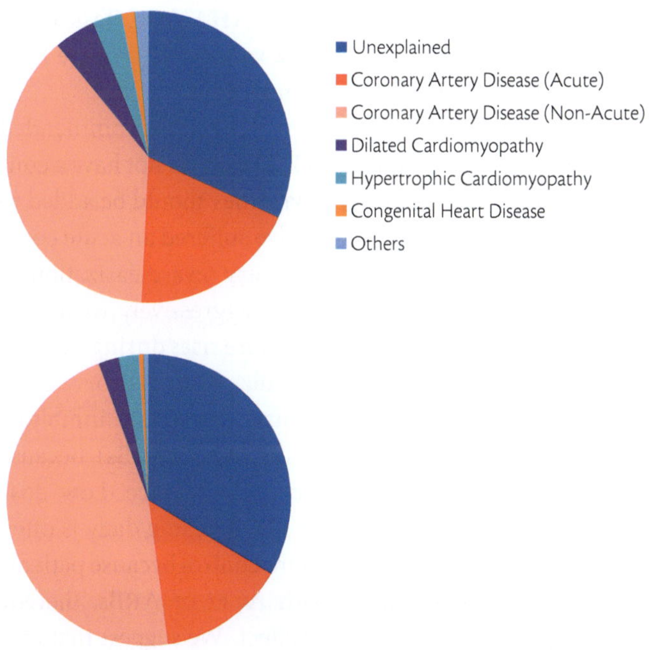

Fig. 6.3.2 The cardiovascular abnormalities found in 63 individuals suffering cardiac arrest during sporting activities (top) and in 1184 individuals with non-exercise-related cardiac arrest (bottom).
Reproduced with permission from Eloi Marijon et al. Sudden cardiac arrest during sports activity in middle age clinical perspective. *Circulation*, Volume 131, Issue 16, pp.1384–91. Copyright © 2015 Wolters Kluwer Health, Inc.

In 1975 Asher Black described 12 cases of exercise-related cardiac events which he attributed to 'Black's crack in the coronary plaque' due to acute plaque rupture from the increased excursion, bending, and flexing of the coronary arteries during vigorous exercise [16]. Exercise induces increases in heart rate and end-diastolic volume, the reduction in end-systolic volume increases the frequency and flexing of the coronary arteries, and the rise in systolic blood pressure increases endothelial shear rates. All could contribute to acute plaque disruption. Exercise-induced platelet aggregation [17] and haemoconcentration probably increase the thrombotic risk from any plaque disruption.

Clinical features of exercise-related acute myocardial infarction

There are few studies reporting the clinical characteristics of athletes or other individuals suffering an exercise-related AMI. One study examined the clinical characteristics of consecutive patients selected for acute angioplasty treatment of their AMI [1]. Of the 640 patients included, 64 (10%) had their AMI during or promptly after physical exertion. Patients with an exercise-related AMI were more likely to be male (86% vs 68%), to have hyperlipidaemia (62% vs 40%), and to be smokers (59% vs 37%). They also presented with ventricular fibrillation more often (20% vs 11%). Despite their higher risk factors, they were more likely to have single-vessel disease (50% vs 20%) and less likely to have three-vessel disease (8% vs 40%). They more frequently had a large thrombus (>2mm) on angiography (64% vs 35%). The relative risk (RR) of having an AMI with exercise was 10.1 times greater than at other times (CI, 1.6–65.6), confirming that exercise increases AMI risk. Despite suffering their AMIs with exercise, the exercise-related AMI victims were more often characterized as very low or low active, and the risk of an exercise-related AMI was greatest among those who were classified as habitually very low active (30.5%; CI, 4.4–209.9) and low active (20.95; CI, 3.1–142.1).

These results are not directly applicable to adult athletes, but suggest that exercise provokes AMI in those with less atherosclerosis, probably by inducing acute plaque disruption and thrombosis.

Clinical features of exercise-related sudden cardiac death in adult athletes

There are a plethora of studies examining SCD in young athletes, but few studies have examined SCD in adult athletes. The Oregon Sudden Unexpected Death Study examined the clinical features of 1247 individuals, aged from 35 to 65, who suffered a cardiac arrest in the period 2002–2013 [11]. Of these, 5% or 63 SCAs occurred during (76% of exercise SCAs) or within an hour (24%) of sports participation. Many of the exercise-related SCA victims had historical evidence of CAD. Specifically, 16% had diagnosed CAD, and an additional 33% had typical cardiac complaints including chest pain, dyspnoea or influenza-like symptoms before their arrest. The sports-related SCAs occurred in sports facilities 58% of the time, and were more often witnessed (87% vs 51%), received cardiopulmonary resuscitation (CPR) (44% vs 25%), and had a shockable rhythm (84% vs 51%). These individuals were also more likely to reach hospital discharge (23.2% vs 13.5%), but this advantage disappeared when the results were adjusted for CPR and cardiac rhythm.

These results demonstrate the importance of informing active subjects about the nature of prodromal symptoms of heart disease, and also the value of CPR and prompt resuscitation.

Prevention of acute cardiac events in adult athletes

Management of athletes with known coronary artery disease

The American Heart Association/American College of Cardiology (AHA/ACC) created a Task Force to provide recommendations on eligibility and disqualification from competitive sport for athletes with CAD [8]. This Task Force divided athletes with CAD into those with clinically manifest or symptomatic CAD and those with clinically concealed or asymptomatic CAD [8]. Those with manifest disease include patients who have suffered an acute event or who have myocardial ischaemia identified by provocative testing. Patients with concealed CAD are previously and presently asymptomatic, and have been found to have coronary artery calcification (CAC) by computed tomography or to have non-calcified plaque by coronary computed tomography angiography.

These recommendations are based on expert opinion and deductive reasoning using published evidence, but are not truly evidence based because they have never been subjected to controlled trial evaluation. The recommendations assume that the risk of an exercise-related AMI or SCD is greatest in those with symptomatic disease and increases with the severity and extent of CAD, the amount of ventricular (LV) dysfunction, the degree of myocardial ischaemia, and the presence and degree of electrical instability [8].

The most critical elements of managing the adult athlete with CAD are guideline-based medical management of the CAD and aggressive reduction of risk factors. Central to this is an aggressive reduction in serum lipids, focusing on low density lipoprotein cholesterol (LDL-C). LDL-C reduction with statins has been repetitively documented as reducing initial and subsequent CAD events. Unstable plaques are characterized by a rich lipid core, probably because lipid enrichment incites an inflammatory reaction and recruits white blood cells which synthesize matrix metalloproteinases and destabilize the coronary plaque [18]. Aggressive LDL-C reduction decreases the size of carotid, coronary, and aortic artery plaques [19]. The average duration of studies showing regression is 19.7 months and the average reduction in LDL-C was 40.4% [19]. The greatest reduction in plaque lipid content, at least in the carotid artery, occurs within the first 2 years of therapy [20]. The goal for LDL-C for CAD plaque regression is not clear, but lower appears to be progressively better [21]. A value of <2.0mmol (80mg/dl) has been suggested as the level at which progression is minimal and regression likely [21]. The AHA/ACC Task Force suggested that athletes consider 2 years of aggressive lipid reduction before returning to competition.

Low dose aspirin therapy (81mg daily) is recommended for all patients with established CAD who do not have a contraindication to its use. Thienopyridines should be added to aspirin therapy in patients who have suffered an acute coronary syndrome or undergone coronary revascularization.

Resting hypertension should be aggressively treated in athletes because systolic blood pressure rises during exercise and hypertension accelerates vascular disease progression. We initiate therapy with angiotensin convertase inhibitors (ACEi) or angiotensin receptor blockers (ARBs) because these agents do not reduce exercise tolerance. Low dose diuretics such as chlorthalidone 12.5 or 25mg daily is often necessary to achieve blood pressure control because patients can expand plasma volume with ACEi or ARBs, thereby mitigating the antihypertensive effect. We suggest that athletes stop their diuretic two days before endurance events to avoid dehydration. We avoid beta-adrenergic blocking agents in athletes because they often interfere with athletic performance and are not good antihypertensive agents unless they also provide some alpha adrenergic blockade (e.g. carvedilol). Beta-adrenergic blocking agents are recommended for the first 3 years after AMI and should be continued indefinitely in patients with reduced LV function [21,22].

Returning athletes with CAD to competition

The AHA/ACC Task Force recommends that all athletes with either manifest or concealed CAD have their LV function assessed and undergo exercise stress testing while taking their usual medications, including beta-adrenergic blockers [8,21] (see Box 6.3.1).

Ideally, the test should be designed to mimic the athlete's sport. The Task Force also recommends that the patient participates in the decision of when and if to return to competition because some adults consider the psychological benefits and enjoyment of competition to be worth the cardiovascular risks. The Task Force considered it reasonable to allow athletes with either symptomatic or asymptomatic CAD, normal left ventricular ejection function, no inducible ischaemia, and no evidence of electrical instability to return to competition, whereas symptomatic athletes not satisfying these criteria were recommended to engage only in sports with low dynamic and low static demands. It was also considered reasonable to restrict patients from competition for three months after an acute event and when there were changes in symptoms.

Box 6.3.1 American Heart Association/American College of Cardiology eligibility and disqualification recommendations for competitive athletes with coronary artery disease

1. Athletes with CAD should undergo maximal exercise testing to evaluate exercise tolerance, the presence of inducible ischaemia, and the presence of exercise-induced electrical instability. Testing should be performed on the subject's standard medical regimen, including beta-adrenergic blocking medications.
2. Athletes with atherosclerotic CAD should undergo an evaluation of left ventricular function.
3. Once informed of the results of the evaluations contained in recommendations 1 and 2, adult patients with atherosclerotic CAD should participate in the decision as to whether the health and psychological benefits of exercise for them outweigh the risk.
4. Athletes with atherosclerotic CAD should undergo aggressive risk factor reduction with high intensity statin therapy to reduce the chance of plaque disruption.
5. It is reasonable for athletes with clinically concealed CAD to participate in all competitive activities if their resting left ventricular ejection fraction is >50% and they have no inducible ischaemia or electrical instability.
6. It is reasonable for patients with clinically manifest CAD to participate in all competitive activities if their resting left ventricular ejection fraction is >50%, they are asymptomatic, and they have no inducible ischaemia or electrical instability.
7. It may be reasonable to restrict patients with clinically manifest CAD that does not fulfill the criteria in recommendation 6 to sports with low dynamic and low to moderate static demands.
8. It may be reasonable to prohibit patients with clinically manifest CAD from competitive sport participation:

   (a) for at least 3 months after an AMI or coronary revascularization procedure;

   (b) if they have increasing frequency or worsening symptoms of myocardial ischaemia.

Adapted from Thompson PD, Myerburg RJ, Levine BD, Udelson JE, Kovacs RJ. Eligibility and disqualification recommendations for competitive athletes with cardiovascular abnormalities: Task Force 8: Coronary Artery Disease: A Scientific Statement from the American Heart Association and American College of Cardiology. *Circulation* 2015 Dec 1; 132(22): e310–14.

Increases in coronary calcification scores in adult athletes

Several reports suggest that long-term endurance athletes may have increased CAC scores compared with sedentary contemporaries with similar risk factors [23]. Clinicians who treat adult athletes have also seen long-term endurance athletes with surprising high CAC scores and no symptoms of CAD. The significance of this increased CAC is unclear. Increasing CAC scores are associated with increased cardiac events in the general population, but increasing density of CAC is associated with reduced events [24]. In addition, statin therapy increases CAC scores [25], a finding that may indicate plaque stabilization. Athletes with high CAC scores should be evaluated as suggested by the Task Force for asymptomatic CAD patients and have their risk factors treated aggressively until the significance of this increased CAD is clear.

Routine exercise, testing, and screening in adult athletes

The AHA's scientific statement on standards for exercise testing acknowledges that the requirement for exercise testing before vigorous exercise is controversial, but recommends such testing in diabetics, men aged over 45, women aged over 55, and those with major CAD risk factors [26]. This recommendation was adopted largely to be consistent with prior recommendations.

There is some justification for such recommendations since ~60% of exercise-related SCA in one study did not show evidence of acute cardiac events, suggesting that the SCA was due to exercise-induced ischaemia [11]. A study of SCA during long-distance running also noted that none of the victims had evidence of an acute coronary lesion on angiography or autopsy [27]. On the other hand, the risk of SCD during exercise is very small, and most exercise-related AMIs are due to acute plaque disruption, often in previously insignificant coronary lesions which would not have been detected by exercise testing. Routine exercise testing of asymptomatic healthy athletes would generate a preponderance of false-positive results, possibly leading to inappropriate interventions. It would also serve as a barrier to exercise. We suggest that a selective use of exercise testing to evaluate adult athletes is more appropriate than a routine screening strategy.

Perhaps more important than exercise testing is ensuring that adult athletes know the prodromal symptoms of heart disease. Approximately 36% of SCAs in one study had symptoms of chest pain before their arrest [11]. Athletes and clinicians often do not know that epigastric distress is a common symptom of cardiac ischaemia. Similarly, many athletes and clinicians dismiss classical warm-up angina because it appears early in exercise, but subsequently relents and allows normal or near-normal performance. It is also important for clinicians evaluating prospective adult athletes to know why the individual wants to participate in sports or to start a vigorous exercise programme because many such patients are symptomatic and seek to exercise to prove to themselves that their symptoms are not cardiac disease. Education for both clinicians and athletes about such issues may help to reduce exercise-related acute cardiac events.

Conclusions

CAD is responsible for the majority of acute exercise-related cardiac events in adult athletes. Such events can occur in athletes with or without known CAD, although many athletes who suffered exercise-related events had prior prodromal symptoms which they ignored. Clinicians managing athletes with known disease should evaluate the athlete's cardiac risk using exercise testing, a measure of LV function, and an assessment of cardiac electrical stability. Clinicians should pursue aggressive risk factor reduction and ensure that the athlete knows the signs and symptoms of worsening CAD and the need for prompt medical attention.

Further reading

Eijsvogels TM, Fernandez AB, Thompson PD. Are there deleterious cardiac effects of acute and chronic endurance exercise? *Physiol Rev* 2016; 96: 99–125.

Marijon E, Uy-Evanado A, Reinier K, et al. Sudden cardiac arrest during sports activity in middle age. *Circulation* 2015; 131: 1384–91.

Thompson PD, Myerburg RJ, Levine BD, et al. Eligibility and disqualification recommendations for competitive athletes with cardiovascular abnormalities: Task Force 8: Coronary Artery Disease. *Circulation* 2015; 132: e310–14.

References

1. Giri S, Thompson PD, Kiernan FJ, et al. Clinical and angiographic characteristics of exertion-related acute myocardial infarction. *JAMA* 1999; 282: 1731–6.
2. Mittleman MA, Maclure M, Tofler GH, et al. Triggering of acute myocardial infarction by heavy physical exertion: protection against triggering by regular exertion. Determinants of Myocardial Infarction Onset Study Investigators. *N Engl J Med* 1993; 329: 1677–83.
3. Willich SN, Lewis M, Lowel H, et al. Physical exertion as a trigger of acute myocardial infarction. Triggers and Mechanisms of Myocardial Infarction Study Group. *N Engl J Med* 1993; 329: 1684–90.
4. Albert CM, Mittleman MA, Chae CU, et al. Triggering of sudden death from cardiac causes by vigorous exertion. *N Engl J Med* 2000; 343: 1355–61.
5. Siscovick DS, Weiss NS, Fletcher RH, Lasky T. The incidence of primary cardiac arrest during vigorous exercise. *N Engl J Med* 1984; 311: 874–7.
6. Thompson PD, Funk EJ, Carleton RA, Sturner WQ. Incidence of death during jogging in Rhode Island from 1975 through 1980. *JAMA* 1982; 247: 2535–8.
7. Whang W, Manson JE, Hu FB, et al. Physical exertion, exercise, and sudden cardiac death in women. *JAMA* 2006; 295: 1399–1403.
8. Thompson PD, Myerburg RJ, Levine BD, et al. Eligibility and disqualification recommendations for competitive athletes with cardiovascular abnormalities: Task Force 8: Coronary Artery Disease. *Circulation* 2015; 132: e310–14.
9. Rai M, Thompson PD. The definition of exertion-related cardiac events. *Br J Sports Med* 2011; 45: 130–1.
10. Thompson PD, Franklin BA, Balady GJ, et al. Exercise and acute cardiovascular events placing the risks into perspective: a scientific statement from the American Heart Association Council on Nutrition, Physical Activity, and Metabolism and the Council on Clinical Cardiology. *Circulation* 2007; 115: 2358–68.
11. Marijon E, Uy-Evanado A, Reinier K, et al. Sudden cardiac arrest during sports activity in middle age. *Circulation* 2015; 131: 1384–91.
12. Eijsvogels TM, Molossi S, Lee DC, et al. Exercise at the extremes: the amount of exercise to reduce cardiovascular events. *J Am Coll Cardiol* 2016; 67: 316–29.
13. Thompson PD, Buchner D, Pina IL, et al. Exercise and physical activity in the prevention and treatment of atherosclerotic cardiovascular disease. *Circulation* 2003; 107: 3109–16.

14. Anderson L, Oldridge N, Thompson DR, et al. Exercise-based cardiac rehabilitation for coronary heart disease: Cochrane systematic review and meta-analysis. *J Am Coll Cardiol* 2016; 67: 1–12.
15. Albano AJ, Thompson PD, Kapur NK. Acute coronary thrombosis in Boston marathon runners. *N Engl J Med* 2012; 366: 184–5.
16. Black A, Black MM, Gensini G. Exertion and acute coronary artery injury. *Angiology* 1975; 26: 759–83.
17. Kestin AS, Ellis PA, Barnard MR, et al. Effect of strenuous exercise on platelet activation state and reactivity. *Circulation* 1993; 88: 1502–11.
18. Libby P. Molecular and cellular mechanisms of the thrombotic complications of atherosclerosis. *J Lipid Res* 2009; 50(Suppl): S352–7.
19. Noyes AM, Thompson PD. A systematic review of the time course of atherosclerotic plaque regression. *Atherosclerosis* 2014; 234: 75–84.
20. Zhao XQ, Dong L, Hatsukami T, et al. MR imaging of carotid plaque composition during lipid-lowering therapy a prospective assessment of effect and time course. *JACC Cardiovasc Imaging* 2011; 4: 977–86.
21. Nissen SE, Nicholls SJ, Sipahi I, et al. Effect of very high-intensity statin therapy on regression of coronary atherosclerosis: the ASTEROID trial. *JAMA* 2006; 295: 1556–65.
22. Smith SC Jr, Benjamin EJ, Bonow RO, et al. AHA/ACCF Secondary prevention and risk reduction therapy for patients with coronary and other atherosclerotic vascular disease: 2011 update. A guideline from the American Heart Association and American College of Cardiology Foundation. *Circulation* 2011; 124: 2458–73.
23. Eijsvogels TM, Fernandez AB, Thompson PD. Are there deleterious cardiac effects of acute and chronic endurance exercise? *Physiol Rev* 2016; 96: 99–125.
24. Criqui MH, Denenberg JO, Ix JH, et al. Calcium density of coronary artery plaque and risk of incident cardiovascular events. *JAMA* 2014; 311: 271–8.
25. Kataoka Y, Wolski K, Balog C, et al. Progression of coronary atherosclerosis in stable patients with ultrasonic features of high-risk plaques. *Eur Heart J Cardiovasc Imaging* 2014; 15(9): 1035–41.
26. Fletcher GF, Ades PA, Kligfield P, et al. Exercise standards for testing and training: a scientific statement from the American Heart Association. *Circulation* 2013; 128: 873–934.
27. Kim JH, Malhotra R, Chiampas G, et al. Cardiac arrest during long-distance running races. *N Engl J Med* 2012; 366: 130–40.

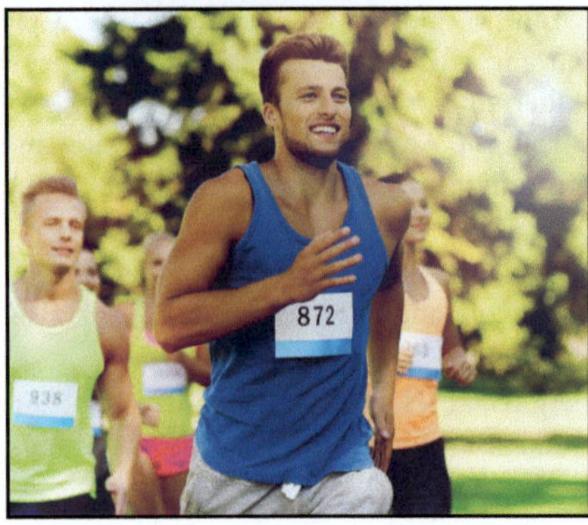

6.4

Less frequent causes of sudden cardiac death

Contents

6.4.1 **Less frequent causes of SCD (commotio cordis): non-cardiac causes (drug abuse, hyperpyrexia, rhabdomyolysis, sickle cell anaemia) —Part 1**
Erik Ekker Solberg and Paolo Emilio Adami 328

6.4.2 **Less frequent causes of SCD (aortic rupture): non-cardiac causes (asthma, extreme environmental conditions (heat, cold, altitude))—Part 2**
Erik Ekker Solberg and Paolo Emilio Adami 332

6.4.1 Less frequent causes of SCD (commotio cordis): non-cardiac causes (drug abuse, hyperpyrexia, rhabdomyolysis, sickle cell anaemia)—Part 1

Erik Ekker Solberg and Paolo Emilio Adami

Commotio cordis

What is commotio cordis?

The term 'commotio cordis' (CC) denotes a severe cardiac arrhythmia, leading to sudden cardiac arrest, triggered by a blow to the area of the chest directly over the heart. Unlike 'contusio cordis', cardiac tissue is not damaged by CC [1]. Thus sudden cardiac arrest (SCA) may occur in a healthy heart.

Clinical features of commotio cordis

If there is a malignant arrhythmic response to the blow, the person affected may rapidly become unconscious, pulseless, cyanotic, and, if there is cerebral ischaemia, develop convulsions. It is important that people recognize the possibility of CC when SCA or another malignant cardiac arrhythmia has occurred following a recent blow to the chest. As CC is rare, there is a risk that it will not be recognized and that the first part of chain of survival [2], namely early recognition of the situation, will not be in place.

Who is at risk?

CC is most likely to occur in healthy young men in their late teens (average age 16–18 years, age range about 10 years to about 25–30 years) [3]. The vulnerability of young men to CC is ascribed to the high degree of elasticity of the chest wall and that they are more likely than young women to participate in sports and violent behaviour. This finding is supported by the incidence in sudden deaths in sport which in general is much greater in men than in women [4]. Research also suggests that there may be individual vulnerability to the risk of acquiring CC (3).

Where does it happen?

CC occurs more in organized sports than in general play, and more frequently in sports that may cause blows to the chest, either in the form of a projectile (baseball, hockey, lacrosse) or, in contact sports, by collisions between knee and chest in football, fists in boxing, trauma to the chest from bicycle accidents, or kicks from horses [3]. CC due to physical struggle, falls [5], and criminal situations [6] has also been reported. It should be noted that, in rare cases, seemingly innocent collisions during play can trigger CC. For example, in one reported case CC was triggered by a snowball [3].

Incidence

Data on the occurrence of CC has primarily been taken from the US Commotio Cordis Registry which now contains more than 250 cases of CC. About 10–20 cases are added to the registry each year. Data from other countries, although sparse, largely confirm the American pattern, except that the types of sport that can trigger CC depend on how popular various sports are in different countries. Internationally, it appears that CC most frequently occurs in football, which is the most common sport in the world. In a US study of sudden deaths in sport, CC accounted for ~20% of cases [7]. It is possible that CC is under-recognized in Europe [8].

Treatment

When a cardiac arrest or other malignant cardiac arrhythmia is suspected following a previous blow to the chest, cardiopulmonary resuscitation (CPR) should be initiated immediately. Standard guidelines for CPR and use of automated external defibrillators (AEDs) should be followed.

Survival

Previous studies of survival from CC have shown that the risk of a fatal outcome is high, and a low survival rate of ~15% has been described [9]. Survival has improved in recent years, perhaps because of the increased public awareness of SCA in sport. More recent observations report survival from CC in more than 50% of cases [10]. Better physical protection against CC may also have made sport safer. As expected, research shows a clear correlation between survival and early CPR and defibrillation [10].

Pathophysiology

Several factors can affect the risk of triggering malignant arrhythmia after an impact on the chest, including the exact position of impact on the chest wall (the contour of the heart), the speed of the projectile hitting the chest (not necessarily the highest speed), and the characteristics of the projectile (a higher risk if the item is compact) [3]. The timing of the hit in relation to the heart rhythm seems to be particularly important.

The result of an unfortunate combination of these factors may induce a malignant arrhythmia. A strike against the chest leading to CC may cause the intra-ventricular pressure in the left ventricle to rise. This results in increased wall stress and eventually to cell membrane deformation and activation of the ATP-sensitive potassium channel, which may trigger a malignant arrhythmia.

Experimental CC model

Current understanding of CC is mainly based on from experimental American studies. In 1998 Link et al. [11] described a model where projectiles were shot at an ECG-monitored pig's heart, and the intra-ventricular cavity pressure and the velocity of the projectile were measured. Researchers also administered drugs that could double block the animal's autonomic nervous system (beta-blocker to block the sympathetic nervous system, and acetylcholine to block the parasympathetic nervous system). They also administered the anti-diabetic drug glibenclamide, which blocks the ATP-sensitive K^+ channel, and colchicine, which can destroy the cell membrane. The findings of various studies using this model, which also took its weaknesses into account (i.e. a pig's heart is not a human heart, anaesthetics may be pro-arrhythmic), showed that a shock to the chest most likely triggers dangerous cardiac arrhythmia (VT degenerating into VF), leading to SCA and asystole, when the collision occurs 10–30ms before the peak T wave in ECG in the repolarization period. Less malignant arrhythmias (bundle branch block, VT, AV block, atrial fibrillation) are more likely to occur when the impact is in the repolarization period, slightly before the most vulnerable time window. CC is most likely under the following conditions.

- The impact results in an average pressure of about 350mmHg in the left ventricle (higher and lower pressure reduces the risk of induction of VF). Significantly higher pressure may cause contusio cordis (crushing heart tissue).
- Impact is at a velocity of about 60 km/h [12] (somewhat surprisingly, a higher velocity reduced the chance of VF).

The properties of the projectile are also important. A compact projectile increases the risk of malignant arrhythmia (e.g. a spherical projectile with a relatively small diameter). Similarly, a direct perpendicular impact on the cardiac silhouette (most vulnerable to shock in the middle of the left ventricle) is necessary to produce VF [13]. Mechanical deformation of the cell membrane appears to be essential for activation of the ATP-sensitive K^+ channel via mechano-electrical coupling. This is the underlying arrhythmic mechanism. Blocking this ion channel with glibenclamide has been shown to reduce the risk of VF, which supports the hypothesis that the ATP-sensitive K^+ channel is involved in the generation of malignant arrhythmias. Cell membranes are affected and destroyed by CC. When administering colchicine, which can destroy the cell membrane, the chance of VF was increased [14]. However, double blockage of the autonomic nervous system does not appear to affect the probability of VF, indicating that the induction of malignant arrhythmias is not due to an abrupt change in the autonomic balance [15]. Cardiac responses to CC are similar to the R-on-T phenomenon in ECG, which has been described in the literature as a mechanism that could trigger VF.

Prevention

Sports and crowd behaviour

Experimental research has identified a number of factors that can trigger CC and has been successful in identifying aspects of CC that can be used clinically. It has been shown that soft rather than hard compact baseballs reduce the incidence of VF (16). Applying softballs in baseball have decreased the risk of CC. Similarly, certain contact sports have introduced penalties for impacts on the left ribcage. The media-driven increased awareness of SCA in sports has probably led to speedier identification of the condition and faster and more accurate action.

Protection

The use of chest protectors in some sports has led to a reduction in CC [16]. However, CC has been shown to cause SCA even when chest protectors are used. The results of chest protection do not appear to have lived up to expectations. This may be because the protectors were not good enough or had not been properly placed and had slipped out of position when the impact occurred. Research on improved protectors is ongoing.

Cardiac arrest in society

Cardiac arrest in or out of sport is a major public health problem. It is very tragic for the families affected and an economic burden when unnecessary lives are lost. CC may be increasingly relevant because the escalating intensity and speed of modern sport enhances the likelihood of CC. Although the media focus on SCA in elite athletes, it may be forgotten that cardiac arrest in wider society is a major medical problem with respect to the numbers of people affected. Therefore it is important to recognize the existence of CC. If CC is not recognized when it actually happens, the risk is that it will not be treated. Similarly, the natural, but wrong, belief that CC could not have occurred because the impact was not severe enough can also lead to an absence of appropriate treatment. Therefore dissemination of information about CC is essential to reduce the number of sudden cardiac deaths.

Drug abuse

Drug abuse in relation to sport (doping) has been defined in several ways, most commonly as the use of performance-enhancing drugs defined by the World Anti-Doping Agency (WADA) (https://www.wada-ama.org/en/what-we-do/the-code).

Despite a number of circumstantial reports on a possible association between drug abuse and SCA in sport during the last five decades, there is no clear scientific and unequivocal evidence supporting or invalidating the widespread perception of the influence of doping on SCA in sports. Thus it is not known whether doping plays an insignificant, minor, or major role in SCA in sports.

However, there is indirect evidence linking the abuse of illicit drugs to SCA in sports. These drugs may trigger a wide range of exercise-related cardiac arrhythmias which can be lethal [17]. Abuse of performance-enhancing substances is associated with ventricular hypertrophy and repolarization changes [18]. There is a large body of information on the cardiovascular side effects of anabolic steroids, including lipoprotein profile abnormalities, thrombotic diathesis, coronary vasoconstriction, cardiac arrhythmias, hypertrophy, and increased blood pressure [19,20], which may predispose to SCA. Case studies suggest that abuse of anabolic steroids is linked to cardiac events such as acute myocardial infarction and fatal ventricular arrhythmias [21]. Other substances, such as stimulants (amphetamines, cocaine, ephedrine alkaloids) and erythropoietin (EPO) have also been associated with sudden death in sport [17, 21–23].

Clarification of the role of doping either as a single factor or as a confounding causal factor in lethal and non-lethal cardiac events is an important challenge. Only systematic registration over time of toxicological agents in registries of SCA in sports will elucidate the actual role of doping in SCA. Such registration of SCA/SCD in sports should include toxicology screen for illicit substances prior to attributing the cause of death to a primary cardiomyopathy [24].

Exercise-induced rhabdomyolysis

The word ‘rhabdomyolysis’ comes from the Greek rhabdo myo (striated muscle) and lysis (degradation). Exercise-induced rhabdomyolysis is the breakdown of skeletal muscle, which may occur during specific strenuous exercise when the energy requirements of the myocytes are not satisfied. The result is muscular necrosis, and the athlete may experience swelling, pain and weakness in the affected muscles. Other clinical features are marked increases of the muscle enzyme creatine kinase (CK) and myoglobin, which in part is responsible for the complications that can result from rhabdomyolysis. Thus the diagnosis of rhabdomyolysis is made by a typical history of illness, examination in the clinic, and measurement of a markedly elevated CK serum sample and myoglobinuria.

A problem when studying the literature of rhabdomyolysis in sports is that many of the diagnoses of rhabdomyolysis are based on other factors such as ‘traumatic’ (muscle trauma), ‘non-traumatic’ (elderly lying on a floor, seizures) and 'non-traumatic, not activity mediated' (toxic, drugs, hereditary, infections, electrolyte imbalance). Exercise-induced rhabdomyolysis in healthy athletes is a fairly benign condition and does not lead to SCA. However, there is report of SCA in sports [25] in which rhabdomyolysis has appeared as the only pathological marker. Rhabdomyolysis in conjunction with other diseases (e.g. sickle cell disease) leading to SCA is well known [25].

Exercise-induced rhabdomyolysis, which is a sign of dysfunctional training, can be avoided by exercising wisely, using a reasonable progression of the training load, and being aware of the increased risk due to eccentric exercise, excessive heat, dehydration, and many repetitions without sufficient warm-up and restitution.

Sickle cell trait

Sickle cell trait (SCT) is a genetic disorder of the red blood cells and is found in 8% of African Americans [26]. In a very large American collegiate athletic register of SCA in sports, SCT was associated with a relative risk of SCD that was 37 times normal [7]. This high figure has led to a discussion of whether screening for SCT (e.g. in specific athletic groups is justified) [27–29].

Unlike SCA in sports due to other conditions, an SCT-associated death occurs as a non-instantaneous collapse with gradual deterioration over time. It is associated with vigorous exercise, heat, and is largely unpredictable [25]. Most frequently it occurs in younger male football players during conditioning training early in the season [25].

The pathophysiology is not quite clear, but may be sickling of the red blood cells during exertion, which may start a cascade of vascular occlusion, endothelial damage, and impaired blood flow to the muscles which promotes rhabdomyolysis and disseminated intravascular coagulation. Rhabdomyolysis leads to hyperkalaemia and acidosis, which in the setting of hypoxia adversely affects cardiac function and lowers the threshold for lethal cardiac arrhythmia [25]. If an SCT-associated collapse occurs, oxygen, intravenous hydration, and cooling should be administered.

To prevent SCT-associated death, in addition to screening, athletes should be educated to avoid vigorous exercise during excessive heat, avoid dehydration, and be extra aware of initial symptoms of SCT-associated cardiac arrest and factors leading to rhabdomyolysis [29].

Further reading

Classie JA, Distel LM, Borchers JR. Safety baseballs and chest protectors: a systematic review on the prevention of commotio cordis. *Phys Sportsmed* 2010; 38: 83–90.

Deligiannis A, Bjornstad H, Carré F, et al. ESC Study Group of Sports Cardiology position paper on adverse cardiovascular effects of doping in athletes. *Eur J Cardiovasc Prev Rehabil* 2006; 13: 687–94.

Furlanello F, Serdoz LV, Cappato R, De Ambroggi L. Illicit drugs and cardiac arrhythmias in athletes. *Eur J Cardiovasc Prev Rehabil* 2007; 14: 487–94.

Harmon KG, Drezner JA, Casa DJ. To screen or not to screen for sickle cell trait in American football? *Br J Sports Med* 2012; 46: 158.

Link MS, Wang PJ, Pandian NG, et al. An experimental model of sudden death due to low-energy chest-wall impact (commotio cordis). *N Engl J Med* 1998; 338: 1805–11.

Link MS, Maron BJ, VanderBrink BA, et al. Impact directly over the cardiac silhouette is necessary to produce ventricular fibrillation in an experimental model of commotio cordis. *J Am Coll Cardiol* 2001; 37: 649–54.

Maron BJ. Sudden death in young athletes. *N Engl J Med* 2003; 349: 1064–75.

Maron BJ, Estes NA III Commotio cordis. *N Engl J Med* 2010; 362: 917–27.

Maron BJ, Gohman TE, Kyle SB, et al. Clinical profile and spectrum of commotio cordis. *JAMA* 2002; 287: 1142–6.

Maron BJ, Ahluwalia A, Haas TS, et al. Global epidemiology and demographics of commotio cordis. *Heart Rhythm* 2011; 8: 1969–71.

Montisci M, El Mazioum R, Cecchetto G, et al. Anabolic androgenic steroids abuse and cardiac death in athletes: morphological and toxicological findings in four fatal cases. *Forensic Sci Int* 2012; 217: e13–18.

Solberg EE, Embrå BI, Börjesson M, et al. Commotio cordis under recognised in Europe? *Eur J Cardiovasc Prev Rehabil* 2011; 18: 378–83

References

1. Nesbitt AD, Cooper PJ, Kohl P. Rediscovering commotio cordis. *Lancet* 2001; 357: 1195–7.
2. Newman M. The chain of survival revisited. The emergence of early recognition as the unsung vital link. *JEMS* 1998; 23: 46.
3. Maron BJ, Estes NA, III Commotio cordis. *N Engl J Med* 2010; 362: 917–27.
4. Harmon KG, Asif IM, Klossner D, Drezner JA. Incidence of sudden cardiac death in National Collegiate Athletic Association athletes. *Circulation* 2011; 123: 1594–1600.
5. Tibballs J, Thiruchelvam T. A case of commotio cordis in a young child caused by a fall. *Resuscitation* 2008; 77: 139–141.
6. Maron BJ, Mitten MJ, Greene BC. Criminal consequences of commotio cordis. *Am J Cardiol* 2002; 89: 210–13.
7. Maron BJ. Sudden death in young athletes. *N Engl J Med* 2003; 349: 1064–75.
8. Solberg EE, Embra BI, Borjesson M, et al. Commotio cordis—under-recognized in Europe? A case report and review. *Eur J Cardiovasc Prev Rehabil* 2011; 18: 378–83.
9. Drezner JA, Chun JS, Harmon KG, Derminer L. Survival trends in the United States following exercise-related sudden cardiac arrest in the youth: 2000-2006. *Heart Rhythm* 2008; 5: 794–9.
10. Maron BJ, Haas TS, Ahluwalia A, et al. Increasing survival rate from commotio cordis. *Heart Rhythm* 2013; 10: 219–23.
11. Link MS, Wang PJ, Pandian NG, et al. An experimental model of sudden death due to low-energy chest-wall impact (commotio cordis). *N Engl J Med* 1998; 338: 1805–11.

12. Link MS, Maron BJ, Wang PJ, et al. Upper and lower limits of vulnerability to sudden arrhythmic death with chest-wall impact (commotio cordis). *J Am Coll Cardiol* 2003; **41**: 99–104.
13. Link MS, Maron BJ, VanderBrink BA, et al. Impact directly over the cardiac silhouette is necessary to produce ventricular fibrillation in an experimental model of commotio cordis. *J Am Coll Cardiol* 2001; 37: 649–54.
14. Madias C, Maron BJ, Supron S, et al. Cell membrane stretch and chest blow-induced ventricular fibrillation: commotio cordis. *J Cardiovasc Electrophysiol* 2008; 19: 1304–9.
15. Stout C, Maron BJ, VanderBrink BA, et al. Importance of the autonomic nervous system in an experimental model of commotio cordis. *Med Sci Monit* 2007; 13: BR11–15.
16. Classie JA, Distel LM, Borchers JR. Safety baseballs and chest protectors: a systematic review on the prevention of commotio cordis. *Phys Sportsmed* 2010; 38: 83–90.
17. Furlanello F, Serdoz LV, Cappato R, De Ambroggi L. Illicit drugs and cardiac arrhythmias in athletes. *Eur J Cardiovasc Prev Rehabil* 2007; 14: 487–94.
18. Papadakis M, Carré F, Kervio G, et al. The prevalence, distribution, and clinical outcomes of electrocardiographic repolarization patterns in male athletes of African/Afro-Caribbean origin. *Eur Heart J* 2011; 32: 2304–13.
19. Angell PJ, Chester N, Sculthorpe N, et al. Performance enhancing drug abuse and cardiovascular risk in athletes: implications for the clinician. *Br J Sports Med* 2012; 46(Suppl 1): i78–84.
20. Deligiannis A, Bjornstad H, Carré F, et al. ESC study group of sports cardiology position paper on adverse cardiovascular effects of doping in athletes. *Eur J Cardiovasc Prev Rehabil* 2006; 13: 687–94.
21. Achar S, Rostamian A, Narayan SM. Cardiac and metabolic effects of anabolic-androgenic steroid abuse on lipids, blood pressure, left ventricular dimensions, and rhythm. *Am J Cardiol* 2010; 106: 893–901.
22. Nascimento JH, Medei E. Cardiac effects of anabolic steroids: hypertrophy, ischemia and electrical remodelling as potential triggers of sudden death. *Mini Rev Med Chem* 2011; 11: 425–9.
23. Montisci M, El Mazioum R, Cecchetto G, et al. Anabolic androgenic steroids abuse and cardiac death in athletes: morphological and toxicological findings in four fatal cases. *Forensic Sci Int* 2012; 217: e13–18.
24. Solberg EE, Borjesson M, Sharma S, et al. Sudden cardiac arrest in sports—need for uniform registration: a Position Paper from the Sport Cardiology Section of the European Association for Cardiovascular Prevention and Rehabilitation. *Eur J Prev Cardiol* 2016; 23: 657–67.
25. Harris KM, Haas TS, Eichner ER, Maron BJ. Sickle cell trait associated with sudden death in competitive athletes. *Am J Cardiol* 2012; 110: 1185–8.
26. Tsaras G, Owusu-Ansah A, Boateng FO, Amoateng-Adjepong Y. Complications associated with sickle cell trait: a brief narrative review. *Am J Med* 2009; 122: 507–12.
27. Harmon KG, Drezner JA, Klossner D, Asif IM. Sickle cell trait associated with a RR of death of 37 times in National Collegiate Athletic Association football athletes: a database with 2 million athlete-years as the denominator. *Br J Sports Med* 2012; 46: 325–30.
28. Shephard RJ. Sickle cell trait: what are the costs and benefits of screening? *J Sports Med Phys Fitness* 2016; 56: 1562–73.
29. Harmon KG, Drezner JA, Casa DJ. To screen or not to screen for sickle cell trait in American football? *Br J Sports Med* 2012; 46: 158.

6.4.2 Less frequent causes of SCD (aortic rupture): non-cardiac causes (asthma, extreme environmental conditions (heat, cold, altitude))—Part 2

Erik Ekker Solberg and Paolo Emilio Adami

Aortic diseases

Aortic diseases account for about 1–5% of SCD in athletes [1–3]. The acute manifestations of aortic diseases may represent a life-threatening emergency and include aortic dissection, intra-mural haematoma and penetrating atherosclerotic ulcer. Increases in blood pressure, and consequently stress on aortic walls during intense physical activity, put subjects with aortic disease at risk for aortic dissection or rupture. Therefore the presence of aortic diseases must be taken into account when screening athletes and establishing their eligibility to practise sport.

Aortic dissection

Aortic dissection is the most common manifestation of an acute aortic disease, with an estimated annual incidence of 2.6–3.5 per 100,000 person-years [4]. Data derived from the International Registry of Acute Aortic Dissection (IRAD) show that mean age for aortic dissection is 63 years and a large majority of patients are male [5]. In patients younger than 40 years, aortic dissection is more frequently associated with genetic syndromes or congenital conditions. In patients older than 40 years, hypertension is the most common risk factor [6]. There is also an age difference regarding the type of dissection, which is more proximal (i.e. at the sinuses of Valsalva or the sino-tubular junction, Type A dissection) in younger patients [6].

Measuring the aortic root and ascending aorta

Echocardiographic measurements of the aorta should be taken at the end-diastolic phase and at several locations, including the aortic annulus, the sinuses of Valsalva, the sino-tubular junction, the maximal diameter of the proximal ascending tract, and the aortic arch. Measurements should be taken perpendicular to the blood flow and include the largest measured diameter [7].

Factors influencing aortic dimension in athletes

Height, weight, body surface area (BSA), age, gender, and exercise training influence aortic root dimensions. Healthy athletes generally have a slightly larger aortic root diameter than the non-athletic population. Aortic diameters in athletes are on average 3.2mm larger at the sinuses of Valsalva and 1.6mm larger at the aortic valve annulus compared with non-athletes [8].

Body size and height

BSA and height seem to be the two most relevant determinants of aortic diameter and must be taken into consideration, particularly when assessing very small or very tall subjects. The most common nomogram adopted [9] uses BSA to predict normal aortic dimensions. The formula assumes linearity between BSA and aortic diameter, but more recent studies have shown a non-linear relationship, especially in subjects above the 95th percentile for height (>189 cm in men, >175 cm in women), in whom the relationship seems to plateau [10–12]. Therefore, to avoid under-estimating aortic root dimensions in very tall athletes, it is important not to rely solely on height or BSA, but to take into consideration all aspects determining the dimension. Tall athletes with large aortic diameters (≥40mm for males, and ≥34 for females), showing no signs of systemic diseases or valvular abnormalities, should be closely monitored, since these values are uncommon in highly trained athletes and are unlikely to be the expression of a cardiac adaptation to exercise [13]. Avoidance of intense weight training may be advised [8].

Influence of exercise training on aortic diameter

The larger aortic root diameter in athletes has been hypothetically attributed to increased haemodynamic stress on the aorta caused by exercise [14]. In particular, it has been hypothesized that certain sports disciplines, such as weightlifting [15,16], might enlarge the aorta more than endurance sports [17,18] because of the the extremely high values of blood pressure (peak systolic blood pressure, 320mmHg; diastolic blood pressure, 250mmHg) reported during weightlifting [19] and the association between weightlifting training and aortic dissection [20]. However, studies of larger populations of athletes have not demonstrated a significant difference in aorta dimensions among sports disciplines. Power disciplines have only a trivial impact on aortic remodelling [11,12]. Therefore weightlifting training remains a safe exercise, since pre-existing enlargement of the aorta is already present when the weightlifting-related aortic dissection occurs [20,21]. In conclusion, sport per se does not seem to have a major influence on aortic dimension, with a very small difference existing among different types of sports.

Age and gender

Aortic root dimensions are 1–3mm larger in men than in women [22], and tend to increase with increasing age in the general population, with a predicted increase of 0.89mm in men and 0.68mm in women for each successive decade of life, starting in mid-adulthood [23]. Athletes do not differ from the general population. Interestingly, the largest increase with ageing seems to occur after the cessation of the athletic career [12], suggesting that aortic dilation might be the consequence of a combination of intrinsic pathological changes, ageing, and possibly strenuous exercise.

Associated conditions

The conditions most frequently associated with aortic diseases are bicuspid aortic valve (BAV), Marfan syndrome, Ehlers–Danlos syndrome, Loeys–Dietz syndrome, and familial thoracic aortic aneurysm.

Bicuspid aortic valve

BAV is the most common cardiovascular malformation in humans, with a prevalence of 1–2% in the general population; it is twice as frequent in males as in females [24–26]. It is an autosomal dominant disorder with reduced penetrance and a prevalence of approximately 10% in first-degree relatives of an individual with a BAV [27,28]. BAV may evolve progressively in valve dysfunction (stenosis or regurgitation) and is associated with aortopathy [29]. Altered valve and annular geometry impose abnormal stress on the aortic wall, predisposing to abnormal elasticity which contributes to aortic dilation and risk of dissection [30].

Baseline aortic root diameter is an important predictor of the rate of aortic expansion, ranging between 0.2 and 1.9mm per year in patients with BAV [30–32]. The relative risk of aortic dissection is increased compared with the general population, but the absolute risk appears to be low. Patients with BAV incur excess morbidity over a 25 year period, with a clearly increased risk of aortic and valve surgery and aneurysm formation [30]. It should be noted that exercise in subjects with BAV does not appear to accelerate the increase in aortic size [32,33].

Advice to athletes with BAV on eligibility to participate in competition should be based on the presence of valvular disease and/or aortic root dilation (see also Chapter 4.2.2). Athletes with BAV showing no signs of significant aortic regurgitation or stenosis and normal aortic root dimensions can participate in sport without restrictions [13]. These athletes should be assessed by trans-thoracic echocardiography at least every 12 months for progressive valve dysfunction and aortic dilation.

Marfan syndrome

Marfan syndrome (MFS) is a systemic connective tissue, autosomal dominant disorder, characterized by mutations in the fibrillin-1 gene (*FBN1*). It has an estimated prevalence of 1 in 3000–5000 individuals and no predilection for sex or ethnicity [34]. Approximately 25% of cases have no previous family history, thus representing de novo mutations. MFS affects the cardiovascular, ocular, and skeletal systems and, despite the effective treatment of aortic root disease, cardiovascular mortality remains high due to arrhythmia, heart failure, complications at the distal aorta, and valvular dysfunction [35]. In the '2010 Revised Ghent Nosology' for the diagnosis of MFS [35], great importance is given to aortic dilation/dissection, ectopia lentis, family history, and genetic testing for mutations of *FBN1*. All other manifestations contribute to a 'systemic score' which supports the diagnosis when major features are not present [36–38]. In addition to aortic dilation these diagnostic criteria (systemic *z*-score) incorporate height, weight, age, and sex. This score is particularly useful when evaluating young subjects [22]. Aortic dissection is the main cause of mortality; 50% of undiagnosed patients less than 40 years old die from aortic dissection. However, if treated, they have a near-normal life expectancy [39].

Athletes with MFS are advised to avoid high intensity sports activities, weightlifting, and contact sports [3].

Other syndromes associated with aortic diseases

Other syndromes, such as Ehlers–Danlos syndrome, Loeys–Dietz syndrome, and familial thoracic aortic aneurysm are also associated with aortic dilation/dissection. These genetically transmitted conditions present an altered structure of the aorta, and rupture or dissection can occur without previous vascular dilation. Therefore all subjects diagnosed with these conditions are usually advised not to participate in competitive sport.

Asthma in athletes

Asthma is a very rare cause of sudden death in athletes, with an estimated mortality rate of 0.23 per million competitive athletes [40,41]. It is the most common chronic disease among elite athletes, with a prevalence of 23% in athletes competing in summer sports and reportedly even higher in winter sports [42]. Olympic athletes reported a prevalence of 15% over a 12-year period [43]. It appears to be more frequent in male and black populations, and has a higher prevalence among endurance athletes, specifically cross-country skiers, swimmers, speed skaters, figure skaters, ice-hockey players, long distance runners, and cyclists, compared with athletes competing in other sports disciplines [44].

Asthma should be suspected if cough, wheezing and phlegm occur together with expiratory dyspnoea and audible rhonchi or sibilating rhonchi on lung auscultation after intense exercise of at least 5 min duration [45].

Sports that require high minute ventilation for a prolonged period of time expose athletes to environmental factors, contributing to develop a damage to the airways and resulting in airways hyper-responsiveness [46,47]. Heavy ventilation during endurance training represents an early local respiratory injury that induces and maintains airway mucosal inflammation and delays epithelial repair. Environmental factors such as cold dry air, particulate matter, and by-products of chlorine produce further damage to the already inflamed mucosa [48]. The hyper-vagal (parasympathetic) tone induced by endurance training, whose connection has been clearly demonstrated [49], seems to play a leading role in the development of the exercise-induced bronchoconstriction [46]. All these factors combined contribute to the development of asthma in athletes. Intense ventilation induces respiratory epithelial damage, causing airway inflammation with cell recruitment and production of cytokines, leukotrienes, mucous and cholinergic substances, all on the epithelial surface. Frequent high intensity exercise maintains the inflammation status, perpetuating the condition which is complicated by external environmental factors and the parasympathetic hyper-tone [47]. These mechanisms are partially reversible at the end of the athletic career [50,51]. The exact pathophysiological pathway leading to sudden death by asthma is not clear. Several theories have been hypothesized for a fatal asthma attack, including asphyxia, reduced chemosensitivity to hypoxia, or reduced perception of dyspnoea. In this context, exercise seems to induce a more severe sudden exacerbation [52–54].

Sport in extreme environments

Extreme environments are defined as those environments characterized by extraordinary microclimatic conditions critical for the physiological homeostasis. These environments can be extreme in terms of high or low temperature (i.e. heat or cold), pressure (i.e. underwater), oxygen concentration (i.e. high altitude), or gravity (i.e. microgravity). Living and exercising in these settings is becoming more frequent as a consequence of the improvements in human performance, supporting materials and technologies. Up to a certain extent, the human body can adapt to these extreme conditions through physiological mechanisms. In this section we will limit the discussion of extreme environments to sport in heat, in cold, and at high altitude. For a full understanding of the effects of exercising in extreme conditions, its consequences, and the related risks, we refer readers to specific manuals and textbooks.

Heat stress

The human body normally regulates core temperature to near 37°C and even small fluctuations within the narrow range of 35 to 41°C can impair exercise performance. Larger fluctuations, outside that range, can be lethal and are associated with morbidity and mortality [55].

The autonomic nervous system regulates the body's core temperature through physiological mechanisms including the rate of metabolic heat production (e.g. shivering), body heat distribution via the blood from the core to the skin (e.g. cutaneous vasodilation and constriction), and sweating.

Exercise causes an immediate metabolic heat production, eliciting heat-dissipating responses as the core temperature increases until heat loss responses are sufficient to match heat production and a new thermal balance is achieved. When exercise stops, heat loss exceeds heat production, so the core temperature declines to baseline levels and the pre-exercise conditions are established [56]. Circumstances or conditions that in any way impair this fine-control mechanism can cause pathological manifestation such as dehydration or exertion heat illness (e.g. heat exhaustion, heat injury, heat stroke). Risk factors for serious heat illness include lack of heat acclimatization, low physical fitness, dehydration, high body fat or mass, and certain medications.

Individuals suspected of having an exertional heat injury or stroke must receive early assistance in the field. Delay in cooling is the most important factor leading to death or residual serious disability. The patient should lie down, and as much as clothing as possible should be removed. Body cooling should be initiated by the most practical means and as quickly as possible, and continued until the core temperature is less than 38.5°C. Immersion of the body in cold or iced water while massaging the skin is the most rapid method, but particular care should be adopted in these situations [57].

Cold stress

The main determinants of cold stress during outdoor events in cold weather are air temperature and wind speed. Heat loss occurs even more rapidly with water immersion or wet clothing.

Upon exposure to cold, the human body reacts with a decrease in peripheral blood flow (peripheral vasoconstriction) resulting in a reduced transfer of heat from the body core to the skin, subcutaneous fat, and skeletal muscles, increasing insulation [57]. Vasoconstriction begins when the skin temperatures drop below 35°C and becomes maximal when temperature is about 31°C or less [58]. As the temperature continues to fall, vasoconstriction response extends beyond the extremities of the limbs, spreading to the entire body periphery and probably contributing to peripheral cold injuries. Exposure to cold also elicits increased metabolic heat production through modifying behaviour (i.e. increasing physical activity, exercise, fidgeting) and by shivering. Shivering may start immediately or after several minutes of exposure to cold. It consists of involuntary repeated rhythmic muscle contractions in which most of the metabolic energy is used to generate heat and very little external work is performed. It usually starts in the torso, and then spreads to the limbs.

Hypothermia may occur in athletes or exercising individuals, with a systemic involvement in extreme cases or limited to extremities. Systemic hypothermia is defined as a core body temperature less than 35°C with signs and symptoms that are generally non-specific and are strictly dependent on the subject's health and hypothermic circumstances [59]. In mild hypothermia (between 35 and 32°C) symptoms include tachycardia, hypertension, shivering, impaired coordination, and apathy. As the temperature drops further (between 32 and 28°C), the body slows down—no shivering, bradycardia, dilated pupils, slowed reflexes, cold diuresis, confusion, and lethargy. When the body core temperature drops below 28°C the skin may appear blue or puffy, and coma, apnoea, loss of reflexes, asystole, or ventricular fibrillation may occur. Ventricular fibrillation or asystole is usually the final cause of death.

The electrocardiogram (ECG) may show a high J wave or Osborn waves, defined as positive deflection in the terminal portion of the QRS complex, mostly visible in leads II, V_5 and V_6 [60,61].

Hypothermia of extremities may occur in different forms and seriousness, including frostnip, chilblain, trench foot, and frostbite. In all situations, warm up is the imperative treatment. Methods for warming up depend upon the degree of hypothermia and the resources available [62].

High altitude

The main feature of living and exercising in high altitude is the reduction in oxygen concentration. The decrease in atmospheric pressure reduces the oxygen concentration in the lungs, creating the conditions for hypoxia. Hypoxia is defined as an 'Oxygen deficiency caused by a reduction in the partial pressure of oxygen (PO_2) in ambient air because of a decrease in either the ambient barometric pressure (P_B) or the oxygen concentration of the inspired gas' [63]. Exposure to altitude reduces the PO_2 in the lungs with a consequent decrease in oxygen concentration in the arterial circulation. The physiological mechanisms activated involve ventilatory, haemodynamic, haematological, neural, hormonal, metabolic, acid–base, and body water responses. Depending on the altitude, non-acclimatized individuals, who are not properly prepared or have health issues, may find it difficult to adapt to the reduced oxygen concentration and counteract hypoxia, resulting in an altitude-related illness. Rate and height of ascent and individual variability determine the severity of the altitude-related illness, which comprises a range of conditions based on organ involvement [65]: acute mountain sickness (AMS), high altitude pulmonary oedema (HAPE), high altitude cerebral oedema (HACE), sub-acute mountain sickness, and chronic mountain sickness (Monge disease). In all manifestations of altitude-related illness the initial key treatments are immediate descent to lower altitudes and oxygen administration [59].

Further reading

Aslam AF, Aslam AK, Vasavada BC, Khan IA. Hypothermia: evaluation, electrocardiographic manifestations, and management. *Am J Med* 2006; 119: 297–301.

Bonini M, Gramiccioni C, Fioretti D, et al. Asthma, allergy and the Olympics: a 12-year survey in elite athletes. *Curr Opin Allergy Clin Immunol* 2015; 15: 184–92.

Cheng A, Owens D. Marfan syndrome, inherited aortopathies and exercise: What is the right answer? *Heart* 2015; 101: 752–7.

Hatzaras I, Tranquilli M, Coady M, et al. Weightlifting and aortic dissection: more evidence for a connection. *Cardiology* 2007; 107: 103–6.

Iskandar A, Thompson PD. A meta-analysis of aortic root size in elite athletes. *Circulation* 2013; 127: 791–8.

Iskandar A, Thompson PD. Diseases of the aorta in elite athletes. *Clin Sports Med* 2015; 34: 461–72.

Mayercik C, Carré F, Elefteriades J. Aortic dissection and sport: physiologic and clinical understanding provide an opportunity to save young lives. *J Cardiovasc Surg* 2010; 51: 669–81.

Pelliccia A, Di Paolo FM, De Blasiis E, et al. Prevalence and clinical significance of aortic root dilation in highly trained competitive athletes. *Circulation* 2010; 122: 698–706.

Pelliccia A, Di Paolo FM, Quattrini FM. Aortic root dilation in athletic population. *Prog Cardiovasc Dis* 2012; 54: 432–7.

Plant T, Aref-Adib G. Travelling to new heights: practical high altitude medicine. *Br J Hosp Med (Lond)* 2008; 69: 348–52.

References

1 Maron BJ, Doerer JJ, Haas TS, et al. Sudden deaths in young competitive athletes: analysis of 1866 deaths in the United States 1980-2006. *Circulation* 2009; 119: 1085–92.

2 Maron BJ, Haas TS, Murphy CJ, et al. Incidence and causes of sudden death in U.S. college athletes. *J Am Coll Cardiol* 2014; 63: 1636–43.

3 Basso C, Corrado D, Thiene G. Cardiovascular causes of sudden death in young individuals including athletes. *Cardiol Rev* 1999; 7: 127–35.

4 Tsai TT, Nienaber CA, Eagle KA. Acute aortic syndromes. *Circulation* 2005; 112: 3802–13.

5 Hagan PG, Nienaber CA, Isselbacher EM, et al. The International Registry of Acute Aortic Dissection (IRAD): new insights into an old disease. *JAMA* 2000; 283: 897–903.

6 Januzzi JL, Isselbacher EM, Fattori R, et al. Characterizing the young patient with aortic dissection: results from the International Registry of Aortic Dissection (IRAD). *J Am Coll Cardiol* 2004; 43: 665–9.

7 Otto CM. Disease of the great arteries. In Otto CM, (ed.), *Textbook of Clinical Echocardiography* (4th edn). Philadelphia, PA: WB Saunders 2009, pp. 397–417.

8 Iskandar A, Thompson PD. Diseases of the aorta in elite athletes. *Clin Sports Med* 2015; 34: 461–72.

9 Lang RM, Badano LP, Mor-Avi V, et al. Recommendations for cardiac chamber quantification by echocardiography in adults: an update from the American Society of Echocardiography and the European Association of Cardiovascular Imaging. *Eur Heart J Cardiovasc Imaging* 2015; 16: 233–70.

10 Reed CM, Richey PA, Pulliam DA, et al. Aortic dimensions in tall men and women. *Am J Cardiol* 1993; 71: 608–10.

11 Kinoshita N, Mimura J, Obayashi C, et al. Aortic root dilation among young competitive athletes: echocardiographic screening of 1929 athletes between 15 and 34 years of age. *Am Heart J* 2000; 139: 723–8.

12 Pelliccia A, Di Paolo FM, De Blasiis E, et al. Prevalence and clinical significance of aortic root dilation in highly trained competitive athletes. *Circulation* 2010; 122: 698–706.

13 Braverman AC, Harris KM, Kovacs RJ, Barry JM. Eligibility and disqualification recommendations for competitive athletes with cardiovascular abnormalities: Task Force 7: Aortic Diseases, Including Marfan Syndrome. *J Am Coll Cardiol* 2015; 66: 2398–405.

14 Babaee Bigi MA, Aslani A. Aortic root size and prevalence of aortic regurgitation in elite strength trained athletes. *Am J Cardiol* 2007; 100: 528–30.

15 Copeland SR, Mills MC, Lerner JL, et al. Hemodynamic effects of aerobic vs. resistance exercise. *J Hum Hypertens* 1996; 10: 747–53.

16 Hill DW, Butler SD. Hemodynamic responses to weightlifting exercise. *Sports Med* 1991; 12: 1–7.

17 Clifford PS, Hanel B, Secher NH. Arterial blood pressure response to rowing. *Med Sci Sports Exerc* 1994; 26: 715–19.

18 Palatini P. Exercise hemodynamics: field activities versus laboratory test. *Blood Press Monit* 1997; 2: 133–7.

19 MacDougall JD, Tuxen D, Sale DG, et al. Arterial blood pressure response to heavy resistance exercise. *J App Physiol* 1985; 58: 785–90.

20 Hatzaras I, Tranquilli M, Coady M, et al. Weight lifting and aortic dissection: more evidence for a connection. *Cardiology* 2007; 107: 103–6.

21 Mayerick C, Carré F, Elefteriades J. Aortic dissection and sport: physiologic and clinical understanding provide an opportunity to save young lives. *J Cardiovasc Surg* 2010; 5: 669–81.

22 Devereux RB, de Simone G, Arnett DK, et al. Normal limits in relation to age, body size and gender of two-dimensional echocardiographic aortic root dimensions in persons ≥15 years of age. *Am J Cardiol* 2012; 110: 1189–94.

23 Lam CS, Xanthakis V, Sullivan LM, et al. Aortic root remodeling over the adult life course: longitudinal data from the Framingham Heart Study. *Circulation* 2010; 122: 884–90.

24 Roberts WC. The congenitally bicuspid aortic valve: a study of 85 autopsy cases. *Am J Cardiol* 1970; 26: 72–83.

25 Hoffman JI, Kaplan S. The incidence of congenital heart disease. *J Am Coll Cardiol* 2002; 39: 1890–1900.

26 Ward C. Clinical significance of the bicuspid aortic valve. *Heart* 2000; 83: 81–5.

27 Cripe L, Adelfinger G, Martin LJ, et al. Bicuspid aortic valve is heritable. *J Am Coll Cardiol* 2004; 44: 138–43.

28 Huntington K, Hunter AG, Chan KL. A prospective study to assess the frequency of familial clustering of congenital bicuspid aortic valve. *J Am Coll Cardiol* 1997; 30: 1809–12.

29 Verma S, Siu SC. Aortic dilatation in patients with bicuspid aortic valve. *N Engl J Med* 2014; 370: 1920–9.

30 Michelena HI, Khanna AD, Mahoney D, et al. Incidence of aortic complications in patients with bicuspid aortic valves. *JAMA* 2011; 306: 1104–12.

31 Shimada I, Rooney SJ, Pagano D, et al. Prediction of thoracic aortic aneurysm expansion: validation of formulae describing growth. *Ann Thorac Surg* 1999; 67: 1968–70.

32 Tadros TM, Klein MD, Shapira OM. Ascending aortic dilatation associated with bicuspid aortic valve: pathophysiology, molecular biology, and clinical implications. *Circulation* 2009; 119: 880–90.

33 Galanti G, Stefani L, Toncelli L, et al. Effects of sports activity in athletes with bicuspid aortic valve in the community. *Circulation* 2008; 117: 2776–84.

34 Judge DP, Dietz HC. Marfan's syndrome. *Lancet* 2005; 47: 476–85.

35 von Kodolitsch Y, Rybczynski M, Detter C, Robinson PN. Diagnosis and management of Marfan syndrome. *Future Cardiol* 2008; 4: 85–96.

36 Loeys RM, Dietz HC, Braverman AC, et al. The revised Ghent nosology for the Marfan syndrome. *J Med Genet* 2010;47 : 476–85.

37 Radonic T, de Witte P, Groenink M, et al. Critical appraisal of the revised Ghent criteria for diagnosis of Marfan syndrome. *Clin Genet* 2011; 80: 346–53.

38 Chandra A, Patel D, Aragon-Martin JA, et al. The revised Ghent nosology: reclassifying isolated ectopia lentis. *Clin Genet* 2015; 87: 284–7.

39 Ammash NM, Sundt TM, Connolly HM. Marfan syndrome diagnosis and management. *Curr Probl Cardiol* 2008; 33: 7–39.

40 Nishimura RA, Otto CM, Bonow RO, et al. 2014 AHA/ACC guideline for the management of patients with valvular heart disease: a report of the American College of Cardiology/American Heart Association Task Force on Practice Guidelines. *J Thorac Cardiovasc Surg* 2014; 148: e1–132.

41 Center for Disease Control and Prevention. Asthma mortality and hospitalization among children and young adults: United States, 1980-1993. *MMWR Morb Mortal Wkly Rep* 1996; 45: 350–3.

42 Becker JM, Rogers J, Rossini G, et al. Asthma deaths during sports: report of a 7-year experience. *J Allergy Clin Immunol* 2004; 113: 264–7.

43 Helenius I, Haahtela T. Allergy and asthma in elite summer sport athletes. *J Allergy Clin Immunol* 2000; 106: 444–52.

44 Bonini M, Gramiccioni C, Fioretti D, et al. Asthma, allergy and the Olympics: a 12-year survey in elite athletes. *Curr Opin Allergy Clin Immunol* 2015; 15: 184–92.

45 McKenzie DC, Fitch KD. The asthmatic athlete: inhaled beta-2 agonists, sport performance, and doping. *Clin J Sport Med* 2011; 21: 46–50.

46 Del Giacco SR, Firinu D, Bjermer L, Carlsen KH. Exercise and asthma: an overview. *Eur Clin Respir J* 2015; 2: 279–84.

47 Deal EC Jr, McFadden ER Jr, Ingram RH Jr, et al. Airway responsiveness to cold air and hyperpnea in normal subjects and in those with hay fever and asthma. *Am Rev Respir Dis* 1980; 121621–8.

48 Carlsen KH. Asthma in Olympians. *Paediatr Respir Rev* 2016; 17: 34–5.

49 Carlsen KH. Sports in extreme conditions: the impact of exercise in cold temperatures on asthma and bronchial hyper-responsiveness in athletes. *Br J Sports Med* 2012; 46: 796–9.

50 Goldsmith RL, Bigger JT Jr, Bloomfield DM, Steinman RC. Physical fitness as a determinant of vagal modulation. *Med Sci Sports Exerc* 1997; 29(6): 812–7.

51 Price OJ, Ansley L, Menzies-Gow A, et al. Airway dysfunction in elite athletes—an occupational lung disease? *Allergy* 2013; 68: 1343–52.

52 Bougault V, Turmel J, Boulet LP. Airway hyperresponsiveness in elite swimmers: is it a transient phenomenon? *J Allergy Clin Immunol* 2011; 127: 892–8.

53 Molfino NA, Nannini LJ, Martelli AN, Slutsky AS. Respiratory arrest in near-fatal asthma. *N Engl J Med* 1991; 324: 285–8.

54 Wasserfallen JB, Schaller MD, Feihl F, Perret CH. Sudden asphyxic asthma: a distinct entity? *Am Rev Respir Dis* 1990; 142: 108–11.

55 Kikuchi Y, Okabe S, Tamura G, et al. Chemosensitivity and perception of dyspnea in patients with a history of near-fatal asthma. *N Engl J Med* 1994; 330: 1329–34.

56 Katschinski DM. On heat and cells and proteins. *News Phyiol Sci* 2004; 19: 11–15.

57 Sawka MN, Wenger CB, Pandolf KB. Thermoregulatory responses to acute exercise heat stress and heat acclimation. In Fregly MJ, Blatteis CM (eds), *Handbook of Physiology, Section 4: Environmental Physiology*. New York: Oxford University Press; 1996, pp. 379–418.

58 Sawka MN, Young AJ. Physiological systems and their responses to conditions of heat and cold. In Tipton CM, (ed.), *ACSM's Advanced Exercise Physiology*. Baltimore, MD: Lippincott-Williams & Wilkins; 2006, pp. 535–63.

59 Veicstenas A, Ferretti G, Rennie DW. Superficial shell insulation in resting and exercising men in cold water. *J Appl Physiol* 1982; 2: 1557–64.

60 Nemer JA, Moelleken BRW. Disorders due to physical agents. In McPhee SJ, Papadakis MA (eds), *Current Medical Diagnosis and Treatment* (49th edn). San Francisco, CA: University of California-McGraw-Hill; 2010, pp. 1403–19.

61 Aslam AF, Aslam AK, Vasavada BC, Khan IA. Hypothermia: evaluation, electrocardiographic manifestations, and management. *Am J Med* 2006; 119: 297–301.

62 Aslan S, Erdem AF, Uzkeser M, et al. The Osborn wave in accidental hypothermia. *J Emerg Med* 2007; 32: 271–3.

63 Castellani JW, Young AJ, Ducharme MB, et al. American College of Sports Medicine position stand: prevention of cold injuries during exercise. *Med Sci Sports Exerc* 2006; 38: 2012–29.

64 Mazzeo RS, Fulco CS. Physiological systems and their responses to conditions of hypoxia. In Tipton CM, (ed.), *ACSM's Advanced Exercise Physiology*. Baltimore, MD: Lippincott-Williams & Wilkins; 2006, pp. 564–580.

65 Plant T, Aref-Adib G. Travelling to new heights: practical high altitude medicine. *Br J Hosp Med (Lond)* 2008; 69: 348–52.

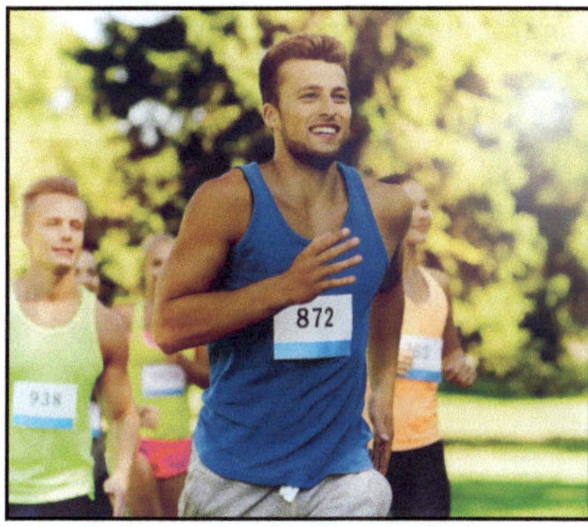

6.5

Pre-participation screening of young competitive athletes

Domenico Corrado and Alessandro Zorzi

Introduction

The catastrophic nature of sudden death (SD) during sports activity mandates the medical community to develop and implement effective preventive strategies [1–4]. Pre-participation screening offers the potential to identify those athletes who have life-threatening cardiovascular abnormalities before onset of symptoms and to reduce the risk of SD [5–7]. However, there is a significant debate among cardiologists about the efficacy, the impact of false-positive results, and the cost-effectiveness of routine pre-participation screening [8,9].

This chapter presents an appraisal of the available data concerning the efficacy of pre-participation screening programmes to reduce cardiovascular risk in young competitive athletes.

Risk of sudden death in the athlete

The risk of SD among athletes or during sports activity varies in the different series reported in the literature [10–33]. It generally increases with age and is greater in men. In apparently healthy adults (>35 years), joggers, or marathon runners, the estimated rate of SD ranges from 1:15,000 to 1:50,000 per year [3,4,10,16]. In comparison, a significantly lower incidence of fatal events, in the range of 0.5–1 in 100,000 per year, has been reported in young athletes (≤35 years) (➲ Table 6.5.1).

In a nationally based survey carried out between 1983 and 1993, Van Camp et al. [34] estimated the prevalence of SD in high school and college athletes in the USA to be 0.4 in 100,000 athletes per year. Over a 26-year study period Maron et al. [32] found the prevalence of SD in high school athletes from Minnesota (age 12–19 years, mean 16) to be 0.7 in 100,000 per year [32]. More recently, Harmon et al. [23] reported a higher incidence of SD (2.28 in 100,000 per year) in athletes of the National Collegiate Athletic Association. A prospective population-based study in the Veneto region of Italy reported an incidence of sudden death of 2.3 (2.62 in males and 1.07 in females) per 100,000 athletes per year from all causes, and 2.1 in 100,000 athletes per year from cardiovascular diseases [10].

The different SD rates found in different studies can be explained by a variety of factors, including age range, the proportion of men, the estimation of the denominator, and the methodology of data collection (prospective collection versus retrospective analysis of data from public media reports and insurance claims). In this respect, Harmon et al. [23] found that nowadays, with the use of the internet, only about half of SD cases would have been identified relying on media reports only.

The risk of SD in athletes increases with age and is greater in men [12]. A recent French study reported an incidence of SD during moderate or vigorous exercise of 1 in 100,000 per year among males and of 0.05 in 100,000 per year among females [35]. A variety of explanations for the striking male predominance (male-to-female ratio of up to 10:1) of SD in athletes have been proposed, including the higher participation rate of males than females in competitive sports, the more intensive training load and higher level of athletic achievement of males, and the greater prevalence and/or phenotypic expression in young males of cardiac diseases at risk of arrhythmic cardiac arrest, such as cardiomyopathies and premature coronary artery disease.

Atherosclerotic coronary artery disease accounts for the vast majority of fatalities in adults (>35 years), while the most common causes of SD in younger athletes are

Table 6.5.1 Main studies reporting the incidence of cardiac arrest/sudden death in the young and/or during sports activity.

Study	Study period	Region	Population	Results
Maron et al. 1998 [11]	1985/1986–1996/1997	Minnesota, USA	651,695 High School athletes 13–19 years	SD among athletes during competition or training: 0.46/100,000/year
Corrado et al. 2003 [11]	1979–1999	Veneto, Italy	1,386,600 people, 12–35 years 112,970 athletes, 12–35 years	SD in the general population: 0.9/100,000/year SD among athletes: 2.3/100,000/year
Gerein et al. 2006 [13]	1991–2002	Ontario, Canada	500,000 people 0–18 years	OHCA: 9.1/100,000/year
Corrado et al. 2006 [10]	1979–2004	Veneto, Italy	2,938,730 athletes 12–35 years 33,205,370 non athletes 12–35 years	Cardiovascular SD among athletes: 1.9/100,000/year Cardiovascular SD among non-athletes: 0.79/100,000/year SD rate reduction after screening implementation: 89%
Ong et al. 2006 [14]	1992–2002	Ontario, Canada	800,000 people 0–19 years	OHCA: 5.97/100,000/year
Maron et al. 2009 [15]	2001–2006	USA	10,700,000 athletes 13–25 years	Cardiovascular SD among athletes: 0.61/100,000/year
Chugh et al. 2009 [16]	2002–2005	Multnomah County, Oregon, USA	Estimated number of children 0–14 years	SD rate 1–13 years: 7.5/100,000/year SD rate <1 year: 96.0/100,000/year
Atkins et al. 2009 [17]	2005–2007	Canada	Canadian population 0–19 years	OHCA rate <1 year: 72.71/100,000/year OHCA rate 1–11 years: 3.73/100,000/year OHCA rate 12–19 years: 6.73/100,000/year OHCA rate 0–19 years: 8.04/100,000/year
Solberg et al. 2010 [18]	1990–1997	Norway	Norwegian population 15–34 years	Sports-related SD: 0.9/100,000/year
Holst et al. 2010 [19]	2000–2006	Denmark	Danish population 12–35 years	Sports-related SD: 1.21/100,000/year SD in the general population: 3.76/100,000/year
Donohoe et al. 2010 [20]	2003–2007	London, UK	4,000,000 people 0–35 years	OHCA rate 0–35 years: 19.3/100,000/year OHCA rate in the general population: 131.2/100,000/year
Park et al. 2010 [21]	2006–2007	South Korea	South Korean population 0–20 years	OHCA rate <1 year: 67.1/100,000/year OHCA rate 1–11 years: 2.5/100,000/year OHCA rate 12–20 years: 3.5/100,000/year OHCA rate 0–20 years: 4.2/100,000/year
Deasy et al. 2010 [22]	1999–2007	Melbourne, Australia	810,400 people 0–16 years	OHCA rate: 3/100,000/year
Harmon et al. 2011 [23]	2004–2008	USA	1,969,663 athletes/year 17–23 years	Cardiovascular SD among athletes: 2.28/100,000/year
Winkel et al. 2011 [24]	2000–2006	Denmark	2,380,000 people 1–35years	Cardiovascular SD rate: 2.8/100,000/year
Margey et al. 2011 [26]	2005–2007	Ireland	Irish population 15–35 years	Cardiovascular SD rate: 2.85/100,000/year
Eckart et al. 2011 [27]	1998–2008	US military training base	US military recruits	SD rate <20 years: 3.3/100,000/year SD rate >50 years: 106/100,000/year
Meyer et al. 2012 [25]	1980–2009	King County, Washington, USA	620,000 people 0–35 years	Overall OHCA rate: 2.28/100,000/year OHCA rate 0–2 years: 2.1/100,000/year OHCA rate 3–13 years: 0.61/100,000/year OHCA rate 14-24 years: 1.44/100,000/year OHCA rate 25–35 years: 4.40/100,000/year
Roberts et al. 2013 [28]	1993/1994–2011/2012	Minnesota, USA	1,666,509 high school athletes	Cardiovascular SD among athletes: 0.24/100,000/year

Table 6.5.1 Main studies reporting the incidence of cardiac arrest/sudden death in the young and/or during sports activity. *(Continued)*

Pilmer et al. 2013 [30]	2008	Ontario, Canada	6,602,680 people 2–40 years	Cardiovascular SD rate 2–18 years: 0.7/100,000/year Cardiovascular SD rate 19–29 years: 2.4/100,000/year Cardiovascular SD rate 30–40 years: 5.3/100,000/year
Berdowski et al. 2013 [31]	2006–2008	North Holland	2,400,000 people 10–90 years 1,000,000 people 10–35 years	Exercise-related OHCA during the study period: 5.7% Exercise related OHCA rate 10–90 years: 2.1/100,000/year Exercise-related OHCA rate 10–35 years: 0.3/100,000/year At rest OHCA rate 10–90 years: 35.5/100,000/year At rest OHCA rate 10–35 years: 2.8/100,000/year
Maron et al. 2013 [32]	1986–2011	Minnesota, USA	1,930,504 high school athletes	SD rate among athletes: 0.7/100,000/year
Risgaard et al. 2014 [33]	2007–2009	Denmark	3,470,000 people 1–49 years	Overall cardiovascular SD rate: 8.6/100,000/year Cardiovascular SD rate: 31–49 years: 21.7/100,000/year Cardiovascular SD rate: 1–35 years: 2.3/100,000/year
Pilmer et al. 2014 [29]	2005–2009	Ontario, Canada	14,893,860 people 1–19 years	Cardiovascular SD rate 1–2 years: 3.1/100,000/year Cardiovascular SD rate 2–4 years: 1.3/100,000/year Cardiovascular SD rate 5–9 years: 0.4/100,000/year Cardiovascular SD rate 10–14 years: 0.5/100,000/year Cardiovascular SD rate 15–19 years: 1.0/100,000/year

OHCA, out-of-hospital cardiac arrest.

genetic or congenital cardiovascular abnormalities, including cardiomyopathies and coronary artery anomalies (see ➔ Chapter 6.2). Hypertrophic cardiomyopathy (HCM) has been reported to account for more than a third of fatal cases in the USA [34,36], and arrhythmogenic right ventricular cardiomyopathy (ARVC) for approximately one fourth in the Veneto Region of Italy [10,12]. A sizeable proportion of young people and athletes who die suddenly have no evidence of structural heart disease, and the cause of their cardiac arrest is probably related to a primary electrical heart disease, such as inherited cardiac ion-channel defects (channelopathies), including long and short QT syndromes, Brugada syndrome, and catecholaminergic polymorphic ventricular tachycardia [37]. Sudden death may also be caused by a non-arrhythmic mechanism (e.g. spontaneous aortic rupture complicating Marfan syndrome or bicuspid aortic valve) as well was by diseases not related to the heart (e.g. bronchial asthma or rupture of a cerebral aneurysm). Blunt, non-penetrating, and often apparently innocent blows to the precordium may trigger ventricular fibrillation without structural injury to the ribs, the sternum, or the heart itself (commotio cordis) (see ➔ Chapter 6.4.1) [38].

The risk–benefit ratio of physical exercise differs between adults and young competitive athletes because of the different nature of the cardiovascular causes of death. Several epidemiological studies have assessed the relationship between physical exercise and the risk of acute myocardial infarction/SD in middle-aged/senior individuals engaged in leisure sports activity, in which physical exercise can be regarded as a 'two-edged sword'. The available evidence indicates that vigorous exercise acutely increases the incidence of both cardiac arrest and acute myocardial infarction in those who do not exercise regularly. However, epidemiological studies support the concept that habitual sports activity may offer protection against cardiovascular events over the long term [4,39,40]. Adolescents and young adults involved in competitive sports activity have an estimated risk of SD approximately three times greater than their non-athletic counterparts [10, 12] (➔ Fig. 6.5.1). Sport acts as a trigger of arrhythmic cardiac arrest in those athletes with predisposing cardiovascular conditions.

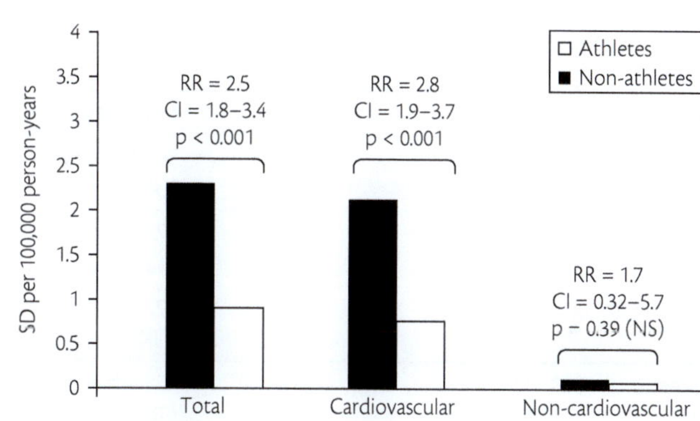

Fig. 6.5.1 Incidence and relative risk (RR) of sudden death among young athletes and non-athletes: total, cardiovascular, and non-cardiovascular causes.

Adapted from *Herz*. Exercise and the risk of sudden cardiac death, Volume 31, Issue 6, 2006, pp. 553–8. Domenico Corrado, with permission from Springer.

Pre-participation screening of competitive athletes

The primary purpose of pre-participation screening is to identify athletes affected by unsuspected cardiovascular diseases and to prevent SD occurring during sports by appropriate interventions [5–7]. Thus, from a screening perspective, knowledge of the prevalence of cardiovascular conditions with the potential for SD among adolescents and young adults is of the utmost importance. In contrast with the disparities in SD rates, the overall prevalence of cardiovascular diseases that predispose to SD in young competitive athletes has been estimated to range from 0.2% to 0.7% [10, 41–45] (➲ Table 6.5.2).

The vast majority of 'at risk-athletes' do not experience premonitory symptoms and thus pre-participation screening is the only strategy capable of identifying the underlying cardiovascular disorder. The importance of early identification of clinically silent cardiovascular diseases at a pre-symptomatic stage relies on the specific possibility of SD prevention by lifestyle modification, including restriction of competitive sports activity (if necessary), prophylactic treatment with drugs, and an implantable defibrillator [7].

Both the American Heart Association (AHA) and the European Society of Cardiology (ESC) consensus panel recommendations agree that cardiovascular screening for young competitive athletes is justifiable and compelling on ethical, legal, and medical grounds [46,47]. However, there is considerable discordance in the consensus guidelines on the pre-participation screening protocols used between European and US cardiologists/sports medicine physicians.

The AHA recommends pre-participation cardiovascular evaluation using history (personal and family history) and physical examination alone, although this screening protocol has a recognized limited power (<10%) to detect potentially lethal cardiovascular abnormalities [47,48]. Glover and Maron [49] found that only 3% of 134 high-school and collegiate athletes who died suddenly after they underwent pre-participation screening were suspected of having cardiac disease, and eventually less than 1% received an accurate diagnosis. Twelve-lead ECG enhances the sensitivity of the screening process by allowing early detection of cardiovascular conditions which distinctively manifest with ECG abnormalities, such as cardiomyopathies, pre-excitation syndromes, and cardiac ion-channel disorders [7,46] (➲ Table 6.5.3). Based on published series from the USA and Italy, these ECG-detectable conditions are present in approximately two-thirds of young competitive athletes who suffered SD.

In Italy the law mandates that every individual engaged in competitive sports activity must undergo a clinical evaluation to obtain eligibility. A nationwide mass pre-participation screening programme, essentially based on ECG, has been operating since 1982 (➲ Fig. 6.5.2). The efficacy of ECG screening in the identification of cardiomyopathies has been demonstrated in a large population-based prospective study in the Veneto region of Italy [10,50]. Among 33,735 athletes undergoing ECG screening at the Center for Sports Medicine in Padua, 22 (0.07%) were identified with HCM, based predominantly on an abnormal ECG [50]. An absolute value of ECG screening sensitivity for HCM cannot be derived from this study because systematic echocardiographic findings were not available; however, this 0.07%

Table 6.5.2 Prevalence of cardiovascular disease at risk of sudden cardiac death in the athletes

Study	Population	Prevalence (%)
Fuller et al. 1997 [71]	5617 high school athletes (USA)	0.4
Corrado et al. 2006 [10]	42,386 athletes aged 12–35 (Italy)	0.2
Wilson et al. 2008 [42]	2720 athletes and children aged 10–17 (UK)	0.3
Bessem et al. 2009 [43]	428 athletes aged 12–35 (The Netherlands)	0.7
Baggish et al. 2010 [44]	510 collegiate athletes (USA)	0.6
Sheik et al. 2014 [45]	3210 elite athletes aged 14–35 (U.K.)	0.5

Table 6.5.3 ECG features of cardiac diseases detectable during pre-participation screening in young competitive athletes

Disease	QTc interval	P wave	PR interval	QRS complex	ST interval	T wave	Arrhythmias
Hypertrophic cardiomyopathy	Normal	(Left atrial enlargement)	Normal	Increased voltages in mid- left precordial leads; abnormal Q waves in inferior and/or lateral leads; (LAD, LBBB); (delta wave)	Down-sloping (up-sloping)	Inverted in mid- left- precordial leads; (giant and negative in the 'apical' variant)	(Atrial fibrillation); (PVB); (VT)
Arrhythmogenic right ventricular cardiomyopathy/ Dysplasia	Normal	Normal	Normal	Prolonged >110ms in right precordial leads; epsilon wave in right precordial leads; reduced voltages ≤0.5mV in frontal leads; (RBBB)	(Up-sloping in right precordial leads)	Inverted in right precordial leads	PVB with LBBB pattern; (VT with LBBB pattern)
Dilated cardiomyopathy	Normal	(Left atrial enlargement)	(Prolonged ≥0.21s)	LBBB	Down-sloping (up-sloping)	Inverted in inferior and/or lateral leads	PVB; (VT)
Myocarditis	(Prolonged)	Normal	Prolonged ≥0.21 sec	(Abnormal Q waves)	Down- or up- sloping	Inverted in ≥2 leads	(Atrial arrhythmias); (PVB); (second- or third-degree AV block); (VT)
Long QT syndrome	Prolonged >470ms in males, >480ms in females	Normal	Normal	Normal	Normal	Bifid or biphasic in all leads	(PVB); (torsade de pointes)
Brugada syndrome	Normal		Prolonged ≥0.21s	S1S2S3 pattern; (RBBB/LAD)	Up-sloping 'coved-type' in right precordial leads	Inverted in right precordial leads	(Polymorphic VT); (atrial fibrillation) (sinus bradycardia)
Lenègre disease	Normal	Normal	Prolonged ≥0.21s	RBBB; RBBB/LAD; LBBB	Normal	Secondary changes	(Second- or third-degree AV block)
Short QT syndrome	Shortened <300ms	Normal	Normal	Normal	Normal	Normal	Atrial fibrillation (polymorphic VT)
Pre-excitation syndrome (WPW)	Normal	Normal	Shortened<0.12s	Delta wave	Secondary changes	Secondary changes	Supraventricular tachycardia; (atrial fibrillation)
Coronary artery diseases*	(Prolonged)	Normal	Normal	(Abnormal Q waves)	(Down- or up-sloping)	Inverted in ≥2 leads	PVB; (VT)

Less common or uncommon ECG findings are reported in brackets.*Coronary artery diseases, either premature coronary atherosclerosis or congenital coronary anomalies. QTc, QT interval corrected for heart rate by Bazett's formula; LBBB, left bundle branch block; RBBB. right bundle branch block; LAD, left axis deviation of −30° or more; PVB, either single or coupled premature ventricular beats; VT, either non-sustained or sustained ventricular tachycardia; WPW, Wolff–Parkinson–White.

prevalence of HCM is similar to that (0.10%) observed in a population-based study using echocardiography in the USA [51]. This indicates that an ECG may be as sensitive as an echocardiogram in detecting HCM in the context of a young athletic population.

A recent meta-analysis by Harmon et al. [48] evaluated the sensitivity and specificity of ECG for pre-participation screening compared with history and physical examination. The study found that the sensitivity of ECG (80%) was superior to history (50%) and physical examination (33%), and that the false-positive rates of history (8%) and physical examination (10%) were higher than that of ECG (6%).

Impact on mortality

The Italian experience provides the most compelling evidence of the efficacy of ECG screening to save lives by identifying and disqualifying athletes with at-risk heart diseases. A time-trend analysis of the incidence of SD in

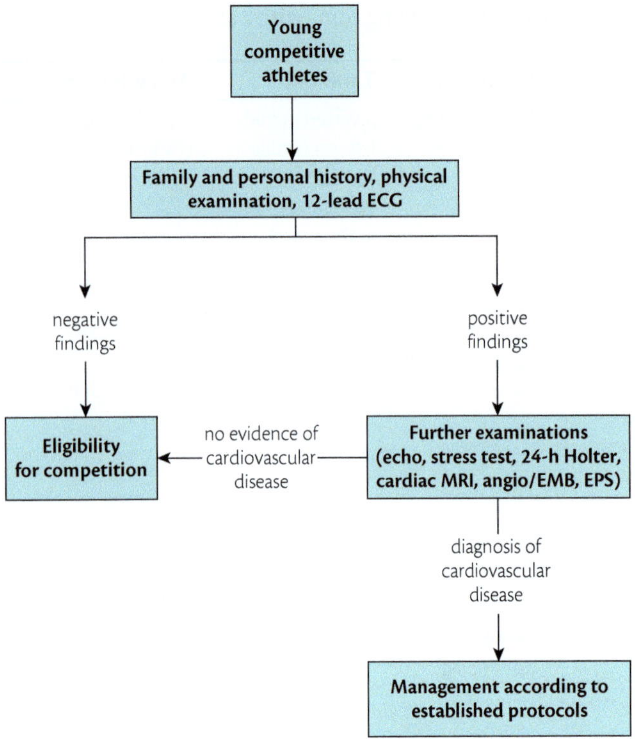

Fig. 6.5.2 Flowchart of the Italian protocol for pre-participation screening. First-line examination includes family history, physical examination, and 12-lead ECG; additional tests are requested only for subjects who have positive findings at the initial evaluation. The screening starts at the beginning of competitive athletic activity, which for the majority of sports disciplines corresponds to an age of 12–14 years. Because the phenotypic manifestations, both ECG abnormalities and arrhythmic substrates of most inherited heart diseases, are age dependent and occur during adolescence or young adulthood, screening of children is expected to have a low sensitivity for detection of cardiomyopathies and cardiac ion-channel diseases, except for long QT syndrome. It is essential to repeat screening on a regular basis every 1–2 years, mostly in teenagers, to ensure the timely identification of delayed phenotypic manifestations, disease progression, or substrate worsening over time. Athletes identified as being affected by cardiovascular conditions potentially responsible for sudden death in association with participation in exercise and sport are managed according to the recommendations available for sports eligibility. Screening for cardiac disease is part of a more comprehensive medical evaluation which includes a general clinical history, physical examination, orthopaedic examination, spirometry, and urinalysis. In addition, athletes undergo a Montoye step test, which is limited to evaluation of heart rate recovery after exercise, although it may occasionally unmask effort-dependent arrhythmias. Exercise-induced ST-T abnormalities are appropriately assessed by maximal exercise testing, which is reserved for competitive athletes aged ≥35 years. Angio/EMB, contrast angiography/endomyocardial biopsy; EPS, electrophysiologic study with programmed ventricular stimulation; MRI, magnetic resonance imaging.

young competitive athletes in the Veneto region of Italy over 26 years (1979–2004) showed a sharp decline in mortality rates after the introduction of the nationwide screening programme [10]. Fifty-five SDs occurred in screened athletes (1.9 deaths per 100,000 person-years) and 265 deaths occurred in non-screened non-athletes (0.79 deaths per 100,000 person-years). The annual incidence of SD in athletes decreased by 89%, from 3.6 per 100,000 person-years in the pre-screening period to 0.4 per 100,000 person-years in the late screening period (➲ Fig. 6.5.3).

These data have generated a number of concerns [52–54]. The main criticism is that the study was not a randomized trial comparing screened versus non-screened young competitive athletes, and thus it was not possible to draw a definitive conclusion that the reduced mortality was solely the consequence of the screening process. However, the strong cause–effect relationship between ECG screening and the substantial reduction of SD in this prospective population-based investigation is supported by the following findings.

1 The timing of the decline of SD in young competitive athletes coincided with the implementation of the screening programme in Italy.
2 Most of the reduced incidence of SD was due to fewer deaths from cardiomyopathies (HCM and ARVC), and over the same period there was a concomitant increase in the proportion of athletes who were identified with these cardiomyopathies at the Centre for Sports Medicine in Padua and disqualified from competition.
3 The incidence of SD in the unscreened non-athletic population of the Veneto region of the same age range did not change during the study period.

Although additional factors (environmental, socio-economic, or medical/surgical) may have contributed to the reduction in mortality, such factors are expected to impact mortality in a similar fashion in screened athletes and unscreened non-athletes, and hence are unlikely to explain the declining trend in SD *selectively* recorded in the screened athletic population [10,55].

During the time period 1993–2004 the annual rate of SD among screened Italian athletes was roughly similar to that of unscreened US high school and college competitors (0.87 vs 0.93 per 100,000 athlete-years, respectively) [36]. Thus, it has been argued that SD in young competitive athletes is a low rate event which is unlikely to be influenced by pre-participation ECG screening. However, as discussed in ➲ Chapter 6.2, the Italian and US athletic populations were clearly non-comparable with regard to age and gender,

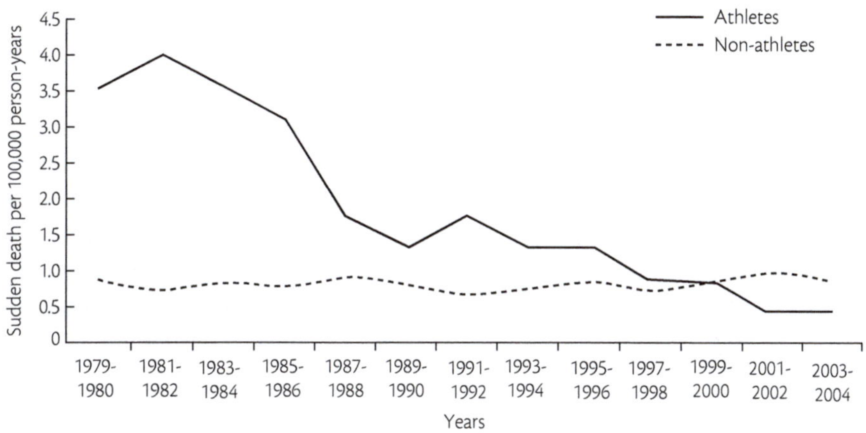

Fig. 6.5.3 Annual incidence rates of SD per 100,000 people for screened competitive athletes and unscreened non-athletes 12–35 years of age in the Veneto region of Italy from 1979 to 2004. During the study period (the nationwide pre-participation screening programme was initiated in 1982), the annual incidence of SD declined by 89% in screened athletes (P <0.001). In contrast, the incidence of SD in unscreened non-athletes did not demonstrate consistent changes in the same period.
Modified from Corrado D, Basso C, Pavei A, Michieli P, Schiavon M, Thiene G. Trends in sudden cardiovascular death in young competitive athletes after implementation of a preparticipation screening program. *JAMA* 2006; 296: 1593–1601.

with the Italian athletes being older and including more males. Moreover, the US mortality rates were unavoidably under-estimated because of the lack of a reliable reporting system and the use of retrospective data based on reviews of public media reports and insurance claims. In contrast, the SD database in the Veneto region of Italy is unique, in so far as cases are collected according to a prospective study design with systematic investigation of all young people (≤35 years) who die suddenly and undergo a standardized post-mortem investigation of the heart by a team of cardiovascular pathologists. The heart specimens, as well as the clinical records of all SD victims since 1979, are stored at the Registry of Cardiovascular Pathology, University of Padua, allowing retrieval and review of each case This accounts for the greater reliability of data on causes and trends of SD in Italian young people and athletes compared with reports from other countries which are based on a less rigorous data collection.

An Israeli group reported an incidence of SD in athletes of 2.6 per 100,000/years, but failed to demonstrate a decline in SD rate after pre-participation screening became legally mandatory in Israel in 1997 [56]. However, the study used media reports as the sole source of data, and this may have led to an under-estimation of the true incidence of arrhythmic death among athletes in Israel [23,57,58].

False-positive results

Changes in the ECG of trained athletes usually develop as a consequence of the heart's adaptation to sustained physical exercise ('athlete's heart') [59]. There is a misconception that such physiological ECG changes overlap significantly with ECG abnormalities seen in cardiovascular diseases which cause SD in the young. Therefore the ECG has traditionally been considered to be a poor screening test in the athlete, because of its presumed high level of false-positive results [52–54]. Several studies have disproved the idea that ECG is a non-specific and non-cost-effective test. Among 42,386 athletes initially screened by history, physical examination, and ECG, 3,914 (9%) had positive findings which required further examination, 879 (2%) were diagnosed with cardiovascular disorders, and 91 (0.2%) were ultimately disqualified from competition because of potentially lethal heart diseases [10]. The percentage of false-positive results, i.e. athletes with a normal heart but positive screening findings, was 7% for all cardiovascular disorders and 8.8% for heart diseases at high risk of SD during sports. Likewise, ECG screening of highly trained competitive athletes in the UK was associated with a false-positive rate of only 3.7% [42].

However, recent data in black athletes have shown a higher prevalence of ECG abnormalities, indicating a varying ECG specificity among athletes of different ethnicity [60]. An increase in the accuracy of ECG screening is expected as new studies emerge and are translated into updated guidelines for ECG interpretation in the athlete, such as the recent recommendations of the ESC Section of Sports Cardiology [59], the Stanford criteria [61], and the Seattle criteria [62]. Defining which ECG changes are physiological (common and training-related ECG abnormalities) and which are pathological (uncommon and training-unrelated ECG abnormalities) (➲ Fig. 6.5.4) has significant favourable effects on the athlete's cardiovascular management, including clinical diagnosis, risk stratification, and cost savings. The specificity of ESC, Stanford and Seattle Criteria was compared in a series of 1417 healthy US athletes (62% white, mean age 20±4 years). The study found that the rate of false positive ECG abnormalities requiring further evaluation decreased when applying the Stanford (8%) or Seattle (6%) criteria compared to the older ESC

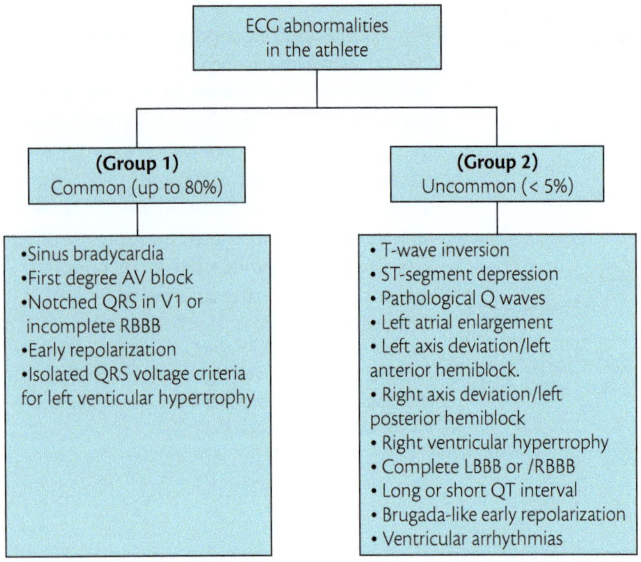

Fig. 6.5.4 Classification of ECG abnormalities in the athlete.
Common ECG abnormalities: Up to 80% of trained athletes exhibit ECG changes such as sinus bradycardia, first-degree AV block, early repolarization, incomplete right bundle branch block, and pure increase of QRS voltages (Group 1). Such common ECG changes are the consequence of the physiological cardiovascular adaptation to sustained physical exertion and do not reflect the presence of an underlying cardiovascular disease. Therefore they are not associated with an increase of cardiovascular risk and allow eligibility to participate in competitive sports without additional evaluation.
Uncommon ECG abnormalities: This subset includes uncommon ECG patterns (<5%) such as ST-segment and T-wave repolarization abnormalities, pathological Q waves, intraventricular conduction defects, and ventricular arrhythmias (Group 2). These ECG abnormalities are unrelated to athletic conditioning and should be regarded as an expression of possible underlying cardiovascular disorders, notably cardiomyopathies and cardiac ion-channel diseases and thus are associated with an inherent increased risk of sudden arrhythmic death.
Reproduced with permission from Corrado, Domenico; Pelliccia, Antonio. Recommendations for interpretation of 12-lead electrocardiogram in the athlete. *European Heart Journal*, Volume 31, Issue 2, pp.243–259. Copyright © 2009 Oxford University Press and the European Society of Cardiology.

(26%) criteria [63]. Similar results were obtained by Brosnan et al, who tested 1197 Australian elite athletes and found a 12.8% lower rate of false positives (from 17.3 to 4.5%) when applying the Seattle instead of the ESC criteria. The rate of false positives mostly decreased in the sub-population of endurance athletes (from 29.9% to 11.15%) [64]. However, none of these two studies performed echocardiography to all athletes to assess the number of false negatives. Instead, Berge et al. examined 595 male Norwegian professional soccer players with both ECG and echocardiogram. The authors confirmed that the Seattle criteria resulted in a significantly lower number of athletes with false positive ECG findings (11.2%) compared with the ESC criteria (29.3%), mostly because of re-definition of right precordial T-wave inversion, atrial enlargement and intraventricular conduction delay, without increasing the number of false-negative test [65]. Other studies on various athletic populations have confirmed that the use of the Seattle criteria, compared with the ESC criteria, significantly decreased the number of false-positive ECG findings [66,67]. A new revision of the Seattle ECG criteria has recently been proposed by British authors (the Cardiac Risk in the Young (CRY) Criteria). Compared with the Seattle and ESC criteria, these refined criteria improve ECG specificity in both white athletes (CRY = 94.1% vs ESC = 73.8% and Seattle = 92.1%) and black athletes (CRY = 84.2% vs ESC = 40.3% and Seattle = 79.3%). The reduction of false positives was the result of interpretation as normal of the ECG patterns of isolated atrial enlargement, axis deviation, voltage criteria for right ventricular hypertrophy, and (limited to black athletes) T-wave inversion in leads V1–V4 preceded by ST-segment elevation [45].

Costs of screening

There is compelling evidence that early identification of young athletes/patients affected by genetic disease carrying a risk of SD is associated with a good prognosis over a long-term follow-up. Unlike older patients with coronary artery diseases or heart failure, young individuals are likely to survive for many decades with normal or nearly normal life expectancy if detected by pre-participation cardiovascular evaluation because of restriction from competition, individualized risk assessment, and appropriate prophylactic therapy for life-threatening arrhythmias [68]. The large number of life-years saved favourably influences analysis of the cost-effectiveness of the screening process, with cost estimates per year of life saved consistently below $50,000 [69–71], which is the traditional threshold for considering a health intervention to be cost-effective.

The benefit of pre-participation evaluation goes beyond the detection of index athletes with an inherited heart disease because it enables cascade screening of relatives, which results in a multiplier effect for identifying other affected family members, thus saving additional lives [7,72].

Individual cost

Disqualification of a young athlete diagnosed with a heart disease from competition may be associated with important *individual costs* in terms of health, contentment, and even future opportunity for professional sport. The risk of SD during sport inherent to many cardiovascular disorders is still unknown, difficult to assess, and relatively low. A number of disqualified athletes would not die or experience any other consequences because of their physical activity. However, the screening perspective is that the risk of SD associated with competitive sports in the setting of potentially life-threatening cardiovascular disease is a controllable factor, and the devastating impact of even infrequent fatal events in the young athletic population justifies appropriate restriction from competition [7,73].

Screening athletes for cardiomyopathies and ion-channel disorders is expected to be very productive in preventing SD on sports fields, whereas exclusion of other young athletes with non-lethal diseases from competition is more arbitrary and probably not as productive. The prevalence of Italian athletes who were diagnosed and disqualified because of cardiovascular diseases was approximately 2%; however, true potentially lethal conditions such as cardiomyopathies, rhythm and conduction disturbances, long QT syndrome, valvular heart disease, premature coronary artery disease, and Marfan syndrome were identified in a smaller subgroup not exceeding 0.2% [10] (➔ Table 6.5.3). This has significant implications for optimizing sports eligibility guidelines and management of young competitive athletes with cardiovascular diseases in the future. The main objective should be to reduce the number of unnecessary disqualifications and to adapt (rather than restrict) sports activity in relation to the specific cardiovascular risk.

Other preventive strategies

The ability of screening to detect young competitive athletes with either premature coronary atherosclerosis or congenital coronary anomalies is limited by the lack of baseline ECG signs for myocardial ischaemia [7,46,74]. Moreover, SD during sport may be the result of non-penetrating chest injury (commotio cordis) which cannot be prevented by screening [8]. This justifies the increasing efforts to implement additional strategies for preventing sudden cardiac arrest based on early external defibrillation [38]. The presence of a free-standing automated external defibrillator (AED) at sports events may be a valuable intervention for conditions unrecognized by screening. However, AED should not be considered as either a substitute for pre-participation evaluation or a justification for allowing athletes with at-risk heart diseases to participate in competitive sports.

On-field cardiopulmonary resuscitation may be unsuccessful even if manoeuvres are started immediately and defibrillation equipment is readily available. Drezner et al. [75] initially reported a 90% mortality rate from athletic-field cardiac arrest due to underlying cardiomyopathy, despite a witnessed collapse, timely cardiopulmonary resuscitation, and prompt defibrillation.

A subsequent report from the same authors on a cohort of 1710 US high schools with free-standing AED programmes demonstrated an improved survival rate (i.e. 64%) in young athletes with sudden cardiac arrest if early defibrillation is achieved [76]. Compared with previous studies, this higher survival rate reported in high school athletes may be explained by the higher proportion of sudden cardiac arrest victims treated with AED and the smaller proportion of victims with HCM.

Conclusions

The available evidence, based on the long-running Italian experience, indicates that ECG screening has to be considered an efficient health strategy for prevention of sudden death of young competitive athletes. It meets the most important Wilson–Jungner criteria [77] for appraising the validity of a screening strategy:

(1) safe sports activity represents an important health issue;
(2) asymptomatic athletes with at-risk heart diseases may be successfully identified;
(3) an effective management strategy based on restriction of life-threatening training/competition and subsequent clinical treatment of at-risk athletes does exist;
(4) early identification/management of the underlying disease favourably modifies the outcome and leads to substantial reduction in mortality.

It is noteworthy that an interval of 25 years was required to generate the Italian data showing the actual success of the pre-participation ECG screening programme. Until data from other studies of comparable prospective study design, size of the athletic cohort, and follow-up duration are obtained, the existing Italian data provide good evidence that pre-participation screening does work. If the principle, sanctioned by both the AHA and the ESC, that cardiovascular screening for young competitive athletes is justifiable and compelling is accepted, the available evidence suggests adopting a screening protocol including ECG, which is the only screening tool that has been proved to be effective. Hence, pre-participation ECG screening of young competitive athletes has been recommended by the ESC [46], by the International Olympic Committee (Lausanne Recommendations) [78] and by most European Cardiology Societies and Sports Medical Federations (➔ Table 6.5.4). According to a recent consensus document on cardiovascular evaluation of athletes by the European Heart Rhythm Association and the European Association of Preventive Cardiology, pre-participation screening should be considered as a strategy not just to prevent SD but also to identify in a timely manner cardiovascular conditions

Table 6.5.4 Pre-participation athletic screening of young competitive athletes in European countries

Country	Medical/sports associations	Target athletic population	Screening protocol
Luxembourg	National Sports Ministry, Olympic Medical Committee, National Association of Sports Physicians	Competitive athletes of all sports	History, physical examination, ECG (required)
Sweden	National Board of Health and Welfare, National Federation of Sports	Elite athletes of all sports	History, physical examination, ECG (recommended)
Norway	Norwegian Football Association Medical Committee	Professional football players	History, physical examination, ECG, echocardiography (required)
Germany	German Association of Sports Medicine, National Sports Federations	Elite athletes of all sports	History, physical examination, ECG, echocardiography, exercise testing (required)
Poland	Ministry of Sports and Tourism, Ministry of Health, Polish Cardiac Society, Sports Federations	Competitive athletes (age <23 years) of all sports and national team members	History, physical examination, ECG (required)
France	National Sports Ministry, French Society of Cardiology	Professional athletes of all sports	History, physical examination, ECG, echocardiography, exercise testing (required)
		Competitive athletes of all sports	History, physical examination, ECG (recommended)
Scotland	Government, Department of Health	Football, competitive athletes 16 years old	History, physical examination, ECG (required)
England	British Lawn Tennis and Football Associations	Competitive athletes	History, physical examination, ECG (required)
Greece	Hellenic College of Sports Medicine, National Sports Federations	Competitive athletes of all sports	History, physical examination, ECG (recommended)
Belgium	National Sports Federations	Athletes of cycling and motocross sports	History, physical examination, ECG (required)
Spain	High Sports Government Council	Competitive athletes of all sports	History, physical examination, ECG (recommended)
The Netherlands	Working group of Cardiovascular Prevention and Rehabilitation, National Olympic Committee, National Sports Federations, Netherlands Society of Cardiology	Elite competitive athletes (age <35 years) of all sports	History, physical examination, ECG (required)
		Professional football players	History, physical examination, ECG, echocardiography (required)
		Elite athletes of cycling, motor and flying sports and diving	History, physical examination, ECG (required)

that might benefit from appropriate medical management (including exercise restriction). Therefore pre-participation screening is considered by the panel of experts as justifiable on ethical, social, and medical grounds. Moreover, the consensus is that the protocol of pre-participation screening should include the 12-lead ECG, which has been demonstrated to have superior diagnostic capability, as well as just clinical history and physical examination [79]. However, the 2014 AHA statement for screening young people and athletes, while not disputing the incremental value of ECG screening, argues that it is not applicable to the US system because of the logistics, manpower, and financial resources required for a national screening programme [53].

Interestingly, in 2014 *The New England Journal of Medicine* promoted an online poll which received 1266 votes from 86 countries; the majority (56%) were in favour of an ECG-based pre-participation screening, 24% believed that screening should include history and physical examination only, and 18% believed that screening should not be performed. The majority (66%) of European voters favoured screening with ECG, whereas just under half of US voters (45%) shared this opinion [80].

Further reading

Corrado D, Basso C, Pavei A, et al. Trends in sudden cardiovascular death in young competitive athletes after implementation of a preparticipation screening program. *JAMA* 2006; 296: 1593–601

Van Brabandt H, Desomer A, Gerkens S, Neyt M. Harms and benefits of screening young people to prevent sudden cardiac death. *BMJ* 2016; 353: i1156.

Corrado D, Basso C, Schiavon M, et al. Reply to Van Brabandt and colleagues. *BMJ* 2016; 354: i3631.

Corrado D, Basso C, Thiene G. Pros and cons of screening for sudden cardiac death in sports. *Heart* 2013; 99: 1365–73.

Corrado D, Pelliccia A, Bjornstad HH, et al. Cardiovascular pre-participation screening of young competitive athletes for prevention of sudden death: proposal for a common European protocol. *Eur Heart J* 2005; 26: 516–24.

Drezner JA, Rao AL, Heistand J, et al. Effectiveness of emergency response planning for sudden cardiac arrest in United States high schools with automated external defibrillators. *Circulation* 2009; 120: 518–25.

Harmon KG, Asif IM, Klossner D, Drezner JA. Incidence of sudden cardiac death in National Collegiate Athletic Association athletes. *Circulation* 2011; 123: 1594–1600

Maron BJ, Thompson PD, Ackerman MJ, et al. Recommendations and considerations related to preparticipation screening for cardiovascular abnormalities in competitive athletes: 2007 update. *Circulation* 2007; 115: 1643–55.

Maron BJ, Doerer JJ, Haas TS, et al. Sudden deaths in young competitive athletes: analysis of 1866 deaths in the United States, 1980-2006. *Circulation* 2009; 119: 1085–92.

Mont L, Pelliccia A, Sharma S, et al. Pre-participation cardiovascular evaluation for athletic participants to prevent sudden death. *Europace* 2017; 19: 139–63.

References

1 Corrado D, Thiene G, Nava A, et al. Sudden death in young competitive athletes: clinicopathologic correlations in 22 cases. *Am J Med* 1990; 89: 588–96.

2 Schmied C, Borjesson M. Sudden cardiac death in athletes. *J Intern Med* 2014; 275: 93–103.

3 Schwartz PJ, Corrado D. Sudden cardiac death in young competitive athletes. *Eur Heart J* 2012; 33: 1986–8.

4 Corrado D, Basso C, Thiene G. Essay: Sudden death in young athletes. *Lancet* 2005; 366(Suppl 1): S47–8.

5 Corrado D, Basso C, Thiene G. Sudden cardiac death in athletes: what is the role of screening? *Curr Opin Cardiol* 2012; 27: 41–8.

6 Pelliccia A, Corrado D. Can electrocardiographic screening prevent sudden death in athletes? Yes. *BMJ* 2010; 341: c4923.

7 Corrado D, Basso C, Schiavon M, Pelliccia A, Thiene G. Preparticipation screening of young competitive athletes for prevention of sudden cardiac death. *J Am Coll Cardiol* 2008; 52: 1981–9.

8 Corrado D, Basso C, Thiene G. Pros and cons of screening for sudden cardiac death in sports. *Heart* 2013; 99: 1365–73.

9 Sharma S, Estes NA 3rd, Vetter VL, Corrado D. Clinical decisions. Cardiac screening before participation in sports. *N Engl J Med* 2013; 369: 2049–53.

10 Corrado D, Basso C, Pavei A, et al. Trends in sudden cardiovascular death in young competitive athletes after implementation of a preparticipation screening program. *JAMA* 2006; 296: 1593–1601.

11 Maron BJ, Gohman TE, Aeppli D. Prevalence of sudden cardiac death during competitive sports activities in Minnesota high school athletes. *J Am Coll Cardiol* 1998; 32: 1881–4.

12 Corrado D, Basso C, Rizzoli G, et al. Does sports activity enhance the risk of sudden death in adolescents and young adults? *J Am Coll Cardiol* 2003; 42: 1959–63.

13 Gerein RB, Osmond MH, Stiell IG, et al. What are the etiology and epidemiology of out-of-hospital pediatric cardiopulmonary arrest in Ontario, Canada? *Acad Emerg Med* 2006; 13: 653–8.

14 Ong ME, Stiell I, Osmond MH, et al. Etiology of pediatric out-of-hospital cardiac arrest by coroner's diagnosis. *Resuscitation* 2006; 68: 335–42.

15 Maron BJ, Doerer JJ, Haas TS, et al. Sudden deaths in young competitive athletes: analysis of 1866 deaths in the United States, 1980–2006. *Circulation* 2009; 119: 1085–92.

16 Chugh SS, Reinier K, Balaji S, et al. Population-based analysis of sudden death in children: The Oregon Sudden Unexpected Death Study. *Heart Rhythm* 2009; 6: 1618–22.

17 Atkins DL, Everson-Stewart S, Sears GK, Daya M, Osmond MH, Warden CR, Berg RA. Epidemiology and outcomes from out-of-hospital cardiac arrest in children: the Resuscitation Outcomes Consortium Epistry-Cardiac Arrest. *Circulation* 2009; 119: 1484–91.

18 Solberg EE, Gjertsen F, Haugstad E, Kolsrud L. Sudden death in sports among young adults in Norway. *Eur J Cardiovasc Prev Rehabil.* 2010; 17: 337–41.

19 Holst AG, Winkel BG, Theilade J, Kristensen IB, Thomsen JL, Ottesen GL, Svendsen JH, Haunso S, Prescott E, Tfelt-Hansen J. Incidence and etiology of sports-related sudden cardiac death in Denmark—implications for preparticipation screening. *Heart Rhythm* 2010; 7: 1365–71.

20 Donohoe RT, Innes J, Gadd S, et al. Out-of-hospital cardiac arrest in patients aged 35 years and under: a 4-year study of frequency and survival in London. *Resuscitation* 2010; 81: 36–41.

21 Park CB, Shin SD, Suh GJ, et al. Pediatric out-of-hospital cardiac arrest in Korea: a nationwide population-based study. *Resuscitation* 2010; 81: 512–17.

22 Deasy C, Bernard SA, Cameron P, et al. Epidemiology of paediatric out-of-hospital cardiac arrest in Melbourne, Australia. *Resuscitation* 2010; 81: 1095–1100.

23 Harmon KG, Asif IM, Klossner D, Drezner JA. Incidence of sudden cardiac death in National Collegiate Athletic Association athletes. *Circulation* 2011; 123: 1594–1600.

24 Winkel BG, Holst AG, Theilade J, et al. Nationwide study of sudden cardiac death in persons aged 1-35 years. *Eur Heart J* 2011; 32: 983–L 90.

25 Meyer L, Stubbs B, Fahrenbruch C, et al. Incidence, causes, and survival trends from cardiovascular-related sudden cardiac arrest in children and young adults 0 to 35 years of age: a 30-year review. *Circulation* 2012; 126: 1363–72.

26 Margey R, Roy A, Tobin S, et al. Sudden cardiac death in 14- to 35-year olds in Ireland from 2005 to 2007: a retrospective registry. *Europace* 2011; 13: 1411–18.

27 Eckart RE, Shry EA, Burke AP, et al. Sudden death in young adults: an autopsy-based series of a population undergoing active surveillance. *J Am Coll Cardiol* 2011; 58: 1254–61.

28 Roberts WO, Stovitz SD. Incidence of sudden cardiac death in Minnesota high school athletes 1993–2012 screened with a standardized pre-participation evaluation. *J Am Coll Cardiol* 2013; 62: 1298–1301.

29 Pilmer CM, Kirsh JA, Hildebrandt D, et al. Sudden cardiac death in children and adolescents between 1 and 19 years of age. *Heart Rhythm* 2014; 11: 239–45.

30 Pilmer CM, Porter B, Kirsh JA, et al. Scope and nature of sudden cardiac death before age 40 in Ontario: a report from the Cardiac Death Advisory Committee of the Office of the Chief Coroner. *Heart Rhythm* 2013; 10: 517–23.

31 Berdowski J, de Beus MF, Blom M, et al. Exercise-related out-of-hospital cardiac arrest in the general population: incidence and prognosis. *Eur Heart J* 2013; 34: 3616–23.

32 Maron BJ, Haas TS, Ahluwalia A, Rutten-Ramos SC. Incidence of cardiovascular sudden deaths in Minnesota high school athletes. *Heart Rhythm* 2013; 10: 374–7.

33 Risgaard B, Winkel BG, Jabbari R, et al. Burden of sudden cardiac death in persons aged 1 to 49 years: nationwide study in Denmark. *Circ Arrhythm Electrophysiol* 2014; 7: 205–11.

34 Van Camp SP, Bloor CM, Mueller FO, et al. Nontraumatic sports death in high school and college athletes. *Med Sci Sports Exerc* 1995; 27: 641–7.

35 Marijon E, Bougouin W, Perier MC, et al. Incidence of sports-related sudden death in France by specific sports and sex. *JAMA* 2013; 310: 642–3.

36 Maron BJ, Haas TS, Doerer JJ, et al. Comparison of U.S. and Italian experiences with sudden cardiac deaths in young competitive athletes and implications for preparticipation screening strategies. *Am J Cardiol* 2009; 104: 276–80.

37 Basso C, Carturan E, Pilichou K, et al. Sudden cardiac death with normal heart: molecular autopsy. *Cardiovasc Pathol* 2010; 19: 321–5.

38 Link MS. Pathophysiology, prevention, and treatment of commotio cordis. *Curr Cardiol Rep* 2014;16; 495.

39 Corrado D, Drezner J, Basso C, et al. Strategies for the prevention of sudden cardiac death during sports. *Eur J Cardiovasc Prev Rehabil* 2011; 18: 197–208.

40 Mittleman MA, Maclure M, Tofler GH, et al. Triggering of acute myocardial infarction by heavy physical exertion. Protection against triggering by regular exertion. Determinants of Myocardial Infarction Onset Study Investigators. *N Engl J Med* 1993; 329: 1677–83.

41 Fuller CM, McNulty CM, Spring DA, et al. Prospective screening of 5,615 high school athletes for risk of sudden cardiac death. *Med Sci Sports Exerc* 1997; 29: 1131–8.

42 Wilson MG, Basavarajaiah S, Whyte GP, et al. Efficacy of personal symptom and family history questionnaires when screening for inherited cardiac pathologies: the role of electrocardiography. *Br J Sports Med* 2008; 42: 207–11.

43 Bessem B, Groot FP, Nieuwland W. The Lausanne recommendations: a Dutch experience. *Br J Sports Med* 2009; 43: 708–15.

44 Baggish AL, Hutter AM Jr, Wang F, et al. Cardiovascular screening in college athletes with and without electrocardiography: a cross-sectional study. *Ann Intern Med* 2010; 152: 269–75.

45 Sheikh N, Papadakis M, Ghani S, et al. Comparison of electrocardiographic criteria for the detection of cardiac abnormalities in elite black and white athletes. *Circulation* 2014; 129: 1637–49.

46 Corrado D, Pelliccia A, Bjornstad HH, et al. Cardiovascular pre-participation screening of young competitive athletes for prevention of sudden death: proposal for a common European protocol. *Eur Heart J* 2005; 26: 516–24.

47 Maron BJ, Thompson PD, Ackerman MJ, et al. Recommendations and considerations related to preparticipation screening for cardiovascular abnormalities in competitive athletes: 2007 update. *Circulation* 2007; 115: 1643–5.

48 Harmon KG, Zigman M, Drezner JA. The effectiveness of screening history, physical exam, and ECG to detect potentially lethal cardiac disorders in athletes: a systematic review/meta-analysis. *J Electrocardiol* 2015; 48: 329–38.

49 Glover DW, Maron BJ. Profile of preparticipation cardiovascular screening for high school athletes. *JAMA* 1998; 279: 1817–19.

50 Corrado D, Basso C, Schiavon M, Thiene G. Screening for hypertrophic cardiomyopathy in young athletes. *N Engl J Med* 1998; 339: 364–9.

51 Maron BJ, Gardin JM, Flack JM, et al. Prevalence of hypertrophic cardiomyopathy in a general population of young adults. Echocardiographic analysis of 4111 subjects in the CARDIA Study. Coronary Artery Risk Development in (Young) Adults. *Circulation* 1995; 92: 785–9.

52 Thompson PD, Levine BD. Protecting athletes from sudden cardiac death. *JAMA* 2006; 296: 1648–50.

53 Maron BJ, Friedman RA, Kligfield P, et al. Assessment of the 12-lead ECG as a screening test for detection of cardiovascular disease in healthy general populations of young people (12–25 years of age): a scientific statement from the American Heart Association and the American College of Cardiology. *Circulation* 2014; 130: 1303–34.

54 Van Brabandt H, Desomer A, Gerkens S, Neyt M. Harms and benefits of screening young people to prevent sudden cardiac death. *BMJ* 2016; 353: i1156.

55 Corrado D, Basso C, Schiavon M, et al. Reply to Van Brabandt and colleagues. *BMJ* 2016; 354: i3631.

56 Steinvil A, Chundadze T, Zeltser D, et al. Mandatory electrocardiographic screening of athletes to reduce their risk for sudden death proven fact or wishful thinking? *J Am Coll Cardiol* 2011; 57: 1291–6.

57 Higgins JP, Laing ST, Chen Z. Media reporting bias affects reported sudden death rates. *J Am Coll Cardiol* 2011; 58: 990–1; author reply 1-2.

58 Pelliccia A, Corrado D. The Israel screening failure analyzing the data to understand the results. *J Am Coll Cardiol* 2011; 58: 989–L 90; author reply 991-2.

59 Corrado D, Pelliccia A, Heidbüchel H, et al. Recommendations for interpretation of 12-lead electrocardiogram in the athlete. *Eur Heart J* 2010; 31: 243–59.

60 Basavarajaiah S, Boraita A, Whyte G, et al. Ethnic differences in left ventricular remodeling in highly-trained athletes relevance to differentiating physiologic left ventricular hypertrophy from hypertrophic cardiomyopathy. *J Am Coll Cardiol* 2008; 51: 2256–62.

61 Uberoi A, Stein R, Perez MV, et al. Interpretation of the electrocardiogram of young athletes. *Circulation* 2011; 124: 746–57.
62 Drezner JA, Ackerman MJ, Anderson J, et al. Electrocardiographic interpretation in athletes: the 'Seattle criteria'. *Br J Sports Med* 2013; 47: 122–4.
63 Pickham D, Zarafshar S, Sani D, et al. Comparison of three ECG criteria for athlete pre-participation screening. *J Electrocardiol.* 2014; 47: 769–74.
64 Brosnan M, La Gerche A, Kalman J, et al. Comparison of frequency of significant electrocardiographic abnormalities in endurance versus nonendurance athletes. *Am J Cardiol* 2014; 113: 1567–73.
65 Berge HM, Gjesdal K, Andersen TE, et al. Prevalence of abnormal ECGs in male soccer players decreases with the Seattle criteria, but is still high. *Scand J Med Sci Sports* 2014; 25: 501–8.
66 Bessem B, de Bruijn MC, Nieuwland W. The ECG of high-level junior soccer players: comparing the ESC vs. the Seattle criteria. *Br J Sports Med* 2015; 49: 1000–6.
67 Wasfy MM, DeLuca J, Wang F, et al. ECG findings in competitive rowers: normative data and the prevalence of abnormalities using contemporary screening recommendations. *Br J Sports Med* 2015; 49: 200–6.
68 Corrado D, McKenna WJ. Appropriate interpretation of the athlete's electrocardiogram saves lives as well as money. *Eur Heart J* 2007; 28: 1920–2.
69 Wheeler MT, Heidenreich PA, Froelicher VF, et al. Cost-effectiveness of preparticipation screening for prevention of sudden cardiac death in young athletes. *Ann Intern Med* 2010; 152: 276–86.
70 Tanaka Y, Yoshinaga M, Anan R, et al. Usefulness and cost effectiveness of cardiovascular screening of young adolescents. *Med Sci Sports Exerc* 2006;38 : 2–6.
71 Fuller CM. Cost effectiveness analysis of screening of high school athletes for risk of sudden cardiac death. *Med Sci Sports Exerc* 2000; 32: 887–90.
72 Myerburg RJ, Vetter VL. Electrocardiograms should be included in preparticipation screening of athletes. *Circulation* 2007; 116: 2616–26.
73 Maron BJ, Zipes DP, Kovacs RJ. Eligibility and disqualification recommendations for competitive athletes with cardiovascular abnormalities: preamble, principles, and general considerations. *J Am Coll Cardiol* 2015; 66: 2343–9.
74 Basso C, Maron BJ, Corrado D, Thiene G. Clinical profile of congenital coronary artery anomalies with origin from the wrong aortic sinus leading to sudden death in young competitive athletes. *J Am Coll Cardiol* 2000; 35: 1493–1501.
75 Drezner JA, Rogers KJ. Sudden cardiac arrest in intercollegiate athletes: detailed analysis and outcomes of resuscitation in nine cases. *Heart Rhythm* 2006; 3: 755–9.
76 Drezner JA, Rao AL, Heistand J, et al. Effectiveness of emergency response planning for sudden cardiac arrest in United States high schools with automated external defibrillators. *Circulation* 2009; 120: 518–25.
77 Wilson JMG, Jungner G. Principles and practice of screening for disease. Geneva: WHO; 1968.
78 Hamilton B, Jaques R, Budgett R. Observations on the 'Lausanne Recommendations' on sudden cardiovascular death in sport. *Br J Sports Med* 2007; 41: e1.
79 Mont L, Pelliccia A, Sharma S, et al. Pre-participation cardiovascular evaluation for athletic participants to prevent sudden death. *Europace* 2017; 19: 139–63.
80 Colbert JA. Clinical decisions. Cardiac screening before participation in sports—polling results. *N Engl J Med* 2014; 370: e16.

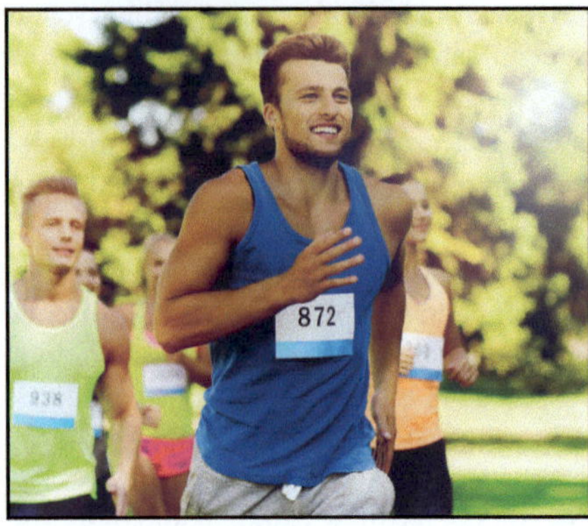

6.6

Cardiovascular screening of adult/senior competitive athletes

Luc Vanhees and Mats Börjesson

Introduction

It is well established that exercise reduces total and cardiovascular mortality [1,2]. The phenotype of high cardiovascular fitness is strongly associated with a decrease in all-cause and cardiovascular mortality, mediated through its association with a favourable risk factor profile for cardiovascular disease (CVD), including insulin sensitivity, lipid profile, blood pressure, and overweight [3–5]. Other beneficial effects of physical activity (PA) and exercise training have been reported on endothelial function, autonomic balance, and blood coagulation [6–8], also contributing to the preventive effect of exercise. Therefore in recent decades physical activity has been recognized as an important tool for prevention and treatment of coronary artery disease (CAD) by both the American Heart Association (AHA) [9–11] and the European Society of Cardiology (ESC) [4,5,12,13]. Whereas earlier guidelines focused mainly on the duration of PA, more recently the importance of intensity (moderate to strenuous) exercise has been emphasized.

Unfortunately acute bouts of high intensity exercise may themselves trigger cardiac events. Reports indicate a four- to fivefold higher risk of acute cardiovascular events in association with exercise, even in trained athletes [10]. The prevalence of SCD in joggers and marathon runners has been reported to be 1 one in 15,000 and one in 50,000, respectively [14,15], which is much higher than the incidence in young athletes (one in 100,000–300,000 per year in young high school or college-aged athletes). In a review of studies of SCD in marathon runners, James et al. [15] reported an incidence of SCD varying between 0.54 and 2.1 in 100,000 athletes, with a higher incidence of death mainly observed in full marathons and often in experienced runners.

In young athletes, the cause of sudden cardiac arrest (SCA) is dominated by inherited/congenital disease, such as hypertrophic cardiomyopathy, whereas in adult/senior individuals known or unknown underlying CAD is by far the most common aetiology [16]. Indeed, 95% of the cause of SCD in athletes aged >45 years has been reported to be CAD [17]. Although the mechanisms are not fully elucidated, acute intense exercise activates the sympathetic nervous system, increases circulating catecholamines, which may increase the risk of ventricular fibrillation, and increases platelet adhesion and the risk of atherosclerotic plaque rupture [18–20]. In subjects not accustomed to performing intense exercise, vigorous exercise increases the risk for SCD by a factor of 56 [21]. Importantly, the average age of participants in events such as marathons is increasing [15,22]. Consequently, James et al. [15] reported an average age of SCD or survivors of SCA ranging from 37 to 56 years.

Recommendations to increase the physical activity pattern of the population, and more specifically the middle-aged/senior population, for preventive reasons should also address the safety of exercise and the risk–benefit ratio. This ratio for exercise depends not only on the properties of the activity performed (intensity, duration, type of activity [4,5]), but also on the individual risk profile, i.e. for sedentary individuals [23], subjects with an increased risk profile for CAD, and older subjects compared with younger individuals. As participation in competitive and recreational sports increases throughout the world, a greater number of individuals and athletes are being enrolled in intensive training programmes or competition, often without pre-participation medical evaluations. Occult cardiovascular disease, of different degrees, with the potential to cause sudden cardiac death, stroke, acute coronary syndromes, or heart failure, may exist in these non-screened individuals. Furthermore, many athletes with known cardiovascular disease also continue to participate in intense activities or competition [24]. Many of these may have vague, diffuse, or even no symptoms of underlying disease. Since an asymptomatic status does not guarantee immunity from cardiac events, specific attention should be paid to screening adults or senior athletes, since they may be at higher risk than believed in relation to their age and the intensity of exercise.

In the present chapter, we will review the existing recommendations regarding cardiovascular evaluation of adult and senior competitive athletes or individuals, with or without known CAD, intending to participate in intense competitive or leisure-time sporting activities. This chapter will not cover recommendations for screening in young competitive athletes, which are covered in ➲ Chapter 7.1.

Definition of adult/senior competitive athlete

An athlete is a person who is trained or skilled in exercises, sports, or games requiring physical strength, agility, or endurance. In a more general context, an adult or senior athlete could also mean someone participates in organized sport or competition. This chapter considers apparently healthy adults, aged ≥35, who are either conditioned experienced competitive athletes who continue to compete after the end of their formal careers, or individuals with only sporadic training regimens performing a competitive sport or intense recreational activity, such as soccer, cycling, long-distance running, or triathlon. It may also include subjects who resume competition after long periods of physical inactivity, or who want to start intense sporting activities from a preventive perspective.

Existing screening recommendations

The principle of existing screening recommendations in senior/adult individuals is that any screening should interfere as little as possible, so as to not decrease the willingness to be physically active, but at the same time to be able to identify relevant underlying disease. Therefore existing recommendations invariably advocate some kind of stepwise screening, targeting mainly high(er) risk individuals.

AHA/ACSM screening of participants of health/fitness facilities

In 1998, American Heart Association (AHA) and the American College of Sports Medicine (ACSM) published recommendations for cardiovascular screening of persons of all ages enlisting for training at health/fitness facilities [25]. Before 1997, 40% of the fitness facilities stated that they did not routinely use a screening interview or questionnaire to evaluate new members [26]. Importantly, 50% of health club/fitness facility members were older than 35 years, and the fastest growing group of users were those aged 35–54 and over 55 [26]. Thus these recommendations may have been aimed primarily at middle-aged/senior leisure-time athletes. The AHA/ACSM recommendation use self-administered screening questionnaires (PAR-Q/AHA pre-participation screening questionnaire) to identify individuals with known cardiovascular disease, symptoms of cardiovascular disease, and/or risk factors for disease development who need further medical evaluation before starting an exercise programme [25]. After completion of the initial health appraisal and (when needed) the additional medical evaluation, participants can be further classified into groups as follows: Class A (apparently healthy), Class B (presence of known stable cardiovascular disease with low risk during vigorous exercise), Class C (those at moderate to high risk of cardiac complications during exercise and/or unable to self-regulate activity), and Class D (unstable conditions with activity restrictions). These groups then provide the basis for giving appropriate individual advice on exercise and eligibility.

Screening of master athletes (AHA)

The AHA Science Advisory Committee also recommends pre-participation screening for all master athletes (defined as >40 years old) [14]. They recommend cardiovascular evaluation consisting of history and physical examination, including a routine standard 12-lead ECG for the evaluation of all master athletes, of both sexes, over 40 years old. In addition, they recommend that master athletes with a moderate to high cardiovascular risk profile for CAD, who want to enter vigorous master competitions, undergo symptom-limited maximal ECG exercise testing (treadmill or cycle ergometer). This includes all men aged over 40 and all women aged over 50 years with one additional coronary risk factor (hyperlipidaemia, hypertension, smoking, diabetes mellitus or insulin resistance, positive family history) as well as all master athletes with symptoms suggestive of underlying coronary artery disease and all participants aged over 65.

Eligibility after screening: ESC/EACPR and AHA/ACC

In 2005–2006 a series of papers were published by the ESC/EACPR Study Group of Sports Cardiology, on both screening and eligibility for participation in competitive athletes [27,28] and for competitive and leisure-time sports in subjects with various cardiovascular disorders, such as cardiomyopathies [29], arrhythmias [30,31], valvular heart disease (HD) [32], congenital HD [33], hypertension [34], and ischaemic HD [35]. These recommendations included the evaluation, criteria for eligibility, recommendations for sports, and follow-up of persons with these CV disorders participating in competitive or leisure-time sports. The recommendations for sports participation in subjects with ischaemic heart disease [35] will be discussed in more detail in the next section.

Recently, the AHA and American College of Cardiology (ACC) released a series of documents from 15 task forces, dealing with eligibility recommendations for competitive athletes with various cardiovascular abnormalities [36]. Similarly to the European recommendations, most of these different task force reports deal with cardiovascular abnormalities in young competitive athletes (HCM [37], congenital defects [38]. channelopathies [39], WPW syndrome [40], etc.) and therefore will not be discussed further here. However, other task forces discussed eligibility and disqualification recommendations for competitive athletes with hypertension [41], aortic diseases [42], valvular disease [43], and coronary artery disease [44], which are most relevant for the adult/senior population. Classes of recommendations and levels of evidence are described for diagnostic evaluation recommendations and qualifications for the type/intensity of competitive/leisure sports in athletes with these pathologies [36].

In general, if the pathology is clinically stable, not acute, well treated, and without manifestations during exercise, competitive sports are allowed. If this is not the case, more conservative recommendations regarding the type, intensity, and competitive nature of sports are formulated, in both the European and US recommendations [27–44].

Recommendations for participation in leisure-time exercise and competitive sports for patients with CAD

Recommendations from the European Association of Cardiovascular Prevention and Rehabilitation (EACPR) [35] focus on the evaluation and eligibility for exercise and sports in patients with risk factors for CAD and with established CAD. The recommendations state that patients with CAD will profit from individually prescribed leisure-time PA (LTPA), achieving both functional and preventive benefits. Competitive sports for these patients, however, may be contraindicated or restricted, depending on the probability of cardiac events and the demands of the sport [28].

Patients with CAD can be divided into a lower risk and a higher risk group according to the profile of risk factor, age, the results of an exercise test (exercise capacity, exercise-induced ischaemia, arrhythmias during exercise), ejection fraction on echocardiography, the presence of any ventricular arrhythmias, and the result of coronary angiography (if performed) [35]. However, competitive sports is generally severely restricted in patients with established CAD [35,44].

In the ESC recommendations, patients without evidence of CAD, but with one or more classical risk factors for CAD, may be classified as having a high risk profile or a low risk profile. The higher risk factor profile for developing a fatal cardiovascular event is defined as one of the following [35]:

(1) the presence of various multiple risk factors, resulting in a 10-year risk greater than 5% immediately or if extrapolated to 60 years of age in the SCORE chart;
(2) markedly raised levels of total cholesterol (>8mmol/L = 320mg/dL) and LDL cholesterol (>6mmol/L = 240mg/dL) or blood pressure >180/110mmHg;
(3) diabetes mellitus type 2 or type 1 with microalbuminuria;
(4) a strong family history of premature CVD in first-degree relatives aged less than 50 years, or individuals having a BMI greater than 28kg/m^2 [35].

Importantly, individuals without CAD but with a high risk profile and a negative exercise test and those with a low risk profile (SCORE <5%) are allowed to participate in competitive sports with a few exceptions (see also ➔ Chapter 7.1)

Cardiovascular evaluation of middle-aged/senior individuals engaged in leisure-time sport activities

Complementing earlier recommendations, in 2011 the EACPR published recommendations regarding middle-aged or senior individuals who wished to participate in competitive or recreational sporting activities [16,45].

The rationale for these recommendations is that the extent of the cardiovascular evaluation needed in middle-aged/senior individuals before starting leisure-time physical and sports activities depends on the individual risk profile, as well as the intended level of PA. The individual risk profile is estimated from the burden of the known classical cardiovascular risk factors and the current level of fitness or habitual PA undertaken by the individual [4,45] The identification of risk factors for CAD can be achieved in several ways. The recommended first-line risk evaluation is self-assessment (by the individual or by non-physician health professionals) using validated questionnaires such as the

AHA Pre-participation Questionnaire [46] or the PAR-Q [47] This method of self-assessment can easily be used for large groups of individuals, thereby constituting a minimal obstacle to exercise. In addition, as a secondary step in individuals with positive answers in the first-line evaluation, a more thorough risk assessment could be performed by a qualified physician using the ESC Risk SCORE [45,48,49].

Middle-aged/senior individuals can be categorized into two major groups according to their habitual PA level: Sedentary individuals are defined as individuals who are not regularly engaged in PA or exercise (<2 MET-hours per week). This low activity level has been associated with higher coronary event rates and a poorer prognosis. Active individuals are defined as individuals regularly engaged in leisure-time, even intense, non-competitive sport activities, including master athletes.

Competitive athletes typically engage in intensive/very intensive physical activity. Different types of sport are classified into four main categories: endurance, power, skill, and mixed (see also ➲ Chapter 7.1). High intensity PA includes endurance events such as long distance cycling, city marathons, long distance cross-country skiing, and triathlons, corresponding to more than 6 METs. However, it is the relative intensity of any PA undertaken by the middle-aged/senior individual that influences the burden on the cardiovascular system. Any categorization of the intensity of exercise as 'moderate' or 'vigorous' has to be related to the individual exercise tolerance rather than using absolute measures such as metabolic equivalentss. For example, walking at a speed of 6km/h may represent a vigorous, rather than a low to moderate intensity of exercise, for an obese individual with low fitness. Physically active senior/master individuals, willing to participate in moderate intensity (3–6 METs) PA, or to continue being active at that level, should be evaluated using self-assessment questionnaires (➲ Fig. 6.6.1). Individuals with symptoms or a history of CVD, identified by a self-assessment questionnaire, should be evaluated by a physician including reassessment of the personal and family history, physical examination, risk SCORE, and 12-lead resting ECG. All individuals (regardless of being active or sedentary) over 35 years old, contemplating or engaged in high intensity (>6 METS) activity are subject to the same detailed evaluation by a qualified physician even in the absence of symptoms or other known risk factors for CAD. If positive, these individuals are advised to undergo additional maximal exercise testing. Subjects are advised as being eligible for moderate to high intensity exercise training if the exercise test is normal.

Very rarely, sedentary individuals decide to take up competitive sports. Although this is discussed in the recommendations, it is not highlighted in this chapter [45].

Patients may have associated comorbidities that could affect their ability to achieve an adequate level of activity, including orthopaedic problems [50]. In addition, the use of

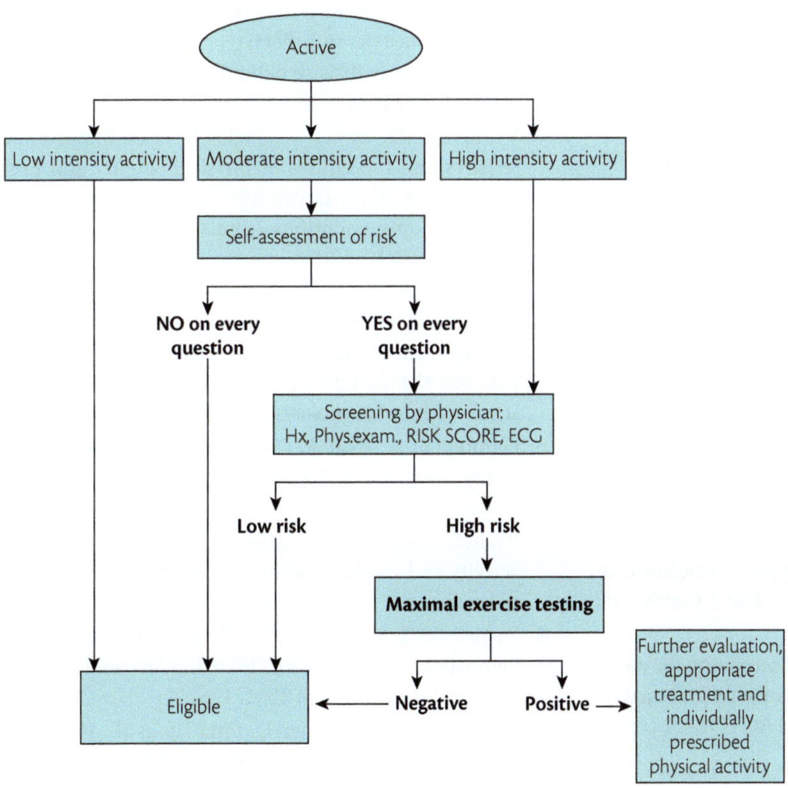

Fig. 6.6.1 Proposed pre-participation evaluation protocol for asymptomatic *active* adult/senior individuals: PA, physical activity.

Adapted with permission from Borjesson M, Urhausen A, Kouidi E, et al. Cardiovascular evaluation of middle-aged/senior individuals engaged in leisure-time sport activities: position stand from the sections of exercise physiology and sports cardiology of the European Association of Cardiovascular Prevention and Rehabilitation. *European Journal of Preventive Cardiology*, Volume 18, pp.446–58. Copyright 2011 SAGE.

medication (beta-blockers, diuretics) could affect the ability to reach maximal pulse[51]. In the event of a positive exercise test, further evaluation is necessary to confirm/refute the presence of CAD or another cardiovascular abnormality and to advise appropriate management. A reassessment of the risk factor profile on an individual basis is also recommended. The exercise test is important to aid the prescription of PA at the optimal intensity for each individual. Regular reassessment of the cardiorespiratory fitness level by a suitable evaluation method should be part of the regular follow-up of these individuals.

Recently, an update of the ACSM's recommendations for exercise participation health screening became available [52]. These recommendations, in contrast with the older ones [25], take into account (1) the individual's current level of physical activity, (2) the presence of symptoms, and (3) the desired exercise intensity. This update is very similar to the existing ESC recommendations on screening [45] and therefore will not be repeated in detail here.

Summary

The number of older/senior athletes is increasing worldwide, including those participating in competition. This is viewed as a favourable development, since the level of physical activity is too low in a majority of the world population. While the benefits of regular activity are well established, there is a risk of occurrence of adverse cardiac events with increased intensity of the activity, as well as with the high risk profile (and age) of the individual. This forms the rationale for cardiac screening of senior/older athletes prior to intensive sports participation. However, any such screening must be adapted to the individual, according to the total risk profile and the intended activity, with the aim of achieving maximal healthy active behaviour at the lowest possible risk.

Further reading

Aagaard P, Sahlén A, Braunschweig F. Performance trends and cardiac biomarkers in a 30-km cross-country race, 1993-2007. *Med Sci Sports Exerc* 2012; 44: 894–9.

Borjesson M, Urhausen A, Kouidi E, et al. Cardiovascular evaluation of middle-aged/senior individuals engaged in leisure-time sport activities: position stand from the sections of exercise physiology and sports cardiology of the European Association of Cardiovascular Prevention and Rehabilitation. *Eur J Cardiovasc Prev Rehabil* 2011; 18: 446–58.

Muhlestein JB, Lappé DL, Lima JC, et al. Effect of screening for coronary artery disease using CT angiography on mortality and cardiac events in high-risk patients with diabetes: the FACTOR-64 ranfomized clinical trial. *JAMA* 2014; 312: 2234–43.

Douglas PS, Hoffmann U, Patel MR, et al. Outcomes of anatomical versus functional testing for coronary artery disease. *N Engl J Med* 2015; 372: 1291–1300.

Genders TSS, Petrsen SE, Pugliese F, et al. The optimal imaging strategy for parients with stable chest pain: a cost-effectiveness analysis. *Ann Intern Med* 2015; 162: 474–84.

Riebe D, Franklin BA, Thompson PD, et al. Updating ACSM's recommendations for exercise preparticipation health screening. *Med Sci Sports Exerc* 2015; 47: 2473–9.

Siskovick DS, Weiss NS, Fletcher RH, et al. Habitual vigorous exercise and primary cardiac arrest: effect of other risk factors on the relationship. *J Chronic Dis* 1984; 37 : 625–31.

Thompson PD, Franklin BA, Balady GJ, et al. Exercise and acute cardiovascular events: placing the risks into perspective. A scientific statement from the American Heart Association Council on Nutrition, Physical Activity, and Metabolism and the Council on Clinical Cardiology. *Circulation* 2007; 115: 2358–68.

Vanhees L, Rauch B, Piepoli M, et al. Importance of characteristics and modalities of physical activity and exercise in the management of cardiovascular health in individuals with cardiovascular disease (Part III). *Eur J Prev Cardiol* 2012; 19: 1333–56.

Vrints CJM, Senior R, Crea F, Sechtem U. Assessing suspected angina: requiem for coronary computed tomography angiography or exercise electrocardiogram? *Eur Heart J* 2017; 38: 1792–1800.

References

1. Blair SN, Kohl HW, Pattenbarger RS Jr, et al. Physical fitness and all-cause mortality: a prospective study of healthy men and women. *JAMA* 1989; 262: 2395–401.
2. Paffenbarger RS Jr, Hyde RT, Wing AL, et al. The association of changes in physical activity and other lifestyle characteristics with mortality among men. *N Engl J Med* 1993; 328: 538–45.
3. Iestra JA, Kromhout D, van der Schouw YT, et al. Effect size estimates of lifestyle and dietary changes on all-cause mortality in coronary artery disease patients: a systematic review. *Circulation* 2005; 112: 924–34.
4. Vanhees L, De Sutter J, Geladas N, et al. Importance of characteristics and modalities of physical activity and exercise in the mangement of cardiovascular health within the general population: recommendations from the EACPR (part I). *Eur J Prev Cardiol* 2012; 19: 670–86.
5. Vanhees L, Geladas N, Hansen D, et al. Importance of characteristics and modalities of physical activity and exercise in the management of cardiovascular health in individuals with cardiovascular risk factors: recommendations from the EACPR (part II). *Eur J Prev Cardiol* 2012; 19: 1005–33.
6. Hambrecht R, Wolf A, Gielen S, et al. Effect of exercise on coronary endothelial function in patients with coronary artery disease. *N Engl J Med* 2000; 342: 454–60.
7. Panagiotakos DB, Kokkinos P, Manios Y, Pitsavos C. Physical activity and markers of inflammation and thrombosis related to coronary artery disease. *Prev Cardiol* 2004; 7: 190–4.
8. Yarnell JWG, Sweetnam PM, Rumley A, Lowe GD. Lifestyle and hemostatic risk factors for IHD: the Caerphilly study. *Arterioscler Thromb Vasc Biol* 2000; 20: 271–9.
9. Thompson PD, Buchner D, Pina IL, et al. AHA scientific statement: exercise and physical activity in the prevention and

treatment of atherosclerotic cardiovascular disease. *Circulation* 2003; 107: 3109–16.

10. Thompson PD, Franklin BA, Balady GJ, et al. Exercise and acute cardiovascular events: placing the risks into perspective. A scientific statement from the American heart Association Council on Nutrition, Physical Activity, and Metabolism and the Council on Clinical Cardiology. *Circulation* 2007; 115: 2358–68.
11. Williams MA, Haskell WL, Ades PA, et al., American Heart Association Council on Clinical Cardiology, American Heart Association Council on Nutrition, Physical Activity and Metabolism. Resistance exercise in individuals with and without cardiovascular disease: 2007 update. *Circulation* 2007; 116: 572–84.
12. Perk J, deBacker G, Gohlke H, et al. European Guidelines on Cardiovascular Disease Prevention in Clinical Practice (Version 2012): the Fifth Joint Task Force of the European Society of Cardiology and other Societies on cardiovascular disease prevention in clinical practice. *Eur Heart J* 2012; 33: 1635–1701.
13. Vanhees L, Rauch B, Piepoli M, et al. Importance of characteristics and modalities of physical activity and exercise in the management of cardiovascular health in individuals with cardiovascular disease (Part III). *Eur J Prev Cardiol* 2012; 19: 1333–56.
14. Maron BJ, Araujo CG, Thompson PD, et al. Recommendations for preparticipation screening and the assessment of cardiovascular disease in master athletes: an advisory for healthcare professionals from the working group PFS of the World Heart Federation, the International federation of Sports Medicine and the American Heart Association Committe on Exercise, Cardiac Rehabilitation and Prevention. *Circulation* 2001; 103: 327–34.
15. James J, Merghani A, Sharma S. Sudden death in marathon runners. *Card Electrophysiol Clin* 2013; 5: 43–51.
16. Corrado D, Schmied C, Basso C, et al. Risk of sports. Do we need a pre-participation screening for competitive and leisure athletes? *Eur Heart J* 2011; 32: 934–44.
17. Mathews SC, Narotsky DL, Bernholt DL, et al. Mortality among marathon runners in the United States, 2000-2009. *Am J Sports Med* 2012; 40: 1495–500.
18. Burke AP, Farb A, Malcolm GT, et al. Plaque rupture and sudden death related to exertion in men without coronary artery disease. *JAMA* 1999; 281: 921–6.
19. Peronnet F, Cleroux J, Perreault H, et al. Plasma norepinephrine response to exercise before and after training in humans. *J Appl Physiol* 1981; 51: 812–15.
20. Willich SN, Lewis M, Lowel H, et al. Physical exertion as a trigger of acute myocardial infarction. *N Engl J Med* 1993; 329: 1684–90.
21. Siskovick DS, Weiss NS, Fletcher RH, et al. Habitual vigorous exercise and primary cardiac arrest: effect of other risk factors on the relationship. *J Chronic Dis* 1984; 37: 625–31.
22. Aagaard P, Sahlén A, Braunschweig F (2012) Performance trends and cardiac biomarkers in a 30-km cross-country race, 1993-2007. *Med Sci Sports Exerc* 44: 894–899
23. Maron BJ. The paradox of exercise. *N Engl J Med* 2000; 343: 1409–11.
24. Sahlén A, Gustafsson TP, Svensson JE, et al. Predisposing factors and consequences of elevated biomarker levels in long-distance runners aged >or = 55 years. *Am J Cardiol* 2009; 104: 1434–1440
25. Balady GJ, Chaitman B, Driscoll D, et al. AHA/ACSM scientific statement: recommendations for cardiovascular screening, staffing, and emergency policies at health/fitness facilities. *Circulation* 1998; 97: 2283–93.
26. McInnis KJ, Hayakawa S, Balady GJ. Cardiovascular screening and emergency procedures at health clubs and fitness centers. *Am J Cardiol* 1997; 80: 380–3.
27. Corrado D, Pelliccia A, Bjørnstad HH, et al. Cardiovascular pre-participation screening of young competitive athletes for prevention of sudden death: proposal for a common European protocol. *Eur Heart J* 2005; 26: 516–24.
28. Pelliccia A, Fagard R, Bjornstad H, et al. Recommendations for competitive sports participation in athletes with cardiovascular disease. *Eur Heart J* 2005; 26: 1422–45.
29. Pelliccia A, Corrado D, Bjørnstad HH, et al. Recommendations for participation in competitive sport and leisure-time physical activity in individuals with cardiomyopathies, myocarditis and pericarditis. *Eur J Cardiovasc Prev Rehabil* 2006; 13: 876–85
30. Heidbüchel H, Panhuyzen-Goedkoop N, Corrado D, et al. Recommendations for participation in leisure-time physical activity and competitive sports in patients with arrhythmias and potentially arrhythmogenic conditions. Part I: Supraventricular arrhythmias and pacemakers. *Eur J Cardiovasc Prev Rehabil* 2006; 13: 475–84.
31. Heidbüchel H, Corrado D, Biffi A, et al. Recommendations for participation in leisure-time physical activity and competitive sports of patients with arrhythmias and potentially arrhythmogenic conditions Part II: Ventricular arrhythmias, channelopathies and implantable defibrillators. *Eur J Cardiovasc Prev Rehabil* 2006; 13: 676–86.
32. Mellwig KP, van Buuren F, Gohlke-Baerwolf C, Bjørnstad HH. Recommendations for the management of individuals with acquired valvular heart diseases who are involved in leisure-time physical activities or competitive sports. *Eur J Cardiovasc Prev Rehabil* 2008; 15: 95–103.
33. Hirth A, Reybrouck T, Bjarnason-Wehrens B, et al. Recommendations for participation in competitive and leisure sports in patients with congenital heart disease: a consensus document. *Eur J Cardiovasc Prev Rehabil* 2006; 13: 293–9
34. Fagard RH, Bjornstad HH, Borjesson M, et al. ESC Study Group of Sports Cardiology recommendations for participation in leisure-time physical activities and competitive sports for patients with hypertension. *Eur J Cardiovasc Prev Rehabil* 2005; 12: 326–31.
35. Borjesson M, Assanelli D, Carré F, et al. ESC Study Group of Sports Cardiology: recommendations for participation in leisure-time physical activity and competitive sports for patients with ischaemic heart disease. *Eur J Cardiovasc Prev Rehabil* 2006; 13: 137–49.
36. Maron BJ, Zipes DP, Kovacs RJ, et al. Eligibility and disqualification recommendations for competitive athletes with cardiovascular abnormalities: preamble, principles, and general considerations. *Circulation* 2015; 132: e256–61.
37. Maron BJ, Udelson JE, Bonow RO, et al. Eligibility and disqualification recommendations for competitive athletes with cardiovascular abnormalities. Task Force 3: Hypertrophic Cardiomyopathy, Arrhythmogenic Right Ventricular Cardiomyopathy and Other Cardiomyopathies, and Myocarditis. *Circulation* 2015; 132: e273–80.
38. Van Hare GF, Ackerman MJ, Evangelista JA, et al. Eligibility and disqualification recommendations for competitive athletes with

cardiovascular abnormalities: Task Force 4: Congenital Heart Disease. *Circulation* 2015; 132: e281–91.

39. Ackerman MJ, Zipes DP, Kovacs RJ, Maron BJ. Eligibility and disqualification recommendations for competitive athletes with cardiovascular abnormalities. Task Force 10: The Cardiac Channelopathies. *J Am Coll Cardiol* 2015; 66: 2424–8.
40. Zipes DP, Link MS, Ackerman MJ, et al. Eligibility and disqualification recommendations for competitive athletes with cardiovascular abnormalities. Task Force 9: Arrhythmias and Conduction Defects. *Circulation* 2015; 132: e315–25.
41. Black HR, Sica D, Ferdinand K, et al. Eligibility and disqualification recommendations for competitive athletes with cardiovascular abnormalities. Task Force 6: Hypertension. *Circulation* 2015; 132: e298–302.
42. Braverman AC, Harris KM, Kovacs RJ, et al. Eligibility and disqualification recommendations for competitive athletes with cardiovascular abnormalities. Task Force 7: Aortic Diseases, Including Marfan Syndrome. *Circulation* 2015; 132: e303–9.
43. Bonow RO, Nishimura RA, Thompson PD, et al. eligibility and disqualification recommendations for competitive athletes with cardiovascular abnormalities. Task Force 5: Valvular Heart Disease. *Circulation* 2015; 132: e292–7.
44. Thompson PD, Myerburg RJ, Levine BD, et al. Eligibility and disqualification recommendations for competitive athletes with cardiovascular abnormalities. Task Force 8: Coronary Artery Disease. *Circulation* 2015; 132: e310–14
45. Borjesson M, Urhausen A, Kouidi E, et al. Cardiovascular evaluation of middle-aged/senior individuals engaged in leisure-time sport activities: position stand from the sections of exercise physiology and sports cardiology of the European Association of Cardiovascular Prevention and Rehabilitation. *Eur J Cardiovasc Prev Rehabil* 2011; 18: 446–58.
46. Balady GJ, Larson MG, Vasan RS, et al. Usefulness of exercise testing in the prediction of coronary disease risk among asymptomatic persons as a function of the Framingham risk score. *Circulation* 2004; 110: 1920–5.
47. Thomas S, Reading J, Shephard RJ. Revision of the Physical Activity Readiness Questionnaire (PAR-Q). *Can J Sports Sci* 1992; 17: 338–45.
48. Conroy RM, Pyörälä K, Fitzgerald AP, et al. Estimation of ten-year risk of fatal cardiovascular disease in Europe: the SCORE project. *Eur Heart J* 2003; 24: 987–1003.
49. Laukkanen JA, Rauramaa R, Salonen JT, Kurl S. The predictive value of cardiorespiratory fitness combined with coronary risk evaluation and the risk of cardiovascular and all-cause death. *J Intern Med* 2007; 262: 263–72.
50. Anandacoomarasamy A, Fransen M, March L. Obesity and the musculoskeltal system. *Curr Opin Rheumatol* 2009; 21: 71–7.
51. Guidry MA, Blanchard BE, Thompson PD, et al. The influence of short and long duration beta blockade on the blood pressure response to an acute bout of dynamic exercise. *Am J Cardiol* 2006; 151: 1322–7.
52. Riebe D, Franklin BA, Thompson PD, et al. Updating ACSM's Recommendations for Exercise Preparticipation Health Screening. *Med Sci Sports Exerc* 2015; 47: 2473–9.

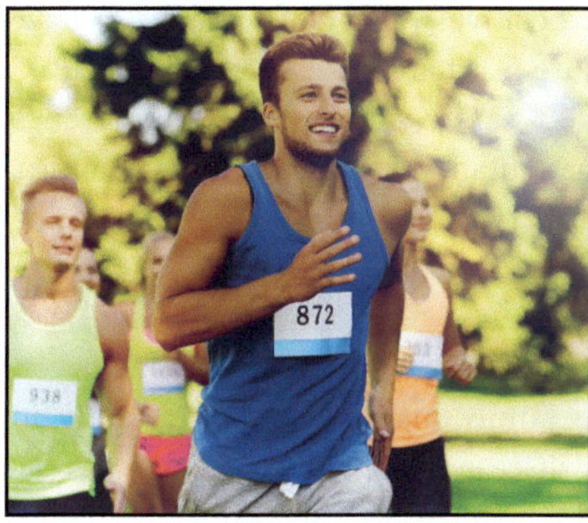

6.7

Cardiovascular screening of children and adolescent athletes (<14 years)

Massimo Chessa, Werner Budts, and Javier Fernandez Sarabia

Introduction

Sudden cardiac death (SCD) in young athletes is rare, but remains a tragic and counterintuitive event, subject to persistently high public visibility, triggering of emotion, and media attention, with potential legal liability considerations. The widely held perception is that athletes are examples of health and vitality, so that SCD of an athlete can evoke strong emotions and disbelief.

Regular physical activity improves cardiorespiratory fitness, body composition, and psychosocial well-being, and reduces the overall risk of atherosclerotic cardiovascular disease; however, sport, particularly when practised vigorously, has been shown to increase the risk of SCD in predisposed individuals.

The aim of CV pre-participation screening (PPS) is to identify high risk athletes with potentially lethal genetic or congenital diseases, so that can be withdrawn from competitive sports to decrease their risk and make the athletic field a safer environment. Moreover, during this process some high risk individuals may be recognized as candidates for medical treatment or surgical intervention, or for implantable defibrillators as primary prevention.

Definitions

- **Sudden cardiac death** is defined as an unexpected death, usually occurring within an hour of onset of symptoms in cases where the death is witnessed, and within 24 hours of the individual last being seen alive and well when the death is not witnessed [1].
- **Exercise-associated SCA/SCD** There is no standard definition. It is arbitrarily defined as SCA/SCD occurring during or within an hour of exercise/sport activity [2].
- Athlete An individual who participates in an organized team or individual sport that requires regular competition against others as a central component, places a high premium on excellence and achievement, and requires some form of systematic (and usually intense) training [3]. This definition generally includes students aged over 14 and those participating in professional sports, but there is no reason why children and adolescents younger than 14 years who satisfy this definition should not be considered as athletes.

SCD, sport, and risk factors

Sport is not itself the cause of enhanced mortality. During strenuous physical activity, physiological changes, such as increased catecholamine levels, acidosis, and dehydration, can trigger cardiac arrest in those athletes who are affected by underlying cardiovascular disorders predisposing to life-threatening ventricular arrhythmia [4].

The most frequent underlying cardiovascular condition [5] in young competitive athletes are cardiomyopathies, with hypertrophic cardiomyopathy [6,7] being the most common form. Other predisposing conditions are congenital coronary anomalies, myocarditis, aortic valve stenosis, aortic dissection/rupture (including cases of the Marfan phenotype), atherosclerotic coronary artery disease, arrhythmogenic right ventricular cardiomyopathy and ion channelopathies.

Epidemiological data place SCD in athletes in the range of approximately 1 in 50,000 to 1 in 80,000 participants per year, although a wide range has been reported [8–10] from 1 in 3000 in some sub-populations to 1 in 1,000,000 in others. SCD risk varies with age, gender, race, and the intensity of activity. The incidence increase with age (there is a paucity of data for children under 12 years old), male gender (5–10:1) and African-American/black athletes. The incidence also increases with intensity of activity, with the rate in athletes three to five times higher than in non-athletes, and the rate in athletes competing in Division I basketball 2.5 to 3.3 times higher than that in Division III [11]. Finally, it is noteworthy that SCD often occurs without warning signs or symptoms, and represents the first clinical presentation of the inherent disease in up to 50% of children [12].

Screening programmes

Because sports can reveal underlying severe cardiac disease, PPS has an important role in prevention of SCD in competitive athletes. Scientific committees such as the American Heart Association (AHA) [6] and the European Society of Cardiology (ESC) [13], and international sports associations such as the International Olympic Committee (IOC) Medical Commission recommend a PPS programme to provide medical clearance for participation in competitive sports.

Currently, broad-based PPS is practised systematically for athletes at all levels of performance in several countries: in the USA, with personal/family history and physical examination (but without ECGs), and in both Italy [14] and Israel [15], with 12-lead ECGs in addition to history and physical examination. The need for a systematic resting 12-lead ECG is a matter of scientific debate [16]. Conditions that can be identified by the ECG (such as cardiomyopathies and channelopathies) represent a substantial proportion of the causes of SCA in the young. Therefore ESC recommends that the first PPS for competitive sports in subjects aged 12–35 should include a resting 12-lead ECG [13].

Nowadays participation in competitive athletics begins even earlier. We believe that it is appropriate for all children (over 6 years old) who participate in competitive sports, independently of the type of sport, race, or sex, to be part of a PPS programme. According to the recommendations of the ESC and IOC, evaluations should be repeated every 2 years if the initial evaluation is negative.

PPS of children and adolescent athletes can be done by an experienced specialist (paediatrician, family doctor, cardiologist, or asports medicine specialist), and should include family and personal history, physical examination (with blood pressure), and resting 12-lead ECG [13,17].

Cardiovascular screening in paediatric patients

Family history

Because most diseases responsible for sudden death in the young are genetic/familial, a thorough family history may raise suspicion for the presence of CV disease. The family history is considered positive when close relative(s) have experienced a premature heart attack or sudden death (<55 years old in men and <65 years in women), or in the presence of a family history of hereditary diseases (cardiomyopathies, channelopathies, etc.) [12].

Congenital heart disease

Between 5% and 10% of people with congenital heart diseases have a positive family history, more frequently in cases were the cardiac disease is associated an extra-cardiac anomaly, for example upper-limb deformities in Holt–Oram syndrome or skeletal and ocular anomalies in Alagille syndrome [18]. In these cases cardiac assessment should be performed with ECG and echocardiography.

Sudden cardiac death/arrest

Drezner et al. [12] studied a population of children and young adults (5–30 years old) who suffered sudden cardiac arrest (SCA). About 27% of patients reported a family member who had died because of a heart condition before the age of 50. A small number of families knew of a specific cardiac condition in their family before their child's SCA.

In cases of positive family history, comprehensive cardiac assessment should be performed, with ECG and echocardiography.

Premature cardiovascular disease

Atherosclerosis, the pathological basis for clinical cardiovascular disease (CVD), originates in childhood, and remains one of the leading causes of mortality in adults. Risk factors and risk behaviours that accelerate the development of atherosclerosis begin in childhood, and there is increasing evidence that risk reduction delays progression towards a clinically overt disease.

In cases of positive family history (parent, grandparent, aunt, uncle, or sibling) of premature atherosclerotic disease, or SCD (<55 years in males and <65 years in females), or defined dyslipidaemias, measurement of apolipoprotein B, apolipoprotein A-1, LDL cholesterol, and HDL cholesterol levels, are recommended. If these are normal, screening every 3–5 years is recommended [19,20].

Cardyomiopathies

In case of hypertrophic cardiomyopathy, or other cardiomyopathies where molecular genetic data are available, genetic testing of the child may be advised. If genetic testing is not available, early identification of clinically affected relatives should be performed, including those without any symptoms [21].

In cases of positive family history for cardiomyopathies, cardiac assessment should be performed with ECG, echocardiography, and/or cardiac magnetic resonance (CMR). Other examinations (signal-averaged ECG, exercise testing, Holter-ECG monitoring) may be necessary to define diagnosis and risk stratification.

Arrhythmia syndromes

Ion channelopathies represent one of the most frequent predisposing cardiovascular conditions to SCD/SCA. Long QT syndrome (LQTS), short QT syndrome (SQTS), Brugada syndrome (BrS), and catecholaminergic polymorphic ventricular tachycardia (CPVT) are the most important channelopathies.

In cases of positive family history (family members of individuals in whom the diagnosis of a channelopathy is clinically possible, likely, or established, or family members who suffer from arrhythmias) cardiac assessment should include ECG, echocardiography, Holter-ECG monitoring, and/or an exercise test [22].

Personal history

The personal history is aimed at identifying symptoms that raise suspicion of the presence of a potentially lethal cardiovascular disease. It is considered positive in the case of exertional chest pain or discomfort, syncope or near-syncope, irregular heartbeat or palpitations, and the presence of shortness of breath or fatigue out of proportion to the degree of exertion [6].

Syncope

Syncope is a transient loss of consciousness (TLOC) due to transient global cerebral hypoperfusion characterized by rapid onset, short duration, and spontaneous complete recovery. Many forms of syncope exist: neurally mediated syncope (vasovagal, carotid sinus, situational), orthostatic syncope, syncope of cardiac origin (arrhythmic or structural disease), and cerebrovascular syncope.

The initial assessment should distinguish syncope from other TLOCs, such as epilepsy, transient ischaemic attack, and drop attack. Secondly, it should distinguish a cardiac from a non-cardiac syncope [23].

Neurally mediated syncope is by far the most common form of syncope, and has typical warning symptoms caused by a fall in arterial blood pressure and impaired cerebral perfusion (weakness and visual disturbances), autonomic activation (pallor, nausea, sweating), and finally loss of consciousness. Recovery is typically prompt (usually less than 15–30s) and complete without any need for medical intervention. Syncope occurring during exercise is more likely of cardiac aetiology [24]: cardiomyopathies, valvular heart disease, arrhythmias in channelopathies, or anomalous coronary artery origin. If syncope occurs during swimming, consider long QT syndrome.

When the initial assessment is not diagnostic for distinguishing cardiac from non-cardiac origin, further investigations are indicated. Echocardiography and CMR are suggested in order to exclude the presence of structural heart diseases, and maximal stress test ECG is indicated for exercise-related syncope.

Chest pain

Chest pain (CP) is a common complaint referred to paediatric cardiologists and among paediatric patients, but it is generally non-cardiac in origin [25]. It is often self-limiting, independent of exercise, and not associated with other symptoms. Common benign causes of chest pain in children and teenagers include costo-chondritis, precordial catch syndrome (pleural pain with breathing), stress, and anxiety.

CP triggered by intense exercise and associated with other concerning symptoms, such as radiating pain, lightheadedness, syncope, and/or tachycardia, is more suggestive of a cardiac aetiology [26]. In these cases it is necessary to exclude anomalous coronary artery origin or Kawasaki disease.

When initial assessment is not diagnostic for distinguishing cardiac from non-cardiac origin, beyond the ECG, imaging testing (echocardiography or CMR) should be performed. If CP is triggered by effort, a maximal stress test electrocardiogram is indicated.

Palpitations

Palpitations are another common complaint in children and teenagers presenting to paediatric cardiologists, and are usually benign. The history should focus on the timing of the palpitations (day, night, during exercise, at rest), the heart rate reported during the episode, associated symptoms (particularly syncope or near syncope), a precise description of sensation, including sudden onset and/or cessation, and the duration of the symptoms [27].

When palpitations are triggered by exercise or stress, cardiac arrhythmia must be excluded (and specifically CPVT, LQTS, HCM, or ARVC). If arrhythmia is suspected, cardiac assessment should be performed with ECG, echocardiography, and Holter-ECG, and if palpitations are related to physical effort, a maximal stress test electrocardiogram is indicated.

Shortness of breath or fatigue during exertion

Fatigue is a common non-specific complaint. The history should focus on characterizing the nature and severity of the symptom: whether it is associated with a decrease in exercise capacity, is episodic or predictable, is severe relative to other children, occurs in the setting of wheezing or coughing, or is associated with rapid or slow heart rate during physical activity. It is commonly due to exercise-related asthma and/or deconditioning, and less frequently to cardiac disease (HCM, DCM) [27].

If cardiac disease is suspected, ECG and echocardiography or CMR are recommended. Cardiopulmonary exercise testing may be indicated in selected patients. Suspected pulmonary causes of dyspnoea can be explored using pulmonary function tests at rest and, if necessary, with a provocative test.

Physical examination

The physical examination in paediatric athletes is usually normal. A careful clinical examination is needed to detect abnormalities or risk factors for physical exercise. The physical examination includes anthropometry, measurement of blood pressure (BP), cardiopulmonary auscultation, pulse assessment, and assessment of clinical signs related to Marfan syndrome.

Anthropometry

All paediatric patients should be weighed and have their height measured. The body mass index (BMI = weight in kilograms/(height in metres)^2) should be calculated and plotted on appropriate BMI centile charts. BMI is a relatively easy, low cost, and non-invasive measurement [28].

Obesity is defined as BMI above the 98th percentile, and overweight as BMI between the 85th and 98th percentiles. Childhood obesity is considered as one of the greatest public health problems in developed countries. Obesity increases cardiovascular risk, hyperlipidaemia, hypertension, abnormal glucose tolerance, and reduced quality of life. Patients with BMI above the 98th percentile must be referred to a specialist.

Blood pressure

Normal BP is defined as systolic BP (SBP) and diastolic BP (DBP) that are below the 90th percentile for sex, age, and height. If the SBP or DBP levels are above or equal to the 90th percentile, but less than the 95th percentile, the condition is known as pre-hypertension, and if SBP and/or DBP is above or equal to the 95th percentile on three or more occasions, it is known as hypertension [29].

The BP tables are based on auscultatory measurements; therefore auscultation is the preferred method. Measurements obtained by oscillometric devices that exceed the 90th percentile should be confirmed by auscultation. The proper method to measure BP is as follows: the child should sit quietly for a few minutes with his/her back supported, feet on the floor and right arm supported, and cubital fossa at heart level [30]. Correct measurement requires a cuff that is appropriate to the size of the child's upper arm. Normal data for BP are available in the literature [31].

If the BP is above the 90th percentile for sex, age, and height, or above 120/80mmHg in adolescents, the measurement should be repeated after 10min. If the second measurement confirms the first one, cardiovascular assessment is indicated to confirm the diagnosis of hypertension and exclude secondary causes (aortic coarctation, renal artery stenosis, chronic renal disease, pheochromocytoma, etc.). Ambulatory BP monitoring, blood analysis, and an echocardiogram may be necessary.

Cardiopulmonary auscultation (heart murmurs)

Heart murmurs should be evaluated in terms of intensity (graded from I to VI), timing (systolic, diastolic, or continuous), location, transmission, and quality (soft, harsh, vibratory, etc.) [32]. The patient has to be examined in the supine and standing positions. The initial assessment should first try to distinguish innocent murmurs from pathological murmurs due to structural heart disease. Innocent murmurs are frequently found during childhood (in 50–70% of cases) and most commonly are the crescendo–decrescendo mid-systolic type, low intensity (grade I–II/VI), and soft, vibratory, or musical, being audible at the (lower) left sternal border, non-radiating, and increasing in intensity in the supine position [33]. Innocent murmurs are usually associated with normal variable splitting of the second heart sound. Pathological murmurs have different characteristics, including a long systolic murmur, diastolic or continuous, of high intensity (>II/VI), harsh quality, and/or irradiating (to the back, apex, neck, etc.). The presence of clicks, fourth heart sound, or fixed second heart sound are also characteristics of pathological murmurs [34]. Echocardiography is indicated in cases of suspected pathological murmurs.

Arterial pulses

Pulse rate should be assessed, noting regularity and quality of the pulsations, and capillary refill time [33]. Bounding pulses (aortic insufficiency, arterial duct, or arteriovenous malformations) or diminished and delayed femoral artery pulses with normal brachial pulses (aortic coarctation) need cardiovascular assessment with echocardiography or CMR.

Marfan syndrome

Marfan syndrome is a systemic heritable (autosomal dominant) connective tissue disorder which affects many different organ systems, and is mainly caused by defects in the gene that codes for the protein fibrillin. Approximately a quarter of cases occur as a result of a new mutation [35,36].

The diagnosis of Marfan syndrome is clinically based on well-defined criteria, but the problem in the paediatric age range is that many of the specific clinical features are age dependent (e.g. ectopic lentis or dural ectasia). For this reason, younger patients suspected of Marfan syndrome (positive family history but incomplete clinical criterial) should be evaluated periodically.

The clinical features that should be examined during physical examination are [35,37]:

- musculoskeletal—joint hypermobility (wrist sign, thumb sign), pectus deformity (carinatum, excavatum, chest asymmetry), hind foot deformity, pes planus, reduced upper to lower segment ratio and increased arm span to height ratio, scoliosis or thoracolumbar kyphosis, reduced elbow extension;
- craniofacial features—three of dolichocephaly, downward-slanting palpebral fissures, enophthalmos, retrognathia, and malar hypoplasia);
- skin striae.

The cardiovascular system is the major source of morbidity and mortality in Marfan syndrome. Near 25% of patients have cardiovascular anomalies detected during childhood. Cardiovascular manifestations include dilatation of the aorta, aortic valve insufficiency, a predisposition for aortic tear and rupture, mitral valve prolapse with or without regurgitation, tricuspid valve prolapse, and enlargement of the proximal pulmonary artery.

In cases of clinical suspicion or positive family history, evaluation by specialist is indicated. Initial cardiac assessment with echocardiography or CMR is recommended.

The electrocardiogram in cardiovascular screening

Changes in the ECG pattern are related to age, stage of development (especially puberty), gender, and race. The intense systematic training undertaken by athletes induces structural, functional, and electrical remodelling of the heart, which is termed 'athlete's heart'. These changes are not generally detrimental but represent physiological adaptions that aid athletic performance. Athletes frequently have increased vagal tone and enlarged cardiac dimensions (mild left and right ventricular dilatation and mild concentric left ventricular hypertrophy).

Distinguishing the physiological changes related to exercise training from pathological ECG changes is important to enable timely identification of cardiac disease and minimize the risk of SCD [38–42]. There are limited paediatric data regarding athlete's heart, but participation in an endurance sports discipline has been shown to be significantly associated with physiological ECG changes, such as sinus bradycardia and increase of QRS voltages.

Heart rate and cardiac rhythm

Heart rate should be determined after at least 5min rest, with the child calm and relaxed. Because of the increased vagal tone, child athletes usually present with sinus bradycardia. Only when there is marked bradycardia (less than 40 bpm in adolescents, or 50bpm in children) or other symptoms, is CV assessment needed (24-hour Holter monitoring and maximal exercise test).

The normal origin of the cardiac rhythm is the sinus node, which manifests at ECG with the P-wave axis between 0° and 90°. A P-wave axis between 0° and 90°, indicates an origin in the low right atrium and is considered normal during childhood with no need for cardiac assessment. A wandering atrial pacemaker (presence of more than two types of P-wave morphology) is also common and isrelated to increased vagal tone. Other P-wave origins, atrial enlargement, and/or hypertrophy should be investigated to exclude heart disease.

Atrioventricular conduction

The PR interval is measured from the onset of the P wave to the Q wave, or to the R wave if no Q wave is present. It increases with age and decreases with heart rate. It is frequently prolonged in athletes because of the increased vagal tone (first-degree atrioventricular block) and does not need further cardiological evaluation if it resolves with exercise or hyperventilation but only a follow-up. If it doe not resolve, echocardiography is recommended. Higher degrees of atrioventricular block (Mobitz type 2 or third_degree atrioventricular block) need cardiovascular assessment (including echocardiography or CMR, ECG-Holter monitoring, and maximal exercise test).

QRS complex

QRS voltages

The ECG patterns of physiological LVH in trained athletes usually manifests as an isolated increase of QRS amplitude (with normal QRS axis, normal atrial and ventricular activation patterns, and normal ST-segment T-wave repolarization). If it is associated with one or more additional non-voltage criteria (such as left atrial enlargement, left axis deviation, ST-segment depression, T-wave inversion, or pathological Q waves) an echocardiographic or CMR evaluation is required to rule out underlying pathological hypertrophy [38,40,43].

QRS morphology

- Incomplete right bundle branch block: the prevalence of incomplete right bundle branch block has been estimated as 35–50% in athletes as compared with 10% in young healthy controls. This ECG pattern does not require investigation in asymptomatic athletes. Particular attention should be paid to excluding atrial septal defect (systolic ejection murmur, usually soft, and fixed split of the second tone).
- Complete right/left bundle branch block and/or left anterior/posterior fascicular block [44]: when this is present, cardiac assessment with echocardiography or CMR, Holter-ECG monitoring, and maximal stress test ECG is indicated.
- Ventricular pre-excitation: most individuals with pre-excitation syndrome remain asymptomatic throughout their lives, but others can develop supraventricular tachycardia or atrial fibrillation, which could degenerate into ventricular fibrillation and cause SCD [45]. Sport has been reported to be associated with an increased risk of developing ventricular fibrillation. In cases of ventricular pre-excitation in 12-lead ECG, evaluation of risk (echocardiography, Holter-ECG, and maximal exercise test) is indicated. If the patient is symptomatic (Wolff–Parkinson–White syndrome), evaluation in an arrhythmic unit and eventual ablation procedure are indicated.

ST segment and T wave

- Early repolarization (ER) is a common ECG variant in the general population and more frequent in young trained athletes. It does not require further clinical evaluation if the patient has a negative personal and family history. In athletes presenting with syncope which remains unexplained after cardiovascular assessment, the ECG pattern of ER in the inferior and/or lateral leads with a horizontal or downward-sloping ST segment should raise suspicion of an underlying disease predisposing to SCD, and should be investigated [46–48].
- T-wave morphology: T waves in anterior leads (V1–V3) are negative after the first week of life and remain negative until at least the age of 10 years. T waves in the left lateral precordial leads (V5–V6) become positive after 48 hours of life. Positive T waves in V1 suggest right ventricular hypertrophy, and cardiac assessment should be performed. Negative T waves in anterior leads (V1–V3) after adolescence are also a possible manifestation of ARVC [49] and, less commonly, HCM. Inverted T waves in the inferior (L2, L3, aVF) and/or lateral (L1, aVL, V5–V6) leads raise the suspicion of cardiomyopathy, aortic valve disease, systemic hypertension, or left ventricular non-compaction [50,51]. Cardiac assessment should include echocardiogram and/or CMR. In the case of negative work-up, continued clinical surveillance and follow-up by serial ECG and imaging evaluations are recommended.
- ST-segment depression on resting ECG, either isolated or associated with T-wave inversion, should be evaluated to exclude heart disease.

QT interval

The QT interval should be measured from the beginning of the QRS complex to the end of the T wave. Leads II or V5 aremost commonly used to measure the QT interval. Bazett's formula

$$QT_C = QT/\sqrt{(\text{RR interval})}$$

corrects the QT duration for heart rate [52]. The normal QTc interval is 330–450ms. Athletes generally have slightly longer QT intervals than the general population, which may be due to profound bradycardia and/or an increase in left ventricular mass [53,54]. If a prolonged QT interval is seen, either acquired or congenital LQTS should be ruled out. If LQTS is suspected, the patient should be referred to a specialist.

Further reading

Asif IM, Yim ES, Hoffman JM, Froelicher V. Update: Causes and symptoms of sudden cardiac death in young athletes. *Phys Sportsmed* 2015; 43: 44–53.

Beaumont A, Grace F, Richards J, et al. Left ventricular speckle tracking-derived cardiac strain and cardiac twist mechanics in athletes: a systematic review and meta-analysis of controlled studies. *Sports Med* 2017; 47: 1145–70.

Chatard JC, Mujika I, Goiriena JJ, Carré F. Screening young athletes for prevention of sudden cardiac death: practical recommendations for sports physicians. *Scand J Med Sci Sports* 2016; 26: 362–74.

Kropa J, Close J, Shipon D, et al. High prevalence of obesity and high blood pressure in urban student-athletes. *J Pediatr* 2016; 178: 194–9.

Maron BJ, Friedman RA, Kligfield P, et al. Assessment of the 12-lead electrocardiogram as a screening test for detection of cardiovascular disease in healthy general populations of young people (12-25 years of age): a scientific statement from the American Heart Association and the American College of Cardiology. *J Am Coll Cardiol* 2014; 64: 1479–1514.

Maron BJ, Levine BD, Washington RL, et al. Eligibility and disqualification recommendations for competitive athletes with cardiovascular abnormalities: Task Force 2: Preparticipation Screening for Cardiovascular Disease in Competitive Athletes. *J Am Coll Cardiol* 2015; 66: 2356–61.

Mazzanti A, Ng K, Faragli A, et al. Arrhythmogenic right ventricular cardiomyopathy: clinical course and predictors of arrhythmic risk. *J Am Coll Cardiol* 2016; 68: 2540–50.

Sharma S, Drezner JA, Baggish A, et al. International recommendations for electrocardiographic interpretation in athletes. *J Am Coll Cardiol* 2017; 69: 1057–75.

Stephens P. Sudden cardiac death in the young: the value of exercise testing. *Cardiol Young* 2017; 27(S1): S10–18.

References

1 Myerburg RJ, Castellanos A. Cardiac arrest and sudden cardiac death. In Braunwald E (ed), *Heart Disease: A Textbook of Cardiovascular Medicine*. Philadelphia, PA: WB Saunders, 1992; pp. 756–89.

2 Rai M, Thompson PD. The definition of exertion-related cardiac events. *Br J Sports Med* 2011; 45: 130–1.

3 Maron BJ, Zipes DP. 36th Bethesda Conference: Introduction. Eligibility recommendations for competitive athletes with cardiovascular abnormalities. *J Am Coll Cardiol* 2005; 45: 1318–21.

4 Corrado D, Basso C, Rizzoli G, et al. Does sports activity enhance the risk of sudden death in adolescents and young adults? *J Am Coll Cardiol* 2003; 42: 1959–63.

5 Corrado D, Basso C, Pavei A, et al. Trends in sudden cardiovascular death in young competitive athletes after implementation of a pre-participation screening program. *JAMA* 2006; 296: 1593–1601.

6 Maron BJ, Thompson PD, Ackerman MJ, et al. Recommendations and considerations related to preparticipation screening for cardiovascular abnormalities in competitive athletes: 2007 update. *Circulation* 2007; 115: 1643–55.

7 Maron BJ, Shirani J, Poliac L, et al. Sudden death in young competitive athletes: clinical, demographic, and pathological profiles. *JAMA* 1996; 276: 199–204.

8 Harmon KG, Asif IM, Klossner D, Drezner JA. Incidence of sudden cardiac death in National Collegiate Athletic Association athletes. *Circulation* 2011; 123: 1594–1600.

9 Roberts WO, Stovitz SD. Incidence of sudden cardiac death in Minnesota high school athletes 1993-2012 screened with a standardized pre-participation evaluation. *J Am Coll Cardiol* 2013; 62: 1298–1301.

10 Harmon KG, Drezner JA, Wilson MG, Sharma S. Incidence of sudden cardiac death in athletes: a state- of-the-art review. *Heart* 2014; 100: 1227–34.

11 Harmon KG, Asif IM, Maleszewski JJ, et al. Incidence, cause, and comparative frequency of sudden cardiac death in National Collegiate Athletic Association athletes. *Circulation* 2015; 132: 10–19.

12 Drezner JA, Fudge J, Harmon KG, et al. Warning symptoms and family history in children and young adults with sudden cardiac arrest. *J Am Board FamMed* 2012; 25: 408–15.

13 Corrado D, Pelliccia A, Bjørnstad HH, et al. Cardiovascular pre-participation screening of young competitive athletes for prevention of sudden death: proposal for a common European protocol. *Eur Heart J* 2005; 26: 516–24.

14 Pelliccia A, Maron BJ. Preparticipation cardiovascular evaluation of the competitive athlete: perspectives from the 30-year Italian experience. *Am J Cardiol* 1995; 75: 827–9.

15 Steinvil A, Chundadze T, Zeltser D, et al. Mandatory electrocardiographic screening of athletes to reduce their risk for sudden death: proven fact or wishful thinking? *J Am Coll Cardiol* 2011; 57: 1291–6.

16 Harmon KG, Zigman M, Drezner JA. The effectiveness of screening history, physical exam, and ECG to detect potentially lethal cardiac disorders in athletes: a systematic review/meta-analysis. *J Electrocardiol* 2015; 48: 329–38.

17 Crespo Marcos D, Pérez-Lescure Picarzo FJ, Boraita Pérez A, et al. *Guía clínica de Evaluación Cardiovascular Previa a la Práctica Deportiva en Pediatría*. Madrid: Consejo Superior de Deportes; 2015 (in Spanish).

18 Pierpont ME, Basson CT, Benson DW Jr, et al. Genetic basis for congenital heart defects: current knowledge. *Circulation* 2007; 115: 3015–38.

19 Haney EM, Huffman LH, Bougatsos C, et al. Screening and treatment for lipid disorders in children and adolescents: systematic evidence review for the US Preventive Services Task Force. *Pediatrics* 2007; 120: 189–214.

20 Expert Panel on Integrated Guidelines for Cardiovascular Health and Risk Reduction in Children and Adolescents: ummary report. *Pediatrics* 2011; 128(Suppl.5): S213–56.

21 Biffi A, Delise P, Zeppilli P, et al. Italian cardiological guidelines for sports eligibility in athletes with heart disease: part 1. *J Cardiovasc Med (Hagerstown)* 2013; 14: 477–99.

22 Priori SG, Wilde AA, Horie M, et al. HRS/EHRA/APHRS expert consensus statement on the diagnosis and management of patients with inherited primary arrhythmia syndromes. *Heart Rhythm* 2013; 10: 1932–63.

23 Moya A, Sutton R, Ammirati F, et al. (2009). Guidelines for the diagnosis and management of syncope. *Eur Heart J* 2009; 30, 2631–71.

24 Tretter JT, Kavey RW. Distinguishing cardiac syncope from vasovagal syncope in a referral population. *J Pediatr* 2013; 163: 1618–23.

25 Danduran MJ, Earing MG, Sheridan DC, et al. Chest pain: characteristics of children/adolescents. *Pediatr Cardiol* 2008; 29: 775–81.

26 Kane DA, Fulton DR, Saleeb S, et al. Needles in hay: chest pain as the presenting symptom in children with serious underlying cardiac pathology. *Congenit Heart Dis* 2010; 5: 366–73.

27 Behera SK, Pattnaik T, Luke A. Practical recommendations and perspectives on cardiac screening for healthy pediatric athletes. *Curr Sports Med Rep* 2011; 10: 90–8.

28 Daniels SR, Hassink SG and Committee on Nutrition. The role of the pediatrician in primary prevention of obesity. *Pediatrics* 2015; 136; e275.

29 National High Blood Pressure Education Program Working Group on High Blood Pressure in Children and Adolescents. The fourth report on the diagnosis, evaluation, and treatment of high blood pressure in children and adolescents. *Pediatrics* 2004; 114(Suppl 2): 555–76.

30 Prineas RJ. Blood pressure in children and adolescents. In Bulpitt CJ, (ed.), *Epidemiology of Hypertension*. New York: Elsevier; 2000, pp. 86–105.

31 Task Force on Blood Pressure Control in Children. Report of the Second Task Force on Blood Pressure Control in Children—1987. National Heart, Lung, and Blood Institute, Bethesda, Maryland. *Pediatrics* 1987;79:1–25.

32 Pelech AN. The physiology of cardiac auscultation. *Pediatr Clin North Am* 2004; 51: 1515–35.

33 Biancaniello T. Innocent murmurs. *Circulation* 2005; 111: e20–2.

34 McCrindle BW, Shaffer KM, Kan JS, et al. Cardinal clinical signs in the differentiation of heart murmurs in children. *Arch Pediatr Adolesc Med* 1996; 150: 169–74.

35 Loeys BL, Dietz HC, Braverman AC, et al. The revised Ghent nosology for the Marfan syndrome. *J Med Genet.* 2010; 47: 476–85.

36 Tinkle BT, Saal HM, and the Committee on Genetics. Health supervision for children with Marfan syndrome. *Pediatrics* 2013; 132: e1059–72.

37 Dean JC Marfan syndrome: clinical diagnosis and management. *Eur J Hum Genet* 2007; 15: 724–33.

38 Corrado D, Pelliccia A, Heidbüchel H, et al. Recommendations for interpretation of 12-lead electrocardiogram in the athlete. *Eur Heart J* 2010; 31: 243–59.

39 Drezner JA, Fischbach P, Froelicher V, et al. Normal electrocardiographic findings: recognising physiological adaptations in athletes. *Br J Sports Med* 2013; 47: 125–36.

40 Drezner JA, Ashley E, Baggish AL, et al. Abnormal electrocardiographic findings in athletes: recognising changes suggestive of cardiomyopathy. *Br J Sports Med* 2013; 47: 137–52.

41 Drezner JA, Ackerman MJ, Cannon BC, et al. Abnormal electrocardiographic findings in athletes: recognising changes suggestive of primary electrical disease. *Br J Sports Med* 2013; 47: 153–67.

42 Rodday AM, Triedman JK, Alexander ME, et al. Electrocardiogram screening for disorders that cause sudden cardiac death in asymptomatic children: a meta-analysis. *Pediatrics* 2012; 129: e999–1010.

43 Konno T, Shimizu M, Ino H, et al. Diagnostic value of abnormal Q waves for identification of preclinical carriers of hypertrophic cardiomyopathy based on a molecular genetic diagnosis. *Eur Heart J* 2004; 25: 246–51.

44 Kim JH, Noseworthy PA, McCarty D, et al. Significance of electrocardiographic right bundle branch block in trained athletes. *Am J Cardiol* 2011; 107: 1083–9.

45 Maron BJ, Doerer JJ, Haas TS, et al. Sudden deaths in young competitive athletes: analysis of 1866 deaths in the United States, 1980-2006. *Circulation* 2009; 119: 1085–92.

46 Rosso R, Glikson E, Belhassen B, et al. Distinguishing 'benign' from 'malignant early repolarization': the value of the ST-segment morphology. *Heart Rhythm* 2012; 9: 225–9.

47 Macfarlane PW, Antzelevitch C, Haissaguerre M, et al. The early depolarization pattern. *J Am Coll Cardiol* 2015; 66: 470–7.

48 Patton KK, Ellinor PT, Ezekowitz M, et al. Electrocardiographic early repolarization. *Circulation* 2016; 133: 1520–9.

49 Zaidi A, Sheikh N, Jongman JK, et al. Clinical differentiation between physiological remodeling and arrhythmogenic right ventricular cardiomyopathy in athletes with marked electrocardiographic repolarization anomalies. *J Am Coll Cardiol* 2015; 65: 2702–11.

50 Wilson MG, Sharma S, Carré F, et al. Significance of deep T-wave inversions in asymptomatic athletes with normal cardiovascular examinations: practical solutions for managing the diagnostic conundrum. *Br J Sports Med* 2012; 46(Suppl 1): i51–8.

51 Migliore F, Zorzi A, Michieli P, et al. Prevalence of cardiomyopathy in Italian asymptomatic children with electrocardiographic T-wave inversion at preparticipation screening. *Circulation* 2012; 125: 529–38.

52 Martin AB, Perry JC, Robinson JL, et al. Calculation of QTc duration and variability in the presence of sinus arrhythmia. *Am J Cardiol* 1995; 75: 950–2.

53 Basavarajaiah S, Wilson M, Whyte G, et al. Prevalence and significance of an isolated long QT interval in elite athletes. *Eur Heart J* 2007; 28: 2944–9.

54 Johnson JN, Ackerman MJ. QTc: how long is too long? *Br J Sports Med* 2009; 43: 657–62.

SECTION 7

Sports eligibility in athletes with cardiac abnormalities

7.1 **Criteria and considerations relative to safe participation in sport for athletes with cardiac abnormalities** *369*
Antonio Pelliccia, Hein Heidbüchel, Domenico Corrado, Sanjay Sharma, and Mats Börjesson

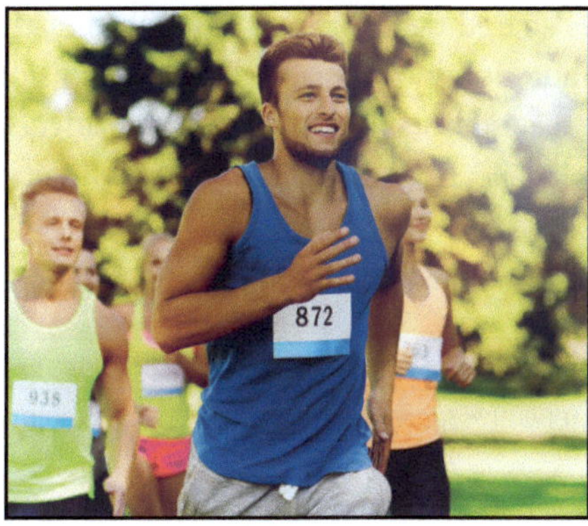

7.1

Criteria and considerations relative to safe participation in sport for athletes with cardiac abnormalities

Antonio Pelliccia, Hein Heidbüchel, Domenico Corrado, Sanjay Sharma, and Mats Börjesson

Introduction

The aim of this chapter is to provide guidance for the appropriate evaluation of athletes with CV abnormalities and the criteria for advising safe participation in sport, based on updates from previous ESC consensus documents [1–3]. This chapter is also intended to address individuals with CV abnormalities that do not necessarily increase the risk of sudden cardiac death/cardiac arrest (SCD/CA), but may deteriorate due to the effect of inappropriate long-term exercise training and participation in sport. These recommendations assume that the cardiac diagnosis has already been made, so that issues related to the modalities and diagnostic setting of CV disease is beyond the scope of this chapter.

The rationale for this expert consensus document is based on the clinical perception, substantiated by scientific evidence, that athletes with underlying (or even clinically silent) CV disease are exposed to an increased risk of SCD/CA and progression of their underlying CV disease in association with intensive exercise training and participation in sport [4–6]. Modification of the type/intensity of sport or abstinence from competition may reduce the risk for these athletes [7].

The recommendations for participation in competitive sport produced by the Sport Cardiology Section of the ESC/EAPC [1–3] have been in place for more than 10 years, and have facilitated medical advice relative to sport prescription in athletes with CV diseases. Over the past decade, there have been substantial developments relevant to participation in exercise and sport by patients with cardiac diseases, such as improved understanding of the clinical features and natural history of several CV diseases, the emerging role of cardiovascular magnetic resonance (CMR) imaging in diagnosis and risk stratification, the clarification of genotype–phenotype relationships in cardiomyopathies and other genetic diseases, and the potential role of the implanted cardioverter defibrillator (ICD) in patients engaged in competitive sport.

For the most part, the recommendations discussed here are the same as those reported in the previous position papers [1–3). However, in certain areas where our knowledge has improved over time, the current recommendations are much more liberal than previously. Nevertheless, there are numerous 'grey areas' where knowledge regarding the impact of participation in sport on the clinical progression and outcome of CV diseases is scarce, creating difficulties in formulating the best evidence-based medical advice.

Nature of the recommendations

The present recommendations are based on published scientific evidence and personal experience, as well as on the consensus of experts. However, since there have been few scientific investigations concerning the impact of sport activities on the clinical course of several CV diseases and arrhythmic outcomes, we acknowledge the difficulties inherent in formulating arbitrary recommendations. Therefore, in the absence of robust evidence, these recommendations cannot be considered as legally binding. They should not discourage individual physicians from practice outside the remit of this document, based on their scientific and professional experiences in sports cardiology. In contrast with the previous document, and in line with developments in good clinical practice, the present document encourages shared decision-making with the athlete and respects the autonomy of the athlete after provision of detailed information about the potential risks of an adverse event. See ➲ Tables 7.1.1–7.1.5 for these recommendations.

Table 7.1.1. Recommendation for competitive sport participation in athletes with arrhythmias and primary arrhythmogenic conditions

Lesion	Evaluation	Criteria for eligibility	Recommendations	Follow-up
Marked sinus bradycardia (≤30 bpm) and/or sinus pauses ≥3s with symptoms	History, ECG, ET, 24-h Holter, Echo	(a) If no symptoms[2], no cardiac disease, with resolution during exercise	(a) All competitive sports	(a) Not required
		(b) If symptoms[2] are present	(b) Temporary interruption of sport and re-evaluation	(b) Yearly
		(c) After symptom resolution and off therapy	(c) All sports	(c) Yearly
(a) AV block first and second degree, type 1	History, ECG, ET, 24-h Holter, Echo, (CMR, EP study selectively)	(a) If no symptoms[2], no cardiac disease, with resolution during exercise	(a)All competitive sports	(a)Not required
(b) AV block second degree, type 2 or advanced		(b) In the absence of symptoms, cardiac disease, ventricular arrhythmias during exercise, and if resting heart rate is >40 bpm	(b) All sport (endurance discouraged)	(b) Yearly
Supraventricular premature beats	History, ECG, 24-h Holter, thyroid function	No symptoms[2], no cardiac disease	All competitive sports	Not required
Supraventricular paroxysmal tachycardia (AVNRT or AVRT over a concealed accessory pathway)	History, ECG, Echo, EP study	(a) Ablation is usually done After catheter ablation: if no recurrences for >1 month, and no cardiac disease	(a) All competitive sports	(a) Not required
		(b) If ablation is not performed and SVT is sporadic, without cardiac disease, short duration and without haemodynamic consequences	(b) All competitive sports, except those with increased intrinsic risk[1]	(b) Yearly
Ventricular pre-excitation (WPW syndrome) in association with:	History, ECG, Echo, EP study			
(a) paroxysmal AV re-entry tachycardia		(a) Ablation is advised After catheter ablation: if no recurrences, for >1 month, no cardiac disease	(a) All competitive sports after ablation	Yearly
(b) atrial fibrillation or flutter		(b) Ablation is advised After catheter ablation: if no recurrences, for >1 month, no cardiac disease		Yearly
(c) only pre-excitation pattern in asymptomatic athlete		(c) Ablation dependent on risk assessment (including EP study if competitive athlete)	(c) Asymptomatic athletes at low risk: all competitive sports	Yearly
Atrial fibrillation (paroxysmal, permanent)	History, ECG, Echo, ET, 24-h Holter	(a) After paroxysmal AF: if no cardiac disease, no WPW, and stable sinus rhythm >1–3 months	(a) All competitive sports	(a) Yearly
		(b) after successful AF ablation; if no symptoms for > 1 month	(b) All competitive sports	(b) 6–12 months
		(c) permanent AF in the absence of cardiac disease or WPW: assess heart rate and haemodynamic response to exercise	(c) Assessed on individual basis	(c) 6–12 months
Atrial flutter	History, ECG, Echo, EP study	Ablation is advised. After ablation: if no symptoms[2] for >1 month, no cardiac disease, and off therapy	All competitive sports	Yearly
Premature ventricular beats	History, ECG, Echo, ET, 24-h Holter, CMR	*In the absence of*: cardiac disease or arrhythmogenic condition,[3] family history of SD, symptoms[2], increasing complexity (i.e. increased frequency ±shorter coupling interval, couplets, triplets, or non-sustained VT) during exercise	All competitive sports	Yearly

Table 7.1.1. Recommendation for competitive sport participation in athletes with arrhythmias and primary arrhythmogenic conditions *(Continued)*

Non-sustained ventricular tachycardia	History, ECG, Echo, ET, 24-h Holter, CMR	*In the absence of*: cardiac disease or arrhythmogenic[3] condition, symptoms[2], familial SCD	All competitive sports	Every 6 months
Slow ventricular tachycardia, fascicular ventricular tachycardia, right ventricular outflow tachycardia	History, ECG, Echo, CMR, ET, 24-h Holter (in selected cases EP study)	*In the absence of*: cardiac disease or arrhythmogenic[3] condition, family history of SD, symptoms[2]	All competitive sports, except those with increased intrinsic risk[3]	Every 6–12 months
Syncope	History, ECG, Echo, ET, 24-h Holter (tilt test in selected cases)	(a) Neurocardiogenic	(a) All competitive sports (except those with increased intrinsic risk[1])	(a)Not required
		(b) Arrhythmic or primary cardiac	(b) See specific cause	(b) 6–12 months
Long QT syndrome	History, ECG, ET, 24-h Holter, genetic testing	(a) Phenotype-positive LQTS (QTc ≥490ms)	(a) No competitive sports; sport only as leisure-time activity; avoidance of specific triggers (diving, swimming, auditory)	Yearly
		(b) LQT1 silent gene carrier	(b) All competitive sports except swimming/diving	Yearly
		(c) Other genotype-positive, phenotype-negative LQTS ('silent gene carrier')	(c) All competitive sports	Yearly
Short QT syndrome	History, ECG, (24-h Holter, genetic testing)	Phenotype-positive SQTS	Only leisure-time activities	Yearly
Brugada syndrome	History, ECG, ET, 24-h Holter, EP study	(a) Phenotype-positive Brugada syndrome or others considered ***high risk***	(a) No competitive sports; only leisure time activities	Yearly
		(b) Phenotype-positive Brugada type 1 pattern, but otherwise considered ***low risk*** (asymptomatic; no family history; no QRS widening; non-VF inducible at EP study)	(b) All competitive sports	Yearly
		(c) Genotype-positive, phenotype-negative	(c) All competitive sports	Yearly
Catecholaminergic polymorphic ventricular tachycardia	History, ECG, ET, 24h Holter, provocative test, genetic testing	Positive catecholaminergic polymorphic ventricular tachycardia	No competitive sports; only leisure-time activities if arrhythmia-free under treatment, or with ICD	Every 6 months
Implanted pacemaker	ECG, Echo, ET, 24-h Holter	Normal heart rate increase during exercise, no significant arrhythmias, normal cardiac function	All competitive sports, except those with risk of bodily collision	Yearly
Implantable cardioverter defibrillator	ECG, Echo, ET, 24-h Holter as dictated by the underlying arrhythmic condition	Normal cardiac function at least 8 weeks after the implantation, after assessment of maximal sinus rhythm and risk for SV arrhythmias	Dictated by underlying arrhythmic condition All competitive sports, except those with risk of bodily collision. Guidance based in accordance with the athlete after he/she is fully informed	Every 6 months

Evaluation of a patient with complex arrhythmias at risk of SCA/SD wishing to participate in competitive sport should be preferentially performed on an individual basis in experienced centres.

[1] Increased risk if syncope occurs (scuba diving, mountain climbing, motor racing).

[2] Symptoms include presyncope, lightheadedness, and exertional fatigue.

[3] Arrhythmogenic conditions include cardiomyopathies, ischaemic heart disease, and channelopathies.

NB. For athletes with structural heart disease, see the recommendations of the specific disease.

ECG, 12-lead electrocardiogram; Echo, echocardiography; ET, exercise testing; 24-h Holter, 24-hour Holter monitoring; EP, Electrophysiological; CMR, cardiac magnetic resonance; WPW, Wolff–Parkinson–White syndrome.

Derived from: (1) Heidbuchel H, Panhuyzen-Goedkoop N, Corrado D, et al. Recommendations for participation in leisure-time physical activity and competitive sports in patients with arrhythmias and potentially arrhythmogenic conditions. Part I: Supraventricular arrhythmias and pacemakers. *Eur J Cardiovasc Prev Rehabil*. 2006;13(4):475-84. (2) Heidbuchel H, Corrado D, Biffi A, et al. Recommendations for participation in leisure-time physical activity and competitive sports of patients with arrhythmias and potentially arrhythmogenic conditions. Part II: ventricular arrhythmias, channelopathies and implantable defibrillators. *Eur J Cardiovasc Prev Rehabil*. 2006;13(5):676-86.

Table 7.1.2. Recommendations for competitive sport participation in athletes with cardiomyopathies, myocarditis, and pericarditis

Lesion	Evaluation	Criteria for eligibility	Recommendations	Follow-up
Athletes with definite diagnosis of HCM	History, PE, ECG Echo, CMR	Asymptomatic with low risk score (<4 ES(C)) If symptoms, LVOT obstruction, arrhythmias or abnormal BP at exercise, and/or risk score >4 ESC	All competitive sport on individual assessment Only leisure-time sport	Yearly
Athletes positive with gene abnormalities of HCM, but phenotype negative	History, PE, ECG, Echo, CMR[1]	Asymptomatic, no evidence of LVH	All competitive sports	Yearly
Athletes with definite diagnosis of DCM	History, PE, ECG, Echo, CMR	Asymptomatic: near normal LV function, no exercise-induced arrhythmias	All competitive sport on individual assessment	Yearly
Athletes with definite diagnosis of AC	History, PE, ECG Echo, CMR	Asymptomatic; no major ventricular arrhythmias	No competitive sport; only leisure-time sport	Yearly
Athletes positive with gene abnormalities for AC but phenotype negative	History, PE, ECG, Echo, CMR	Asymptomatic; no major ventricular arrhythmias	No competitive sport; only leisure-time sport	Yearly
Athletes with definite diagnosis of LVNC	History, PE, ECG, Echo, CMR	Asymptomatic; near normal LV function, no exercise-induced arrhythmias	All competitive sport on individual assessment	Yearly
Athletes with CMPs and ICD	As required by the underlying CMP	Asymptomatic	Dictated by underlying CMP	Yearly
Athletes with active myocarditis, or pericarditis	History, PE, ECG, Echo, CMR		Temporary interruption of all competitive sports for 3-6 months	
Athletes after complete resolution of myocarditis	History, PE, ECG, Echo, CMR[1], ET	No symptoms, Normal LV function, No major ventricular arrhythmias,	All competitive sports	First control within 3–6 months
Athletes after complete resolution of pericarditis	History, PE, ECG, Echo, ET	No symptoms, no relapses	All competitive sports	First control within 3–6 months

Evaluation of a patient with CMP, wishing to participate in competitive sport should be preferentially performed on an individual basis in experienced centres.

[1] Subsequent controls according to the individual case. Athletes with LGE (myocardial scarring) on CMR should be assessed annually with an echocardiogram and exercise stress test.

ARVC, arrhythmogenic right ventricular cardiomyopathy; BP, blood pressure; CMR, cardiac magnetic resonance; DCM, dilated cardiomyopathy; HCM, hypertrophic cardiomyopathy; Echo, echocardiography; EF, ejection fraction; ET, exercise testing; 24-h Holter, 24-hour Holter ECG monitoring; LV, left ventricular; LVH, left ventricular hypertrophy; LVNC, left ventricular non-compaction; PE, physical examination; SD, sudden death;

Derived from Pelliccia, Solberg E, Papadakis M. et al. Recommendations for participation in competitive and leisure time sport in athletes with cardiomyopathies, myocarditis and pericarditis. Position statement of the Sport Cardiology and Exercise Nucleus of the European Association of Preventive Cardiology (EAPC). *Eur Heart J* 2018; (in press).

Table 7.1.3. Recommendation for competitive sport participation in athletes with hypertension according to the cardiovascular risk profile

Lesion	Evaluation	Criteria for eligibility	Recommendations	Follow-up
BP: well controlled Further RF: none TOD: none ACC: none	History, PE, ECG, ET; Echo	Well-controlled BP	All competitive sports	Yearly
BP: well controlled Further RF: well controlled TOD: none ACC: none	History, PE, ECG, ET; Echo	If well-controlled BP and risk factors	All competitive sports	6–12 months

Table 7.1.3. Recommendation for competitive sport participation in athletes with hypertension according to the cardiovascular risk profile (*Continued*)

BP: well controlled Further RF: well controlled TOD: present ACC: none	History, PE, ECG, ET; Echo	If well-controlled BP and risk factors, and without associated clinical conditions	All sports, except power sports known to severely increase BP	6 months
BP: well controlled Further RF: well controlled TOD: none or present ACC: present	History, PE, ECG, ET; Echo	If well-controlled BP and risk factors	All sports, except power sports known to severely increase BP	6 months

Echocardiography will be performed once every 1–2 years according to the individual clinical condition.
Depending on the type and severity of ACC and/or TOD, individuals with coexisting hypertension may selectively participate in competitive sports.
ACC, associated clinical condition; BP, blood pressure; ET, exercise testing; LVH, left ventricular hypertrophy; PE, physical examination, including repeated BP measurements according to guidelines; RF, risk factors; TOD, target organ damage.
Derived from Niebauer J, Börjesson M, Carre F, et al. Recommendations for participation in competitive sports of athletes with arterial hypertension: a position statement from the sports cardiology section of the European Association of Preventive Cardiology (EAPC). *Eur Heart J*. 2018;39 (40):3664-71.

Table 7.1.4. Recommendation for competitive sport participation in athletes with ischaemic heart disease (IHD)

Lesion	Evaluation	Criteria for eligibility	Recommendations	Follow-up
High-risk CV profile, (likelihood of CAD/ subclinical CAD)	MExT	Normal test	All competitive sports Active risk profile management	Yearly
High-risk CV profile + borderline or pathological MExT (high probability of CAD/subclinical CAD)	CT scan and/or stress-echo/CT scan/SPECT, coro	No evidence of significant CAD	All competitive sports Active risk profile management	6 months
Documented CAD (with ***low probability*** of exercise-induced adverse cardiac events)	MExT, stress-echo/CT scan/SPECT, coro	Absence of critical coronary stenosis + EF >55% + absence of exercise-induced ischaemia at peak exercise + absence of relevant VTs + near-normal age-adjusted exercise capacity	All competitive sports after individual assessment Active risk profile management	6 months
Documented CAD (with ***high probability*** of exercise-induced adverse cardiac events)	MExT, CT scan, stress-echo/CT scan/SPECT coro,	Presence of critical coronary stenosis and/or EF <50%, and/or exercise-induced ischaemia and/or exercise-induced pathological dyspnoea (angina equivalent), and/or syncope, and/or VTs at rest and/or during stress testing	Revascularization advised After 3 months from successful revascularization, re-evaluation needed All competitive sports after individual assessment Active risk profile management	
Congenital coronary artery anomalies (of wrong origin with inter-arterial course)	CT scan, MRI MexT + scintigraphy, or IVUS, FFR	(a) Anomalous origin from PA	(a) No competitive sports; only leisure-time sport	
		(b) Anomalous origin from wrong sinus and inter-arterial course between Ao and PA	(b) No competitive sports; only leisure-time sport	
		(c) All other variants, if no evidence of exercise ischaemia	(c) Competitive sport after individual assessment	
Myocardial bridging	CMR, CT scan, MexT + scintigraph, or FFR, IVUS	Absence of exercise- induced ischaemia	All competitive sports	Yearly

Critical coronary stenosis: >70% of major coronary arteries or >50% left main stem on coronary angiography
Exercise-induced ischaemia: >0.1 mV horizontal or down-sloping ST depression (80ms after the J point) in two chest leads, or ST elevation >0.1 mV (in a non-Q-wave lead and excluding aortic valve replacement), or new LBBB on exercise testing at lower steps or immediately after exercise
High risk profile: presence of multiple risk factors, which result in a 10 year mortality risk of >5% at present, or if extrapolated to the age of 60.
CAD, coronary artery disease; coro, coronary angiography; MRI, magnetic resonance maging; MexT, maximal exercise testing; VT, ventricular tachyarrhythmia; EF, ejection fraction, Ao, aorta; PA, pulmonary artery.
Derived from: Borjesson M, Dellborg M, Niebauer J, et al. Recommendations for participation in leisure time or competitive sports in athletes-patients with coronary artery disease: a position statement from the Sports Cardiology Section of the European Association of Preventive Cardiology (EAPC). *Eur Heart J*. 2018 Jul 19.

Table 7.1.5. Recommendation for competitive sport participation in athletes with valvular disease

Lesion	Evaluation	Criteria for eligibility	Recommendations	Follow-up
Mitral valve stenosis	History, PE, ECG, ET, Echo (or CMR)	Mild stenosis, stable sinus rhythm	All competitive sports after individual assessment	Yearly
		Mild stenosis in atrial fibrillation, and anticoagulation	Skill and mixed sport after individual assessment No contact sports	Yearly
		Moderate and severe stenosis(either in atrial fibrillation or sinus rhythm)	Skill sport advised on individual assessment No contact sports	Yearly
Mitral valve regurgitation	History, PE, ECG, ET, Echo (or CMR)	Mild to moderate regurgitation, stable sinus rhythm, normal LV size/function, normal exercise testing	All competitive sports	Yearly
		Mild to moderate regurgitation, normal LV size and function, normal exercise testing If atrial fibrillation, in anticoagulation	All competitive sports, with exception of contact sports	Yearly
		Mild to moderate regurgitation, mild LV dilatation (end-systolic volume <55ml/m²), normal LV function, in sinus rhythm	Skill and mixed sport after individual assessment	Yearly
		Mild to moderate regurgitation, LV enlargement (end-systolic volume >55ml/m²) or LV dysfunction (ejection fraction <50%)	Only leisure-time sport	
		Severe regurgitation	No competitive sports Valve repair advised	
Bicuspid aortic valve	History, PE, ECG, ET, Echo (or CMR)	No or mild stenosis, absence of severe regurgitation, ascending aorta not enlarged (by **z** score), normal LV size and function, no symptoms, no significant arrhythmia	All competitive sport	Yearly
Aortic valve stenosis	History, PE, ECG, ET, Echo (or CMR)	Mild stenosis, normal LV size and function at rest and under stress, no symptoms, no significant arrhythmia	Skill and mixed sport after individual assessment	Yearly
		Moderate stenosis, normal LV function at rest and under stress, frequent/complex arrhythmias	Only competitive skill sport	Yearly
		Moderate stenosis, LV dysfunction at rest or under stress, symptoms	Only leisure-time sport	
		Severe stenosis	No competitive sport Valve repair advised	
Aortic valve regurgitation:	History, PE, ECG, ET, Echo (or CMR)	Mild to moderate regurgitation, normal LV size and function, normal exercise testing, no significant arrhythmia	All competitive sports	Yearly
		Mild to moderate regurgitation, evidence of progressive LV dilatation	Skill and mixed sport after individual assessment	Yearly
		Mild to moderate regurgitation, significant ventricular arrhythmia at rest or under stress, dilatation of the ascending aorta	Skill sport after individual assessment	
		Severe regurgitation	No competitive sports Valve repair advised	
Tricuspid valve stenosis	History, PE, ECG, ET, Echo (or CMR)	No symptoms	Skill and mixed sport after individual assessment	Yearly
Tricuspid valve regurgitation	History, PE, ECG, ET, Echo (or CMR)	Mild to moderate regurgitation	Skill and mixed sport after individual assessment	Yearly
		Any degree, with right atrial pressure more than 20mmHg	No competitive sports Only leisure-time sport	
Poly-valvular diseases	History, PE, ECG, ET, Echo (or CMR)	See most relevant defect	Individual recommendation	
Bioprosthetic aortic or mitral valve	History, PE, ECG, ET, Echo (or CMR)	Normal valve function and normal LV function, in stable sinus rhythm	Skill and mixed sport after individual assessment	Yearly
		Normal valve function and normal LV function, in atrial fibrillation	Skill and mixed sport after individual assessment	Yearly

Table 7.1.5. Recommendation for competitive sport participation in athletes with valvular disease *(Continued)*

Prosthetic (artificial) aortic or mitral valve	History, PE, ECG, ET, Echo (or CMR)	Normal valve function and normal LV function, and anticoagulation	Skill and mixed sport after individual assessment No contact sports	Yearly
Post valvuloplasty	History, PE, ECG, ET, Echo (or CMR)	See the residual severity of the mitral valve stenosis or mitral valve regurgitation	Skill and mixed sport after individual assessment. No contact sports	Yearly
Mitral valve prolapse	History, PE, ECG, ET, Echo, CMR	In the absence of recurrent syncope, family history of sudden death, complex ventricular arrhythmias in association with scars on CMR, or long QT interval, or severe mitral regurgitation	All competitive sports	Yearly

CMR, cardiac magnetic resonance; ECG, 12-lead electrocardiography; Echo, echocardiography; ET, exercise stress testing; PE, physical examination; sport type, see Fig. 7.1.1.

Derived from: Mellwig KP, van Buuren F, Gohlke-Baerwolf C, et al. Recommendations for the management of individuals with acquired valvular heart diseases who are involved in leisure-time physical activities or competitive sports. *Eur J Cardiovasc Prev Rehabil*. 2008;15(1):95-103.

Targets of the recommendations

The main targets of this document are *competitive athletes*, defined here as both young and adult individuals who are engaged in intensive exercise training on a regular basis and participate in official sports competition. Official sports competitions (local, regional, national, or international) are defined as those events organized and scheduled in the agenda of athletic associations and national sport federations, either as organized team or individual sport disciplines, which place a high premium on excellence and achievement.

Participation in competitive events is regarded as a regular activity which characterizes the athlete's lifestyle. A common characteristic of competitive athletes, regardless of their level of achievement, is a strong proclivity to exert themselves to their physical limit with the aim of improving performance and results.

An important consideration is the age of the competitive athlete. Although most are young adult adults, others start their competitive career very early (e.g. gymnastics or swimming) or prolong their competitive activities to an advanced age (e.g equestrian events, yachting, or even endurance disciplines).

Although this chapter essentially focuses on competitive athletes, we assume that the principles of these recommendations can also be applied to individuals engaged in *amateur and leisure-time sports activities*. In fact, it should be emphasized that many young and adult individuals choose to engage in recreational physical activities that involve vigorous training programmes, similar (or even harder) in intensity, duration, and frequency than those of competitive athletes.

Role of the physician in decision-making process

The medical interest in formulating advice for participation in competitive sport is dictated by the awareness that elite and professional competitive athletes are a special subset of our society, not only because of their outstanding performances, perceived as models for achievement and success, but also because of the substantial economic interests they attract and the intense pressure they are under from sponsors, athletic associations, and the media.

Historically, the unpredictable nature of SCD/CA has necessitated a cautious approach regarding advice on intense exercise and competitive sport in individuals with CV diseases. This attitude has inevitably affected several athletes who would never have experienced an adverse event during an entire sporting career and has been challenged as an intrusion into the personal freedom of the patient, rather than a precautionary measure aimed at reducing the unpredictable risk associated with sporting competition.

Competitive athletes, especially professionals with clinically silent CV abnormalities, may be driven by the desire to accept possible future risks in order to achieve the immediate benefits associated with a lucrative athletic career, including (but not limited to) the economic, societal, and visibility correlates. Several actors involved in the athlete's life, including sponsors, media, athletic association, school, and relatives/partner, may also contribute to the athlete's decision to pursue a competitive/professional career regardless of the severity of the risk.

In this context, we believe that the first priority of the advising physician is the athlete's health, regardless of other considerations with respect to the athlete's visibility and the potential for substantial financial revenues. The relevant role of the examining physician is to make an appropriate assessment of the risk associated with the specific cardiac condition of the individual athlete and report this to the athlete in a clear, comprehensive, and plain fashion. Based on the evolving knowledge in this field, we advocate the adoption of an individualized approach, taking into account symptoms, established risk factors for

SCD/CA, the natural history of the disease, the age of the athlete, and the characteristics of the sport discipline when advising participation in or precautionary disqualification from competitive sport.

We believe that it is correct to involve the athlete in the decision-making process, which should include detailed information about the disease and a candid discussion about the potential risks associated with ongoing competitive sport and high intensity exercise. The examining physician should not be prejudiced by athletes who, with full judgement and complete understanding, decide to participate in competitive sport despite contrary medical advice.

The role of the examining physician is crucial when the perceived cardiac risk is disproportionately high and/or in case of a minor athlete. In this scenario, the physician should not only exhaustively inform the candidate-athlete, but also share the information with competent parties (i.e. the relatives or tutor of the athlete) in order to ensure that full understanding of the clinical picture is achieved and a proper decision will be made.

Finally, we should acknowledge that this process is conducted differently in different countries depending on the local cultural and societal rules and the medical competencies [8–13]. The relative weights of the physician advice and the athlete's autonomy are largely influenced by the different legal systems in place, and therefore shared decision-making should be viewed in the context of the existing medical and legal rules.

Implementation of the recommendations

At present, there is a variety (or lack) of regulations worldwide, with only a few countries mandating medical clearance of competitive athletes [10]. This is particularly true for regulations and practices regarding participation in sport for individuals with CV diseases. Most of these regulations are the responsibility of the medical teams of national and international sport organizations, which often do not include specific recommendations for athletes with CV diseases. Therefore the present recommendations are a proposed framework for a common international protocol for the evaluation and management of competitive athletes with CV disease. Implementation of the recommendations reported in this chapter is of relevant medical value to physicians examining athletes, and they provide a uniform method for managing elite and professional athletes participating in international competitions.

Legal implications of implementing the recommendations

Implementation of the recommendations may differ depending on the legal framework where the physician is operating. For instance, adherence to the recommendations is direct and undisputed in countries, such as Italy where the physician is mandated by the legal framework and/or sport regulations to be the final decision-maker of the eligibility/disqualification [13].

However, in most countries no such legal/sport framework exists, and the recommendations for the appropriate management will guide physicians advising eligibility/disqualification in a consistent fashion by ensuring that the athlete is fully informed, completely aware of the risk, and states whether he/she is willing to accept the risk (preferably in writing) [12]. It should be noted that no liability waiver can exonerate the physician from the duty to provide medical advice consistent with good medical practice and coherent with the primary aim of protecting the athlete's cardiovascular health [12,13].

Addendum

Cardiac classification of sports

Sports activities are classified according to the cardiovascular changes associated with the exercise training and the long-term impact on cardiac morphology. In this regard, sport disciplines may be schematically classified in four major groups: skill, power, mixed, and endurance.

- ***Skill sports*** are disciplines with prominent technical characteristics, where the achievement is mostly based on the athlete's neuromuscular coordination and skill (i.e. low dynamic, low static). The cardiovascular response to regular exercise is characterized by an increase in heart rate, which may be substantial, with only modest changes in blood pressure and cardiac output. The long-term cardiac adaptation to these disciplines is characterized by minimal or no morphological cardiac remodelling.
- *Power sports* are disciplines with a prominent muscle strength component, where achievement is due to the generation of explosive muscle power (i.e. high static). The cardiovascular response to power exercise is characterized by substantial increases in blood pressure and heart rate for several short repetitive bursts. The long-term cardiac adaptation to power disciplines is characterized by an increase in left ventricular (LV) wall thickness and a modest change in LV cavity size.

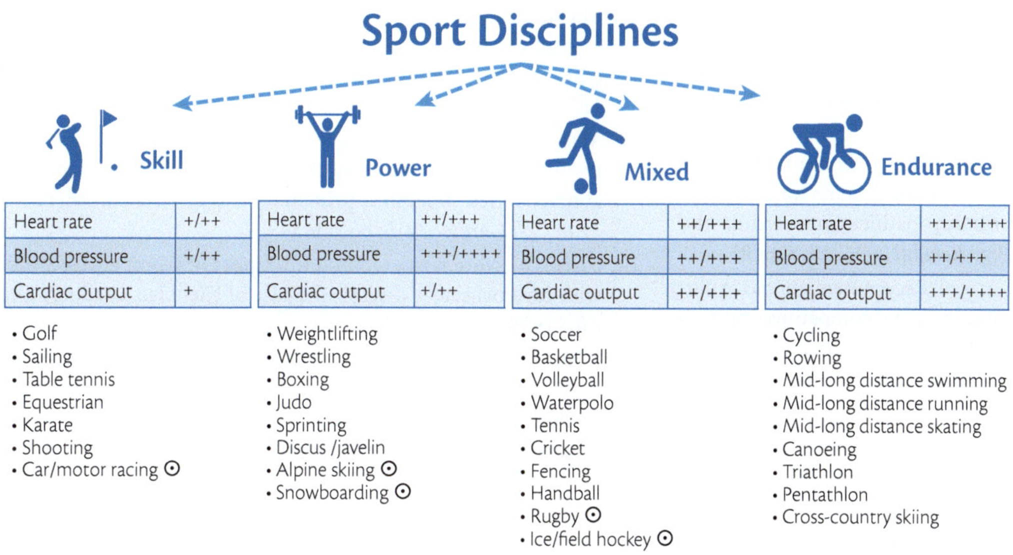

Fig. 7.1.1 Schematic classification of different sports. Symbol indicates sport with increased risk of bodily collision.

- *Mixed sports* present alternating phases of work (dynamic and/or static) and recovery periods. Typical examples are ball games and team disciplines. The duration and intensity of work varies greatly according to the type of discipline, the role of the athlete, and the trend of the game. The cardiovascular response to mixed exercise includes phasic increases in heart rate and blood pressure, which may reach near-maximum values, alternating with recovery phases when the heart rate, blood pressure, and cardiac output decrease. The long-term cardiac adaptation to mixed disciplines is characterized by an increase in LV cavity size and a modest change in LV wall thickness.
- *Endurance sports* are disciplines characterized by prolonged intensive dynamic exercise (i.e. high dynamic, often associated with high static exercise), where the achievement is related to the athlete's capability to attain and maintain a very high cardiac output through persistent increase in heart rate and blood pressure. The duration of the haemodynamic load is usually prolonged for 1–2 hours, with habitually 6–12 session a week for elite athletes. Cardiac remodelling with increased LV cavity size and wall thickness characterizes cardiac adaptation to endurance disciplines. The degree of cardiac remodelling may be marked, depending on the type of discipline, gender, ethnic origin, and body size and composition.

The CV changes for each group are indicated schematically in ➲ Fig. 7.1.1.

Further reading

Di Luca TR. Medical malpractice and the modern athlete: a whole new ballgame. Or is it? *Westchester Bar J* 2008; 35: 17–26.

Maron BJ, Mitten MJ, Quandt EF, Zipes DP. Competitive athletes with cardiovascular disease: the case of Nicholas Knapp. *N Engl J Med* 1998; 339: 1632–5.

Maron BJ, Chaitman BR, Ackerman MJ, et al. Recommendations for physical activity and recreational sports participation for young patients with genetic cardiovascular diseases. *Circulation* 2004; 109: 2807–16.

Maron BJ, Zipes DP. 36th Bethesda Conference. Introduction: eligibility recommendations for competitiveathletes with cardiovascular abnormalities. *J Am Coll Cardiol* 2005; 45: 1318–21.

Maron BJ, Friedman RA, Kligfield P, et al. Assessment of the 12-lead ECG as a screening test for detection of cardiovascular disease in healthy general populations of young people (12–25 years of age): a scientific statement from the American Heart Association and the American College of Cardiology. *J Am Coll Cardiol* 2014; 64: 1479–1514.

Mitchell JH, Haskell W, Snell P, Van Camp SP. Task Force 8: classification of sports. *J Am Coll Cardiol* 2005; 45: 1364–7.

Mitten MJ, Zipes DP, Maron BJ, Bryant WJ. Eligibility and disqualification recommendations for competitive athletes with cardiovascular abnormalities. Task Force 15: Legal aspects of medical eligibility and disqualification recommendations. *J Am Coll Cardiol* 2015; 66: 2447–50.

Pelliccia A, Fagard R, Bjornstad HH, et al. Recommendations for competitive sports participation in athletes with cardiovascular disease. *Eur Heart J* 2005; 26: 1422–45.

Sharma S, Drezner JA, Baggish A, et al. International recommendations for electrocardiographic interpretation in athletes. *Eur Heart J* 2018; 39: 1466–80.

References

1. Pelliccia A, Fagard R, Bjornstad HH, et al. Recommendations for competitive sports participation in athletes with cardiovascular disease. *Eur Heart J* 2005; 26: 1422–45.
2. Pelliccia A, Corrado D, Bjørnstad HH, et al. Recommendations for participation in competitive sport and leisure-time physical activity in individuals with cardiomyopathies, myocarditis and pericarditis. *Eur J Cardiovasc Prev Rehabil* 2006; 13: 876–85.
3. Heidbüchel H, Corrado D, Biffi A, et al. Recommendations for participation in leisure-time physical activity and competitive sports of patients with arrhythmias and potentially arrhythmogenic conditions. Part II: Ventricular arrhythmias, channelopathies and implantable defibrillators. *Eur J Cardiovasc Prev Rehabil* 2006; 13: 676–86.
4. Corrado D, Basso C, Rizzoli G, et al. Does sports activity enhance the risk of sudden death in adolescents and young adults? *J Am Coll Cardiol* 2003; 42: 1959–63.
5. Maron BJ. Sudden death in young athletes. *N Engl J Med* 2003; 349: 1064–75.
6. Maron BJ, Doerer JJ, Haas TS, et al. Sudden deaths in young competitive athletes: analysis of 1866 deaths in the United States, 1980–2006. *Circulation* 2009; 119: 1085–92
7. Biffi A, Maron BJ, Verdile L, et al. Impact of physical deconditioning on ventricular tachyarrhythmias in trained athletes. *J Am Coll Cardiol* 2004; 44: 1053–8.
8. Maron BJ, Zipes DP. 36th Bethesda Conference. Introduction: eligibility recommendations for competitive athletes with cardiovascular abnormalities. *J Am Coll Cardiol* 2005; 45: 1318–21.
9. Maron BJ, Zipes DP, Kovacs RJ. Eligibility and disqualification recommendations for competitive athletes with cardiovascular abnormalities: preamble, principles, and general considerations. *J Am Coll Cardiol* 2015; 66: 2343–9.
10. Maron BJ, Mitten MJ, Quandt EF, Zipes DP. Competitive athletes with cardiovascular disease: the case of Nicholas Knapp. *N Engl J Med* 1998; 339: 1632–5.
11. Mitten M, Zipes D, Maron BJ, Bryant W. Eligibility and disqualification recommendations for competitive athletes with cardiovascular abnormalities. Task Force 15: Legal aspects of medical eligibility and disqualification recommendations. *J Am Coll Cardiol* 2015; 66: 2447–50.
12. Mitten MJ. Team physicians and competitive athletes: allocating legal responsibility for athletic injuries. *Univ Pitt Law Rev* 1993; 55: 129–60.
13. Antoniotti F, di Luca N. *Medicina Legale e Delle Assicurazioni Nello Sport*. Rome: Società Editrice Universo; 1996.

SECTION 8

Exercise prescription for cardiovascular health

8.1 **Physical activity and leisure-time exercise prescription for sedentary/untrained individuals** *381*
Massimo F. Piepoli, Mikael Dellborg, and Mats Börjesson

8.2 **Monitoring exercise programmes and improving cardiovascular performance** *389*
Stephan Mueller, Flavia Baldassarri, Julia Schoenfeld, and Martin Halle

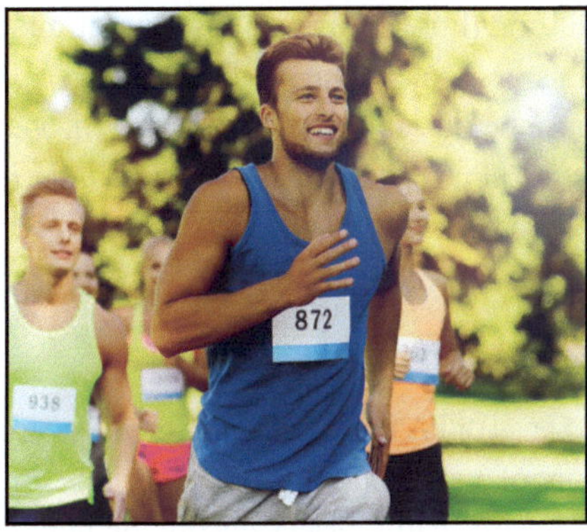

8.1

Physical activity and leisure-time exercise prescription for sedentary/untrained individuals

Massimo F. Piepoli, Mikael Dellborg, and Mats Börjesson

Introduction

Life in the twenty-first century has many 'advantages', including all the comforts of modern life that contribute to limited physical demands. Societal change has made travel, work, and free time physically less demanding. Physical inactivity is an obvious side effect of these changes in leisure time, school time, and occupational behaviours. Modern life does a poor job of promoting health and well-being in general, particularly in the Western world, and is also associated with overweight, stress, unhealthy eating habits, and tobacco use.

The distribution of physical activity (PA) is not uniform across Europe. The Eurobarometer questionnaire on self-reported PA shows that the amount of exercise varies widely, with countries with a high socio-economic standard, associated with a higher degree of office employment, showing the largest self-reported PA level, but at the same time the largest amount of sedentary time [1]. Importantly, this development is expected to continue in the future, with studies predicting decreased PA in a variety of forms (occupational, leisure time, travelling) and a concurrent increase in sedentary time [2]. As a consequence, as part of a widespread unhealthy lifestyle, only a minority of European citizens are involved in regular aerobic leisure time and/or occupational activities [1].

Causes and consequences of physical inactivity

Why are so many people sedentary? Are there some benefits associated with a sedentary lifestyle? The potential benefits of a sedentary lifestyle include a lower short-term risk of musculoskeletal injuries and possibly the false belief of avoidance of acute cardiovascular events. In modern life, there are several barriers to increasing the level of PA; for example, PA takes time, it often involves costs, and there are also educational and social barriers. In addition, PA may limit short-term well-being as it makes the individual sweaty and tired, and may also be associated with feeling uncomfortable immediately after exercising. However, in the long run, there are no obvious long-term benefits of being physically inactive, as opposed to the multiple negative effects. When assessing the totality of evidence, the risk–benefit ratio of a sedentary lifestyle is severely tilted towards an increased risk for the individual.

Indeed, physical inactivity is associated with several negative effects on health and well-being. The increasing prevalence of obesity worldwide, which is perhaps the most highlighted effect, is associated with a sedentary lifestyle [3]. Physical inactivity has also been shown to be related to an increased risk of many adverse health outcomes over a wide age range: all-cause and cardiovascular disease (CVD) mortality in healthy individuals [4–6], in subjects with coronary risk factors [6], and in patients with heart failure [7]. The risks of cancer of the large bowel, prostate, and breast are increased in a dose–response fashion [8,9]. This effect is mediated, in part, by the negative effect of physical inactivity on cardiovascular risk factors. Being sedentary or relatively inactive results in an increase in blood pressure, an increase in low density lipoprotein cholesterol (LDL-C) and a decrease in non-HDL-C, an increase in body weight, and an increase in the risk of developing type 2 diabetes mellitus [5]. This applies to both men and women and across a broad range of ages from childhood to the very elderly. Physical inactivity is also negatively related to quality of life for patients with malignancies [10], renal dysfunction, and muscuoskeletal disorders, as well as for children and young adults with congenital heart disease [11].

A healthy lifestyle

When a sedentary individual decides to modulate an unhealthy lifestyle several changes are involved. Stopping tobacco use, changing unhealthy eating habits, losing weight, and increasing PA level are all important steps in improving health. Importantly, they interact with and enhance each other; for example, eating habits aree changed to lose weight and PA level is increased for the same reason. Stopping tobacco use is often a prerequisite for taking up PA. While it is of great value to change your overall lifestyle, it is important to point out that increasing PA level has its own merits. For instance, it may aid weight loss and also help to lower blood pressure and cholesterol [12]. Thus, patients should be encouraged to pursue a physically active lifestyle, whether they actually manage to lose weight or not, independent of the effect on blood pressure and other risk factors.

A physically active lifestyle includes habitual PA in several areas of life: at work, while commuting, and in free time. The strongest predictor of cardiovascular health is still cardiorespiratory fitness [13], which includes a genetic component. Non-exercise PA is also associated with health [14]. This is clinically relevant, since not all patients can be expected to be motivated to be physically active at a sufficient level to increase their fitness. In recent years, a third component of PA, or rather inactivity, has been gaining scientific evidence as a risk factor for cardiovascular health, i.e. sedentary time [15]. A sedentary lifestyle is a risk factor for CVD, independently of participation in PA [3]. Thus, all components of the PA pattern (fitness, PA, and sedentary time) are independently associated with the metabolic syndrome in middle-aged Europeans [16].

It is important to define what we mean by 'sedentary' in this chapter. Watching television, playing video games, sitting, and reading for most of free time involves very little physical effort, and is traditionally considered to be a sedentary lifestyle. Before the introduction of accelerometers, 'sedentary' was typically defined as the least active group in various PA questionnaires. For example, in the widely used SGPALS questionnaire, the most inactive group (sedentary group) is defined as 'being almost completely inactive: reading, TV watching, movies, using computers or doing other sedentary activities during leisure time' [17].

However, this definition is not the same as the definition of 'sedentary' in recent studies using accelerometry, where only sitting/lying/being still, and thus acquiring a very low number of 'counts', is defined as being sedentary. In this chapter we use a broader definition: being sedentary refers to '*somebody who is physically inactive most of the time, and thus could be expected to have a low mean respiratory fitness*' (i.e. untrained).

Physical activity prescription

Although an increased level of PA for the population in general can be considered more of a societal issue, the close relationship between PA and health firmly places encouragement of PA within the responsibilities of the health care system. Despite an increased knowledge and awareness of the disadvantages of inactivity, most people still remain physically inactive, and PA is still not considered to be a proper, important, and generally accepted 'treatment' for CV risk factors or CVD. Although tens of thousands of patients are participating in randomized trials of lipid lowering, blood pressure reducing, and blood thinning drugs, there is still a shortage of large long-term randomized trials which clearly demonstrate a mortality benefit of PA increments. Despite this, PA has accumulated sufficient scientific evidence for its efficacy in health care to be uniformly recommended as a primary and secondary preventive measure of CVD, regardless of whether the individual is healthy (untrained or trained) [18], has risk factors [19], established CAD [20], or heart failure [21]. The challenge is still the implementation of an understanding of the benefits of PA, as well as national and international recommendations, into regular health care. In parallel with this, routine documentation of PA levels in medical records has been gaining in importance as a mean of identifying sedentary/untrained individuals suitable for targeted exercise intervention.

One reason why PA is still under-utilized as a treatment modality in regular cardiac care is that there are few effective methods of increasing PA in patients, and in the population at large. Different 'exercise on prescription' regimes have been tried in various countries, with varying results [22]. Importantly, the differing methods used vary greatly in their content and must be evaluated separately. The concepts of 'exercise prescription' and 'exercise is medicine' have been launched in Europe and the USA, respectively. The Swedish PA on prescription (PAP) has been shown to increase the level of activity at 6 and 12 months [23], as well as improving quality of life and cardiometabolic markers [24]. This method comprises the following:

(1) individualized patient-centred counselling;

(2) activity guidelines, according to scientific evidence collected in the FYSS book (PA in the prevention and treatment of diseases) [25];

(3) written PA prescription;

(4) follow-up assessments;

(5) collaboration between the health-care system and facilities where the activity is performed (i.e. sports clubs or municipal facilities).

In other countries, such as Italy, sports medicine specialists, operating in selected community-based sports medicine centres in collaboration with specially trained physiotherapists have developed dedicated programms for exercise-based rehabilitation, follow-up, and care, typically in low risk patients.

How to prescribe activity

The clinician prescribing activity has to consider the risks/benefits of any given activity for a sedentary/untrained individual. In this context, it is important to consider being sedentary/untrained, in itself, as a risk factor for cardiovascular events when deciding on suitable PA prescriptions for this group. Subclinical atherosclerotic disease is more advanced in sedentary individuals, as the degree of atherosclerotic disease is associated with the total risk factor burden, regardless of symptoms. Atherosclerosis typically progresses over many years, with age being an important risk factor in addition to the other classical risk factors (hypertension, diabetes, hyperlipidaemia, diet, and physical inactivity).

The individual risk–benefit ratio for a sedentary/untrained subject will vary according to the anticipated gain of any given exercise in relation to the total risk burden of the individual. The benefits of activity can be categorized as positive effects on functional status (strength, fitness and mobility, balance) and positive effects on any underlying disease [26]. The risks are defined according to the risk burden of the individual (disease, risk factors) and the intended PA (type, intensity, duration of activity). The aim of any exercise recommendation is to be as active as possible and to achieve the greatest degree of health benefits at the lowest risk, i.e. safe participation. As part of the assessment of the total risk profile, the health provider should assess the PA level in any subject (how many days and minutes per day are spent, on average, performing physical activities at light, moderate, or vigorous intensity.

The exercise prescription could be divided into major parts as shown in ➲ Box 8.1.1.

It deserves to be stressed that prescription of PA is not and should not be considered in isolation. Most subject want and should be given advice also on other aspects of an unhealthy lifestyle. It should also be stressed that it is not 'either/or' but rather 'both'. Increasing the PA could be leverage to any other lifestyle changes achieved.

Box 8.1.1 Exercise prescription

1 As a starting point, identify the 'ideal' activity for the target disease or for general functional capacity.

2 Consider any contraindications or somatic barriers to this activity (risk assessment).

3 Identify any simultaneous diseases necessitating further adjustment of the prescription. For example, the sedentary individual may have two diseases or conditions at the same time, which may have slightly different ideal prescriptions. Typically, this means that the lowest common level of intensity should be recommended initially.

4 Identify any psychological barriers to activity (motivation, fear of movement).

5 Finally, communicate the activity prescription.

Subjects should be advised on appropriate types of activities (see next section) and ways of progressing, and should be helped to set personal goals to achieve and maintain the benefits. To this end, individuals should be encouraged to find either an activity they either enjoy and/or one they could include in their daily routines, as such activities are more likely to be sustainable. For a more effective behaviour change, clinicians should explore practical ways of overcoming barriers to exercise. Thus, the link between primary care and local community-based structures for activity, recreation, and sport is crucial [27] The amount of time spent being sedentary should be minimized by active travelling (cycling or walking), taking breaks from extended periods of sitting, and reducing screen time [28]. Brief exercise advice is more cost-effective than supervised gym-based exercise classes or instructor-led walking programmes [29].

Recommended ideal activity for the sedentary/untrained individual

Aerobic physical activity

Although the intensity of recommended activity for a given individual will vary, some general statements regarding aerobic activity for sedentary/untrained individuals can be made. Since the fitness level of the sedentary/untrained individual per se is low or relatively low, an increase in fitness is one of the major goals of exercise prescription in this group of individuals. Normally, this is achieved by at least moderate intensity aerobic activity, but in unfit individuals, this level of (relative) activity can be achieved by aerobic activities which are normally considered as low to medium intensity, such as walking [30]. If the sedentary/unfit individual has a specific disorder, the prescription must be adjusted accordingly.

Aerobic PA, which is the most studied and recommended modality with a beneficial dose–response effect on prognosis [8,9,31], consists of movements of large muscle mass in a rhythmic manner for a sustained period. It includes everyday activities, such as active travel (cycling or walking), heavy household work, gardening, occupational activity, and leisure-time activity or exercise such as brisk walking, Nordic walking, hiking, jogging or running, cycling, cross-country skiing, aerobic dancing, skating, rowing, and swimming.

The prescription outlined below is primarily intended for healthy unfit individuals and, similarly to all other interventions, can and should be adjusted in terms of intensity, frequency, and duration according to individual needs and risk assessment.

Moderate or vigorous aerobic exercise should be recommended. It can be expressed either in absolute or relative terms. However, practising PA even below the lowest recommended levels should be encouraged in individuals unable to meet these requirements or in sedentary individuals who have just started to be active. These individuals are recommended to increase the intensity level gradually. Although activity leading to increased fitness may be most effective on an individual level, moving from being sedentary to performing low intensity activity (LPA) may confer the greatest health benefits on a population level.

Absolute intensity is the amount of energy expended per minute of activity, assessed by oxygen uptake per unit of time (ml/min or L/min) or metabolic equivalent (MET), which is estimated as the rate $\dot{V}O_2$ of energy expenditure while sitting at rest. By convention this corresponds to $3.5 mlO_2/kg/min$) [19]. A list of PA intensities in MET values is available [32]. An absolute measure does not take into account individual factors such as body weight, sex, and fitness level; older people exercising at a vigorous intensity of 6 METs may be exercising at near maximal intensity, while a younger person working at the same absolute intensity may be exercising 'moderately'.

Relative intensity is the level of effort required to perform an activity. By definition, less fit individuals require a higher level of effort than fitter people to perform the same activity. It is determined relative to the individual's level of cardiorespiratory fitness ($\dot{V}O_2max$) or as a percentage of their measured or estimated maximum heart rate (HR), which is 220 – age (%HRmax). It also can be expressed as an index of the individual rate of effort (how hard the person feels that they are exercising), i.e. the rating of perceived exertion (RPE) [33], or by frequency of breathing (the 'talk test'). For individuals on medication it is important to consider possible modification of HR response and to refer to other relative intensity parameters. A relative measure of intensity is more appropriate, particularly for older and deconditioned individuals. In fact, relative intensity may be more important to health outcomes than absolute intensity [30]. Classifications of both absolute and relative intensity, with examples, are presented in ➲ Table 8.1.1.

Table 8.1.1 Classification of physical activity intensity and examples of absolute and relative intensity levels

	Absolute intensity		Relative intensity		
Intensity	**METs**	**Examples**	**%HRmax**	**RPE (Borg scale score)**	**Talk test**
Light	1.1–2.9	Walking <4.7km/h, light household work, painting/decorating	50–63	10–11	No change in breathing rate
Moderate	3–5.9	Brisk walking (4.8–6.5km/h), slow cycling (15km/h), vacuuming, gardening (mowing lawn), golf (pulling clubs in trolley), tennis (doubles), ballroom dancing, water aerobics	64–76	12–13	Breathing is faster but compatible with speaking full sentences
Vigorous	≥6	Race-walking, jogging or running, cycling >15km/h, heavy gardening (continuous digging or hoeing), swimming laps, tennis (singles)	77–93	14–16	Breathing very hard, incompatible with carrying on a conversation comfortably

MET (metabolic equivalent) is estimated as the energy cost of a given activity divided by resting energy expenditure: 1 MET = 3.5mlO2/kg/min oxygen consumption ($\dot{V}O2$).
RPE, rating of perceived exertion (20 value Borg score).
%HRmax, percentage of measured or estimated maximum heart rate (220 – age).
Adapted with permission from Edward Howley. Type of activity: resistance, aerobic and leisure versus occupational physical activity. *Medicine & Science in Sports & Exercise*, Volume 33, Issue 6, S364–9. Copyright © 2001 Wolters Kluwer Health Inc.
Adapted with permission from Michael Pollock, Glenn Gaesser, Janus Butcher, et al., ACSM Position Stand: The Recommended Quantity and Quality of Exercise for Developing and Maintaining Cardiorespiratory and Muscular Fitness, and Flexibility in Healthy Adults. *Medicine & Science in Sports & Exercise*, Volume 30, Issue 6, pp.975–91. Copyright © 1998 Wolters Kluwer Health Inc.
Reproduced with permission from Borg G. Perceived exertion as indicator of somatic stress. *Scandinavian Journal of Rehabilitation Medicine*, Volume 2, pp.92–98. Copyright © 1970 *Journal of Rehabilitation Medicine.*

Frequency should bet least three to five sessions per week, but preferably every day.

Duration should be an accumulation of at least 30min/day, 5 days/week of moderate intensity exercise (i.e. 150min/week), or 15min/day, 5 days/week of vigorous intensity exercise (75min/week), or a combination of both, performed in sessions of at least 10min duration is recommended [18]. Shorter bouts of exercise (i.e. <10min) may also be appropriate, especially in highly deconditioned individuals (5, 34, 35) Longer durations of exercise (40 and 60–90min/day, respectively) have been proposed for lipid control or body weight management [36].

Aerobic interval training and high intensity interval training (HIIT) must be recommended on an individual basis only until further data on safety and efficacy are available [37]. HIIT may have a higher yield in terms of effect for some health parameters (fitness, insulin resistance, lipids, etc.) [38], but has a potentially greater risk in sedentary individuals (if underlying CAD exists). Therefore HIIT has to be individualized in detail for risk–benefit, and lower compliance must be taken into consideration.

Muscle strength/resistance physical activity

Isotonic PA stimulates bone formation and reduces bone loss, and preserves and enhances muscle mass, strength, power and functional ability, with some evidence of benefit in lipid and BP control and insulin sensitivity, especially in combination with aerobic exercise [5,39]. It should target the major muscle groups (agonist and antagonist) and include multi-joint or compound movements through the full range of joint motion, such as working with resistance bands, calisthenic exercises using body weight for resistance, carrying heavy loads, and heavy gardening. For each exercise session, the suggested prescription is two or three sets of 8–12 repetitions at an intensity of 60–80% of the individual's one repetition maximum (1-RM), i.e. the maximum load that can be lifted one time, at a frequency of least 2 days/week. Older adults or very deconditioned individuals should start with one set of 10–15 repetitions at 60–70% of 1RM [40].

Neuromotor physical activity

Neuromotor exercise helps to maintain and improve balance and motor skills (balance, agility, coordination, and gait) in older adults at risk of falls,. This includes multifaceted activities such as tai chi and yoga, and recreational activities using paddles or sport balls to challenge hand–eye coordination. The optimal volume is not known [34].

Contraindications/barriers to exercise: risk assessment

The sedentary/unfit individual may have another simultaneous disease or condition which contraindicates some or all of the exercise modalities or intensities. For example, an individual with underlying hypertrophic cardiomyopathy (HCM) should not participate in high intensity aerobic activity or sport [41]. Therefore the prescription has to be adjusted accordingly, recommending low-medium (non-competitive) intensity activity instead.

Importantly, the risk of an adverse CV response during PA is extremely low for apparently healthy adults (5–17 sudden deaths per million population per year) [42] The risk of participation is outweighed by the substantial health benefits conferred by PA [5]. Risk during light or moderate intensity exercise is lower than during vigorous activity [5]; thus a preliminary medical evaluation is not needed for healthy individuals who wish to undertake moderate PA, such as a walking programme [36]. This is an important message for any individual who is considering increasing their PA level: there is a suitable activity for everyone.

Before an individual starts more intensive leisure-time activities (i.e. structured or competitive activity, amateur sport, exercise and fitness training), risk assessment should be tailored to their clinical (i.e. metabolic, musculoskeletal condition/disease) and cardiac risk profile, the current level of habitual PA, and the intended level of PA [43]. Individuals who exercise only occasionally appear to have an increased risk of acute coronary events and sudden cardiac death during or after high intensity exercise [44]. Sedentary subjects and those with CV risk factors should start aerobic PA at low intensity and progress gradually. Clinical evaluation, including exercise testing, may be considered for sedentary people with CV risk factors who intend to engage in vigorous PA and sports. The information gathered from exercise tests may be useful for establishing a safe and effective exercise prescription. Simple validated self-assessment questionnaires have been proposed for sedentary individuals starting low intensity leisure-time sport activity or at least moderate intensity activities [43] (see also Chapter 6.6).

Simultaneous diseases

An individual may have two or more concomitant diseases that would potentially benefit from increased PA, but perhaps ideally not the same activity. For instance, if an individual has increased cholesterol, where high intensity aerobic activity is recommended, but also a chronic pain problem, where high intensity activity may not be deemed ideal, at least initially, the final prescription has to be adjusted accordingly. For individuals with certain conditions (e.g complex congenital heart disease) it may be appropriate to consult physicians specialized within that particular field.

Psychological barriers to exercise

As in every doctor–patient relationship, the prescription of activity must consider the need, motivation, and other possible barriers to exercise. Depression [45], fear of movement, low self-efficacy [46], and low motivation for lifestyle change all have the potential to negatively affect both the compliance with and the success of any given prescription.

Individual prescription

Points 1-4 in Box 8.1.1 lead to the final adjusted prescription of activity for the sedentary/untrained individual.

Phases and progression of physical activity

Ideally, PA sessions should include the following phases: warm up, conditioning phase (aerobic, muscle strength/resistance, and neuromotor exercise), cool down, and stretching/flexibility. A progressive warm up before and cool down after exercise may prevent injuries and adverse cardiac events. Inactive adults should start gradually at light or moderate intensity for short periods of time (even less than 10min), with sessions spread throughout the week. With improvement in exercise tolerance, each subject progresses in the level of PA, but the increase in any component (i.e. frequency, duration, and intensity) should be gradual to minimize risks of muscle soreness, injury, fatigue, and the long-term risk of overtraining [34]. Following any adjustments, the individual should check for adverse effects (e.g. excessive shortness of breath), and if there are any such effects, downward adjustments should be made [33].

Follow-up

Any given prescription should be followed up, preferably by the same health-care provider who provided the initial prescription. The follow-up should include evaluation of the level of PA, similarly to the standard follow-up of blood pressure or cholesterol levels. This PA assessment can be performed by validated questionnaires, simple functional tests (submaximal exercise tests, such as 6min walking tests), or more objective measurements (accelerometers). Ideally, maximal exercise testing should be performed for assessment of cardiorespiratory fitness, but this may be limited by availability and resources. The 6min walking test is easy to perform, does not need ECG monitoring, and is suitable for following up a sedentary individual, with or without underlying cardiovascular disease. However, in the modern era of cardiology, exercise testing for risk evaluation is under-utilized, probably because of a change in the focus of acute cardiac care, but is suitable for both exercise prescription and follow-up of a given prescription [47]. In practical terms, in clinical practice we often only have the option of using a simple, but validated, PA questionnaire to assess the level of PA. At present, no available PA questionnaire shows more than poor to medium concurrent validity compared with accelerometry or fitness testing [48]. However, many still provide a more than adequate validity in predicting future morbidity and mortality [17].

Follow-up of the PA level and/or fitness should also include assessment of any underlying CV risk factor (cholesterol levels, obesity, etc.) or disease condition, as well as quality of life and functional capacity evaluation. It should also address any alteration in motivation towards lifestyle behavioural change. All these aspects must be summarized and could lead to adjustments of the exercise prescription.

If indicated, it is vital that follow-up of a PA prescription is also done in relation to changes in the concomitant disease and medications, where progression or regression may significantly influence the prescription.

Further reading

ACSM's Guidelines for Exercise Testing and Prescription. Philadelphia, PA: Wolters Kluwer/Lippincott Williams & Wilkins Health; 2014.

Börjesson M, Sundberg CJ. FYSS (physical activity book for prevention and treatment): behavioural change also for the physician? *Br J Sports Med* 2013; 47: 937–8.

Lee IM, Shiroma EJ, Lobelo F, et al. Effect of physical inactivity on major non-communicable diseases worldwide: an analysis of burden of disease and life expectancy. *Lancet* 2012; 380: 219–29.

Myers J, Prakash M, Froelicher V, et al. Exercise capacity and mortality among men referred for exercise testing. *N Engl J Med* 2002; 346: 793–801.

Piepoli MF, Hoes AW, Agewall S, Albus C, et al. 2016 European Guidelines on cardiovascular disease prevention in clinical practice. *Eur J Prev Cardiol* 2016; 23: NP1–96.

Ten Harkel AD, Takken T. Exercise testing and prescription in patients with congenital heart disease. *Int J Pediatr* 2010; doi: 10.1155/2010/791980.

Vanhees L, De Sutter J, Gelada SN, et al. Importance of characteristics and modalities of physical activity and exercise in defining the benefits to cardiovascular health within the general population: recommendations from the EACPR: Part I. *Eur J Prev Cardiol* 2012; 19: 670–86.

Vanhees L, Geladas N, Hansen D, et al. Importance of characteristics and modalities of physical activity and exercise in the management of cardiovascular health in individuals with cardiovascular risk factors: recommendations from the EACPR: Part II. *Eur J Prev Cardiol* 2012; 19: 1005–33.

Vanhees L, Rauch B, Piepoli M, et al. Importance of characteristics and modalities of physical activity and exercise in the management of cardiovascular health in individuals with cardiovascular disease: Part III. *Eur J Prev Cardiol* 2012; 19(6): 1333–56.

Whitfield GP, Pettee Gabriel KK, Rahbar MH, Kohl HW 3rd. Application of the American Heart Association/American College of Sports Medicine Adult Preparticipation Screening Checklist to a nationally representative sample of US adults aged >=40 years from the National Health and Nutrition Examination Survey 2001 to 2004. *Circulation* 2014; 129: 1113–20.

References

1. European Union. Standard Eurobarometer 2015. Available at: http://ec.europa.eu/commfrontoffice/publicopinion/archives/eb/eb83/eb83_first_en.pdf
2. Ng SW, Popkin BM. Time use and physical activity: a shift away from movement across the globe. *Obes Rev* 2012; 13: 659–80.
3. Lee IM, Shiroma EJ, Lobelo F, et al. Effect of physical inactivity on major non-communicable diseases worldwide: an analysis of burden of disease and life expectancy. *Lancet* 2012; 380: 219–29.
4. Lollgen H, Bockenhoff A, Knapp G. Physical activity and all-cause mortality: an updated meta-analysis with different intensity categories. *Int J Sports Med* 2009; 30: 213–24.
5. US Department of Health and Human Services. 2008 Physical Activity Guidelines for Americans. Available at: https://health.gov/paguidelines/pdf/paguide.pdf
6. Talbot LA, Morrell CH, Fleg JL, Metter EJ. Changes in leisure time physical activity and risk of all-cause mortality in men and women: the Baltimore Longitudinal Study of Aging. *Prev Med* 2007; 45: 169–76.
7. Piepoli MF, Davos C, Francis DP, et al. Exercise training meta-analysis of trials in patients with chronic heart failure (ExTraMATCH). *BMJ* 2004; 328: 189.
8. Moore SC, Patel AV, Matthews CE, et al. Leisure time physical activity of moderate to vigorous intensity and mortality: a large pooled cohort analysis. *PLoS Med* 2012; 9: e1001335.
9. Sattelmair J, Pertman J, Ding EL, Kohl HW 3rd, et al. Dose response between physical activity and risk of coronary heart disease: a meta-analysis. *Circulation* 2011; 124: 789–95.
10. Gerritsen JK, Vincent AJ. Exercise improves quality of life in patients with cancer: a systematic review and meta-analysis of randomised controlled studies. *Br J Sports Med* 2016; 50: 796–803.
11. Kahr PC, Radke RM, Orwat S, et al. Analysis of associations between congenital heart defect complexity and health-related quality of life using a meta-analytic strategy. *Int J Cardiol* 2015; 199: 197–203.
12. Piepoli MF, Hoes AW, Agewall S, et al. 2016 European Guidelines on Cardiovascular Disease Prevention in Clinical Practice. *Eur J Prev Cardiol* 2016; 23: NP1–96.
13. Myers J, Prakash M, Froelicher V, et al. Exercise capacity and mortality among men referred for exercise testing. *N Engl J Med* 2002; 346: 793–801.
14. Ekblom-Bak E, Ekblom B, Vikstrom M, et al. The importance of non-exercise physical activity for cardiovascular health and longevity. *Br J Sports Med* 2014; 48: 233–8.
15. Katzmarzyk PT, Lee IM. Sedentary behaviour and life expectancy in the USA: a cause-deleted life table analysis. *BMJ Open* 2012; 2: e000828
16. Ekblom O, Ekblom-Bak E, Rosengren A, et al. Cardiorespiratory fitness, sedentary behaviour and physical activity are independently associated with the metabolic syndrome: results from the SCAPIS pilot study. *PLoS One* 2015; 10: e0131586.
17. Grimby G, Borjesson M, Jonsdottir IH, et al. The 'Saltin–Grimby Physical Activity Level Scale' and its application to health research. *Scand J Med Sci Sports* 2015; 25(Suppl4): 119–25.
18. Vanhees L, De Sutter J, Gelada SN, et al. Importance of characteristics and modalities of physical activity and exercise in defining the benefits to cardiovascular health within the general population: recommendations from the EACPR (Part I). *Eur J Prev Cardiol* 2012; 19: 670–86.
19. Vanhees L, Geladas N, Hansen D, et al. Importance of characteristics and modalities of physical activity and exercise in the management of cardiovascular health in individuals with cardiovascular risk factors: recommendations from the EACPR (part II). *Eur J Prev Cardiol* 2012; 19: 1005–33.
20. Vanhees L, Rauch B, Piepoli M, et al. Importance of characteristics and modalities of physical activity and exercise in the management of cardiovascular health in individuals with cardiovascular disease: Part III. *Eur J Prev Cardiol* 2012; 19: 1333–56.
21. Ponikowski P, Voors AA, Anker SD, et al. 2016 ESC Guidelines for the diagnosis and treatment of acute and chronic heart failure. *Eur J Heart Fail* 2016; 18: 891–975.
22. Pavey TG, Taylor AH, Fox KR, et al. Republished research: Effect of exercise referral schemes in primary care on physical activity and improving health outcomes: systematic review and meta-analysis. *Br J Sports Med* 2013; 47: 526.
23. Kallings LV, Leijon M, Cnius ML, Stahle A. Physical activity on prescription in primary health care: a follow-up of physical activity level and quality of life. *Scand J Med Sci Sports* 2008; 18: 154–61.
24. Kallings LV, Sierra-Johnson J, Fischer RM, et al. Beneficial effects of individualized physical activity on prescription on body composition and cardiometabolic risk factors: results from a randomized controlled trial. *Eur J Cardiovasc Prev Rehabil* 2009; 16: 80–4.
25. Borjesson M, Sundberg CJ. FYSS (physical activity book for prevention and treatment): behavioural change also for the physician? *Br J Sports Med* 2013; 47: 937–8.
26. *Physical Activity on Prescription–FYSS*. Stockholm: Swedish National Institute of Public Health, 2018.
27. Campbell FBL, Messina J, Day M, et al. *National Institute for Health and Clinical Excellence (NICE) public health intervention guidance physical activity: BA for adults in primary care. Review of effectiveness evidence*. London: NICE; 2012.
28. *Start Active, Stay Active: A Report on Physical Activity for Health from the Four Home Countries, Chief Medical Officers*, 2011. Available from: www.gov.uk/government/uploads/system/uploads/attachment_data/file/216370/dh_128210.pdf
29. Garrett S, Elley CR, Rose SB, et al. Are physical activity interventions in primary care and the community cost-effective? A systematic review of the evidence. *Br J Gen Pract* 2011; 61: e125–33.
30. Lee IM, Sesso HD, Oguma Y, Paffenbarger RS. Relative intensity of physical activity and risk of coronary heart disease. *Circulation* 2003; 107: 1110–16.

31. Lee DC, Pate RR, Lavie CJ, et al. Leisure-time running reduces all-cause and cardiovascular mortality risk. *J Am Coll Cardiol* 2014; 64: 472–81.
32. Ainsworth BE, Haskell WL, Herrmann SD, et al. 2011 Compendium of Physical Activities: a second update of codes and MET values. *Med Sci Sports Exerc* 2011; 43: 1575–81.
33. Borg G. Perceived exertion as indicator of somatic stress. *Scand J Rehabil Med* 1970; 2: 92–8.
34. Garber CE, Blissmer B, Deschenes MR, et al. American College of Sports Medicine Position Stand. Quantity and quality of exercise for developing and maintaining cardiorespiratory, musculoskeletal, and neuromotor fitness in apparently healthy adults: guidance for prescribing exercise. *Med Sci Sports Exerc* 2011; 43: 1334–59.
35. Glazer NL, Lyass A, Esliger DW, et al. Sustained and shorter bouts of physical activity are related to cardiovascular health. *Med Sci Sports Exerc* 2013; 45: 109–15.
36. Donnelly JE, Blair SN, Jakicic JM, et al. American College of Sports Medicine Position Stand. Appropriate physical activity intervention strategies for weight loss and prevention of weight regain for adults. *Med Sci Sports Exerc* 2009; 41: 459–71.
37. Fletcher GF, Ades PA, Kligfield P, et al. Exercise standards for testing and training: a scientific statement from the American Heart Association. *Circulation* 2013; 128: 873–934.
38. Weston K, Wislöff U, Coombes J. High-intensity interval training in patients with lifestyle-induced cardiometabolic disease: a systematic review and meta-analysis. *Br J Sports Med* 2014; 48: 1227–34.
39. Schwingshackl L, Missbach B, Dias S, et al. Impact of different training modalities on glycaemic control and blood lipids in patients with type 2 diabetes: a systematic review and network meta-analysis. *Diabetologia* 2014; 57: 1789–97.
40. *ACSM's Guidelines for Exercise Testing and Prescription.* Philadelphia, PA: Wolters Kluwer/Lippincott Williams & Wilkins Health; 2014.
41. Pelliccia A, Fagard R, Bjornstad H, et al. Recommendations for competitive sports participation in athletes with cardiovascular disease. *Eur Heart J* 2005; 26: 1422–45.
42. Marijon E, Tafflet M, Celermajer DS, et al. Sports-related sudden death in the general population. *Circulation* 2011; 124: 672–81.
43. Borjesson M, Urhausen A, Kouidi E, et al. Cardiovascular evaluation of middle-aged/senior individuals engaged in leisure-time sport activities. *Eur J Cardiovasc Prev Rehabil* 2011; 18: 446–58.
44. Thompson PD, Franklin BA, Balady GJ, et al. Exercise and acute cardiovascular events placing the risks into perspective. *Circulation* 2007; 115: 2358–68.
45. Chipperfield K, Fletcher J, Millar J, et al. Factors associated with adherence to physical activity guidelines in aptients with prostate cancer. *Psychooncology* 2013; 22: 2478–86.
46. Zelle D, Corpeleijn E, Klaassen G, et al. Fear of movement and low self-efficacy are important barriers in physical activity after renal transplantation. *PLos One* 2016; 11: e0147609.
47. Börjesson M, Dellborg M. The role of exercise testing in the interventional era: a shift of focus. *Interv Cardiol* 2012; 4: 577–83.
48. Ekblom O, Ekblom-Bak E, Bolam KA, et al. Concurrent and predictive validity of physical activity measurement items commonly used in clinical settings—data from SCAPIS pilot study. *BMC Public Health* 2015; 15: 978.

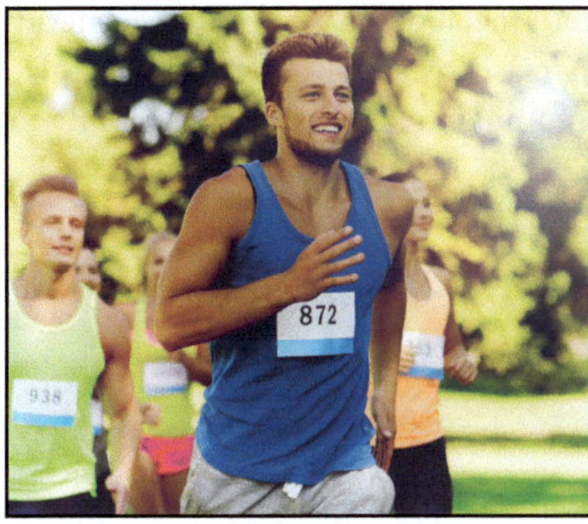

8.2

Monitoring exercise programmes and improving cardiovascular performance

Stephan Mueller, Flavia Baldassarri, Julia Schoenfeld, and Martin Halle

Introduction

A high cardiovascular exercise performance is one of the key components associated with lower morbidity and mortality of chronic disease such as diabetes, cardiovascular disease, cancer and dementia [1–8]. Moreover, a high muscular strength seems to be an independent risk predictor [9,10]. The elderly, in particular, benefit from muscular strength when accompanied by a high level of coordination and balance capacity [11]. Therefore the following three components determine global exercise performance:

- endurance capacity
- muscular strength
- flexibility and coordination.

Endurance capacity and muscular strength are the primary components of cardiovascular performance.

Exercise training intervention programmes are aimed at improving these three components. Key parameters for endurance capacity are maximal, aerobic, and anaerobic capacity. Key parameters for muscular strength are maximal or submaximal power. As flexibility and coordination are not as important for overall cardiocirculatory performance as endurance and strength, they will not be discussed in this chapter.

Endurance exercise capacity

Maximal endurance exercise capacity depends on four major components determining the transport of oxygen from the atmosphere to the muscle fibre mitochondria to produce energy in form of adenosine triphosphate (ATP): Oxygen is transported from the air via (1) the upper respiratory tract to the bronchial tree and the lung alveoli across the basal membrane to (2) erythrocytes where it binds to haemoglobin and is then (3) transported via the arterial vasculature to (4) the muscle fibres where it enters the energy production cycle, which depends on energy substrates, primarily glucose and fatty acids [12,13]. These endurance exercise components can best be assessed by maximal exercise testing accompanied by lactate measurements (lactate testing) or spirometry (cardiopulmonary exercise testing (CPET)). In this way both physiological and pathophysiological responses to exercise can be detected, including heart rate and blood pressure response, aerobic and anaerobic capacity, oxygen transport, and the interaction between and impairment of any one of the four key components of energy production [13].

Energy systems during physical activity

Energy metabolism can be divided into different components, as energy is not provided by a single pathway but a combination of pathways. These pathways differ in substrate availability, flow rate, necessity of oxygen for energy production, and energy per mmol of substrate (➲ Fig. 8.2.1).

Intense physical activity requires an *immediate energy release*. Most of the energy for short and intense physical activity comes from the intramuscular high energy phosphate ATP and anaerobic splitting of phosphocreatine

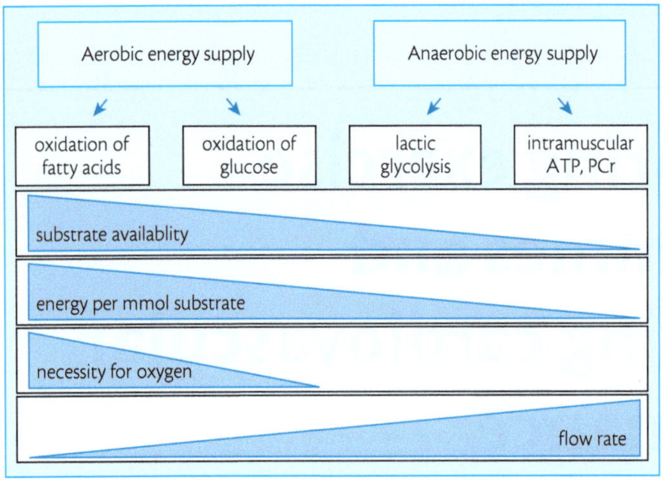

Fig. 8.2.1 Pathways of energy supply with the corresponding substrate availability: energy per mmol substrate, flow rate, and necessity of oxygen for energy production. ATP, adenosine triphosphate; PCr, phosphocreatine.

(PCr), which is the fastest way to resynthesize ATP. This energy is stored directly in working muscles and is independent of oxygen. It fully depletes within 5–8s of all-out exercise. For exercise lasting up to 2min (at maximum speed), high energy phosphates have to be restored immediately by the *short-term glycolytic energy system.* Synthesization of ATP depends on intramuscular glucose, and is also independent of oxygen. This leads to an accumulation of lactate, limiting the maximal duration for this pathway. *Long-term aerobic energy systems* can be divided into two pathways, oxidation of glucose and oxidation of fatty acids. Oxidation of glucose is limited by storages in muscle fibre and the hepatocytes, and lasts for a maximum of 60–90min. In contrast, the fatty acid storage is almost unlimited. Energy production per mmol of fatty acids is four times higher than energy per mmol of glucose. However, oxidation of fatty acids requires more oxygen and has a lower flow rate, which limits this energy pathway to low intensity physical activity [14].

These energy components can be assessed by CPET or lactate testing during maximal and submaximal continuous ramp (CPET) or stepwise (lactate testing) exercise protocols before, during, and after exercise intervention programmes. In this assessments, the following components are of particular interest:

- primary *aerobic* metabolism without accumulation of lactate, reflected by a high oxygen uptake ($\dot{V}O_2$) and a lower to equal carbon dioxide output ($\dot{V}CO_2$)
- *aerobic–anaerobic* metabolism with mild accumulation of lactate and increased CO_2 output, remaining in a steady state of lactate production and elimination
- increasing *anaerobic* metabolism, where the energy demand has to be increasingly supplied by anaerobic glycolysis leading to accumulation of lactate and inability to adequately exhale CO_2.

Exercise testing for assessment and prescription of exercise intervention programmes

Exercise testing procedures differ with respect to validity, reliability, test duration, and cost of equipment. Performance, prescription of exercise intensities, and monitoring of improvement are based on maximal and also sub-maximal exercise parameters. The exercise prescription (e.g. mode, duration, frequency, and intensity) determines the improvement during exercise intervention and depends on genetics, age, gender, and level of exercise capacity [15,16].

Assessment of maximal exercise parameters

Maximal exercise performance can be measured as maximal or peak oxygen consumption ($\dot{V}O_2$max/$\dot{V}O_2$peak) or maximum power (in Watts or km/h) achieved during subjective or objective maximal exercise testing. $\dot{V}O_2$max is defined by no further increase in $\dot{V}O_2$ despite a further increase in load. Adapted from multiple constant load tests, $\dot{V}O_2$max is displayed as a plateau of oxygen consumption at the end of the incremental test, and is primarily seen in athletes. Non-athletes and patients do not often reach this plateau ($\dot{V}O_2$peak) [17].

The only direct method of measuring $\dot{V}O_2$peak or $\dot{V}O_2$max is CPET [13]. During increasing exercise, ventilation ($\dot{V}E$), $\dot{V}O_2$ and $\dot{V}CO_2$, heart rate, and blood pressure are continuously measured. Determination of blood gases and O_2 saturation can be added for a more detailed investigation. CPET is usually performed using a ramp protocol, in which the intensity is continuously increased until exhaustion within 8–12min. $\dot{V}O_2$peak is used to differentiate between trained and untrained or healthy and diseased individuals, and also depends on gender and age. Values range from <10ml/min/kg in patients with severe heart failure to 85ml/min/kg in highly trained elite endurance athletes (➔ Table 8.2.1) [14,18]. This parameter has a significant prognostic value for disease progression and survival [4,8]. For better interpretation, values are compared with evaluations for healthy populations. The evaluations most frequently applied for $\dot{V}O_2$max are the Hansen–Wasserman equations [17] or the equations given in the Study of Health in Pomerania (SHIP) [19].

Table 8.2.1 Fitness categories for relative $\dot{V}O_2$max (ml/kg/min) values for non-athletes

Gender	Age	Poor	Fair	Average	Good	Excellent
Men	≤29	≤24.9	25–33.9	34–43.9	44–52.9	≥53
	30–39	≤22.9	23–30.9	31–41.9	42–49.9	≥50
	40–49	≤19.9	20–26.9	27–38.9	39–44.9	≥45
	50–59	≤17.9	18–24.9	25–37.9	38–42.9	≥43
	60–69	≤15.9	16–22.9	23–35.9	36–40.9	≥41
Women	≤ 29	≤23.9	24–30.9	31–38.9	39–48.9	≥49
	30–39	≤19.9	20–27.9	28–36.9	37–44.9	≥45
	40–49	≤16.9	17–24.9	25–34.9	35–41.9	≥42
	50–59	≤14.9	15–21.9	22–33.9	34–39.9	≥40
	60–69	≤12.9	13–20.9	21–32.9	33–36.9	≥37

From McArdle WD, Katch FI, Katch VL. *Exercise Physiology: Nutrition, Energy, and Human Performance* (8th edn). Philadelphia: Lippincott Williams & Wilkins; 2015.

Other ways of testing maximal exercise capacity are field tests, which are simple to perform and require less equipment; however, they are less standardized. One of these tests is the Cooper 12min run, which measures the maximal distance covered in 12min. This simple test is commonly used in schools, the military, and amateur sport clubs. If performed at maximum speed, the distance covered allows $\dot{V}O_2$max to be approximated by the equation:

$$\dot{V}O_{2max}\,(\text{ml/kg/min}) = 3.126 * (\text{metres covered in 12 min}) - 11.3\ [20].$$

The methods used most frequently for exercise prescription based on maximal values (➔ Table 8.2.2) are percentage of maximum heart rate (%HRmax), %$\dot{V}O_2$peak, percentage of heart rate reserve (%HRR), and percentage of $\dot{V}O_2$ reserve (%$\dot{V}O_2$R). However, these values do not provide information on aerobic or anaerobic metabolism, and therefore may be more inaccurate with respect to exercise prescription and monitoring than sub-maximal thresholds derived from CPET or lactate testing [21,22]. In addition, the method of prescribing exercise intensity by %HRmax is particularly inaccurate in atrial fibrillation, chronotropic incompetence, or heart-rate-lowering medication such as beta-blockers.

Table 8.2.2 Prescription of exercise intensity according to maximal exercise parameters [85].

	Low (%)	Moderate (%)	Vigorous (%)
HR_{max}	<55	55–70	70–90
$\dot{V}O_2$peak	<40	40–60	60–80
HRR	<40	40–60	60–85
$\dot{V}O_2$R	<40	40–60	60–85

HR, heart rate; $\dot{V}O_2$peak, peak oxygen consumption; HRR, heart rate reserve; $\dot{V}O_2$R, $\dot{V}O_2$reserve)

Adapted from Vanhees L, De Sutter J, Gelada SN, et al. Importance of characteristics and modalities of physical activity and exercise in defining the benefits to cardiovascular health within the general population: recommendations from the EACPR (Part I). *Eur J Prev Cardiol*, Aug 2012; 19(4): 670–86.

Assessment of submaximal exercise parameters

Determining the transition from mostly oxidative energy metabolism to the steady state condition (*first threshold*) and the transition from the steady state condition to the increasing anaerobic condition (*second threshold*) yields detailed information for prescribing exercise intensity and monitoring improvement beyond maximal parameters.

The first threshold from CPET (ventilatory threshold (VT1)) and lactate testing (lactate threshold (LT1)) can be used interchangeably because of a strong physiological association. When the mitochondrial proton shuttle fails to re-oxidize the reduced nicotinamide adenine dinucleotide ($NADH + H^+$) to NAD^+, this happens by reducing pyruvate to lactate (pyruvate + $NADH + H^+ \rightarrow$ lactate + NAD^+). As the associated proton (H^+) of lactic acid is buffered by bicarbonate (HCO_3^-), there is a disproportionate increase in $\dot{V}CO_2$ ($HCO_3^- + H^+ \rightarrow H_2O + CO_2$) [17]. Even though the methodologies for the second thresholds (VT2 and LT2) do not have a physiological association, both have been shown to be correlated with the maximal lactate steady state (MLSS), also referred to as the critical power (CP). [23–25]. MLSS and CP represent the upper limits for prolonged exercise without further increase of blood lactate levels [26–29]. This intensity has also been shown to be safe in patient populations [30–33]. Several investigators have shown that the submaximal thresholds and MLSS are additional, and sometimes stronger, predictors for exercise performance than $\dot{V}O_2$max [34–39]. For example, studies of well-trained athletes [38,39] have shown that time to exhaustion varies significantly between subjects with a comparable $\dot{V}O_2$max exercising at 80–88% $\dot{V}O_{2max}$. This variation is related to the %$\dot{V}O_2$max at LT1 and the ability to tolerate high lactate levels [18].

It is often believed that the greater the training intensity, the greater is the effect on exercise performance. However, the question as to which exercise intensity reveals the greatest improvements in exercise capacity cannot be unequivocally answered. and depends, among other factors, on the individual submaximal performance parameters and the training goals.

For untrained individuals and patients, higher intensities and threshold training at intensities up to VT2/LT2 seem to be the best way to increase exercise performance and decrease the risk of cardiovascular events [40–45]. However, in elite athletes, the distribution of training sessions is most likely to accord with the polarized training model, which comprises about 80% of training sessions below VT1/LT1 and about 20% near or above VT2/LT2 [46–50].

Stated simply, to increase aerobic capacity (especially fatty acid oxidation during exercise) exercise training has to be performed at lower intensities for longer times (slightly below VT1/LT1) [47,51,52]. To increase the capability for lactate clearance or a better anaerobic capacity with a higher lactate tolerance, exercise training has to be performed at intensities that lead to at least moderate levels of lactate (between VT1/LT1 and VT2/LT2) or consist of intermittent bouts of very high intensities (higher than VT2/LT2) leading to extreme lactate concentrations. Either way, a mixed model with different exercise training stimuli will most likely lead to the greatest effects.

Determining thresholds by cardiopulmonary exercise testing

As described above, the first threshold reflects the zone where there is a disproportionate increase in $\dot{V}CO_2$, known as excess CO_2. When plotted against $\dot{V}O_2$, the disproportionate increase in $\dot{V}CO_2$ versus $\dot{V}O_2$ in Wasserman graph 5 (Fig. 8.2.2, central) identifies the *first ventilatory threshold (VT1)* and is termed the V-slope method [53]. The excess CO_2 can also be identified in Wasserman graphs 6 and 9. Because of the increased ventilation for exhaling CO_2, the ratio $\dot{V}E/\dot{V}O_2$ increases while the ratio $\dot{V}E/\dot{V}CO_2$ remains constant (Fig. 8.2.2, central right). Graph 9 shows the end-tidal partial pressure of oxygen ($P_{ET}O_2$) and carbon dioxide ($P_{ET}CO_2$). At VT1, the slope of $P_{ET}O_2$ increases while $P_{ET}CO_2$ remains constant (➲ Fig. 8.2.2, lower right) [17].

When the intensity exceeds the *second ventilatory threshold (VT2)*, HCO_3^- fails to fully buffer lactic acidosis. The increased H^+ concentration stimulates ventilation, leading to a disproportionate increase of $\dot{V}E$ over $\dot{V}CO_2$ [17]. This can be identified in Wasserman graph 4 (Fig, 8.2.2, central left), where $\dot{V}E$ is plotted against $\dot{V}CO_2$. This is in accordance with an increase in the $\dot{V}E/\dot{V}CO_2$ ratio in Wasserman graph 6 (Fig. 8.2.2, central right) and a decrease in $P_{ET}CO_2$ in graph 9 (Fig. 8.2.2, lower right). Furthermore, there is a second increase in the $\dot{V}CO_2/\dot{V}O_2$ slope in graph 5 (Fig. 8.2.2, central) and a disproportionate increase in $\dot{V}E$ in graph 1 (Fig. 8.2.2, top left) [17]. As none of these parameters are measured at the muscle but at the mouth, defining ventilatory thresholds can be difficult owing to pathophysiological breathing patterns (e.g. exercise oscillatory ventilation, inability to adequately increase ventilation in severe COPD) or volitional control.

Exercise training programmes may produce an improvement in $\dot{V}O_2$peak and maximal power or an increase in power or $\dot{V}O_2$ at VT1 and VT2. In addition to $\dot{V}O_2$peak, VT1 is of particular interest in the clinical setting as it is unaffected by the individual's motivation for maximal testing, has a low variability, and is of clinical significance [13,54]. As for $\dot{V}O_2$peak, $\dot{V}O_2$ at VT1 should be compared with predicted values of $\dot{V}O_2$max with the lower limit of normality being 40% of predicted $\dot{V}O_2$max. In the majority of cases VT1 is reached at 40–60% of $\dot{V}O_{2max}$ [17], but can be as high as 80% of $\dot{V}O_2$max [18].

Figure 8.2.2 shows the evaluation of a 26-year-old leisure-time sportsman with a good $\dot{V}O_{2peak}$ of 49ml/kg/min which corresponds to 113% of the predicted $\dot{V}O_2$max. $\dot{V}O_2$ at VT1 corresponds to 43% of the predicted $\dot{V}O_2$max and only 38% of the measured $\dot{V}O_{2peak}$. This reveals that the basic endurance capacity of this individual is rather low compared with a high maximal exercise capacity ($\dot{V}O_2$peak). This demonstrates the potential of assessing submaximal thresholds for improving exercise prescription and guidance for a tailored time-efficient exercise training programme.

Determining thresholds by lactate testing

During graded exercise testing with increasing workloads lasting for at least 3min, lactate is measured in capillary blood from the earlobe or fingertip at the end of each workload. Lactate increases with increasing anaerobic energy metabolism, only moderately at first but exponentially at high intensities. Accordingly, the *first lactate threshold (LT1)* is defined as the first increase in blood lactate above the resting level [45,55]. The accumulating lactate is eliminated in adjacent muscles, liver, heart, brain, or kidney [56,57], and the associated H^+ is buffered by HCO_3^- [17]. The *second lactate threshold (LT2)* should represent the maximal lactate steady state, where lactate synthesis by anaerobic glycolysis exceeds lactate elimination. Several methods of determining

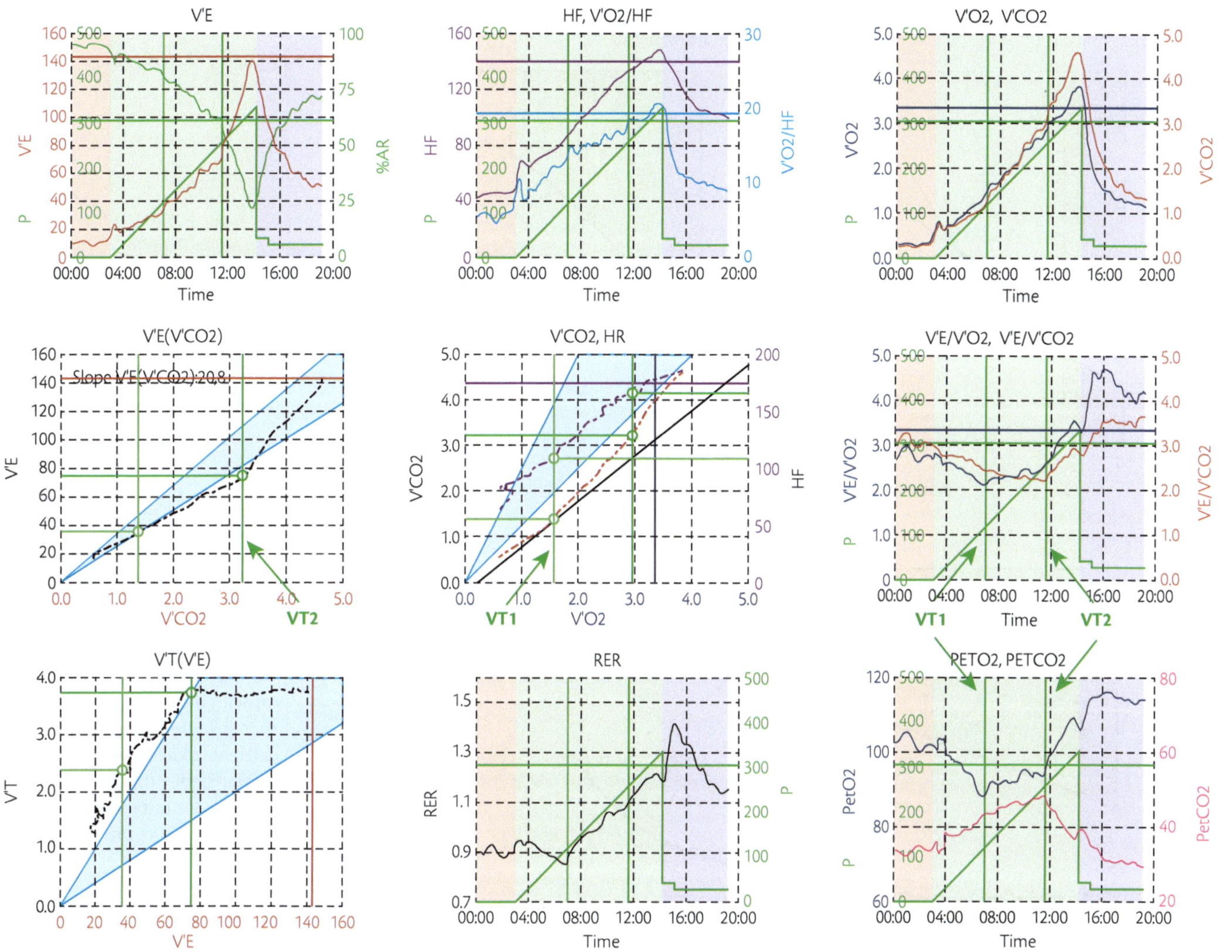

Fig. 8.2.2 Nine Wasserman graphs for a 26-year-old amateur athlete. $\dot{V}O_2$peak is 49ml/min/kg, which corresponds to 113% of the predicted $\dot{V}O_2$max. VT1 is reached at 43% of the predicted $\dot{V}O_2$max and 38% of the achieved $\dot{V}O_2$peak, which is at the lower end of normal values. Consequently, subsequent training recommendation will have to focus on a more pronounced basic endurance training programme. VT1 can be identified by a disproportionate increase in $\dot{V}CO_2$ vs $\dot{V}O_2$ in graph 5 (middle), an increase in $\dot{V}E/\dot{V}O_2$ without a concomitant increase in $\dot{V}E/\dot{V}CO_2$ in graph 6 (middle right) and an increase of $PETO_2$ without a concomitant decrease in $PETCO_2$ in graph 9 (lower right). VT2 can be identified by a disproportionate increase in $\dot{V}E$ vs $\dot{V}CO_2$ in graph 4 (middle left), an increase in the $\dot{V}E/\dot{V}CO_2$ ratio in graph 6 (middle right), and a decrease in $PETCO_2$ in graph 9 (lower right). This is reflected in a second increase in the $\dot{V}CO2/\dot{V}O2$ slope in graph 5 (centre) and a disproportionate increase in $\dot{V}E$ in graph 1 (upper left).

LT2 are used, and all reflect the exercise intensity when lactate levels increase exponentially [24].

Differences in aerobic endurance exercise capacity can easily be determined. In a trained individual lactate levels remain low or do not increase even after several incremental increases in workload, whereas in untrained individuals lactate levels increase even at low exercise intensities. Improvements in lactate thresholds can be obtained by intensifying endurance training (➔ Fig. 8.2.3) and reveal improved oxidative capacity.

An advantage of lactate testing over a maximal test is best explained by an example (Fig. 8.2.4). A 48-year-old leisure-time sportsman presented with the following history: regular exercise training for the last two years, weight reduction of 25 kg, non-smoker for the last four months after 30 years of smoking, blood pressure 150/100mmHg, no medical complaints but a stagnating performance despite increasing exercise volume (seven times a week) with three spinning sessions (1–1.5h, 170bpm), two long cycle rides (3h, 130bpm) and two fitness gym sessions (1.5h workout, including 30min cycling) per week. Despite this high volume of exercise his lactate curve (➔ Fig, 8.2.4, broken lines) shows no basic lactate plateau, but a slight increase from the beginning of the test. The early increase in lactate values reveals a non-optimal basic aerobic endurance capacity due to training at too high an intensity and insufficient

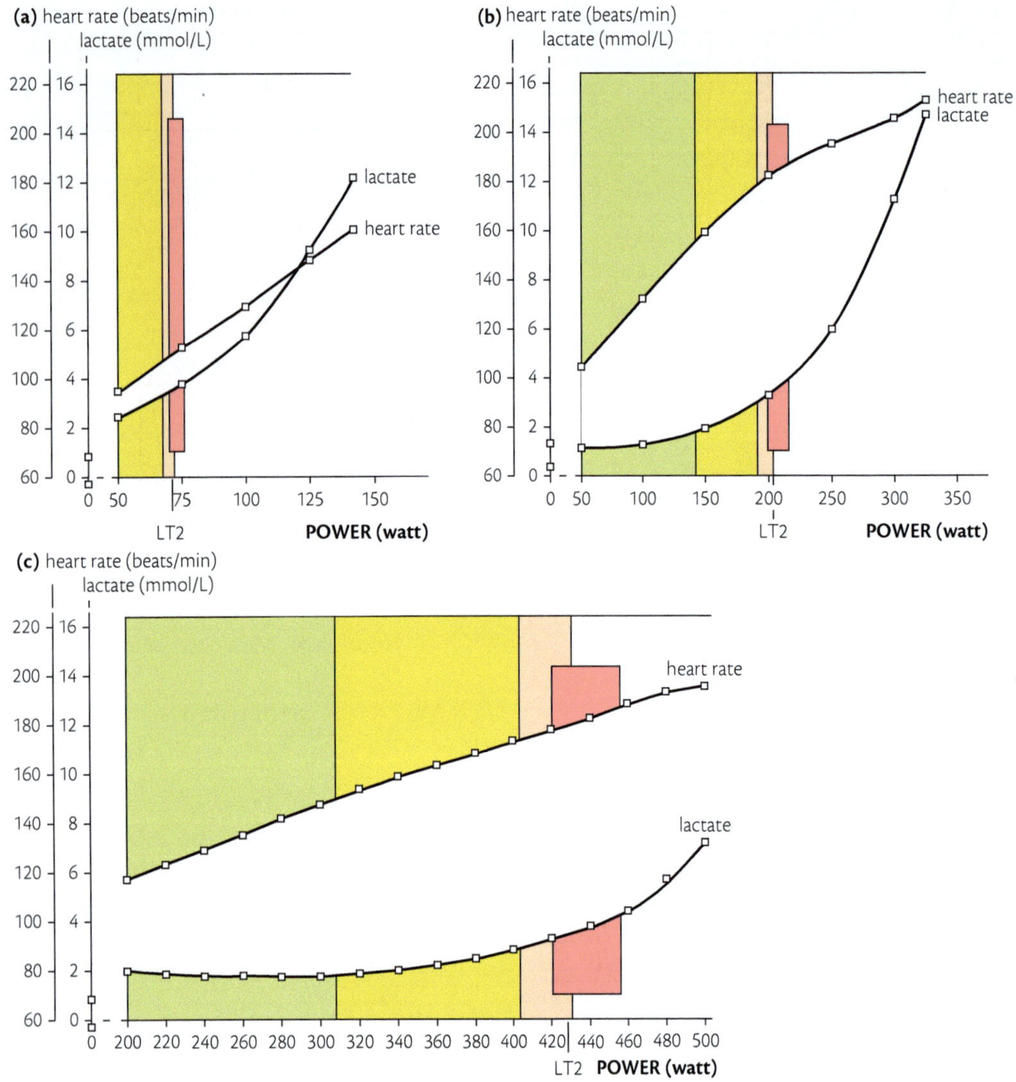

Fig. 8.2.3 Lactate test curves for (a) an untrained individual, (b) an amateur sportsman, and (c) an elite world-class endurance athlete. The higher the aerobic exercise capacity, the flatter and more right-shifted is the lactate curve. The different colours correspond to the recommended training intensities based on the test for basic endurance 1/recovery (lower than LT1, green), basic endurance 2 (between LT1 and LT2, yellow), threshold training (at LT2, light pink), and the supra-threshold intensity for interval training (beyond LT2, pink).

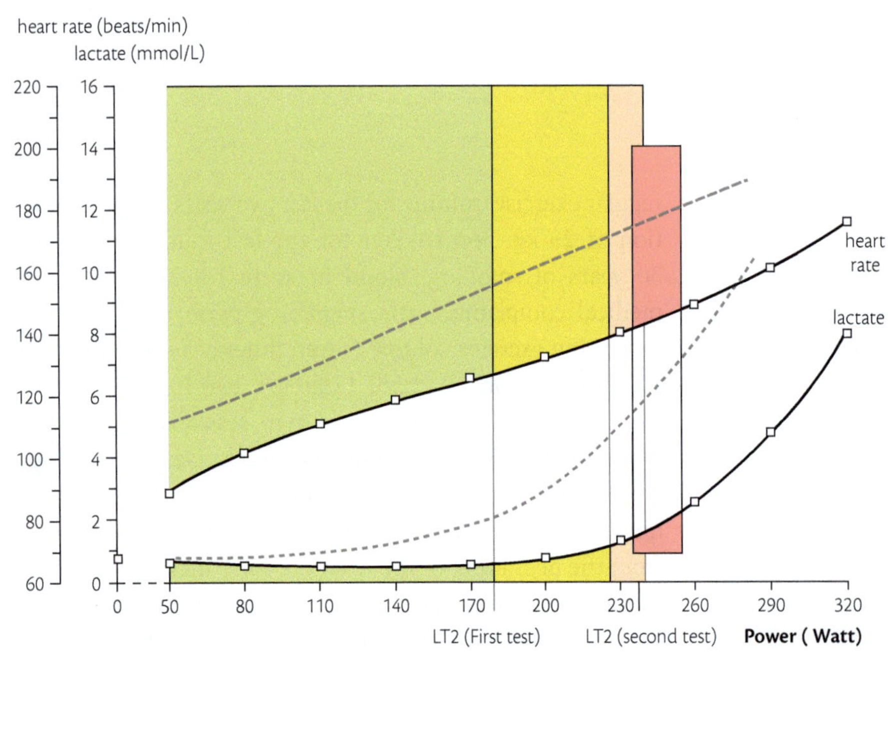

Fig. 8.2.4 The broken lines (baseline) show the lactate and heart rate curves of a 48-year-old leisure-time athlete training intensively seven times a week with a stagnating performance. The early increase in lactate concentration reveals non-optimal basic endurance. After adjusting the training programme for pronounced basic endurance intensities and a day of rest, the retest after 3 months (solid lines) showed a clearly flatter and right-shifted lactate curve with lower heart rates on corresponding workloads and a significantly higher maximal performance.

recovery periods. Consequently, training recommendations were changed to low intensity training with less spinning and a day of rest. Furthermore, a pharmaceutical treatment for arterial hypertension was initiated. The new training plan consisted of three long cycle rides slightly below LT1 (2.5–4h), one or two rides between LT1 and LT2 (1–1.5h) and one session at LT2 (1h) per week. A retest after 3 months (➔ Fig. 8.2.4, solid lines) revealed a clearly flatter and right-shifted lactate curve with a pronounced basic plateau and a concomitant reduction of heart rate on each workload as well as a significantly higher maximum power.

Lactate testing is not only valuable in elite and leisure time athletes, but also in untrained individuals starting an exercise programme. In an obese middle-aged woman (➔ Fig. 8.2.5) lactate analysis during exercise testing revealed an immediate increase of lactate beyond 4mmol/L, indicating that even brisk walking for 3min would be too high for a basic exercise programme. Prescribing a lower intensity guided by heart rate and a successive increase in duration and later in intensity improved her aerobic and maximal exercise capacity substantially.

In summary, analysis of submaximal thresholds allows a more differentiated view on performance and aids in prescribing an optimal training schedule that is based on the individual's submaximal and maximal performance capacity.

Assessment of strength

Strength testing is important for pre and post analysis of resistance exercise training programmes. Strength performance improves significantly during early stages of training[58] and strength assessment has to be repeated for adaptation of intensity. This is mandatory for a continuation of training success. For longitudinal analyses a standardized protocol is necessary. Importantly the strength test battery should be aligned according to the training programme. The higher the difference between training and testing, the less changes can be identified by the test protocol. Consequently, the use of a maximal strength test (e.g. 1-RM, one repetition maximum) assessing different muscle strength capacities is necessary for prescribing and following a training programme in athletes [58].

Maximum strength testing

Maximum strength is the greatest force generated by a muscle during a maximal voluntary contraction [59] and can be assessed by several methods, termed iso-inertial and isokinetic testing [60]. In all strength testing the length–tension and force–velocity relationships must be respected: an unfavourable joint angle (e.g. a deep squat) and higher velocities of muscle shortening are inversely related to the force output generated [60].

Iso-inertial testing

Single or multiple repetition maximum (RM) testing is an iso-inertial method and the simplest and most accessible method involving the gravitational force; maximum 1-RM is the weight that can be lifted once. In multiple RM, a submaximal weight is lifted three to ten times. For example, a

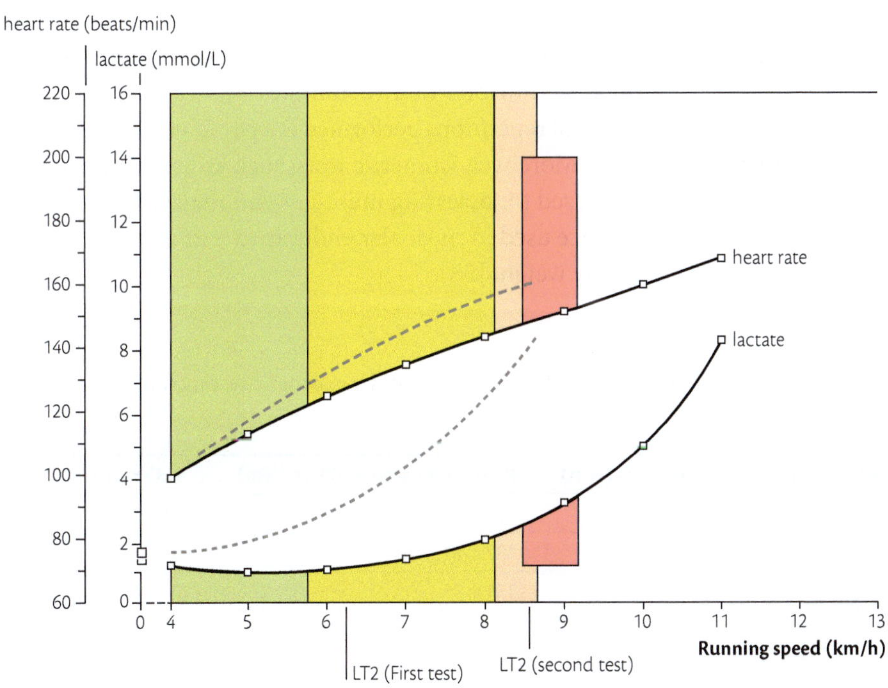

Fig. 8.2.5 The broken lines (baseline) show the lactate and heart rate curves of an obese middle-aged woman. The immediate increase of lactate reveals a very low endurance capacity. After 12 weeks of exercise training (solid lines) a flatter right-shifted lactate curve and lower heart rates on corresponding workloads as well as a higher maximum speed reveals a significantly improved submaximal and maximal exercise capacity.

Table 8.2.3 Effects of 12 weeks specific resistance training (mean ± SD) on bench press and squat (1-RM) on American football players

	Pre-training	Post-training
1-RM bench press (kg)	124.7 ± 21.0	123.9 ± 18.6
1-RM squat (kg)	155.0 ± 31.8	163.3 ± 30.0*

*Significant change. 1-RM, one repetition maximum.
Adapted from Hoffman JR, Kang J. Strength changes during an in-season resistance-training program for football. *J Strength Cond Res* Volume 17, Issue 1, 109–114. Copyright © 2003 Wolters Kluwer Health, Inc.

bench press assesses upper-body strength and is commonly used because of the large muscle mass recruited [58,60]. For lower-body strength more variance can be found in test exercises, but squats or leg presses are frequently used as they also recruit a large muscle mass [58]. The results of a training programme are outlined in ➲ Table 8.2.3, which shows the effect of 12 weeks resistance training (2 days/week, starting in pre-season and ending in the final week of regular season) on trained American football players [61].

Isokinetic testing

Isokinetic testing is a reliable and precise method of strength diagnostics [62] and describes the sequence of motion under constant velocity through the whole range of motion [58]. Force–velocity and length–tension issues are quantifiable and controlled by a dynamometer. They are expressed in torque units such as newton metres (Nm) (force due to the body segment rotating around its axis) [58,60]. According to the force–velocity–power relationship, the torque decreases with increasing angle velocity [14].

A common method for identifying potential muscle weaknesses to prevent injuries compares agonist and antagonist muscle groups as well as muscle groups from bilateral limbs. The most prevalent agonist–antagonist relationship is the hamstring–quadriceps ratio (H:Q), which is normally 2:3 [58]. Isokinetic testing is commonly used in various sports with common angle velocities of 60°/s and 180°/s [63–65] (➲ Table 8.2.4).

Ballistic testing

The underlying mechanism in motor tasks requiring high movement speeds (e.g. jumping, running, or throwing) is the stretch–shortening cycle (SSC) of the muscle–tendon unit (MTU). The MTUs have to be stretched before subsequent rapid shortening (eccentric versus concentric). SSC is an important mechanism for improving performance, as the kinetic energy stored in the MTUs during the eccentric phase is used in the subsequent concentric phase [60].

Vertical jump performance can best be determined using a force plate, and assessing the jump height by impulse measurements [66] with squat jumps (SJs), counter-movement jumps (CMJs), and drop jumps (DJs). SJs analyse the ability to performing a concentric jump without any counter-movement (no SSC), whereas CMJs use the SSC (kinetic energy) and should lead to a higher jump height. Next to higher joint moments [67], arm–leg coordination during take-off while performing a CMJ requires higher technical demands than SJ. Therefore similar jump heights in SJ and CMJ within the same athlete may indicate poor arm–leg coordination. DJs assess two important parameters: on one side the height of the jump after a drop from different heights (20, 40, 60, or 80 cm) and on the other side the contact time between landing and the subsequent jump. The higher the jump and the shorter the contact time, the better the performance [68].

Muscular endurance

Muscular endurance is defined as the fatigue resistance of a muscle or muscle group against repeated movements with submaximal resistance [58]. To test this, an individual performs as many repetitions as possible in a specific time frame; for example, repetitions of sit-ups or press-ups performed within one or two minutes (➲ Table 8.2.5). The number of repetitions performed is a parameter for dynamic testing. Moreover, isometric tests, such as flexed-arm hang, can be used for assessing muscular endurance. The primary resistance used in muscular endurance tests is the individual's body weight [58].

Table 8.2.4 Values (mean ± SD) obtained for knee flexion (hamstrings) and extension (quadriceps) by isokinetic testing (angle velocity, 60°/s) and the resulting hamstring–quadriceps ratio (H:Q ratio) for different competitive sports.

Population	Gender (age)	Knee flexion at 60°/s (Nm)	Knee extension at 60°/s (Nm)	H:Q ratio
Basketball [86] (dominant leg)	F (19–22)	74± 11	127 ± 18	0.58 ± 0.05
Basketball [86] (dominant leg)	M (19–22)	120 ± 29	187 ± 31	0.64 ± 0.12
Figure skating* (right leg)	F (20–28)	91 ± 15	131 ± 15	0.70 ± 0.11
Figure skating* (right leg)	M (20–28)	160 ± 25	232 ± 42	0.69 ± 0.21

* Own data, Flavia Baldassarri, 2015.

Table 8.2.5 Number of repetitions (mean ± SD) to assess for muscular endurance in high school athletes (press-ups and sit-ups).

Sport	Gender (age)	Press-ups	Sit-ups
Field hockey	F (16–17)	20.0 ± 6.7	40.3 ± 7.7
Soccer	M (16–17)	35.7 ± 9.5	50.1 ± 7.2
Swimming	M (16–17)	42.0 ± 7.3	43.3 ± 5.3

Data from Hoffman J. *Norms for Fitness, Performance, and Health*. Champaign, IL: Human Kinetics, 2006.

New technologies for monitoring training and health

New technologies can be used by athletes and patients to monitor parameters of physical fitness and training modalities. These gadgets provide a broad spectrum of tracking possibilities. In order to improve performance and thus to be successful in physical activity, training can be controlled using parameters and procedures under realistic conditions. CPET and lactate testing are useful tools for prescribing and evaluating exercise performance, and these results can also be used to monitor training progress by new methods such as digital assistance systems, innovative gadgets, and mobile applications. These non-invasive systems monitor and control training continuously using special physiological and biological markers [69,70].

Wearable and gadget technology

Wearable technology devices have increased in popularity, with a sales volume of $6 billion in 2016 [71]. Wearables are small and lightweight [70], and must be worn directly on the body [72] (e.g. smartwatches, wristbands/activity trackers, chest straps, or smart garments). They incorporate sensors or microcomputers, which provide immediate biofeedback, via apps on a smartphone or tablet, to athletes, coaches, and patients, and therefore provide additional information about exercise training performance.

- Wearables can measure body position, movement velocity, distance travelled, and acceleration by analysing GPS data [73,74].
- Accelerometers are used to measure any distance covered (e.g. steps completed, sleep time, and sleep quality) [75,76].
- Pulse oximetry can constantly monitor the oxygen saturation of arterial blood by absorbing near-infrared light at different wavelengths [77].
- Heart rate and blood pressure sensors such as chest belts, wrist bands, or photoplethysmography enable assessment of pulse rate and blood pressure by detection of near-infrared radiation [78,79].
- Gadgets include smart garments, such as shirts, shorts, helmets, and socks, which monitor a wide variety of internal and external training and health parameters (e.g. duration, distance covered, velocity, changes in elevation, HR, HR variability, HR recovery, and neuromuscular fatigue).
- Complete training/body suits are able to track muscle strain and contraction so that athletes know exactly which muscles were exercised most during workouts. Smart clothing utilizes accelerometers, electrocardiography and/or conductive fibres woven into the fabric.

Telemonitoring

Adequate measurements of vital signs, such as blood pressure, heart rate, and weight, can also be made via mobile applications (apps, smartphone) with or without additional external hardware. Apps without external hardware use photoplethysmography which determines the amount of infrared radiation detected by a photodetector (smartphone camera) [80,81]. Thus training or health parameters, such as blood pressure, can be measured by simply placing a finger in front of the smartphone camera. Together with external hardware (e.g. heart rate sensors), telemonitoring can be seen as another tool for controlling or monitoring training interventions with athletes and patients at a distance [82]. Using wearables as well as standalone apps, data are recorded and transmitted to a platform. A coach, supervisor, or a sports scientist can evaluate the training data and, if necessary, send new instructions to the athlete or patient [83].

Virtual Reality

Emerging technologies, such as Virtual Reality (VR), are innovating the training experience for athletes. Some VR companies promise to improve athletes' decision-making capabilities, cycling time, distance, and caloric expenditure by putting them repeatedly in realistic visual training scenarios [84]. If real-life training is limited due to environmental factors, VR training can be an alternative. Because of its relatively recent emergence in training and health, VR is not yet extensively used. Several start-up companies and studies have already investigated VR training and analysed the first results, but further evidence-based research is needed [84].

In view of the large number of devices that currently dominate the market, every user should be aware that personal data are generated. Furthermore, many devices have not yet been scientifically tested for reliability and validity [70]. Devices should be used to support exercise training, but not as a diagnostic tool. In summary, new technologies facilitate collection of objective parameters for training management and can be seen as tools for training assistance. These devices can motivate, promote social skills, and increase quality of life.

Further reading

Carvalho VO, Mezzani A. Aerobic exercise training intensity in patients with chronic heart failure: principles of assessment and prescription. *Eur J Cardiovasc Prev Rehabil* 2011; 18: 5–14.

Hansen D, Dendale P, Coninx K, et al. The European Association of Preventive Cardiology Exercise Prescription in Everyday Practice and Rehabilitative Training (EXPERT) tool: a digital training and decision support system for optimized exercise prescription in cardiovascular disease. Concept, definitions and construction methodology. *Eur J Prev Cardiol* 2017; 24: 1017–31.

McArdle WD, Katch FI, Katch VL. *Exercise Physiology: Nutrition, Energy, and Human Performance* (8th edn). Philadelphia, PA: Lippincott Williams & Wilkins; 2015.

Patel S, Park H, Bonato P, et al. A review of wearable sensors and systems with application in rehabilitation. *J Neuroeng Rehabil* 2012; 9: 21.

Pescatello LS, Arena R, Riebe D, et al. (eds). *ACSMS Guidelines for Exercise Testing and Prescription*. Philadelphia, PA: Wolters Kluwer-Lippincott Williams & Wilkins Health; 2013.

Wasserman K, Hansen JE, Sue D, et al. *Principles of Exercise Testing and Interpretation: Including Pathophysiology and Clinical Applications* (5th edn.). Philadelphia, PA: Lippincott Williams & Wilkins; 2012.

References

1. Lee DC, Sui X, Church TS, et al. Changes in fitness and fatness on the development of cardiovascular disease risk factors hypertension, metabolic syndrome, and hypercholesterolemia. *J Am Coll Cardiol* 2012; 59: 665–72.
2. Lee DC, Sui X, Artero EG, et al. Long-term effects of changes in cardiorespiratory fitness and body mass index on all-cause and cardiovascular disease mortality in men: the Aerobics Center Longitudinal Study. *Circulation* 2011; 124: 2483–90.
3. Sui X, Hooker SP, Lee IM, et al. A prospective study of cardiorespiratory fitness and risk of type 2 diabetes in women. *Diabetes Care* 2008; 31: 550–5.
4. Myers J, Prakash M, Froelicher V, et al. Exercise capacity and mortality among men referred for exercise testing. *N Engl J Med* 2002; 346: 793–801.
5. Kokkinos P, Myers J, Faselis C, et al. Exercise capacity and mortality in older men: a 20-year follow-up study. *Circulation* 2010; 122:790–7.
6. Nyberg J, Aberg MA, Schioler L, et al. Cardiovascular and cognitive fitness at age 18 and risk of early-onset dementia. *Brain* 2014; 137: 1514–23.
7. Ravaglia G, Forti P, Lucicesare A, et al. Physical activity and dementia risk in the elderly: findings from a prospective Italian study. *Neurology* 2008; 70: 1786–94.
8. Barry VW, Baruth M, Beets MW, et al. Fitness vs. fatness on all-cause mortality: a meta-analysis. *Prog Cardiovasc Dis* 2014; 56: 382–90.
9. Volaklis KA, Halle M, Thorand B, et al. Handgrip strength is inversely and independently associated with multimorbidity among older women: results from the KORA-Age study. *Eur J Intern Med* 2016; 31: 35–40.
10. Volaklis KA, Halle M, Meisinger C. Muscular strength as a strong predictor of mortality: a narrative review. *Eur J Intern Med* 2015; 26: 303–10.
11. Siegrist M, Freiberger E, Geilhof B, et al. Fall prevention in a primary care setting. *Dtsch Arztebl Int* 2016; 113: 365–72.
12. Wasserman K, Beaver WL, Whipp BJ. Gas exchange theory and the lactic acidosis (anaerobic) threshold. *Circulation* 1990; 81(1 Suppl): Ii14–30.
13. Guazzi M, Arena R, Halle M, et al. 2016 Focused update: clinical recommendations for cardiopulmonary exercise testing data assessment in specific patient populations. *Circulation* 2016; 133: e694–711.
14. McArdle WD, Katch FI, Katch VL. *Exercise Physiology: Nutrition, Energy, and Human Performance* (8th edn). Philadelphia, PA: Lippincott–Williams & Wilkins; 2015.
15. Neufer PD, Bamman MM, Muoio DM, et al. Understanding the cellular and molecular mechanisms of physical activity-induced health benefits. *Cell Metab* 2015; 22: 4–11.
16. Bouchard C, Antunes-Correa LM, Ashley EA, et al. Personalized preventive medicine: genetics and the response to regular exercise in preventive interventions. *Prog Cardiovasc Dis* 2015; 57: 337–46.
17. Wasserman K, Hansen JE, Sue D, et al. *Principles of Exercise Testing and Interpretation: Including Pathophysiology and Clinical Applications* (5th edn.). Philadelphia, PA: Lippincott Williams & Wilkins; 2012.
18. Joyner MJ, Coyle EF. Endurance exercise performance: the physiology of champions. *J Physiol* 2008; 586: 35–44.
19. Koch B, Schaper C, Ittermann T, et al. Reference values for cardiopulmonary exercise testing in healthy volunteers: the SHIP study. *Eur Respir J* 2009; 33: 389–97.
20. Cooper KH. A means of assessing maximal oxygen intake: correlation between field and treadmill testing. *JAMA* 1968; 203: 201–4.
21. Scharhag-Rosenberger F, Meyer T, Gassler N, et al. Exercise at given percentages of VO2max: heterogeneous metabolic responses between individuals. *J Sci Med Sport* 2010; 13: 74–9.
22. Meyer T, Gabriel HH, Kindermann W. Is determination of exercise intensities as percentages of VO_2max or HRmax adequate? *Med Sci Sports Exerc* 1999; 31: 1342–5.
23. Dekerle J, Baron B, Dupont L, et al. Maximal lactate steady state, respiratory compensation threshold and critical power. *Eur J Appl Physiol* 2003; 89: 281–8.
24. Faude O, Kindermann W, Meyer T. Lactate threshold concepts: how valid are they? *Sports Med* 2009; 39: 469–90.
25. Smith CG, Jones AM. The relationship between critical velocity, maximal lactate steady-state velocity and lactate turnpoint velocity in runners. *Eur J Appl Physiol* 2001; 85: 19–26.
26. Hill DW. The critical power concept: a review. *Sports Med* 1993; 16: 237–54.
27. Heck H, Mader A, Hess G, et al. Justification of the 4-mmol/l lactate threshold. *Int J Sports Med* 1985; 6: 117–30.
28. Beneke R. Anaerobic threshold, individual anaerobic threshold, and maximal lactate steady state in rowing. *Med Sci Sport Exerc* 1995; 27: 863–7.

29. Mezzani A, Corra U, Giordano A, et al. Upper intensity limit for prolonged aerobic exercise in chronic heart failure. *Med Sci Sport Exerc* 2010; 42: 633–9.
30. Dubach P, Myers J, Dziekan G, et al. Effect of high intensity exercise training on central hemodynamic responses to exercise in men with reduced left ventricular function. *J Am Coll Cardiol* 1997; 29: 1591–8.
31. Roveda F, Middlekauff HR, Rondon MU, et al. The effects of exercise training on sympathetic neural activation in advanced heart failure: a randomized controlled trial. *J Am Coll Cardiol* 2003; 42: 854–60.
32. Beckers P, Vanstraelen N, Possemiers C, et al. Exercise intensity in chronic heart failure: should we use individual ergospirometric data or stick to the Karvonen formula? *Eur J Cardiovasc Rehabil.* 2007; 14(1 suppl): S42.
33. Mezzani A, Hamm LF, Jones AM, et al. Aerobic exercise intensity assessment and prescription in cardiac rehabilitation. *Eur J Prev Cardiol* 2013; 20: 442–67.
34. Beneke R, Hutler M, Leithauser RM. Maximal lactate-steady-state independent of performance. *Med Sci Sport Exerc* 2000; 32: 1135–9.
35. Haverty M, Kenney WL, Hodgson JL. Lactate and gas exchange responses to incremental and steady state running. *Br J Sports Med* 1988; 22: 51–4.
36. Lucia A, Pardo J, Durantez A., Physiological differences between professional and elite road cyclists. *Int J Sports Med* 1998; 19: 342–8.
37. Sjodin B, Jacobs I. Onset of blood lactate accumulation and marathon running performance. *Int J Sports Med* 1981; 2: 23–6.
38. Coyle EF. Integration of the physiological factors determining endurance performance ability. *Exerc Sport Sci Rev* 1995; 23: 25–63.
39. Coyle EF, Coggan AR, Hopper MK, Walters TJ. Determinants of endurance in well-trained cyclists. *J Appl Physiol (Bethesda Md 1985)* 1988; 64: 2622–30.
40. Dickstein K, Cohen-Solal A, Filippatos G, et al. ESC guidelines for the diagnosis and treatment of acute and chronic heart failure 2008. *Eur J Heart Fail* 2008; 10: 933–89.
41. Piepoli MF, Conraads V, Corra U, et al. Exercise training in heart failure: from theory to practice. *Eur J Heart Fail* 2011; 13: 347–57.
42. Swain DP, Franklin BA. Comparison of cardioprotective benefits of vigorous versus moderate intensity aerobic exercise. *Am J Cardiol* 2006; 97: 141–7.
43. Gaskill SE, Walker AJ, Serfass RA, et al. Changes in ventilatory threshold with exercise training in a sedentary population: the HERITAGE Family Study. *Int J Sports Med* 2001; 22: 586–92.
44. Gormley SE, Swain DP, High R, et al. Effect of intensity of aerobic training on VO_2max. *Med Sci Sport Exerc J* 2008; 40: 1336–43.
45. Kindermann W, Simon G, Keul J. The significance of the aerobic–anaerobic transition for the determination of work load intensities during endurance training. *Eur J Appl Physiol Occup Physiol* 1979; 42: 25–34.
46. Seiler KS, Kjerland GO. Quantifying training intensity distribution in elite endurance athletes: is there evidence for an 'optimal' distribution? *Scand J Med Sci Sports* 2006; 16: 49–56.
47. Guellich A, Seiler S. Lactate profile changes in relation to training characteristics in junior elite cyclists. *Int J Sports Physiol Perform* 2010; 5: 316–27.
48. Steinacker JM, Lormes W, Lehmann M, Altenburg D. Training of rowers before world championships. *Med Sci Sport Exerc* 1998; 30: 1158–63.
49. Billat VL, Demarle A, Slawinski J, et al. Physical and training characteristics of top-class marathon runners. *Med Sci Sport Exerc* 2001; 33: 2089–97.
50. Schumacher YO, Mueller P. The 4000-m team pursuit cycling world record: theoretical and practical aspects. *Med Sci Sport Exerc* 2002; 34: 1029–36.
51. Jeppesen J, Kiens B. Regulation and limitations to fatty acid oxidation during exercise. *J Physiol* 2012; 590: 1059–68.
52. Horowitz JF, Klein S. Lipid metabolism during endurance exercise. *Am J Clin Nutr* 2000; 72(2 Suppl): 558–63S.
53. Beaver WL, Wasserman K, Whipp BJ. A new method for detecting anaerobic threshold by gas exchange. *J Appl Physiol (Bethesda Md, 1985)* 1986; 60: 2020–27.
54. Kunutsor SK, Kurl S, Khan H, et al. Associations of cardiovascular and all-cause mortality events with oxygen uptake at ventilatory threshold. *Int J Cardiol* 2017; 236: 444–50.
55. Beaver WL, Wasserman K, Whipp BJ. Improved detection of lactate threshold during exercise using a log-log transformation. *J Appl Physiol (Bethesda Md, 1985)* 1985; 59: 1936–40.
56. van Hall G. Lactate kinetics in human tissues at rest and during exercise. *Acta Physiol* Aug 2010; 199: 499–508.
57. Brooks GA. Cell-cell and intracellular lactate shuttles. *J Physiol* 2009; 587(Pt 23): 5591–600.
58. Hoffman J. *Norms for Fitness, Performance, and Health*: Champaign, IL: Human Kinetics; 2006.
59. Knuttgen HG, Kraemer WJ. Terminology and measurement in exercise performance. *J Strength Cond Res* 1987; 1: 1–10.
60. Cardinale M, Newton R, Nosaka K. *Strength and Conditioning: Biological Principles and Practical Applications*. Chichester: John Wiley.
61. Hoffman JR, Kang J. Strength changes during an in-season resistance-training program for football. *J Strength Cond Res* 2003; 17: 109–14.
62. Pincivero DM, Lephart SM, Karunakara RA. Reliability and precision of isokinetic strength and muscular endurance for the quadriceps and hamstrings. *Int J Sports Med* 1997; 18: 113–17.
63. Wu X, Zhang S, Liu Y, et al. Do knee concentric and eccentric strength and sagittal-plane knee joint biomechanics differ between jumpers and non-jumpers in landing? *Hum Mov Sci* 2013; 32: 1299–1309.
64. Sattler T, Sekulic D, Spasic M, et al. Isokinetic knee strength qualities as predictors of jumping performance in high-level volleyball athletes: multiple regression approach. *J Sports Med Phys Fitness* 2016; 56: 60–9.
65. Gonzalez-Rave JM, Juarez D, Rubio-Arias JA, et al. Isokinetic leg strength and power in elite handball players. *J Hum Kinet* 2014; 41: 227–33.
66. Hatze H. Validity and reliability of methods for testing vertical jumping performance. *J Appl Biomech* 1998; 14: 127–40.
67. Bobbert MF, Gerritsen KG, Litjens MC, Van Soest AJ. Why is countermovement jump height greater than squat jump height? *Med Sci Sport Exerc* 1996; 28: 1402–12.
68. Walsh M, Arampatzis A, Schade F, Bruggemann GP. The effect of drop jump starting height and contact time on power, work

performed, and moment of force. *J Strength Cond Res* 2004; 18: 561–6.

69. Halson SL. Monitoring training load to understand fatigue in athletes. *Sports Med* 2014; 44(Suppl 2): S139–47.

70. Düking P, Hotho A, Holmberg HC, et al. Comparison of non-invasive individual monitoring of the training and health of athletes with commercially available wearable technologies. *Front Physiol* 2016; 7: 71.

71. Thompson W. Worldwide survey of fitness trends for 2015. What's driving the market? *ACSMs Health Fit J* 2014; 18: 8–17.

72. Hanuska A, Chandramohan B, Bellamy L, et al. *Smart Clothing Market Analysis*. Available at: https://scet.berkeley.edu/wp-content/uploads/Smart-Clothing-Market-Analysis-Report.pdf

73. Schutz Y, Chambaz A. Could a satellite-based navigation system (GPS) be used to assess the physical activity of individuals on earth? *Eur J Clin Nutr* 1997;51(5):338–339.

74. Cummins C, Orr R, O'Connor H, West C. Global positioning systems (GPS) and microtechnology sensors in team sports: a systematic review. *Sports Med* 2013; 43: 1025–42.

75. Kavanagh JJ, Menz HB. Accelerometry: a technique for quantifying movement patterns during walking. *Gait Posture* 2008; 28: 1–15.

76. Yang S, Li Q. Inertial sensor-based methods in walking speed estimation: a systematic review. *Sensors (Basel)* 2012; 12: 6102–16.

77. Chan ED, Chan MM, Chan MM. Pulse oximetry: understanding its basic principles facilitates appreciation of its limitations. *Respir Med* 2013; 107: 789–99.

78. Schafer A, Vagedes J. How accurate is pulse rate variability as an estimate of heart rate variability? A review on studies comparing photoplethysmographic technology with an electrocardiogram. *Int J Cardiol* 2013; 166: 15–29.

79. Spierer DK, Rosen Z, Litman LL, Fujii K. Validation of photoplethysmography as a method to detect heart rate during rest and exercise. *J Med Eng Technol* 2015; 39: 264–71.

80. Treskes RW, van der Velde ET, Barendse R, Bruining N. Mobile health in cardiology: a review of currently available medical apps and equipment for remote monitoring. *Expert Rev Med Devices* 2016; 13: 823–30.

81. Gregoski MJ, Mueller M, Vertegel A, et al. Development and validation of a smartphone heart rate acquisition application for health promotion and wellness telehealth applications. *Int J Telemed Appl* 2012; 2012: 696324.

82. Meystre S. The current state of telemonitoring: a comment on the literature. *Telemed J E Health* 2005;11: 63–9.

83. Du K., Privacy-aware remote mobile health and fitness monitoring: extending the functionality of the Berkeley Telemonitoring Framework. Berkeley: EECS Department, University of California; 2017. Available at: https://www2.eecs.berkeley.edu/Pubs/TechRpts/2017/EECS-2017-36.html

84. Chuang T-Y, Chen C-H, Chang H-A, et al. Virtual reality serves as a support technology in cardiopulmonary exercise testing. *Presence* 2003; 12: 326–31.

85. Vanhees L, De Sutter J, Gelada SN, et al. Importance of characteristics and modalities of physical activity and exercise in defining the benefits to cardiovascular health within the general population: recommendations from the EACPR (Part I). *Eur J Prev Cardiol* 2012; 19: 670–86.

86. Buchanan PA, Vardaxis VG. Lower-extremity strength profiles and gender-based classification of basketball players aged 9–22 years. *J Strength Cond Res* 2009; 23: 406–19.

SECTION 9

Cardiac safety at sports facilities

9.1 Resuscitation on the field: basic and advanced life support and automatic external defibrillators *403*
Mark S. Link and Mark Estes III

9.2 Cardiac safety at sports events: the medical action plan *411*
Luis Serratosa, Efraim Kramer, and Mats Börjesson

9.3 Cardiac safety at fitness centres *419*
Erik Ekker Solberg, Jakob Johansson, and Alessandro Biffi

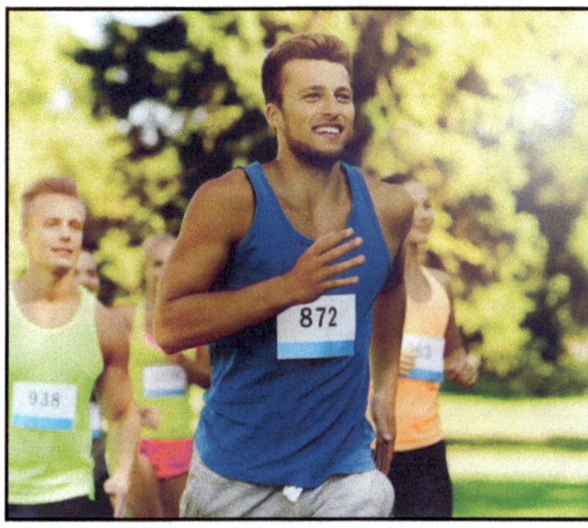

9.1

Resuscitation on the field: basic and advanced life support and automatic external defibrillators

Mark S. Link and Mark Estes III

Introduction

Resuscitation on the playing field is at least as important as screening for the prevention of sudden death. Even with a screening strategy which is effective, there will still be individuals with undetected structural heart disease who will suffer sudden cardiac arrest (SCA) [1]. In addition, there will be cardiac arrests in those athletes following undetectable cardiac conditions [2] and commotio cordis (sudden death with chest wall impact) [3–5]. An effective resuscitation strategy requires more than the presence of automated external defibrillators (AEDs) [6,7]. The most effective resuscitation strategies are pre-cardiac arrest planning and a comprehensive emergency action plan [7] (see Chapter 9.2). Coaches, training staff, and in our opinion all athletes should be able to provide cardiopulmonary resuscitation (CPR), and utilize AEDS [6]. AEDs and other appropriate equipment must be readily available and an emergency action plan must be in place to activate and call external emergency medical services [6,7]. For effective survival, the American Heart Association (AHA) and the European Society of Cardiology (ESC) call for immediate recognition of SCA, early CPR, rapid defibrillation, effective advanced life support, and integrated post-cardiac care [8–13]. Inadequacy in any one of these facets will reduce the chances of survival.

The likelihood of survival with good neurological status is directly related to the time between onset of cardiac arrest, implementation of CPR, and defibrillation. In the adequately prepared athletic environment, including both trained staff and appropriate equipment, and with a witnessed SCA, it is a reasonable goal to begin CPR within 60–90 seconds and deliver an initial shock in those with a shockable rhythm in less than 3–5 minutes. Indeed, in commotio cordis, survival has increased from less than 5% to more than 60% (➲ Fig. 9.1.1), due not only to increased recognition of SCA, but also to improved resuscitation attempts [14].

Initial response

Collapse on the field is a medical emergency and requires immediate assessment (➲ Fig. 9.1.2). The differential diagnosis of collapse is extensive, and includes exertional heat stroke, exertional hyponatraemia, exercise-associated collapse, seizure, syncope, and SCA. The initial assessment of a collapsed athlete includes the level of consciousness. Victims of exertional heat stroke, exertional hyponatraemia and exercise associated collapse will have an impaired level of consciousness, but will still be conscious. Athletes with syncope will generally wake up quickly, but those with seizure and SCA will remain unconscious. It is not generally difficult to differentiate seizure and SCA because of the increased muscular tone of the former and the flaccid tone of the latter. Occasionally, however, it is difficult to make the sometimes subtle distinctions between epilepsy-related seizures and the involuntary seizure-like movements associated with cardiac arrest. However, myotonic jerks associated with SCA will only last for a short time, while seizure activity will continue for some time. Although exertional heat stroke, exertional hyponatraemia, exercise-associated collapse, syncope, and seizure are all medical

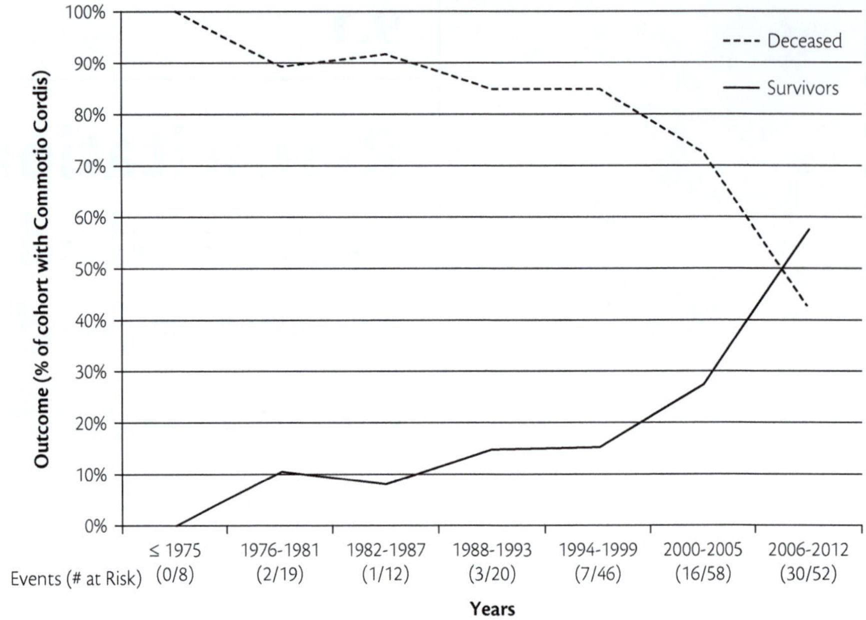

Fig. 9.1.1 Resuscitation in the commotio cordis registry has improved from less than 5% to over 60%. This improvement is probably a result of both improved recognition of sudden cardiac arrest and resuscitiation.

Reprinted from *Heart Rhythm*, Volume 10, Issue 2. Barry J. Maron, Tammy S. Haas, Aneesha Ahluwalia, Ross F. Garberich, N.A. Mark Estes, Mark S. Link. Increasing survival rate from commotio cordis, pp.219–223. Copyright (2013) with permission from Elsevier.

emergencies, it is the athlete with SCA who requires immediate attention or death will occur within minutes. Since sport-related cardiac arrest has a higher probability of being witnessed by appropriately trained bystander staff than does cardiac arrest in many other situations, a beneficial outcome is more likely if delays in recognition and responses are avoided.

A player/athlete who collapses on the field, without any preceding body contact (trauma), must be suspected of having an SCA, until proved otherwise. FIFA, for example, now allows the team physician to enter the field immediately in such cases, without asking the referee's permission (as previously was necessary), which is a new rule since 2014 (after the World Cup).

It is critical to determine quickly whether impaired consciousness is associated with loss of pulse and respiration, and if so to institute appropriate resuscitative therapy immediately. Distinguishing between true spontaneous respirations and gasping respirations is also important, as the are part of cardiac arrest physiology [15] that supports the recognition of true cardiac arrest and implies better survival probability.

Comprehensive emergency response plans are important [7] (see Chapter 9.2). The initial recognition of an arrest and immediate CPR must cascade into activation of the emergency response plan, which includes early access to a defibrillator and calls to the local emergency medical services. An emergency response plan includes preparation for cardiac arrests including anticipation of events, placement of AEDs and training of individuals to use them, access to emergency services, and simulations of real life events. Monthly AED checks for integrity and battery life are included in emergency response plans.

Basic life support for the athlete in cardiac arrest

If the pulse and spontaneous respirations are absent, a cardiac arrest is in progress. Critical initial steps in resuscitation are initiation of cardiopulmonary resuscitation (CPR) (➲ Fig. 9.1.3), activation of the emergency action plan, and calls for an AED. On the playing field there is rarely a shortage of individuals to perform these various actions. Current recommendations for CPR include a rate of 100–120 and compression depths of 5–6cm (2–2.5 inches) [8,16]. Additionally, full recoil of the chest should be allowed. Rescue breathing is not generally needed early in resuscitation because of the pre-arrest oxygenation of the blood and agonal breathing, which is frequent during the initial 5 minutes, especially with adults. Compression-only CPR has been shown to be as effective as a combination of compression and respiration, and certainly is more palatable to many first responders [17]. Compression-only CPR also has the advantage of simplicity, and thus mental and physical retention of technique. High quality CPR has the capacity to provide blood and oxygen flow to the brain for quite some time, as was exhibited in the resuscitation of Fabrice Muamba who had CPR for 78 minutes—both he and his brain survived. It is our opinion that all involved with sports,

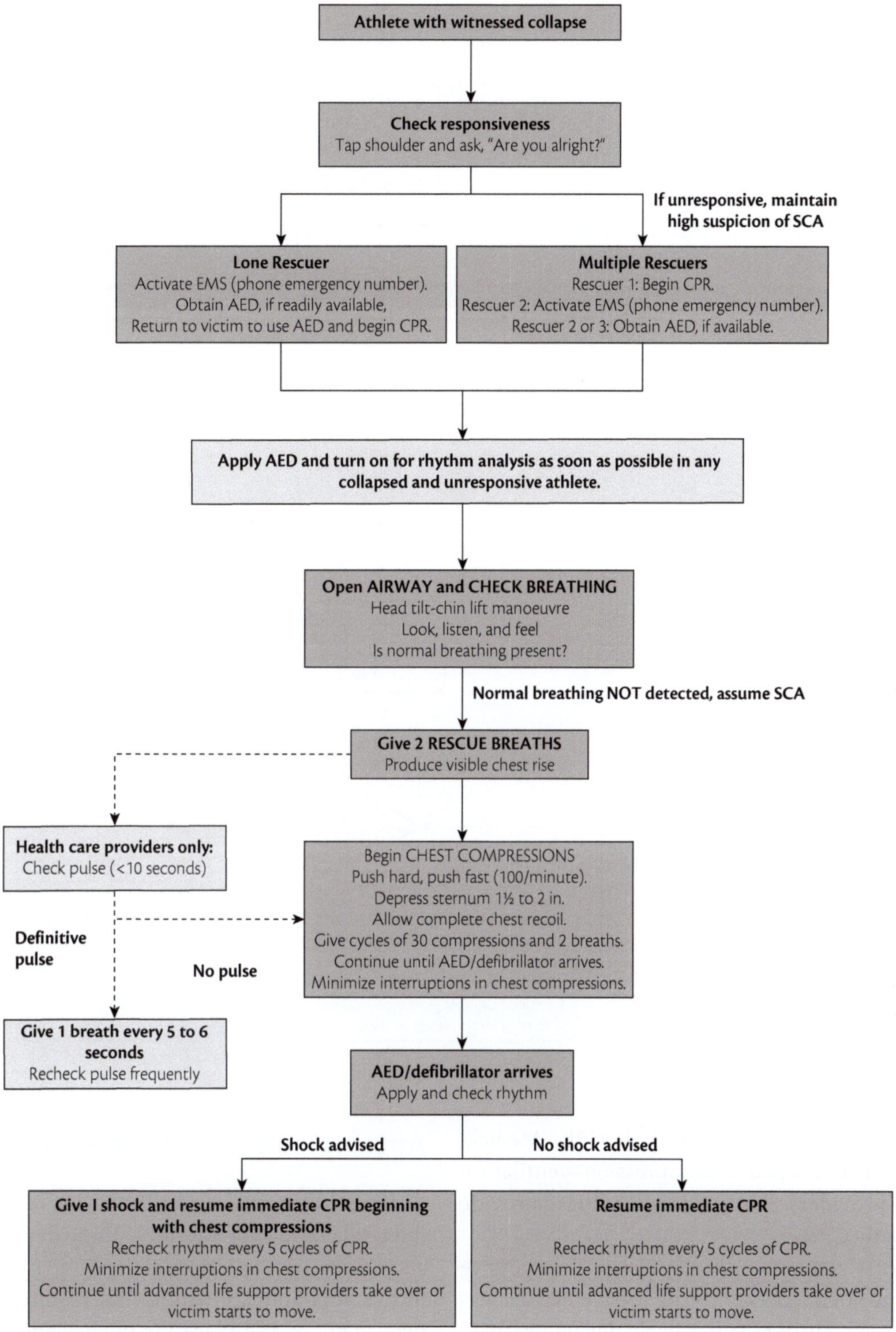

Fig. 9.1.2 Flow diagram of the approach to a collapsed athlete.

Reprinted from *Heart Rhythm*, Volume 4, Issue 4, Jonathan A. Drezner, Ron W. Courson, William O. Roberts, Vincent N. Mosesso, Mark S. Link, Barry J. Maron. Inter-Association Task Force Recommendations on Emergency Preparedness and Management of Sudden Cardiac Arrest in High School and College Athletic Programs: A Consensus Statement, pp.549–565. Copyright (2007) with permission from Elsevier.

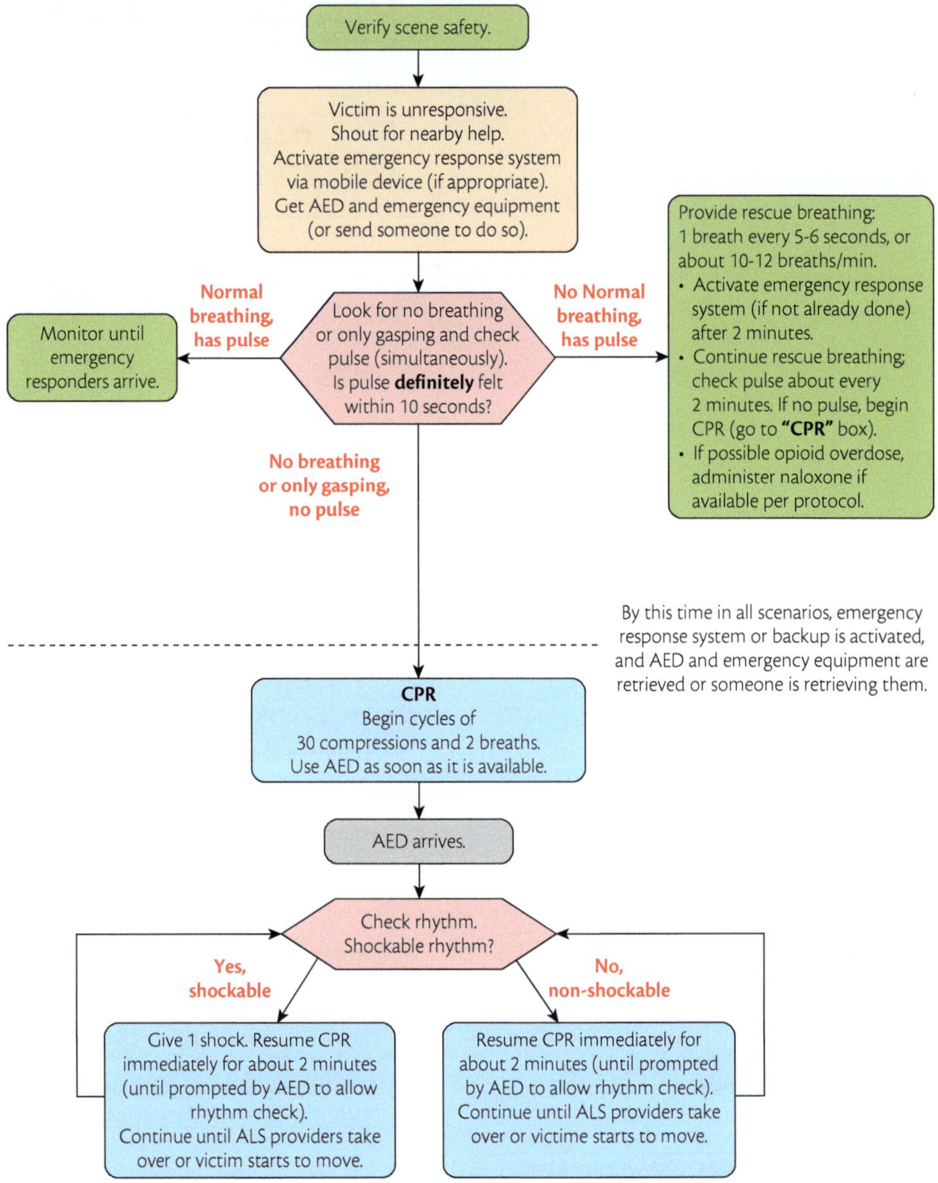

Fig. 9.1.3 BLS Adult Cardiac Arrest Algorithm 2015

Copyright American Heart Association 2010, Fig 1. http://circ.ahajournals.org/content/122/18_suppl_3/S685.figures-only

including players, should be trained in CPR. Medical providers should be trained in compression–ventilation CPR, while lay providers should at least be able to provide compression-only CPR.

In some sports settings, primarily during competitive events with large attendances, a rescue vehicle may be stationed at the scene, but that is less likely during practices or sports events in small facilities. In any cardiac arrest, both security personnel and fire rescue should be contacted immediately.

It is our opinion that all coaches, trainers, and even athletes should be trained in recognition of SCA and performance of CPR. Certification of Basic Life Support is provided by many organizations, including the American Heart Association and the International Red Cross.

Automated external defibrillators

Automated external defibrillators are increasingly becoming available at sports venues. These devices have excellent success in the detection and termination of ventricular tachycardia and fibrillation. All require human input to turn them on and place the defibrillation pads. Some are fully automated, i.e. they analyse the rhythm and shock if the arrhythmia is deemed shockable. However, most are semi-automated in that analysis of the rhythm requires human activation and then further activation if the arrhythmia is deemed shockable. Evidence of their efficacy in resuscitation comes from casinos and airlines, with successful resuscitation in up to 74% of individuals with a shockable rhythm [18,19]. AEDs are now available in up to

90% of high school and collegiate sporting venues in the USA [20,21].

The sensitivity and specificity of AEDs is excellent, and almost certainly better than physician analysis [16]. In ventricular arrhythmia libraries, the sensitivity and specificity of most devices approaches 100% [16,22]. Although manufacturers' algorithms are proprietary and thus not directly comparable, the accuracy appears similar. Correction for CPR artefact is a goal, as then CPR could continue during analysis of the rhythm. Some devices will also analyse for the quality of the CPR, including compression depth and rate. Although energy outputs and waveforms differ among manufacturers, it is not clear if one is superior to the other; defibrillation efficacy is generally excellent.

AED use in children is recommended, using paediatric dose attenuator systems and paediatric pads, if available, for children aged 1–8 years [16,22]. However, if these are not available, using an adult AED is preferable to waiting for a paediatric AED to arrive. AEDs can be used in wet environments without concern for injury or shock to bystanders. In these situations the major limiting factor is adhesion of the pads to a wet torso. Drying the skin with towels is necessary prior to the placement of the pads. AEDs cannot be placed in isolation but rather must be part of a resuscitation programme. They require routine maintenance, including monthly battery life and system integrity checks; in addition, pads have a limited shelf-life span of approximately two years.

As soon as possible the AED is turned on, pads are placed, and rhythm analysis is performed [11]. If a shockable rhythm is found, a single shock should be delivered followed immediately by CPR [13.23]. After 2 minutes of CPR, rhythm analysis by the AED should be performed again, with additional shock if called for. A pulse check should also be attempted during the AED analysis. If the initial AED analysis does not call for a shock, CPR should be performed with repeat AED analysis every 2 minutes.

Advanced cardiac life support

Once emergency rescue personnel and equipment are on the scene, advanced life support activities are implemented as needed (➲ Fig. 9.1.4). These will include pharmacological interventions and respiratory management. European and American guidelines were updated in 2015 [12,24]. It is important to recognize that there is very little evidence that pharmacological management improves survival in SCA. Epinephrine (adrenaline) is perhaps the best studied drug in cardiac arrest but, despite a multitude of studies, the evidence of its benefit in cardiac arrest is scant. One randomized controlled trial (RCT) of standard dose epinephrine found improved survival to hospital admission and improved return of spontaneous circulation (ROSC) when it was used; however, there was no benefit in survival to discharge and survival to discharge with good neurological outcome [25]. Observational studies which evaluated epinephrine in SCA provided conflicting results [26,27]. There is a little more evidence for epinephrine in non-shockable rhythms in that early administration improves survival [28,29]. Therefore epinephrine remains in resuscitation algorithms. However, vasopressin has been dropped from the American and European guidelines because it has no benefit compared with epinephrine [24,30]. Blinded RCTs in patients with refractory SCA demonstrated that amiodarone improved survival to hospital admission, but there was no difference in hospital discharge or neurological survival [31,32]. However, amiodarone remains in both sets of guidelines.

In observational studies individuals with bag–mask ventilation generally had a higher survival rate than intubated patients, but this clearly could be biased [22]. Current guidelines recommend either bag–mask or advanced airways if the provider is comfortable with their insertion. If intubation is performed, continuous waveform capnography after intubation is the most accurate means of assessing placement of the airway.

Post-resuscitation care

Post-arrest care has developed into a field of its own. Targeted temperature management in comatose patients resuscitated from a shockable rhythm has been demonstrated to improve survival. While targeted temperature management once referred to hypothermia, cooling to 32°C, a recently published large RCT demonstrated no difference in survival between those cooled to 36°C and 32°C. Given the benefit of cooling, most resuscitated comatose patients, including those resuscitated from asystole and pulseless electrical activity (PEA), should be cooled to at least 36°C.

Conclusion

Appropriate recognition and treatment of a cardiac arrest victim will increase the odds of survival. It is our opinion that athletes, trainers, and coaches should all be trained in CPR and AED use. An emergency action plan is critical in order to render advanced life support as soon as possible.

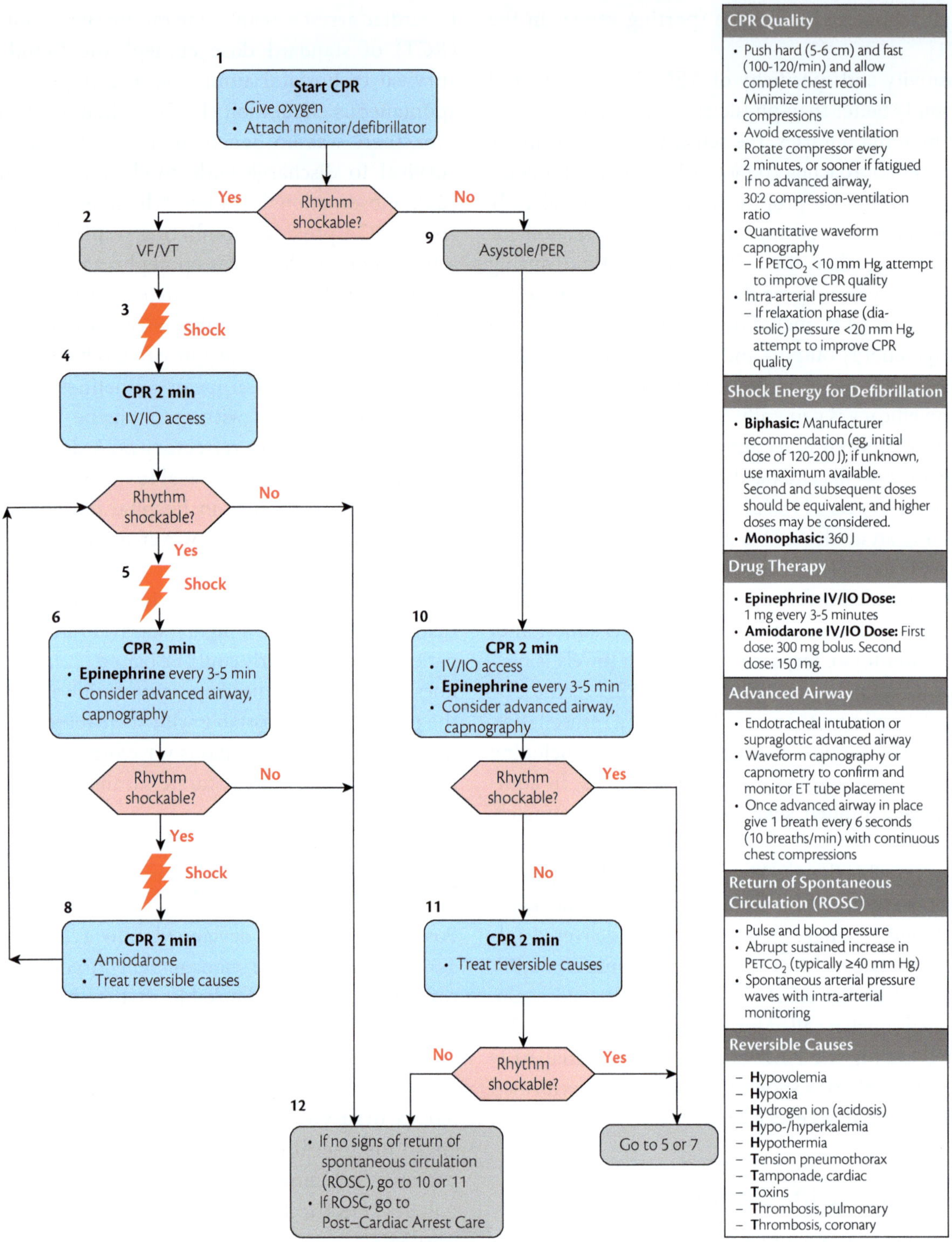

Fig. 9.1.4 Adult Cardiac Arrest Algorithm.

Further reading

Drezner JA, Courson RW, Roberts WO, et al. Inter-association task force recommendations on emergency preparedness and management of sudden cardiac arrest in high school and college athletic programs: a consensus statement. *Heart Rhythm* 2007; 4: 549–65.

Drezner JA, Rogers KJ, Horneff JG. Automated external defibrillator use at NCAA Division II and III universities. *Br J Sports Med* 2011; 45: 1174–8.

Kleinman ME, Brennan EE, Goldberger ZD, et al. Part 5: Adult basic life support and cardiopulmonary resuscitation quality. 2015 American Heart Association guidelines update for cardiopulmonary resuscitation and emergency cardiovascular care. *Circulation* 2015; 132: S414–35.

Lawless CE, Asplund C, Asif IM, et al. Protecting the heart of the American athlete. *J Am Coll Cardiol* 2014 ;64: 2146–71.

Link MS, Berkow LC, Kudenchuk PJ, et al. Part 7: Adult advanced cardiovascular life support. 2015 American Heart Association guidelines update for cardiopulmonary resuscitation and emergency cardiovascular care. *Circulation* 2015; 132: S444–64.

Link MS, Myerburg RJ, Estes NA 3rd. Eligibility and disqualification recommendations for competitive athletes with cardiovascular abnormalities. Task Force 12: Emergency action plans, resuscitation, cardiopulmonary resuscitation, and automated external defibrillators. *J Am Coll Cardiol* 2015; 66: 2434–8.

Neumar RW, Shuster M, Callaway CW, et al. Part 1: Executive summary: 2015 American Heart Association guidelines update for cardiopulmonary resuscitation and emergency cardiovascular care. *Circulation* 2015; 132: S315–67.

Perkins GD, Handley AJ, Koster RW, et al. European Resuscitation Council guidelines for resuscitation 2015. Section 2. Adult basic life support and automated external defibrillation. *Resuscitation* 2015; 95: 81–99

References

1. Lawless CE, Asplund C, Asif IM, et al. Protecting the heart of the American athlete. *J Am Coll Cardiol* 2014 ;64: 2146–71.
2. Krahn AD, Healey JS, Chauhan V, et al. Systematic assessment of patients with unexplained cardiac arrest: Cardiac Arrest Survivors with Preserved Ejection Fraction Registry (CASPER). *Circulation* 2009; 120: 278–85.
3. Link MS, Wang PJ, Pandian NG, et al. An experimental model of sudden death due to low-energy chest-wall impact (commotio cordis). *N Engl J Med* 1998; 338: 1805–11.
4. Maron BJ, Estes NA 3rd. Commotio cordis. *N Engl J Med*. 2010; 362: 917–27.
5. Link MS, Estes NA 3rd, Maron BJ. Eligibility and disqualification recommendations for competitive athletes with cardiovascular abnormalities. Task Force 13: Commotio cordis. *Circulation* 2015; 132:e339–42.
6. Link MS, Myerburg RJ, Estes NA 3rd. Eligibility and disqualification recommendations for competitive athletes with cardiovascular abnormalities. Task Force 12: Emergency action plans, resuscitation, cardiopulmonary resuscitation, and automated external defibrillators. *J Am Coll Cardiol* 2015; 66: 2434–8.
7. Drezner JA, Courson RW, Roberts WO, et al. Inter-association task force recommendations on emergency preparedness and management of sudden cardiac arrest in high school and college athletic programs: a consensus statement. *Heart Rhythm* 2007; 4: 549–65.
8. Field JM, Hazinski MF, Sayre MR, et al. Part 1: Executive summary. 2010 American Heart Association guidelines for cardiopulmonary resuscitation and emergency cardiovascular care. *Circulation* 2010; 122: S640–56.
9. Travers AH, Rea TD, Bobrow BJ, et al. Part 4: CPR overview: 2010 American Heart Association guidelines for cardiopulmonary resuscitation and emergency cardiovascular care. *Circulation* 2010; 122: S676–84.
10. Monsieurs KG, Nolan JP, Bossaert LL, et al. European Resuscitation Council guidelines for resuscitation 2015. Section 1. Executive summary. *Resuscitation* 2015; 95: 1–80.
11. Jacobs I, Sunde K, Deakin CD, et al. Part 6: Defibrillation: 2010 international consensus on cardiopulmonary resuscitation and emergency cardiovascular care science with treatment recommendations. *Circulation* 2010; 122: S325–37.
12. Neumar RW, Shuster M, Callaway CW, et al. Part 1: Executive summary: 2015 American Heart Association guidelines update for cardiopulmonary resuscitation and emergency cardiovascular care. *Circulation* 2015; 132: S315–67.
13. Kleinman ME, Brennan EE, Goldberger ZD, et al. Part 5: Adult basic life support and cardiopulmonary resuscitation quality. 2015 American Heart Association guidelines update for cardiopulmonary resuscitation and emergency cardiovascular care. *Circulation* 2015; 132: S414–35.
14. Maron BJ, Haas TS, Ahluwalia A, et al. Increasing survival rate from commotio cordis. *Heart Rhythm*. 2013; 10: 219–223
15. Bobrow BJ, Zuercher M, Ewy GA, et al. Gasping during cardiac arrest in humans is frequent and associated with improved survival. *Circulation* 2008; 118: 2550–4.
16. Link MS, Atkins DL, Passman RS, et al Part 6: Electrical therapies: automated external defibrillators, defibrillation, cardioversion, and pacing. 2010 American Heart Association guidelines for cardiopulmonary resuscitation and emergency cardiovascular care. *Circulation* 2010; 122: S706–19.
17. Rea TD, Fahrenbruch C, Culley L, et al. CPR with chest compression alone or with rescue breathing. *N Engl J Med* 2010; 363: 423–33.
18. Valenzuela TD, Roe DJ, Nichol G, et al. Outcomes of rapid defibrillation by security officers after cardiac arrest in casinos. *N Engl J Med* 2000; 343: 1206–9.
19. Page RL, Joglar JA, Kowal RC, et al. Use of automated external defibrillators by a u.S. Airline. *N Engl J Med* 2000; 343: 1210–16.
20. Drezner JA, Rogers KJ, Horneff JG. Automated external defibrillator use at NCAA Division II and III Universities. *Br J Sports Med* 2011; 45: 1174–8.
21. Toresdahl BG, Rao AL, Harmon KG, Drezner JA. Incidence of sudden cardiac arrest in high school student athletes on school campus. *Heart Rhythm* 2014; 11: 1190–4
22. Link MS, Berkow LC, Kudenchuk PJ, et al. Part 7: Adult advanced cardiovascular life support. 2015 American Heart Association guidelines update for cardiopulmonary resuscitation and emergency cardiovascular care. *Circulation* 2015; 132: S444–64.
23. Perkins GD, Handley AJ, Koster RW, et al. European Resuscitation Council guidelines for resuscitation 2015. Section 2: Adult basic life support and automated external defibrillation. *Resuscitation* 2015; 95: 81–99.
24. Soar J, Nolan JP, Bottiger BW, et al. European Resuscitation Council guidelines for resuscitation 2015. Section 3: Adult advanced life support. *Resuscitation* 2015; 95: 100–47
25. Jacobs IG, Finn JC, Jelinek GA, et al. Effect of adrenaline on survival in out-of-hospital cardiac arrest: a randomised double-blind placebo-controlled trial. *Resuscitation* 2011; 82: 1138–43
26. Hagihara A, Hasegawa M, Abe T, et al. Prehospital epinephrine use and survival among patients with out-of-hospital cardiac arrest. *JAMA* 2012; 307: 1161–8.

27. Machida M, Miura S, Matsuo K, et al. Effect of intravenous adrenaline before arrival at the hospital in out-of-hospital cardiac arrest. *J Cardiol* 2012; 60: 503–7
28. Goto Y, Maeda T, Goto Y. Effects of prehospital epinephrine during out-of-hospital cardiac arrest with initial non-shockable rhythm: an observational cohort study. *Crit Care* 2013; 17: R188.
29. Nakahara S, Tomio J, Nishida M, et al. Association between timing of epinephrine administration and intact neurologic survival following out-of-hospital cardiac arrest in Japan: a population-based prospective observational study. *Acad Emerg Med* 2012; 19: 782–92.
30. Mukoyama T, Kinoshita K, Nagao K, Tanjoh K. Reduced effectiveness of vasopressin in repeated doses for patients undergoing prolonged cardiopulmonary resuscitation. *Resuscitation* 2009; 80: 755–61.
31. Kudenchuk PJ, Cobb LA, Copass MK, et al. Amiodarone for resuscitation after out-of-hospital cardiac arrest due to ventricular fibrillation. *N Engl J Med* 1999; 341: 871–8.
32. Dorian P, Cass D, Schwartz B, et al. Amiodarone as compared with lidocaine for shock-resistant ventricular fibrillation. *N Engl J Med* 2002; 346: 884–90.

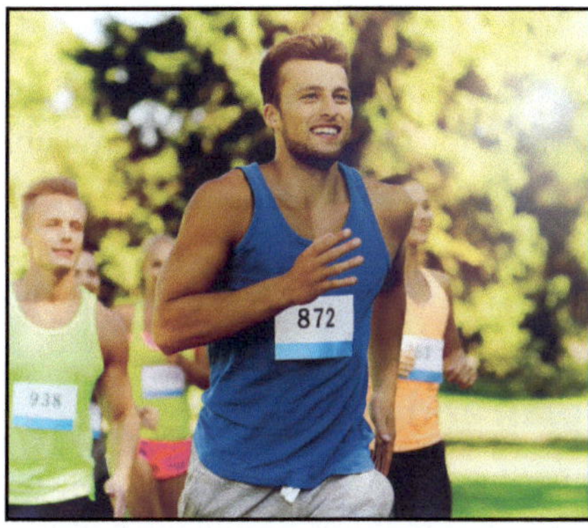

9.2

Cardiac safety at sports events: the medical action plan

Luis Serratosa, Efraim Kramer, and Mats Börjesson

Introduction

The aim of all sport arena safety measures is to ensure safe participation for the athlete, as well as caring for the spectators in this complex environment. Specifically, the present chapter deals with cardiac medical services planning, in and around a sports stadium or arena, in order to provide safe, effective, efficient, and coordinated management of any sudden cardiac arrest (SCA). The general recommendations presented are broad based in order to allow the reader to adapt them to the size and specifics of the sports environment concerned. Thus it is important to individualize the specific needs of both small and large arenas, with the common aim of providing adequate emergency care measures within the first few minutes of an SCA, without attempting to provide 'one recipe for all'.

Mass gathering medical care is defined as emergency health-care services provided to spectators and participants in events where at least 1000 persons are gathered at a specific location for a defined period of time [1]. As in other mass gathering events, sports arenas usually gather several thousands of people during a specific period of time, creating challenges not only related to medical care for both athletes and spectators inside the stadium, but also affecting local (non-event-related) health-care resources (pre-hospital emergency medical services and hospitals).

Because of the increased physical and/or emotional stress, the risk of cardiac events may be increased in both athletes [2] and spectators [3–6], typically in those with underlying cardiovascular disease. However, the effect of emotional stress on the incidence of cardiac events among spectators remains controversial [7,8]. The reported incidence of SCA among spectators ranges from 0.17 [9] to 0.25 [10], or even 0.38 [11], per 100.000 spectators. This means that a medium to large sports arena is likely to have a number of SCA events per season [12].

A coordinated response with early and effective CPR and defibrillation is key to improving survival from out-of-hospital SCA [13]. Placing automated external defibrillators (AEDs) in areas where one cardiac arrest per 5 years can be expected is considered to be cost-effective [13], and AED programmes should be actively implemented in public places such as sports arenas. By introducing the 'chain of survival', having trained rescuers able to deliver early and effective CPR, and providing access to early defibrillation within 3–5 minutes of collapse, survival rates from out-of-hospital SCA can be as high as 70% [13–15].

Hence, in the clinical context of sports arenas, the German Football League's study showed impressive resuscitation success rates, with 96% of the 52 patients who suffered an SCA being transported to hospital with spontaneous circulation [10]. These results were related to well-organized and adequately trained emergency medical services, able to provide short response times and support the need to implement effective strategies for emergency cardiac care in large sporting arenas. Disappointingly, the 2005–2006 season European Arena study showed that as many as 28% of the participating First and Second Division football clubs did not have an AED available in the arena, 36% did not have a written medical action plan (MAP), and 35% did not have a CPR training programme for personnel [9].

As a result of these findings, in 2011 the Section of Sports Cardiology of the European Association for Cardiovascular Prevention and Rehabilitation (EACPR) published a consensus document regarding cardiovascular safety at sports arenas [16], which is expected to be implemented by major sporting bodies. Before this, the only comprehensive document available was that published in 2000 by the National Association of Emergency Medical Services Physicians (NAEMSP) of the USA to assist emergency medical service (EMS) physicians with planning emergency medical care at mass gathering events [17]. More recently, FIFA has published recommendations on mass gathering football emergency medicine, in the second edition of the *Football Emergency Medicine Manual* [18]. Based on existing scientific data and expert consensus, all these documents propose minimum standards for the delivery of emergency medical services at sports mass gathering events.

Ensuring an adequate and timely response to life-threatening cardiac events, for both athletes and spectators in sports arenas, is a common aim of all recommendations and thus for the present chapter.

Unique characteristics of sport mass gathering emergency medical care

There are several aspects that make mass gathering medical care in arenas different from standard emergency medical services, and these have to be considered in planning:

- medical personnel will usually need to navigate large crowds and architectural barriers (fences, lifts, ramps, etc.) that will interfere with providing adequate emergency medical care and meet response times (➲ Fig. 9.2.1);
- architectural barriers may prevent use of motorized transport (➲ Fig. 9.2.2);
- weather conditions (i.e. rain, snow, extreme temperatures);
- patients refusing to receive medical care and hostility from surrounding spectators or between rival fans may complicate the working environment;
- VIP medical care;
- potential for terrorist acts and mass casualty incidents needing greater demand for medical care than available resources and initial triage of casualties;
- communication challenges.

Medical action plan and event planning

As in any mass gathering event, organizing emergency medical care in sports arenas requires producing a written description of the medical resources available and providing detailed plans for its use. This MAP should be specifically tailored to each venue and ideally adjusted for each event.

For practical purposes, the majority of medium-sized or larger sport stadiums and arenas can be divided into two specific functional areas, namely the competitions area (CA) and the non-competitions area (NCA). Because of security considerations, the CA comprises those areas of a stadium where the particular sports are actually undertaken and the area inside the stadium structure comprising changing rooms, officials' offices, doping control room, VIP lounges, etc. Specific accreditation passes are generally required in order to gain access to these areas. The NCA comprises the spectator seating area (SSA), commercial vendor areas, hospitality areas, and public display areas, and in certain locations the parking areas in and around the stadium.

Any stadium medical emergency planning, specifically that related to the response and initial management of an SCA, is critically time dependent, must ensure safety of the patient, rescuers, and surrounding spectators, and ensure the safe and efficient transfer of the patient away from the site of collapse to the nearest and most appropriate medical facility.

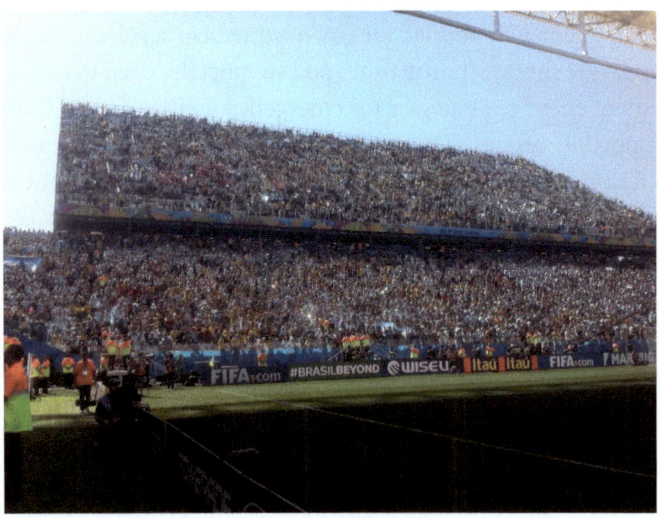

Fig. 9.2.1 Large arena, full-capacity crowd.

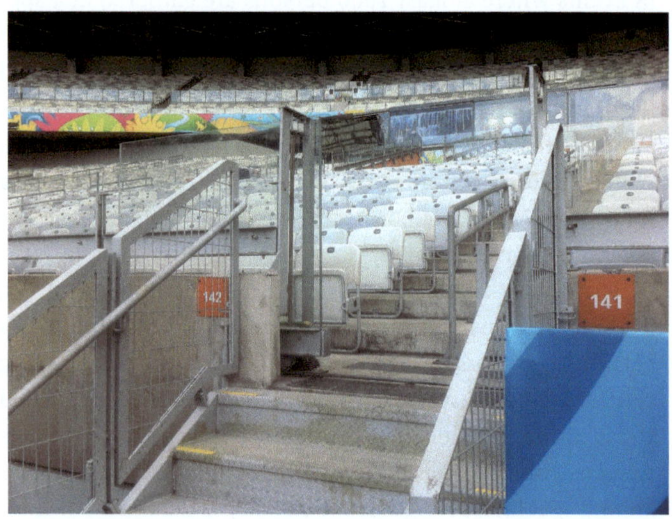

Fig. 9.2.2 Stairs and other obstacles may be present in the arena.

Minimally, the MAP should address the following aspects:

- responsibilities and contact information, of the appointed event medical director
- roles and responsibilities of all medical and healthcare human resources
- medical equipment including AEDs
- treatment facilities
- transportation
- communications
- documentation
- continuous quality improvement and training
- coordination with local health-care resources.

A licensed physician, experienced in out-of-hospital medical care and familiar with the local health-care resources (EMS and hospitals), acting as medical director, will positively impact decision-making and transportation and should be mandated for every arena of sufficient size. The medical director should always be available via some form of communication modality, especially to all EMS personnel. He or she should maintain open and continuous communication with the EMS representative located inside the venue operations centre (VOC) of large arenas (➔ Fig. 9.2.3).

The distance and predicted transport times to the nearest hospital should be timed and stated in the MAP. Open communication and collaboration with the local EMS and nearest hospital will improve patient outcomes and allow for follow-up of critically ill patients transported to the hospital.

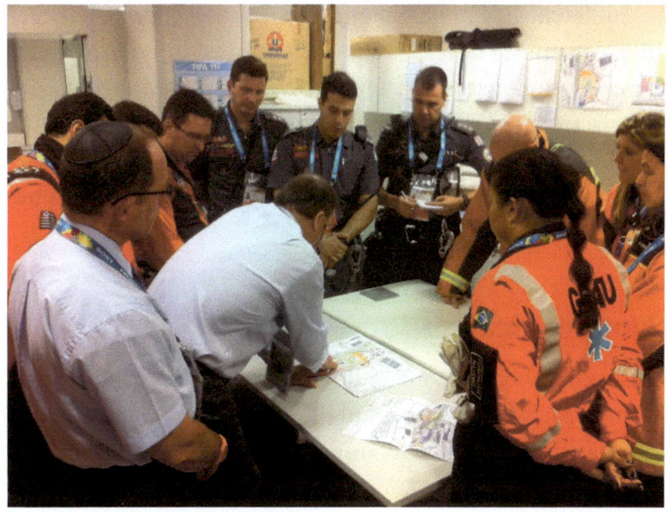

Fig. 9.2.3 Medical director at work with his crew.

A map of the venue with locations of all health-care resources (mobile medical teams (MMTs), medical care posts, advanced life support (ALS) medical centres, basic life support (BLS) and ALS ambulances, and AEDs) may be very useful for all the EMS personnel, as both a guide during the event and for pre- and post-event debriefing sessions (➔ Fig. 9.2.4).

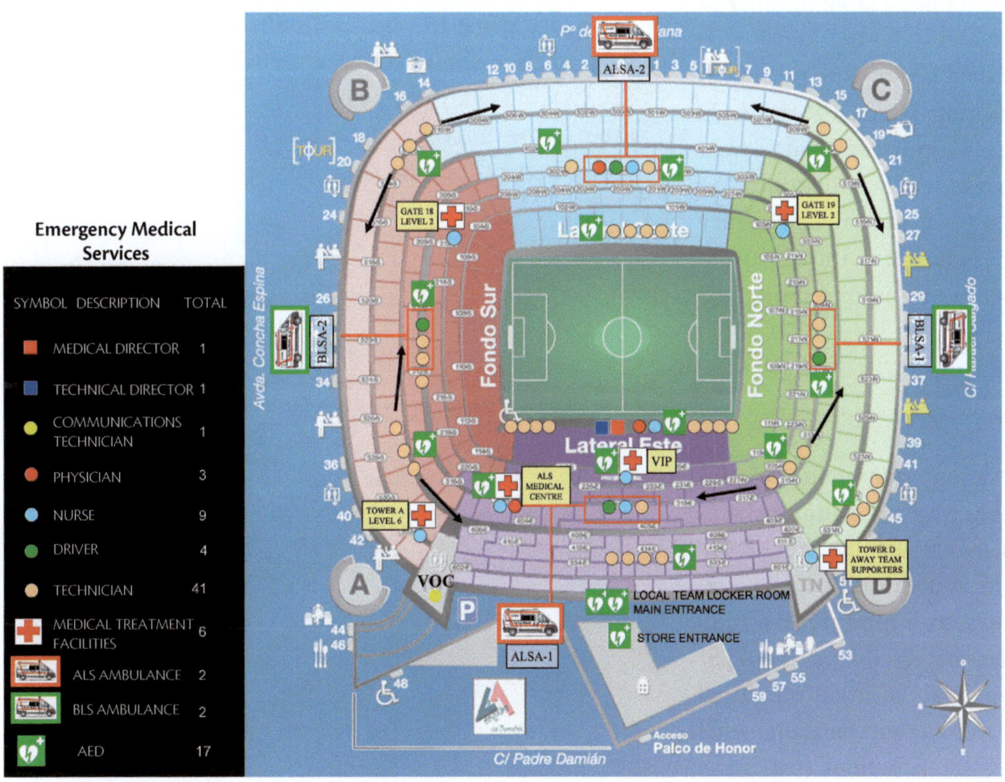

Fig. 9.2.4 EMS map of a football stadium with a capacity of 80,000 spectators.

Sufficient EMS general and professional (personnel) liability insurance coverage should be agreed upon in advance by event organizers and EMS providers. When media contact is required, the medical director could be designated as the spokesperson. All EMS personnel should remember that their duty to protect confidentiality remains at all times, including after a patient's death.

Time-critical response

It is recognized that one of the single most important determining factors for successful SCA management is the time from patient collapse to initiation of CPR and first AED shock, when indicated. Within a sports stadium, the overwhelming majority of SCA events will probably be witnessed, potentially allowing for almost immediate CPR activation and basic life support (BLS) (CPR + AED competent medical team) response within the required goal of 3–5 minutes.

Medical and health-care personnel

Timely response to a collapsed, possible SCA, patient with initial cardiac resuscitation and subsequent transfer from the site of collapse, with or without return of spontaneous circulation (ROSC), requires an adequate number of medical and allied health-care personnel who are sufficiently qualified, skilled, and experienced. They must be well adapted to the pre-hospital medical environment and also to that of a large multi-level arena, designed to hold a large number of participants.

The majority of medical and allied health-care personnel on duty will be BLS-qualified, encompassing CPR and AED training. These initial responders to a collapse need to wear appropriately visible uniforms for immediate identification by spectators and should be equipped with the necessary BLS medical and communication equipment, thus ensuring expeditious medical team recognition, response, and BLS treatment (➔ Fig. 9.2.5).

Medical equipment

The appropriate cardiac resuscitation equipment required for management of an SCA within a sports stadium structure encompasses the equipment carried by the MMTs and the equipment within the fixed medical posts or centres of larger arenas. This requires, as a minimum, a fully functional AED and, where necessary, such as in the ALS/ICU medical centre, an ALS type manual multifunctional defibrillator/synchronized cardioverter/transcutaneous pacemaker with accessory diagnostic functions (e.g. pulse oximetry) (➔ Fig. 9.2.6). If only older monophasic defibrillators are available for use within the sports stadium, this is practically and logistically acceptable, as is the use of defibrillator paddles and gel, rather than self-adhesive pads, as long as adequate safety precautions are undertaken during defibrillator shocks.

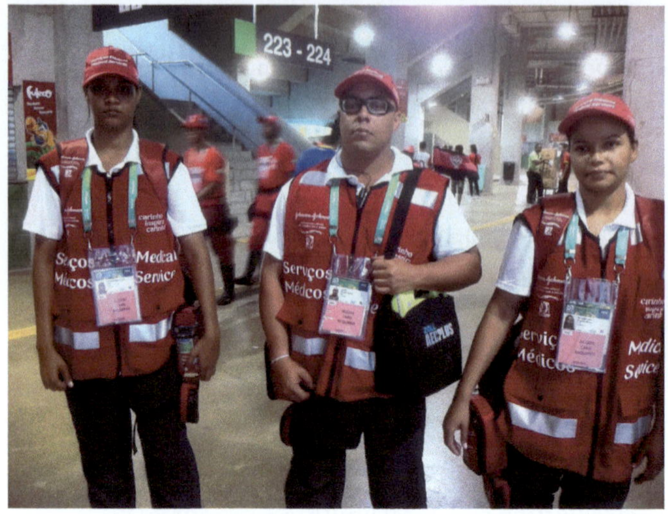

Fig. 9.2.5 Medical personnel.

The use of emergency medical cardiac equipment for the management of SCA within a sports stadium may have to be adapted, in specific conditions, in order to ensure safety.

- CPR + AED use in wet conditions (rain) is considered safe [19].
- Adequate space to position the patient horizontal on a hard surface for effective external chest compressions (ECCs). This may not be possible if a patient collapses in their seat within the SSA because of the minimal available space. It may then be necessary to speedily transfer the

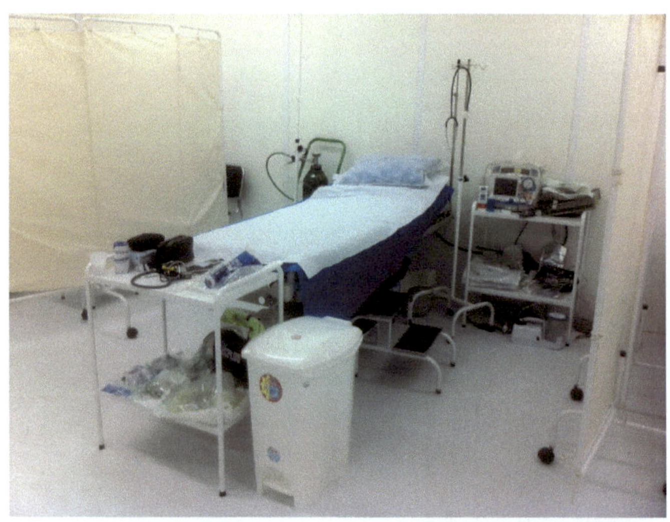

Fig. 9.2.6 Equipment for medical room.

SCA patient from their seat or collapsed area to the nearest steps and lay them down horizontally before ECC can be effectively initiated and AED pads applied for rhythm analysis. The technique for lifting an unconscious pulseless patient from within the seated area requires training and regular practice.

- Consideration must be given to limited exposure of the chest in females, particularly in certain locations, especially when there is no privacy or confidentiality in a crowded SSA. It is recommended that a small towel is added to the BLS medical bag for use on female SCA patients.
- Consideration must be given to the presence of vomiting during cardiac resuscitation, its appropriate waste removal, and infection control. The same applies to the establishment of peripheral venous access and the safe removal of all items and body waste.
- Consideration should be given to the various causes of cardiac arrest, particularly within a sports stadium, which may require various adaptations to the normal clinical protocol practised, namely lightning strike cardiac arrest, multiple patient cardiac arrest during a stadium stampede, insect envenomation with anaphylactic cardiac arrest, etc.

Mobile medical teams

Although it is common practice to establish a hierarchy of medical care within a stadium structure (encompassing everything from MMTs and primary health-care medical posts to advanced life support/intensive medical care centres), the main overall SCA response and resuscitation will be performed by the MMTs within the stadium environment.

Therefore, for any resuscitation to be successfully undertaken safely, practically, and logistically, the appropriate number of highly visible, currently certified, adequately equipped, stadium-orientated, and well-rehearsed teams of BLS responders should be calculated, according to each arena (size, geography, barriers). They must be on site when activated by a patient collapse. These MMTs should be able to speedily and safely respond to and gain access to the collapsed patient anywhere within the stadium structure, including the crowded spectator seating stands. Once on site, the MMT should be able to safely and immediately initiate CPR + AED or efficiently transfer the SCA patient to a nearby area which is both safe and sufficient for CPR + AED application. To be able to safely, satisfactorily, and successfully respond, resuscitate, and if necessary remove the SCA patient in an often crowded stadium structure, while carrying a BLS medical bag, an AED, and a rigid patient-carrying device, involves planning, training, and regular rehearsals.

Depending on the size and architectural design of the sports stadium and any external environmental medical service responsibility (e.g. parking areas, hospitality tents, public displays, etc.), additional MMTs using bicycles, motorcycles, or modified motorized stretcher-carrying carts (simple or off-road) may also be considered.

Patient transfer/transport

Once cardiac resuscitation has been in progress for a period of time, it is necessary to plan the evacuation of the patient from the site of CPR and/or AED use. This may require transfer of the patient who has attained ROSC to the stadium ALS medical centre for immediate post-resuscitation stabilization and care, or alternatively direct referral to the nearest and most appropriate medical facility, the latter typically in smaller arenas. However, it may also be necessary to transfer a patient who has not yet attained ROSC for reasons which may include safety, crowd considerations, need for upgraded clinical management at the ALS medical centre, or termination of resuscitation in privacy.

In a patient who has gained ROSC, transfer logistics include use of an immobilizing patient carriage device so that CPR + AED use can be restarted immediately if ROSC is lost during transfer. This entails considering various potential difficulties, namely stairs, ramps, and lifts which, if not considered during the planning and practice phase, may cause major logistical problems, to ensure safe and appropriate patient transfer within or out of the stadium to waiting ambulances which cannot directly access the patient because of structural limitations (➲ Fig. 9.2.7). Carriage of an unconscious patient from the SSA, using a long spinal board type device, maintaining a constant horizontal position whilst negotiating a 33° or 45° incline, should be planned and practised beforehand in order to determine the required manpower. The traditional four-person team required to carry a patient horizontally on a long trauma spinal board may in fact need to be increased to 10 persons to undertake the same task down inclined SSA steps.

Furthermore, if the SCA patient has not successfully achieved ROSC and transfer is thought to be most appropriate, this will not only entail carriage of the pulseless patient horizontally on a long trauma spinal board, but will also require mandatory continuous competent chest compressions, rescue ventilation, and AED analysis and shocks. This requires coordination and control, ensuring that ECC and rescue ventilations are undertaken continuously,

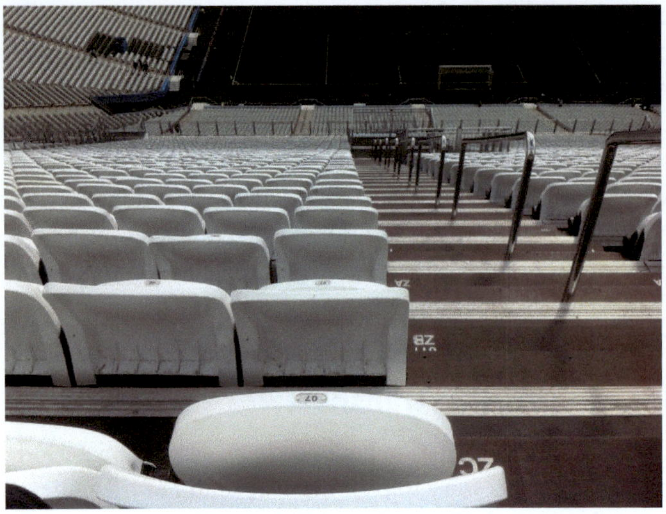

Fig. 9.2.7 Geographical barriers to moving a patient on a stretcher.

interspersed with AED analysis breaks, and timed carriage of the patient, with interruption of CPR for no longer than 10 seconds. This logistically challenging undertaking can only effectively and efficiently be undertaken if the MMT personnel have been adequately trained with regular rehearsals beforehand.

Arena inspection

Because of the many different architectural designs of sports stadiums, it is always important to inspect the arena before writing a definitive MAP in order to ascertain which modes of patient transport are possible in an emergency in a particular arena. It is important to ascertain whether an ambulance can enter the field of play, so that appropriate plans can be made in advance. Likewise, it is important to establish whether the stadium ramps or lifts are accessible for ambulance stretchers, ambulances, or modified motorized stretcher-carrying carts, all of which need adequate access if they are to be used to convey the patient safely and appropriately away from the site.

The presence of an ambulance does not guarantee that the appropriate level of care will be undertaken en route to the designated receiving medical facility, unless the ambulance, its crew, its medical equipment, and its medical protocols have been audited and inspected to ensure that, if required, safe, effective, and efficient CPR can be undertaken in the moving ambulance. Manual or mechanical CPR requires regular preparation and training if it is to be safe and procedurally sound.

Many larger sport arenas will have a designated helicopter landing area, approved by the local civil aviation authority, for use in life-threatening medical emergencies. Because of the hazardous nature of helicopter landings and take-offs, particularly in the context of a full-capacity arena, all standard operating procedures regarding this mode of emergency transfer must be assessed, inspected, and adequately rehearsed, so that all members of the medical and health-care team who will access the helicopter landing zone in an actual situation are familiar with the various safety and operational aspects concerned.

Planning, coordination, and continuous training

The effective and efficient management of any life-threatening cardiac emergency requires good coordination, cooperation, and communication in order to recognize in a timely manner any patient who has collapsed, anywhere within and/or around the stadium area of responsibility. In addition, speedy response to the scene of the collapse by the nearest MMT, immediate resuscitation, and, where indicated, ALS back-up response within the approved required critical time frame are necessary.

This sequence of life-saving events can only be successfully accomplished if the approved, and regularly audited emergency MAP is known to all members of the medical and health-care services, and is regularly rehearsed using lifelike scenarios with critical debriefing sessions in order to correct, update, modify, or adapt any weakness in the system.

Such clinical training scenarios, should include practical response to and evaluation of resuscitation and transfer of the victim in a crowded SSA, or in other areas of difficult access inside the venue. In this way, the difficulties likely to be encountered in these incidents can be fully appreciated and effective safe management can be adequately practised. These training scenarios additionally bond the various team members together into a fully functioning cohesive unit, which is the ultimate aim of training.

Communications

It is an accepted principle that no emergency can be effectively managed without adequate communications. It is vital that all members involved with a medical emergency to have up-to-date information necessary for a speedy response, both primary and secondary. Whatever form the relevant stadium communication system may take—two-way mobile radios, cellphones, pager messages, or similar devices—it is imperative that all members of the medical and health-care services on duty in and around the stadium are contactable whenever necessary. Likewise, any cardiac emergency that is being managed must relay the necessary information to the VOC in large stadiums, or to a person with these responsibilities in a smaller arena, so that medical assistance can be dispatched if necessary, transport arranged as required, and other allied emergency services briefed or alerted (e.g. traffic police, referral hospital, air ambulance helicopter response). Communication training must be integral to any of the clinical simulated scenario training to familiarize all medical and health-care team members with the designated communication devices being used.

Documentation

All patient contacts at the arena should be registered, ideally in a standardized electronic medical records database, ensuring confidentiality and safety of all the patient's information. If possible a signed copy of the report should be delivered to the patient or those accompanying him/her. An 'against medical advice' section or specific form for patients who refuse treatment will help in reducing the event and/or venue liability. If the patient is transferred to a hospital, written documentation is a necessary part of the transfer and should include information on the patient's condition, investigations, treatment, method, and timing of transfer, as well as any problems incurred during transport [20]. The medical record may also be used for continuous quality improvement of the EMS, research purposes, and, more importantly, as a legal document, possibly with varying requirements in different national settings.

Signage and information related to access to care

Easily discernible signs should be strategically placed throughout the arena to facilitate rapid location of medical care posts/centres and AEDs (➔ Fig. 9.2.8).

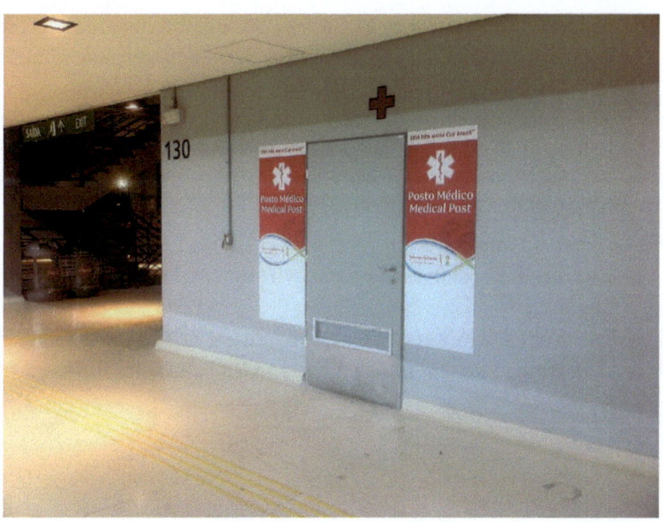

Fig. 9.2.8 Signs showing the location of the medical rooms.

Information including a map with the location of treatment facilities (BLS and ALS), MMTs, AEDs, and ambulances should also be provided in event programmes/guides, as well as in visible posters/wall charts located in the teams' and referees' locker rooms, in the doping control and delegates rooms, and in VIP lounges in the competitions area (➔ Fig. 9.2.4). To maximize visibility, signs, posters, and programme information should be designed with pictograms, bold text, and bright colours.

The map must also be distributed to the opposing teams, well before the competitive game or tournament.

Local/national adaptations

There is no current validated, internationally accepted, medical mass gathering system, although the basic principles are accepted by expert opinion and consensus. Individual countries may promulgate laws and regulations that legally mandate the various aspects of medical mass gathering, including the composition of medical staff, minimum levels of medical equipment availability, prescribed minimum time critical interventions and mutual emergency services assistance, etc. Additionally, architectural variations in the size, shape, location, and functionality of a sports stadium may require adaptations and modifications to any standard generic sport stadium emergency medical plan, failure of which may compromise the emergency medical plan logistically and practically.

National regulations may also prescribe the scope and range of pre-hospital emergency medical practice by specific medical and allied health-care professionals, influencing who may undertake which particular out-of-hospital emergency medical treatment in and around the sport stadium. This legislative, and hence logistical, prerequisite may be further influenced by the basic requirements of participation recommended by different international sports federations (e.g. FIFA) [18]. This multiplicity of regulatory requirements needs to be considered, with practical adaptations or modifications where necessary.

Conclusions

Medical mass gathering medicine does not adhere to a *one size fits all* policy, but to *a plan must fit all sizes*. The medical action plan for a sports stadium or arena aims to support safe, coordinated, and efficient management of any acute life-threatening event, most commonly sudden cardiac arrest. This is ensured by individually tailoring the number of health-care and related personnel, as well as the medical equipment, communication system, and emergency transportation logistics, with the aim of achieving CPR and defibrillation, if needed, in the first 3–5 minutes of SCA, regardless of the characteristics of any given arena.

Further reading

Börjesson M, Serratosa L, Carré F, et al. Consensus document regarding cardiovascular safety at sports arenas. *Eur Heart J* 2011; 32: 2119–24.

De Lorenzo RA. Mass gathering medicine: a review. *Prehosp Disaster Med* 1997; 12: 68–72.

Drezner JA, Toresdahl BG, Rao AL, et al. Outcomes from sudden cardiac arrest in US high schools: a 2-year prospective study from the National Registry for AED Use in Sports. *Br J Sports Med*. 2013; 47: 1179–83.

Dvorak J, Kramer EB, Mandelbaum B, et al. Mass-gathering football medicine. In Dvorak J, Kramer EB (eds), *Football Emergency Medicine Manual* (2nd edn). Zurich: Fédération Internationale de Football Association (FIFA); 2015: pp.72–109.

Gordon J, Nordström A (eds). *Encyclopedia of Football Medicine*. Vol 1, *Trauma and medical emergencies*. New York: Thieme Verlag; 2017.

Jaslow D, Yancey A 2nd, Milsten A. Mass gathering medical care. National Association of EMS Physicians Standards and Clinical Practice Committee. *Prehosp Emerg Care* 2000; 4: 359–60.

Kramer E, Botha M. Emergency cardiac care in the athletic setting. In Wilson MG, Drezner JA, Sharma S (eds), *IOC Manual of Sports Cardiology*. Chichester: John Wiley; 2016: Chapter 45.

Perkins GD, Handley AJ, Koster RW, et al. European Resuscitation Council Guidelines for Resuscitation 2015: Section 2. Adult basic life support and automated external defibrillation. *Resuscitation* 2015; 95: 81–99.

Toresdahl B, Courson R, Börjesson M, et al. Emergency cardiac care in the athletic setting: from schools to the Olympics. *Br J Sports Med* 2012; 46(Suppl 1): i85–9.

Truhlar A, Deakin CD, Soar J, et al. European Resuscitation Council Guidelines for Resuscitation 2015: Section 4. Cardiac arrest in special circumstances. *Resuscitation* 2015; 95: 148–201.

References

1. De Lorenzo RA. Mass gathering medicine: a review. *Prehosp Disaster Med* 1997; 12: 68–72.
2. Corrado D, Basso C, Rizzoli G, et al. Does sports activity enhance the risk of sudden death in adolescents and young adults? *J Am Coll Cardiol* 2003; 42: 1959–63.
3. Carroll D, Ebrahim S, Tilling K, et al. Admissions for myocardial infarction and World Cup football: database survey. *BMJ* 2002; 325: 1439–42.
4. Katz E, Metzger JT, Schlaepfer J, et al. Increase of out-of-hospital cardiac arrests in the male population of the French speaking provinces of Switzerland during the 1998 FIFA World Cup. *Heart* 2005; 91: 1096–7.
5. Leeka J, Schwartz BG, Kloner RA. Sporting events affect spectators' cardiovascular mortality: it is not just a game. *Am J Med* 2010; 123: 972–7.
6. Wilbert-Lampen U, Leistner D, Greven S, Pohl T, et al. Cardiovascular events during World Cup soccer. *N Engl J Med* 2008; 358: 475–83.
7. Barone-Adesi F, Vizzini L, Merletti F, Richiardi L. It is just a game: lack of association between watching football matches and the risk of acute cardiovascular events. *Int J Epidemiol* 2010; 39: 1006–13.
8. Niederseer D, Thaler CW, Egger A, et al. Watching soccer is not associated with an increase in cardiac events. *Int J Cardiol* 2013; 170: 189–94.
9. Börjesson M, Dugmore D, Mellwig KP, et al. Time for action regarding cardiovascular emergency care at sports arenas: a lesson from the Arena study. *Eur Heart J* 2010; 31: 1438–41.
10. Luiz T, Preisegger T, Rombach D, Madler C. Cardiac arrest in spectators in German football stadiums: precautionary measures, frequency and short-term outcome. *Anaesthesist* 2014; 63: 636–42.
11. Leusveld E, Kleijn S, Umans VA. Usefulness of emergency medical teams in sport stadiums. *Am J Cardiol* 2008; 101: 712–14.
12. Serra Grima R, Carreno MJ, Tomas Abadal L, et al. Acute coronary events among spectators in a soccer stadium. *Rev Esp Cardiol* 2005; 58: 587–91.
13. Perkins GD, Handley AJ, Koster RW, et al. European Resuscitation Council Guidelines for Resuscitation 2015: Section 2. Adult basic life support and automated external defibrillation. *Resuscitation* 2015; 95: 81–99.
14. Berdowski J, Blom MT, Bardai A, et al. Impact of onsite or dispatched automated external defibrillator use on survival after out-of-hospital cardiac arrest. *Circulation* 2011;124(20): 2225–32.
15. Drezner JA, Rao AL, Heistand J, Bloomingdale MK, Harmon KG. Effectiveness of emergency response planning for sudden cardiac arrest in United States high schools with automated external defibrillators. *Circulation* 2009; 120: 518–25.
16. Börjesson M, Serratosa L, Carré F, et al. Consensus document regarding cardiovascular safety at sports arenas. *Eur Heart J* 2011; 32: 2119–24.
17. Jaslow D, Yancey A 2nd, Milsten A. Mass gathering medical care. National Association of EMS Physicians Standards and Clinical Practice Committee. *Prehosp Emerg Care* 2000; 4: 359–60.
18. Dvorak J, Kramer EB, Mandelbaum B, et al. Mass-gathering football medicine. In Dvorak J, Kramer EB (eds), *Football Emergency Medicine Manual* (2nd edn). Zurich: Fédération Internationale de Football Association (FIFA); 2015: pp.72–109.
19. Lyster T, Jorgenson D, Morgan C. The safe use of automated external defibrillators in a wet environment. *Prehosp Emerg Care* 2003; 7: 307–11.
20. Dunn MJ, Gwinnutt CL, Gray AJ. Critical care in the emergency department: patient transfer. *Emerg Med J* 2007; 24: 40–4.

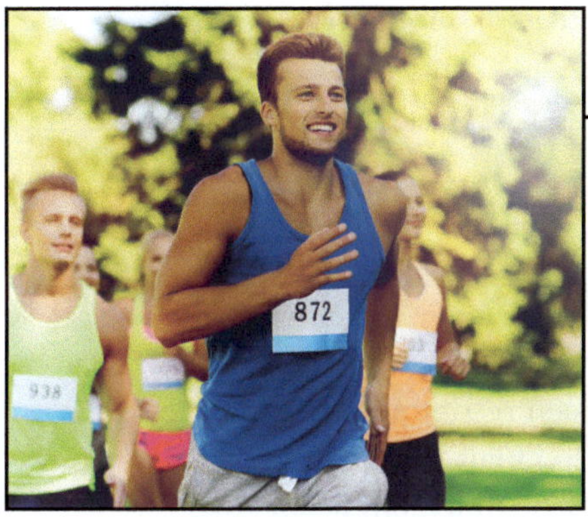

9.3

Cardiac safety at fitness centres

Erik Ekker Solberg, Jakob Johansson, and Alessandro Biffi

Introduction

Science has demonstrated that exercise benefits health in both primary and secondary prevention [1], and the concept 'Exercise is medicine' has spread worldwide. Many people now exercise in fitness centres, which have grown into a huge industry. According to the organization Euroactive, the European health and fitness sector serves over 44 million consumers, generates €25.2 billion in revenue, employs 400.000 people, and consists of 48,000 facilities [2]. While the benefit of exercise for health has been extensively proved, there is less clarity about its safety. There is no official European recommendation on cardiac safety at fitness centres, which is the subject of this chapter.

Terminology

The terms gym, health, training, or fitness centres, clubs, or facilities are used to denote such centres. In this chapter we have adopted the terms 'fitness centre' or 'fitness facility' because these seem to be the terms most frequently used.

Physical activities in fitness centres

How many centres are there and who trains at them?

Training at fitness centres is one of the most common, and thus most important, methods of exercising. However, precise European data on how many fitness centres exist and who is training at fitness are lacking. For example, 16% of those practising sports activities in Italy do so in fitness facilities, which thus rank second after soccer clubs as the most frequently used sports arena [3]. Data on fitness industry derived from the European Health Club Report of the IHRSA (➲ Table 9.3.1) shows a large number of members and clubs, and a substantial market size in various European countries [4]. It is noteworthy that there has been a dramatic increase in fitness centre activity in subjects aged over 55 [4].

Types of activity

Various types of physical activity take place at fitness centres. The most common training modalities are aerobic, strength, and coordination training. Assorted aerobic exercises, such as step, bicycle, treadmill, dance, cardio-funk, interval circuit training, and weight training in various forms—gravity (weight stacks, plates, and dumbbells) or training machines which oppose muscular contractions—are well established practices for the fitness centre customer. Activities which take place at fitness centres, such as high intensity interval training, strength training, fitness programmes for the elderly, and the use of personal trainers, are all included in annual worldwide top ten list of fitness trends produced by the American College of Sports Medicine [5].

Incidence of cardiac events at fitness centres

The incidence rate of sudden cardiac arrest (SCA) in sports in general has been extensively studied. The results vary, but it is estimated to be about 1 in 50,000 in those aged under 35 [6,7].

Neither the exact incidence of SCA, nor the occurrence of a cardiac event such as syncope during training at a fitness centre, is precisely known. SCA occurs rarely (the absolute risk is low), but if it takes place, it is frequently at a fitness centre (the relative risk is high). In France 27% of SCAs in sports between 2005 and 2010 occurred in a fitness centre [8]. Fitness centres were also found to be one of the major locations for SCA in sports in The Netherlands (11% registered between 2006 and 2009) [9]. A British study showed that 24% of exercise-related SCAs between 2010 and 2012 occurred in gyms or leisure centres [10]. Among fitness centres in Ohio, 17% had experienced an SCA over a five-year

Table 9.3.1 Number of fitness centres, number of members, and market size generated from fitness in European countries

	UK	Germany	Spain	France	Italy	Russia	Netherlands	Sweden	Belgium	Denmark	Norway
Members (million)	7.9	7.8	6.4	4.2	4.2	2.5	2.1	1.2	0.8	0.8	0.8
Fitness centres	6.019	7.566	4.7	2.97	6.5	3.45	1.9	1.3	850	970	903
Market size (million €)	4.79	4.09	3.84	2.52	2.117	1.643	1.235	0.566	0.558	0.562	0.581

period [11]. These data indicate that about a fifth of SCA in sports is expected to occur at fitness centres, justifying a specific focus on cardiovascular protection at such centres.

Predictors of sudden cardiac arrest: individual and systemic factors

The incidence rate of SCA at fitness centres depends on the following exercising at the centre: gender (males are more frequently exposed); age (the elderly are more frequently exposed); participants in special programmes offered to a clinical population (e.g. programmes for the elderly or for individuals with specific medical conditions) [12]; the types of exercise practised at the centre; and the specific country. The incidence of SCA in sports in general is higher in the elderly (>35 years) [10,13], among men [14], and during vigorous exercise [6].

Subjects at risk

Physical exercise can trigger acute cardiac events in the presence of silent and asymptomatic cardiovascular abnormalities, especially in untrained subjects. These findings can be explained by the phenomenon of the 'paradox of exercise' [15]. Although exercise has a long-term protective action against coronary artery disease (CAD), it can also trigger an adverse or even lethal event. The paradox of exercise also raises the question of screening people using fitness centres and the role of physicians in prescribing physical activity ('exercise is medicine'). Attention to cardiovascular warning symptoms, such as pre-syncope and syncope, palpitations, chest pain, and exertion fatigue is a possible suitable approach to the fitness centre safety. Many victims of SCA in sport in general have had symptoms prior to the event [16] or have a positive family history of premature SCA [17,18]. The increased number of older patients who exercise probably also results in increased risk of SCA. This could be prevented by evaluating the cardiovascular risk profile of individuals who use gym facilities with regard to coronary risk factors such as hyperlipidaemia, hypertension, diabetes, smoking, overweight, and a family history of CAD [19]. Self-assessment of the habitual level of physical activity and any risk factors has been recommended for screening large populations [20]. Individuals deemed to be at risk require further evaluation by a qualified physician [20].

Survival rate

The survival rate from SCA will depend on the underlying disease leading to the event, the age and individual features of the victim, and the environment in which the SCA occurs. SCA in sports has a substantially higher survival rate than SCA out of sports. The French dataset showed an almost threefold higher survival rate in sports facilities [8]. The reasons were that the victims were younger and less likely to have underlying cardiovascular disease, the events were more often witnessed, cardiopulmonary resuscitation (CPR) was initiated faster, and the rhythm was more often shockable [8]. CAD accounts for the majority of exercise-related SCAs in older people, and this is reflected by the high rate of coronary revascularization (70% in victims surviving SCA). However, only a third received bystander CPR prior to arrival of the ambulance and only a minority were defibrillated [8,21]. The large Netherlands study supports a markedly higher survival rate (unadjusted odd ratio = 4) in exercise-related SCA compared with non-exercise-related SCA [9]. This may also be due to relatively less advanced CAD in individuals who are regularly engaged in physical activity. Intense exercise may trigger SCA in relatively healthier subjects affected with CAD. Therefore, although exercise may trigger SCA, these results suggest that the favourable impact of exercise training and a healthier lifestyle can mitigate the 'paradox of exercise'.

Although these studies are comprehensive, the number of cardiac arrests is relatively small which hampers statistical comparisons. The survival rate also depends on health personnel and public access to automated external defibrillators (AEDs) which may not be easily available for most victims of out-of-hospital cardiac arrest (OHCA) [22]. In addition, most countries do not report figures on SCAs. Thus a large variation between countries may exist. To date, no study has examined the expected effect on survival rate of CPR training for fitness centre employees.

Table 9.3.2 Facility characteristics

Type of facility	Unsupervised exercise room	Single exercise leader	Fitness centre for healthy clients	Fitness centre offering special programmes for clinical populations	Medically supervised clinical exercise programme (e.g. cardiac rehabilitation)
Emergency equipment	Telephone in room Signs Encouraged: PAD plan with AED as part of composite PAD plan in the host facility (e.g. hotel, commercial building, apartment complex)	Telephone Signs Encouraged: blood pressure kit; stethoscope; PAD plan with AED	Telephone Signs Encouraged: blood pressure kit; stethoscope; PAD plan with AED*	Telephone Signs Blood pressure kit Stethoscope Strongly encouraged: PAD plan with AED	Telephone Signs Blood pressure kit Stethoscope Oxygen Crash cart AED

At all levels it is recommended that an emergency plan is in place.
*AED is strongly encouraged in facilities with >2500 customers and those in which the EMS response time is expected to be >5min from recognition of arrest.
AED, automate external defibrillator; PAD, public access to defibrillation.
AED strongly encouraged in facilities with membership
Table modified from Balady GJ, Chaitman B, Foster C, Froelicher E, Gordon N, Van Camp S. Automated external defibrillators in health/fitness facilities: supplement to the AHA/ACSM Recommendations for cardiovascular screening, staffing, and emergency policies at health/fitness facilities. *Circulation* 2002; 105: 1147–50.

Emergency preparedness

The American Heart Association (AHA) and American College of Sports Medicine (ACSM) have together published recommendations for how fitness centres should be prepared for cardiovascular events [12,23]. These recommendations include emergency equipment on site, regular training in basic life support for staff members, and development of an emergency plan. The recommended level of emergency preparedness will differ depending on the type of fitness facility, which can range from an unsupervised exercise room to a medically supervised exercise programme (see ➲ Table 9.3.2). No European recommendations are currently available.

Chain of survival

In the event of an OHCA, it is of vital importance that prompt medical action is provided and that the response is coordinated from alarm to hospital care. This is often referred to as 'the chain of survival' [24].The four links in the chain are (1) early recognition and call for help, (2) early bystander CPR, (3) early defibrillation, and (4) early advanced life support and standardized post-resuscitation care. In the event of a cardiac arrest in a fitness centre, the first two or three of these links will occur at the centre. The first three links, and the critical importance of rapid interaction between them, are highlighted in the international CPR guidelines published in 2015 [24]. Knowledge and effective practice of these three links by staff members and customers of the fitness centre are of utmost importance in improving outcome.

Reasons for higher survival rate at fitness centres

In contrast with the setting of, for example, a large arena, a fitness centre has some advantages regarding compliance with the chain of survival. A fitness centre is far less disseminated, and thus it is easier to handle the logistics at the scene of the event. Obstacles such as large arena crowds are not present. Communication is easier, there are fewer personnel, and they are familiar with the surroundings, making it easier to carry out regular basic life support training, in particular on-site practice. The distance to an AED (if on site) is usually shorter. In addition, the fitness centre may have prior knowledge of their customers through health appraisal questionnaires or cardiovascular screening.

Emergency plan

Every fitness centre should have written emergency policies and procedures. A written medical action plan for fitness centres should include the following information:

- emergency medical dispatcher number
- the location and how emergency transport teams can access the fitness centre
- importantly, upon arrival emergency personnel must quickly find the fastest way to the patient
- medical equipment at the centre
- staff training in basic life support
- name of general manager/executive director
- name of medical liaison.

Staff training in basic life support should include strategies to recognize early warning signs of a cardiac event so that they may even be able to prevent an SCA. The regular skill practice in CPR should focus not only on how to perform CPR, but also on the importance of bystander CPR delivered promptly after the arrest and continued uninterrupted until an AED is in place. Despite the increase in access to CPR training for lay people, there is still an unwillingness to perform CPR. This has been demonstrated among bystanders at sports facilities [8]. The reasons for this could be the fear of getting it wrong, fear of infection, and legal implications [25]. Legal actions such as the enactment of Good Samaritan laws have been taken in order to increase the willingness to interfere [26].

Defibrillation

In cardiac arrests in fitness centres, as in any OHCA, the majority of cases initially present as a shockable rhythm. In these cases, the single greatest determinant of survival is the time to defibrillation [4]. In order to reduce this, AEDs must be present close to where the cardiac arrest occurs. the number of publicly accessible AEDs have increased dramatically i recent decades, but their usage by lay people is still quite low in some settings [27]. However, it has been demonstrated that the usage of public-access AEDs is relatively high in sports facilities [28], but there is still room for improvement [8]. In 2002, the AHA and the ACSM recommended to that there should be an AED in all fitness centres [12]. As noted in ➲ Table 9.3.2, the importance of an on-site AED is specifically emphasized for larger facilities, for those running programmes for clinical populations (the elderly or those with medical conditions), and where the estimated time from cardiac arrest to the first defibrillation by emergency medical personnel is more than 5 minutes. However, there have not been any studies evaluating the cost–benefit of AEDs in fitness centres. Since SCA in fitness centres are often witnessed, often present with a shockable rhythm, have favourable patient characteristics, and the circumstances are often clearly identified, AEDs may well be cost effective.

Suggestions for safety at fitness centres

Currently there are no European recommendations for how fitness centres should be prepared for cardiovascular events, but some suggestions can be made.

- Every fitness centre should have a written emergency plan.
- Staff members should receive regular training in basic life support (at least once every three months, and more often when there are staff changes).
- AED is strongly encouraged in fitness centres with membership >2500 and where the emergency medical system response time is expected to be >5 minutes from recognition of cardiac arrest.
- Self-assessment of risk factors for customers of fitness centres may be recommended, and those with a higher risk should undergo further evaluation by a qualified physician.

Future perspectives

Data on cardiac safety at fitness centres are scarce. An American joint position statement recommends written emergency policies and regularly reviewed emergency procedures. No common European statement exists, although a position statement regarding AED at sports arenas is available [29]. Exercising in fitness centres is a major and growing aspect of exercise, particularly for the elderly and those with a medical condition. Thus it is likely that the number of cardiac events at fitness centres will increase. The survival rate for SCAs in fitness centres is relatively high, but there is room for improvement. Both staff members and customers of fitness centres could be a resource for detecting warning signals and performing adequate CPR. The effect of screening customers has not been tested, but may be of value especially in higher-risk groups. Many fitness centres are part of larger chains. Therefore improved cardiovascular safety within one centre can easily spread to many other centres in the chain. These potentials for improvement require practically oriented studies examining the risk of exercise at fitness centres.

References

1 Pedersen BK, Saltin B. Exercise as medicine—evidence for prescribing exercise as therapy in 26 different chronic diseases. *Scand J Med Sci Sports* 2015; 25(Suppl 3): 1–72.

2 http://www.europeactive.eu/

3 Italian Institute of Statistics and Italian National Olympic Committee report on 'Sports Activity in Italy'. 2011.

4 www.ihrsa.org/

5 https://www.acsm.org/about-acsm/media-room/news-releases/2015/10/26/annual-survey-reveals-new-1-fitness-trend-in-2016.

6 Harmon KG, Asif IM, Klossner D, Drezner JA. Incidence of sudden cardiac death in national collegiate athletic association athletes. *Circulation* 2011; 123: 1594–1600.

7 Corrado D, Basso C, Schiavon M, Thiene G. Screening for hypertrophic cardiomyopathy in young athletes. *N Engl J Med* 1998; 339: 364–9.

8 Marijon E, Bougouin W, Karam N, et al. Survival from sports-related sudden cardiac arrest: In sports facilities versus outside of sports facilities. *Am Heart J* 2015; 170: 339–345.

9 Berdowski J, de Beus MF, Blom M, et al. Exercise-related out-of-hospital cardiac arrest in the general population: incidence and prognosis. *Eur Heart J* 2013; 34: 3616–23.

10 Edwards MJ, Fothergill RT. Exercise-related sudden cardiac arrest in London: incidence, survival and bystander response. *Open Heart* 2015; 2: e000281.

11 McInnis K, Herbert W, Herbert D, et al. Low compliance with national standards for cardiovascular emergency preparedness at health clubs. *Chest* 2001; 120: 283–8.

12 Balady GJ, Chaitman B, Foster C, et al. Automated external defibrillators in health/fitness facilities: supplement to the AHA/ACSM Recommendations for Cardiovascular Screening, Staffing, and Emergency Policies at Health/Fitness Facilities. *Circulation* 2002; 105: 1147–50.

13 Marijon E, Tafflet M, Celermajer DS, et al. Sports-related sudden death in the general population. *Circulation* 2011;124: 672–81.

14 Harmon KG, Drezner JA, Wilson MG, Sharma S. Incidence of sudden cardiac death in athletes: a state-of-the-art review. *Heart* 2014;100: 1227–34.

15 Diller GP, Baumgartner H. Sudden cardiac arrest during execrcise in patients with congenital heart disease: the exercise paradox and the challenge of approriate counselling. *Eur Heart J* 2016; 37: 627–9.

16 Margey R, Roy A, Tobin S, et al. Sudden cardiac death in 14- to 35-year olds in Ireland from 2005 to 2007: a retrospective registry. *Europace* 2011; 13: 1411–18.

17 Drezner JA, Fudge J, Harmon KG, et al. Warning symptoms and family history in children and young adults with sudden cardiac arrest. *J Am Board Fam Med* 2012; 25: 408–15.

18 Wisten A, Messner T. Symptoms preceding sudden cardiac death in the young are common but often misinterpreted. *Scand Cardiovasc J* 2005; 39: 143–9.

19 M.Borjesson LV. Cardiovascular evaluation of master athletes and middle-aged/senior individuals engaged in leisure-time sport activities. In Corrado D, Basso C, Thiene G (eds), *Arrhythmias in Athletes*. Elsevier e-book; 2013.

20 Borjesson M, Urhausen A, Kouidi E, et al. Cardiovascular evaluation of middle-aged/senior individuals engaged in leisure-time sport activities: position stand from the sections of exercise physiology and sports cardiology of the European Association of Cardiovascular Prevention and Rehabilitation. *Eur J Cardiovasc Prev Rehabil* 2011; 18: 446–58.

21 Malta HC, Al-Khatib SM. Better survival for victims of cardiac arrest occurring in sports facilities: from speculations to facts. *Am Heart J* 2015; 170: 200–1.

22 Deakin CD, Shewry E, Gray HH. Public access defibrillation remains out of reach for most victims of out-of-hospital sudden cardiac arrest. *Heart* 2014;100: 619–23.

23 Balady GJ, Chaitman B, Driscoll D, et al. Recommendations for cardiovascular screening, staffing, and emergency policies at health/fitness facilities. *Circulation* 1998; 97: 2283–93.

24 Perkins GD, Handley AJ, Koster RW, et al. European Resuscitation Council Guidelines for Resuscitation 2015: Section 2. Adult basic life support and automated external defibrillation. *Resuscitation* 2015; 95: 81–99.

25 Savastano S, Vanni V. Cardiopulmonary resuscitation in real life: the most frequent fears of lay rescuers. *Resuscitation* 2011; 82: 568–71.

26 Gilchrist S, Schieb L, Mukhtar Q, et al. A summary of public access defibrillation laws, United States, 2010. *Prev Chronic Dis* 2012; 9: E71.

27 Agerskov M, Nielsen AM, Hansen CM, et al. Public access defibrillation: great benefit and potential but infrequently used. *Resuscitation* 2015; 96: 53–8.

28 Murakami Y, Iwami T, Kitamura T, et al. Outcomes of out-of-hospital cardiac arrest by public location in the public-access defibrillation era. *J Am Heart Assoc* 2014; 3: e000533.

29 Borjesson M, Serratosa L, Carré F, et al. Consensus document regarding cardiovascular safety at sports arenas: position stand from the European Association of Cardiovascular Prevention and Rehabilitation (EACPR), section of Sports Cardiology. *Eur Heart J* 2011; 32: 2119–24.

SECTION 10

Cardiovascular effects of substances of abuse/doping

10.1 World Anti-Doping Agency (WADA) and International Olympic Committee (IOC) list of prohibited substances and methods and their cardiovascular effects *427*
Josef Niebauer and Carl Johan Sundberg

10.2 Nutrition and ergogenic aids prescription for competitive athletes *433*
Ronald J. Maughan and S.M. Shirreffs

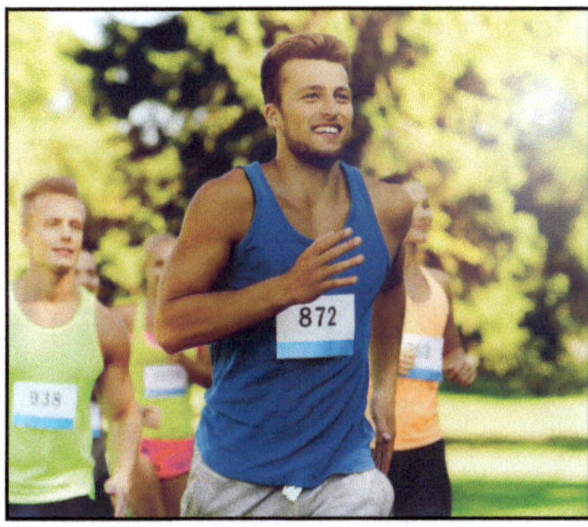

10.1

World Anti-Doping Agency (WADA) and International Olympic Committee (IOC) list of prohibited substances and methods and their cardiovascular effects

Josef Niebauer and Carl Johan Sundberg

Introduction

The history of doping is as old as that of mankind. According to reports from ancient times, athletes used herbal remedies to increase their own power to outperform their competitors. The word 'doping' appears for the first time in an English dictionary in 1889 and refers to a mixture of opium and narcotic substances used to stimulate horses in the hippodrome. Indeed, doping was and is not limited to use in humans. Horses and dogs are given substances with the aim of getting the edge over competitors, i.e. for the purpose of doping.

However, it is not only the athlete who apparently benefits from doping by winning competitions and gaining popularity and wealth, it is also the team, support staff, family, and friends who benefit from it and therefore are as vulnerable as the athlete when facing the temptation of doping. Since winning is supposedly easier when using performance-enhancing substances, doping continues to be popular despite increased anti-doping efforts. In fact, since the internet has led to increased accessibility, even leisure-time athletes take performance-enhancing substances and use prohibited methods as part of their daily routine. Even though modifications in training efficiency, nutrition, and equipment may lead to success, athletes often believe that performance-enhancing substances are necessary, regardless of ethical issues and deleterious effects on their health.

Definition of doping in sports

Doping in sports is the administration of active substances or their metabolites or using methods that are on the World Anti-Doping Agency (WADA) list of prohibited substances and/or the use of prohibited methods.

To combat doping, WADA was founded in 1999 in Lausanne and has had its headquarters in Montreal since 2001. For its fight against doping it receives funding from governments, the International Olympic Committee (IOC), non-governmental organizations, public authorities, and other public and private bodies.

Before the institution of WADA, there was a lack of coordination and leadership in the anti-doping field. The IOC rules were applicable only every four years at the Olympic Games. Thus, the creation of WADA established uniform regulation, responsibilities, controls, and sanctions in the fight against doping worldwide.

It is the aim of the WADA to protect the right of athletes to take part in a doping-free sport and to protect their health. Coordinated and targeted anti-doping checks are now performed in increasing proportion of the athlete population in order to promote and ensure fairness in sport. Even though most countries accept the WADA code, not all of them have implemented effective anti-doping programmes. Obviously, the financial cost is also an issue, as millions of dollars are needed for the implementation of an effective anti-doping programme [1].

Since anti-doping checks are expensive and cannot be conducted in very large numbers, more subtle measures have to be taken. Currently, databases are being created in which laboratory results are stored with the aim of collecting sufficient data to finally provide athletes with their own individual 'biological passport'. This includes the athlete's normal range of blood values, so that outliers can be identified and additional tests can be performed if suspicion arises. Testing dates, medication, and results can also be entered into such passports [2]. At the Olympic Games in Rio de Janeiro in 2016 a more targeted testing approach was used to obtain a higher yield than by random selection only. The athlete's age, type of sport, results development, and other factors were used in this approach.

Every year WADA's Executive Committee meets and approves the current List of Prohibited Substances and Methods, which is available on WADA's website (https://www.wada-ama.org/en/media/news/2018-09/wada-publishes-2019-list-of-prohibited-substances-and-methods).

With regard to prohibited substances and methods the WADA code distinguishes:

- Substances (S0-5) and methods (M1-3) prohibited at all times (in and out of competition)
- Substances (S6-9) and methods prohibited in competition
- Substances prohibited in particular sports (P1)

Substances and methods prohibited at all times include:

- Non-approved substances (S0) (i.e. substances currently not approved by any governmental regulatory health authority for human therapeutic use, e.g. drugs under pre-clinical or clinical development or discontinued, designer drugs, substances approved only for veterinary use)
- Anabolic agents (S1)
- Peptide hormones, growth factors, related substances, and mimetics (S2)
- Beta-2 agonists (S3)
- Hormone and metabolic modulators (S4)
- Diuretics and masking agents (S5)
- Manipulation of blood and blood components (M1)
- Chemical and physical manipulation (M2)
- Gene doping (M3)

In addition to the items listed above, certain substances and methods are prohibited in competition or in particular sports.

Substances and methods prohibited in competition:

- Stimulants (S6)
- Narcotics (S7)
- Cannabinoids (S8)
- Glucocorticoids (S9)

Substances prohibited in particular sports:

- Beta-blockers (P1)

Also included in the list of prohibited substances:

- Beta-2 agonists for inhalation
- Certain stimulants
- Cannabinoids
- Glucocorticoids
- Meldonium

Doping is very prevalent

Unfortunately, athletes continue to enhance their performances with an ever-growing arsenal of banned methods and substances. Indeed, owing to the internet, it has never been easier to gain access to banned substances. Fortunately, the increasing number of anti-doping tests, in both training and competition, has made it more difficult even for the high-performance athletes and their coaches to commit doping offences without being caught. Neverthless, the re-analysis during 2016 of samples from the Beijing and London Games has shown that the percentage of positive tests is markedly increased when more sensitive test methods are applied.

Critics often say that athletes will always dope and find ways to not get caught. Therefore, the paradoxical conclusion is that doping should be legalized. However, this is not an option for ethical as well as medical reasons. It would also have disastrous consequences for children, adolescents, and adults. For instance, it has been shown in a recent study that 1% of 11-year-old children who exercised daily in France took substances present on the WADA list of prohibited substances, even though 44% of these children experienced side effects [3]. The effect that legalization of doping would have on these children can easily be imagined. Parents would be even more hesitant to let their children participate in competitive sports, since they would fear for the health of their loved ones. This would lead to deleterious consequences for both competitive sports and public health. The majority of children, adolescents, and adults do not meet current recommendations for physical activity. With the risk of easy access to drugs if doping were legalized, many children, adolescents, and adults would find it even harder to become motivated to exercise, resulting in an even larger number of sedentary children and adults. Therefore legalizing doping is not a reasonable option.

Doping agents can have severe side effects

Quite often the dangers of doping are downplayed. However, this is wrong. More often than not, drugs are being used that have not been tested and are not approved for use in humans.

- Most data have been obtained from animal studies.
- Relevant clinical studies have been conducted only for therapeutic reasons, and not for doping.
- Substances or methods are developed for patients with disease, not for healthy people/athletes.
- Illegal and counterfeit substances may contain impurities or additives.
- Athletes using prohibited substances:
  - are not necessarily monitoreded by health professionals
  - often take higher doses than patients
  - often use drugs in combination with (many) other substances.

It is inherently difficult to draw firm scientific conclusions about the side-effect profile of several of the doping agents used because of the ethical aspects of exposing volunteers to drugs at dosages and durations employed by users of doping substances. Therefore, very few tightly controlled, randomized, prospective, and blinded studies have been conducted with supra-physiological doses over a long period of time to assess adverse effects. Thus, most findings are based on uncontrolled natural observations of doping substance abusers or on animal studies. As a consequence, there are methodological limitations such as selection or information bias, confounding factors including the concurrent use of other drugs or supplements (sometimes of unknown composition), and/or important lifestyle factors such as extreme dietary or training regimens [4].

As the prevalence of the use of doping agents in sports and in society at large is almost certainly under-estimated, it is very likely that many side effects are either undetected or are not interpreted as being linked to the use of such substances.

In this chapter, the main focus is on the side effects of androgenic anabolic steroids (AAS), erythropoietin, and stimulants, but some comments on growth hormones, diuretics, beta-2 agonists, and meldonium are also included. The overall possible side effects of banned drugs include a variety of effects on the cardiovascular system, which are summarized in ➔ Table 10.1.1.

Consideration of the side effects of well-studied substances such as anabolic steroids, growth hormones (human growth hormone (HGH)), and erythropoietin (EPO) clearly demonstrate the danger that lies in the use of these drugs not only in the clinical setting but specifically in athletes. Indeed, of the 700 tonnes of anabolic steroids sold annually worldwide, the vast amount is not used in medicine, but is mainly consumed by body-builders and strength athletes The side effects can be severe and include myocardial hypertrophy, diastolic dysfunction, arterial hypertension, hypercoagulability, and a pro-atherogenic lipid profile [6,7] which may lead to premature atherosclerosis, myocardial infarction, and thus increased mortality [8,9]. Awareness has to be raised, even among physicians, about which effects are due to training and which are side effects of prohibited substances. For instance, cardiac hypertrophy in power athletes and body-builders has often been misclassified as 'athlete's heart', but more recent data question these initial findings [10].

The most severe cardiovascular side effects, which are sometimes lethal (see ➔ Table 10.1.1), are linked to abuse of anabolic steroids, stimulants, and narcotics (for case examples, see Chapter 11.1).

Androgenic anabolic steroids

Regardless of the methodological limitations discussed above, it seems that AAS markedly reduces HDL cholesterol levels, possibly in the range of 40–70%, with a concurrently increase in LDL. These lipid effects seem to be reversible and normalize within 5 months. It is also possible that AAS promote monocyte adhesion to endothelial cells.

The side effects of newer groups of substances, such as selective androgen receptor modulators (SARMs) or insulin-like growth factor 1 (IGF-1), can be expected to be severe and are currently impossible to assess to their full extent.

Erythropoietin and blood doping

The side effects of erythropoietin, which leads to an increase in red blood cells and thus to improved endurance performance, are better known. There is a risk of thrombus formation, fatal cerebral and cardiac embolism, and renal and splenic infarction [4,11]. Equally dangerous is blood

Table 10.1.1 The most important doping substances that are taken with the objective of abuse by leisure-time, amateur, and professional athletes

Doping substance	General effects	Cardiovascular effects
Anabolic agents (S1) (e.g. dianabol, nandrolone, stanozolol)	Anabolic: increase in muscle mass and strength*** reduced fat mass*** erythropoiesis (higher blood count)*** Androgenic: virilizing properties*** maintenance of masculine characteristics***	Dyslipidaemia***: HDL↓, HDL2↓, LDL↑ Endothelial dysfunction, vasospasm* Coronary artery disease* Thromboembolic episodes* Myocardial infarction* Arterial hypertension* LV hypertrophy***, fibrosis**, destruction of mitochondria*, and systolic and diastolic dysfunction** Increased QT dispersion, short QT intervals* Tachyarrhythmias including ventricular fibrillation and SCD*
Peptide hormones, growth factors, related substances and mimetics (S2) (e.g. somatrotropic hormone (STH), human growth hormone (hGH), erythropoietin (EPO), IGF-1, insulin)	GH: cell and body growth*** Erythropoetin: increased production of red blood cells*** Corticotropin regulates cortisone and cortisol production	Hypercoagulability**, thrombosis, emboli to heart, lung, brain Progression of cardiovascular diseases* Increase in collagen, fibrosis, and myocardial necrosis** Cardiomegaly*** Arrhythmias* Arterial hypertension*** Oedema*** Diabetes**
Beta-2 agonists (S3) (e.g. clenbuterol, salbutamol, terbutaline, salmeterol)	Anabolic* Bronchospasmolytic*** Vasodilation***	Positive chronotropic and inotropic effects*** QT prolongation** Palpitations, arrhythmias, SCD** Acute myocardial infarction**
Hormone and metabolic modulators (S4) (e.g. aromatase inhibitors, oestrogen receptor antagonists)	Suppression of biomedical side effects caused by an abuse of anabolic androgenic steroids in males***	Non-specific side effects*
Diuretics (S5) (e.g. acetazolamide, furosemide)	Increased urine production*** Reduced reabsorption of urine*** Loss of fluids and weight***	Arterial hypotension*** Electrolyte imbalance including hypokalaemia*** Prolonged QT** Arrhythmias*
Stimulants (S6) (e.g. amphetamine, cocaine, ephedrine, modafinil)	Cardiostimulation*** Energy substrate mobilization** Bronchodilation** Decreased feeling of fatigue*** Enhanced performance***	Arterial hypertension*** Cardiac arrhythmias*** Coronary artery spasm resulting in acute myocardial infarction*** Cardiogenic shock*** SCD***
Narcotics (S7) (e.g. morphine, heroin, codeine, methadone)	Reduced pain*** Induced sleep*** Altered mood from euphoria and excitation***	Bradycardia*** Depression of respiratory activity and death***

***Clear proven effect.**Effect with some evidence.*Possible/less proven evidence.
Data from Schänzer and Thevis 2007 [5], and http://www.doping-prevention.sp.tum.de/doping-in-general.html.

doping with autologous or homologous blood administration, which is being performed by some endurance athletes. It can lead to disabling side effects such as hypertension, embolism, or death due to infections or haemolytic or anaphylactic transfusion reactions.

Beta-2 agonists

Drugs such as clenbuterol and salbutamol may contribute to cardiac ischaemia, congestive heart failure, arrhythmias, myocardial infarction, and sudden death [11].

Stimulants

The use of amphetamine and ephedrine has been linked to tachycardia, vasoconstriction, hypertension, cardiomyopathy, arrhythmias, myocardial infarction and stroke (15]. The drug has been shown to improve performance in such patients [12–14).

Meldonium

Meldonium is registered and prescribed in several former Soviet republics for the management of, for example, ischaemic cardiovascular diseases [15]. The drug has been shown to improve performance in such patients [16]. Unexpected meldonium effects (side effects) may include irregular heartbeat, changes in blood pressure, irregular skin conditions, an allergic reaction, and/or indigestion.

A long list of doping cases in cycling alone, with many athletes dying as a consequence, can be found at https://en.wikipedia.org/wiki/List_of_doping_cases_in_cycling.

Doping does not involve the athlete alone

Reports in the media often imply that athletes use doping agents all by themselves. However, blood doping often requires a fully trained team and professional equipment, such as a centrifuge, a deep freeze, and blood-drawing kits. Not just in blood doping, but in many other forms of doping, it is not only the athlete but also their team, or even country, that largely benefits from successes and therefore supports athletes with manpower, knowledge, and financial resources. Even though it is laudable that athletes are being banned from competition for some time after having tested positive, coaches, medical staff, and possibly third parties should be severely fined and possibly banned from sport as well.

Therapeutic use exemption (TUE)

WADA and the national anti-doping agencies allow athletes to apply for and obtain a therapeutic use exemption (TUE) when there is a legitimate medical need for a prohibited substance. TUE applications are reviewed by a TUE Committee consisting of independent physicians and medical experts, and permission to use the banned drug is allowed in individual cases when there is a clear indication for that drug and no alternatives exist.

Conclusions

Use of banned substances and methods in sports is doping, and this is prohibited, unethical, and dangerous. Furthermore, it is fraud, and not only puts the athlete's health at risk but is also unfair to other athletes and spectators. Physicians, and everybody else, should do all they can to discourage doping. Legalization of doping would drive an even greater number of athletes into substance abuse and would expose them to an incalculable risk to their health. Furthermore, research efforts in sports sciences and sports medicine need to be increased in order to help athletes be successful without the need for doping.

Further reading

Howman D. The way forward. *Play True* 2007; 1: 3–8.

Kamber M, Mullis P-E. Doping im Jugendalter. *Ther Umschau* 2007; 64: 83–9.

Melnik B, Jansen T, Grabbe S. Abuse of anabolic-androgenic steroids and bodybuilding acne: an underestimated health problem. *J Dtsch Dermatol Ges* 2007; 5: 110–17.

Santos MA, Oliveira CV Silva AS. Adverse cardiovascular effects from the use of anabolic-androgenic steroids as ergogenic resources. *Subst Use Misuse* 2014; 49: 1132–7.

Vanberg P, Atar D. Androgenic anabolic steroid abuse and the cardiovascular system. *Handb Exp Pharmacol* 2010;(195):411–57.

NADA Deutschland: Jahresbericht 2006, Pressekonferrenz 12 July 2007. Available at: www.nada-bonn.de

OEDAC (Österreichisches Antidoping Comite) Statistik 2006. Available at:www.oeadc.org.com

WADA: World Antidoping Agency, www.wada-ama.org http://www.doping-prevention.sp.tum.de/doping-in-general.html

References

1. Striegel H, Simon P. Doping, High-Tech-Betrug im Sport. *Internist* 2007; 10: 1842–9.
2. Schmidt W, Prommer N, Steinacker JM, Böning D. Sinn und Unsinn von hämatologischen Grenzwerten im Ausdauersport: Folgerung aus den Dopingskandalen von Turin 2006. *Dtsch Zeitschr Sportmed* 2006; 57: 54–7.
3. Laure P, Binsinger C. Doping prevalence among preadolescent athletes: a 4-year follow up. *Br J Sports Med* 2007; 41: 660–3.
4. Pope HG Jr, Wood R, Rogol A, Nyberg F, et al. Adverse health consequences of performance-enhancing drugs: an Endocrine Society scientific statement. *Endocr Rev* 2014; 35: 341–75.
5. Schänzer W, Thevis M. Doping im Sport. *Med Klin* 2007; 102: 631–46.
6. Grace F, Sculthorpe N, Baker J, et al. Blood pressure and rate pressure product response in males using high-dose anabolic androgenic steroids (AAS). *J Sci Med Sport* 2003; 6: 307–12.
7. Achar S, Rostamian A, Narayan SM. Cardiac and metabolic effects of anabolic-androgenic steroid abuse on lipids, blood pressure, left ventricular dimensions, and rhythm. *Am J Cardiol* 2010; 106: 893–901.
8. Kindermann W. Kardiovaskuläre Nebenwirkungen von anabolandrogenen Steroiden. *Herz* 2006; 31: 566–73.
9. Petersson A, Garle M, Granath F, Thiblin I. Morbidity and mortality in patients testing positively for the presence of anabolic androgenic steroids in connection with receiving medical care. A controlled retrospective cohort study.*Drug Alcohol Depend* 2006; 81: 215–20.
10. Urhausen A, Albers T, Kindermann W. Are the cardiac effects of anabolic steroid abuse in strength athletes reversible? *Heart* 2004; 90: 496–501.
11. Deligiannis A, Björnstad H, Carré F, Heidbüchel H, et al. ESC Study Group of Sports Cardiology position paper on adverse cardiovascular effects of doping in athletes. *Eur J Cardiovasc Prev Rehabil* 2006; 13: 687–94.
12. Angell PJ, Chester N, Sculthorpe N, et al. Performance enhancing drug abuse and cardiovascular risk in athletes: implications for the clinician. *Br J Sports Med* 2012; 46(Suppl 1): i78–84.

13. Haller CA, Benowitz NL Adverse cardiovascular and central nervous system events associated with dietary supplements containing ephedra alkaloids. *N Engl J Med* 2000; 343: 1833–8.
14. Deligiannis AP, Kouidi EI. Cardiovascular adverse effects of doping in sports. *Hellenic J Cardiol* 2012; 53: 447–57.
15. Stuart M, Schneider C, Steinbach K. Meldonium use by athletes at the Baku 2015 European Games. *Br J Sports Med* 2016; 50: 694–8.
16. Schobersberger W, Dünnwald T, Gmeiner G, Blank C. Story behind meldonium—from pharmacology to performance enhancement: a narrative review. *Br J Sports Med* 2017; 51: 22–5.

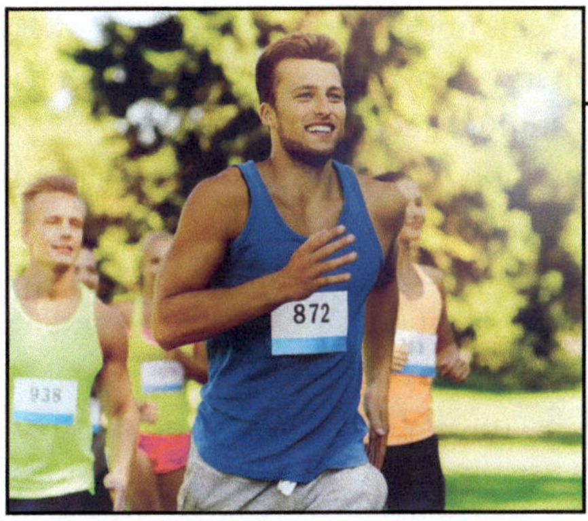

10.2

Nutrition and ergogenic aids prescription for competitive athletes

Ronald J. Maughan and S.M. Shirreffs

Introduction

Competitive athletes by definition are characterized by participation in a competitive sports event and by implication undergo a systematic programme of preparation for those competitions. These activities, in both training and competition, have significant nutritional implications, but the effects will depend on many factors including the nature of the sports event and the competitive level and training load of the individual athlete. Many athletes, whatever their competitive level and their aspirations, look to nutrition to provide a short cut to success. However, it is only one of the many different factors that contribute to successful performance in sport, and is far from the most important. Genetic endowment is undoubtedly the primary determinant of success, but the innate sporting talent conferred by the individual genotype can be modified by various factors. Among these, training probably plays the greatest role; in general, the greater the training load in terms of intensity, duration, and frequency, the better the performance outcome. Successful athletes will possess the motivation to undertake this training, and tactics and other factors will also contribute. However, when all else is equal, as it usually is in elite sport which is structured in such a way that the outcome is always in doubt, an assortment of minor factors can determine who will be successful. Good food choices will not make a mediocre athlete into a champion, but poor food choices may prevent the potential champion from realizing his or her potential. Adequate nutrition support can help the athlete sustain consistent intensive training without succumbing to chronic fatigue, illness, and injury, and can also help to promote the adaptations in muscle and other tissues that occur in response to the training stimulus [1].

Energy balance

Exercise increases the metabolic rate above the resting level, so an exercise programme must result in either an increased food intake to balance the increased energy expenditure or a loss of body mass (or some combination thereof). However, there is also scope for a change in physique, and many sports participants use a combination of exercise and dietary manipulation to induce changes in their proportions of lean and fat tissue.

The primary factors which determine the energy requirement of athletes in training are body size and training load. The importance of body mass is often under-estimated, but athletes range in size from the female gymnast or marathon runner who may weigh less than 40kg to the heavyweight weightlifter who may exceed 120kg. At the extreme, sumo wrestlers may weigh in excess of 200kg. The total training load will increase energy requirements above those of normal daily living; the three important components of any training programme are intensity, duration, and frequency. All these components will influence the energy expenditure, but, as with the general population, there is likely to be a large inter-individual variability in energy requirements even when body mass and training load are similar. The reasons for this variability remain obscure, and several factors probably contribute. In sports involving prolonged strenuous exercise on a regular basis, participation has a significant effect on energy balance. Metabolic rate during running or cycling at 70-80% of the individual's maximal oxygen uptake (VO_2max), for example, may be 10-15 times the resting rate, and such levels of activity may be sustained for several hours by trained athletes [2]. Even for events which last only a few seconds, such as sprinting or weightlifting, the top performers may spend several hours per day training, resulting in very high levels of energy expenditure and a need for a correspondingly high energy intake. Among swimmers, it is common for athletes competing in events lasting no more than 1–2 minutes to train at least twice a day with each training session lasting 1–2 hours. Similarly, rowers, whose competitive event lasts about 6–7 minutes, may spend several hours per day in training, resulting in high energy demands.

There are many reports in the published literature of energy intake and some of energy expenditure in athletes at various levels of competition and at different times of the annual training–competition cycle. However, these reports must be treated with caution, as they are prone to the usual errors associated with dietary recording. In addition to these errors, other factors must also be considered:

- athletes may deliberately manipulate energy balance to alter body mass and physique;
- athletes periodize their training across the season, and energy demands fluctuate accordingly;
- injury or illness may curtail training, causing temporary imbalance between intake and expenditure.

The principal effect of exercise is to increase the rate of energy expenditure during the exercise period itself, but the metabolic rate may remain elevated for at least 12 and possibly up to 24 hours afterwards if the exercise is both prolonged and intense [3]. The effect of this sustained elevation of metabolic rate will be to further increase the energy cost of training. Unfortunately, the recreational exerciser, whose aim is often to lose weight, is unlikely to benefit from this effect because the duration and intensity of exercise will be too short for it to be significant, but the elite athlete who trains once or more daily at the limits of the tolerable load will incur an additional energy cost which may be unwelcome. If body weight and performance levels are to be maintained, the high rate of energy expenditure must be matched by an equally high energy intake.

Most studies reporting the dietary habits of athletes show high levels of energy intake; after correction for body weight (BW), there is, perhaps, a tendency for higher energy intakes among the endurance athletes and males as opposed to females [4]. Available data for most athletes suggest that they are in energy balance within the limits of the techniques used for measuring intake and expenditure. This is to be expected, as a chronic deficit in energy intake would lead to a progressive loss of body mass and a reduced capacity to tolerate high training loads; therefore the process is self-limiting to a large degree. However, data for women engaged in sports where a low body weight, and especially a low body fat content, are important consistently show a lower than expected energy intake [5]; such sports include gymnastics, distance running, and ballet. There is no obvious physiological explanation for this finding, which has led to the suggestion that it is a result of methodological errors in the calculation of energy intake. Many of these women athletes have a very low body fat content; a total fat content of less than 10% of body weight is not uncommon in female long distance runners. Secondary amenorrhoea is common in these women, but is usually reversed when training stops [6], suggesting that the menstrual cycle disturbances may be related more to the training load than to the low body fat content. Loucks [7] introduced the concept of 'energy availability' and suggested that when the dietary energy intake remaining after allowing for energy expended in training is low, and remains low for prolonged periods, adverse health outcomes may result. This area remains controversial [5,8].

Other factors which influence the athlete's energy requirement include the requirement for growth when dealing with young athletes who have not reached full maturity; energy intake must exceed expenditure if growth is to take place. Some athletes, mostly in events where a high power output is an important part of successful performance, will also benefit from an increased body mass, and an increase in muscle mass rather than fat mass is usually desired. In some events, such as the heaviest weight categories in weightlifting and in combat sports, and the throwing events in track and field, a high absolute mass may be important, and a high body fat content is often seen in the most successful competitors. If the body mass is to increase, there must be an excess of energy intake over expenditure. The reverse situation, a need to reduce body mass and especially to reduce the body fat content, is also frequently encountered. Here there are particular problems in reducing the energy intake to a level that will result in a loss of body mass without compromising the ability to sustain the training load. In seasonal sports, such as soccer or rugby, a gain in body fat is not unusual in the off-season, and the pre-season training for these athletes often involves a combination of sudden increases in the training load in combination with a restriction on energy intake.

Modest levels of physical activity may be sufficient exercise to confer some protection against cardiovascular disease, although it is increasingly recognized that leisure-time physical activity may not be sufficient to prevent the growing public health problem of obesity in the general population [9]. However, even a small daily contribution from exercise to total daily energy expenditure can have a cumulative effect on a long- term basis, although questions remain as to whether active individuals simply compensate for increased energy expenditure by an increased intake [10]. For obese individuals, whose exercise capacity is low, the role of physical activity in raising energy expenditure is necessarily limited. This effect is offset to some degree by the increased energy cost of weight-bearing activity, but exercise programmes are likely to have limited success until sufficient weight is lost by dietary restriction to allow exercise to be tolerable.

In the general population, there is some evidence that hypo-energetic diets with a high protein content may promote the loss of body fat and retention of lean mass [11–13]. Other potentially beneficial strategies include an emphasis on carbohydrate-rich foods with a low glycaemic index [11] and an increased intake of dairy foods [14]. The evidence for these strategies comes from observational studies, animal trials, and some clinical trials in overweight populations. Investigation in athletic populations seems warranted, although some modifications or periodization may be needed when these strategies are in opposition to the athlete's sports nutrition goals (e.g. carbohydrate needs for refuelling or performance). The potential benefits of increased intake of dairy foods on fat loss via both calcium-dependent and calcium-independent mechanisms are of interest, however, since dairy protein may also assist with the athlete's goals for protein synthesis related to training adaptations. There is currently a high level of interest in dairy products in sports nutrition; flavoured milk products can provide useful quantities of fluid, electrolytes, protein, and carbohydrate in a practical form for consumption in the athlete's diet [15].

Fuels for energy

Carbohydrate, fat, protein (and alcohol) can all be used as energy sources during exercise, and considerable debate exists as to the appropriate proportions of these different fuels in the athlete's diet. At rest, all these fuels are used, and over a period of 24 hours or longer, substrate use will generally reflect the dietary intake. Eating a high carbohydrate diet increases carbohydrate oxidation, and a low carbohydrate diet will result in increased fat oxidation. From a weight-control perspective, the energy intake is far more relevant than the macronutrient composition of the diet; high protein diets may suppress appetite and may increase post-ingestion metabolic rate, but the long-term effects of dietary protein content on weight control are not clear [16]. During exercise, however, protein normally contributes little to energy metabolism. Fat is the primary fuel at low exercise intensities, but the fractional contribution of carbohydrate increases as exercise intensity increases [17,18]. Therefore high carbohydrate intakes are generally recommended for athletes in endurance sports [19].

Although it is an essential fuel for high intensity exercise performance, the total amount of carbohydrate stored in the body is small, with a maximum of about 100g in the liver and 400–500g in the muscles. These amounts depend on the energy and carbohydrate content of the preceding diet, and will be reduced by fasting and exercise, although the muscle glycogen content is well maintained in the absence of exercise [20]. Liver glycogen can be broken down to glucose and released into the bloodstream, where it is available to all tissues to act as a fuel. This is particularly important for the brain, which relies heavily on blood glucose as a fuel, and for other tissues such as the red blood cells which, lacking mitochondria, use blood glucose as their only substrate. The muscle store of glycogen is more immediately available when the muscles are called on to do work, but it is not so readily available to other tissues. Resting muscle can meet the majority of its energy demand by the oxidation of any available fuels, including fat, amino acids, and ketone bodies as well as carbohydrate. During exercise, the rate of carbohydrate utilization and its contribution to the total fuel mix vary according to a range of factors, including the intensity and duration of exercise, the training state of the athlete, the composition of the prior diet, and whether carbohydrate is ingested immediately prior to and during the exercise session [21].

Total body carbohydrate stores are often substantially less than the daily fuel requirements of intensive training and competition sessions, so athletes are guided to consume dietary sources of carbohydrates to avoid or delay the depletion of body carbohydrate stores during exercise [22]. A summary of current recommendations for carbohydrate intake by athletes is provided in ➲ Table 10.2.1. It should be noted from this summary that sports nutrition guidelines no longer promote a 'high carbohydrate' diet for all athletes. Instead, general targets are provided to allow athletes to meet the carbohydrate fuel requirements for their specific training and competition schedules, with suggestions for total amounts of carbohydrate that might be consumed over a day, as well as goals for intake before and during exercise, or in the recovery period between one session and the next. There is a sound body of evidence that carbohydrate intake strategies which maintain high carbohydrate availability during exercise and prevent carbohydrate depletion are associated with enhanced endurance and performance. Such strategies include glycogen super-compensation prior to endurance and ultra-endurance events, the intake of a carbohydrate-rich meal in the hours before events of prolonged (>90min), sustained, or intermittent exercise,

Table 10.2.1 Summary of current guidelines for carbohydrate intake by athletes

Situation	Recommended carbohydrate intake
Acute situation	Maximize daily muscle glycogen storage (e.g. for post-exercise recovery or carbohydrate load before an event)
7–12g/kg body mass/day	Rapid post-exercise recovery of muscle glycogen, where recovery between sessions is <8h
1–1.2g/kg immediately after exercise; repeated each hour until meal schedule is resumed There may be some advantages to consuming carbohydrate as a series of small snacks every 15–60min in the early recovery phase.	Pre-event meal to increase carbohydrate availability before prolonged exercise session
1–4g/kg eaten 1–4h before exercise	Carbohydrate intake during moderate intensity or intermittent exercise of >1h
Exercise of 1h: small amounts of carbohydrate (including even mouth rinsing with a carbohydrate drink) Exercise of >90min: 0.5–1.0g/kg/h (30–60g/h) Exercise of >4h: maximal rates of oxidation of ingested carbohydrate occur with intakes of ~1.5–1.8g/min of multiple transportable carbohydrates	Chronic or everyday situation
Daily recovery or fuel needs for athletes with very light training programmes (low intensity exercise or skill-based exercise); these targets may be particularly suited to athletes with large body mass or a need to reduce energy intake to lose weight	3–5g/kg/day*
Daily recovery or fuel needs for athletes with moderate exercise programme (i.e. 60–90min)	5–7g/kg/day*
Daily recovery or fuel needs for endurance athletes (i.e. 1–3h of moderate to high intensity exercise)	7–12g/kg/day*
Daily recovery or fuel needs for athlete undertaking extreme exercise programme (i.e. >4–5h of moderate to high intensity exercise such as Tour de France)	≥10-12 g/kg/day*

*Note that this carbohydrate intake should be spread over the day to promote fuel availability for key training sessions, i.e. consumed before, during, or after these sessions
Source data from Louise M Burke, Bente Kiens, John L Ivy. Carbohydrates and fat for training and recovery. *Journal of Sports Sciences*, Volume 22, Issue 1. Copyright © 2004 Taylor & Francis.

the intake of carbohydrate during sustained high intensity exercise lasting ~60min or in prolonged sustained/intermittent exercise, and the intake of carbohydrate in the recovery period between two bouts of carbohydrate-demanding exercise. Carbohydrate is an essential ingredient of effective sports drinks, and water and carbohydrate have independent and additive performance-enhancing effects when ingested during endurance exercise [23]. Even small amounts of carbohydrate ingested at regular intervals during prolonged exercise may benefit performance [24]. Ingestion of large amounts of carbohydrate (up to 90g/h or even more) may be beneficial if these include varied carbohydrate types that can take advantage of the different intestinal transport mechanisms to maximize absorption and if the gut has been trained by repeated exposure to high carbohydrate concentrations [25].

Low carbohydrate, high fat diets have been promoted for athletes in recent years [26,27], but the evidence of benefits to performance is not clear. Training with restricted carbohydrate availability may enhance the capacity for fat oxidation during exercise, but it seems that a performance benefit does not result [28,29].

The primary source of carbohydrate comes from the diet, although small amounts can be synthesized from the carbon skeleton of some amino acids and the glycerol moiety of triglycerides, and sugar-rich and starch-rich foods can contribute to energy and fuel needs as well as providing other useful nutrients for health and performance [30]. However, special sports products containing substantial amounts of carbohydrate provide a valuable nutrition aid in some situations. The advantages or value of these products include taste appeal, provision of a known amount of carbohydrate to meet a specific sports nutrition goal, simultaneous provision of other important nutrients for sports nutrition goals, and gastrointestinal characteristics promoting quick digestion and absorption. Other benefits relate to characteristics that make the products practical for consumption around exercise sessions (low bulk, conveniently packaged) or in the athlete's lifestyle (portable, non-perishable, minimal preparation). When these sports products are used by an athlete to meet the sports nutrition situations outlined above, they are likely to enhance performance. The performance benefits achieved by addressing a situation that would otherwise result in low carbohydrate availability are robust, ranking carbohydrate supplements among the performance enhancers with the strongest evidence base in sports nutrition.

Protein needs for muscle adaptation and growth

Protein has been considered a key nutrient for sporting success by athletes of all eras. Whereas ancient Olympians were reported to eat unusually large amounts of meat, today's athletes are provided with a vast array of protein and amino acid supplements to increase their protein intakes. Protein plays an important role in the response to exercise. Amino acids from proteins form building blocks for the manufacture of new tissue, including muscle, and the repair of damaged tissue. They are also the building blocks for hormones and enzymes that regulate metabolism and support the immune system and other body functions. Protein provides a small source of fuel for the exercising muscle. Endurance and resistance-training exercise may increase daily protein needs up to a maximum of 1.3–1.8g/kg BW [31], compared with the estimated average requirement of 0.6g/kg/day for the sedentary person. To allow for individual variability, the recommended daily intake is generally set at about 0.8 g/kg BW for a sedentary person, although this does vary between countries, reflecting the uncertainties in the setting of all dietary recommendations. The evidence for this increase in protein needs is not clear and universal. Part of the confusion is caused by problems involved in the scientific techniques used to measure protein requirements [32].

The debate over the protein needs of athletes is largely unnecessary. Dietary surveys show that most athletes already consume diets providing protein intakes above 1.2–1.6g/kg BW, even without the use of protein supplements [33]. Therefore most athletes do not need to be encouraged or educated to increase their protein intakes. Rather, athletes who consume adequate total energy intake from a variety of nutrient-rich foods should be confident of meeting their protein needs, including any increases that could arise from high-level training. Athletes at risk of failing to meet their protein needs are those who severely restrict their energy intake or dietary variety. Some resistance-trained athletes and body builders routinely consume protein intakes in excess of 2–3g/kg BW/day, but there is no evidence that intakes of more than about 1.8g/kg BW/day are ever necessary to enhance the response to training or increase the gains in muscle mass and strength. While such diets are not necessarily harmful, they are expensive, and can cause athletes to fail to meet other nutritional goals such as replacing important fuel sources (carbohydrates) needed to optimize training and performance. The exception, as mentioned earlier, is that increased daily protein intakes, as high as 1.8–2.7g/kg BW depending on the energy deficit, may help to prevent loss of muscle mass during periods of energy restriction [13,34].

There is evidence that about 20–25g of high quality protein ingested after training will maximize the response of the muscles; whey protein, easily obtained by drinking milk or milk-based products, seems to be more effective than many other protein source [35,36]. Frequent intakes of small amounts of protein over the course of the day may be more effective in stimulating protein synthesis and promoting metabolic adaptations than consuming the same total amount of protein in fewer meals [37,38]. Each athlete must fine tune guidelines for the optimum amount, type, and timing of intake of these nutrients, and to confirm that these eating strategies lead to better achievement of the goals of training. In the meantime, it appears sensible to focus on the total balance of the diet and the timing of protein–carbohydrate meals and snacks in relation to training, rather than on high protein intakes per se. Special sports foods, such as sports bars and liquid meal supplements, can provide a compact and convenient way to consume carbohydrate and protein when everyday foods are unavailable or are too bulky and impractical. There is little justification for using very expensive protein powders or amino acid supplements, which are not superior in quality to foods and do not contain valuable nutrients that are found in protein foods (➲ Box 10.2.1).

Box 10.2.1 Protein-rich foods

Ten grams of protein is provided by:

- 300ml cow's milk
- 20g skim milk powder
- 30g cheese
- 200g yoghurt
- two small eggs
- 35–50g meat, fish, or chicken
- four slices bread—90g breakfast cereal
- two cups cooked pasta or three cups rice
- 400ml soy milk, 60g nuts or seeds
- 120g tofu or soy meat
- 150g legumes or lentils
- 200g baked beans
- 150ml fruit smoothie or liquid meal supplement

Vitamins, minerals, and antioxidants

Long hard training sessions, particularly those involving aerobic exercise, stress the body both physically and mentally. Adequate intakes of energy, protein, iron, calcium, copper, manganese, magnesium, selenium, sodium, potassium, zinc, and vitamins A, C, E, B6, and B12 are particularly important to health and performance. All these nutrients, as well as others, can be obtained from a varied and wholesome nutrient-rich diet based largely on vegetables, fruits, beans, legumes, grains, lean meats, fatty fish, dairy foods, and healthy oils, provided that energy intake is sufficient. Because of their generally high energy intakes, most athletes achieve adequate nutrient intakes, but some do not, and deficiencies of various micronutrients are more or less common in different groups of athletes.

Despite claims in the popular media that food quality has deteriorated substantially in recent years as a consequence of intensive farming practices, there is no evidence of widespread nutrient deficiences in the general population when total energy intake is adequate. This may in part be the result of the fortification of many foods with essential nutrients. Dietary surveys consistently show that most athletes are well able to meet the recommended intakes for vitamins and minerals by eating everyday foods; their increased energy intake generally helps to ensure an adequate intake of all essential nutrients. Not all of the ingested nutrients are absorbed, however, and nutrient status is more relevant than intake. Although a low intake may be an indication of an inadequate intake, deficiency cannot be diagnosed on the basis of intake alone, and requires fuller investigation of nutrient status. Those at risk of sub-optimal status of micronutrients include:

- athletes who restrict their energy intake, especially over long periods, to meet weight-loss goals;
- athletes who follow eating patterns with restricted food variety and reliance on foods with a poor nutrient density—this includes vegetarians who fail to appreciate the consequences of excluding animal products;
- athletes with clinical conditions that restrict nutrient absorption.

When food intake cannot be adequately improved—for example, when the athlete is travelling in a country with a limited food supply—or if an individual is found to be suffering from a lack of a particular vitamin or mineral, short-term supplementation can be warranted. In general, a broad-range multivitamin/mineral supplement is the best choice to support a restricted food intake, although targeted nutrient supplements may be necessary to correct an established nutrient deficiency (e.g. iron deficiency). Routine supplementation with a low dose, broad spectrum supplement is generally not harmful, but neither is it generally necessary.

Antioxidant nutrients

Many different antioxidant nutrients help the body neutralize harmful oxidizing products, including reactive oxygen radicals and reactive nitrogen species, and there is a complex interplay between these antioxidant nutrients and the body's endogenous defence mechanisms [39,40]. Free-radical species are a concern to the athlete because they accumulate during intense or prolonged training and potentially damage healthy tissues and impair proper recovery [39]. It is not known whether hard training increases the need for dietary antioxidants, as the body's endogenous antioxidant enzymes naturally develop an effective defence in response to regular training. Free radicals are also a concern in the general population, as there is evidence of a strong relationship between oxidative stress and vascular disease [40,41]. Supplementation with dietary antioxidants cannot be recommended because there is little evidence of benefit, while it is known that over-supplementation can diminish the body's natural defence system and there is some evidence that this may interrupt many of the beneficial adaptations that occur in tissues in response to training [42]. Antioxidants are safest and most effective when consumed in abundance as plant-derived foods from a wide variety of sources (e.g. fruits, vegetables, nuts, seeds, whole grains, teas, non-medicinal herbs, etc.). However, there may be some specific situations where supplementation is warranted. Selenium has antioxidant functions, and dietary intake is low in some parts of the world including much of Europe. In a small study involving a 10-year follow-up of a group of healthy elderly individuals living in rural Sweden, four years of supplementation with a combination of selenium and coenzyme Q10 significantly reduced cardiovascular mortality, with the effect persisting during the follow-up period [43]. Other similar small studies also sometimes find positive outcomes from studies involving supplementation of a wide range of nutrients with antioxidant properties. However, confirmation of these results is needed before nutrient supplementation can be recommended.

Special concerns

Iron

Iron-deficiency anaemia is the most common and widespread nutrient deficiency in the general population and affects about 3% of the population—adults and children, athletes and non-athletes. It must be recognized that iron plays many important biological roles other than its central role in oxygen transport, and modest depletion of iron stores may be a concern for the athlete even though it has no effect on the non-athlete [44]. High iron losses and impaired absorption, rather than an inadequate dietary intake, must also be considered as possible factors contributing to poor iron status. It has recently been reported that iron deficiency is a common finding in young women with heavy menstrual bleeding, and that this is accompanied by symptoms of fatigue. However, Sandstrom et al. [45] reported that the prevalence of iron deficiency and iron-deficiency anaemia was similar in adolescent female athletes and non-athletes, despite factors that should favour a better iron status in the athlete group, such as higher iron intake and less menstrual bleeding.

Notwithstanding the widespread concern over iron status, supplementation should be considered only if impaired status is diagnosed and an effective food-based solution cannot be implemented. Routine supplemenation with iron is not warranted as it may do more harm than good [46]. The risk of haemochromatosis from excess iron intake is well recognized, but there are several other potentially adverse consequences. It is well known that high levels of free iron catalyse the formation of oxygen free radicals, leading to oxidation of low density lipoprotein, which is a well-established risk factor for vascular damage. Free iron may also promote synthesis of homocysteine, and has been proposed as an independent risk factor for cardiovascular disease (CVD) [47]. However, the picture is complex: haem iron is much better absorbed than non-haem iron, and a recent review and meta-analysis found evidence that a higher dietary intake of haem iron is associated with an increased risk of CVD, but there was no association between CVD and non-haem iron intake or total iron intake [48].

Calcium and vitamin D

The key roles of calcium and vitamin D, which promotes intestinal calcium absorption and regulates calcium metabolism in bone, muscle, and other tissues, are widely recognized, but both of these nutrients play many other roles in the body. Bone growth and remodelling occur at high rates during the early adolescent years and are also stimulated by any exercise that imposes stress on the skeleton [49]. There is evidence from dietary surveys and assessments of bone mineral content that the calcium intake of many adolescent athletes is less than the recommended amount and that bone health may be compromised at this crucial stage of development. This may be because of the avoidance of dairy produce in this population, and should be addressed by an appropriate education programme to identify good food sources of calcium and encouragement to consume these products. There is a growing interest in the role of vitamin D, with insufficiency reported in many athletic groups, especially in those who live at high latitudes, in the winter and spring months, and in those who train indoors [50]. In addition to its key role in calcium metabolism, it is now recognized that vitamin D affects many tissues including muscle. There is some evidence to support a link between vitamin D status and aspects of athletic performance, but it is inconsistent, although there is some evidence that supplementation can increase muscle strength [51]. Nevertheless, a review of the evidence by Sports Medicine Australia [52] concluded that 'Correction of any vitamin D deficiency or insufficiency through supplementation may be necessary to ensure optimal performance and bone health in adolescent athletes'. As always, this should be an informed decision which takes account of the individual circumstances.

Recent evidence suggests that vitamin D deficiency may be associated with an increased cardiovascular risk [53]. Low magnesium intakes have also been implicated in CVD and in chronic metabolic and musculoskeletal disorders, and concerns have been raised about the implications of the coexistence of poor magnesium and vitamin D status [54]. These results may suggest the need for an increased awareness in the general population of the need for a diet that contains a range of foods, rather than a need for specific supplementation.

Water and electrolyte balance

Few situations represent such a challenge to the body's homeostatic mechanisms as that posed by prolonged strenuous exercise in a warm environment. Only about 20–25% of the energy available from substrate catabolism is used to perform external work, with the remainder appearing as heat. At rest, the metabolic rate is low; oxygen consumption is about 250ml/min, corresponding to a rate of heat production of about 60W. Heat production increases in proportion to metabolic demand, and reaches about 1kW in strenuous activities such as marathon running (for a 70kg runner at a speed that takes about 2.5 hours to complete the race). To prevent a catastrophic rise in core temperature, heat loss must be increased correspondingly and this is achieved primarily by an increased rate of evaporation of sweat from the skin surface. In hard exercise in hot conditions, sweat rates can reach 3L/h, and trained athletes can sustain sweat rates in excess of 2L/h for many hours. This represents a much higher fractional turnover rate of water than that of most other body components. In the sedentary individual living in a temperate climate, about 5–10% of total body water may be lost and replaced on a daily basis. When prolonged exercise is performed in a hot environment, 20–40% of total body water can be turned over in a single day. Despite this, the body water content is tightly regulated, and regulation by the kidneys is closely related to osmotic balance.

Along with water, a variety of minerals and organic components are lost in variable amounts in sweat [55]. Sweat is often described as an ultrafiltrate of plasma, but it is invariably hypotonic. The main electrolytes lost are sodium and chloride, at concentrations of about 15–80mmol/L, but a range of other minerals, including potassium and magnesium, are also lost, as well as small amounts of trace elements. Some athletes may lose up to 10g of salt (sodium chloride) in a single training session, and may train in these conditions twice per day [56]. These substantial salt losses must be replaced from food and drink, although the use of salt supplements is seldom necessary.

Failure to maintain hydration status has serious consequences for the active individual. A body water deficit of as little as 1–2% of total body mass can result in a significant reduction in exercise capacity [57], although this is disputed by some authors [58,59], reflecting the variability that results from individual differences, different exercise tasks, different environments, and different methods of altering hydration status. Endurance exercise is affected to a greater extent than high intensity exercise, and muscle strength may not be adversely affected until water losses reach 5% or more of body mass. Hypohydration greatly increases the risk of heat illness, and also abolishes the protection conferred by prior heat acclimatization [60].

Many studies have shown that the ingestion of fluid during exercise can significantly improve performance lasting longer than about 60min [57]. Adding an energy source in the form of carbohydrate confers an additional benefit by providing additional fuel for the working muscles. Addition of small amounts (perhaps about 2–8%) of carbohydrate, in the form of glucose, sucrose, or maltodextrin, will promote water absorption in the small intestine as well as providing exogenous substrate that can spare stored carbohydrate [57]. The addition of too much carbohydrate will slow gastric emptying and, if the solution is strongly hypertonic, may promote secretion of water into the intestinal lumen, thus delaying fluid availability. Voluntary fluid intake is seldom sufficient to match sweat losses, and therefore palatability of fluids is an important consideration. It is not necessary to consume enough fluid during exercise to match sweat losses, as a body mass deficit of 1–2% is unlikely to have adverse consequences. If exercise is prolonged and sweat losses high, the addition of sodium to drinks may help to prevent the development of hyponatraemia [60]. Ingestion of large volumes of plain water is also likely to limit intake because of a fall in plasma osmolality, leading to suppression of thirst.

Replacement of water and electrolyte losses incurred during exercise is an important part of the recovery process in the post-exercise period. This requires ingestion of fluid in excess of the volume of sweat lost to allow for ongoing water losses from the body [61]. Re-establishment of water balance requires replacement of solute, especially sodium, losses as well as volume replacement. If food containing electrolytes is not consumed at this time, electrolytes, especially sodium, must be added to drinks to prevent diuresis and loss of the ingested fluid [62].

Alcohol

Many individuals who would describe themselves as serious athletes consume alcohol—sometimes in large amounts—on a regular basis, and there are many examples of successful elite athletes who suffer from alcohol dependency. This makes it clear that alcohol consumption is not incompatible with athletic success for some individuals, but nevertheless there are some compelling reasons why athletes should only drink alcohol in moderation, if at all. The aim of athletic training is to induce changes in muscle and other tissues that lead to improved performance. These adaptations involve selective stimulation of protein synthesis and degradation. Provided that sufficient essential amino acids are available, exercise increases the rate of muscle protein synthesis in the few hours after exercise. Ingestion of alcohol at this time blunts this response by causing an impairment of muscle protein synthesis [63]. However, this study required subjects to drink a relatively large amount of alcohol (1.5g/kg, which is equivalent to about 12 standard drinks). There is now also evidence that alcohol, consumed in the same amount as in the protein synthesis study, can impair muscle glycogen repletion in the post-exercise period, thus compromising recovery [64]. Contrary to popular belief, however, ingestion of dilute alcohol solutions in the form of weak beer does not compromise restoration of fluid balance after exercise-induced dehydration [65,66]. Therefore ingestion of small amounts of alcohol after training is probably not harmful.

The health effects of moderate alcohol use are controversial, suggesting that any effects are generally small, but there is evidence of some protection against CVD [67]. This is very different from the chronic abuse of alcohol, which has clear adverse effects including an increased cancer risk [68], defective cardiac muscle contractility, dilated cardiomyopathy, and low output heart failure [67]. These are only some of the many health reasons to avoid excess alcohol consumption.

Dietary supplements

A wide range of supplements are on sale to athletes, often with exaggerated claims of efficacy in enhancing performance in competition [69]. Many of these claims are not supported by evidence of either their effects on performance or their safety when taken in high doses for prolonged periods [70]. Sports supplements which may be useful in helping the athlete meet nutritional goals during training and competition include sports drinks, high carbohydrate supplements, and liquid meal supplements. These are more expensive than everyday foods, but often provide a convenient and practical way of meeting dietary needs in a specific situation. There is good evidence for an ergogenic effect of some supplements in some specific situations, including caffeine, creatine, and bicarbonate or other buffering agents, possibly including beta-alanine. Caffeine in relatively small doses (typically 2–4mg/kg) can improve performance in a variety of exercise tasks, with greater effects generally seen in prolonged exercise, probably by action on adenosine receptors in the central nervous system rather than on lipolysis as was previously thought [71]. Creatine, in the form of creatine phosphate, acts as an energy source for ATP resynthesis in high intensity exercise. Meat eaters normally obtain about 1g of creatine per day from their diet, which is about 50% of the daily requirement, with the remainder synthesized from amino acids. Ingestion about 10–20g of creatine for a period of 4–6 days can increase the muscle creatine content by 10–20%, leading to improvements in strength and sprint performance [72]. The biggest improvements in performance are generally seen in repeated sprints with limited recovery. Acute ingestion of large doses of sodium bicarbonate (about 0.3g/kg) can increase the extracellular buffering capacity and improve performance in exercise lasting from about 30s to about 10min. Similar benefits may be seen after a few days of beta-alanine supplementation, which leads to an increase in muscle carnosine content and hence in buffer capacity [73]. Recent data suggest a beneficial effect on exercise performance of large doses of dietary nitrate, which have been shown to reduce the oxygen cost of exercise [74,75] and to improve performance [76]. Both inorganic nitrate and vegetable sources, such as beetroot juice, have been shown to be effective.

Dietary supplements are generally safe, but this is not always the case and it seems sensible to exercise caution with regard to their use [77]. Most supplements in common use are safe when used in the recommended doses, but any compound that has the potential to alter physiological function so as to enhance exercise performance or achieve other goals must also have the potential for adverse effects in some individuals. Prospective consumers should see good evidence of a performance or other benefit before accepting the financial cost and the health or performance risks associated with any supplement. Some of these problems arise from poor quality control and poor hygiene in manufacturing, processing, and storage facilities. The websites of the US Food and Drugs Administration (FDA) and the UK Food Standards Agency (FSA) contain daily notices of food product recalls because of manufacturing issues. In a 14-day period in January 2013, the FDA issued recall notices for food products because of undeclared milk (two products from different companies), peanuts, and eggs, the presence of metal fragments (two products from different companies), and the presence of *Listeria* (two products from different companies) and *E.coli* (http://www.fda.gov/Safety/Recalls/ucm2005683.htm). In the corresponding period, the UK Food Standards Agency notified recalls of products because of the presence of salmonella and *Bacillus cereus*, and because of inspections that revealed poor standards of hygiene in two separate factory premises (http://www.food.gov.uk/news-updates/recalls-news/).

Some pharmaceuticals are sold inappropriately as dietary supplements. Many steroid-related compounds and stimulants are on sale as dietary supplements; some are likely to be effective in achieving physiological effects, although those that are may have adverse effects on health [78]. Dinitrophenol (DNP) is used as a weight-loss agent, but it acts by uncoupling mitochondrial respiration, leading to up to twofold increases in metabolic rate and resulting in large rises in body temperature. Its use as a dietary supplement has been prohibited, but it continues to be used, despite well-publicized fatalities, because of its high potency in reducing body fat levels [79]. The use of body-building supplements has been identified as the most common cause of liver injury in some populations (http://www.internalmedicinenews.com/cme/click-for-credit-articles/single-article/liver-injury-from-herbal-and-dietary-supplements-on-the-rise/d4dfaf68b00193e60bf80ae86a9c97fa.html). Using data from the Drug-Induced Liver Injury Network (DILIN), which was established in 2003 by the National Institute of Diabetes and Digestive and Kidney Diseases to collect and analyse cases, it was found that, in the period from September 2004 to March 2013, 845 cases of liver injury were thought to be 'definitely, highly likely, or probably' from a herbal or dietary supplement, or from prescription drugs. In 2004–2005, 7% of all liver injuries were attributed to herbal and dietary supplements, and this figure increased to 20% in 2010–2012.

A further concern with many supplements on sale, apart from the lack of evidence of efficacy and safety, is the emergence in the last 15 years of numerous reports of contamination of supplements with prohibited substances, including stimulants and anabolic steroids [80]. The amounts present are generally, although not always, too small to be effective in improving performance or to pose a risk to health, but can cause a positive drug test [81]. However, in some cases high doses, even higher than the normal therapeutic dose, of steroids, stimulants, and anorectic agents have been found in supplements, with not only potential performance benefits but with a real risk of adverse health effects.

Vegetarian considerations

Many athletes, often endurance athletes and/or female athletes, adopt a vegetarian lifestyle. This personal choice can be very healthy and is in no way incompatible with success in sport. However, it does mean that vegetarian athletes must be more aware of the food choices that they make in order to maintain energy levels, meet training and recovery needs, and support proper immune function. Plant-based high fibre diets may reduce energy availability, and athletes should monitor body weight and body composition to ensure that energy needs are being met.

Some female athletes may use vegetarianism as a means of restricting calorie intake in order to achieve a desired physique. Female athletes should seek help from a trusted health professional if they feel out of control with calorie restriction and/or trying to achieve excessive leanness. Severe calorie restriction may compromise performance as well as reproductive and bone health. Although most vegetarians meet or exceed their protein requirements, plant protein quality and digestion is decreased and often requires an intake of approximately 10% more protein than if consuming animal proteins. Therefore, protein recommendations for vegetarian athletes are approximately 1.3–1.8g/kg/day from a variety of plant protein sources. This fact may be of more concern for vegans, who avoid all animal proteins, such as meat, eggs, and milk.

Those who avoid animal products in their diets generally have lower intakes of some key nutrients, especially vitamins B_{12} and D, and may show lower status of some key micronutrients [82]. A recent survey of Danish vegans [83] showed that their average intake of macro- and micronutrients (including supplements) did not reach the Nordic Nutrition Recommendations for protein, vitamin D, iodine, and selenium; vegan women's intake also failed to reach the recommendations for vitamin A. Some vegan food products, such as meat substitutes, are commonly fortified with vitamin B_{12}, but avoiding red meat means that special attention must be paid to ensuring that the diet contains enough iron, especially in women and adolescents. Iron intake from plant sources should be combined with other foods that aid iron absorption; for example, iron-fortified breakfast cereals, consumed in a meal containing vitamin C (a glass of orange juice). Dairy produce should be included in the diet to ensure an adequate calcium intake, but many calcium-fortified foods are also available. Vegetarian athletes may also be at risk of low intakes of fat (essential fatty acids are especially important), riboflavin, vitamin D, and zinc, which should be monitored and supplemented in the diet if necessary.

Further reading

Academy of Nutrition and Dietetics (AND), Dietitians of Canada (DC), and American College of Sports Medicine (ACSM). Nutrition and athletic performance. *Med Sci Sports Exerc* 2016; 48: 543–68.

References

1. Maughan RJ, Burke LM. Practical nutritional recommendations for the athlete. In Maughan RJ, Burke LM (eds), *Sports Nutrition: More Than Just Calories—Triggers for Adaptation*. Basel: Karger AG 2011, pp.131–49.
2. Maughan RJ, Leiper JB. Aerobic capacity and fractional utilisation of aerobic capacity in elite and non-elite male and female marathon runners. *Eur J Appl Physiol* 1983; 52: 80–7.
3. Bahr R (1992) Excess postexercise oxygen consumption: magnitude, mechanisms and practical implications. *Acta Physiol Scand Suppl* 1992; 605: 1–70.
4. Burke LM, Deakin V (eds). Energy requirements and energy availability. *Clinical Sports Nutrition* (5th edn). Sydney: McGraw-Hill 2015, Chapter 5.
5. Mountjoy M, Sundgot-Borgen J, Burke L, et al. The IOC consensus statement. Beyond the female athlete triad-relative energy deficiency in sport (RED- S). *Br J Sports Med* 2014; 48: 491–7.
6. Drinkwater BL, Nilson K, Ott S, Chesnut CH. Bone-mineral density after resumption of menses in amenorrheic athletes. *JAMA* 1986; 256: 380–2.
7. Loucks AB. Energy availability, not body fatness, regulates reproductive function in women. *Exerc Sport Sci Rev* 2003; 31: 144–8.
8. Joy E, De Souza MJ, NattivA, et al. 2014 Female Athlete Triad Coalition consensus statement on treatment and return to play of the female athlete triad. *Curr Sports Med Rep* 2014; 13: 219–32.
9. Bauman A, Allman-Farinell M, Huxley R, et al. Leisure-time physical activity alone may not be a sufficient public health

approach to prevent obesity: a focus on China. *Obes Rev* 2008; 9(Suppl 1): 119–26.

10. Hazell TJ, Islam H, Townsend LK, et al. Effects of exercise intensity on plasma concentrations of appetite regulating hormones: potential mechanisms. *Appetite* 2016; 98: 80–8.
11. Abete I, Astrup A, Martinez JA, et al. Obesity and the metabolic syndrome: role of different dietary macronutrient distribution patterns and specific nutritional components on weight loss and maintenance. *Nutr Rev* 2010; 68: 214–31.
12. Krieger JW, Sitren HS, Daniels MJ, et al. Effects of variation in protein and carbohydrate intake on body mass and composition during energy restriction: a meta-regression. *Am J Clin Nutr* 2006; 83: 260–74.
13. Murphy CH, Hector AJ, Phillips SM. Considerations for protein intake in managing weight loss in athletes. *Eur J Sport Sci* 2015; 15: 21–8
14. Zemel MB, Shi H, Greer B, et al. Regulation of adiposity by dietary calcium. *FASEB J* 2000; 14: 1132–8.
15. Roy BD. Milk: the new sports drink? A review. *J Int Soc Sport Nutr* 2008; 5: 15.
16. Li J, Armstrong CLH, Campbell WW. Effects of dietary protein source and quantity during weight loss on appetite, energy expenditure, and cardio-metabolic responses. *Nutrients* 2016; 8: 63.
17. Romijn JA, Coyle EF, Sidossis LS, et al. Substrate metabolism during different exercise intensities in endurance-trained women. *J Appl Physiol* 2000; 88: 1707–14.
18. an Loon LJC, Greenhaff PL, Teodosiu DC, et al. The effects of increasing exercise intensity on muscle fuel utilisation in humans. *J Physiol* 2001; 536: 295–304.
19. Burke LM, Hawley JA, Wong SHS, Jeukendrup AE. Carbohydrates for training and competition. *J Sports Sci* 2011; 29(Suppl 1); S17–27.
20. Hultman E. Studies on muscle metabolism of glycogen and active phosphate in man with special reference to exercise and diet. *Scand J Clin Lab Invest* 1967; 94(Suppl): 1–63.
21. Maughan R, Gleeson M. *The Biochemical Basis of Sports Performance* (2nd edn). Oxford: Oxford University Press 2010.
22. Academy of Nutrition and Dietetics (AND), Dietitians of Canada (DC), and American College of Sports Medicine (ACSM). Nutrition and athletic performance. *Med Sci Sports Exerc* 2016; 48: 543–68.
23. Coyle EF. Fluid and fuel intake during exercise. *J Sports Sci* 2004; 22: 39–55.
24. Maughan RJ, Bethell L, Leiper JB. Effects of ingested fluids on homeostasis and exercise performance in man. *Exp Physiol* 1996; 81: 847–59.
25. Jeukendrup AE, McLaughlin J. Carbohydrate ingestion during exercise: effects on performance, training adaptations and trainability of the gut. In Maughan RJ, Burke LM (eds), *Sports Nutrition: More Than Just Calories—Triggers for Adaptation*. Basel: Karger AG 2011, pp.1–17
26. Brukner P. Challenging beliefs in sports nutrition. Are two 'core principles' proving to be myths ripe for busting? *Br J Sports Med* 2013; 47: 663.
27. Volek JS, Noakes T, Phinney SD. Rethinking fat as a fuel for endurance exercise. *Eur J Sport Sci* 2015; 15; 13–20.
28. Hawley JA. Nutritional strategies to modulate the adaptive response to endurance training. In Tipton KD, van Loon LJC (eds). *Nutritional Coaching Strategy to Modulate Training Efficiency*. Basel: Karger AG 2013, pp.1–14
29. Burke LM. Re-Examining high-fat diets for sports performance: did we call the 'nail in the coffin' too soon? *Sports Med* 2015; 45: S33–49.
30. Burke LM. *Practical sports nutrition*. Champaign, IL: Human Kinetics 2007, p.12.
31. Phillips SM, van Loon L. Dietary protein for athletes: from requirements to optimum adaptation. *J Sports Sci* 2011; 29: S29–38.
32. Phillips SM. Dietary protein requirements and adaptive advantages in athletes. *Br J Nutr* 2012; 108(Suppl 2): S158–67.
33. Moore D, Phillips S, Slater G. Protein. In Burke L, Deakin V (eds), *Clinical Sports Nutrition* (5th edn). Sydney: McGraw-Hill, pp.94–113.
34. Helms ER, Zinn C, Rowlands DS, et al. A systematic review of dietary protein during caloric restriction in resistance trained lean athletes: a case for higher intakes. *Int J Sport Nutr Exerc Metab* 2014; 24: 127–38.
35. Moore DR, Robinson MJ, Fry JL, et al. Ingested protein dose response of muscle and albumin protein synthesis after resistance exercise in young men. *Am J Clin Nutr* 2009; 89: 161–8.
36. Devries MC, Phillips SM. Supplemental protein in support of muscle mass and health: advantage whey. *J Food Sci* 2015; 80(Suppl 1): A8–15.
37. Areta JL, Burke LM, Ross ML, et al. Timing and distribution of protein ingestion during prolonged recovery from resistance exercise alters myofibrillar protein synthesis. *J Physiol* 2013; 591; 2319–31.
38. Moore DR, Areta J, Coffey VG, et al. Daytime pattern of post-exercise protein intake affects whole-body protein turnover in resistance-trained males. *Nutr Metab (Lond)* 2012; 9: 91
39. Powers SK, Talbert EE, Adhihetty PJ. Reactive oxygen and nitrogen species as intracellular signals in skeletal muscle. *J Physiol* 2011; 589: 2129–38.
40. Conti V, Izzo V, Corbi G, et al. Antioxidant supplementation in the treatment of aging-associated diseases. *Front Pharmacol* 2016; 7: 24.
41. Santilli F, D'Ardes D, Davi G. Oxidative stress in chronic vascular disease: from prediction to prevention. *Vasc Pharmacol* 2015 74; 23–37
42 Mankowski RT, Anton SD, Buford TW et al. Dietary antioxidants as modifiers of physiologic adaptations to exercise. *Med Sci Sports Exerc* 2015; 47: 1857–68.
43. Alehagen U, Aaseth J, Johansson P. reduced cardiovascular mortality 10 years after supplementation with selenium and coenzyme Q10 for four years: follow-up results of a prospective randomized double-blind placebo-controlled trial in elderly citizens. *PLoS One* 2015; 10: e0141641.
44. Deakin V, Peeling P. Prevention, detection and treatment of iron depletion and deficiency in athletes I. In Burke L, Deakin V (eds), *Clinical Sports Nutrition* (5th edn). Sydney: McGraw-Hill 2015, pp.266–309.
45. Sandstrom G, Borjesson M, Rodjer S. Iron deficiency in adolescent female athletes. Is iron status affected by regular sporting activity? *Clin J Sports Med* 2012; 22: 495–500

46. Papanikolaou G, Pantopoulos K. Iron metabolism and toxicity. *Toxicol Appl Pharmacol* 2005; 202: 199–211.
47. Baggott JE, Tamura T. Homocysteine, iron and cardiovascular disease: a hypothesis. *Nutrients* 2015; 7: 1108–18.
48. Fang X, An P, Wang H, et al. Dietary intake of heme iron and risk of cardiovascular disease: a dose-response meta-analysis of prospective cohort studies. *Nutr Metab Cardiovasc Dis* 2015; 25; 24–35.
49. Dalsky GP. The role of exercise in the prevention of osteoporosis. *Comp Ther* 1989; 15; 30–7.
50. Farrokhyar F, Tabasinejad R, Dao D, et al. Prevalence of vitamin D inadequacy in athletes: a systematic review and meta-analysis. *Sports Med* 2015; 45: 365–78.
51. Tomlinson PB, Joseph C, Angioi M. Effects of vitamin D supplementation on upper and lower body muscle strength levels in healthy individuals. A systematic review with meta-analysis. *J Sci Med Sport* 2015; 18: 575–80.
52. Desbrow B, McCormack J, Burke LM, et al. Sports Dieticians Australia position statement: sports nutrition for the adolescent athlete. *Int J Sport Nutr Exerc Metab* 2014; 24: 570–84.
53. Bi Xinyan, Tey SL, Leong C, et al. Prevalence of vitamin D Deficiency in Singapore: its implications to cardiovascular risk factors. *PLoS One* 2016; 11: e0147616
54. Rosanoff A, Dai Q, Shapses SA. Essential nutrient interactions. Does low or suboptimal magnesium status interact with vitamin D and/or calcium status? *Adv Nutr* 2016; 7; 25–43.
55. Shirreffs SM, Maughan RJ. Whole body sweat collection in man: an improved method with some preliminary data on electrolyte composition. *J Appl Physiol* 1997; 82: 336–41.
56. Shirreffs SM, Aragon-Vargas LF, Chamorro M, et al. The sweating response of elite professional soccer players to training in the heat. *Int J Sports Med* 2005; 26, 90–5,
57. Sawka MN, Burke LM, Eichner ER, et al. Exercise and fluid replacement. *Med Sci Sports Exerc* 2007; 39: 377–90.
58. Goulet EDB. Effect of exercise-induced dehydration on endurance performance: evaluating the impact of exercise protocols on outcomes using a meta-analytic procedure. *Br J Sports Med* 2013; 47: 679–86.
59. Wall BA, Watson G, Peiffer JJ, et al. Current hydration guidelines are erroneous: dehydration does not impair exercise performance in the heat. *Br J Sports Med* 2015; 49; 1077–83.
60. Hew-Butler T, Rosner MH, Fowkes-Godek S, et al. Statement of the 3rd International Exercise-Associated Hyponatremia Consensus Development Conference, Carlsbad, California, 2015. *Clin J Sports Med* 2015; 25: 303–20.
61. Shirreffs SM, Taylor AJ, Leiper JB, Maughan RJ. Post-exercise rehydration in man: effects of volume consumed and sodium content of ingested fluids. *Med Sci Sports Exerc* 1996; 28: 1260–71.
62. Maughan RJ, Leiper JB, Shirreffs SM. Restoration of fluid balance after exercise-induced dehydration: effects of food and fluid intake. *Eur J Appl Physiol* 1996; 73: 317–25.
63. Parr EB, Camera DM, Areta JL, et al. (2014) Alcohol ingestion impairs maximal post-exercise rates of myofibrillar protein synthesis following a single bout of concurrent training. *PLoS One* 2014; 9: e88384.
64. Burke LM, Collier GR, Broad EM, et al. (2003) Effect of alcohol intake on muscle glycogen storage after prolonged exercise. *J Appl Physiol* 2003; 95: 983–90.
65. Shirreffs SM, Maughan RJ. Restoration of fluid balance after exercise-induced dehydration: effects of alcohol consumption. *J Appl Physiol* 1997: 83; 1152–8
66. Hobson RM, Maughan RJ. Hydration status and the diuretic action of a small dose of alcohol. *Alcohol Alcohol* 2010; 45: 366–73
67. George A, Figueredo VM. Alcoholic cardiomyopathy: a review. *J Card Fail* 2011; 17: 844–9.
68. Praud D, Rota M, Rehm J, et al. Cancer incidence and mortality attributable to alcohol consumption. *Int J Cancer* 2016; 138: 1380–7.
69. Maughan RJ. Risks and rewards of dietary supplement use by athletes. In Maughan RJ (ed.), *Sports Nutrition*. Oxford: Wiley-Blackwell 2014, pp.291–300.
70. Maughan RJ, Depiesse F, Geyer H. The use of dietary supplements by athletes. *J Sports Sci* 2007; 25: S10313.
71. Davis JM, Zhao ZW, Stock HS. Central nervous system effects of caffeine and adenosine on fatigue. *Am J Physiol* 2003; 284: R399–404.
72. Kreider RB. Effects of creatine supplementation on performance and training adaptations. *Mol Cell Biochem* 2003; **244**: 89–94.
73. Sale C, Saunders B, Harris RC. Effect of beta-alanine supplementation on muscle carnosine concentrations and exercise performance. *Amino Acids* 2010; 39: 321–33.
74. Larsen FK, Ekblom B, Sahlin K, et al. Effects of dietary nitrate on oxygen cost during exercise. *Acta Physiol* 2007; 191: 59–66.
75. Larsen FJ, Schiffer TA, Bourniquet S, et al. Dietary inorganic nitrate improves mitochondrial efficiency in humans. *Cell Metab* 2011; 13: 149–59.
76. Bailey SJ, Winyard P, Vanhatalo A, et al. Dietary nitrate supplementation reduces the O_2 cost of low-intensity exercise and enhances tolerance to high-intensity exercise in humans. *J Appl Physiol* 2009; 107: 1144–55.
77. Maughan RJ (2015) Dietary supplement (and food) safety for athletes. In Rawson ES, Volpe SL (eds). *Nutrition for Elite Athletes*. Boca Raton, FL: CRC Press 2015, pp.193–204.
78. Granados J, Gillum TL, Christmas KM, Kuennen MR. Prohormone supplement 3β-hydroxy-5α-androst-1-en-17-one enhances resistance training gains but impairs user health. *J Appl Physiol* 2014; 16: 560–9.
79. Petróczi A, Ocampo JA, Shah I, et al. (2015) Russian roulette with unlicensed fat-burner drug 2,4-dinitrophenol (DNP): evidence from a multidisciplinary study of the internet, bodybuilding supplements and DNP users. *Subst Abuse Treat Prev Pol* 2015; 10; 39.
80. Maughan RJ. Contamination of dietary supplements and positive drugs tests in sport. *J Sports Sci* 2005; 23: 883–9.
81. Watson P, Houghton E, Grace PB, et al. The effect of delivery mode on excretion patterns of nandrolone metabolites after ingestion of a nandrolone pro-hormone. *Med Sci Sports Exerc* 2010; **42**, 754–61.
82. Elorinne A-L, Alfthan G, Erlund I, et al. Food and nutrient intake and nutritional status of Finnish vegans and non-vegetarians. *PloS One* 2016; 11: e0148235.
83. Kristensen NB, Madsen ML, Hansen TH, et al. Intake of macro- and micronutrients in Danish vegans. *Nutr J* 2015; 14: 115.

SECTION 11

Hypertension in athletes

11.1 **Diagnosis and management of hypertension in athletes** *447*
Stefano Caselli and Josef Niebauer

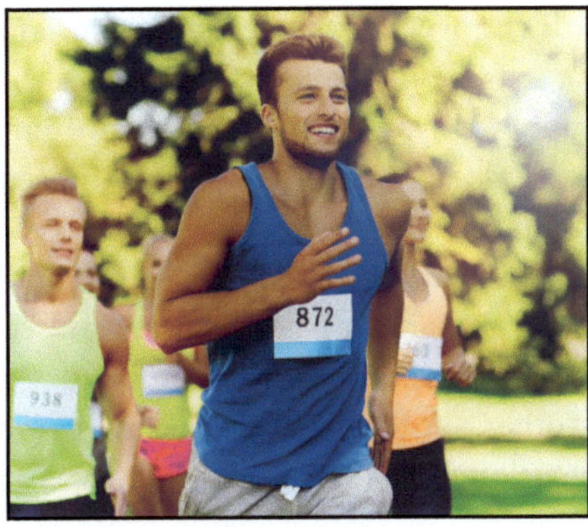

11.1

Diagnosis and management of hypertension in athletes

Stefano Caselli and Josef Niebauer

Introduction

Hypertension is the most prevalent risk factor worldwide and has been associated with increased mortality and overall burden of cardiovascular (CV) diseases [1]. The prevalence of hypertension in 2000 was estimated to be 26% of the adult population, with 972 million people affected worldwide, and the projected prevalence in 2025 is 29%, with 1.5 billion people affected [2]. This is a major health issue and the focus of intense scrutiny regarding the most efficient means of reducing blood pressure in order to decrease the burden of CV diseases.

In this context, regular exercise training has been demonstrated to be effective in lowering blood pressure and reducing the CV risk profile [3]. Indeed, current guidelines recommend lifestyle modification including 30 minutes of moderate intensity aerobic exercise for 5–7 days per week [4]. The mechanisms leading to a long-term decrease in blood pressure are mainly associated with an improved peripheral vascular structure and function [5].

While the beneficial effects of moderate intensity exercise have been extensively proven, the acute increase in blood pressure associated with bursts of strenuous exercise may lead to potentially harmful complications. Indeed, increased blood pressure during effort has also been considered as contributing determinants of cardiac events, such as coronary plaque rupture and cerebral arterial aneurysm rupture [6]. Therefore timely identification of hypertensive individuals is important in the setting of pre-participation CV screening, in order to implement appropriate management and follow-up [7–10]. Recommendations for participation in competitive sports by athletes with arterial hypertension have recently been published by the sports cardiology section of the European Association of Preventive Cardiology (EAPC) [7b].

Prevalence of hypertension in athletes

Paricipation in competitive sport usually involves individuals between 20 and 40 years of age. The prevalence of hypertension in this age range is lower than in older individuals [11]. In the US population, prevalence of hypertension in young adults is reported to be between 4% and 19% [12,13]. In European countries, the prevalence of hypertension in the age group 35–44 years was reported as up to 27% [14]. In Italy, a national cross-sectional study of individuals aged 18–35 (evaluated during the 2014 World Hypertension Day) showed that 11% of young adults had high blood pressure [15].

High blood pressure is one of the most common CV disorders reported within the young athletic population in the setting of pre-participation screening [16,17]. Certain sport disciplines, such as American football, baseball and weightlifting, seem to be associated with a greater prevalence of high blood pressure. Karpinos et al. [18] reported that football players had a higher prevalence of hypertension compared with other sports (19% vs 7%), and Tucker et al. [19] found that the average blood pressure in National Football League players was higher than that of age- and race-matched individuals [19].

However, a meta-analysis by Berge et al. [16] indicated that there is a high variability within athletes, with mean systolic blood pressure ranging from 109±11mmHg to 138±7mmHg and diastolic blood pressure ranging from 57±12mmHg to 92±10mmHg. The prevalence of hypertension also differs significantly among studies, ranging from 0% to 83% (in heavy weightlifters) [16]. Part of the variability observed among the studies is related to differences of methods: either the definition of hypertension was not uniform (with 11 different definitions among studies), or the methods for blood pressure measurement were poorly standardized.

Preliminary data from the Institute of Sports Medicine and Science in Rome suggest that in a large cohort of more than 2000 young competitive athletes (mean age, 24 years) the prevalence of hypertension averages 3%, including a small minority (<0.4%) of individuals with secondary hypertension.

Diagnosis

Hypertension is defined by values of resting blood pressure: ≥140mmHg for systolic blood pressure and/or ≥90mmHg for diastolic blood pressure [4]. Classification of blood pressure according to the European Society of Cardiology guidelines is shown in ➲ Table 11.1.1. The approach to measuring blood pressure in athletes should be rigorous and follow the recommendations, especially if the initial measurement is above 120/80mmHg. The measurement should be performed in a quiet room, with the athlete in a sitting position, after at least 5 minutes rest. The athlete's arm should be horizontal and supported at heart level, and an appropriate cuff-size should be selected to fit it. Korokoff I and V phases of cardiac sound should be recorded for systolic and diastolic blood pressure, respectively. An average of two or more measurements should be taken [4].

In selected cases, such as when 'white coat' hypertension is suspected, 24-hour ambulatory blood pressure monitoring is advised [4,20]. This technique has the advantage of avoiding the mental stress of the medical environment and providing a large number of measurements including daily variations. The current cut-off values for defining hypertension on 24-hour ambulatory blood pressure monitoring are ≥130mmHg for systolic and/or ≥80mmHg for diastolic blood pressure (≥135mmHg and/or ≥85mmHg for day-time blood pressure and/or ≥120mmHg and/or ≥70 mmHg for night-time blood pressure) [4]. Moreover, serial self-measurements at home are useful for ultimately defining the blood pressure profile of the candidate athlete.

Table 11.1.1 Classification of blood pressure according to the European Society of Cardiology Guidelines

	Systolic		Diastolic
Optimal	<120	and	<80
Normal	120–129	and/or	80–84
High normal	130–139	and/or	85–89
Grade 1 hypertension	140–159	and/or	90–99
Grade 2 hypertension	160–179	and/or	100–109
Grade 3 hypertension	≥180	and/or	≥110
Isolated systolic hypertension	≥140	and	<90

Source: Williams B, Mancia G, Spiering W, et al. 2018 ESC/ESH Guidelines for the management of arterial hypertension. *Eur Heart J*, 2018; 39: 3021–3104.

An accurate clinical history, physical examination, and subsequent diagnostic tests should be performed in athletes with the occasional finding of hypertension at physical examination in order to exclude secondary causes [6]. Indeed, 5–10% of patients with hypertension may have an underlying disorder which can be treated appropriately, if promptly identified [21]. The clinical characteristics suggesting a secondary cause of hypertension are early onset (<30 years of age) in the absence of other risk factors and a positive family history, severe hypertension (180/110mmHg), or hypertensive emergencies (i.e. sudden increase in blood pressure in a previously normotensive individual or resistant hypertension despite medical treatment) [21]. The use of supplements, energy drinks, or medications (such as anti-inflammatory drugs) should be specifically investigated, as they may be an under-estimated cause of secondary hypertension in athletes. Symptoms such as anxiety, sweating, flushing, headache, and paroxysmal hypertension may suggest phaeochromocytoma; palpitations, changes in body weight, or fatigue may suggest a thyroid dysfunction; weight gain, fatigue, muscle weakness, hirsutism, skin atrophy, and striae rubrae may be symptoms and signs of Cushing's syndrome; fatigue, constipation, polyuria, and muscle weakness may be indicative of primary aldosteronism; abdominal bruits on physical examination may suggest a renal artery stenosis [4,21].

When there are signs or symptoms of an underlying cardiac disorder, additional examinations should be performed according to the specific case, and the athlete should be referred to a competent specialist.

Blood tests that may be indicated for clinical evaluation of an athlete with hypertension are listed in ➲ Box 11.1.1. Additional tests, such as plasma renin activity, aldosterone,

Box 11.1.1. Routine laboratory tests to be performed in athletes with hypertension

Baseline blood tests

- Haemoglobin and blood count
- Sodium and potassium
- Serum creatinine
- Total cholesterol
- LDL-cholesterol
- HDL-cholesterol
- Triglycerides
- Uric acid
- Thyroid hormones
- Urinalysis
- In selected instances: plasma renin activity, aldosterone, urinary catecholamine

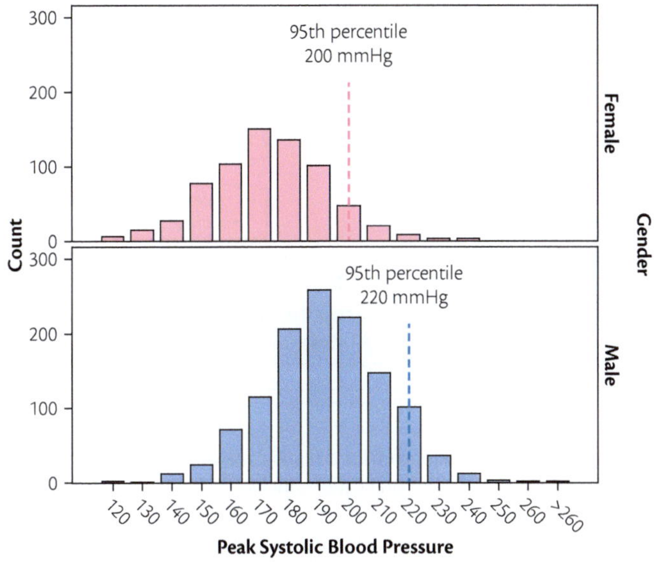

Fig. 11.1.1 Upper limits of peak systolic blood pressure on exercise testing in normotensive male (bottom) and female (top) Olympic athletes.
Adapted from Caselli S, Vaquer Segui A, Quattrini F, et al. Upper normal values of blood pressure response to exercise in Olympic athletes. *Am Heart J* 2016, Volume 177, pp.120–8. Copyright (2016) with permission from Elsevier.

and urinary catecholamine, may be selectively requested to confirm the suspected diagnosis [21].

Exercise testing may provide additional information for evaluating the CV adaptation to exercise and assessing the increase in blood pressure during effort. In a recent study of a large population of Italian Olympic athletes [22], the blood pressure profile was evaluated during exercise, and a substantial increase in the systolic blood pressure during effort compared with the baseline (average, +70mmHg) was observed. Conversely, the diastolic blood pressure did not change (average, +1mmHg,). The upper values (defined by the 95th percentile) for the systolic and diastolic blood pressures in the overall athlete population were 220mmHg and 85mmHg, respectively. The upper value for systolic blood pressure was 220mmHg for male and 200mmHg for female athletes, and the upper value for diastolic blood pressure was 85mmHg ifor-male and 80mmHg for female athletes (➲ Fig. 11.1.1).

The prognostic role of high blood pressure response to exercise is still under debate. A previous meta-analysis showed that exercise-induced hypertension is associated with a higher risk of future cardiac events in healthy volunteers and patients with isolated systemic hypertension [23]. Weiss et al. [24] showed that elevated blood pressure at rest, at low level exercise, or at maximal exercise were all associated with larger incidence of future CV events in a 20-year follow-up. However, a more recent meta-analysis failed to confirm these observations and reported conflicting results [25]. It is possible that a high blood pressure response may be an initial sign of vascular functional impairment and that its clinical utility relies on the identification of pre-hypertensive subjects. Consequently, athletes presenting with isolated high blood pressure response to exercise should be advised to have a periodical follow-up, with special attention to CV risk factors, but without restriction from competitive sport [22].

Echocardiography may provide useful information in assessing the CV risk of hypertensive athletes. An increase in LV wall thickness and mass beyond the expected values (considered the age, gender, and type of sport) may suggest pathological hypertrophy [26]. The LV geometry in hypertensive athletes more frequently shows a concentric hypertrophy, characterized by an increase in mass (>110g/m^2 in men and 95g/m^2 in women) associated with increased relative wall thickness (RWT) of >0.42,

(RWT= (interventricular septum + posterior wall)/end-diastolic diameter).

Hypertensive individuals may also show initial signs of impaired relaxation (measured on tissue Doppler imaging echocardiography as global longitudinal strain), or a subclinical reduction in systolic function different from normotensive athletes with physiological LV remodelling [27–30].

Finally, the assessment of hypertension should depend not only on blood pressure measurements, but also on the presence of other risk factors, target organ damage, diabetes mellitus, and CV and/or renal complications. ➲ Table 11.1.2 shows the criteria for stratification of the CV risk in hypertensive athletes based on the degree of hypertension and associated clinical characteristics. According to clinical data and blood pressure stage, the 10-year risk of CV mortality is defined as low (<1%), moderate (1–4%), high (5–10%) or very high (>10%) [20] (➲ Table 11.1.3).

Management and sport participation

Athletes with hypertension should be managed according to the current guidelines [4,20,31]. After secondary causes of hypertension have been excluded, the athlete should be advised on lifestyle modifications including salt restriction, weight reduction, low alcohol consumption, increased consumption of vegetables and fruits, smoking cessation, and discontinuation of supplements and anti-inflammatory drugs. The athlete is then reassessed periodically, and if these lifestyle changes fail to normalize blood pressure or the athlete is considered to have a high-risk profile, pharmacological treatment should be promptly initiated [4] (➲ Fig. 11.1.2).

Current guidelines recommend several drug classes for the control of high blood pressure, including preferentially angiotensin-converting enzyme inhibitors, angiotensin receptor blockers, beta-blockers, calcium antagonists and diuretics.

Table 11.1.2. Relevant clinical characteristics for risk stratification of patients with hypertension

Risk factors	◆ Men >55 years; women >65 years ◆ Smoking ◆ Dyslipidaemia ◆ Abdominal obesity ◆ Premature CV disease in family (men <55years, women<65 years)
Target organ disease	◆ LV hypertrophy induced by hypertension ◆ Ultrasound evidence of arterial wall thickening or atherosclerotic plaque ◆ Slight increase in serum creatinine (men 1.3–1.5mg/dl, women 1.2–1.4mg/dl) ◆ Microalbuminuria
Associated clinical conditions	◆ Cerebrovascular disease ◆ Ischaemic heart disease ◆ Heart failure ◆ Peripheral vascular disease ◆ Renal impairment ◆ Proteinuria ◆ Advanced retinopathy

Adapted with permission from Giuseppe Mancia, Robert Fagard, Krzysztof Narkiewicz, et al., 2013 ESH/ESC Guidelines for the management of arterial hypertension: The Task Force for the management of arterial hypertension of the European Society of Hypertension (ESH) and of the European Society of Cardiology (ESC), *J Hypertens*, Volume 31, Issue 7, pp.1281–1357. Copyright © 2013 Wolters Kluwer Health, Inc.

However, the physician responsible for the athlete's care should be aware that some of these medications are included in WADA's 'List of Prohibited Substances and Methods', which can easily be consulted online (http://list.wada-ama.org), and should not be prescribed. For example, diuretics are always prohibited and beta-blockers may be banned in certain sport disciplines (such us shooting and archery) in which control of muscular tremors is of ultimate importance. If the prohibited drug is deemed to be essential for blood

Table 11.1.3. Stratification of risk according to clinical characteristics and grade of hypertension

	Grade 1	Grade 2	Grade 3
No risk factors	Low	Moderate	High
1–2 risk factors	Moderate	Moderate	Very high
≥3 risk factors or target organ damage or diabetes	High	High	Very high
Associated clinical conditions	Very high	Very high	Very high

Adapted with permission from Giuseppe Mancia, Robert Fagard, Krzysztof Narkiewicz, et al., 2013 ESH/ESC Guidelines for the management of arterial hypertension: The Task Force for the management of arterial hypertension of the European Society of Hypertension (ESH) and of the European Society of Cardiology (ESC), *J Hypertens*, Volume 31, Issue 7, pp.1281–1357., Copyright © 2013 Wolters Kluwer Health, Inc.

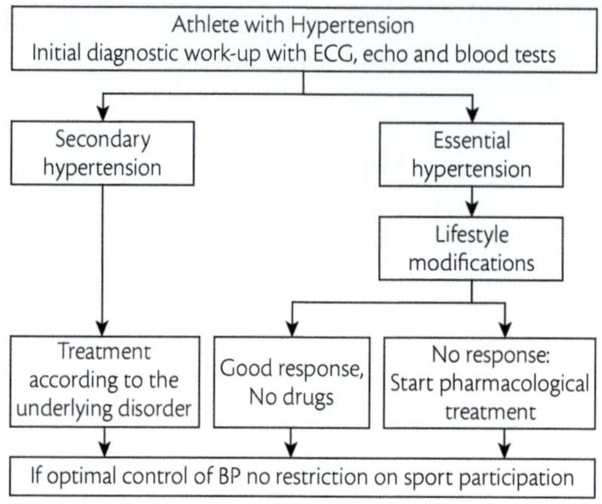

Fig. 11.1.2 Simplified algorithm for the initial management of athletes with hypertension. Lifestyle modifications, including salt restriction, weight reduction, low alcohol consumption, increased consumption of vegetables and fruits, smoking cessation, and discontinuation of supplements and anti-inflammatory drugs are generally sufficient to achieve optimal control of blood pressure levels. Pharmacological treatment is only rarely necessary.

pressure control and cannot be changed, a Therapeutic Use Exemption should be presented to the athlete's national anti-doping agency for appropriate authorization.

When blood pressure is only mildly elevated and the overall CV risk profile is low, which is the common scenario in a young athlete, a single drug regimen with angiotensin-converting enzyme inhibitors or angiotensin receptor blockers will usually control the blood pressure profile. However, in other cases a drug combination may be necessary [4].

With regard to the recommendations for participation in sport, the decision should be taken after careful consideration of blood pressure control, overall cardiovascular risk profile, and type of sport. ➲ Tables 11.1.2 and 11.1.3 give the criteria for stratification of CV risk used to advise hypertensive athletes on sport participation in [20].

Based on these criteria, the hypertensive athlete can be classified as low, moderate, high, and very high risk. The advice for participation in competitive sport depends on control of the blood pressure profile. Usually, there is no contraindication participation in for competitive sport if the athlete's blood pressure is well controlled by appropriate treatment and the overall CV profile is low to high. Certain restrictions may be necessary when the overall CV is very high (see Chapter 7.1). Evaluation of the athlete, with reassessment of the CV risk, should be performed annually or every six months in the case of high or very high risk.

Further reading

Caselli S, Vaquer Seguì A, Lemme E, et al. Prevalence and management of systemic hypertension in athletes. *Am J Cardiol* 2017; 119: 1616–22.

Williams B, Mancia G, Spiering W, et al. 2018 ESC/ESH Guidelines for the management of arterial hypertension. *Eur Heart J* 2018; 39: 3021–3104.

Rimoldi SF, Scherrer U, Messerli FH. Secondary arterial hypertension: when, who, and how to screen? *Eur Heart J* 2014; 35: 1245–54.

References

1. Whitworth JA. 2003 World Health Organization (WHO)/ International Society of Hypertension (ISH) statement on management of hypertension. *J Hypertens* 2003; 21: 1983–92.
2. Kearney PM, Whelton M, Reynolds K, et al. Global burden of hypertension: analysis of worldwide data. *Lancet* 2005; 365: 217–23.
3. Naci H, Ioannidis JP. Comparative effectiveness of exercise and drug interventions on mortality outcomes: metaepidemiological study. *BMJ* 2013; 347: f5577.
4. Mancia G, Fagard R, Narkiewicz K, et al. 2013 ESH/ESC Guidelines for the management of arterial hypertension. *J Hypertens* 2013; 31: 1281–1357.
5. Sabbahi A, Arena R, Elokda A, Phillips SA. Exercise and hypertension: uncovering the mechanisms of vascular control. *Prog Cardiovasc Dis* 2016; 59: 226–34.
6. Black HR, Sica D, Ferdinand K, White WB. Eligibility and disqualification recommendations for competitive athletes with cardiovascular abnormalities: Task Force 6: Hypertension. *Circulation* 2015; 132: e298–302.
7. Selden MA, Helzberg JH, Waeckerle JF. Early cardiovascular mortality in professional football players: fact or fiction? *Am J Med* 2009; 122: 811–14.

7b. Niebauer J, Börjesson M, Carre F, et al. Recommendations for participation in competitive sports of athletes with arterial hypertension: a position statement from the sports cardiology section of the European Association of Preventive Cardiology (EAPC). *Eur Heart J* 2018; 39(40): 3664–71.

8. Baron SL, Hein MJ, Lehman E, Gersic CM. Body mass index, playing position, race, and the cardiovascular mortality of retired professional football players. *Am J Cardiol* 2012; 109: 889–96.
9. Hurst RT, Burke RF, Wissner E, et al. Incidence of subclinical atherosclerosis as a marker of cardiovascular risk in retired professional football players. *Am J Cardiol* 2010; 105: 1107–11.
10. Sundstrom J, Neovius M, Tynelius P, Rasmussen F. Association of blood pressure in late adolescence with subsequent mortality: cohort study of Swedish male conscripts. *BMJ* 2011; 342: d643.
11. Battistoni A, Canichella F, Pignatelli G, et al. Hypertension in young people: epidemiology, diagnostic assessment and therapeutic approach. *High Blood Press Cardiovasc Prev* 2015; 22: 381–8.
12. Chiolero A, Bovet P, Paradis G. Screening for elevated blood pressure in children and adolescents: a critical appraisal. *JAMA Pediatr* 2013; 167: 266–73.
13. Liu J, Wade TJ, Tan H. Cardiovascular risk factors and anthropometric measurements of adolescent body composition: a cross-sectional analysis of the Third National Health and Nutrition Examination Survey. *Int J Obes (Lond)* 2007; 31: 59–64.
14. Wolf-Maier K, Cooper RS, Banegas JR, et al. Hypertension prevalence and blood pressure levels in 6 European countries, Canada, and the United States. *JAMA* 2003; 289: 2363–9.
15. Bruno RM, Pucci G, Rosticci M, et al. Association between lifestyle and systemic arterial hypertension in young adults: a national, survey-based, cross-sectional study. *High Blood Press Cardiovasc Prev* 2016; 23: 31–40.
16. Berge HM, Isern CB, Berge E. Blood pressure and hypertension in athletes: a systematic review. *Br J Sports Med* 2015; 49: 716–23.
17. Corrado D, Basso C, Pavei A, et al. Trends in sudden cardiovascular death in young competitive athletes after implementation of a preparticipation screening program. *JAMA* 2006; 296: 1593–1601.
18. Karpinos AR, Roumie CL, Nian H, et al. High prevalence of hypertension among collegiate football athletes. *Circ Cardiovasc Qual Outcomes* 2013; 6: 716–23.
19. Tucker AM, Vogel RA, Lincoln AE, et al. Prevalence of cardiovascular disease risk factors among National Football League players. *JAMA* 2009; 301: 2111–19.
20. Pelliccia A, Fagard R, Bjornstad HH, et al. Recommendations for competitive sports participation in athletes with cardiovascular disease. *Eur Heart J* 2005; 26: 1422–45.
21. Rimoldi SF, Scherrer U, Messerli FH. Secondary arterial hypertension: when, who, and how to screen? *Eur Heart J* 2014; 35: 1245–54.
22. Caselli S, Vaquer Segui A, Quattrini F, et al. Upper normal values of blood pressure response to exercise in Olympic athletes. *Am Heart J* 2016; 177: 120–8.
23. Smith RG, Rubin SA, Ellestad MH. Exercise hypertension: an adverse prognosis? *J Am Soc Hypertens* 2009; 3: 366–73.
24. Weiss SA, Blumenthal RS, Sharrett AR, et al. Exercise blood pressure and future cardiovascular death in asymptomatic individuals. *Circulation* 2010; 121: 2109–16.
25. Schultz MG, Otahal P, Cleland VJ, et al. Exercise-induced hypertension, cardiovascular events, and mortality in patients undergoing exercise stress testing: a systematic review and meta-analysis. *Am J Hypertens* 2013; 26: 357–66.
26. Baggish AL, Weiner RB, Yared K, et al. Impact of family hypertension history on exercise-induced cardiac remodeling. *Am J Cardiol* 2009; 104: 101–6.
27. Caselli S, Di Paolo FM, Pisicchio C, et al. Patterns of left ventricular diastolic function in olympic athletes. *J Am Soc Echocardiogr* 2015; 28: 236–44.
28. Caselli S, Montesanti D, Autore C, et al. Patterns of left ventricular longitudinal strain and strain rate in Olympic athletes. *J Am Soc Echocardiogr* 2015; 28: 245–53.
29. Galderisi M, Lomoriello VS, Santoro A, et al. Differences of myocardial systolic deformation and correlates of diastolic function in competitive rowers and young hypertensives: a speckle-tracking echocardiography study. *J Am Soc Echocardiogr* 2010; 23: 1190–8.
30. Lin J, Wang F, Weiner RB, et al. Blood pressure and LV remodeling among American-style football players. *JACC Cardiovasc Imaging* 2016; 9: 1367–76.
31. Piepoli MF, Hoes AW, Agewall S, et al. 2016 European Guidelines on cardiovascular disease prevention in clinical practice. *Atherosclerosis* 2016; 252: 207–74.

Index

Note: *b*, *f*, and *t* afer locators denote boxes, figures and tables

A

ablation (ventricular arrhythmias) 119, 278–82
  of accessory pathway 281–2
  catheter ablation 119, 284, 291
  cryo-ablation, vs radiofrequency (RF) ablation 280
accessory pathways
  Kent bundle 281–2, 288
  mitral valve, tricuspid valve and inter-atrial septum 289*t*
acetazolamide 430*t*
acute mountain sickness 336
adrenergic stress 257
'adult' age, variously defined 321
advanced life support, European and American guidelines 407
aerobic capacity, increase, exercise training 392
aerobic glycolysis 4, 390
  fatty acids 390
aerobic training, *see also* exercise training
aerobic–anaerobic energy metabolism 390*f*
African/Afro-Caribbean ethnicity *see* black athletes; ethnicity of athletes
Ajmaline test, suspected Brugada syndrome 115*f*
Alagille syndrome 360
alcohol 440–1
alpha-actinin-3 (ACTN3), polymorphisms 170
altitude effects
  Fontan palliation 245
  SCA/SCD in athletes 336
alveolar ventilation 7–8
ambulatory ECG, arrhythmia registration 107–13
American College of Sports Medicine (ACSM), new recommendations for exercise participation health screening 356
American Heart Association (AHA), AHA/ACC Task Force 324–5
amphetamine 430*t*
anaerobic glycolysis 390*f*
anaerobic speed reserve (ASR) 94*f*
anaerobic threshold 93
  oxygen debt 4–5
androgenic anabolic steroids (AAS)
  cardiovascular effects 430*t*
  production, consumption data 429
  severe side effects 429
aneurysm, Ehlers–Danlos syndrome, Loeys–Dietz syndrome, and familial thoracic aortic aneurysm 334
aneurysm of descending aorta 247*f*, 314
angiotensin I converting enzyme (ACE)
  BP control 324
  genetic screening 170
angiotensin II 11
angiotensin receptor blockers (ARBs) 324
anomalous left coronary artery from the pulmonary artery (ALCAPA) 217–18, 222
anterograde refractory period of Kent bundle, predicting risk of SCD 290–1
anthropometry, paediatric 362
anti-arrhythmic drug provocation test 114–15
antidromic atrioventricular re-entrant tachycardia 288
antioxidant nutrients 438–9
aorta
  aortopathy, increased risk 236
  coarctation and other abnormalities 247
  dimension in athletes 333
  rate of aortic expansion 333
  vascular adaptation 42
    isometric vs endurance exercise 42
aortic dissection 314–15
  Marfan syndrome 334
  SCA/SCD in athletes 332–3
aortic remodelling 17
aortic root
  and ascending aorta 332–3
  diameter 42, 333
  dilation, echocardiography 133–4
  see also bicuspid aortic valve (BAV)
aortic stenosis, cause of SCD 247, 314
aortic stiffness 42
aromatase inhibitors 430*t*
arrhythmias
  commotio cordis 328–30
  ESC/EAPC recommendation for competitive sport participation 370–1*t*
  evaluation during exercise tests 99–100
  genetics 166–9, 187–8
  inducing 278
  inherited arrhythmogenic disorders 166
  paediatric 361
  primary arrhythmogenic disorders/syndromes 166, 371*t*–2
  registration 107–19
    ambulatory ECG 107–13
arrhythmogenic cardiomyopathy (AC) 145–7, 184–200
  2010 Task Force criteria for 193*t*–4
  classic right ventricular AC 190*f*
  CMR 145–7
  consensus statements regarding AC and participation in exercise 198*t*
  desmoplakin mutation in mouse model 188*f*, 196
  detection of AC in athletes 191–3
  differential diagnosis 190*f*
  ECG abnormalities 189
  ECG and echocardiographic findings (14-year-old male) 194*f*
  genetics 166–9, 187–8
  ICD
    indications, flowchart of risk stratification 196*f*
    main life-saving tool 198
  incidence, relative risk (RR) of sudden death 195*f*
  induced by exercise? 196
  Kaplan–Meier analysis of actual AC patient survival 196*f*
  morpho-functional abnormalities of RV 189–90
  participation in competitive sport 196–7
  pre-participation screening 197
  recommendation for competitive sport participation 372*t*
  risk stratification and prevention 193–4, 196*f*
  SCD, during exercise 185*f*, 311–12
  transgenic mouse model, Wnt/β-catenin signalling 188
  see also arrhythmogenic right ventricular cardiomyopathy (ARVC)

arrhythmogenic right ventricular cardiomyopathy (ARVC) 166–71
AHA/ACC Task Force criteria 272
clinical diagnosis 190*f*
prevalence, associated genes, contribution, and yield of genetic testing 171*t*
strenuous exercise and development of phenotype 168*f*
arterial pulse rate, paediatric 362
arteries
hypothesized response to increased flow and shear stress exercise training 44*f*
luminal diameter 42
ARVC
ARVC Task Force diagnostic criteria 272
exercise–ARVC spectrum
diagnosis 272–3
epidemiology 272
evidence 272
predominant role of RV 272
aspirin therapy 324
asthma, SCA/SCD in athletes 334
asymptomatic ventricular pre-excitation 281
risk assessment, competitive and recreational athletes 281
atherosclerosis
childhood 360
coronary artery disease, athletes 309–10
Kaplan-Meier event-free survival curves 155*f*
underestimation in older athletes 154
'athlete's heart'
arrhythmia registration 107–19
cardiomyopathies 77–80
cardiovascular remodelling 41–9
in children and adolescents 32–41
differential diagnosis, vs inherited arrhythmogenic disorders 167
ECG 57–85
overlap patterns 77–85
exercise testing 87–106
genetic testing 166–74
history and physical examination 51–6
imaging 120–65
long-term adaptation to exercise 9–11
sporting discipline, gender, ethnicity and genetics 20–31
structural and functional adaptations 11–20
syndrome 107, 161
ATP levels 3
ATP production in muscle 4–5*f*, 389–90
atrial fibrillation (AF) 99–100, 281–4
first onset, paroxysmal, or persistent 283
high frequency 290
radiofrequency catheter ablation 284, 291
recommendation for competitive sport participation 370*t*
stroke risk 285
treatment and exercise recommendations 283–4
WPW pattern 288
atrial flutter (AFL) 282–3
catheter ablation of the isthmus 284
cavotricuspid isthmus dependent 118
recommendation for competitive sport participation 370*t*
stroke risk 285
atrial premature beats (APBs) 278–9
atrial septal defects (ASD) 246–7
echocardiography 135–6
atrioventricular (AV) block 246
competitive sport participation 370*t*
first-degree 108, 291
second-degree AV block Mobitz 100, 108, 291
third-degree 100
Wenckebach 108
atrioventricular conduction, paediatric 363
atrioventricular re-entrant tachycardia (AVRT), orthodromic/antidromic 288
atrioventricular septal defects (AVSD) 246–7
Australian Government Department of Health, paediatric exercise activity 33*t*
automatic external defibrillators (AEDs) 406–7, 411
cost-effective placement rate, sports arenas 411
European Arena study 411
autopsy, sudden cardiac death 170

B

ballistic testing 396
Barlow's disease 226
basic life support (BLS)
certification 404–5
sudden cardiac arrest (SCA) 404–5
bench press and squat, specific resistance training 396
beta-2 agonists 430*t*
beta-adrenergic blocking agents, in athletes 324–5
beta-alanine supplementation 441
bicarbonate, supplementation 441
bicarbonate ions, carbonic acid 5, 6–7
bicuspid aortic valve (BAV) 134–5*f*, 233–7
clinical course of patients 235–6
echocardiography 134–5*f*
epidemiology 234
legal concerns 237
pathophysiology 234, 234–5
sport risks 236
black athletes
Brugada syndrome 28
distribution of LV wall thickness 14*f*, 15
and HCM 179
incidence of SCD 300, 315
long QT syndrome (LQTS) 28
range of mild LV hypertrophy 15*f*
see also ethnicity of athletes
blood flow capacity, functional adaptive changes 41–2
blood pressure
evaluation during exercise 100–1
inadequate decrease in BP during recovery 101
interpretation of maximal systolic BP 101
paediatric 362
Rost's formula 101
specificities of BP responses to exercise 101
upper limits, exercise testing 449*f*
body size and height, aortic dissection 332–3
body-building supplements, liver injury 441
brachial artery diameter 42
brachial artery flow-mediated dilation (FMD) 42
breathing reserve, calculation 93
Bruce treadmill protocol 159
Brugada syndrome 114–15, 258–60
black population 28
defined 253
pre-participation and eligibility screening protocol 260
prevalence, associated genes, contribution, and yield of genetic testing 171*t*, 292
recommendation for competitive sport participation 371*t*
risk of SCD 259

C

C-reactive protein 205
caffeine 441
calcified plaque 153
calcium *see* coronary artery calcium (CAC)
calcium channels, PKC signalling, response to stretch 44
calcium and vitamin D 439
Canadian Society for Exercise Physiology (CSEP), paediatric exercise activity 33*t*
capillaries
density, maintenance in cardiac hypertrophy 45
diameters, transit time and 44*f*
exchange capacity, product of permeability and surface area 45
full perfusion, maximal exchange capacity 46
see also skeletal muscle
carbohydrate
body stores 435
carbohydrate-rich foods, low glycaemic index 435
current guidelines for intake by athletes 436*t*
fuel requirements 435
low, in diet 436
RQ 4
carbon dioxide
output (VCO_2) and heart rate (HR) vs oxygen uptake ($\dot{V}O_2$) 6*f*
production, acidosis 7
ventilatory equivalent (VE/VCO_2) 93
carbonic acid 5
cardiac abnormalities
safe participation in sport 369–80
cardiac arrhythmias *see* arrhythmias
'cardiac classification of sports' 376
cardiac enlargement, history 21
cardiac hypertrophy
capillary density maintenance 45
determinants 12–13
cardiac magnetic resonance imaging (CMR) 140–52
acquisition and post-processing 141–3
advantages 141
athletes 140–1*f*
balanced steady state free precession (bSSFP) 141
cine imaging 141
delayed gadolinium enhancement (DGE) 141, 143
clinical importance 206*b*
phase-contrast velocity encoding 142–3
cardiac myocyte, 'beneficial' adaptive changes 11–12
cardiac output
normal resting and maximal 3
stroke volume and 6
cardiac rhythm, paediatric 363
cardiac safety, sports facilities 403–26
cardiomyopathies 166
defined 166
genetics of 171
paediatric 360–1

recommendation for competitive sport participation 372*t*
sudden cardiac arrest/death 311–12
see also arrhythmogenic cardiomyopathy (AC); dilated cardiomyopathy (DCM); hypertrophic cardiomyopathy (HCM)
cardiopulmonary auscultation, paediatric 362
cardiopulmonary exercise test (CPET) *see* exercise testing; exercise training
cardiovascular adaptations, historical 9–11
cardiovascular disease, risk factor profile 352
cardiovascular effects, prohibited substances and methods 427
cardiovascular performance, endurance capacity and muscular strength 389
cardiovascular protection with exercise 352, 434
cardiovascular remodelling 41–9
adaptation of aorta and peripheral circulation 42–3
diastolic LV function 15
functional adaptive changes in the blood flow capacity 41
impact of various sport disciplines 12*f*
integrative coronary vascular function 45–6
structural adaptations in cardiac and skeletal muscle vascular beds 41
vascular adaptation of coronary system 43–4
cardiovascular screening *see* pre-participation screening; screening
carotid bodies 7
catecholaminergic polymorphic ventricular tachycardia (CPVT) 166, 167, 257–8
abstinence from competitive performances 169
concept of 'phenotype negative' 174
defined 253
genetics 257
polymorphic ventricular tachycardia 273
pre-participation and eligibility screening protocol 260
prevalence, associated genes, contribution, and yield of genetic testing 171*t*
prevention of SCD 173, 257
recommendation for competitive sport participation 371*t*
catheter ablation
isthmus, atrial flutter (AFL) 284
ventricular arrhythmias 119
cavotricuspid isthmus dependent atrial flutter 118
channelopathies 166, 253–64
electrophysiological study 261
exercise stress testing and Holter monitoring 205–6, 260
genetics of 171, 261
imaging with echocardiography and MRI 261
management 261–2
eligibility decision-making 261–2
oral drug therapy and ICD implantation 261
paediatric 361
pre-participation and eligibility screening protocol 260
see also Brugada syndrome; catecholaminergic polymorphic ventricular tachycardia (CPVT); long QT syndrome (LQTS); short QT syndrome (SQTS)
chemoreceptors, carotid bodies 7
chest protection 330
children/adolescents
adaption to exercise training in child athletes: comparison with adults 37*t*
age-related changes in the ECG 35*f*
approach to CV evaluation 38*t*
assessing child athletes 38
cardiomyopathies 39
chest pain 361
CV conditions, young competitive athletes 359
CV remodelling in peri-pubertal child athletes 36*t*–7
CV screening 359–66
questionnaire, history, and examination 38
early childhood and puberty 34
echocardiography screening 39
effect of exercise training 35–6
electrocardiography 39
elite training 32
ethnicity 34–5
infancy 33
physical activity daily 32
screening programmes 360
summary of recommendations 33*t*
cholesterol (HDL-C), increases with activity 323
cholesterol (LDL-C), reduction with statins 324
chronotropy, positive 5, 6
coarctation *see* aorta
cocaine 430*t*
related myocarditis 313–14
cold stress, SCA/SCD in athletes 335
collagen diseases 227
collapse
BLS Adult Cardiac Arrest Algorithm 406*f*
differential diagnosis 403
flow diagram/algorithm 405*f*
initial response 403–4
see also sudden cardiac arrest (SCA)
commotio cordis 328–30
communications, emergency 416–17
conduction abnormalities 291–6
AV, left fascicular, right and left bundle branch blocks 291
paediatric 364
see also atrioventricular (AV) block; Wolff–Parkinson–White syndrome
congenital coronary artery anomalies (CAAs) 217–22
of anatomy, CA fistula 221–2
clinical management 221–4
guidelines for sport eligibility 222
of origin and course 217
ALCAPA 217–18, 222
myocardial bridge 220–2
wrong sinus CAA 218*f*–20, 222
congenital heart disease 238–50, 360
arrhythmias 244
assessment
age-specific assessment 243–4
cardiopulmonary exercise testing 243
exercise stress echocardiography 244*f*
functional and dynamic assessment 242–3
imaging 242
RV 245
children, exercise advice 239–40
competition guidelines 248–9
cyanosis 247
defined 238
epidemiology of athletes 238–9
exercise pathophysiology 241
exercise prescription, stepwise assessment approach 240*t*
heart failure 244–5
high altitude effects 245–6
interventions, timing and risk stratification 246
physical activity and sport 239
risks of sudden cardiac death 240–1
specific lesions 246–8
congenitally corrected transposition of the great arteries (ccTGA) 248
Cooper 12min run 391
coronary angiography 162–5
CT angiography 156–7
coronary artery calcium (CAC) 153–4*f*
scores 159, 161*f*, 325
severe calcification 160*f*, 325
long-term follow-up data 159
coronary artery disease
aetiology 322–3
AHA/ACC Task Force recommendations 325*b*
angiography 162–5
atherosclerotic 309–10
Kaplan–Meier event-free survival curves 155*f*
CMR 148–9
coronary plaque 323
eligibility and disqualification recommendations for competitive athletes (AHA/ACC) 325*b*
exercise-related sudden cardiac events 322–3
false-positive detection of asymptomatic 98
known, athletes 309–10
management 324–5
magnitude of ischaemia 88
non-atherosclerotic 311–12
participants of leisure exercise and competitive sports 354
recommendation for competitive sport participation 373*t*
returning to competition 325
coronary computed tomography 153–8
identification of candidate athletes 153
pathophysiological and prognostic implications 156–7
coronary computed tomography angiography 156
coronary system
blood flow (CBF), capillaries fully perfused with maximal exchange capacity 46
epicardial conduit arteries 43–4
integrative vascular function 45–6
resistance vessels, densities and diameters 44, 45*f*
structural and functional adaptations to chronic exercise 45*f*
vascular adaptation 43–4
countries
cardiac arrest/sudden death in the young and/or during sports activity 340–1*t*
pre-participation screening in young competitive athletes 348*t*
CPR, compression-only, effectiveness 404–5
creatine 441
cyanosis, congenital heart disease 247

D

defibrillator/synchronized cardioverter/ transcutaneous pacemaker 414
desmoplakin, mutation in mouse model 188*f*–9*f*, 196

desmosomal gene transfer 195
Determinants of Myocardial Infarction Onset Study (ONSET) 321
diagnosis 134, 228
dilated cardiomyopathy (DCM)
  cause of SCD 167
  CMR 147
  echocardiography 131–2
  prevalence, associated genes, contribution, and yield of genetic testing 171*t*
  recommendation for competitive sport participation 372*t*
dinitrophenol (DNP) 441
diuretics 430*t*
  BP control 324
doping
  defined 427
  dinitrophenol (DNP) 441
  list of prohibited substances and methods 427–8
  prevalence 428
  and SCA 330
  severe side effects 429
  substances and cardiovascular effects 430*t*
  substances and methods
    prohibited at all times 428
    prohibited in competition 428
  taken with the objective of abuse 430*t*
  therapeutic use exemption (TUE) 431
  use of team and professional equipment 431
  World Anti-Doping Agency (WADA), list of prohibited substances and methods 427
Doppler imaging, septal *e'* velocity 8.0cm/s 16
drug abuse *see* doping
Drug-Induced Liver Injury Network (DILIN) 441–2
dyspnoea 8

E

Ebstein anomalies 248, 280, 314
ECG
  abnormalities
    athlete, classification 346*f*
    unselected large young population 289*t*
  ambulatory ECG, arrhythmia registration 107–13
  anti-arrhythmic drug provocation test 114–15
  common ECG patterns 68–76
  interventricular dispersion of repolarization 103
  most common alterations in athletes 167
  new technologies 112–13
  paediatric 362–4
  pre-participation screening programmes 265
  signal-averaged ECG 111–12
    time-domain parameters 112*f*
  training-related and training-unrelated 21*t*
  Wolff–Parkinson–White pattern, sudden cardiac death 289
echocardiography 121–40
  2D speckle tracking 15, 127*f*, 128*t*–30
  3D 11*f*, 130
    duration of mechanical systole 15
  apical four-chamber view 124*f*
  apical two- and three-chamber views 125–6
  indications 121*b*
  morphological and functional evaluation 120–39
  new echo modalities 127
  parasternal long axis view 122
  parasternal short axis view 123*f*
  reference values 122*t*
  specific abnormalities 131–6
  standard examination protocol 121–2
  stress echocardiography 126
  subcostal view 126
  suprasternal view 126
  trans-oesophageal echocardiography 230–1
  trans-thoracic echocardiography 134, 228
education of athletes, prodromal symptoms of heart disease 326
Ehlers–Danlos syndrome 227, 314, 334
  aortic dilation/dissection 334
ejection fraction, measured by echocardiography using Simpson's rule 16*f*
electrical remodelling 20–4, 37–8
electrolyte balance 439–40
electrophysiological (EP) study 116–19
  arrhythmia therapy 118*f*
  atrial vulnerability 290
  degeneration of AVRT into atrial fibrillation 290
  diagnostic EP 116–17
  endocavitary (E-EPS) and trans-oesophageal (T-EPS) 291
  Europe vs US approach 281
  inducibility of AVRT 290
  Kent bundle
    anterograde effective refractory period 290–1
    retrograde conduction 290
  risk assessment 116–17
  ventricular stimulation 117*f*
elite athletes
  functional adaptive changes in the blood flow capacity 41
  no common DNA variants associated with physical performance 170
  structural adaptations in cardiac and skeletal muscle vascular beds 41
emergency medical service (EMS) physicians, mass gathering events 412
emergency responses, *see also* sudden cardiac arrest (SCA)
end-tidal carbon dioxide levels 8
endocarditis, antibiotic prophylaxis 246
endothelial function, brachial artery flow-mediated dilation (FMD) 42
endothelium-dependent vasodilatation 42–4
endurance, muscular 396–7
endurance capacity, muscular strength 389
endurance exercise capacity 389, 393
endurance sports, LV enlargement 21
energy metabolism
  aerobic–anaerobic 390*f*
  transitions, first and second thresholds 391
energy requirements 433–5
  growth in young athletes 434
energy sources 435–6
  substrate availability 4, 390*f*
energy systems, physical activity 389–90
ephedrine 430*t*
epilepsy-related seizures, differential diagnosis 403
ergogenic aids prescription 433
erythropoietin (EPO) 430*t*
  side effects 429–30
ethnicity of athletes 24–7, 300
  Arabic (Middle Eastern), South Asian and East Asian ethnicity 27
  ECG
    abnormal ECG patterns 26*f*
    other ECG changes 25–6
    T-wave inversion 24–5*f*
  LV cavity dimensions 26
  LV hypertrophy 26–7
    range of mild 15*f*
  RV adaptations 27
  training-related and training-unrelated ECG changes 21*t*
  see also black athletes
European Association for Cardiovascular Prevention and Rehabilitation (EACPR) 354, 411
European countries
  cardiac arrest/sudden death in the young and/or during sports activity 340–1*t*
  pre-participation screening in young competitive athletes 348*t*
European Society of Cardiology (ESC) 352
event monitors 110*t*
  external real-time continuous event recorder patch 110
  implantable event recorders 110
  post-event non-looping event monitors (PER900) 109
exercise capacity
  aerobic endurance exercise capacity 393
  Cooper 12min run 391
exercise hypertension 101, 102
exercise intensity, prescription according to maximal exercise parameters 391*t*
exercise performance, components 389
exercise physiology 3–8
exercise testing 87–106
  AHA recommendations 325–6
  cardiopulmonary (CPET) 87, 389, 390
  determining thresholds by CPET 392
  in diabetics, men of 45+, women of 55+, and those with major CAD risk factors 325
  diagnostic 87–8
  ECG changes and arrhythmic disorders 98*f*
  functional 88
  gas exchange analysis assessment of repeated sprint sequences (RSSs) 94–5
  graded 90
  implications for high intensity training 94
  indications 87
    contraindications 326
  interest and limitations of 98
  metabolic equivalents (METs) 95
  modalities 89
  parameters measured 90–2
  prognostic 88
  protocols 89–90
    increasing/constant work rates 90*f*
  upper limits of peak systolic blood pressure 449*f*
  ventilatory equivalents for oxygen and carbon dioxide 93–5
exercise training
  acute response 11–13
  aortic diameter 333
  arrhythmias during 99–100
  beneficial changes in CAD risk factors 322–3
  blood pressure during 100–1
  cardiac structural and electrical remodelling processes 166–8
  determining thresholds by CPET 392
  increase in aerobic capacity 392
  intervention programmes 389
  maximal exercise parameters 390, 391

prescription for cardiovascular health 381–402
prescription of intensity according to maximal exercise parameters 391*t*
principal effect 434
QT interval adaptations 102–5
respiratory system and 6–8, 389–90
see also physical activity
exercise-induced cardiac remodelling *see* athlete's heart
exercise-induced rhabdomyolysis 330–1
exercise-related cardiac events in adults 322–3
arrhythmias 278
ARVC-like cardiomyopathy 272
exercise-related SCD 321–4
absolute risk 322
aetiology of cardiac events 322–3
clinical features
AMI 323–4
SCD in adult athletes 323–4
Nurses' Health Study 321
prevention 324
aggressive reduction of risk factors 324
exertional heat stroke, differential diagnosis 403
exertional hyponatraemia, differential diagnosis 403
extreme environments, sport in 334–5

F

familial thoracic aortic aneurysm 334
aortic dilation/dissection 334
fascicular blocks 291
fatigue during exertion, paediatric 361–2
fatty acids, as energy substrate 4, 390
FDG-positron emission tomography (PET) 159
femoral artery diameter 42
Fick equation 4
FIFA, rule on possible SCA 404
fitness categories, relative $V{\cdot}O_2$max (ml/kg/min) values for non-athletes 391*t*
fitness centres 419–25
defibrillation 422
emergency policies and procedures 421
preparedness, UK and Europe 421, 422
facility characteristics 421*t*
incidence rate of sudden cardiac events 419–20
predictors of SCA 420
survival rate of SCA 420
numbers, members, market size: European countries 420*t*
terminology and types of physical activity 419
flow-mediated dilation (FMD) 42
Fontan palliation, effects of high altitude 245
Football Emergency Medicine Manual (FIFA) 412
Frank–Starling relationship, intrinsic force 6
functional adaptive changes, blood flow capacity 41–2
furosemide 430*t*

G

GAMES consortium, genetic profiling of athletes 170
gas exchange analysis, assessment of repeated sprint sequences (RSSs) 94
gender
electrical remodelling 23–4
structural remodelling 23–4
genetic testing of athletes 166–76
current expert recommendations 171
established clinical diagnosis 168–9
first-degree relatives of person with inherited CV disease 169–70
hypertrophic cardiomyopathy (HCM) 182
impact of positive result on sports eligibility 171–3
indications 166–7, 168
inherited arrhythmogenic disorders 166–9
requests 171
role for genetic screening 170
sudden cardiac death autopsy 170
cascade screening of relatives 170
suspected clinical diagnosis 169
genetics 166–9, 187–8
electrical remodelling 27–8, 37–8
LV remodelling 27–8
primary determinant of success in sport 433
structural remodelling 37–8
gluconeogenesis 4
glucose
as energy substrate 4, 390
storage as glycogen 4
glycaemic index 435
glycogen, body store of carbohydrate 4, 435
glycogenolysis 4
glycolytic energy system 390
growth factors 430*t*

H

hamstring–quadriceps ratio (H:Q ratio), different sports 396
Hansen–Wasserman equations 390
healthy lifestyle 382
heart disease, prodromal symptoms 326
heart murmurs, paediatric 362
heart output *see* cardiac output
heart rate (HR)
and lactate curves 394–5*f*
and oxygen pulse (VO_2/HR) vs time 6*f*
paediatric 363
heat stress, SCA/SCD in athletes 335
heat stroke, differential diagnosis 403
'Heidbüchel syndrome' 272–3
high altitude cerebral oedema (HACE) 336
high altitude pulmonary oedema (HAPE) 336
high fibre diets 442
high intensity training (HIT) 94
rating of perceived exertion (RPE) 94
Holt–Oram syndrome 360
Holter monitoring
24-h 205–6, 260
event recorders and 107–9
human growth hormone (hGH) 430*t*
human-induced pluripotent stem cells (hiPSCs) 195
hypertension in athletes 100–2, 447–51
classification 448*t*
diagnosis and management 447–52
European Society of Cardiology Guidelines 448*t*
inadequate decrease in BP during recovery 101
management and sport participation 449–50
algorithm 450*f*
'masked' 100
physical training and 101
prevalence 447
recommendation for competitive sport participation 372*t*
risk stratification 450*t*
routine laboratory tests 448*t*
specificities of BP responses to exercise 101
stratification of risk 450*t*
hypertrophic cardiomyopathy (HCM) 179–83
abnormal T-wave inversion (TWI) 180
cause of SCD 167, 311–12
CMR 143–5
features 182
commonest cause of SCD in young athletes 179
diagnosis 180
diastolic function 181
differentiation of physiological LVH from HCM 180
ECG 180
echocardiography 131
exercise guidelines for athletes 182–3
genetic testing 182
HCM Risk-SCD calculator to estimate the 5-year SCD risk 118
LV cavity size 181
LV outflow tract obstruction 182
normalization of wall thicknesses after long-term detraining 21
prevalence 179–80
associated genes, contribution, and yield of genetic testing 171*t*
recommendation for competitive sport participation 372*t*
response to exercise 182
role of detraining 182
hyponatraemia, differential diagnosis 403
hypothermia 334, 335

I

impact of various sport disciplines 12*f*
implantable cardioverter defibrillator (ICD) 196*f*, 198, 261
recommendation for competitive sport participation 371*t*
inherited arrhythmogenic disorders 166–7
characteristics 167
genetic testing 166–9
vs athlete's heart 167
see also arrhythmogenic right ventricular cardiomyopathy (ARVC)
inotropy 5
International Olympic Committee (IOC) 427
intra-coronary Doppler ultrasound (ICD) 164
ion-channel disease *see* Brugada syndrome; catecholaminergic polymorphic ventricular tachycardia (CPVT); channelopathies; long QT syndrome (LQTS); short QT syndrome (SQTS)
iron, supplemenation 439
iron-deficiency anaemia 439
ischaemia
detection *see* exercise testing
indications for complementary tests 99
positive or false positive test? 98–9*f*
recommendation for competitive sport participation 373*t*
isokinetic strength testing 396
Israel, pre-participation screening in young competitive athletes 345
isthmal coarctation 314
Italy, pre-participation screening in young competitive athletes 344*f*–5

J

junior sport pre-participation screening 339–51
see also young competitive athletes

K

Kaplan–Meier analysis
  actual AC patient survival 196*f*
  event-free survival curves, coronary atherosclerosis 155*f*
Kawasaki disease 361
Kent bundle
  abnormal accessory pathways 288, 315
  anterograde refractory period, predicting risk of SCD 290–1
  retrograde conduction 290
knee flexion (hamstrings) and extension (quadriceps) 396*t*

L

lactate and heart rate curves 394–5*f*
lactate/lactic acid
  accumulation 6, 390
  advantage of lactate testing 393
  buffering capacity of the blood 7
  generation 4–5
  lactate threshold (LT1)
    determining threshold 392
    energy metabolism threshold 391
  maximal lactate steady state (MLSS) 391
  production and muscle hypoxia 93
Laplace law 11
left atrium (LA), remodelling 16–17
left bundle branch block (LBBB) 291, 293*f*–4
  prevalence 288
left heart dimensions and function in athletes 13–15
  distribution of aortic root dimensions, trained athletes 13*f*
  distribution of LV wall thickness, large population 13*f*
  prevalence and clinical significance of aortic root dilation 14*f*
  prevalence and clinical significance of left atrial remodelling 14*f*
left ventricle (LV)
  distribution of left ventricular end-diastolic cavity dimensions 22*f*
  end-diastolic chamber diameter 21
    and wall thicknesses, upper limits of normal 22*f*
  end-diastolic volume in endurance athletes 14
  function in athletes, no different from that in untrained subjects 15
  hypertrophy
    differentiation from HCM 180–1*f*
    idiopathic 312
  mass, maximal exercise systolic BP and 102
  outflow tract obstruction 182
  trabeculation, physiological increases, differentiation from left ventricular non-compaction (LVNC) 215
  volume and mass, measured by 3D echocardiography 15*f*
  wall thickness, athletes 21
left ventricular non-compaction (LVNC) 209–17
  algorithm, differentiation from physiological increases of LV trabeculation 215
  classification 209
  clinical presentation 211–12
  CMR 147, 212*t*
  diagnosis
    CMR criteria 213–14
    CV imaging criteria 212
    echocardiographic criteria 132–3, 212–13
    summary 214*t*
  differentiating from athlete's heart 209–15
  evaluation of athlete 214–15
  genetics 210–11
  pathogenesis 210–12
  prevalence 211
left ventricular tachycardia, first-line therapy 119
Lenègre disease 292, 295
liver injury, body-building supplements 441
Loeys–Dietz syndrome 314, 334
  aortic dilation/dissection 334
long QT syndrome (LQTS) 254–6
  Bazett's formula 255, 364
  black population 28
  cause of SCD 167
  defined 253
  genetic counselling 256
  genetic testing 168–70
  pre-participation and eligibility screening protocol 260
  prevalence, associated genes, contribution, and yield of genetic testing 171*t*
  prevention of SCD 173
  recommendation for competitive sport participation 371*t*

M

magnesium, low intake 439
marathon runners
  incidence of SCD 352
  middle-aged amateur 102
  pre-syncope 280*f*
Marfan syndrome 38, 52, 54, 134, 227, 231, 334, 347
  genetics 362–3
mass gathering medical care
  defined 411
  local/national adaptations 417–18
  unique characteristics 412
maximum strength testing 395
medical action plan (MAP), event planning 412–13
medical personnel, uniform requirement in sports arena 414
meldonium 430–1
metabolic equivalents (METs) 95
  definition of activity 321
  estimates of VO_2 95
metabolic syndrome 382
MIBG scintigraphy 159
minerals 438–9
minute ventilation (VE) and work, vs time 7*f*
mitochondrial proton shuttle 391
mitochondrial respiration 441
  limiting factor 4
mitral regurgitation 228–9
mitral valve prolapse (MVP) 226–32
  and arrhythmias 227
  classification 226
  diagnosis 228–30
    CMR 230
    trans-oesophageal echocardiography 230–1*f*
    trans-thoracic echocardiography 134, 228
  management 230–1
  prevalence 227
  in relation to sport 227
  sudden cardiac death 227, 314
    risk factors 228
mobile medical teams 415
modafinil 430*t*
Monge disease 336
monitoring
  exercise programmes 389–400
  training and health, new technologies 397–8
mountain sickness, acute and chronic 336
multifunctional defibrillator/synchronized cardioverter/transcutaneous pacemaker 414
muscle *see* skeletal muscle
muscular endurance 396–7
  press-ups and sit-ups 397*t*
muscular strength, cardiovascular performance 389
myocardial bridging 162, 220–2, 373*t*
myocardial capillary density 45
myocardial contractile force 6
myocardial and coronary diseases 179–224
myocardial infarction, acute (AMI) 309, 321–8
  definitions 321
  Determinants of Myocardial Infarction Onset Study (ONSET) 321
  exercise-related, clinical features 323–4
  risk of exertion-related AMI 321–2*f*
  Triggers and Mechanisms of Myocardial Infarction Study (TRIMM) 321
myocardial perfusion imaging 159, 161
myocarditis 201–8
  24-h Holter monitoring 205–6
  aetiology 201–2
    viral myocarditis 203*b*
  AHA/ACC Task Force recommendations 209*b*
  clinical and diagnostic work-up 207*b*
  clinical presentation 203–4
  CMR 148, 206
  cocaine-related cardiovascular complication 313
  diagnostics 205–6
  echocardiography 205–6
  endomyocardial biopsy 207
  exercise 202–3
    recommendations 207–8
  inferolateral T waves 204*f*
  pathophysiology and phases of inflammation 202
  recommendation for competitive sport participation 372*t*
  recommendations for return to sport 208
  special aspects in athletes 202
  sudden cardiac death 313–14*f*
  therapy 207

N

Naxos disease 187–8
new technologies for monitoring training and health 397–8
  ergogenic aids prescription 433
  wearable and gadget technology 397
nicotinamide adenine dinucleotide (NADH) 391
nitric oxide (NO) production, eNOS phosphorylation 43–4
non-sustained ventricular tachycardia (NSVT) 108
Noonan syndrome, ventricular hypertrophy 38
noradrenaline, nerve conduction 6
nuclear imaging 159–61

Nurses' Health Study (NHS), risk of exercise-related SCD in nurses 322
nutrition 433–44
body-building supplements, liver injury 441
dietary supplements 441
energy requirements 433–5
errors associated with dietary recording 434
vitamins, minerals, and antioxidants 438–9

O

obesity
paediatric 362
and physical inactivity cancer risks 381
role of physical activity in raising energy expenditure 435
oestrogen receptor antagonists 430*t*
orthodromic atrioventricular re-entrant tachycardia (O-AVRT) 288
osteogenesis imperfecta 227
ostium primum 135
ostium secundum 135
overtraining and burnout, paediatric 32
oxygen
end-tidal oxygen levels 8
transfer from air to tissues 88*f*
ventilatory equivalent (VE/VO_2) 93
oxygen debt, anaerobic threshold 4
oxygen pulse (surrogate of stroke volume) 6
oxygen uptake
maximal (VO_2max) 433
peak oxygen consumption 4
($V{\cdot}O_2max/V{\cdot}O_2peak$), maximal/peak 390

P

pacemaker, recommendation for competitive sport participation 371*t*
palpitations
paediatric 361
WPW ECG pattern 290*f*
paroxysmal supraventricular tachycardias (PSVT) without pre-excitation 279
patent arterial duct (PDA) 246
patient documentation 417
patient transfer/transport 415
peptide hormones 430*t*
performance-enhancing substances 427–8
therapeutic use exemption (TUE) 431
see also doping
pericarditis, recommendation for competitive sport participation 372*t*–3
peripheral blood vessels
arterial luminal diameter 42
conduit arteries
adaptations mediated by exercise 42–3
changes in compliance 43
vascular adaptation 42
vasoconstriction 5
pharmaceuticals, inappropriate sale as dietary supplements 441
phosphocreatine 389–90
physical activity
beneficial effects 352
causes and consequences of physical inactivity 381–2
definition 321
energy systems 389–90
heavy physical exertion defined 321
how to prescribe activity 383*b*
increased risk of AMI and SCD 323
individual prescription 386
intensity, classification and examples of absolute and relative intensity levels 384*t*
muscle strength/resistance 385
neuromotor exercise 385
phases and progression 386
prescription of intensity according to maximal exercise parameters 391*t*
prescription for sedentary/untrained individuals 381–402
psychological barriers to exercise 386
recommended ideal activity 383–4
simultaneous diseases 385–6
underutilization as treatment modality 382
see also exercise training
physical examination, paediatric 362
physical fitness
categories, relative $V{\cdot}O_2max$ (ml/kg/min) values for non-athletes 391*t*
defined 87
Physicians' Health Study, risk of exertion-related AMI 322
physiology of exercise 3–8
playing field resuscitation 403–10
collapse, initial response 403–4
sudden cardiac arrest (SCA) 403–10
polymorphic ventricular tachycardia
associated conditions 273
eligibility for competitive sport 273
post-event non-looping event monitors (PER900) 109*f*
pre-excitation and conduction abnormalities 288–96
paediatric 364
see also Wolff–Parkinson–White syndrome
pre-participation screening (PPS)
aim 359
asymptomatic ventricular pre-excitation 281
evaluation protocol for asymptomatic active adult/senior 355*f*
programmes 265, 359–60
in young competitive athletes 339–51
costs 346–7
ECG features of cardiac diseases detectable 343*t*
European countries 348*t*
false-positive results 345
flowchart/findings of Italian protocol 344*f*–5
impact on mortality 343–4
other preventive strategies 347
primary purpose 342
screening protocols used 342
see also screening
premature ventricular beats, recommendation for competitive sport participation 370*t*
premature ventricular contractions (PVCs) 99
prodromal symptoms of heart disease 326
prohibited substances 427–8
cardiovascular effects 427, 430*t*
therapeutic use exemption (TUE) 431
see also doping
protein
hypo-energetic diets 435
requirements, muscle adaptation and growth 437–8
unnecessary debate on intake 437
protein kinase C (PKC) signalling, calcium-dependent 44
protein-rich foods 437
pseudoxanthoma elasticum 227
pulmonary atresia with ventricular septal defect 248*f*
pulseless electrical activity (PEA), targeted temperature management 407

Q

QRS complex, paediatric 363
QT interval
Bazett's formula 255, 364
paediatric 364
see also long QT syndrome (LQTS); short QT syndrome (SQTS)
QT interval adaptations during exercise 102–5
in athletes 103–4
diagnosis of long QT 102–3
burst cyclo-ergometer protocol 103
normal/abnormal 102–3

R

ramp-like incremental running/cycling tests 89
rating of perceived exertion (RPE) 94
repaired tetralogy of Fallot, ventricular tachycardia unmasked 241*f*
repeated sprint sequences (RSSs) 94–5
respiratory exchange ratio 4, 5
respiratory quotient 4
respiratory system, exercise 6–8, 389–90
resuscitation
commotio cordis registry 404*f*
on the playing field 403–10
post-resuscitation care 407
targeted temperature management 407
resuscitation equipment, sports stadium 414–15
rhabdomyolysis 330–1
rhythm disorders 253–96
right atrium (RA), remodelling 17
right bundle branch block (RBBB) 291–2, 294*f*
prevalence 288
right heart remodelling 17
see also cardiovascular remodelling
right ventricle (RV)
adaptation to exercise 21
end-diastolic cavity dimensions and wall thicknesses, upper limits of normal 22*f*
outflow tract diameter measured by echocardiography 17*f*
right ventricular outflow tract obstruction (tetralogy of Fallot) 246–7
risk–benefit ratio of physical exercise, adults and young athletes 341
risks of exercise-related SCD 321–4
absolute risk 322
aetiology of cardiac events 322–3
clinical features
AMI 323–4
SCD in adult athletes 323–4
Nurses' Health Study (NHS) 321
prevention 324
aggressive reduction of risk factors 324
Rost's formula, blood pressure 101
ryanodine receptor gene (RyR2) 257

S

safe participation in sport 369–80
legal implications of implementing the recommendations 376–7
role of physician in decision-making process 375
targets of the recommendations 375
scintigraphy, myocardial perfusion 159, 161
SCN5A, deletion and substitution 293*f*, 295

screening
  adult/senior competitive 352–9
    CV abnormalities 354
    defined 353
    master athletes (AHA) 353–4, 355
  children and adolescent athletes 359–66
    anthropometry 362
    ECG pattern 363–4
    epidemiological data 359–60
    frequent underlying CV conditions 359–60
    physical examination 362
    programmes 360
  eligibility after screening: ESC/EACPR and AHA/ACC 353–4
  evaluation of middle-aged/seniors in leisure and sport activities 354
  existing screening recommendations 353
  participants with CAD, leisure exercise and competitive sports 354
  participants of health/fitness facilities 354–5
  programmes 360
  self-assessment methods 354–5
  summary 356
  in young competitive athletes 359–64
  see also children/adolescents; pre-participation screening
sedentary/untrained individuals 381–401
  defined 382
  exercise prescription 382–4
selenium and coenzyme Q10 438
short QT syndrome (SQTS) 103, 256–7
  defined 253
  genetic testing 168–70
  pre-participation and eligibility screening protocol 260
  prevalence, associated genes, contribution, and yield of genetic testing 171*t*
  QTc cut-off in athletes 256
  recommendation for competitive sport participation 371*t*
shortness of breath, paediatric 361–2
shunt lesions 246–8
sickle cell trait 331
signage and information related to access to care 417
sinus bradycardia, marked, recommendation for competitive sport participation 370*t*
skeletal muscle
  acid–base homeostasis 4
  capillaries
    increase in density 43
    local vasodilatation 5
  exercise physiology 3–8
  hypertrophy, decrease in capillary density 43
  hypoxia, lactate production and 93
  preferred limb vs non-preferred limb 43
  resistance arteries 43
smoking 382
  atherosclerosis, underestimation in older athletes 154
somatrotropic hormone (STH) 430*t*
SPECT imaging, athletes 159
spectators, reported incidence of SCA 411
sports
  cardiac classification 376, 377*f*
  eligibility
    athletes with cardiac abnormalities 369–80
    patients with CVD 236
  extreme environments 334–5
  main categories 355
  named, impacts on CV remodelling in athletes 12*f*
sports arenas 411–18
  cost-effective placement rate of AEDs 411
  field resuscitation 403–10
  inspection 416
  map of the venue 413*f*
  stairs and other obstacles 412*f*
  see also mass gathering medical care
sprint running, repeated sprint sequences (RSSs) 94–5
stadium medical emergency planning *see* mass gathering medical care
statins 324
stem cells, human-induced pluripotent stem cells (hiPSCs) 195
sternotomies, cyanotic CHD 241
stimulants 430*t*
strength testing 395
  iso-inertial testing 395–6
  isokinetic testing 396
stroke volume
  oxygen pulse 6
  vagal tone, and low heart rates 14
structural remodelling 9–20, 21–4
  dynamic nature 18
substances of abuse/doping 427–32
success, primary determinants 433
sudden cardiac arrest (SCA) 352–3, 403–10
  adult algorithm (AHA) 408*f*
  advanced life support, European and American guidelines 407
  basic life support 404–5
  commotio cordis 328–30
  differential diagnosis 403
  exercise-induced ischaemia 326
  exercise-related vs non-exercise-related 323*f*
  incidence of arrest and death 299
  prevention 324–5
  in society 330
  sports-related, clinical features 324
  suspicion/action 404
  time-critical response 414
sudden cardiac arrest/sudden death in the young and/or during sports activity 339–41*t*, 352
sudden cardiac death (SCD) in adults 305*t*, 306*f*, 340*t*, 352
  aetiology 323
  leading cause 167
sudden cardiac death (SCD) in athletes 290–5, 297–366
  associated electrophysiological parameters 281
  autopsy 170
    cascade screening of relatives 170
  cardiac conditions most frequently responsible 265
  clinical features, exercise-related 324
  CV causes 309–20
    atherosclerotic coronary artery disease 309–10
  defined 359
  epidemiology 359–60
  impact of gender, race, and sport 300–1
  impact of study methodology 299
  incidence 300–8
    geographical differences 300–4*t*
    versus other populations 304–5, 306*f*
  incidence and relative risk (RR) 341*f*
  less frequent causes 328–36
    altitude effects 336
    aortic dissection 332–3
    asthma 334
    bicuspid aortic valve 333
    cold/heat stress 335
    commotio cordis 328–30
    doping 330
    exercise-induced rhabdomyolysis 330–1
    hyperpyrexia 328
    sickle cell trait 331
  risk of exertion-related SCD 322–4
  sports activity, published series 316*t*–17
  structurally normal heart 315
supraventricular tachyarrhythmias (SVT) 277–87
  atrial premature beats (APBs) 278–9
    recommendation for competitive sport participation 370*t*
  diagnostic evaluation: general framework 277–8
  paroxysmal supraventricular tachycardias (PSVT)
    recommendation for competitive sport participation 370*t*
    with ventricular pre-excitation 280
    without pre-excitation 279–80
  treatment and exercise recommendations 282
sympathetic vasoconstriction, venous filling pressure, increased venous return 5
syncope
  defined 361
  differential diagnosis 403
  paediatric 361
  recommendation for competitive sport participation 371*t*

T

Tako–Tsubo cardiomyopathy 162
targeted temperature management 407
  pulseless electrical activity (PEA) 407
Task Force (AHA/ACC) recommendations 325*b*
technologies for monitoring training and health 397–8
  virtual reality 397–8
  wearable and gadget technology 397
telemonitoring 397
tetralogy of Fallot 246–7
thallium-201 perfusion imaging 159
thienopyridines 324
thoracotomies, cyanotic CHD 241
tidal volume 7
transposition of the great arteries (TGA) 247–8
  congenitally corrected 248
Triggers and Mechanisms of Myocardial Infarction Study (TRIMM) 321

U

UK Department of Health (DoH), paediatric exercise activity 33*t*
US Department of Health and Human Services (HHS), paediatric exercise activity 33*t*

V

valvular and aortic disease 226–50, 314–15
  recommendation for competitive sport participation 374*t*–6
Vam-Eval exercise testing 89
vascular remodelling *see* cardiovascular remodelling
vasoconstriction, peripheral blood vessels 5
vasodilation

by muscle capillaries 5
endothelium-dependent 42
vegetarian lifestyle 442
veins, distensible capacitance vessels 5
venous filling pressure, increased venous return of blood 5
ventilation–perfusion matching 7
ventilatory anaerobic threshold (AT) 4–5*f*
ventilatory dead space, ratio to tidal volume (Vd/Vt) 93
ventilatory efficiency 7
ventilatory equivalents, oxygen and carbon dioxide (VE/VO_2 and VE/VCO_2) 93, 94
ventilatory threshold 93–4
ventricular arrhythmias (VA) 265–76
catheter ablation 119
complex ventricular arrhythmias 270–2
fascicular tachycardias 270–1
right/left ventricular outflow-ventricular tachycardia 270
echocardiography 267
electrophysiological (EP) study 117
frequent or complex monomorphic ventricular arrhythmias 268–70
idiopathic 270–1*f*
infrequent ventricular premature beats 267–9
morphology of and origin of ventricular beats 265–6*f*
origin in LV outflow tract 266
polymorphic ventricular tachycardia 273
pre-participation screening programmes 265
in the presence of a cardiomyopathy 271–2
prevalence in the athlete 266
diagnostic tests 266–7
resting 12-lead ECG 267
risk in athletes vs prevalence 265
ventricular pre-excitation 59
asymptomatic 281
paediatric 364
see also Wolff–Parkinson–White syndrome
ventricular septal defects (VSD) 246–8
echocardiography 135–6
pulmonary atresia 248*f*
ventricular tachyarrhythmias *see* ventricular arrhythmias (VA)
ventricular tachycardia
first-line therapy 119
non-sustained (NSVT) 108
recommendation for competitive sport participation 371*t*
ventricular wall thickness by CMR 142*f*
vitamins 438–9
VO_2max
Hansen–Wasserman equations 390
Wasserman graphs 393*f*

W

Wasserman graphs 393*f*
water requirements 439–40
wearable and gadget technology 397
Wnt/β-catenin signalling 195–6
Wolff–Parkinson–White syndrome 279
arrhythmias 288
asymptomatic subjects with WPW pattern
incidence of SCD 289–90
recommendations for competitive sport 291
risk of arrhythmias 290
asymptomatic ventricular pre-excitation 281
clinical characteristics, patients with cardiac arrest 289
defined 280
diagnostics 280
ECG pattern 289*f*
pattern identified at birth 288
pre-excitation ECG pattern 288
prevalence 288
safety of anti-arrhythmic drugs 282
SCD 315
treatment and exercise recommendations 281
WPW pattern identified at birth 288
World Anti-Doping Agency (WADA), list of prohibited substances and methods 427
world, countries
cardiac arrest/sudden death in the young and/or during sports activity 340–1*t*
pre-participation screening in young competitive athletes 348*t*
World Health Organization (WHO), paediatric exercise activity 33*t*

Y

young competitive athletes
cardiac arrest/sudden death in the young and/or during sports activity, main studies 340–1
pre-participation screening 339–51
young endurance athletes, Rost's formula 101

Z

zebrafish, experimental model for investigation of AC 195